DISEASES OF THE
GUT AND PANCREAS

DISEASES OF THE GUT AND PANCREAS

EDITED BY

J. J. MISIEWICZ
BSc, FRCP
Consultant Physician
Department of Gastroenterology
and Nutrition
Central Middlesex Hospital
London

R. E. POUNDER
MA, MD, FRCP
Reader in Medicine and
Clinical Sub-Dean
Royal Free Hospital
School of Medicine,
London

C. W. VENABLES
MS, FRCS
Consultant in Surgical Gastroenterology
Freeman Hospital, Newcastle-upon-Tyne

BLACKWELL SCIENTIFIC PUBLICATIONS

OXFORD LONDON EDINBURGH

BOSTON PALO ALTO MELBOURNE

© 1987 by Blackwell Scientific Publications
Editorial offices:
Osney Mead, Oxford, OX2 oEL
8 John Street, London, WC1N 2ES
23 Ainslie Place, Edinburgh, EH3 6AJ
52 Beacon Street, Boston Massachusetts 02108, USA
667 Lytton Avenue, Palo Alto California 94301, USA
107 Barry Street, Carlton Victoria 3053, Australia

First published 1987

Printed and bound in Great Britain by
Butler & Tanner Ltd Frome and London

DISTRIBUTORS

USA
  Year Book Medical Publishers
  35 East Wacker Drive
  Chicago, Illinois 60601

Canada
  The C.V. Mosby Company
  5240 Finch Avenue East,
  Scarborough, Ontario

Australia
  Blackwell Scientific Publications (Australia) Pty Ltd
  107 Barry Street
  Carlton, Victoria 3053

British Library
Cataloguing in Publication Data

Diseases of the gut and pancreas.
  1. Digestive organs——Diseases
  I. Misiewicz. JJ   II. Pounder, R.E.
  III. Venables, C.W.
  616.3   RC801

ISBN 0-632-01121-1

Contents

Contents

Contents

Contributors

M. ATKINSON MD, FRCP
Special Professor in Gastroenterology, University of Nottingham, Consultant Physician, University Hospital, Queens Medical Centre, Nottingham, Department of Surgery, University Hospital, Queens Medical Centre, Nottingham NG7 2UH

A. T. R. AXON MD, FRCP
Consultant Physician, Gastroenterology Unit, The General Infirmary, Great George Street, Leeds LS1 3EX

K. D. BARDHAN DPhil, MB, BS, FRCP
Consultant Physician, District General Hospital, Moorgate Road, Oakwood, Rotherham S60 2UD

P R. H. BARNES MD(SYD), FRACP
Consultant Gastroenterologist, Repatriation General Hospital Concord, Hospital Road, Concord, N.S.W. 2139, Australia

J. H. BARON MA, DM, FRCP
Senior Lecturer and Consultant, Royal Postgraduate Medical School and Hammersmith Hospital, London, Consultant Physician, St Charles Hospital, Sub-Dean, St Mary's Hospital Medical School, London, Royal Postgraduate Medical School, Du Cane Road, London W12 0HS

J. F. W. M. BARTELSMAN MD
Consultant in Gastroenterology, Academic Medical Centre, Meibergdreef 9, Amsterdam 1105 AZ, The Netherlands

J. R. BENNETT MD, FRCP
Consultant Physician, Hull Royal Infirmary, Anlaby Road, Hull HU3 2JZ

J. N. BLACKWELL MB, ChB, MRCP
Consultant Physician and Gastroenterologist, Whiteabbey Hospital, 95 Doagh Road, Newtownabbey BT37 9RH, Northern Ireland

L. BLESOVSKY MB, BS
Registrar in Anaesthesia, St Mary's Hospital, Praed Street, London W2 1PG

A. L. BLUM MD
Division de Gastro-enterologie, Département de Médecine Interne, Chuv Centre Hospitalier Universitaire Vaudois, 1011 Lausanne, Switzerland

E. J. S. BOYD MB, MRCP
Senior Registrar, Western General Infirmary, Glasgow

B. N. BROOKE MD, MChir, FRCS, Hon FRACS
Emeritus Professor of Surgery, University of London (St George's Hospital), 112 Balham Park Road, London SW12 8EA

A. K. BURROUGHS MB, ChB, MRCP
Lecturer in Medicine and Honorary Senior Registrar, Royal Free Hospital and School of Medicine, Pond Street, London NW3 2QG

D. C. CARTER MD, FRCS(Ed), FRCS(Glasg)
St Mungo Professor of Surgery, University Department of Surgery, Royal Infirmary, Glasgow G31 2ER

D. O. CASTELL MD
Professor of Medicine, Chief of Gastroenterology, Bowman Gray School of Medicine, 300 S Hawthorne Road, Winston-Salem, N.C. 27103, USA

M. B. CLAGUE MD, FRCS
Consultant General Surgeon, Newcastle General Hospital, Westgate Road, Newcastle-upon-Tyne NE4 6BE

R. COCKEL MA, MB, FRCP
Consultant Physician, Selly Oak Hospital Birmingham, Senior Clinical Lecturer, University of Birmingham, Selly Oak Hospital, Raddlebarn Road, Birmingham B29 6JD

M. M. COHEN MB, ChB, FRCS(Ed), FRCS(C), FACS
Professor of Surgery, University of Toronto, Mount Sinai Hospital, 440–600 University Avenue, Toronto, Ontario M5G 1X5, Canada

D. G. COLIN-JONES MD, FRCP
Consultant Physician and Gastroenterologist, Honorary Senior Lecturer, University of Southampton, Queen Alexandra Hospital, Southwick Hill Road, Portsmouth PO6 3LY

G. C. COOK MD, DSc, FRCP, FRACP
*Consultant Physician, Hospital for Tropical Diseases,
London NW1 0PE, and School of Hygiene and Tropical
Medicine, London WC1E 7HT*

J. L. CRAVEN BSc, MBChB, MD, FRCS
*Consultant General Surgeon, York District Hospital,
Wigginton Road, York YO3 7HE*

J. H. CUMMINGS MA, MSc, MB, ChB,
FRCP
*Clinical Scientific Staff, DCNC & Hon. Consultant
Physician, Addenbrooke's Hospital, Cambridge, MRC
Dunn Clinical Nutrition Centre, 100 Tennis Court Road,
Cambridge CB2 1QL*

F. T. DE DOMBAL MA, MD, FRCS
*Reader in Clinical Information Science, Clinical Sciences
Building, St James University Hospital, Beckett Street,
Leeds LS9 7TF*

A. W. DELLIPIANI MD, FRCP, FRCP(Ed)
*Consultant Physician, North Tees General Hospital,
Hardwick, Stockton on Tees, Cleveland TS19 8PE*

H. B. DEVLIN MA, MD, MCh, FRCS,
FACS
*Consultant Surgeon, North Tees General Hospital,
Hardwick, Stockton on Tees, Cleveland TS19 8PE*

M. J. DEW MD, MRCP
*Consultant Physician, Llanelli General Hospital, Llanelli,
Dyfed*

R. J. DICKINSON MD, FRCP
*Consultant Physician, Hinchingbrooke Hospital,
Hinchingbrooke Park, Huntingdon PE18 8NT*

M. W. DRONFIELD DM, MRCP
*Consultant Physician, Peterborough District Hospital,
Thorpe Road, Peterborough PE3 6DA*

M. EASTWOOD MB, ChB, MSc,
FRCP(Ed)
*Consultant Physician, Department of Medicine,
Gastrointestinal Unit, Western General Hospital, Crewe
Road, Edinburgh EH4 2XU*

J. B. ELDER MB, ChB, MD, FRCS(Ed),
FRCVS(Glasg)
*Professor of Surgery, University of Keele, Consultant
Surgeon, North Staffs Royal Infirmary, Hartshill, Stoke on
Trent, University of Keele, Department of Postgraduate
Medicine, North Staffordshire Medical Institute,
Hartshill Road, Hartshill, Stoke on Trent ST4 7NY*

P. D. FAIRCLOUGH MD, MRCP
*Senior Lecturer in Medicine. St Bartholomew's Hospital
Medical College, Consultant Physician, Hackney and St
Bartholomew's Hospitals, St Bartholomew's Hospital,
West Smithfield. London EC1A 7BE*

R. R. FERGUSON MB, ChB, MD, MRCP
*Consultant Physician and Gastroenterologist, Arrowe
Park Hospital, Birkenhead, Merseyside L49 5PE*

J. F. FIELDING BSc, MD, FRCP
*Professor of Medicine, The Charitable Infirmary, Jervis
Street, Dublin 1, Ireland*

L. P. FIELDING MB, FRCS, FACS
*Chief of Surgery, St Mary's Hospital, Waterbury,
Connecticut, USA, Clinical Professor of Surgery, Yale
University School of Medicine, Visiting Clinical Scientist,
St Mary's Hospital, London, St Mary's Hospital,
Department of Surgery, 56 Franklin Street, Waterbury,
Connecticut 06702, USA*

G. R. GILES MD, FRCS
*Professor of Surgery, University of Leeds, Department of
Surgery, St James's Hospital, Leeds LS9 7TH*

J. GILLON MD, MRCP
*Consultant Physician, Blood Transfusion Service, Royal
Infirmary, Lauriston Place, Edinburgh EH3 9HB*

T. G. GIRDWOOD MB, ChB, DMRD,
FRCR
*Consultant Radiologist, Cumberland Infirmary, Carlisle,
Cumbria CA2 7HY*

T. GLEDHILL ChM, FRCS
*Senior Registrar General Surgery, St James's University
Hospital, Beckett Street, Leeds LS9 7TF*

D. G. GRAHAME-SMITH MB, BS, PhD,
FRCP
*Rhodes Professor of Clinical Pharmacology, University of
Oxford, MRC Clinical Pharmacology Unit, Radcliffe
Infirmary, Oxford OX2 6HE*

G. E. GRIFFIN BSc, PhD, MRCP
*Wellcome Trust Senior Lecturer, Consultant Physician,
Department of Communicable Diseases, St George's
Hospital Medical School, Cranmer Terrace, Tooting,
London SW17 0RE*

J. D. HARDCASTLE MA, MChir, FRCS,
FRCP
*Professor of Surgery, Department of Surgery, University
Hospital, Queen's Medical Centre, Nottingham NG7 2UH*

A. D. HARRIES MA, MD, MRCP
*Lecturer in Tropical Medicine, Department of Medicine,
Kamazu Central Hospital, Lilongwe, Malawi, Africa*

R. C. HEADING BSc, MD, FRCP
*Senior Lecturer and Consultant Physician, Royal
Infirmary, Edinburgh EH3 9YW*

M. D. HELLIER MA, MB, BCh, MD, FRCP
Consultant Physician and Gastroenterologist, Princess Margaret Hospital, Okus Road, Swindon SN1 4JU

M. M. HENRY MB, FRCS
Consultant Surgeon, Central Middlesex Hospital, London NW10 7NS

M. HOBSLEY MA, MChir, PhD, FRCS
David Patey Professor of Surgery, Head of Department of Surgical Studies, University of London, the Middlesex Hospital, Medical School, Mortimer Street, London W1N 8AA

C. D. HOLDSWORTH MD, FRCP
Consultant Physician, Royal Hallamshire Hospital, Glossop Road, Sheffield S10 2JF

R. H. HUNT MB, ChB, FRCP, FRCP(Ed), FRCP(C)
Professor and Head, Division of Gastroenterology, McMaster University Medical Centre, 1200 Main Street W, Hamilton, Ontario, L8N 3Z5, Canada

G. H. HUTCHINSON MB, ChB, MD, FRCS, FRCS(Ed)
Consultant Surgeon, Halton General Hospital, Runcorn, Cheshire WA7 2DA

B. T. JACKSON MS, FRCS
Consultant Surgeon, St Thomas' Hospital, London SE1 7EH

O. F. W. JAMES MA, FRCP
Professor of Geriatric Medicine, Consultant Physician, The Medical School, University of Newcastle-upon-Tyne, Newcastle-upon-Tyne NE2

M. G. W. KETTLEWELL MA, MB, MChir, FRCS
Consultant Surgeon, Fellow, Green College, Oxford, John Radcliffe Hospital, Headington, Oxford OX3 9DU

J. G. C. KINGHAM MD, MRCP
Consultant Physician, Morriston Hospital, Heol Maes Eglwys, Morriston, Swansea SA6 6NL

R. M. KIRK MS, FRCS
Consultant Surgeon, Royal Free Hospital, Pond Street, London NW3 2QG

O. KRONBORG MD, PhD
Assistant Professor in Surgery, Senior Lecturer in Surgery, Odense University Hospital, Department of Surgical Gastroenterology, 23 Sdr Boulevard, Odense 5000, Denmark

S. J. LA BROOY MB, BS, MRCP
Consultant Physician, Hillingdon Hospital, Uxbridge, Middlesex UB8 3NN

M. J. S. LANGMAN MD, FRCP
Professor of Therapeutics, University of Nottingham Medical School, Queens Medical Centre, Nottingham NG7 2UH

R. LENDRUM MA, MB, BChir, FRCP
Consultant Physician (Gastroenterology) and Senior Lecturer in Medicine, The University of Newcastle-upon-Tyne, Freeman Hospital, Freeman Road, Newcastle-upon-Tyne NE7 7DN

J. E. LENNARD-JONES MD, FRCP
Consultant Gastroenterologist, St Mark's Hospital, City Road, London EC1 2PS

M. H. LESSOF MD, FRCP
Professor of Medicine, United Medical and Dental Schools of Guy's and St Thomas's Hospital, Hunt's House, Guy's Hospital, St Thomas's Street, London SE1 9RT

S. T. D. MCKELVEY MCh, FRCS(Ed), FRCS(Eng)
Consultant Surgeon, The Ulster Hospital, Dundonald, Belfast BT16 0RH

M. J. McMAHON MB, ChB, ChM, PhD, FRCS
Senior Lecturer in Surgery and Consultant Surgeon, Assistant Director, University Department of Surgery, General Infirmary, Leeds, Great George Street, Leeds LS1 3EX

A. MARSTON MA, DM, MCh, FRCS, MD(Hon.Causa, Nice)
Consultant Surgeon, The Middlesex and University College Hospitals, Bloomsbury Vascular Unit, The Middlesex Hospital, Mortimer Street, London W1N 1PP

J. F. MAYBERRY MD, MRCP
Senior Medical Registrar, City Hospital, Huchnall Road, Nottingham

A. S. MEE MD, MRCP
Consultant Physician and Gastroenterologist, Battle Hospital, Oxford Road, Reading RG3 1AG

J. J. MISIEWICZ Bsc, MBBS, FRCP(Lond), FRCP(Edin)
Co-director Department of Gastroenterology & Nutrition, Consultant Physician, Member of External Scientific Staff Medical Research Council, Honorary Lecturer, St Bartholomew's Hospital, Consultant Gastroenterologist, Royal Navy, Central Middlesex Hospital, Acton Lane, London NW10 7NS

G. NEALE MA, BSc, MB, ChB, FRCP
Consultant Physician, Addenbrooke's Hospital, Hills Road, Cambridge CB2 2QQ

R. NELSON MB, ChB, FRCP, DCH
Consultant Paediatrician, Gateshead and Newcastle Health Authorities, Royal Victoria Infirmary, Queen Victoria Road, Newcastle-upon-Tyne NE1 4LP

Contributors

T. C. NORTHFIELD MA, MD, FRCP
*Consultant Gastroenterologist and Reader in Medicine,
Department of Medicine, St George's Hospital Medical
School, Cranmer Terrace, London SW17 0RE*

E. J. PARKER-WILLIAMS MB, BS,
MRCPath
*Senior Lecturer and Honorary Consultant Haematologist,
St George's Hospital Medical School, Cranmer Terrace,
London SW17 0RE*

R. E. POUNDER MA, MD, FRCP
*Reader in Medicine and Clinical Sub-Dean, Royal Free
Hospital School of Medicine, Pond Street, London NW3
2QG*

S. A. RAIMES FRCS
*Research Associate, University Department of Surgery,
New Medical School, Framlington Place, Newcastle-
upon-Tyne NE2 4HH*

C. O. RECORD DPhil, MB, FRCP
*Consultant Physician in Gastroenterology, Royal Victoria
Infirmary and University of Newcastle-upon-Tyne,
Newcastle-upon-Tyne NE1 4LP*

J. RHODES MD, FRCP
*Consultant Physician, University Hospital of Wales,
Heath Park, Cardiff CF4 4XW*

R. C. G. RUSSELL MS, FRCS
*Consultant Surgeon, The Middlesex Hospital, Mortimer
Street, London W1N 1PP*

F. SABBATINI MD
*Clinical Assistant, Gastroenterology Unit, 2nd School of
Medicine, Via S Pansini 5, Naples 80131, Italy*

R. H. SALTER BSc, MB, BS, FRCP
*Consultant Physician, Cumberland Infirmary, Carlisle,
Cumbria CA2 7HY*

M. SCHACHTER BSc, MB, BS, MRCP
*Clinical Research Fellow, Department of Clinical
Pharmacology, St Mary's Hospital Medical School,
Norfolk Place, London W2 1PG*

J. R. SIEWERT MD
*Director of the Department of Surgery, Technical
University of Munich, Department of Surgery, Technical
University Munich, Ismaningerstrasse 22, D-8000
Munich 80, West Germany*

D. B. A. SILK MD, FRCP
*Consultant Physician and Co-director, Department of
Gastroenterology and Nutrition, Central Middlesex
Hospital, Acton Lane, London NW10 7NS*

G. E. SLADEN MA, DM, FRCP
*Consultant Physician in Gastroenterology, Guy's
Hospital, St Thomas Street, London SE1 9RT*

F. STADIL MD
*Professor of Surgery, Surgical Department C,
Rigshospitalet University Hospital, Blegdamsvej 9, DK-
2100 Copenhagen Ø, Denmark*

E. STONEHILL MD, FRCPsych
*Consultant Psychiatrist, Central Middlesex Hospital,
Department of Psychological Medicine, Acton Lane,
London NW10 7NS*

E. T. SWARBRICK MD, FRCP
*Consultant Physician and Gastroenterologist, New Cross
and Royal Hospitals, Wolverhampton WV10 OPQ*

R. H. TEAGUE MD, FRCP
*Consultant Physician, Torbay Hospital, Lawes Bridge,
Torquay, Devon TQ2 7AA*

J. G. TEMPLE MB, ChM, FRCS, FRCS(Ed)
*Consultant Surgeon, Queen Elizabeth Hospital,
Edgbaston, Birmingham B15 2TH*

M. H. THOMPSON MD, FRCS
*Consultant Surgeon, Southmead Hospital, Bristol BS10
5NB*

J. P. S. THOMSON MS, FRCS
*Consultant Surgeon, St Mark's Hospital and Hackney
Hospital; Honorary Consultant Surgeon, St Mary's
Hospital; Honorary Lecturer in Surgery, The Medical
College of St Bartholomew's Hospital; Civil Consultant in
Surgery (Rectal) to the Royal Air Force, St Mark's
Hospital, City Road, London EC1V 2PS*

L. A. TURNBERG MD, FRCP
*Professor of Medicine, University of Manchester;
Honorary Consultant Physician, Salford Health
Authority; Department of Medicine, Hope Hospital
(University of Manchester School of Medicine), Eccles
Old Road, Salford, Manchester M6 8HD*

G. N. J. TYTGAT MD
*Professor of Medicine (Gastroenterology), Chief of the
Division of Hepatogastoenterology, Academic Medical
Centre, Meibergdreef 9, Amsterdam, 1105 AZ, The
Netherlands*

C. W. VENABLES MS, FRCS, MB, BS
*Consultant in Surgical Gastroenterology, Freeman
Hospital, High Heaton, Newcastle-upon-Tyne NE7 7DJ*

J. WAGGET MB, BS, FRCS
*Consultant Paediatric Surgeon, Newcastle Health
Authority, The Fleming Memorial Hospital, Great North
Road, Newcastle-upon-Tyne NE2 3AX*

A. WATSON MB, ChB, MD, FRCS
*Consultant Surgeon and Surgical Gastroenterologist,
Department of Surgery, Royal Lancaster Infirmary,
Lancaster LR1 4RP*

R. C. N. WILLIAMSON MA, MD, MChir, FRCS
Professor and Head of Department of Surgery, University of Bristol and Honorary Consultant Surgeon, Bristol Royal Infirmary, University Department of Surgery, Bristol Royal Infirmary, Bristol BS2 8HW

K. G. WORMSLEY DSc, MD, FRCP
Consultant Physician, Honorary Reader in Therapeutics, Ninewells Hospital, Dundee DD1 9SY

Preface

Progress in gastroenterology during recent years has been rapid and the increasing use of specialized techniques and new diagnostic tests has led to improvements in the management of patients. At the same time the clinical spectrum of some alimentary disorders has been changing. New diseases have been characterized. It has become increasingly difficult for the general clinician, or even for the specialist, to keep up to date with the torrent of publications which document the expansion of scientific and technological areas in gastroenterology. In addition, alternative treatments for a number of alimentary diseases have become available and the selection of appropriate management may present problems for the non-specialist.

Diseases of the Gut and Pancreas aims to give a practical account of modern gastroenterology. We invited the contributors to present an overview of pathophysiology, diagnosis and treatment of alimentary diseases. The book has been written by a distinguished team of experts and practical clinicians, mainly from the United Kingdom, and provides guidance at the postgraduate level to the management of common, and some uncommon, alimentary diseases. *Diseases of the Gut and Pancreas* has been written in a concise format, providing adequate information in one reasonably easily handled volume. Access to further in-depth information is through references to medical and scientific literature listed at the end of each chapter. These references include review articles, as well as original sources, thus catering for the varying needs of the readers.

Diseases of the Gut and Pancreas should appeal to physicians and surgeons in training, or to those studying for higher professional examinations. The book will also be helpful as a source of practical information, and will provide a guide to further reading. The editors hope that this book will be of particular value to general physicians and surgeons, who may wish to use it to gain access to present knowledge on how best to manage some of the more complicated gastrointestinal problems that face them in clinical practice. While the book has not been written for the undergraduate to use routinely, we trust that some will find it useful and stimulating for reading about their more complex patients, or when studying for honours in medicine.

The book opens with an account of the pathophysiology and significance of common alimentary symptoms, providing a sound practical foundation for the following sections that deal in detail with the aetiology, clinical and laboratory diagnosis, and the treatment of alimentary conditions. Diseases of the alimentary tract are described on an anatomical basis, except when, as in inflammatory bowel disease, this classification is inappropriate. Separate chapters deal with paediatrics, systemic disorders, nutrition, psychiatry and the like where they interact with gastroenterology.

We are very grateful to all our authors for their contributions and for their patience during the preparation and editing of the text. The initial stages were nurtured by Adam Sisman, then of Grant MacIntyre and later of Blackwell Scientific Publications. Our thanks go to him and also to Peter Saugman and John Robson for their support. We thank Ms Rosemary Hope-Hockett who dealt with the major labour of converting the manuscripts into a book and we are grateful to David Sisman for the elegant design of the cover. Needless to say, we are deeply indebted to our secretaries: Ms Lesley Cowen, Ms Julia Semus and Ms Saila Shah who uncomplainingly coped with much extra work. Our wives showed their customary amused forbearance and it is a great pleasure to dedicate this book to them.

October 1986

J.J.M.
R.E.P.
C.W.V.

SECTION I

PATHOPHYSIOLOGY OF GASTROINTESTINAL SYMTPOMS

Chapter 1
Dysphagia

M. ATKINSON

Difficulty in swallowing is a symptom that must always be taken seriously and that demands urgent attention because it often indicates serious disease. Dysphagia is seldom ignored by the patient because at best it is a social embarrassment and at worst it leads to rapid weight loss and life threatening respiratory complications.

In hospital most patients are seen in medical, surgical or ear, nose and throat clinics, but the pulmonary complications may cause referral to the chest physicians, while pharyngeal dysphagia is encountered in neurological clinics.

Normal swallowing

Neural control

The neural control of swallowing rests with the swallowing centre in the brain stem situated in the reticular formation just caudal to the facial nucleus. It is mediated through the lower motor neuron ganglion cells in the nucleus ambiguus in the medulla, which supply the pharyngeal constrictor muscles through the ninth and tenth cranial nerves. The dorsal vagal nucleus controls oesophageal motor activity through the vagus. The upper oesophageal sphincter may also be controlled through this pathway, because this sphincter is usually unaffected by bulbar poliomyelitis which involves the nucleus ambiguus. The resting tone of the striated muscle of the upper oesophageal sphincter is maintained by a constant stream of impulses in its vagal nerve supply and this is temporarily interrupted to allow relaxation during swallowing.

Knowledge of the basic physiology of swallowing is essential for the clinical evaluation of dysphagia. Swallowing is a reflex that is initiated voluntarily, but only the oral phase is wholly under voluntary control. Transit through the oesophagus is normally subconscious, being entirely under autonomic control.

Oral phase

Swallowing is initiated by pressing the tongue upward against the hard palate from before backwards, thus propelling the bolus into the pharynx. This is quite a forceful movement and squirts liquids through the pharynx into the lower oesophagus well ahead of the oesophageal peristaltic wave.

Pharyngeal phase

The pharynx forms part of the alimentary and respiratory tracts and during this phase of swallowing respiration is arrested. The respiratory tract is closed off above by contraction of the upper pharyngeal constrictor muscle separating the nasopharynx. It is closed off below by elevation of the larynx and inversion of the epiglottis, so preventing entry to the respiratory tract. The cricopharyngeus, which forms the upper oesophageal sphincter, relaxes and the passage of solid boluses is effected by rapid and sequential contraction of the upper middle and lower pharyngeal constrictor muscles (Fig.1.1). As respiration is suspended, the passage of the bolus through the pharynx must be fast and this phase of swallowing is completed in under two seconds.

of oesophageal trans-section in experiments on animals. The smooth muscle of the lower oesophagus responds to the interruption of low frequency, electrical stimulation by a contraction termed the 'off' response.

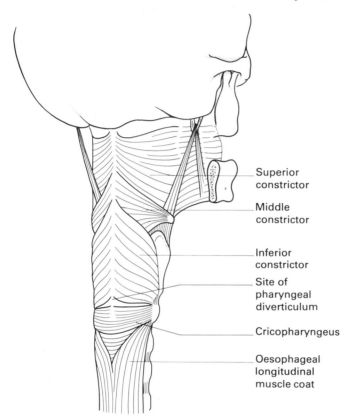

Superior constrictor

Middle constrictor

Inferior constrictor

Site of pharyngeal diverticulum

Cricopharyngeus

Oesophageal longitudinal muscle coat

Fig. 1.1. Diagram of pharyngeal musculature viewed from the right posterior oblique position.

Oesophageal phase

This phase of swallowing lasts eight to 10 seconds and consists of a peristaltic wave sweeping down the oesophagus at a speed of 2–3 cm/sec, propelling the bolus through the relaxed lower oesophageal sphincter. Liquids are squirted into the lower oesophagus ahead of the following peristaltic wave which sweeps the oesophagus clear. The progress of the peristaltic wave is not affected by the transition from striated (upper one-third) to smooth (lower two-thirds) muscle of the oesophageal wall. The peristaltic wave is controlled centrally by the dorsal vagal nucleus, jumping the gap

The latent period of this 'off' response increases progressively in a caudal direction. Hence a single neural stimulus to the whole of the oesophageal circular smooth muscle could result in a progressive peristaltic wave [5]. The tone of the lower oesophageal sphincter appears to be an intrinsic property of its muscle fibres (myogenic tone), but it is modulated by neuronal pathways. The sphincter relaxes ahead of the peristaltic wave and remains open for several seconds. Liquid boluses arrive before this relaxation and are transiently held up in the lower oesophagus [16].

Clinical presentation

At the outset it is essential to establish the exact nature of the patient's difficulty, as disturbance of the oral, pharyngeal or oesophageal phases of swallowing produce different symptoms and are likely to have very different causes.

The oral phase of swallowing is sometimes disturbed in Parkinson's disease, where akinesia can cause difficulty in initiating a swallow. The bolus does not leave the mouth and choking is unusual unless attempts are made to force fluids down. Painful lesions of the mouth and throat cause reluctance to swallow and weakness of the masticatory muscles may impair the ability to form a bolus suitable for swallowing (Table 1.1).

Pharyngeal dysphagia characteristically causes coughing and choking on swallowing, with occasional regurgitation of fluids through the nose. The symptoms occur immediately after swallowing and most commonly result from neurological disease. Because of inability to close off the respiratory tract properly, cough and aspiration pneumonia are common. Pharyngeal dysphagia may be mimicked by an obstructive lesion in the oesophagus, of which the patient is unaware, until the oesophagus is completely filled and spillage into the respiratory tract occurs [15].

Oesophageal dysphagia causes a sensation of food sticking at some point in the chest. The sensation varies from discomfort to severe pain and is usually sufficient to discourage further swallows. It is consistently relieved by the regurgitation of food material into the mouth, or by its eventual passage through the obstruction. The regurgitated material looks and tastes as it did when swallowed, unless it has remained in the oesophagus for many hours or days, when decomposition causes it to have a foul taste and smell. Oesophageal dermatomes are linearly represented on the chest wall, but localization of sensation is variable and many patients are unaware of the site of the obstruction. Sensory localization in the upper oesophagus and the pharyngo-oesophageal junction is more accurate than lower down, so that filling of the obstructed oesophagus tends to cause discomfort above, rather than at the point of obstruction, when the obstruction is in the lower oesophagus, or at the cardia [9, 10].

Associated symptoms

Vomiting and regurgitation

Vomiting is an active ejection of gastric contents with retching and contraction of the abdominal wall muscles. Regurgitation is a passive process of effortless return of gastric or oesophageal contents into the mouth. Patients often describe regurgitation as vomiting. Retching may be caused by contact of regurgitated oesophageal contents with the pharyngeal mucosa. Regurgitation of oesophageal contents into the mouth occurs in recumbency or on bending. The distinction between the two symptoms is provided by the taste of the material entering the mouth. The taste is sour or bitter if material originates in the stomach; it is not unpleasant if it originates from the oesophagus unless it has remained there for long and has undergone decomposition. These symptoms are considered further in Chapter 2 [14].

Cough

Coughing immediately after swallowing suggests either pharyngeal dysphagia, or an oesophago-tracheal fistula. Spillage of oesophageal food residues may cause nocturnal coughing and staining of the pillow.

Odynophagia

Odynophagia is pain experienced within 15 seconds of swallowing and it may or may not be associated with delayed oesophageal transit. Odynophagia without delay occurs sometimes in reflux oesophagitis or in inflammatory disorders of the oesophageal mucosa and mediastinum; for example in mediastinitis and mediastinal abscess. It can occur in the absence of any demonstrable abnormality in the so-called tender oesophagus syndrome, when it can be provoked by swallowing hot fluids or alcohol.

Odynophagia with delay in transit may accompany oesophageal spasm in conditions such as diffuse oesophageal spasm, or

Belching

Troublesome belching is a symptom of gastro-oesophageal reflux. It is absent in complete oesophageal obstruction, but is common when dysphagia results from oesophagitis with spasm.

Differential diagnosis of dysphagia

At the outset it must be decided whether food passes through the throat normally. If

Table 1.1. Causes of oral dysphagia.

Difficulty	Mechanism	Disorder
Difficulty in initiating swallowing Masticatory difficulty with inability to form a bolus	Akinesia Muscular weakness	Parkinson's disease Bulbar poliomyelitis Motor neuron disease Syringomyelia Muscular dystrophy
	Painful mastication	Moniliasis, *Herpes simplex* Tumours of the tongue or jaw Trauma

gastro-oesophageal reflux. More frequently it is associated with mechanical blockage from a peptic stricture secondary to reflux oesophagitis, or a malignant stricture caused by carcinoma. The time interval between swallowing and the onset of pain gives a useful index of the site of the lesion. Pain occurs immediately on swallowing with pharyngeal disorders, while there is a lag of several seconds in oesophageal disease—the lower the lesion the longer the delay. It is useful to ask the patient to time the onset of pain from the moment of swallowing [2].

Hiccough

Hiccough results from irritation of the mucosa of the lower oesophagus and often accompanies dysphagia when the site of obstruction is at or near the cardia. It is induced by distension of the lower oesophagus by swallowed food.

Table 1.2. Causes of pharyngeal dysphagia.

Lesion	Disorder
Bilateral upper motor neuron lesion e.g. stroke	Pseudobulbar dysphagia from spastic muscle weakness
Damage to medulla	Lateral medullary syndrome Motor neuron disease Syringobulbia Poliomyelitis
Striated muscle weakness	Myasthesia gravis Dermatomyositis Dystrophia myotonica
Mechanical block	Postcricoid carcinoma Pharyngeal pouch Cricopharyngeal bar and achalasia Goitre
Inflammation	Tonsillitis Moniliasis *Herpes simplex*
Psychological	Globus hystericus Depression

the patient is uncertain, observation during a swallow is helpful. This will confirm inability to initiate swallowing—choking, or coughing immediately on swallowing points to pharyngeal dysphagia. Regurgitation of fluids through the nose indicates a neuromuscular disorder. The causes of oral, pharyngeal and ocsophageal dysphagia are summarized in Tables 1.1, 1.2 and 1.3.

a lower motor neuron lesion such as motor neuron disease and movements of the soft palate, tongue and facial muscles must be tested. Unilateral weakness, particularly when associated with Horner's syndrome, suggest the lateral medullary syndrome. Variable dysphagia getting worse during a meal and bilateral ptosis characterizes myasthenia gravis. Puffiness of the face and

Table 1.3. Causes of oesophageal dysphagia.

Neural disorders		Achalasia and Chagas' disease
		Diffuse oesophageal spasm
		Hypertensive lower oesophageal sphincter
		Autonomic neuropathy, e.g. diabetes
		Multiple sclerosis
Muscular disorders		Systemic sclerosis (scleroderma)
		Systemic lupus erythematosus
		Dystrophia myotonica
Mechanical block	Webs	Sideropenic dysphagia
	Fibrous stricture	Gastro-oesophageal reflux
		Schatzki ring
		Ingestion of drugs or corrosive poisons
		Behçet's disease
		Radiotherapy
	Foreign bodies	Particularly in children and the mentally subnormal
	Neoplastic	Carcinoma of oesophagus or cardia
		Leiomyoma
	Extrinsic compression	Carcinoma of bronchus
		Enlarged mediastinal glands
		Retrosternal goitre
		Aortic aneurysm. Double or right sided aorta.
		Post-operative: fundoplication
		Angelchik prosthesis
	Oesophageal diverticulum	
Inflammatory disorders		Reflux oespohagitis
		Sideropenic dysphagia
		Moniliasis
		Herpes simplex

Pharyngeal dysphagia (Table 1.2)

When pharyngeal dysphagia is suspected a careful examination of the throat and neck and detailed neurological testing are needed [13]. Infection is usually self evident. Wasting and fasciculation of the tongue point to

a violaceous skin rash point to dermatomyositis.

A palpable swelling in the neck is most probably caused by a pharyngeal pouch or metastatic glands from a post-cricoid carcinoma. If the swelling varies in size and can be emptied by pressure, causing food

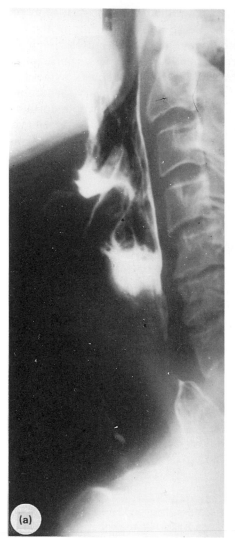 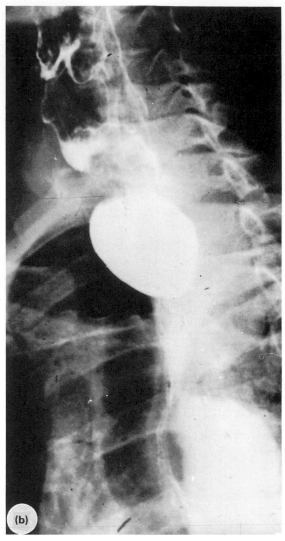

Fig. I.2. (a) Dysphagia in motor neuron disease showing considerable residues of barium in the pharynx. The cricopharyngeus is unaffected and the pharyngo-oesophageal junction remains closed. (b) Pharyngeal pouch distended with barium.

material to return to the throat, a pharyngeal pouch is present (Fig. I.2).

Oesophageal dysphagia

If the pharyngeal phase of swallowing is normal, but hold-up occurs in the chest, then an oesophageal cause of dysphagia must be sought. In deciding the cause, the length of history, the pattern of dysphagia (variable and intermittent or constant and progressive) and the particular articles of diet that cause symptoms are especially helpful.

Fibrous and neoplastic strictures (Fig. I.3)

Carcinoma of the oesophagus or of the cardia causes progressive and unremitting dysphagia which is seldom of more than a few

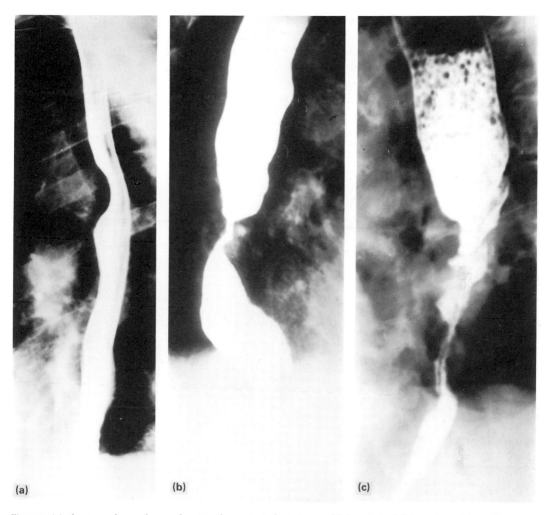

(a)   (b)   (c)

Fig. 1.3. (a) the normal oesophagus showing the aortic indentation and below it the left bronchus. (b) peptic oesophageal stricture just above the oesophagogastric junction in a patient with a hiatal hernia. (c) carcinoma of the lower third of the oesophagus showing shouldering and an irregular narrowing with a residue of food material in the oesophagus above it.

months duration; it is usually associated with rapid loss of weight. Preceding symptoms of heartburn, belching and acid reflux into the mouth are present in most patients with fibrous strictures secondary to reflux, but their absence does not exclude the diagnosis. The earliest symptom in neoplastic and benign strictures is the difficulty in swallowing lumpy solids such as steak, raw apple or crusty bread. Gradually the difficulty extends to softer foods and finally even liquids cannot be swallowed. Failure to swallow liquids strongly suggests a neoplastic lesion, as fibrous strictures seldom progress to this stage.

Neuromuscular disorders (Fig. 1.4)

In the neuromuscular types of dysphagia, the difficulty is less clearly related to the nature of food and often from the outset liquids cannot be swallowed normally. Dysphagia usually starts gradually and has often been present for years before the patient seeks medical advice. Occasionally it starts abruptly after an emotional shock. The severity of dysphagia fluctuates in the early stages but becomes constant with

progression of the disorder. Pain may be severe occurring at night or after food, as a cramping discomfort across the chest—it is the dominant symptom in diffuse oesoph- ageal spasm and is easily mistaken for cardiac pain. Pain is commoner in the early

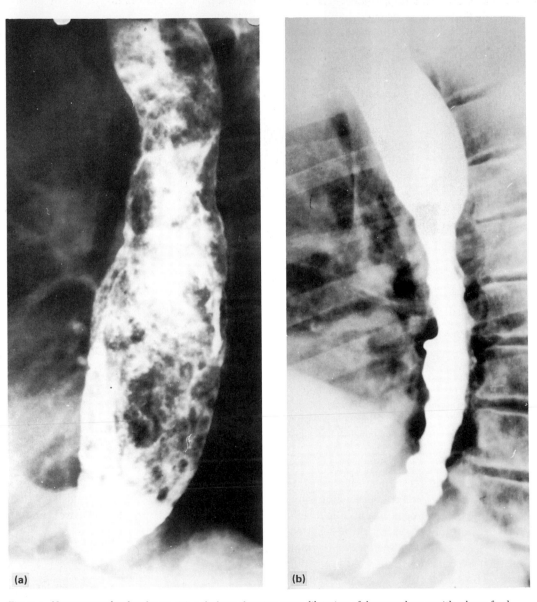

(a)

(b)

Fig. 1.4. Neuromuscular dysphagia. (a) achalasia showing gross dilatation of the oesophagus with a large food residue present in the lumen. Note that the oesophagogastric junction remains tightly closed. (b) diffuse oesophageal spasm characteristically affecting the smooth muscle portion of the oesophagus and causing dysphagia associated with severe chest pain. (c) diffuse oesophageal spasm pushing out a large epiphrenic

rather than in the late stages of achalasia, when the oesophagus has become dilated; it is particularly troublesome in vigorous achalasia. A characteristic feature of achalasia is regurgitation of food into the mouth during recumbency, causing soiling of the pillow at night. This happens because oesophageal dilatation is greater in achalasia than in other types of dysphagia, with a correspondingly greater volume of retained contents in the lumen and at risk of regurgitation. Although peristaltic failure does not in itself cause serious dysphagia, the absence of a peristaltic push from above will often aggravate dysphagia caused by an obstructive lesion.

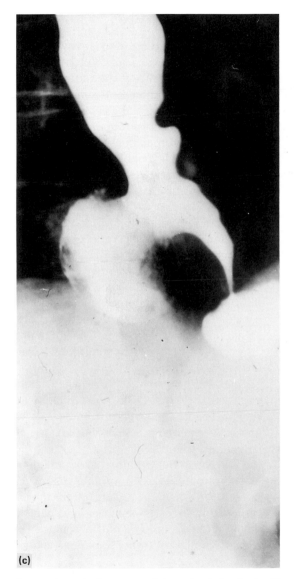

(c)

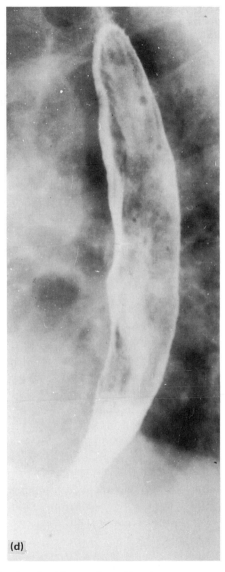

(d)

diverticulum which aggravated the patient's dysphagia. (d) systemic sclerosis with oesophageal involvement, showing the dilated, air-containing oesophagus at rest. This patient had mild dysphagia from lack of propulsive motor activity.

Loss of oesophageal smooth muscle in systemic sclerosis seldom causes troublesome dysphagia, but occasional difficulty may be encountered with dry solids. This can usually be overcome by taking frequent drinks during a meal. Severe dysphagia in a patient with systemic sclerosis suggests a fibrous stricture resulting from reflux oesophagitis secondary to damage of the lower oesphageal sphincter by the disease. Such dysphagia is preceded by reflux symptoms of heartburn and belching [1].

Webs and rings (Fig. 1.5)

Oesophagitis of the proximal oesophagus, with or without web formation, causes dysphagia. As the changes often extend up to the pharyngo-oesophageal junction, attempts to swallow cause choking. Proximal oesophagitis with web formation is commonly, but not always, associated with sideropenia, koilonychia and atrophic changes in the glossal and upper oesophageal mucosa which predispose to post-cricoid carcinoma [4]. Oesophageal moniliasis and oesophageal herpes also involve the upper oesophagus, causing painful dysphagia.

Dysphagia resulting from a Schatzki ring in the distal oesophagus is characteristically sporadic and related to swallowing lumpy foods, which cause bouts of bolus obstruction. Between these the patient is symptom-free and indeed, after an obstructing bolus has been dislodged by washing it through with copious drinks, or by inducing vomiting, the patient may finish the meal without further difficulty. Careful questioning will, however, frequently reveal mild symptoms of gastro-oesophageal reflux. These conditions are discussed further in Chapter 15.

Globus hystericus

This consists of a feeling of a lump in the throat which rarely interferes with swallowing. Weight loss is rare. The terminology is misleading, because this symptom occurs in association not with hysterical, but obsessional and depressive personalities.

Investigation of dysphagia

Radiology

The chest radiograph may show mediastinal masses due to bronchial carcinoma or retrosternal goitre. The outline of a grossly dilated oesophagus is sometimes visible and in it an air-fluid level may be identified in the erect position. Severe dysphagia, notably in achalasia, results in loss of the gastric air bubble. The lung fields may show appearances of aspiration pneumonia or lung abscess.

Contrast studies with barium (or propyliodone suspension (Dionosil) if the risk of aspiration seems great) are essential by helping to identify and localize the underlying disorder. An antigravity swallow is an essential part of the radiological investigation. Video recording of swallowing played back slowly is often helpful in the assessment of pharyngeal dysphagia and of motor disorders of the oesophagus. Neuromuscular disorders causing pharyngeal dysphagia are associated with a baggy pharynx, with slow transit and residues of barium left in the vallecula and pyriform fossae. A localized stricture with an irregular outline is more likely to be neoplastic than fibrous, but retained food material may be confused with tumour tissue. A smoothly tapered narrowing of the lower oesophagus suggests achalasia, but can be mimicked by carcinoma of the stomach infiltrating under an intact squamous epithelium.

If doubt remains after contrast radiography, an attempt should be made to provoke the patient's symptoms and to identify

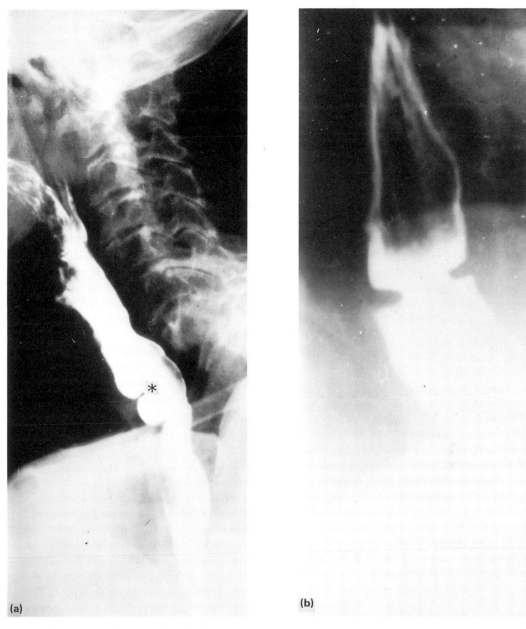

(a)

(b)

Fig. 1.5. (a) upper oesophagitis with web* formation in a patient with sideropenic dysphagia. (b) Schatzki ring in the lower oesophagus.

the site of the hold-up by giving a marsh-mallow with the barium, or barium tablets. Where peristaltic failure is suspected, the ability to swallow barium in the 15° head down position, provides an index of the efficiency of peristalsis.

Endoscopy

An endoscopic examination should always be preceded by contrast radiography to indicate the site and dimensions of any obstructive lesion, to identify endoscopic pitfalls such as a diverticulum or pharyngeal pouch and to show large oesophageal food residues that must be cleared before endoscopy. Mechanical obstructions are usually readily identified at endoscopy, but neuromuscular disorders present few abnormalities—the achalasic cardia appears normal and admits the endoscope without undue resistance. Multiple biopsies and exfoliative brush cytology complete the endoscopic examination.

Manometry

Intraluminal pressure recording in the pharynx and oesophagus is only of diagnostic value in neuromuscular dysphagia. It provides a quantitative measure of the strength of the peristaltic wave and of its coordination, provided the oesophagus is not grossly dilated. It measures resting tone and the presence and timing of relaxation of the oesophageal sphincter.

Radionuclide imaging

This non-invasive technique documents transit through the oesophagus and can quantify oesophageal emptying and gastro-oesophageal reflux. All these topics are discussed in more detail in Chapters 9 and 10.

Effects of dysphagia

Nutritional impairment

The degree and duration of dysphagia determine the magnitude of nutritional loss. Inadequate food intake results in protein-calorie malnutrition with wasting. Serial measurements of body weight are the simplest means of monitoring wasting [3], but hypoalbuminaemia may lead to oedema, which will partially mask weight loss. Skin fold thickness and mid-upper-arm muscle circumference provide indices of body fat and lean body mass respectively [10] (See

Chapter 78). Nutritional depletion causes immunodeficiency with impairment of cell mediated immunity which increases susceptibility to infection [7]. Protein depletion and low serum albumin impair wound healing after operation. When dysphagia is severe, even fluids cannot be taken in adequate amounts and dehydration and uraemia are added to the clinical picture.

Respiratory complications

Aspiration of food into the respiratory tree may occur during swallowing, or may result from regurgitation of oesophageal contents above an obstructive lesion. This leads to cough with episodes of fever, chest pain and shadowing on chest radiographs caused by aspiration pneumonia, which may progress to a lung abscess. The respiratory complications of dysphagia carry a considerable mortality, aggravated by immunodeficiency resulting from nutritional loss. Massive aspiration can cause sudden death and is a constant risk in the patient with a large oesophageal residue.

Iatrogenic oesophageal damage

When transit through the oesophagus is delayed, tablets may be retained for long periods and cause mucosal damage [11]. Non-steroidal anti-inflammatory drugs, potassium tablets, tetracycline and other antibiotics and emepronium bromide are particularly liable to cause trouble and whenever possible should be given in liquid form and washed down with drinks of water [6] (See Chapter 15).

Management of dysphagia

This will obviously depend upon the cause and is dealt with in the succeeding chapters. Enteral feeding through a fine bore tube inserted if necessary at endoscopy, will repair nutritional deficiency and may be so used before surgery. In pharyngeal dysphagia of neurological origin such as the lateral medullary syndrome, enteral feeding is a valuable interim measure until swallowing improves.

References

1 ATKINSON M. Oesophageal motor changes in systemic disease. *Clin Gastroenterol* 1976;**5**:119–133.

2 BLACKWELL JN, CASTELL DO. Oesophageal chest pain: a point of view. *Gut* 1984;**25**:1–6.

3 CAHILL GF. Starvation in man. *Clin Endocrinol Metabol* 1976;**5**:397–415.

4 CHISHOLM M. The association between webs, iron deficiency and post cricoid carcinoma. *Postgrad Med J* 1974;**50**:215–219.

5 CHRISTENSEN J. WINGATE DL. *A guide to gastrointestinal motility.* Edinburgh: Wright Publishing, 1983

6 COLLINS FJ, MATTHEWS HR, BAKER SE, STRAKOVA JM. Drug induced oesophageal injury. *Br Med J* 1979;i:1673–1676.

7 CUNNINGHAM-RUNDLES S. Effects of nutritional status on immunological function. *Am J Clin Nutr* 1973;**26**:912–915.

8 DE CAESTECKER JS, BLACKWELL JN, BROWN J, HEADING RC. The oesophagus as a cause of recurrent chest pain: which patients should be investigated and which tests should be used. *Lancet* 1985;iii:1143–1146.

9 EDWARDS DAW. Discriminatory value of symptoms in the differential diagnosis of dysphagia. *Clin Gastroenterol* 1976;**5**:49–57.

10 GURNEY JM, JELLIFFE DB. Arm anthropometry in nutritional assessment: nomogram for rapid calculation of muscle circumference and cross sectional muscle and fat areas. *Am J Clin Nutr* 1973;**26**:912–915.

11 HELLER SR, FELLOWS IW, OGILVIE AL, ATKINSON M. Non steroidal anti inflammatory drugs and benign oesophageal strictures. *Br Med J* 1982;**285**:167–168.

12 HURWITZ AL, DURANCEAU A, HADDAD JK. The approach to the patient with disordered swallowing. In: *Disorders of oesophageal motility.* Philadelphia: WB Saunders Co. 1979:56.

13 KILMAN WJ, GOYAL RK. Disorders of pharyngeal and upper esophageal motor function. *Arch Intern Med* 1976;**136**:592–601.

14 MALAGELADA J-R, CAMILLERI M. Unexplained vomiting—a diagnostic challenge. *Ann Intern Med* 1984;**101**:211–218.

15 PALMER ED. Disorders of the cricopharyngeus muscle: a review. *Gastroenterology* 1976;**71**:510–519.

16 WEISBRODT GW. Neuromuscular organisation of esophageal and pharyngeal motility. *Arch Intern Med* 1976;**136**:524–531.

Chapter 2
Dyspepsia, Nausea and Vomiting

J. R. BENNETT

Dyspepsia, nausea and vomiting

Symptoms described by the terms dyspepsia, nausea and vomiting occur very frequently and are part of everyday speech, but may be misleading when used loosely by patients or doctors. Absence of agreement on the precise definition of these terms leads to weakness in diagnostic ability [6]. The symptoms can be produced by a wide range of conditions, some trivial but others serious—from psychogenic and functional gut disorders at one extreme to obstruction or inflammation of any part of the gut at the other. Accurate diagnosis of their cause is thus often difficult, especially if organic disease is absent [13]. It may be uncertain which, if any, system or organ to investigate, so that a careful analysis of each symptom is needed in order to avoid mistakes and unnecessary tests.

A phrase often used by doctors 'the patient has vague dyspepsia' should be a target for clarification, or at least clear description, before investigation. Discussion of the mechanisms of symptoms is bound to be imprecise as details of normal gut motility and pathways through which gut sensations are perceived are poorly understood.

Dyspepsia

Definition

Dyspepsia is upper abdominal or lower chest discomfort related to eating, which may be accompanied by other gastrointestinal symptoms such as nausea, anorexia, distension, or vomiting. This term is used at times to describe almost any abdominal discomfort, from heartburn to lower abdominal pain. It is also occasionally used for other symptoms such as flatulence, regurgitation or vomiting. Patients may refer to this symptom as 'indigestion'.

Subjective sensations like abdominal discomfort are difficult to describe because of their lack of reference points. Intelligent and articulate patients are more likely to give clear information but, with assistance, most patients can amplify their description to aid the diagnostician.

Physiological mechanisms of dyspepsia

Pain and soreness

It is remarkable how little is known about the mechanisms by which visceral abdominal pain is produced. Unmyelinated autonomic 'C' nerve fibres transmit painful sensation, partly through the vagi (two-thirds of vagal fibres are said to be afferent) and partly through sympathetic ganglia and the lateral spinothalamic tracts of the spinal cord.

The stimulus to the pain-sensitive sensory nerve endings probably varies in different diseases and anatomical areas. Possibly by local release of prostaglandins, inflammation makes nerve endings more sensitive to pain induced by hydrochloric acid, histamine, kinins or serotonin. Where there is inflammation (for example oesophagitis or gastritis) pain may be produced by many stimuli, even if the particular pain sensors have a normally high pain threshold [26].

Changes of motility or distension may also produce pain. It has long been debated whether in duodenal ulceration and oesophagitis pain results from stimulation of nerve endings by acid or from abnormal muscular contractions, traction and distension. It is possible that pain is produced by any of these factors but, in those conditions in which there is mucosal ulceration, direct chemical contact may be the more usual stimulus [3, 20]. Sometimes motor changes secondary to a mucosal lesion may produce pain at a remote site, for example epigastric pain in some patients with duodenal ulcer appears to originate in the lower oesophagus [7, 8, 14].

As uncertainty exists about mechanisms of pain even in the presence of mucosal abnormality [23], it is even more difficult to offer an adequate account of pain mechanisms in the absence of organic disease, though the assumption that motor factors are important is generally accepted. More sensitive methods of measuring motility are needed before its role can be assessed properly. Stretching or distention of the gut causes pain [2], probably by direct action on nerve endings and also by increasing tension on the mesentery [21]. The threshold at which distension begins to cause pain varies between subjects; e.g. patients with irritable bowel syndrome being more susceptible than controls to colonic distension [22]. The site at which such pain is perceived may have no relation to its anatomical origin, as shown by studies in which various parts of the gut were distended by a balloon [17, 24].

Distension

Many patients complain of bloating and unsightly abdominal protrusion which is often worse late in the day. On investigation there is no change in the gut or abdominal volume, a combination of diaphragmatic contraction and exaggerated lordosis 'pushing' the abdominal contents downwards and forwards [12]. Swallowing excess air makes only a small contribution to abdominal distension. In reality most swallowed air—as in aerophagy—never reaches the stomach, being noisily belched up from the oesophagus instead.

The sensation of fullness or distension in the upper abdomen in the absence of overloading with food or organically delayed gastric emptying, is presumed to be a motor phenomenon. The intragastric volume is usually not different from normal, but gastric emptying measured by scintiscanning after a radionuclide-labelled meal, is delayed in some patients [9].

In a few studies on patients with this type of abdominal discomfort, abnormalities of the gastric electrical rhythm (the swings of electrical potential that are thought to control the rate of muscle contractions) have been shown [27]. Too few patients have been studied to know whether such abnormalities of gastric function are common or whether some perceive normal motor function abnormally.

Apart from organic obstruction and functionally delayed colonic transit, excessive gas in the gut is uncommon. In any form of intestinal malabsorption there is increased gas production because of bacterial action on unabsorbed carbohydrate in the colon; the commonest example of this is lactase deficiency. In this condition undigested lactose passes into the colon where it is fermented to produce carbon dioxide and hydrogen.

Dyspeptic symptoms

Not all dyspepsia is pain, and many other discomforts are often described by patients.

Unease

This description probably refers to nausea

or the abdominal sensation that accompanies nausea. The site is usually unhelpful.

Fullness and distension

These are common complaints. Fullness perceived mainly in the upper abdomen suggests gastroduodenal origin, often without any structural cause, and may be associated with satiety. However, the sensation of distension in colonic disease is sometimes predominantly upper abdominal. Lower abdominal distension may be due to a colonic abnormality (especially disturbed motility), often becoming worse in the evening. Lower abdominal distension, especially without diurnal variation, may be a symptom of gynaecological disease or ascites.

The variation of symptoms with time may be helpful. Rapid and recent distension or persistent and slowly increasing distension, more often indicate organic disease, whereas intermittent distension is more likely to be due to functional causes.

Heaviness

Patients use this term sometimes to describe the sensation caused by overfilling of organic origin (for example gastric distension secondary to pyloric stenosis) but more often it is a manifestation of a functional disorder, as in the flatulent dyspepsia syndrome.

Burning

This is particularly associated with inflammation of oesophageal or gastric mucosa, but functional disorders without epithelial inflammation may also cause a burning sensation. If food or drink causes or exacerbates burning within seconds of swallowing, an inflammatory oesophageal cause is more likely. The best example is odynophagia, a soreness or pain behind the sternum as food or liquid (especially hot or alcoholic drinks or citrus fruits) are swallowed; this is highly suggestive of oesophagitis. Burning, or a hot sensation in the colon after defecation is sometimes a feature of functional colonic disease.

Aching

Patients may use 'aching' to describe a mild, but persistent pain. If localized to a small area of the abdomen it may indicate a mucosal lesion, such as a peptic ulcer. The wider the area the smaller the likelihood of an organic lesion, but the relentless discomfort of pancreatic carcinoma or an enlarged liver (as in metastatic liver disease, fatty liver or infective hepatitis) may be described as an ache. The vague early symptoms of pancreatic cancer are especially likely to be mistakenly ascribed to a functional bowel disorder.

Pain

Unless abnormally hypersensitive, patients use the term 'pain' to describe severe discomfort. Its nature (dull, sharp, gripping etc.), as well as its site and radiation, always need amplification (see chapter 3).

Satiety

Definition

Satiety is the decreased or absent desire to eat during or after a meal.

The hypothalamus is important in regulating appetite and animal studies show that lesions in specific parts of the hypothalamus alter food intake. On the basis of experiments on animals a 'satiety centre' in the ventromedial hypothalamus and a feeding centre in the lateral hypothalamus have been postulated. However, no hypothalamic lesion has been correlated with disordered food intake in humans [18]. The sensation of satiety may be due to inhibition of gastric emptying mediated by ingested fat acting on receptors in the ileum [25].

The sensation of a comfortable fullness and a diminished desire to eat and drink is normal at the end of a meal. When the sensation arises after only a few mouthfuls of food it is abnormal. It is different from, though may be accompanied by, fullness.

Satiety is to be clearly differentiated from anorexia. Abnormal satiety differs from anorexia, in that the appetite (desire to eat) is normal, but is readily satisfied so that eating a normal meal leads to discomfort. Easy satiety often coexists with abdominal fullness and nausea, probably as a consequence of gastroduodenal motor abnormalities. Abnormal satiety may occur in space-occupying lesions of the abdomen, such as ascites.

Anorexia

Definition

Anorexia is a diminished, or absent desire to eat. Anorexia has many causes and, if severe, is accompanied by loss of body weight. It is common in carcinoma of the stomach and in neoplastic disease at other sites, but may be a part of any severe systemic illness. Associated with nausea, it occurs in uraemia, hypercalcaemia and the early stages of infectious hepatitis and is often a feature of alcoholism. It may be a symptom of psychiatric disease, as in anorexia nervosa (see chapter 68).

Nausea

Definition

Nausea may be used by patients to describe a variety of sensations and emotions, from those experienced before vomiting, to anorexia, revulsion of food, abdominal fullness, or satiety. It should be used to describe the feeling of being about to vomit, even though vomiting does not invariably follow. Patients sometimes describe a sensation of nausea lasting for hours or days. More often it increases with waves of growing severity, eventually culminating in retching and finally vomiting. Severe nausea is usually accompanied by hypersalivation.

Mechanism

Nausea may result from stimulation of the labyrinths (for example motion sickness or ear disease), viscera (for example distension of stomach or duodenum; or any severe somatic pain), from psychological causes (for example unpleasant or frightening emotions), or from any sensation—visual, aural, olfactory, or tactile which a person finds unpleasant. It is accompanied by decreased gastric tone, inhibition of gastric peristalsis and increased duodenal tone.

Nausea in the absence of a recognizable stimulus is poorly understood. Sometimes it is presumed to be psychologically determined, but on other occasions local gastric changes may produce motor changes which result in nausea. Reflux of bile into the stomach, for example, may produce rapid and severe nausea.

Nausea as a symptom

Nausea which does not lead to vomiting may be no more than 'abortive emesis'. The stimulus may be insufficiently strong, or too short in duration or the individual may be able to suppress the urge to vomit. A common example is the nausea of motion sickness when vomiting may be avoided either by diverting the attention or by the completion of the voyage.

Persistent, prolonged or frequent nausea without vomiting and in the absence of a recognizable cause is a common functional symptom, often psychologically determined.

Vomiting (emesis)

Definition

Vomiting is the act of forcefully ejecting gastric contents through the mouth by the coordinated contraction of abdominal and gastric muscles during relaxation of the lower oesophageal sphincter. An associated symptom is **retching**, where movements similar to those in vomiting take place, but without ejection of gastric contents.

Mechanisms

A centre in the reticular core of the medulla controls vomiting, initiating the motor changes of the vomiting act. The vomiting centre is anatomically close to the respiratory and salivatory centres, coordinated changes in these areas being part of the vomiting process.

Stimulation of the vomiting centre arises from afferent visceral pathways, mainly transmitted by vagal afferents, or from a chemoreceptor zone in the floor of the fourth ventricle. It is believed that chemical (for example uraemia), or hormonal (for example in pregnancy) stimuli may act by this route. Motion sickness also may be mediated by the chemoreceptor zone [5]. Visceral afferents—from pharynx, heart, peritoneum, pylorus, or duodenum—probably act on the vomiting centre through direct neural connections. It remains uncertain whether vomiting ever results from purely local changes in the alimentary tube without intervention from the medullary centre.

When vomiting is initiated by the vomiting centre, gastric peristalsis is inhibited, the lower oesophageal sphincter relaxes and gastric contents are ejected by forceful contractions of the abdominal muscles and diaphragm. Salivation is increased. Associated changes in small intestinal motility may occur, but this is uncertain [1].

Causes of vomiting

Vomiting is a symptom of many organic and functional disorders. The main categories are listed in Table 2.1 [15]. Meticu-

Table 2.1. Classification of causes of vomiting.

Cause	Clinical example
Cerebral disease	Raised intracranial pressure, migraine.
Centrally acting drugs	Digoxin, apomorphine and other opiates
Chemotherapy	Cytotoxic and immuno-suppressive drugs.
Middle ear disturbance	Motion sickness, Ménière's disease.
Gastric factors	Bile reflux Drugs irritant to the gastric mucosa e.g. sulphasalazine. Overdistension.
Organic obstruction	Pyloric stenosis, Intestinal obstruction (e.g. adhesions).
Peritoneal irritation	Appendicitis.
Metabolic abnormalities	Uraemia, diabetes mellitus, hypercalcaemia.
Endocrine abnormalities	Pregnancy, hypoadrenalism.
Radiation	Cancer therapy.
Psychogenic	Bereavement vomiting. Anorexia nervosa/bulimia. Self-induced.

lous enquiry is needed to establish the colour of vomitus—yellow colour denotes the presence of bile and suggests free patency of the pylorus; coffee–ground pigmentation suggests upper alimentary haemorrhage, while faeculant vomiting indicates prolonged gastric stasis or, rarely, a gastro-colic fistula.

Regurgitation

Regurgitation is the effortless entry of gastric contents into the mouth. The regurgitated material may be swallowed or spat out.

Regurgitation must be differentiated from vomiting. It can result from material retained in the oesophagus, for example in achalasia. Regurgitation is common in the presence of an incompetent gastro-oesophageal anti-reflux mechanism, particularly during stooping or lying down. The volume of regurgitated material is small and the patient is aware of a sour (acid), or bitter (bile) taste. Although the patient may complain of vomiting, careful analysis of the symptom will show the passive nature, the relation to posture, the absence of nausea and abdominal contractions, which characterize vomiting. If oesophageal contents are regurgitated, the patient should be able to differentiate them from vomitus by the absence of the characteristic smell of gastric contents and of the acid taste. However, patients often find it difficult to distinguish acid from bitter tasting fluid.

Rumination

Rumination is the repetitive regurgitation of gastric contents into the mouth after meals.

The regurgitated material is usually swallowed. This may be a variant of simple regurgitation, associated with an incompetent anti-reflux mechanism, but sometimes rumination is an acquired habit with no demonstrable abnormality of the oesophagus or stomach. There is no associated nausea, heartburn or discomfort and some patients appear to find the habit pleasurable.

Causes of dyspeptic symptoms

Organic or functional disease

Any of the foregoing symptoms may be caused by organic disease but they are usually of lesser diagnostic value than other major symptoms that point to a likely diagnosis. Thus gastric or duodenal ulcers, gallstones, reflux oesophagitis, pancreatitis, or carcinoma of the stomach usually have pain as their primary symptom (see Chapter 3), but may also be associated with varying degrees of nausea, vomiting, distension, or regurgitation. In these conditions the associated dyspeptic symptoms are less important and of low discriminatory diagnostic value. Less commonly, the primary symptom of pain is absent or poorly recognized and described by the patient, who emphasizes the dyspeptic symptoms (Table 2.2). Differentiating this group of patients, whose organic disease produces unusual symptoms, from the larger number in whom the dyspeptic symptoms result from disordered function with no organic abnormality, is a common and difficult problem.

Gastritis

Chapter 18 deals with this topic in detail. Although dyspeptic symptoms such as nausea, vomiting, satiety and discomfort are sometimes attributed to gastritis, all detailed studies agree that they correlate poorly with histologically confirmed gastritis. Some patients with gastritis have epigastric discomfort and fullness, or nausea and vomiting, but many with identical symptoms have a normal gastric mucosa. The symptoms may be caused by the motor

Table 2.2. Secondary symptoms associated with organic disease.

Disorder	Secondary symptoms	Possible mechanism
Duodenal ulcer	Vomiting	Delayed gastric emptying, self-induced to relieve pain
Gastric ulcer	Anorexia, nausea and vomiting	Bile reflux, gastritis and disordered gastric motility
Gastric carcinoma	Anorexia, nausea, vomiting, easy satiety	Decreased receptive relaxation of the stomach
Biliary calculi	Distension, heartburn, vomiting	Duodenogastric reflux, entero-enteric reflexes
Pancreatic carcinoma	Vomiting	Duodenal obstruction

Liver disease
  alcoholic
  hepatitis
  metastatic
  malignancy
	Distension
	Nausea
	Retching, vomiting
		Sometimes direct effect on cerebral centres, alcoholic gastritis

Colonic obstruction	Distension, vomiting	Distension of colon and small bowel
Ovarian cyst and neoplasm	Distension	Increased intra-abdominal volume
Metabolic Hypoadrenalism Diabetic ketoacidosis Uraemia	Vomiting Abdominal pain	Direct effect on vomiting centre ?
Intra-abdominal Appendicitis Pancreatitis Cholecystitis	Vomiting	Peritoneal irritation

abnormalities that could lead to gastritis—altered antro-duodenal motility allows increased bile reflux, which causes gastritis. They may be triggered by a common factor such as smoking or alcohol, which may lead to symptoms caused by altered motility but also may produce mucosal damage.

The flatulent dyspepsia syndrome

The flatulent dyspepsia syndrome is an ill-defined condition consisting of abnormal and unpleasant upper abdominal sensations after meals.

Many patients have some or all of the following symptoms—fullness after meals, easy satiety, abdominal distension, excess belching, nausea, vomiting (especially early morning), heartburn, or regurgitation of acid or bile.

Each symptom needs careful analysis.

The patient perhaps complains initially of pain or vomiting, the associated symptoms being disregarded. The complete syndrome is characteristic, and is possibly due to altered gastroduodenal motility, with delayed gastric emptying and duodeno-gastric reflux. The likelihood of structural disease is small, but certain aetiological or associated factors should be considered.

Gallstones

Flatulent dyspepsia may coexist with gallstones, but is common in their absence. After cholecystectomy flatulent dyspepsia may persist and possibly the mechanism lies in disordered antro-duodenal motility, under the influence of cholecystokinin [10]. As the calculous gallbladder may have enhanced sensitivity to cholecystokinin [16], it is possible that the antro-duodenal muscle is also hypersensitive.

Alcoholism

Vomiting and retching, particularly in the early morning, is common in alcoholics. In one study [16] 30% of the female alcoholic patients presented with digestive symptoms.

Smoking

Smoking increases duodenogastric bile reflux, probably by altering antro-duodenal motility and decreasing pyloric pressure. Heavy smokers often experience early morning vomiting, though the classic morning cough must also be a contributing factor.

Psychiatric disease

The flatulent dyspepsia syndrome is often seen in tense, anxious or depressed individuals, or as a consequence of stress. It is regarded by some clinicians as part of the irritable bowel syndrome (see Chapters 67 and 68).

Gastric cancer

The problems of early diagnosis of gastric cancer are considered in Chapter 28, but the outstanding difficulty is the mildness and variability of the symptoms. Abdominal discomfort, post prandial fullness, nausea and vomiting occur in up to three-quarters of patients with gastric cancer, though weight loss, which is uncommon in the flatulent dyspepsia syndrome, occurs in up to 40%. Clearly, if such symptoms persist, or have no likely cause (such as anxiety or stress), or are accompanied by weight loss, the patient needs endoscopic examination. However, endoscopic examination of all dyspeptics is likely to yield only one gastric cancer in every 400 endoscopies.

Drugs

Many drugs have unwanted gastrointestinal effects, which include nausea, vomiting or upper abdominal discomfort. Prominent among them are aspirin, other non-steroidal anti-inflammatory drugs, sulphasalazine and corticosteroids. Abnormalities of the gastroduodenal mucosa such as gastritis or erosions may be found, although they are not invariable. The symptoms usually disappear if the drug is stopped, but a careful history of all medication (prescribed, self-administered and including proprietary medicines) must be taken from patients with these complaints.

Analysis of symptoms

The symptoms of upper gastrointestinal disorders are imprecise, because of the variability of patients' descriptions and because specific causes often cannot be identified. The difference between the symptoms of a gastric ulcer and a non-structural disorder such as flatulent dyspepsia may be small and occasionally nonexistent. The clinician needs experience and care in history taking, if the correct diagnosis is to be made quickly and without unnecessary investigations.

Clarity of description

Even the inarticulate patient's history will become clearer if the doctor takes care to define the symptoms and double-check with later questions to ensure that the patient means what he or she says. This particularly applies to the type of abdominal discomfort experienced.

Timing of symptoms

Particular care is needed to trace symptoms from their onset. What seems at first to be a recent problem may well have started a long time previously. A short history of pain makes an organic cause likely.

Causation and association

With help, the patient may realize that symptoms date from specific life events, or the doctor may discover this when the personal and social history are surveyed in detail. A patient may be reluctant to talk about psychiatric illness or psychogenic symptoms, such as changes of mood, morbid thoughts, anxiety and the like. These may be concealed deliberately, for fear that the doctor may too readily accept them as the cause of the symptoms and thereby fail to discover a dreaded organic disorder. A detailed account of tobacco and alcohol consumption is also very important and, if the patient is suspected of withholding the truth, corroborative information about alcohol should be sought from his or her family, or by appropriate tests—estimations of mean corpuscular volume (MCV) or hepatocellular enzymes (ALT or γGT).

Careful studies show that sociological evidence may give valuable diagnostic information. A male with nausea before breakfast, retching and no abdominal pain has a high likelihood of alcohol-related dyspepsia, for example [4].

Effects of therapy

Therapeutic tests in the diagnosis of dyspepsia are not very helpful, though specific ulcer-healing drugs such as histamine H_2-receptor antagonists are often mistakenly used in this way. Improvement may be due to a placebo response or, more dangerously, to the temporary healing of a malignant ulcer. Lack of response could be due to inadequate dosage or poor compliance. Diagnosis before treatment is the rule. The main exception to this is the patient whose symptoms after careful analysis appear characteristic of a functional (non-structural) disorder, with suitable supportive information concerning personal habits or psychiatric problems. Appropriate advice (for example abstension from alcohol or smoking, improved diet, reassurance or simple psychotherapy) may be used and investigations delayed until it is clear that adequate improvement has not occurred.

Investigations

Some tests will be needed in most patients with upper abdominal symptoms. A test should not be arranged until diagnostic probabilities have been assessed on the basis of the clinical history and physical examination. It is useful to write a list of diagnoses in order of probability—as a computer would [4, 10]—and to determine the sequence of investigations by a combination of likelihood, seriousness and potential therapeutic yield.

This is sound intellectual discipline and a logical and economical way to use tests. It is also comforting to the patient if such an analysis can be presented earlier rather than later—it may be valuable in attaining a good therapeutic outcome, particularly in functional disorders.

If the clinician believes that structural disease is unlikely, but proposes an investigation because of the distant possibility of organic disease, the probability of a negative result should be explained to the patient. This will decrease apprehension, indicate that the clinician is not simply shooting blind and will enable the negative result to be used in a positive way.

References

1 BARNES JH. The physiology and pharmacology of emesis. *Mol Aspects Med* 1984;7:397–508.
2 BLOOMFIELD, AL, POLLARD, WS. Experimental referred pain from the gastro-intestinal tract. *J Clin Invest* 1931; 10: 453–473.
3 BONNEY, GLW, PICKERING, GW. Observations on the mechanism of pain in ulcer of the stomach and duodenum. *Clin Sci* 1946;6: 63–111.
4 CREAN, GP, CARD, WI, BEATTIE, AD, *et al.* Ulcer-like dyspepsia. *Scand J Gastroenterol* Vol. 17, Supp. 79. 9–16.

5 DAVENPORT, HW. *Physiology of the digestive tract.* 3rd ed. Chicago: Year Book Medical Publishers, 1971.

6 DE DOMBAL, FT. Analysis of foregut symptoms. In: Baron JH, Moody, FG, eds. *Foregut.* London: Butterworths, 1982.

7 EARLAM, RJ. Further experience with epigastric pain reproduction test in duodenal ulceration. *Br Med J* 1972;2:683-685.

8 HARRISON, A, ISENBERG, JF, SCHAPIRO, M, HAGUE, L. Most patients with active symptomatic duodenal ulcers fail to develop ulcer type pain in response to gastro-duodenal acidification. *Am J Gastroenterol* 1982; 4:105-108.

9 HEADING, RC. Gastric emptying—a clinical perspective. *Clin Sci* 1982;63:231-235.

10 HORROCKS, JC, DE DOMBAL, FT. Diagnosis of dyspepsia from data collected by a physician's assistant. *Br Med J* 1975;2:421-423.

11 JOHNSON, AG. Cholecystectomy and gall-stone dyspepsia. Clinical and physiological study of a symptom complex. *Ann R Coll Surg* 1975;56: 69-80.

12 JONES, FA. Burbulence. *G.I. for the G.P.* 1980; 1: 8.

13 JONES R. Open access endoscopy. *Br Med J* 1985;291:424-426.

14 JORGENSEN LS, BONLOKKE L, WORMBERG P. Non-ulcer upper dyspepsia. Aspects of pain. *Scand J Gastroenterol* 1985;20:45-50.

15 MALAGELADA, JR, CAMILLENI, M. Unexplained vomiting—a diagnostic challenge. *Ann Int Med* 1984; 101: 211-218.

16 MORGAN, MY, SHERLOCK, S. Sex related differences among 100 patients with alcoholic liver disease. *Br Med J* 1977;1:939-941.

17 MORIARTY, KJ, DAWSON, AM. Functional abdominal pain: further evidence that whole gut is affected. *Br Med J* 1982;1:1670-1672.

18 MORLEY, JE, LEVINE, AS. The central control of appetite. *Lancet* 1983;i:398-401.

19 NORTHFIELD, TC, KUPFER, RM, MAUDGAL, DP, *et al.* Gall bladder sensitivity to cholecystokinin in patients with gall-stones. *Br Med J* 1980;280: 143-144.

20 PALMER, WL, HEINZ, TE. Mechanism of pain in gastric and duodenal ulcers. *Arch Intern Med* 1934; 53:269-308.

21 PAYNE, WW, POULTON, EP. Experiments on visceral sensation: relation of pain to activity in human oesophagus. *J Physiol (Lond)* 1927;63:217-241.

22 RITCHIE, J. Pain from distension of the pelvic colon by inflating a balloon in the irritable colon syndrome. *Gut* 1973;14:125-132.

23 SJODIN I, SVEDLUND J, DOTEVALL G, BILLBERG R. Symptom profiles in chronic peptic ulcer disease. A detailed study of abdominal and mental symptoms. *Scand J Gastroenterol* 1985;20:419-427.

24 SWARBRICK, ET, HEGARTY, JE, BAT, L, WILLIAMS, CB, DAWSON, AM. Site of pain from the irritable bowel. *Lancet* 1980;2:443-446.

25 WELCH I, SAUNDERS K, READ NW. Effects of ileal and intravenous infusions of fat emulsions on feeding and satiety in human volunteers. *Gastroenterology* 1985;89:1293-1297.

26 WOLFF, HG, WOLF, S. *Pain* 2nd ed. Springfield, Illinois: Thomas, 1958.

27 YON, CH, LEE, KY, CHEY, WY, MENGUY, R. Electrogastrographic study of patients with unexplained nausea, bloating and vomiting. *Gastroenterology,* 1980;79: 311-314.

Chapter 3
Patterns of Pain in
Gastrointestinal Disease

F. T. DE DOMBAL

It may seem odd that it should be necessary to defend the concept that pain is important, for the very word dis-ease implies that for most patients, some form of pain is the main reason for seeking help. Yet justification is apparently necessary, and justification is amply contained in the following sequence of facts:

1 *Some 10% of North American and European adults have recognizable digestive disease.* In a single year digestive disorders and their treatment in the United States alone cost $10,000,000,000 and 74,000 lives [1].

2 *Most of these patients complain of pain.* Where a structured enquiry into the symptom is undertaken the correct diagnosis will usually be strongly suspected before anything further is done [7, 8].

3 *Many clinicians ask questions about pain which are irrelevant and fail to ask questions which are relevant.* Worse, questions are often phrased in such a way that the question and/or the patient's reply is unintelligible [13, 16, 17, 20].

4 In consequence, *diagnostic accuracy in patients with abdominal pain is about 50%* [6]. Negative laparotomy rates are as high as 60% in some centres [18]. Half of all patients with dyspepsia or a lower alimentary tract problem are not diagnosed correctly at first hospital visit [10, 14, 23]. In general practice, even fewer patients with gastrointestinal cancer are diagnosed and referred before they develop advanced disease [4, 19].

5 *Increased reliance on high technology that follows from this is understandable, but regrettable.* Excessive reliance on high technology has two important drawbacks. Firstly, it is not universally available [25]. Secondly, high technology consumes time and money. This is well illustrated in the problems of diagnosis of gastrointestinal cancer. Despite the increasing technological sophistication, delays extending often to almost a year can occur before the benefits of this high technology can be brought to bear—the median delay between the onset of symptoms and the diagnosis of gastric or large bowel neoplasm was 24–37 weeks in one study [19].

For these reasons, there has been a revived interest in how best to interview patients and thereby maximize the benefits of new technology. The most frequent symptom in patients with gastrointestinal disease is pain. This chapter gives an account of patterns of pain in several gastrointestinal problems. Initially it is helpful to consider some barriers to our understanding of the patterns of pain.

Geographical variation in patterns of pain

A great deal is made of geographical variation in patterns of pain. While patterns of diseases differ around the world, studies by the Organisation Mondiale de Gastro-Enterologie [6] show that variations in pain are much less pronounced—and they are usually the result of variations in terminology, rather than in the underlying disease (Table 3.1). While geographical variation undoubtedly exists, it can be minimized by careful definition of terms.

Table 3.1. Data from World Organisation of Gastroenterology multi-national survey [6] of acute abdominal pain in 6,097 patients, in 15 countries. Similar pointers emerge as in a smaller, one-centre, series.

	Appendicitis (Appx) $n = 1,800$	Non-specific abdominal pain (NSAP) $n = 2,600$	Comment
Site of pain, right lower quadrant	74%	33%	Favours Appx
Aggravated by movement	50%	26%	Favours Appx
or cough	23%	11%	Favours Appx
Relieved by lying still	34%	18%	Favours Appx
Intermittent pain	11%	24%	Favours NSAP

It is clear that if patterns of pain are to be used to their full advantage, for each particular clinical problem a relevant 'short-list' of questions must be drawn up, the phraseology employed must be defined and agreed, and their discriminative value in diagnosis must be appreciated. In the following sections these principles are discussed in relation to three of the most common categories of problems that face the gastroenterologist—the acute abdomen, the patient with an upper gastrointestinal problem, and the patient with a lower gastrointestinal disorder.

Obstacles to understanding patterns of pain

Pain is a subjective phenomenon, difficult to define precisely [2]. Its value in diagnosis and in measuring the effect of treatment depends on two properties, namely the reliability with which it is elicited and the validity with which it reflects what is going on in the body [15]. The three obstacles to eliciting reliable information about pain are: poor selection of questions, lack of precise terminology and questions that do not discriminate.

Poor selection of questions

Medical students are taught to take a thorough case history, ask every conceivable question and leave no stone unturned.

In clinical practice this is quite unrealistic, partly because of constraints of available time and partly because of limitations of memory which functions 'like an information system of limited channel capacity' [21]. Put more simply, this means that we cannot remember more than about seven things at once. Further studies have shown that doctors (however experienced) are no different in this respect from anyone else [11].

These limitations of our thought processes are relevant to history taking. Studies have shown that experienced clinicians curtail their question list, take short cuts and elicit a much shorter history. This means that they *can* analyse it [5]. Unfortunately, the basis upon which clinicians undergo this transformation is often suspect—relying on personal experience, fallible memory, anecdote, or aphorism, rather than observed fact. The phrase 'in my own experience' is a danger sign! Somewhere between acquiring masses of unanalysable information and developing a personal interview style that ignores valuable clues, lies a happy medium—a reasonable short-list of questions about pain that will neither miss out vital clues, nor overload the mind.

Lack of precise terminology

Perhaps the most surprising data concern the low precision of clinical terminology. In a series of carefully monitored interviews, one in five of all the interviewers' questions was phrased so vaguely that three observers were undecided whether it had been asked or not. One in six patients' responses were so vague that the observers were undecided whether the patient had said 'yes', or 'no' [13]. However, this imprecision is remediable. Detailed discussion about the information and agreement on a common terminology reduce the observer variation by three-quarters [13]. For example, when the site of pain is drawn on a vague abdominal plan (as commonly practised) there

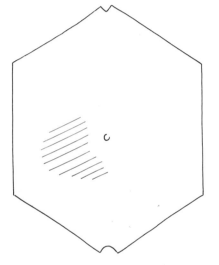

Fig. 3.1. An illustration of a vaguely drawn estimate of pain found in many case records.

is much disagreement as to where the pain really is. When mutually exclusive areas of pain are defined, agreement is easier. In the instance shown (Figs 3.1 and 3.2) observer variation amongst students and junior doctors in describing the site of pain in Fig. 3.1 is 50%, compared with 5% when the framework in Fig. 3.2 is adopted for describing the same pain site.

Nevertheless, categorization of even apparently simple aspects of pain (such as aggravating factors or duration) may turn out to be difficult and unexpectedly complex. For aggravating and relieving factors it is desirable to have the patient do things you can observe—such as to move about in bed, or to cough, and then ask if it hurts. It is also important to distinguish between things that make abdominal pain worse and things that cause pain elsewhere, for example pain in *chest* on coughing. The complexity inherent in the proper elicitation of a history of 'dyspepsia' is illustrated in Fig. 3.3.

On occasion pain cannot be categorized reliably. There is thus little point in carefully classifying pain as mild or moderate, or as a discomfort, or an ache, or as boring, stabbing, knife-like, or by other descriptive terms, if studies of observer variation have shown that it is well nigh impossible to agree on what these terms actually mean.

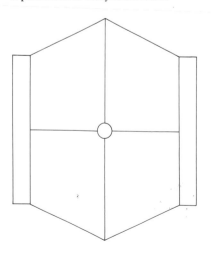

Left upper quadrant
Right upper quadrant
Left lower quadrant
Right lower quadrant

Left half, upper half
Right half, lower half

Left loin, Right loin

Central
General
None

Fig. 3.2. Mutually exclusive system for recording site of abdominal pain under a number of precise headings [13].

History of dyspepsia

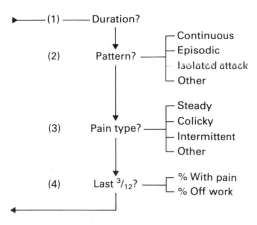

Necessary to specify length and
frequency of episodes/attacks

Fig. 3.3. Classification of interview concerning
dyspepsia. Note complicated series of questions
necessary to deal adequately with the apparently
simple problem of how long discomfort has been
present [13].

Fortunately, such occasions are relatively
rare. During the last decade a number of
centres have developed relatively formal
structures for categorizing pain and clari-
fying this portion of the medical history.

The point is crucial—several studies have
shown that care in asking questions improves the diagnostic accuracy by over
10%.

Questions that do not discriminate

The concept and theory of 'utility of information' has been much discussed. In
clinical practice questions about pain may
be either important in diagnostic terms, or
merely interesting. It is preferable to ask the
former if one wishes to make an accurate
diagnosis [12]. Unfortunately the patterns
of pain in gastrointestinal disease do not fit
precisely into a convenient pathophysiological groove—possibly because patients
find it difficult to translate their disease into
a verbal framework [24]. To the theorist,
this means that patterns of pain are proba-
bilist not determinist and diagnosis usually
rests on a balance of probabilities rather
than on one definitive question.

The inexperienced clinician needs to define for each clinical situation just what are
the most *useful* questions—before the magic
number seven is exceeded and the wood is
obscured by the trees. Consider two possible

Table 3.2. Examples of useful and less useful questions for patients with
acute abdominal pain. The data for each of the seven disease groups
were gathered systematically.

'Pain' aggravated by movement' discriminates for appendicitis or
perforated peptic ulcer, whereas 'vomiting' is so common that it is of
little diagnostic help, as it fails to discriminate among the diagnoses. Yet,
when the patients were interviewed by doctors, 88% were asked about
vomiting and only 46% about pain with movement.

| | % of patients in each diagnostic group | |
Disease category	Pain aggravated by movement	Vomiting
Appendicitis	57	72
Diverticular disease	8	33
Perforated P.U.	24	40
Non-specific pain	9	49
Cholecystitis	6	69
Small bowel obstruction	–	86
Pancreatitis	6	92
% of patients asked	46	88

questions to a patient with acute abdominal pain: 'is the pain aggravated by movement?' and 'have you vomited?' The former question has a high utility. It discriminates well between acute appendicitis, non-specific abdominal pain, and pain due to obstruction of the bowel. The vomiting is actually *more* common in appendicitis—yet this is relatively useless because it occurs in a significant proportion of patients with *any* acute abdominal disorder (Table 3.2). One thus might reasonably suppose that the former question would always be asked, the latter only occasionally. Actually, the reverse is the case—studies in a district general hospital in England showed that the question about vomiting was put to almost 90% of patients with acute abdominal pain, but the more useful question about pain and movement to only 46%. Under such circumstances, small wonder that for many inexperienced clinicians the interview concerning pain leads not to clarity, but to confusion—the magic number seven slips past unnoticed, and the trees crowd in!

Patterns of pain in the acute abdomen

Questions to be asked

Fig. 3.4 shows the questions that should be put to a patient with acute abdominal pain. Developed after consultation with over 100 practising surgeons it represents (at worst) a reasonable starting point for the inexperienced clinician who, by posing these questions, can be reasonably certain that in most instances vital clues are not being missed. It thus represents the minimum acceptable interview concerning pain for all patients with an undiagnosed acute abdomen of less than seven days' duration.

Evaluation of responses

Clearly every patient and each set of responses is unique and can only be properly evaluated by the individual doctor dealing with the patient. This is clinical judgement and no manual or textbook can hope to encompass the problem. However, some general pointers may be helpful.

Typical pain

Fig. 3.5 indicates the commonest site of pain in some of the more common diseases that make up the acute abdomen. At first sight this figure seems unremarkable. However, closer scrutiny shows an important point—that typical pain occurs in less than 75% of patients, whatever the disease, except in renal colic. Indeed, often the stereotype of pain occurs in less than one-third of all patients, as in diverticular disease, where less than one in four patients have the typical lower quadrant pain. In general patients tend to describe pain much more vaguely than textbook descriptions indicate. Thus, while some patients suffer typical pain, a substantial minority describe pain that is more diffuse, or more generalized, or referred to the midline. Whatever the disease suspected, vague, central or general pain in no way rules it out.

Relief and aggravation

Most patients, perhaps surprisingly, claim that very little relieves their acute abdominal pain. By contrast, aggravating factors are of greater importance—especially in the diagnosis of acute appendicitis. The pain of acute appendicitis is much more commonly aggravated by movement, or coughing, than that of any other condition comprising the acute abdomen. To make things more difficult, many patients with perforation fail to claim their pain is made worse by movement because they dare not move. Nevertheless, aggravation by movement and coughing is helpful in diagnosing acute appendicitis from less serious conditions. Pain provoked by inspiration indicates that the

Abdominal Pain Chart

NAME	REG NUMBER
MALE/FEMALE AGE	FORM FILLED BY
PRESENTATION (999, GP, etc)	DATE TIME

PAIN

SITE

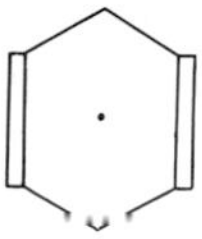

ONSET

PRESENT

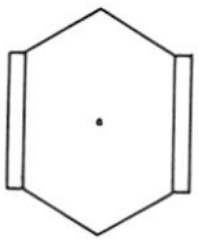

RADIATION

AGGRAVATING FACTORS
  movement
  coughing
  respiration
  food
  other
  none

RELIEVING FACTORS
  lying still
  vomiting
  antacids
  food
  other
  none

PROGRESS
  better
  same
  worse

DURATION

TYPE
  intermittent
  steady
  colicky

SEVERITY
  moderate
  severe

HISTORY

NAUSEA
  yes no

VOMITING
  yes no

ANOREXIA
  yes no

PREV INDIGESTION
  yes no

JAUNDICE
  yes no

BOWELS
  normal
  constipation
  diarrhoea
  blood
  mucus

MICTURITION
  normal
  frequency
  dysuria
  dark
  haematuria

PREV SIMILAR PAIN
  yes no

PREV ABDO SURGERY
  yes no

DRUGS FOR ABDO PAIN
  yes no

LAST MENSTRUAL PERIOD

  pregnant
  vaginal discharge

  dizzy/faint

EXAMINATION

MOOD
  normal
    distressed
    anxious

SHOCKED
  yes no

COLOUR
  normal
  pale
  flushed
  jaundiced
  cyanosed

TEMP   PULSE

BP

ABDO MOVEMENT
  poor/none

  peristalsis

SCAR
  yes no

DISTENSION
  yes no

TENDERNESS

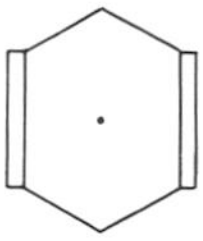

REBOUND
  yes no

GUARDING
  yes no

RIGIDITY
  yes no

MASS
  yes no

MURPHY'S
  +ve −ve

BOWEL SOUNDS
  normal absent +++
RECTAL-VAGINAL EXAM
TENDERNESS
  left
  right
  general
  mass
  none

INITIAL DIAGNOSIS & PLAN

RESULTS
  amylase
  blood count (WBC)
  computer
  urine
  X-ray
  other

DIAG & PLAN AFTER INVEST

(time   )

DISCHARGE DIAGNOSIS

Fig. 3.4 Structured data collection form used in a computer-aided diagnosis trial, showing outline of questions that should be put to patients with acute abdominal pain.

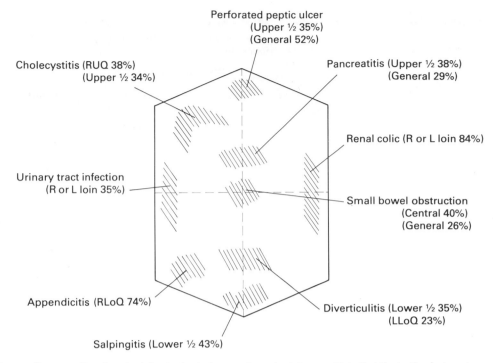

Fig. 3.5 Common sites of acute abdominal pain in some important diseases. Note that the textbook stereotypes of pain occur in relatively few patients. Numbers in parentheses show percentage of patients with the symptom based on a prospective study of more than 1,000 patients (Author's data). RLoQ or LLoQ = right or left lower quadrant.

cause is likely to be above, rather than below, the umbilicus.

Duration, severity and progress

These aspects of pain are of surprisingly little value in the diagnosis of the acute abdomen. Severity and progress are somewhat subjective and perhaps because of this often particularly poorly elicited. This especially applies to mild discomfort or moderate pain—descriptions which seem almost interchangeable to many clinicians and patients. Severe pain, where the patient is in obvious distress, is more helpful and is more commonly found in patients with perforation, pancreatitis, renal colic, cholecystitis, or small bowel obstruction in that order of frequency. The pain of acute ap-

pendicitis is more often described as moderate than severe.

Type of pain

The interviewer should avoid vague descriptive terms such as stabbing or boring. Pain is most helpfully classified as intermittent (with periods of complete relief), colicky or steady. The steadiness of pain due to a perforated ulcer is a useful point of distinction between perforation and high small bowel obstruction. The pain of acute pancreatitis is also surprisingly often colicky—a feature which is useful in discriminating between perforation and acute pancreatitis. Intermittent pain is unlikely to be due to acute appendicitis and this is particularly helpful when this condition is suspected but not certain.

Radiation

Radiation of the pain is also helpful in diagnosis. The pain of appendicitis rarely radiates outside the abdomen. By contrast, pain of urological origin often has a typical loin-to-groin radiation, while gynaecological pain frequently radiates to the back, groin, or down the thigh. The pain of cholecystitis often radiates between the scapulae and to the shoulder tip in about one in seven patients.

Stereotypes of pain

Table 3.3 lists stereotypes of pain patterns in some of the common causes of acute abdominal pain. A disease, (for example, acute appendicitis) *can* present in almost any fashion; but if one wishes to diagnose it with some accuracy, one should look for a patient with pain shifting to the right lower quadrant, aggravated by movement and coughing, relieved by lying still, and so on. Seven aspects of pain for each disease are listed.

Geographical variation

The above stereotypes are based on data from the United Kingdom, mainly from the north of England, and it may be argued that they may not apply elsewhere, but this is not so. Table 3.1 shows data from 1,800 patients with appendicitis and from 2,600 patients with non-specific acute abdominal pain, collated from 15 different countries. The same indicators emerge as useful pointers in this large series. These findings tend to reinforce the conclusion that geographical variation is often the result of poor, or different definitions of the terminology involved. Where, in the World Organisation series, this is remedied, consistent pointers emerge [6].

Patterns of pain in upper gastrointestinal disease

Questions to be asked

The questions that should be put to a patient complaining of non-acute abdominal pain are illustrated in Fig. 3.6. This form was developed after wide consultation and is used in screening and case finding studies. It defines a minimal acceptable interview concerning non-acute abdominal pain in the upper or lower abdomen. If it is to be used by non-medically qualified staff, some of the items are difficult to elicit reproducibly and have to be additionally categorized.* As with acute abdominal pain, the clinician asking this set of questions can be reasonably certain that, most of the time, vital clues are not being missed.

Evaluation of responses

The doctor dealing with patterns of pain in upper gastrointestinal disease should use the history of pain to determine the likely area of the gastrointestinal tract involved. This concept is illustrated in Fig. 3.7 which outlines some of the more helpful features of pain in making this initial anatomical subdivision. This is particularly important because more than one disease can be present in the upper gastrointestinal tract. Thus a patient may have hiatus hernia with reflux oesophagitis, *and* duodenal ulceration, *and* gallstones—the symptom of pain may be the resultant of all three components. In such circumstances the concept outlined in Figure 3.7 is particularly helpful. Pain that has a retrosternal component usually implies that oesophageal disease of some kind is present. In oesophageal disease, perhaps the most important additional questions to ask concern aggravation of pain. In particular, a history of pain pro-

---

* This information is available from Mr F. T. de Dombal, University Department of Surgery, St James Hospital, Leeds LS9 7TF.

Table 3.3. 'Stereotypes' of acute abdominal pain, based on data from over 1,000 patients.

	Acute appendicitis	Non-specific abdominal pain	Cholecystitis	Acute obstruction	Perforation	Acute pancreatitis	Renal colic	Diverticulitis	Salpingitis
Site	Central/ L Symmetrical→RLoQ	Any	Upper ½/RUQ	Symmetrical	Upper½/ general	Upper ½	R/L loin R/L half	Lower ½	Lower ½
Radiation	Nil	Nil	Shoulder/back	Nil	Nil	Nil	Groin	Nil	Groin/back/ thigh
Aggravating factors	Movement cough	Nil	Inspiration	Nil	Movement cough Inspiration	Movement	Nil	Nil	Movement cough
Relieving factors	Lying still	Nil	Nil	Nil	Lying still	Lying still	Nil	Nil	Lying still
Duration	12–48 h	12–48 h	Days	<48 h	<12 h	<48 h	<12 h	Days	Over 24 h
Severity	Moderate	Moderate	Severe	Severe	Severe	Severe	Severe	Moderate	Moderate
Type	Steady	Any	Steady or colicky	Colicky	Steady	Colicky	Colicky	Steady	Steady

R, L = right, left. Lo = lower, upper. Q = quadrant.

NAME: AGE: SEX:

| DURATION OF PAIN/SYMPTOMS: | REFERRING DIAGNOSIS: |

PAIN:

SITE ⬡ ONSET ⬡ CURRENT

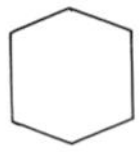

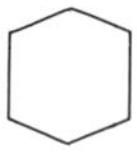

NAUSEA: Yes/No   VOMITING: Yes/No

HAEMATEMESIS: Yes/No   REFLUX: Yes/No

APPETITE: Normal/Decreased

DYSPHAGIA: Yes/No   PREV INDIG: Yes/No

SEVERITY: Moderate/Severe

JAUNDICE: Yes/No   RECTAL PAIN: Yes/No

PROGRESS: Better/Same/Worse

WEIGHT: Steady/Decreased/Increased

AGGRAVATING FACTORS:

BOWELS:

RELIEVING FACTORS:

MICTURITION:

RADIATION:

DETAILS AND/OR OTHER SYMPTOMS:

TYPE OF PAIN:
   Intermittent/Steady/Colicky
   Continuous/Episodic/Cont Attacks

RELATIONS TO MEALS:

NIGHT PAIN: Yes/No

PAST HISTORY: (give details)

SOCIAL HISTORY: (give details)

PREV SIMILAR PAIN: Yes/No

DRUGS:

PREV ABDO SURGERY: Yes/No

FAMILY HISTORY:

OTHER SIG ILLNESS: Yes/No

SMOKING:

PREV ATTENDANCE   Yes/No
AT HOSPITAL

ALCOHOL:

OCCUPATION:

EXAMINATION:

MOOD: Normal/Anxious/Distressed

COLOUR: Normal/Pale/Flushed/Jaundiced

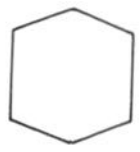

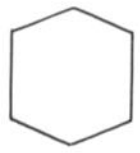

ABDOMINAL MOVEMENT:

TENDERNESS   SWELLINGS

⬡   ⬡

DISTENSION:

RECTAL:

REBOUND:

GUARDING:

HAEMOCCULT: + / − / NP

DIET:

RIGIDITY:

MURPHY:

BOWEL SOUNDS:

OTHER FINDINGS:

DOCTOR'S DIAGNOSIS:

Fig. 3.6 Questions that should be put to a patient complaining of non-acute abdominal pain—a structured form used by physicians' assistants in studies to determine the discriminatory power of various questions.

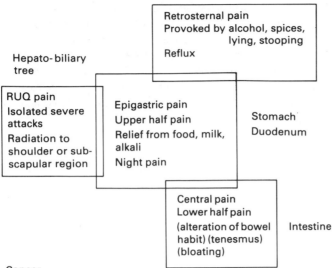

Oesophagus

Fig. 3.7 Patterns of pain in upper gastrointestinal tract disease.

voked by alcohol, hot or spicy food, stooping, or lying down at night, should alert the clinician to the possibility of hiatus hernia, oesophagitis, or perhaps malignancy.

Pain due to disorders in the **stomach** or **duodenum** (it is usually difficult to distinguish between the two) is often epigastric, but may be more vague and perceived throughout the upper half of the abdomen. In this instance it is most helpful to ask about relieving factors. The subject of aggravation by food is mentioned only to be dismissed. Table 3.4 indicates that textbook descriptions of the relationship between eating and pain may not be true. Relief by food, milk, alkali or histamine H_2-receptor antagonists is, however, a useful pointer to a gastroduodenal disorder causing the pain. Such pain often occurs during the night, waking the patient from sleep, as opposed to oesophageal pain which tends to occur as soon as a horizontal posture is adopted.

Hepato-biliary disease is suggested by pain in the right upper quadrant of the abdomen, or which radiates either to the right shoulder, or to the right sub-scapular

Table 3.4. Detailed relationship of timing between ingestion of food and onset of pain in several hundred patients. Note lack of discrimination between diagnostic categories involved.

Timing of pain	Hiatus hernia	Cholecystitis	Duodenal ulcer	Gastric ulcer	Gastric cancer	Non-organic dyspepsia
After food, immediate	20%	10%	2%	15%	16%	15%
After food, delayed	44%	6%	38%	27%	32%	29%
No clear relationship	36%	84%	60%	58%	52%	56%

region. Such pain often occurs in isolated (severe) attacks, rather than continuously, or episodically and may, or may not be accompanied by intolerance of fatty foods.

Confusion may sometimes occur between upper gastrointestinal disease and other disorders such as **diverticular disease, inflammatory bowel disease, irritable bowel syndrome,** or even **large bowel cancer.** In these circumstances it is particularly helpful to remember that central pain, or pain extending into the lower half of the abdomen, or particularly pain which is accompanied by even minor variation in bowel habit may have a lower intestinal cause—even though the patient may assert that he or she suffers from dyspepsia or indigestion.

Stereotypes of pain

As in the acute abdomen, it is profitable to examine stereotypes of pain in some of the common disorders (Table 3.5). This can be instructive, as it indicates how much overlap exists in the patterns of pain resulting from several disorders, reinforcing the concept that study of pain may help determine *where*, rather than *what*, the cause is. In particular the similarity between the pain of gastric ulcer, of gastric cancer and of non-organic dyspepsia is striking. Unless an absolutely classical history is present, the clinician will do well to use the history of pain in upper gastrointestinal disease only to locate the approximate area of the problem, so that further specific questions may follow.

In terms of decision-making, it is worthwhile to point out that the only patients who need an urgent decision are those with cancer. The features which should suggest cancer as a cause for pain are the patient's age and a short history of continuous new symptoms.

Patterns of pain in lower gastrointestinal tract disorders

Questions to be asked

These do not much differ from those to be put to a patient with upper gastrointestinal

Table 3.5. Stereotypes of pain due to common upper GI tract disorders.

	Hiatus hernia	Cholecystitis	Duodenal ulcer	Gastric ulcer	Gastric cancer	'Non organic' dyspepsia
Site	Epigastric	Right upper quadrant	Epigastric	Epigastric	Upper half	Epigastric
Radiation (if present)	Shoulder/back	Shoulder/back	Back	Back	Back	Back
Aggravating factors	Alcohol/food/lying/bending	Food	Food	Food	Food	Food
Relieving Factors	Antacids	Nil	Food, milk antacids	Milk, antacids	Antacids	Antacids
Duration	Any	c. 1 yr	> 1 yr	c. 1 yr	< 1 yr	Any
Type	Continuous	Frequent attacks	Episodic	Frequent attacks	Continuous	Frequent attacks
Progress	Unhelpful	Unhelpful	Unhelpful	Unhelpful	Unhelpful	Unhelpful
Severity	Moderate	Moderate	Moderate	Moderate	Moderate	Moderate
Relationship to food	After eating	Unrelated	Sometimes after eating	Variable	Variable	Variable

symptoms. Indeed, at the first interview it is often impossible to classify the problem; it is quite appropriate that the short list of questions should be similar to those set out in Fig. 3.6.

Evaluation of responses

So far we have studied two types of gastro-intestinal disorders—the acute abdomen, where consideration of pain is crucial and the upper gastrointestinal tract, where consideration of pain may help to localize the disorder anatomically, but not identify the cause. By contrast, in the lower gastro-intestinal tract patterns of pain are much less helpful in diagnosis. This is because many of these patients, even those with colorectal cancer or inflammatory bowel disease, do not complain of pain in the course of their illness, although the presence or absence of pain can itself be a helpful diagnostic feature (Table 3.6). The interviewing clinician normally concentrates upon other symptoms, especially those relating to bowel habit.

Within this overall relatively unhelpful picture, some quite useful diagnostic pointers emerge. Where pain is present, localizing its **site** may be helpful (Table 3.6). **Focal** pain generally indicates diverticular disease in the left lower quadrant and either ileo-caecal Crohn's disease or caecal cancer on the right. Colonic pain in Crohn's disease, ulcerative colitis, rectal cancer or the irrit-

able bowel syndrome is more usually diffuse, central, or vague and general.

Severity and **progress** of pain are of little diagnostic value, but in inflammatory bowel disease, the more severe the pain the more likelihood of Crohn's disease, rather than of ulcerative colitis. If the pain is more important to the patient than altered bowel habit, then Crohn's disease is more likely while the reverse suggests ulcerative colitis.

Enquiring about **aggravating** and **relieving factors** is usually not helpful. The pain of colorectal disease is often relieved by the passage of stool or flatus, but where it is aggravated by this activity a local rectal cause should be suspected—either a minor anorectal condition such as haemorrhoids or fissure, or—more important—a recto-sigmoid cancer.

Unfortunately relief of pain by passage of stool or flatus is a non-specific symptom and may be associated with any of the common conditions affecting the large bowel. This also applies to the sensation of incomplete evacuation. Several textbooks suggest that this symptom is highly suspicious of colorectal cancer. However, studies from a number of centres suggest that a sensation of incomplete evacuation is also common in patients with the irritable bowel syndrome.

As in the upper gastrointestinal tract, **duration** of pain is critical. A short history of continuous pain in middle years is always highly suggestive of a neoplasm. A short history of continuous pain in a

Table 3.6. Location of pain in various common disorders of the lower gastrointestinal tract in 700 patients. Figures are percentages in each disorder.

	Recto-sigmoid cancer	Diverticular disease	Caecal cancer	Ileocaecal Crohn's	Colonic Crohn's	Ulcerative colitis	Irritable bowel syndrome
Focal pain*	5(L)	37(L)	28(R)	46(R)	10(L)	8(L)	14(R)
Diffuse pain†	25	48	38	44	50	47	48
No pain‡	65	10	20	10	40	42	28

*Figures refer to favoured site (R or L lower quadrant).
† Usually lower half.
‡ A small number of patients with unusual or unclassifiable pain are excluded from this table.

patient over 40 years indicates the need for further investigation.

Analysis of pain—humans, mathematics and computers

We have considered in some detail the patterns of pain in several areas of gastrointestinal practice. Finally, as much has been made in recent years of automated decision-making aids and mathematical modelling, it may be worth concluding this chapter by discussing their value.

A number of systems, ranging from simple scoring sheets to complex computer-aided diagnostic systems have been evaluated alongside the clinician in the diagnosis of patients with abdominal pain. Undoubtedly some automated systems have been shown to be associated with a higher diagnostic accuracy than that of the unaided clinician [7]. Various groups demonstrated this in the diagnosis of acute abdominal pain and upper gastrointestinal tract disorders, while the lower gastrointestinal tract has been the subject of a successful attempt by the World Organisation of Gastroenterology Research Committee to develop a simple diagnostic scoring system [3, 22].

Although the potential of these systems seems highly promising, it is likely that in the immediate future they will be available to relatively few clinicians. However, even for clinicians who do not have access to such systems the implications are profound. This is because of the observation that in almost every study the diagnostic accuracy of clinicians improved as terminology was clarified, useful questions were identified and interest in the clinical interview was revived.

Perhaps this is the most important lesson that computer-aided studies can teach and is a suitable point to conclude this chapter. From these studies we learn that an old fashioned approach to patterns of pain,

with careful reproducible questions and considerable attention to detail, improves diagnostic accuracy to an extent which matches that of high technology. It indicates that our present, often lamentable, diagnostic performance is remediable. This is perhaps the most helpful implication of all.

References

1 ALMY TP, MENDELOFF AI, RICE D, *et al.* Prevalence and significance of digestive disease. *Gastroenterology* 1975;**68**:1351–1371.

2 BEECHER PK. *Measurements of subjective responses: Quantitative effects of drugs.* New York: Oxford University Press, 1959.

3 CLAMP SE, MYREN J, BOUCHIER IAD, *et al.* Diagnosis of inflammatory bowel disease: An international multi-centre scoring system. *Br Med J* 1982; **284**:91.

4 CLAMP SE, WENHAM JS. Interviewing by paramedics with computer analysis: Gastro-intestinal cancer. In: *Computer aid in gastroenterology.* Switzerland: S. Karger AG. 1983.

5 DE DOMBAL FT. Surgical diagnosis assisted by a computer. *Proc R Soc Lond [Biol]* 1973;**184**:433.

6 DE DOMBAL FT. Acute abdominal pain. An O.M.G.E. survey. *Scand J Gastroenterol* [*Suppl* 56] 1979;**14**:29–45.

7 DE DOMBAL FT. Computers and the surgeon—A matter of decision. *Surgery Annu* 1979;**11**:33–57.

8 DE DOMBAL FT. Diagnosis of acute abdominal pain. Edinburgh: Churchill Livingstone, 1980.

9 DE DOMBAL FT. The O.M.G.E. acute abdominal pain survey—progress report. *Scand J Gastroenterol* [*Suppl* 25] 1984;**19**:28–41.

10 DE DOMBAL FT, CLAMP SE, HORROCKS JC, *et al.* Computer-aided diagnosis of lower gastrointestinal tract disorders. *Gastroenterology* 1975;**68**,(2) 252–260.

11 DE DOMBAL FT, HORROCKS JC, STANILAND JR. Pattern recognition: A comparison of the performance of clinicians and non-clinicians with a note on the performance of a computer based system. *Meth Inf Med* 1972;**11**:32–37.

12 EDWARDS DAW. Discriminant information in the diagnosis of dysphagia. *J R Coll Physicians Lond* 1975;**9**:257.

13 GILL PW, LEAPER DJ, GUILLOU PJ, *et al.* Observer variation in clinical diagnosis. A computer-aided assessment of its magnitude and importance in 552 patients with abdominal pain. *Meth Inf Medicine* 1973;**12**:108–113.

14 HORROCKS JC, DE DOMBAL FT. Computer-aided diagnosis of dyspepsia. *Amer J Dig Dis* 1975; **20**:397–406.

15 HOUDE RW. Assessment of patients with pain. In: *Pain. New perspectives in measurement and management.* Edinburgh:Churchill Livingstone, 1977:5–12.

16 LEAPER DJ, GILL PW, STANILAND JR, *et al.* Clinical diagnostic process: An analysis. *Br Med J* 1973;3:569.

17 LEAPER DJ, HORROCKS JC, STANILAND JR *et al.* Computer-aided diagnosis of abdominal pain using clinicians estimates of probability. *Br Med J* 1972,4:350–354.

18 LITCHNER S, PFLANZ M. Appendectomy in the Federal Republic of Germany: Epidemiology medical care patterns. *Med Care* 1971;3:911.

19 MACADAM DG. A study in general practice of the symptoms and delay patterns in the diagnosis of gastrointestinal cancer. *J R Coll Gen Pract* 1979,29:723–729.

20 MACADAM WAF. Use of a small desk-top computer to facilitate clinical diagnosis in a district general hospital. Report to the Department of Health & Social Security. 1978.

21 MILLER GA. A magic number seven plus or minus two: some limits on our capacity for processing information. *Psychol Rev* 1966, 81.

22 MYREN J, BOUCHIER JAD, WATKINSON G, DE DOMBAL FT. Inflammatory bowel disease. An O.M.G.E. Survey. *Scand J Gastroenterol [Suppl 56]* 1979; 14:1–27.

23 ROSS P, DUTTON AM. Computer analysis of symptom complexes in patients having upper gastrointestinal examination. *Am J Dig Dis* 1977;17:248.

24 SJÖDIN I, SVEDLUND J, DOTEVALL G, GILLBERG R. Symptom profiles in chronic peptic ulcer disease. *Scand J Gatroenterol* 1985;20:419–427.

25 WILSON G. *A Question of Quality? Roads to assurance in medical care.* Oxford: Oxford University Press, 1976:153.

Chapter 4
Pathophysiology of Diarrhoea

L. A. TURNBERG

Does the patient have diarrhoea?

Although everyone knows what it is, diarrhoea has been surprisingly difficult to define. There is no problem in recognizing its existence in severe cases, but the borderline between normality and diarrhoea can only be agreed arbitrarily. For scientific purposes the passage of stools weighing more than 200 g per day has been a useful indicator. Unfortunately this is not a very helpful definition in clinical practice as few doctors and even fewer patients are likely to weigh their stools.

It is usual therefore to think in terms of frequency of evacuation and consistency of stool; but there are several difficulties with this approach. Not least of these is the setting of limits for frequency and consistency beyond which diarrhoea may be said to occur. A measure of common sense must be applied. A patient who is habitually constipated and who starts evacuating his bowel twice daily might complain of diarrhoea and be right to do so, because it could indicate a serious underlying bowel disease, even though his bowel frequency may not have reached some arbitrarily defined frequency. Similarly, populations consuming diets high in unrefined fibre may pass stools with a consistency which might be regarded in others as indicating diarrhoea, but which clearly is not in those particular populations. Clinical decisions about the occurrence of diarrhoea in a given patient must depend then on the individual patient's usual bowel habit, when a change to a greater frequency or looser consistency

becomes suspicious without the need to define whether the patient has diarrhoea or not.

Another level of difficulty concerns the difference between what patients and what doctors consider as diarrhoea. This is well recognized—for example in patients with carcinoma of the rectum who may pass blood and mucus and complain therefore of diarrhoea, but who also pass normal, formed stools. Less obvious is the patient who has faecal incontinence, but who complains of diarrhoea rather than admits to the incontinence to which some social stigma is attached. In one study of patients complaining of 'diarrhoea', a few were found to have bowel frequencies of only once per day and had incontinence, rather than the diarrhoea of which they complained [21]. Most instances of diarrhoea have an infective cause [22].

These observations only serve to re-emphasize what experienced clinicians know well, that a careful history is essential for accurate diagnosis (see Chapter 3) and definitions of diarrhoea should not be applied slavishly.

Functional definition

The rigorous definition provided by a stool weight of > 200 g/24 h indicates that it is the weight element that is important. As normal stools consist of about 75% water and since the increase in weight in diarrhoea is largely made up of water, another way of defining diarrhoea in a functional sense might be to call it malabsorption of water.

This definition allows consideration of the mechanisms by which water is normally absorbed and the ways in which these processes may be disturbed and diarrhoea result.

Fluid balance in the gut

The duodenum of normal man receives about 7 or 8 l of fluid per day made up of food and endogenous secretions from the salivary glands, stomach, pancreas and biliary tree. Most of this volume is absorbed in the small bowel and only about 1.5 l escapes into the colon. The large bowel absorbs about 90% of the water reaching it, allowing less than 200 ml to escape in the stool of the normal Western man (Fig. 4.1).

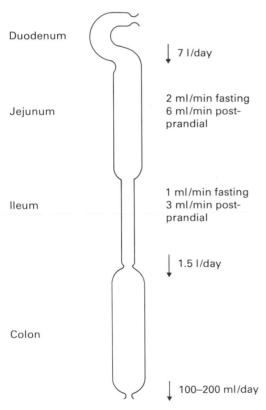

Duodenum

↓ 7 l/day

2 ml/min fasting
6 ml/min post-prandial

Jejunum

Ileum

1 ml/min fasting
3 ml/min post-prandial

↓ 1.5 l/day

Colon

↓ 100–200 ml/day

Fig. 4.1. Average volumes passing through the different regions of the normal human intestinal tract.

Flow rates through the jejunum are about 2 ml/min in the fasting state and may reach 5–6 ml/min after meals. In the ileum flow rates are less and about 1 ml/min and 3 ml/min in the fasting and fed states respectively [11]. Control of gastric emptying influences the flow rate through the upper intestine and hence has an effect on absorption of this large volume of fluid. Among several factors that influence gastric emptying, osmo-receptors in the duodenum detect the presence of hypotonic or hypertonic fluid entering it from the stomach and exert a negative feedback on gastric emptying, allowing time for osmotic equilibration to occur within the duodenum.

Intestinal mucosa acts as a semi-permeable membrane and water absorption occurs as a passive response to physical forces, the most important of which is that derived from osmotic pressure. Osmotic pressure gradients are set up by absorption of solutes and water follows across the mucosa to maintain osmotic equilibrium. Mucosal permeability varies down the length of the intestine. In the jejunum the mucosa is freely permeable to water and small solutes, thus allowing the osmotic pressure of luminal contents to equilibrate rapidly with that of interstitial fluid. Colonic mucosa, on the other hand, is least permeable to water and this characteristic decreases the amount of water that can leak back into the lumen. Ileal permeability lies between that of jejunum and colon. Luminal contents generally remain isotonic throughout the small and large bowel, despite the rapid flux of solutes produced by digestion and absorption of nutrients. In the colon, stool osmolalities may differ from those in plasma because solutes may be absorbed more rapidly than water leaving a hypotonic stool.

Most of the water absorbed passes between epithelial cells rather than through them. The mucosal cells are attached to each other by their so-called 'tight' junctions near to their apical borders, but only loosely applied to each other along their lateral surfaces. The lateral spaces become distended during water absorption. The greater permeability of jejunum than ileum probably reflects differences in permeability of the 'tight' junctions and electron microscopy shows subtle structural differences between the tight junctions in the two regions of the intestine. It has been calculated that the 'pores' in jejunal tight junctions through which water passes are about twice as large as those in the ileum [12]. In the jejunum they are big enough to allow small solutes such as sodium and potassium, as well as water, to pass through readily.

Another force that may influence water transfer is the hydrostatic pressure gradient. It has been shown experimentally that pressure exerted from the luminal side has little effect on transfer of water, but small changes in pressure applied to the serosal aspect of the epithelium markedly influences water absorption [13]. This effect may be responsible for the intestinal secretion induced by experimental portal hypertension and by increasing interstitial pressure with intravenous fluid loading.

Electrolyte absorption

Of the 1000 mmol of sodium chloride that enters the upper intestine each day, only about 3–5 mmol are allowed to escape in the stools. This efficient conservation by the gut helps explain man's ability to survive on a very low salt intake.

Jejunum

In the jejunum, sodium and potassium are absorbed mainly by diffusion down electrical and concentration gradients. In the absence of actively absorbed solutes, salt and water are absorbed sluggishly, but addition of sugars or amino acids markedly stimulates absorption. Here, actively ab-

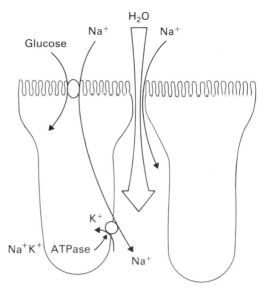

Fig. 4.2. Glucose-stimulated sodium absorption in the jejunum. Glucose and sodium are transported into the cell on a 'common carrier' and the sodium is extruded at the baso-lateral membrane by the ATPase sited there. Water, mainly flowing through the tight junctions in response to the osmotic pressure gradient created by solute movement, sweeps more sodium up in its stream by 'solvent drag'.

sorbed solutes induce water to flow in the same direction to maintain osmotic equilibrium. Because the pores through which water is flowing are large, they allow sodium and potassium ions to be swept up in the stream of water and be 'dragged' across the mucosa between epithelial cells (Fig. 4.2) [12, 35]. In addition sodium is absorbed with organic solutes such as glucose or amino acids on a 'common carrier' protein sited on the brush border membrane. This coupled transfer takes sodium and solute into the cell more efficiently than either alone. Sodium is extruded actively from the other side of the cell by the sodium/potassium sensitive ATPase on the basolateral membrane. This enzyme maintains a low intracellular sodium concentration that encourages sodium entry down its concentration gradient across the apical membrane. This is the driving force for absorption of other solutes, such as glucose, which are coupled to sodium and ride in on its back (Fig. 4.2) [3]. There are thus two routes for sodium transfer across the mucosa, a paracellular and a cellular route. The former is of greater significance in the highly permeable jejunum, while in the ileum 'solvent drag' is of minor importance.

Chloride ions are absorbed passively in the jejunum although in some circumstances chloride may be actively secreted [4].

Bicarbonate is absorbed until its intraluminal concentration is as low as 2–3 mmol/l —well below plasma concentrations. The generation of this concentration gradient for bicarbonate presumably requires metabolic energy and therefore is likely to be an active process. Evidence derived from *in vivo* perfusion studies in man suggests that bicarbonate is 'removed' by secretion of hydrogen ions (Fig. 4.3) [38]. This

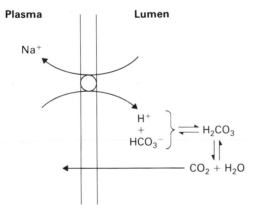

Fig. 4.3. Bicarbonate in the lumen is 'absorbed' by reaction with secreted H+ ions to form carbon dioxide and water. Secreted H+ exchanges for Na+ and thus Na+ absorption is stimulated.

generates carbon dioxide and water and is responsible for the high luminal pCO_2. Since the absorption of bicarbonate also stimulates sodium absorption, it has been postulated that sodium may be absorbed in exchange for the secreted hydrogen ions. It is

interesting that experiments on vesicles derived from isolated brush border membranes also provide evidence of a sodium/hydrogen exchange mechanism [24].

Ileum

The absorption of salt and water in the jejunum is thus dependent on the absorption of nutrients and of bicarbonate secreted in bile and pancreatic juice. A different situation arises in the ileum, where the mucosa is less permeable and there is less nutrient available to stimulate salt and water absorption. Here both sodium and chloride can be absorbed against considerable electrochemical gradients and it is likely that specific active absorptive processes are involved. Luminal chloride concentrations fall while bicarbonate ions accumulate in the lumen and it has been postulated that these changes are compatible with an anion exchange process. In addition there is evidence, as in the jejunum, for a cation (Na^+/H^+) exchange. Thus a double ion exchange may exist with sodium and chloride being absorbed in exchange for bicarbonate and hydrogen secreted, the two secreted ions reacting in the lumen to form carbon dioxide and water (Fig. 4.4) [37]. Evidence in favour of this idea has been derived from *in vivo* perfusion experiments in human ileum, and recent studies of ion transport across vesicles obtained from apical membranes of epithelial cells support this [20]. Whatever the mechanisms involved, absorption of sodium and chloride is achieved by active, energy requiring processes and concentration gradients may be created across ileal mucosa. Since ileal mucosa is less permeable to ions than jejunum, the back flux that might nullify the absorptive process is decreased.

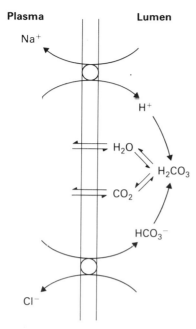

Fig. 4.4. Model for human ileal ion transport. A double ion exchange is depicted as responsible for Na^+ and Cl^- absorption, in exchange for H^+ and HCO_3.

Colon

During the 24 to 48 hours that colonic contents move slowly from the caecum to the anal margin, they are transformed from fluid ileal discharge into semi-solid stools.

The colon is capable of absorbing three to four times its average daily load of some 1.5 l. Infusion of 4 l of saline into the distal ileum during 24 hours hardly affected stool weight, but more rapid infusion of 500 ml over a shorter time did increase stool water [5]. One study suggested that ileal flow rates greater than 6 ml/min are likely to result in diarrhoea, but rates below that are probably compensated for by the colon, providing it functions normally [25]. If the colon is diseased patients may notice diarrhoea when stool volumes increase to only 300 or 400 ml/day and this might occur if water absorption decreased by a small fraction, from say, 1.5 l to 1.1 l per day. Colonic

function is thus critical in determining whether symptomatic diarrhoea will occur.

Large ionic concentration gradients are created by colonic mucosal transport so that stool sodium concentrations reach about 40 mmol/l, potassium concentrations 90 mmol/l and chloride concentrations 16 mmol/l, and these are clearly different from plasma concentrations (Table 4.1). In addition there is a high electrical potential difference across the mucosa with the lumen maintained at about 30–40 mV negative to the interstitial fluid. The mechanisms involved in creating these gradients appear to be an active, current-generating absorption of sodium together with a neutral anion exchange process by which chloride is absorbed in exchange for bicarbonate (Fig. 4.5) [15]. The accumulation of potassium to a high concentration in the lumen results from a combination of passive movement down the electrical gradient, se-

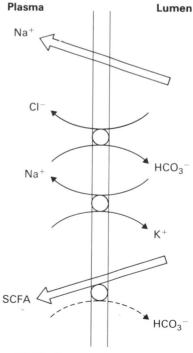

Fig. 4.5. Model of human colonic ion transport. Short chain fatty acids (SCFA) are absorbed passively, possibly in exchange for HCO_3.

Table 4.1. Average concentrations and quantities of electrolytes and water entering and leaving the colon and the amounts absorbed per day. Bicarbonate concentration measurements in stool water are unhelpful, because much of the bicarbonate is removed by reaction with organic acids in the lumen.

	Concentrations (mmol/l)			Quantities (ml or mmol/day)		
	Plasma	Ileal Effluent	Stool Water	Ileal Effluent	Excreted in stool	Absorbed
H_2O	–	–	–	1500	100	1400
Na^+	140	140	40	210	4	206
K^+	5	6	90	9	9	0
Cl^-	100	70	16	105	2	103
HCO_3	25	50	–	75	–	–

cretion in mucus, loss in desquamated epithelial cells and an active secretory process, probably in exchange for some absorbed sodium. The very low permeability of colonic mucosa allows these large ionic concentration gradients to be maintained.

There are regional differences in absorptive activity, the right side dealing with large volumes of ileal effluent, absorbing salt avidly. It is more permeable than the left side and maintains a lower electrical potential difference. The left side of the colon, being less permeable, is capable of maintaining the high concentration gradients with which it is faced.

Short chain or volatile fatty acids are produced from unabsorbed dietary carbohydrates by bacterial fermentation and form about 70% of total stool anions. Acetate, proprionate and butyrate form 85% of these and they have a concentration in stool water of between 100 and 240 mmol/l [41]. Absorption occurs by passive diffusion and is dependent on molecular size and lipid solubility. The larger the molecule and the greater the lipid solubility the more rapid the rate of absorption. As bicarbonate accumulates in the lumen during fatty acid absorption it is possible that there is an anion exchange of fatty acid for bicarbonate. Another possibility is that the fatty acids are absorbed with H^+ ions in the pro-

tonated form, leaving bicarbonate ions in the lumen and causing the observed fall in pCO_2 [31]. Fatty acids stimulate sodium absorption too.

Normally the colon has a large capacity to absorb these fatty acids and the ability to do so may be critically important in determining the likelihood of diarrhoea. Patients with lactase deficiency for example, may not develop diarrhoea, because their colons can compensate by absorbing the volatile fatty acids derived from lactose. It is only if the delicate balance between the fatty acid delivery rate on the one hand, and absorption rate on the other is upset, that diarrhoea may occur. This might happen, for example, if intake of the offending disaccharide was excessive, or if transit rate through the large bowel was increased. This may explain why patients with established lactose intolerance may have intermittent diarrhoea.

Some of these fatty acids can be used by colonic mucosa for its own metabolic needs and some are passed on into the plasma. Their nutritional value is probably less than 1% of calorie requirements in man. It has been calculated however, that where vegetable fibre intake is high, up to 540 kcal might be absorbed per day and this could be of some importance in societies where alternative calorie sources are scarce [23].

Control of absorption

Aldosterone

A number of hormones are capable of influencing intestinal salt and water absorption. Aldosterone and to some extent corticosteroids stimulate colonic sodium and water absorption and have a similar, but less marked influence in the small intestine. Although this effect may be important in some animals its relevance in man is uncertain. The influence of aldosterone on the bowel is trivial compared with its effects on the kidney. Thus even the complete retention of the 5 mmol of sodium which escape in the normal stool will not benefit a salt depleted patient with secondary hyperaldosteronism very much. In patients with diarrhoea however, in whom sodium losses may be much greater, it is possible that secondary hyperaldosteronism will modulate sodium losses and this type of response has been reported in childhood diarrhoea [30]. Patients with chronic purgative addiction may develop secondary hyperaldosteronism which is probably responsible for their excessive potassium losses in the urine and possibly faeces, and which leads to the hypokalaemia so characteristic of this condition (see Chapter 5).

Hormones, peptides and neurotransmitters

As net absorption is the result of a balance between absorption and secretion, control of the net result is achieved by changing the secretory element of this balance. A growing list of hormones, peptides and neurotransmitters have been shown experimentally to be capable of stimulating secretion in the intestine (Table 4.2) [26]. Only some of these are likely to be physiologically important. Cholinergic agonists provoke secretion and α_2 and β adrenergic agonists promote absorption. Relevant nerve fibres close to the intestinal epithelium, and binding receptors for the agonists have been demonstrated on epithelial cells. It is possible therefore that a balance between a cholinergic drive to secretion and an adrenergic

Table 4.2. Agents derived from neuro-endocrine and other cells in the gut shown to be capable of influencing intestinal absorption or secretion under experimental conditions.

Secretory agents	Absorptive agents
Cholinergic (muscarinic)	
VIP	α_2 and β adrenergic
Neurotensin	Cholinergic (nicotinic)
Substance P	Somatostatin
Bombesin	Enkephalin
Bradykinin	Dopamine
Angiotensin II (high concentration)	Angiotensin II (low concentration)
Serotonin	NPY
Secretin	
Glucagon	
Gastrin	
CCK	
GIP	
Motilin	
PHI	
ATP	
Histamine	
Prostaglandins	

drive to absorption exerts fine control over net absorption [27].

Vaso-active intestinal polypeptide (VIP) is found in high concentrations in nerve fibres adjacent to the epithelium and is a potent secretagogue. Its role in control is unknown, but clearly it has a potential for it. Many other peptides found in neuro-endocrine cells in the gut are capable of stimulating secretion. On the other hand, enkephalins and somatostatin stimulate absorption and inhibit secretion and these too are present in neuro-endocrine cells. We are thus faced with a large number of substances that can influence transport and are present at relevant sites within the gut. It has not proved possible, so far, to assign a physiological role to any of these, however.

The possibility that a disturbance of one or more of these agents is responsible for diarrhoeal disease is also worthy of consideration and in some instances a clear association has been demonstrated.

Intracellular events

Many of the biochemical steps involved in mediating intestinal secretion provoked by secretagogues are known and this knowledge is proving valuable in aiding our understanding of the mechanisms of diarrhoea and pointing the direction for therapeutic intervention. After attachment to their selective receptors, agonists stimulate the generation of an intracellular second messenger. The mechanism by which the external trigger is transduced to provoke the intracellular step is uncertain, but in some instances changes in the phospholipids of cell membranes and possibly prostaglandins are involved [1]. In many instances the second messenger is cyclic adenosine monophosphate (cAMP) generated by activation of adenylate cyclase. Activation of protein kinase follows and, after a series of obscure biochemical steps, secretion is stimulated, probably by an increase in mucosal border permeability to chloride

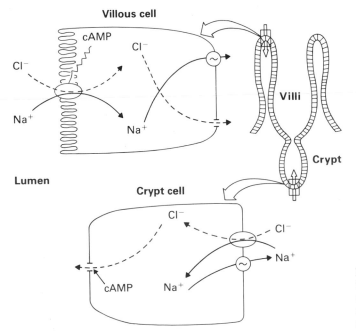

Fig. 4.6. Postulated mechanisms for differential crypt and villous cell function in cyclic AMP mediated secretion (with permission from [8]).

ions [8]. There is indirect evidence to suggest that intestinal secretion arises predominantly by this mechanism from crypt epithelium, while on the villi absorption is simply inhibited in response to cyclic AMP generation (Fig. 4.6) [8].

Another cyclic nucleotide, guanosine monophosphate, has been implicated in mediating secretion provoked by the heat stable toxin of *E. coli*, but not so far in physiological circumstances. Finally, the intracellular free calcium ion concentration seems to be critical for secretion. It is normally held at a very low concentration (10^{-7}M) and transient slight elevations trigger secretion. It may do so by activating a 'calcium-dependent regulator protein', calmodulin [18]. Calcium may also be involved in mediating the response to cyclic nucleotides. Some of these mechanisms are presumed to be operative in physiological circumstances, but more is known about their involvement in toxigenic secretory diarrhoeas.

Mechanisms of diarrhoea

Disturbances of the normal processes by which salt and water are absorbed are liable to result in diarrhoea and it is possible to categorize the mechanisms according to the underlying physiological principles governing water absorption outlined above. Thus malabsorption of any water-soluble nutrient will retain water within the lumen and cause an osmotic diarrhoea. Diseases that interfere with the permeability of intestinal mucosa or that inhibit the active absorption of salt will result in diarrhoea. Finally, the stimulation of secretion of salt and water is an important cause of diarrhoeal disease.

Osmotic diarrhoea

Water moves across intestinal mucosa as a natural consequence of osmotic pressure gradients. It follows therefore that the presence within the lumen of unabsorbed solutes will retain water there to maintain isotonicity. Thus the poorly absorbed magnesium sulphate remains in the lumen in iso-osmotic solution and acts as an osmotic purgative. An osmotic element undoubtedly contributes to the diarrhoea caused by many diseases. A good example is **lactase deficiency,** in which patients do not digest lactose. This disaccharide remains in the lumen, retaining water with it until it reaches the colon. There it is split by colonic bacteria into an increased number of solutes which draw more water into the lumen. Whether such patients develop diarrhoea is dependent to a large extent on the rate at which the short chain fatty acids (produced from lactose) are absorbed, compared with the rate of transit through the colon.

In **coeliac disease** not only is fat malabsorbed, but a number of water-soluble substances such as disaccharides and peptides, may be absorbed poorly too. These add an osmotic load to the steatorrhoea and contribute to the volume of the diarrhoeal stool.

Permeability defects

The high permeability of jejunal mucosa allows the rapid flux of salt and water to accompany the active absorption of nutrients. Diseases which impair jejunal mucosal permeability might therefore have a marked effect on absorption. In **coeliac disease** for example, jejunal permeability is markedly decreased, so that salt and water are only sluggishly transported across it. The gross distortion of mucosal architecture, with a change in the structure of tight-junctions, might be responsible for this disturbance which will enhance the tendency to diarrhoea.

In **inflammatory bowel disease** permeability of the rectosigmoid mucosa to water and small solutes is decreased. On the other hand, studies of small bowel permeability in patients with Crohn's disease suggested an increased permeability when larger probe molecules were used. Thus polyethylene glycols of varying molecular size permeate intestinal mucosa more readily in patients with Crohn's disease than in normal subjects. In order to explain the paradox of increased permeability to large molecules and decreased permeability to small molecules, it is necessary to consider the pathways through which these different molecules pass. Small ions and water pass through innumerable small pores present in tight junctions between every cell and, to a lesser extent, across cell membranes, while large molecules of the size of polyethylene glycol pass through a small number of large pores present, for example, at the tips of villi from where effete cells are shed. These larger holes are likely to be responsible for allowing the normal absorption of very small amounts of very large molecules which are known to enter the body. Decreased permeability to small solutes and increased permeability to large solutes can be explained on the basis of a reduction in the size of the innumerable small pores, but a slightly increased size, or number of the very large pores. The decrease in size is particularly liable to diminish the absorption of salt and water and encourage diarrhoea.

Defects in active transport

Active transport processes for the absorption of sodium and chloride achieve greatest significance in the ileum and colon, where they can generate high concentration gradients across the mucosa. It is likely that a non-specific reduction in transport enzyme activities will accompany a number of inflammatory or destructive diseases of the intestinal mucosa, but there is one rare inherited disease in which a highly specific defect in chloride ion transport results in a profound diarrhoea.

Although rare, **congenital chloride-losing diarrhoea** is an instructive disturbance as it emphasizes the importance of normal intestinal transport. Patients with the disease have severe watery diarrhoea from birth and may die in infancy from the effects of salt and water losses. The diagnostic features of the disease include a remarkably high concentration of chloride ions in the stool water, which usually exceeds plasma chloride concentrations. Diagnostically stool chloride concentrations exceed the sum of the sodium and potassium concentrations, the cation gap being made up of ammonium. It is usual for patients with severe watery diarrhoea to develop a metabolic acidosis, but in chloridorrhoea alkalosis is the abnormality which may alert the paediatrician to the diagnosis. From studies of intestinal function in patients with this disease it has been proposed that the defect is limited to the ileum and colon where chloride absorption and the accompanying bicarbonate secretion are impaired [36]. The most likely biochemical basis for these defects is a deletion of the chloride/bicarbonate exchange in the mucosa. Such a defect would explain why patients are unable to absorb chloride, which will remain in the lumen as an unabsorbed osmotic solute. The failure to secrete bicarbonate results in the development of an alkalosis (Fig. 4.7). The occurrence of this condition lends support to the hypothesis that in the normal intestine an anion exchange mechanism mediates chloride absorption.

If the mucosal changes in patients with **coeliac disease** are severe enough to extend down to the ileum, then it is likely that active ion transport processes normally operative there will be impaired and add to the diarrhoea that these patients suffer. In experimental **viral gastroenteritis** in piglets small intestinal salt and water absorption is impaired and this may be due to the stunt-

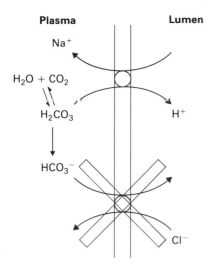

Fig. 4.7. Congenital chloridorrhoea. Model of presumed defect; the absence of a Cl^-/HCO_3 exchange leaves HCl in the lumen and $NaHCO_3$ in the plasma.

ing of villi which occurs. It is likely that this diminution in epithelial cells will reduce the availability of transport enzymes and indeed a reduction in activity of at least one enzyme, sodium potassium ATPase, has been confirmed [19].

In **ulcerative colitis** a defect in active sodium absorption with a concomitant decrease in transmucosal electrical potential difference has been demonstrated [14]. This defect, together with a diminished permeability to chloride ions, may well be important in causing malabsorption of salt and water in inflammatory bowel disease.

Secretory diarrhoea

The most dramatic example of a secretory diarrhoea is that due to **Asiatic cholera** (see Chapter 43). Patients may lose 10–20 l of watery stool per day and the high mortality is directly attributable to the severe degree of dehydration which results. The discovery of the underlying mechanisms by which the cholera toxin stimulates the intestine to secrete these large volumes of fluid has been a major impetus to the understanding of

the pathophysiology of this and other diarrhoeal diseases [7].

Most of the secretion in cholera arises from the jejunum, little or none coming from the colon. There is strong circumstantial evidence to suggest that the crypts, rather than villi, are the source of the secretion [8]. The intriguing early observations that the intestinal mucosa is histologically normal despite the massive secretion of fluid was followed by the demonstration that the mucosa was also functionally normal with respect to absorption of sugars and amino acids. Not only were these nutrients absorbed normally, but they stimulated absorption of salt and water normally too and this observation has had vitally important therapeutic implications. These findings suggested that the disease did not involve a diffuse disturbance of intestinal function, but rather a very specific secretory process was at work.

Although some questions remain, much of the underlying biochemical process responsible for cholera-induced secretion has been elucidated (Fig. 4.8) [10]. The toxin is now known to have one A subunit attached to five B subunits. The B subunits are necessary for the toxin to attach to a selective ganglioside receptor (GM1) on the microvillous cell membrane. Once attached, the A subunit is transferred into the cell membrane where it splits into A_1 and A_2 subunits and the A_1 moiety activates the enzyme adenylate cyclase. This catalyses the generation of cAMP from ATP in the cytoplasm. Cyclic AMP is then believed to act as a second messenger and activates a protein kinase. The subsequent steps leading to secretion are obscure, but involve phosphorylation of intracellular proteins, one or more of which may be directly concerned with mediating ion transport across the apical cell membrane. Considerable experimental evidence supports this proposed mechanism, but work is still needed to clarify several difficulties. Recent work has sug-

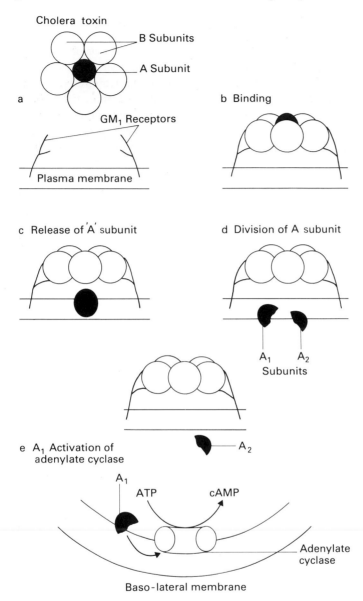

Fig. 4.8. Cholera toxin activation of epithelial adenylate cyclase (adapted from [10]).

gested, for example, that a neurological pathway may be involved in the secretion [2].

Whatever the mechanism, there seems little doubt that cAMP is generated in response to cholera toxin either directly or through a neurological intermediary. Once enterocytes have been triggered they continue to secrete for two to three days, even after a brief exposure to the toxin. It seems likely that activated enterocytes remain in a secretory state during the whole of their life cycle until they are shed at the tips of the villi.

The knowledge that nutrient absorption stimulates the absorption of salt and water even in the presence of cholera-induced secretion has been harnessed to great benefit in oral rehydration therapy. World Health Organization (WHO) programmes widely promulgated in the Indian sub-continent are based on this physiological principle. Initially glucose/salt mixtures were advised, but it now seems likely that the more wi dely available sucrose is just as good as glucose at enhancing absorption of salt and water. The widespread use of oral rehydration therapy is decreasing the need for scarce and expensive intravenous solutions.

Emphasis on oral rehydration has influenced therapy for many other different types of diarrhoea. This has proved particularly important in infants with diarrhoea and in debilitated adults who tolerate dehydration poorly.

It now seems likely that a number of other toxigenic diarrhoeal diseases involve the same mechanism which mediates cholera toxin diarrhoea. Such is the case for the heat labile toxin of *E. coli*, which is responsible for much travellers' diarrhoea. A toxin produced by *Clostridium perfringens* stimulates intestinal adenylate cyclase and there is some suggestive evidence that toxins produced by *Staphylococcus aureus*, *Shigella dysenteriae* and *Klebsiella pneumoniae* may act similarly.

The adenylate cyclase system has also been implicated in a number of non-infective diarrhoeal illnesses. For example, in extensive ileal resection the diarrhoea may be due to stimulation of colonic adenylate cyclase by bile salts that spill over into the colon. Whether this mechanism causes the diarrhoea, or whether a bile salt-induced increase in epithelial cell membrane permeability is responsible has not been resolved. Long chain fatty acids in the colon of patients with **steatorrhoea** have also been shown to be capable of stimulating secretion and the mechanism by which they act is likely to be similar to that underlying bile salt-induced secretion.

Prostaglandins and diarrhoea

A number of prostaglandins have been shown to have profound effects on intestinal transport [16]. Prostaglandin E_2 and $F_{2\alpha}$ provoke intestinal secretion and stimulate adenylate cyclase activity [29]. Since prostaglandins are produced in response to trauma or inflammation, it is reasonable to postulate that in some diseases prostaglandins are liberated locally where they might be the mediators of secretory diarrhoea.

It has been shown recently that prostaglandin E_2 is synthesized predominantly by sub-epithelial tissues and very little is produced in the epithelium. On the other hand prostaglandin E_2 breakdown proceeded at a much greater rate in the epithelial compared with sub-epithelial tissues [34]. This arrangement provides a base for a hypothesis in which prostaglandin production beneath the mucosa influences mucosal function, the prostaglandins then being rapidly broken down at the site of action. Concentrations of prostaglandins in stool water are raised in patients with **ulcerative colitis** and cultured biopsies of colonic mucosa from colitics synthesize prostaglandins at a greater rate than normal mucosal biopsies [33]. Interestingly in this study sulphasalazine and its active constituent 5-aminosalicylic acid inhibited prostaglandin synthesis, suggesting the possibility that part of the mechanism of action of this drug might be through its ability to inhibit prostaglandin synthesis [33]. Unfortunately this potentially interesting line of therapy has not been successful, as treatment of ulcerative colitis with more potent prostaglandin synthesis inhibitors has been fruitless.

Patients with **medullary carcinoma of the thyroid** often have diarrhoea and it is likely that one or more of the substances secreted into the circulation by the tumours are responsible. Prostaglandins have been implicated, but other substances must play a part because diarrhoea persists, even though prostaglandin concentrations are only intermittently raised in many patients. It is not surprising therefore, that inhibitors of prostaglandin synthesis are of only limited benefit in some patients.

Prostaglandin production may be stimulated by a number of infective agents and the observation that aspirin and indomethacin, which inhibit prostaglandin synthesis, decreased secretion provoked by **cholera toxin** and *Salmonella* infection in experimental animals lent support to this idea [40]. However, direct evidence in favour of a role for prostaglandins in these types of secretory diarrhoea has not been forthcoming and the actions of aspirin and indomethacin in enhancing absorption may not involve inhibition of prostaglandin synthesis. Although the action of aspirin is uncertain it has been used in small therapeutic trials in the treatment of cholera where it apparently had a limited effect.

It is possible that prostaglandin synthesis is involved in mediating secretagogue responses at a more subtle level. The prostaglandin precursor, arachidonic acid, is a constituent of phospholipids found in all cell membranes including the intestinal epithelium. Local production of prostaglandins at the cell membrane level may be involved in transducing secretory stimuli [1] and, if this is true, it is unlikely that measurements of prostaglandin concentrations in whole tissues will reveal these subtle changes.

Other secretagogues

A number of the rare peptide-secreting tumour syndromes may be associated with diarrhoea. The classical example of these is the **Verner-Morrison syndrome** due to a VIP secreting adenoma of the islets of Langerhans. It is characterized by severe cholera-like diarrhoea and high circulating concentrations of VIP. Since VIP is a potent secretagogue and activates mucosal adenylate cyclase it seems likely that this is the mechanism by which diarrhoea occurs.

VIP is now recognized to be an important neurotransmitter found in the central and peripheral nervous systems. In the bowel it is present in high concentrations in a network of nerves in the villous core and adjacent to the epithelium [32]. Receptors for VIP have been demonstrated on isolated epithelial cells and since VIP is such a potent secretagogue, it seems reasonable to suppose that it may exert some control over intestinal absorption. It is also conceivable that local production of VIP may mediate secretory diarrhoea provoked by a variety of mechanisms. The observation that nerve blockers inhibit cholera-induced secretion has given rise to the suggestion that a neurological mechanism is activated under these conditions. In favour of this proposal is the observation that VIP is liberated into luminal contents and into venous effluent after exposure of intestinal mucosa to cholera toxin. Direct proof of this involvement of a VIPergic mechanism is lacking, however.

Patients with the **Zollinger-Ellison syndrome** secrete gastrin and some of these patients also have diarrhoea which may be due to a gastrin-induced intestinal secretory process. Gastrin, however, does not stimulate adenylate cyclase activity and another secretory mechanism is presumably involved. A number of other peptides produced in excess by tumours have been described in association with secretory diarrhoea (Table 4.3).

Non-cAMP secretory mechanisms

Secretion can also occur in the absence of changes in mucosal adenylate cyclase activity or cAMP concentrations. For example, the heat-stable toxin of *E. coli*, a potent secretagogue and an important cause of travellers' diarrhoea, stimulates secretion without activating adenylate cyclase. An-

Table 4.3. Neuro-endocrine tumour syndromes and some of the substances presumed to be responsible for the bowel disturbances. In some instances a combination of agents may provoke the diarrhoea [28].

Syndrome	'Hormone'
Pancreatic 'cholera' (Verner-Morrison syndrome)	VIP PHI
Zollinger–Ellison syndrome	Gastrin
Carcinoid syndrome	Serotonin Calcitonin Prostaglandins } less common Histamine
Medullary carcinoma of thyroid	Calcitonin Prostaglandins Serotonin Substance P
Mastocytosis	Histamine
Ganglioneuroma	VIP
Hyperthyroidism	Thyroxine
Glucagonoma	Glucagon (usually constipation)
Somatostatinoma	Somatostatin (steatorrhoea)

other cyclic nucleotide, cyclic guanosine monophosphate increases in response to activation by the toxin of guanylate cyclase, although the exact inter-relationship between cyclic GMP generation and secretion is not yet clear [9]. A toxin produced by *Yersinia enterocolitica* also stimulates secretion through cyclic GMP but other examples of this mechanism remain to be demonstrated.

Recently the toxin of *Clostridium difficile*, the organism held to be responsible for antibiotic-induced pseudomembranous colitis, has also been shown to provoke secretion in the absence of histological damage. Neither cAMP nor cGMP appear to be involved, but it is dependent on the presence of calcium in the bathing medium [17]. A number of secretagogues have been shown to need calcium for their action. Acetyl choline requires calcium to stimulate secretion, but hitherto a diarrhoeal disease associated with an excess cholinergic drive has not been convincingly described. It is tempting to speculate that some patients with the irritable bowel syndrome with watery diarrhoea may have a parasympathetic stimulus to secretion, but there is no direct evidence in favour of this idea.

5-hydroxytryptamine (serotonin, 5-HT) is a secretagogue which is also dependent on calcium for its action [6]. 5-HT is liberated in excess from the tumour of patients with the carcinoid syndrome and this may be responsible for the diarrhoea in this condition.

Combined mechanisms of diarrhoea

It is likely that in any individual a combination of the potential mechanisms described above contributes to the diarrhoea. An osmotic element, decreased permeability, inhibition of active transport processes together with intestinal secretion may all be operative, for example in coeliac disease, and it is likely to be true to a variable degree in other forms of diarrhoea.

The role of disturbances of motility has not been touched upon, but there are considerable difficulties that remain unresolved concerning the part played by motility in the normal and abnormal bowel.

It seems reasonable to assume that if the rate of transit through the intestine was increased by abnormal motility, contact time with the mucosa would be shorter and hence absorption would be impaired. Despite the credibility of this assumption it has been extremely difficult to demonstrate a specific motility defect to which diarrhoea can be ascribed. Certain patterns of motility have been described in some diseases, but they are not constantly present and their relationship to the pathogenesis of the diarrhoea is uncertain [39]. In **scleroderma** for example, a decreased gastro-colic reflex will diminish colonic contractions and thereby decrease resistance to passage of faeces into the rectum. Equally, however, it may be argued that such a disturbance should lead to constipation. In **ulcerative colitis** fewer segmenting contractions, together with increased mass movements will probably promote diarrhoea. Abnormal motor activity has been found in the colon of patients with the **irritable bowel syndrome**, but the defects demonstrated have been as likely to be associated with constipation as with diarrhoea. Such observations do not deny the possibility that motility disturbances can be responsible for diarrhoea, but indicate the inadequacy of current information. It seems likely that a combination of defects in salt and water absorption and of motility disturbances is involved in many diarrhoeal diseases.

Diagnostic value of stool electrolyte concentrations

As the severity of diarrhoea increases so faecal electrolyte concentrations change and increasingly resemble those in plasma. Concentrations of sodium and chloride rise and of potassium fall, approaching concentrations in plasma when stool volumes reach about 1 l per day. This is the case whatever the origin of the diarrhoea, but in those conditions where an osmotic element is present, as for example in lactose malabsorption, sodium concentrations are lower for a given volume of diarrhoea because unabsorbed solute makes up the remainder of the stool osmolality. Rapid transit through the colon presumably reduces contact time between luminal contents and mucosa, thus decreasing the changes in stool electrolyte concentrations normally produced by the colon.

Where stool volumes are moderately large, something can be learned of the underlying cause of diarrhoea from measurements of faecal electrolyte concentrations. It is possible for example, to distinguish osmotic from secretory types of diarrhoea from simple measurements of stool osmolality and sodium and potassium concentrations. In secretory diarrhoea the measured stool osmolality is similar to the sum of the concentrations of the major ions and the simplest method of estimating the latter is to multiply the sum of the sodium and potassium concentrations by two. In osmotic diarrhoea, on the other hand, the measured osmolality far exceeds the total ionic concentration, as much of the osmolality is made up of a non-ionic unabsorbed solute such as lactose, or its bacterial products. Another way of distinguishing osmotic from secretory diarrhoea is on the basis of the response to fasting. Osmotic diarrhoea will cease on a 24 to 48 hours fast, while secretory diarrhoea continues.

These simple stool assessments may indicate the lines for further investigation of difficult cases of watery diarrhoea. It is important to recognize however, that stool electrolyte and osmolality determinations in mild to moderate diarrhoea, where stool volumes may be less than 500 ml/day and stool consistencies less than fluid, are unlikely to be helpful. Determinations on such stools are likely to be inaccurate and the range of concentrations only serve to confuse. Submission of such stools to the chemical pathology department may be met with some resistance.

References

1 BERRIDGE MJ. Phosphotidylinositol hydrolysis: a general transducing mechanism for calcium mobilising receptors. In: Turnberg LA, ed. *Intestinal Secretion*. Welwyn Garden City: Smith, Kline & French, 1983, 23–34.

2 CASSUTO J, JODAL M, TUTTLE R, LUNDGREN O. On the role of intramural nerves in the pathogenesis of cholera toxin-induced intestinal secretion. *Scand J Gastroenterol* 1981;16:377.

3 CRANE RK. Na+ dependent transport in the intestine and other animal tissues. *Fed Proc* 1965;24:1000–6.

4 DAVIS GR, SANTA ANA CA, MORAWSKI S, FORDTRAN JS. Active chloride secretion in the normal human jejunum. *J Clin Invest* 1980;66:1326–33.

5 DEBONGNIE JC, PHILLIPS SF. Capacity of human colon to absorb fluid. *Gastroenterology* 1978;74:698–703.

6 DONOWITZ M, ASARKOF N, PIKE G. Serotonin induced changes in rabbit ileal active electrolyte transport are calcium dependent and associated with increased ileal calcium uptake. *J Clin Invest* 1980;66:341–52.

7 FIELD M. Intestinal Secretion. *Gastroenterology* 1974;66:1063–84.

8 Field M. Regulation of small intestinal ion transport by cyclic nucleotides and calcium. In: Field M, Fordtron JS, Schultz SG, eds. *Secretory diarrhoea*. Bethesda, Maryland: American Physiological Society, 1980:21–31.

9 FIELD M, GRAF LH, LAIRD WJ, SMITH PL. Heat stable enterotoxin of *Escherichia coli*: in vitro effects on guanylate cyclase activity, cyclic GMP concentration and ion transport in small intestine. *Proc Nat Acad Sci USA* 1978;75:2800–4.

10 FISHMAN PH. Mechanism of action of cholera toxin: events on the cell surface. In: Field M, Fordtran JS, Schultz SG, eds. *Secretory diarrhoea*. Bethesda, Maryland: American Physiological Society, 1980:85–107.

11 FORDTRAN JS, LOCKLEAR TW. Ionic constituents and osmolality of gastric and small intestinal fluids after eating. *Am J Dig Dis* 1966;11:503–21.

12 FORDTRAN JS, RECTOR FC JR, EWTON MF, SOTER N, KINNEY J. Permeability characteristics of the human small intestine. *J Clin Invest* 1965;44:1935–44.

13 HAKIM AA, LIFSON N. Effects of pressure on water and solute transport by dog intestinal mucosa in vitro. *Am J Physiol* 1969;216:276–84.

14 HAWKER PC, McKAY JS, TURNBERG LA. Electrolyte transport across colonic mucosa from patients with inflammatory bowel disease. *Gastroenterology* 1980;79:508–11.

15 HAWKER PC, MASHITER KE, TURNBERG LA. Mechanisms of transport of Na, Cl and K in the human colon. *Gastroenterology* 1978;74:1241–7.

16 HAWKEY CJ, RAMPTON DS. Prostaglandins and the gastrointestinal mucosa: are they important in its function, disease or treatment? *Gastroenterology* 1985; 89:1162–88.

17 HUGHES S, WARHURST G, HIGGS NB, GIUGLIANO LG, DRASAR BS, TURNBERG LA. Clostridium difficile cytotoxin induced intestinal secretion in rabbit ileum in vitro. *Gut* 1983;24:94–9.

18 ILUNDAIN A, NAFTALIN RJ. Role of Ca²⁺ dependent regulator protein in intestinal secretion. *Nature* 1979;297:446–8.

19 KERZNER B, KELLY MH, GALL DG, BUTLER DG, HAMILTON JR. Transmissable gastroenteritis: sodium transport and the intestinal epithelium during the course of viral enteritis. *Gastroenterology* 1977;72:457–62.

20 KNICKELBEIN R, ARONSON PS, SCHRON CM, SEIFTER J, DOBBINS JW. Sodium and chloride transport across rabbit ileal brush border. II. Evidence for Cl-HO₃ exchange and mechanisms of coupling. *Am J Physiol* 1985;249:9236–45.

21 LEIGH RJ, TURNBERG LA. Faecal incontinence: the unvoiced symptom. *Lancet* 1982;i:1349–51.

22 LOOSLI J, GYR K, STALDER H, et al. Etiology of acute infectious diarrhoea in a highly industrialized area of Switzerland. *Gastroenterology* 1985;88:75–9.

23 McNEIL NI, CUMMINGS JH, JAMES WPT. Short chain fatty acid absorption by the human large intestine. *Gut* 1978;19:819–22.

24 MURER H, HOPFER U, KINNE R. Sodium/proton antiport in brush border membrane vesicles isolated from rat small intestine and kidney. *Biochem J* 1976;154:597.

25 PALMA P, VIDON N, BERNIER JJ. Maximal capacity for fluid absorption in human bowel. *Dig Dis Sci* 1981;26:929–34.

26 POWELL DW. Neuro-humoral control of intestinal secretion. In: Turnberg LA, ed. *Intestinal secretion*. Welwyn Garden City: Smith, Kline & French, 1983:42–5.

27 POWELL DW, TAPPER EJ. Intestinal ion transport: cholinergic adrenergic interactions. In: Binder HJ, ed. *Mechanisms of intestinal secretion*. New York: Alan R Liss, Inc., 1979:175–93.

28 RAMBAUD JC, MODIGLIANI R. Hormones as potential intestinal secretagogues in health and disease. In: Turnberg LA, ed. *Intestinal secretion*. Welwyn Garden City: Smith, Kline & French, 1983:89–95.

29 RASK-MADSEN J, BUKHAVE K. Prostaglandins and intestinal secretion. In: Turnberg LA, ed. *Intestinal*

secretion. Welwyn Garden City: Smith, Kline & French, 1983:76–83.

30 RUBENS RD, LAMBERT HP. The homeostatic function of the colon in acute gastroenteritis. *Gut* 1972;13:915–9.

31 RUPPIN H, SOERGEL KH. Absorption of volatile fatty acids by the colon. *Clin Res Rev* 1981;1:119–23.

32 SCHULTZBERG M, HOKFELT T, NILSSON G, *et al*. Distribution of peptide and catecholamine containing neurons in the gastrointestinal tract of rat and guinea pig: immunohistochemical studies with antisera to substance P, vasoactive intestinal polypeptide, enkephalins, somatostatin, gastrin/cholecystokinin, neurotensin and dopamin B hydroxylase. *Neuroscience* 1980;5:689–744.

33 SHARON P, LIGUMSKY M, RACHMILEWITZ D, ZOR U. Role of prostaglandins in ulcerative colitis. Enhanced production during active disease and inhibition by sulfasalazine. *Gastroenterology* 1978;75:638–40.

34 SMITH G, WARHURST G, TURNBERG LA. Synthesis and degradation of prostaglandin E2 in the epithelial or sub-epithelial layer of rat small intestine. *Biochim Biophys Acta* 1982;713:684–7.

35 TURNBERG LA. Abnormalities in intestinal electrolyte transport in congenital chloridorrhoea. *Gut* 1971;12:544–52.

36 TURNBERG LA. Potassium transport in the human small bowel. *Gut* 1971;12:811–8.

37 TURNBERG LA, BIEBERDORF FA, MORAWSKI SG, FORDTRAN JS. Interrelationships of chloride, bicarbonate, sodium and hydrogen transport in the human ileum. *J Clin Invest* 1970;49:557–67.

38 TURNBERG LA, FORDTRAN JS, CARTER NW, RECTOR FC JR. Mechanism of bicarbonate absorption and its relationship to sodium transport in the human jejunum. *J Clin Invest* 1970;49:548–56.

39 VANTRAPPEN G, JANSSENS J, ROLEMBERG S, HELLEMANS J. Intestinal motility and diarrhoea. *Clin Res Rev* [suppl 1] 1981;1:83–9.

40 WALD A, GOTTERER GS, RAJENDRA GR, TURJMAN NA, HENDRIX TR. Effect of indomethacin on cholera-induced fluid movements, unidirectional sodium fluxes and intestinal cAMP. *Gastroenterology* 1977;72:107–10.

41 WRONG O, METCALF-GIBSON A, MORRIS RBI, NG ST, HOWARD AV. In vivo dialysis of faeces as a method of stool analysis. I. Techniques and results in normal subjects. *Clin Sci* 1965;28:357–75.

Chapter 5
Constipation

J. H. CUMMINGS

Constipation is a disorder of bowel habit characterized by the passage of small amounts of hard faeces infrequently and with difficulty.

Clinical presentation

The word constipation is used in many different ways, so it is most important to ask the patient to explain exactly the nature of their bowel disorder. Constipation can be quantified in terms of the frequency of defecation, consistency of stool, weight of stool passed daily, presence or absence of discomfort during defecation, or in terms of the transit time.

Average daily stool weight in Western, industrialized countries is 50–250 g/day [10] with most people passing one stool a day. In the British population stool frequency of three a day to three a week seems normal (Fig. 5.1) [4, 13]. The daily weight of stool is subject to many cultural and environmental influences, so that normal ranges differ in different places. For example men aged 40–59 years in rural Finland pass 196 ± 15 (SEM) g/day, but in Copenhagen only 136 ± 13 g/day [7]. Vegetarians have greater stool outputs than non-vegetarians. In many Third World countries stool weights are in the range 250–500 g/day and may be even higher in apparently healthy individuals [10].

Constipation is usually associated with

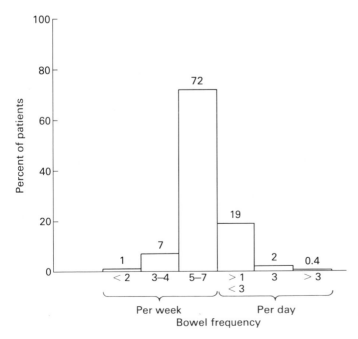

Fig. 5.1. Variation of bowel habit in a general population. Columns and numbers show percentage of subjects at each bowel frequency [4].

59

some discomfort during defecation either due to straining, or to anal discomfort, because of the hard and dry nature of the faecal material. Patients may also complain of a feeling of incomplete evacuation and a useful guide to severity is to ask how long they spend in the toilet each day. It is often more important to ask about a change in bowel habit, than to rely on absolute measurements. In practice stool collections are rarely done and the nature and severity of the symptom is usually assessed from the history and, when possible, confirmed with a transit study.

Prevalence

About one in 100 persons in the United Kingdom consult their family doctor annually because of constipation [19]; that is about 400,000 consultations a year. However, general surveys show that as many as 10% of people consider themselves constipated, or have to strain at stool [4, 26]. The symptom of constipation is commoner in women than men [4, 19] and women tend also to have slower transit time [24, 28]. Constipation is increasingly common over the age of 65, with at least one in five or more of elderly persons suffering from this problem. In a general population, 99% of subjects declared their bowel frequency between three or more bowel actions weekly and up to three actions daily (Fig. 5.1).

Use of laxatives is probably a good index of the prevalence of constipation, although laxatives can be taken probably irrespective of bowel habit, diet or cultural background. In Britain 20% of people use laxatives occasionally with 5–6% taking a dose more often than weekly [4, 26]. Laxative taking increases significantly with age. More than weekly use is very infrequent under the age of 20 years, but increases to 10–15% of the population in middle life and 20–30% at the age of 65.

Causes and pathophysiology (Table 5.1)

There are very many causes of constipation, but most commonly encountered in medical

Table 5.1. Principal causes of constipation.

Diet	Inadequate dietary fibre intake
	'Western' culture
	Old age
	Slimmers
	Anorexia nervosa
	Travel—holidays
	Therapeutic diets
Motor disorders	Slow transit
	Diverticular disease
	Irritable bowel syndrome
	Megacolon
	Hirschprung's disease
	'Outlet obstruction'
	Idiopathic
	Central nervous system
	disorders
	Multiple sclerosis
	Parkinson's disease
	Spinal cord injury and
	tumours
Causes with uncertain or mixed aetiologies	Inactivity
	Pregnancy and menstruation
	(female sex)
	Colorectal disorders
	Bowel cancer
	Haemorrhoids
	Anal fissure/fistula
	Perianal abscess
	Stricture
	Psychiatric
	Depression
	Drugs
	Antacids
	Anticholinergics
	Opiates
	Iron
	Antidepressants
	Endocrine
	Hypothyroidism
	Hypokalaemia
	Diabetes
	Hypercalcaemia
	Dehydration
	Porphyria
	Miscellaneous
	Lead poisoning

practice are an inappropriate diet, inactivity, menstruation or pregnancy, drugs and the irritable bowel syndrome.

Essentially two mechanisms underlie the pathophysiology of constipation. Firstly, there may be insufficient material in the lumen of the bowel to stimulate normal motor activity. This is the constipation of low dietary fibre which leads to decreased fermentation in the colon. Secondly, normal colonic neuromuscular and recto-anal reflex activity may be impaired, as in the irritable bowel syndrome, diverticular disease, Hirschsprung's disease and other types of megacolon (Table 5.1). In most instances it must be remembered that the exact mechanism by which constipation arises has not been defined.

Constipation due to diet

Normal colonic contents consists of cellular material (anaerobic bacteria and plant cells) enmeshed in a gel formed from water, mucus glycoprotein and bacterial exopolysaccharides. The quantity of faeces depends mainly on the presence of microbial and plant cells. The microflora, of which there are 10^{10}–10^{11} organisms per gram of faeces, obtain energy for growth from carbohydrate—either dietary (starch and fibre), or from endogenous sources (mucus). The contribution from mucus is probably small, as subjects maintained on diets free of fibre pass only small amounts of stool [27]. Dietary fibre is principally the polysaccharides of the plant cell wall and includes many carbohydrate polymers made up of hexose sugars (glucose and galactose), pentose (xylose, arabinose) and uronic acids. Dietary carbohydrates that reach the colon are broken down by the colonic anaerobic flora fermentation, with the production of short chain (or volatile) fatty acids—acetic, proprionic and butyric, and also hydrogen, methane and carbon dioxide, and energy [6]. Through fermentation the bacteria obtain energy and grow.

The amount of fibre in the diet contributes to the amount of colonic contents and stool output by four mechanisms. Firstly, fibre that is not degraded retains its cellular structure and holds water in the gut lumen like a sponge and so increases faecal bulk. Secondly, fermented fibre and starch stimulate microbial growth and increase faecal excretion of microbial material. Thirdly, small amounts of fermentation gases become trapped in these materials and so increase the bulk of contents. Finally increased bulk speeds transit through the colon and decreases the dehydration of colonic contents [23].

Low dietary fibre is an important cause of constipation, especially in industrialized countries such as in North America, the United Kingdom, parts of Europe, Australia and New Zealand, where fibre intakes are less than 15 g/day. Fibre intakes are often low and constipation is therefore common in slimmers, in patients with anorexia nervosa, or diabetics, or patients with coeliac disease who omit fibre rich foods for therapeutic reasons. Hospital diets may be low in dietary fibre. Changes in dietary fibre intake leading to constipation also occur during prolonged travel.

Motor disorders

It is widely believed that disorders of colonic motility are a common cause of constipation. Neuronal lesions causing constipation exist in spinal cord injury, Hirschsprung's disease and some recto-anal disorders, but they have not been demonstrated in commoner syndromes, such as colonic diverticular disease or the irritable bowel syndrome [21].

Slow transit

Some patients with constipation eat an adequate diet and have no detectable colonic abnormality other than slow transit. Transit, the time taken for material to pass through the gut, is an important determinant of colonic function. The breakdown of fibre is more complete and microbial growth less efficient during slow transit [22] with the result that stools are drier and der than normal. In some cases slow transit may be associated with an unusually long colon, especially the sigmoid (dolichocolon) or the colon may be dilated (megacolon). No specific motor abnormalities can be detected in this group, although in some increased segmental pressure activity is said to be present in the distal colon [3]. This is not invariable [15] and may be secondary to the constipation. In most patients with slow-transit constipation the barium enema is normal. Experimental studies suggest that difficulty in defecation due to failure of relaxation of the external rectal sphincter and of the striated pelvic floor muscles may contribute to constipation in this predominantly female group of subjects [18].

Colonic diverticular disease and the irritable bowel syndrome
(see also Chapters 62 and 67)

Constipation is prominent in these conditions, both associated with disturbed colonic motility. In colonic diverticular disease there is muscular thickening in the sigmoid colon and in symptomatic patients an increase in intraluminal pressures in response to stimuli from food and drugs [1].

Abnormal colonic (and small bowel) motor activity may be present in the irritable bowel syndrome. Of the two types of basal electric rhythm (BER) which exist in the colon (at frequencies of about six and three cycles per minute), slow waves predominate in irritable bowel syndrome [20]. How these motor abnormalities in diverticular disease and irritable bowel syndrome tie up with the reduced stool output of constipation remains to be shown.

Hirschsprung's disease and outlet obstruction

In Hirschsprung's disease (see Chapter 60) there is in early childhood an aganglionic distal segment, proximal to which the colon is dilated. The recto-anal relaxation reflex is impaired so that rectal distention does not cause relaxation of the internal anal sphincter. It has been suggested recently that some adult forms of constipation may be due to minor disturbances of innervation of the rectum, producing so called 'outlet obstruction' [14] which is characterized by decreased stool frequency, slow transit through the left colon and abnormal anorectal manometry.

Disorders of the central nervous system

Injuries of the spinal cord can produce severe constipation. Injury to the cord above the lumbo-sacral arc (L2) leaves the recto-anal reflexes intact, but anal and rectal sensation is lost. The patient becomes constipated, although reflex emptying of the bowel can be often established with suppositories, or enemas. Injuries of the cauda equina and sacral nerves are a more difficult problem. These patients not only have diminished sensation in the anal canal, but also loss of tone in the external sphincter and of the recto-anal relaxation reflex. Constipation and incontinence follow, with the patient unable to retain or to expel faeces satisfactorily. Bilateral sacral nerve injury during surgery leads to incontinence and constipation, but unilateral division does not usually produce symptoms.

Other disorders of the central nervous system that lead to constipation include multiple sclerosis where there is loss of the normal modulatory effects of colonic motor activity from the higher centres [11], Parkinson's disease and the now uncommon tabes dorsalis.

Uncertain or mixed causes

Inactivity

Although the effect of physical exercise on large bowel function has not been investigated systematically, inactivity almost certainly leads to decreased colonic motor activity, especially mass movements. This is particularly important in the elderly, or in those immobilized because of travel or hospitalization. Constipation is a serious problem in many inpatients, due to a combination of inactivity, dietary change, dehydration, drug treatment and the psychological problems of using a bedpan behind the thin curtains of an open ward.

Menstruation and pregnancy

Constipation occurs in many women just before the onset of menstruation. It is also frequent in early pregnancy, often long before there is any possibility of displacement of the colon by the enlarging uterus. In both, progesterone levels are increased, which may lead to relaxation of gut muscle.

Colorectal disorders

Constipation is associated with haemorrhoids, an anal fissure, a fistula in ano or a perianal abscess. Often the pain simply inhibits defecation. Other colonic disorders such as carcinoma, volvulus and stricture cause constipation, as does ulcerative colitis. In colitis, faecal stasis occurs in the right side of the colon and although the patient may be going to the toilet frequently to pass mucus, blood and some faeces, a plain radiograph of the abdomen or a transit study, will show faecal accumulation in the caecum and ascending colon.

Psychiatric causes

Depressed patients are often constipated, but may not complain of this. Patients with dementia or other chronic psychoses may have faecal incontinence or spurious diarrhoea when the large intestine is loaded with faeces.

Drugs

Drugs commonly cause constipation. So many different drugs can cause it, that it is simplest to assume that constipation following a change in medication is drug-induced. Constipating effects of drugs are listed in the *British National Formulary*. Commonly prescribed drugs causing constipation include aluminium-containing antacids, analgesics, morphine and its derivatives such as codeine, anticholinergics, antidepressants, antihypertensives, iron and some anticonvulsants.

Some patients, usually women, complain of constipation, but do not have it. They take increasing quantities of laxatives to achieve what they believe is a satisfactory bowel habit. After each purge they become constipated largely because the bowel is empty, but instead of allowing it to recover they take ever increasing doses. Alternatively, these patients may present with quite severe diarrhoea, may deny laxative taking and undergo extensive investigation before it is appreciated that the problem is due to laxative abuse. They can be diagnosed by the presence of pseudo-melanosis coli on rectal biopsy, by the barium enema appearance of a dilated featureless colon with pseudo-strictures (the cathartic colon), hypokalemia, by the urine tests for anthraquinones and phenolphthalein, or by the presence of excess magnesium in stools. Sometimes a search of their possessions while in hospital reveals a cache of laxatives [5].

Endocrine

Patients with hypothyroidism, hypercalcaemia or hypokalemia may be constipated.

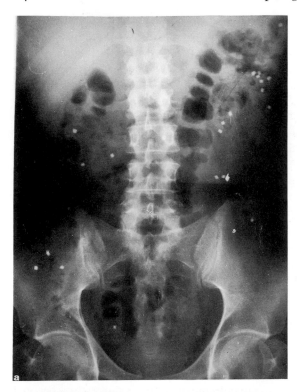

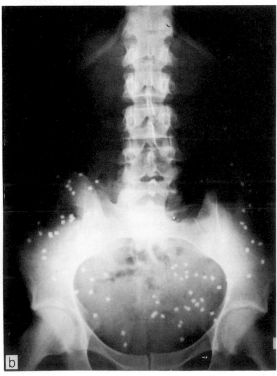

Fig. 5.2(a) measurement of mean transit time in a healthy man taking 10 radio-opaque pellets daily with breakfast for 14 days. Twenty-six pellets are retained and the mean transit time is 2.6 days. Note the descending and sigmoid colon and rectum are empty.

(b) measurement of transit in a constipated 24-year-old woman. One hundred and two pellets are present and the mean transit time is 10.2 days. Note that the pellets are evenly distributed around the large bowel indicating a generalized slowing of transit.

(c) measurement of transit in a 55-year-old woman with constipation due to a tumour of the cauda equina leading to loss of rectal sensation and the recto-anal reflexes. Forty-one pellets are present giving a mean transit time of 4.1 days. Note that most (22) are held up in the recto-sigmoid area.

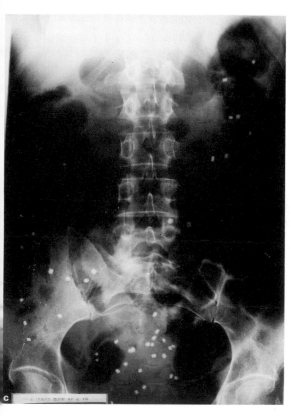

More rarely constipation may be a presenting feature of lead poisoning and porphyria.

Diagnosis

History

Characteristics of the bowel habit are established by asking about the frequency of defecation, the amount of stool passed and its consistency, the time spent on the toilet and the occurrence of straining or anal or abdominal discomfort. The age of onset of the symptoms is important. Life-long constipation usually means that no identifiable cause will be found, except for the rare adult Hirschsprung's type of disorder, while recent onset indicates local or systemic pathology which must be sought. A dietary history should be taken with particular reference to intake of dietary fibre. This is most simply done by asking about consumption of bread, breakfast cereals, fruit and vegetables. A general enquiry to establish any recent changes in the patient's life-style is also important. Evidence of systemic disease should be sought, particularly any neurological condition that may affect recto-anal function. In such circumstances there is often an associated disorder of the bladder, so the constipated patient must always be asked about micturition. Finally a detailed list of medications, including self-prescribed drugs, should be made.

Clinical examination

Careful examination of the rectum and sigmoid is most important. The anus should be inspected for external haemorrhoids, or other perianal disease. Touching the perianal skin produces reflex contraction of the external anal sphincter. If this does not occur, or the sphincter feels slack on digital examination, gapes after the finger is withdrawn, or there is incontinence of faeces, a disorder of anorectal reflex function is likely. Sensation in the perianal region (saddle area) will be decreased in lesions of the cauda equina. Digital examination may show a rectal tumour or hard faeces. Sigmoidoscopy is important and should be combined with rectal mucosal biopsy, which may show pseudo-melanosis coli. Pseudo-melanosis, a brownish discolouration of the colonic mucosa due to the presence of macrophages containing lipofuscin, occurs in patients taking laxatives [16]. It is a good guide to the chronicity and severity of the patient's symptoms. Melanosis affects the right colon predominantly and the rectum may be spared. It regresses spontaneously when laxative taking ceases.

Stool collection

It would be invaluable to have a stool collection in every constipated patient but this is seldom practicable. The weight of stool passed every 24 hours is a useful measure of constipation provided a complete collection is made.

Transit studies

The measurement of intestinal transit time is a more reliable and to the patient more acceptable way of assessing constipation. The most widely used technique is to give orally radio-opaque pellets and either measure their recovery in faeces, or follow their passage through the gut by X-ray. A simple method suitable for outpatients which avoids stool collection, is to give the patient 10 radio-opaque pellets daily with breakfast for 14 days and then take one plain abdominal radiograph and count the number of pellets retained. Mean transit time (days) is calculated from the number of pellets retained divided by 10. The normal range of mean transit time is 1–4 days (Fig. 5.2).

Radiology

If there is any doubt about a patient's constipation a plain abdominal radiograph will show faecal loading of the colon. Barium enema is almost invariably necessary, if only to exclude intrinsic disease of the large bowel such as polyps, cancer or diverticular disease. More often than not, however, the barium enema will be normal, or may show a long sigmoid, or dilated colon. Associated small bowel dilatation may be present in some neurological disorders and in drug-induced constipation.

Motility studies

There is no place for motility studies in routine management of constipation, but it is sometimes useful to assess recto-anal function. The most widely used is the measurement of reflex relaxation of the internal anal sphincter in response to rectal distention by a balloon using a pressure sensitive device in the anal canal. This reflex is absent in aganglionosis and present, but greater than normal, in spinal cord injury. It is also lost in cauda equina and sacral nerve injuries in which external sphincter contraction is also diminished.

Management

It is essential to make a firm diagnosis. If constipation is secondary to colonic, perianal or systemic disorders these must be treated initially. If due to drugs, it may be possible to change to less constipating agents.

General measures

Although it has never been put to the test, patients with constipation probably benefit from increasing fluid intake, taking more exercise and allowing time for unhurried visits to the toilet. Neglecting the call to stool is a frequent cause of constipation [12].

Diet

Fibre is the main component of the diet to benefit the constipated patient. Some other foods, such as prunes, contain cathartic substances and any carbohydrate which escapes absorption in the small bowel, such as lactose in lactase deficient subjects, stachyose and raffinose from legumes and some forms of starch, will have laxative effects. Fibre, especially in the form of wheat bran, has been used for centuries to treat constipation [8, 17, 22].

There is no universal dose, and the amount required is that which will produce a satisfactory bowel habit, usually one soft stool daily, or on alternate days. The aim should be to double the patient's intake from about 12 g per day to 24 g per day, but those who fail to respond to larger doses

Table 5.2. Portions of food that contain about 5 g dietary fibre (measured as non-starch polysaccharides).

Food	Weight (g)	Amount
Bread		
Wholemeal	80	2–3 slices
Brown	120	3–4 slices
White	300	6–10 slices
Bran	10–15	2–3 tablespoonfuls
Weetabix	50	2½ biscuits
All Bran	25	small helping
Muesli (oat based)	75	average helping
Baked beans	140	2 helpings
Peas	100–200	1–2 large helpings
Cabbage	150	2 helpings
Carrots	200	2 helpings
Potatoes	500	3 helpings
Apples	275	3 medium apples
Bananas	500–600	5–6 bananas
Oranges	200–250	2 oranges
Pears	150	1–2 pears

should be looked at carefully for organic causes of the constipation. Simple dietary constipation usually responds to quite modest increases in fibre intake.

Fibre intake can be increased by:
1. Increasing bread intake to about 200 g (six slices) per day and changing to 100% wholemeal.
2. Eating a wholewheat breakfast cereal or one with added bran, or an oat-based muesli.
3. Increasing fruit and vegetable intake.
4. Eating more legumes such as peas, beans and lentils.
5. Using concentrated fibre foods such as bran and All Bran.

Fibre can also be given as a proprietary bulk forming laxative. Table 5.2 shows a list of selected foods that contain 5 g of dietary fibre.

The dangers of eating fibre are small. Because fibre is fermented in the colon gas is produced and therefore patients who increase their fibre intake too quickly will experience abdominal distention, bloating, pain and increased flatus. A slow build up in dose allows the gut to adjust to the pro-

duction of gas. Other complications of fibre therapy such as intestinal obstruction and mineral malabsorption are largely theoretical. However, because of the high phytic acid content of raw bran this product should be used with caution in patients whose mineral balance may be precarious such as the young, the elderly and the pregnant. High fibre diets are not suitable for the treatment of constipation due to neurological disorders, or to obstructive lesions of the gut.

Laxatives

Laxatives are a safe, valuable and effective part of the management of the constipated patient. There are five groups of laxatives, each with differing modes of action (Table 5.3) [5].

Bulk laxatives are the most favoured at present and are a form of purified dietary fibre. They act by retaining water in the gut and by stimulating microbial activity through fermentation. There are three types, those derived from ispaghula (a seed mucilage from the *Plantago* family), stercu-

Table 5.3. Laxatives available for clinical use.

Bulk	Ispaghula, sterculia, methylcellulose
Stimulant	Anthracenes—senna, cascara, danthron, syrup of figs Polyphenolics—bisacodyl, phenolphthalein Sodium picosulphate
Salts	Magnesium sulphate, hydroxide, carbonate, citrate Sodium sulphate Sodium potassium tartrate
Faecal softeners (detergents)	Dioctylsodium sulphosuccinate Poloxamer
Suppositories and enemas	Glycerine, bisacodyl, sodium picosulphate and various salts
Others	Lactulose

lia (a plant gum), or methylcellulose. Tablets of bran are also available. These laxatives are best given with meals starting at a dose of 5 g daily and increasing to 20 g if necessary. No one preparation has been shown to be superior to the rest. It is worth trying patients on each of the three types before abandoning them for more potent agents. They are easier to take if mixed in a carbonated drink.

Stimulants act by stimulating colonic motor activity directly. Some of them (senna, sodium picosulphate) require activation by the colonic microflora and so their efficiency may be reduced in patients on antibiotics. Others (bisacodyl, phenolphthalein) undergo enterohepatic circulation. These laxatives may produce abdominal colic, so initially are best taken as a small dose at night. They are very effective and widely used.

Salts used as laxatives are poorly absorbed from the gut and so attract water into the bowel by osmotic forces leading to an increase in stool output (see Chapter 4). They may also release gut hormones such as cholecystokinin (CCK), which in turn promote muscular activity in the colon and hence a general cathartic effect. Preparations available are mostly sodium or magnesium salts, for example magnesium sulphate (Epsom salts), magnesium hydroxide (milk of magnesia), magnesium citrate,

magnesium carbonate and sodium sulphate (Glauber salts) or sodium potassium tartrate (Rochelle's salt and Seidlitz powder). These preparations are undoubtedly laxative and most valuable when used as a single dose to return bowel function to normal regularity on specific occasions, such as after a period of inactivity or where constipation has occurred due to altered diet or life-style. They are also useful in the right-sided constipation of colitis. The relative efficacy of these preparations varies because of the different potential osmotic effect of each salt. In general those preparations containing the sulphate ion are the most potent and those containing magnesium more so than those with sodium. On theoretical grounds, therefore, magnesium sulphate is the first choice.

Faecal softeners (detergents) are mild aperients which need to be taken throughout the day. Their detergent properties are said to lead to softening of the faecal mass by allowing penetration of water and electrolytes by stimulating their secretion into the gut. However, when taken at the recommended dose they do not increase stool weight [2]. The main danger is the possibility that their detergent action alters drug metabolism by facilitating drug absorption from the gut. They are used mainly for haemorrhoids and anal conditions.

Lactulose, a disaccharide of galactose and

fructose is an effective laxative, but its mode of action makes it difficult to classify. It is not hydrolysed in the small intestine and so has an osmotic action in this part of the gut. On entering the colon it is fermented with the resulting stimulation of colonic function. It lowers pH in the caecum. The combined osmotic, microbial and pH effects lead to increased stool output. Because it stimulates microbial protein synthesis and thus reduces ammonia concentrations, it has been widely used for bowel clearance in hepatic encephalopathy. It is a mild and effective laxative at doses of 15 ml twice daily.

Many **other laxatives** are available, including liquid paraffin, castor oil, bile salts, frangula, rhubarb, podophyllum, etc. Often several are mixed together in a compound tablet. The use of these preparations in the management of constipation is very limited.

A number of laxatives are available as suppositories and enemas. Enemas are particularly valuable as once-only treatment for constipation, while suppositories can be useful in patients with abnormal recto-anal function.

Surgery

Surgery has a very limited place in the management of constipation and may be applicable to severe symptoms of idiopathic megacolon or outlet obstruction (see Chapter 65).

Special problems

Pregnancy

On the principle that the less medication the better in pregnancy, the appropriate management of these patients is a high fibre diet (avoiding raw bran), adequate fluid intake and bulk laxatives. Should these fail, bisacodyl suppositories or oral senna are without danger to mother or foetus.

Old age

Constipation in the elderly occurs for all the same reasons as constipation at other ages and should be managed as such. The elderly are much more likely to suffer faecal impaction, possibly due to diminishing rectal sensation in old age. Faecal impaction leads to faecal incontinence, intestinal obstruction, rectal bleeding, urinary retention and restlessness. It can be diagnosed by digital examination of the rectum. Treatment initially is to empty the bowel with enemas given on successive days, followed by senna which may be needed in large doses. Manual removal of faeces may be necessary. Prevention is best [9].

Spinal cord injuries and disorders of the central nervous system

These patients have disturbances of recto-anal reflex activity and need careful management. They should be encouraged to evacuate their bowels regularly (often they have no rectal sensation). A high fibre diet is not ideal for these conditions and should be tried only with care. Bowel evacuation can be accomplished by the regular use of laxatives given on alternate nights followed by a suppository such as bisacodyl the next day. The use of suppositories is very important especially in those with lesions above the cauda equina, as normal reflex activity is preserved although awareness of this by the higher centres is lacking. Occasionally enemas may be needed, or digital removal of faeces by a district nurse [12].

References

1 ARFWIDSSON S. Pathogenesis of multiple diverticula of the sigmoid colon in diverticular disease. *Acta Chir Scand* 1964; [Suppl] **342**:5–68.
2 CHAPMAN RW, SINERY J, FONTANA DD, MATHYS C,

SAUNDERS DR. Effect of oral dioctyl sodium sulphosuccinate on intake–output studies of human small and large intestine. *Gastroenterology* 1985;**89**:489–493.

3 CONNELL AM. Motor action of the large bowel. In: Code CF, Heidel W, eds. *Handbook of Physiology. Section 6. Alimentary Canal. Vol. IV.* Washington DC: American Physiological Society, 1968:2075–2091.

4 CONNELL AM, HILTON C, IRVINE G, LENNARD-JONES JE, MISIEWICZ JJ. Variation of bowel habit in two population samples. *Br Med J* 1965;**2**:1095–1099.

5 CUMMINGS JH. The use and abuse of laxatives. In: Bouchier IAD, ed. *Recent Advances in Gastroenterology.* London: Academic Press, 1976:124–149.

6 CUMMINGS JH. Dietary fibre. *Br Med Bull* 1981;**37**:65–70.

7 CUMMINGS JH, BRANCH WJ, BJERRUM L, PAERREGAARD A, HELMS P, BURTON R. Colon cancer and large bowel function in Denmark and Finland. *Nutr Cancer* 1982;**4**:61–66.

8 DIMOCK EM. The treatment of habitual constipation by the bran method. (Cambridge University, M.D. Thesis) 1936.

9 EXTON-SMITH AN. Constipation in geriatrics. In: Jones FA, Godding EW eds. *Management of Constipation.* Oxford: Blackwell Scientific Publications, 1972. 156–175.

10 FEACHAM RG, BRADLEY DJ, GARELICK H, MARA DD. Health aspects of *Excreta and Sullage Management— a state-of-the-art-review.* Washington: World Bank 1980, 8–9.

11 GLICK ME, MESHKINPOUR H, HALDEMAN S, BHATIA NN, BRADLEY WE. Colonic dysfunction in multiple sclerosis. *Gastroenterology,* 1982; **83**:1002–1007.

12 JONES FA, GODDING EW. *Management of Constipation.* London: Blackwell Scientific Publications, 1972.

13 MANNING AP, WYMAN JB, HEATON KW. How trustworthy are bowel histories? Comparison of recalled and recorded information. *Br Med J* 1976;**2**:213–214.

14 MARTELLI H, DEVROEDE G, ARHAN P, DUGUAY C. Mechanisms of idiopathic constipation: outlet obstruction. *Gastroenterology* 1978:**75**:623–631.

15 MEUNIER P, ROCHAS A, LAMBERT R. Motor activity of the sigmoid colon in chronic constipation: comparative study with normal subjects. *Gut* 1979;**20**:1095–1101.

16 MORSON BC, DAWSON IMP. *Gastrointestinal Pathology.* Oxford: Blackwell Scientific Publications, 1979: 695–697.

17 OLMSTED WH, WILLIAMS RD, BAUERLEIN T. Constipation: the laxative value of bulking food. *Med Clin North Am* 1936;**20**:449–459.

18 PRESTON DM, LENNARD-JONES JE. Anismus in chronic constipation. *Dig Dis Sci* 1985;**30**:413–418.

19 Royal College of General Practitioners; OPCS: DHSS. *Morbidity Statistics from General Practice, 1971–1972. Second National Study. Studies on Medical and Population Subjects No. 36.* London: HMSO 1979.

20 SNAPE WJ, CARLSON GM, COHEN S. Colonic myoelectric activity in the irritable bowel syndrome. *Gastroenterology* 1976;**70**:326–330.

21 SNOOKS SJ, BARNES PRH, SWASH M, HENRY MM. Damage to the innervation of the pelvic floor musculature in chronic constipation. *Gastroenterology* 1985;**89**:977–981.

22 STEPHEN AM. Dietary fibre and human colonic function. (University of Cambridge, Ph.D. Thesis) 1980.

23 STEPHEN AM, CUMMINGS JH. Mechanism of action of dietary fibre in the human colon. *Nature* 1980;**284**:283–284.

24 STEPHEN AM, WIGGINS HS, ENGLYST HN, COLE TJ, CUMMINGS JH. The effect of age, sex and level of intake of dietary fibre from wheat on large bowel function in 30 healthy subjects. *Br J Nutr* 1986 (in press).

25 STREICHER MH, QUIRK L. Constipation: clinical and roentgenologic evaluation of the use of bran. *Am J Dig Dis* 1943;**10**:179–181.

26 THOMPSON WG, HEATON KW. Functional bowel disorders in apparently healthy people. *Gastroenterology* 1979; **79**:283–288.

27 WINITZ M, SEEDMAN DA, GRAFF J. Studies in metabolic nutrition employing chemical defined diets. I. Extended feeding of normal human adult males. *Am J Clin Nutr* 1970;**23**:525–545.

28 WYMAN JB, HEATON KW, MANNING AP, WICKS ACB. Variability of colonic function in healthy subjects. *Gut* 1978;**19**:146–150.

Chapter 6
Anaemia

E.J. PARKER-WILLIAMS

There is a close association between gastroenterology and haematology [11]. The haematologist becomes involved when anaemia is found during the investigation of a patient with gastrointestinal disease. Alternatively, the symptoms of anaemia may lead the patient to the haematology clinic, and a primary gastrointestinal disorder is found subsequently.

Absorption of haematinics

Iron

Iron has a central role in erythropoiesis and certain enzyme systems [8, 19]. Iron balance in the human is precarious, with iron supply being the limiting factor—iron lack is a dominant feature in many population groups [2, 3]. The gastrointestinal mucosal cell is the keystone in maintaining the balance between the amount of iron absorbed and the amount lost from red cells or desquamated gut cells [12, 14].

At least 1 mg of iron (2 mg in women) needs to be absorbed each day to maintain this balance. The Western diet provides about 15–20 mg daily, but iron absorption is limited to about 10% of iron intake. Luminal and mucosal factors influence the amount absorbed. Non-haem iron is absorbed in small amounts from food and absorption is increased by the presence of gastric acid, ascorbic acid, and some sugars which help the iron to become attached to the mucosal cell. Haem iron, from meat, is easily absorbed and is not interfered with by other constituents of the diet. However, non-haem iron is readily oxidized and, in the presence of dietary phosphates or phytates, absorption is decreased.

The duodenum and upper small intestine are the sites of maximal iron absorption. Iron absorption is under the sensitive regulation of the enterocyte, but details of the process are not known [1]. Mucosal transferrin binds iron in the lumen of the gut and transports it across the brush border of the mucosa. The iron may be held in the mucosal cell or passed rapidly through to be bound by circulating transferrin, the iron transport protein.

The amount of iron absorbed is dictated by the level of iron stores, and is increased in iron deficiency and in conditions that increase erythropoietic activity. Iron absorption is decreased in iron overload and in the presence of infection.

Iron malabsorption classically occurs in **coeliac disease**, but iron deficiency usually occurs either following blood loss due to **parasitic infestation** of the gut [2], or **disease of the gut** itself (see Chapters 30–32).

Vitamin B$_{12}$

Only two biochemical reactions require vitamin B$_{12}$ in man—methionine synthesis, which generates tetrahydrofolate from 5 methyltetrahydrofolate, and the isomerization of methylmalonyl CoA to succinyl CoA providing one of the catabolic pathways via the Krebs' cycle [18].

Vitamin B$_{12}$ exists in different forms (cobalamins). The basic molecule consists of two halves—a planar group containing the essential element cobalt at its centre and a nucleotide. The main form present in the human liver is 5′-deoxyadenosyl cobalamin (coenzyme B_{12}). In plasma, methylcobalamin is the major component [15].

Vitamin B_{12} is synthesized by bacteria. Humans need pre-formed B_{12} and their only dietary source is food of animal origin. Large amounts are present in liver and kidney; smaller are present in shellfish and dairy produce. The normal diet supplies about 5 μg B_{12} daily; the daily requirement is 1–3 μg. Vitamin B_{12} is absorbed in the distal ileum, particularly the last 60 cm. Vitamin B_{12} absorption is invariably impaired if more than 180 cm of the distal ileum is resected, or if the intestinal contents bypass the ileum.

Dietary vitamin B_{12} is released from protein complexes by enzymes in the stomach and upper intestine, and it combines rapidly with intrinsic factor (IF), a glycoprotein secreted by the gastric parietal cells. An excess of intrinsic factor is available, except in pernicious anaemia or after a major gastric resection. There is a limit to the amount of oral vitamin B_{12} that can be absorbed, and this limit is attributed to the saturation of the B_{12}-IF receptor sites in the ileum. This refractory state lasts for some three hours, when no more B_{12} is taken up; the physiological limit is 2–3 μg, irrespective of the amount offered. Specific receptors for the vitamin B_{12}-IF complex are located on the microvillus membrane of the distal ileum; the presence of calcium ions and a pH greater than 5.4 are necessary conditions for the receptors to react with the complex. Precise details of the absorption of B_{12} following this reaction are not clear; in particular it is not known whether or not intrinsic factor enters the intestinal cell with the B_{12}. The vitamin B_{12} is held in the intestinal cell for four to eight hours before it passes from the ileum to the portal blood, attached to transcobalamin II. Peak plasma concentration of B_{12} are found eight to 12 hours after an oral dose, and this can be used as a test of vitamin B_{12} absorption following a radioactive dose of the vitamin.

Serum B_{12} concentration is measured by radioisotope dilution assay [9]. Although the Schilling test is the conventional measure of vitamin B_{12} absorption, tests of protein bound cobalamin absorption are claimed to approximate more closely to the physiological process [9, 10].

A number of factors affect B_{12} absorption. **Deficient intrinsic factor** secretion is found in pernicious anaemia or after major gastric resection, but not during H_2-blockade with cimetidine or ranitidine. The need for calcium ions has been mentioned and hypocalcaemia has been reported to lead to impaired B_{12} absorption. Using the Schilling test, decreased B_{12} absorption occurs in 50% of patients with **chronic pancreatitis**; absorption is usually corrected by performing the Schilling test with a meal or with oral pancreatin. However, it is rare for a patient with chronic pancreatitis to develop vitamin B_{12} deficiency, let alone a megaloblastic anaemia. **Bacterial overgrowth** of the small intestine interferes with the B_{12}-IF complexes, causing vitamin B_{12} malabsorption (see Chapter 44).

A number of **drugs** have been reported to impair the absorption of vitamin B_{12}: phenformin, metformin, para-aminosalicylic acid, potassium supplements, cholestyramine, colchicine and neomycin have been incriminated, not necessarily acting by the same mechanism [24]. **Alcohol** has a direct effect on the ileal cell, and vitamin B_{12} malabsorption has been recorded in alcoholics. **Radiation**, particularly if given to the pelvis, may damage the ileum and malabsorption of vitamin B_{12} is common (see Chapter 74). **Ileal resection** is a common cause of vitamin B_{12} deficiency in Crohn's disease (see Chapter 53). **Dietary** vitamin B_{12} deficiency is common in strict vegetarians (vegans) [20].

Folic acid (Pteroylglutamic acid)

Natural folates exist as polyglutamates in food and are present in large amounts in liver, kidney and yeast and in smaller, but significant amounts in certain beans, nuts and vegetables [18]. About 100 µg are needed each day; more is required in pregnancy. Polyglutamates cannot be absorbed until converted by hydrolysis to monoglutamate by the enzyme folate conjugase (gammaglutamyl carboxypeptidase). This reaction occurs either in the lumen or within the mucosal cell. The principal site for absorption is the upper jejunum and absorption is rapid (20–30 minutes) [22]. The absorptive capacity is almost unlimited. A special mechanism (possibly an active process) probably exists, as there are some persons with a specific defect of folate absorption. During intestinal absorption, all folates are converted to 5-methyltetrahydrofolate and in this form are transferred to the portal blood. Folate concentrations in the portal blood are higher than in the systemic venous blood; the liver is the main organ for storage of folate.

Folate malabsorption occurs particularly in patients with **coeliac disease, tropical sprue** and in those persons with the rare **specific malabsorption of folate.** Lesser degrees of malabsorption may be noted in patients with **Crohn's disease**, with or without extensive gut resection, and sometimes after **partial gastrectomy. Sulphasalazine** may interfere with folate absorption in patients with inflammatory bowel disease [21]. Dietary folate deficiency occurs in **alcoholics** and in **general malnourishment**— for example, prolonged illness.

Assessment of the patient with gastrointestinal disease and anaemia

The main objective is to define the morphological features of the anaemia, particularly the haemoglobin content and size of the red cells, using laboratory tests. The electronic blood cell counter provides quick and accurate measurements of haemoglobin concentration, haemoglobin content (MCH) and red cell size (MCV). Most importantly, the inspection of a well-made, well-stained blood film is the crux of the examination; it provides the clues to the aetiology of the anaemia. An assessment of the white cells and platelets may add valuable information towards the diagnosis. Nothing can replace an expert morphological opinion.

A bone marrow sample may have to be examined before a definitive diagnosis can be made; stained for iron it remains the ultimate method for assessing the iron status. Special tests (for example, measurements of serum iron, ferritin, vitamin B_{12} and folate concentrations) are often done to confirm the diagnosis made from the history, physical examination, blood counts and blood smear. In a few instances, more extensive testing may be required, particularly the Schilling test for vitamin B_{12} absorption.

Anaemia of chronic disease [4]

About one-quarter of the patients presenting with anaemia to a district general hospital are found to have an anaemia secondary to conditions such as infection, malignancy, chronic inflammatory disease or renal disease. Although the anaemia is usually mild, normochromic and normocytic, it can be severe with marked hypochromia and microcytosis, which may make it difficult to distinguish from an iron deficiency anaemia. The activity of the underlying disease and the length of time it has been present are important factors determining the severity and type of anaemia. Inflammation very quickly interferes with iron metabolism, iron utilization is defective, and absorption of non-haem iron is decreased.

Whether the anaemia is mild or severe,

the serum iron and the total iron-binding capacity are decreased, as is the percentage saturation of transferrin, although not usually to the same extent as in iron deficiency. The serum ferritin concentration is increased. A bone marrow sample stained by Perl's method shows that the macrophages are well-filled with iron, but the erythroblasts contain no iron.

The mechanism of this anaemia is not known but a number of factors contribute to it. There is a modest decrease in red cell survival and a failure to increase erythropoietin concentration in response to the anaemia. The most important factor is a metabolic block, with failure of the reticuloendothelial cells to release iron to transferrin. The anaemia does not respond to oral iron therapy, but will respond to successful treatment of the underlying disorder.

In the context of inflammatory bowel disease, the picture can be confusing. Anaemia is common and features of chronic disease and iron deficiency may be present; in such patients a bone marrow stained for iron may be the only way to resolve the issue [6].

Normochromic anaemia (MCV, MCH normal)

Following acute blood loss (see Chapters 30–32) red cell morphology is normal, although increased polychromasia (reticulocytes) will be evident. The microscopist may notice the presence of a small number of hypochromic cells indicating developing iron deficiency; the electronic cell count would not detect this change. Many patients with the anaemia of chronic disease will have a normochromic normocytic blood picture in the early stage; rouleaux of the red cells may be prominent, and the erythrocyte sedimentation rate increased.

Hypochromic anaemia (MCV, MCH decreased)

A hypochromic microcytic anaemia is one of the commonest anaemias associated with diseases of the gut. It is most likely to be due to iron deficiency and could be related to lesions at any site from the mouth to the rectum. In the presence of chronic blood loss there is a marked hypochromic microcytic anaemia with a slight increase in reticulocytes. Platelets will be increased and, if there is a neutrophil leucocytosis, a neoplasm is very likely. A nutritional iron deficiency anaemia can occur in post-gastrectomy patients, and also in adolescent or pregnant women, whose iron balance may be precarious [3].

It can be very difficult to differentiate between iron deficiency and the anaemia of chronic disorders [4]. This is especially true in Crohn's disease or ulcerative colitis. Often there are features of iron deficiency and chronic disease. In these circumstances the serum iron and total iron-binding capacity measurements may not be helpful; a low serum ferritin concentration will confirm iron deficiency but, if in doubt, a bone marrow stained for iron will resolve the matter very quickly.

Macrocytic anaemia (MCV, MCH increased)

The electronic blood cell counter is able to detect minor degrees of macrocytosis much more readily than the microscopist. The observer gains by seeing additional features of the macrocytes—are they round, or oval? Is the slight macrocytosis due to the reticulocytosis following an acute bleed, or is it the result of haemolysis?

A uniform round macrocytosis is characteristic of excess alcohol intake and is the commonest cause of a raised MCV in the United Kingdom. Many patients with pancreatitis have a macrocytosis, reflecting the high prevalence of alcohol as a factor causing this condition. Target cells are also usually present.

In patients with vitamin B_{12} or folate deficiency the macrocytes are oval, with considerable variation in size and shape (anisocytosis and poikilocytosis). The presence of hypersegmented neutrophils provides further support for the lack of these vitamins. Such changes are seen in pernicious anaemia, post-gastrectomy anaemia, resection of distal small bowel, and bacterial overgrowth of the small bowel—the common cause of vitamin B_{12} deficiency. Folic acid deficiency is more likely in coeliac disease or tropical sprue, although vitamin B_{12} deficiency may develop later. The blood picture in most of these conditions may have a superimposed iron deficiency or the anaemia of chronic disorders.

Macrocytic anaemia is not uncommon in Crohn's disease, and folic acid deficiency is more likely than that of vitamin B_{12}, which usually follows ileal resection [17]. Folate stores are sufficient for three months and it is likely that a poor diet and increased folate requirements together account for this deficiency. As patients with Crohn's disease often have the anaemia of chronic disease, the response to folic acid (or to vitamin B_{12} or iron) will be suboptimal. Patients receiving sulphasalazine for chronic inflammatory bowel disorders may develop a macrocytosis, which is not due to vitamin B_{12} or folate deficiency [21].

Dimorphic anaemia

A pure iron deficiency anaemia is only seen in chronic blood loss. In gastrointestinal disorders, such as post-gastrectomy anaemia or coeliac disease, the patient is anaemic and often the MCV is normal. However, on examination of the stained blood film hypochromic microcytic cells and oval macrocytes, as well as hypersegmented neutrophils, will be observed. Treatment of a patient presenting with an iron deficiency anaemia often uncovers the second deficiency. Bone marrow examination confirms the morphological features of a mixed deficiency more easily than the blood film— megaloblastic changes and an absence of iron being the essential features. Any patient with such a picture should be considered to be suffering from malabsorption until proved otherwise.

Some patients with a post-gastrectomy anaemia, or with coeliac disease, may have a dimorphic blood picture and bone marrow examination shows sideroblastic changes [5]. These are usually secondary to the deficiency and disappear with treatmeny.

Anaemia with raised reticulocytes

Following acute blood loss, the reticulocytosis may be sufficiently high ($>10\%$) to result in a transient macrocytosis and should not be confused with a vitamin B_{12} or folate deficiency. A sustained reticulocytosis makes a haemolytic process likely. An autoimmune haemolytic anaemia may complicate ulcerative colitis: the direct Coombs' (antiglobulin) test is positive, and the antibody may show Rhesus specificity. The haemolysis is not usually severe and is related to the diseased bowel, with improvement following bowel resection. The carcinoid syndrome is another condition that may rarely be associated with a Coombs' positive, immune haemolytic process.

Abnormal red cells—fragmentation

The presence of irregularly-contracted and distorted red cells should alert the clinician to a number of rare conditions. A microangiopathic haemolytic anaemia, with thrombocytopenia and the coagulation abnormalities of disseminated intravascular coagulation is sometimes associated with a mucus secreting adenocarcinoma, particularly of the stomach or colon. Widespread bruising and bleeding from venepuncture sites may be present.

Sulphasalazine often causes chemical changes in the red cell leading to their fragmentation [21]. The Coombs' test is negative. These changes are often of little consequence, as severe anaemia occurs infrequently. The beneficial effects of the drug will usually outweigh this unwanted effect. However, it may provoke a severe megaloblastic anaemia in patients who are folate depleted.

The blood film from a patient with hyposplenism (asplenism) will usually have characteristic changes in all three blood elements—target cells, spiculed and irregularly-contracted red cells, as well as the presence of Howell-Jolly bodies and perhaps an occasional erythroblast can be seen on the blood film. The changes become extreme if vitamin B_{12} or folate deficiency develops. A mild lymphocytosis and thrombocytosis may also occur. Hyposplenism may be present in coeliac disease, and less commonly in ulcerative colitis [13, 23].

Severe crenation of the red cells, with marked toxic changes and a shift to the left in the granulocytes (the total count may be very high or very low), can be seen in any very ill patient—for example, the elderly if intestinal obstruction has been present for some days. The blood cells look 'sick'. The patient is usually septicaemic, and may also have disseminated intravascular coagulation.

References

1 AISEN P. Current concepts in iron metabolism. *Clin Haematol* 1982; 11: 241–257.
2 BAKER SJ, DeMAEYER EM. Nutritional anaemia: its understanding and control with special reference to the work of the World Health Organization. *Am J Clin Nutrit* 1979; 32: 368–417.
3 BARBER SA, BULL NL, BUSS DH. Low iron intakes among young women in Britain. *Br Med J* 1985; 290: 743–744.
4 BENTLEY DP. Anaemia and chronic disease. *Clin Haematol* 1982; 11: 465–479.
5 BOTTOMLEY SS. Sideroblastic anaemia. *Clin Haematol* 1982; 11: 389–409.
6 CAVILL I. Diagnostic methods. *Clin Haematol* 1982; 11: 259–273.
7 CHANARIN I, MALKOWSKA V, O'HEA A-M, RINSLER MG, PRICE AB. Megaloblastic anaemia in a vegetarian Hindu community. *Lancet* 1985; ii: 1168–1171.
8 DALLMAN PR, BEUTLER E, FINCH CA. Effects of iron deficiency exclusive of anaemia. *Brit J Haem* 1978; 40: 179–184.
9 DAWSON DW. Diagnosis of vitamin B_{12} deficiency. *Br Med J* 1984; 289: 938–939.
10 DAWSON DW, SAWERS AH, SHARMA RK. Malabsorption of protein bound vitamin B_{12}. *Br Med J* 1984; 288: 675–678.
11 DELAMORE IW. Gastrointestinal disease. *Clin Haematol* 1972; 1: 507–31.
12 EDITORIAL. Gastrointestinal bleeding in long-distance runners. *Ann Int Med* 1984; 101: 127–128.
13 FERGUSON A, HUTTON MM, MAXWELL JD, MURRAY D. Adult coeliac disease in hyposplenic patients. *Lancet* 1970; i: 163–4.
14 FINCH CA, HUEBERS H. Perspectives in iron metabolism. *New Eng J Med* 1982; 306: 1520–1528.
15 GALLAGHER ND. Importance of vitamin B_{12} and folate metabolism in malabsorption. *Clin Gastroenterol* 1983; 12: 437–441.
16 HAMBORG B, KITTANG E, SCHJONSBY H. The effect of ranitidine on the absorption of food cobalamins. *Scand J Gastroenterol* 1985; 20: 756–758.
17 HARRIES AD, HEATLEY RV. Nutritional disturbances in Crohn's disease. *Postgrad Med J* 1983; 59: 690–697.
18 HOFFBRAND AV. Vitamin B_{12} and folate malabsorption. In: Hardisty RM, Weatherall DJ, eds. *Blood and its disorders*, 2nd ed. Oxford: Blackwell Scientific Publications, 1982: 199–263.
19 MARX JJM. Molecular aspects of iron kinetics. *Eur J Clin Invest* 1984; 14: 408–410.
20 MATTHEWS JH, WOOD JK. Megaloblastic anaemia in vegetarian Asians. *Clin Lab Haematol* 1984; 6: 1–7.
21 PEPPERCORN MA. Sulfasalazine—pharmacology, clinical use, toxicity and related new drug development. *Ann Intern Med* 1984; 101: 377–386.
22 ROSENBERG IH. Absorption and malabsorption of folates. *Clin Haematol* 1976; 5: 589–618.
23 RYAN AB, SMART RC, HOLDSWORTH CD, PRESTON FE. Hyposplenism in inflammatory bowel disease. *Gut* 1978; 19: 50–55.
24 SCOTT JM, WEIR DG. Drug-induced megaloblastic change. *Clin Haematol* 1980; 9: 587–606.

SECTION II

DISEASES OF THE MOUTH AND SALIVARY GLANDS

Chapter 7
Diseases of the Mouth

R.R. FERGUSON

Diseases of the mouth are common and may be associated with diseases in the remainder of the gastrointestinal tract, other systemic disease, or occur in immunocompromised patients. These potential associations should always be considered when a patient presents with oral disease.

Aphthous ulceration

Up to 20% of the population may have recurrent aphthae, the condition being more common in females. Onset is usually the second or third decades of life (Table 7.1).

Aetiology

The aetiology is uncertain: most investigations have studied the role of viruses, streptococcal hypersensitivity and autoimmune disease [5, 6, 12, 16]. Cross-reactivity between food or bacterial antigens and the oral mucosa may be a possible cause of autoimmune phenomena.

Other causative factors are local trauma, folate and vitamin B_{12} deficiency, iron deficiency, coeliac disease, Crohn's disease and ulcerative colitis [6], all of which may be occult at the time of presentation of the oral problems.

Pathology

Initially, there is an intense infiltration with lymphocytes and monocytes. Tissue necrosis occurs and is associated with a polymorphonuclear infiltration. Healing of minor aphthae usually occurs without formation of scar tissue.

Clinical features

Oral ulcers may be classified according to the criteria of Lehner [12] (Table 7.1). Initially the patient notices localized pain and hyperaesthesia, although only an indurated erythematous area about 5 mm in diameter is visible on examination. The

Table 7.1. Recurrent aphthous ulceration (adapted from [12]).

	Minor	Major	Herpetiform
Sex ratio F:M	1.3:1	0.8:1	2.6:1
Age of onset (years)	10–19	10–19	20–29
Number of ulcers	1–5	1–10	10–100
Ulcer diameter	10 mm	10 mm	1–2 mm
Duration	4–14 days	10–30 days	7–10 days
Healing by scar (%)	8	64	32
Recurrence	1–4 months	within a month	within a month
Sites	Lips, cheeks, tongue	Lips, cheeks, tongue, pharynx, palate	Lips, cheeks, tongue, palate, pharynx, floor, gum
Total duration	5 years	15 years	5 years
Associated oral lesions	—	Erythema migrans	—

ulcer develops over the next 1–3 days. **Minor aphthous ulcers** are often multiple, gradually increasing in size, but rarely exceeding one centimetre in diameter. They are extremely painful in the first 4–6 days, but this pain subsides as the ulcer becomes covered with a greyish membrane. They heal without a scar in two weeks. By contrast, **major aphthous ulcers** are solitary, have a longer course, heal by scarring and may be associated with submandibular lymphadenopathy.

Minor aphthous ulcers tend to recur every 1–4 months; major ulcers recur more frequently. It is unusual for episodes of minor ulceration to persist for more than 15 years, but major ulcers recur over a longer period.

Herpetiform ulcers are usually multiple, each ulcer being 1–2 mm in size and surrounded by a thin band of erythema. They heal more rapidly than minor ulcers and tend not to recur after five years.

Investigations

Haematological investigations are of value, bearing in mind the possible associated diseases, and should consist of a haemoglobin, MCV, white cell count and differential, serum iron and total iron binding capacity, red cell folate and vitamin B_{12}. Routine biochemistry is usually of no value, but a low serum albumin may alert the physician to the possibility of occult inflammatory bowel or coeliac disease. A jejunal biopsy is essential if a patient has recurrent ulcers, because of the association with coeliac disease [7]. Routine microbiology, immunology and histopathology are unnecessary.

Treatment

If a dietary factor can be identified, it should be avoided. Nutritional deficiencies should be corrected [19]. Local treatment is aimed at protecting the ulcerated mucosa to relieve pain and inflammation. Pain relief is important, using either systemic simple analgesia or topical anaesthesia such as benzocaine lozenges or lignocaine gel. Choline salicylate dental pastes, such as Bonjela, are of value. Carboxymethylcellulose gelatin paste or powder (Orabase and Orahesive) have a mechanical protective effect. Topical carbenoxolone, in the form of Pyrogastrone tablets or Bioral gel, may speed ulcer healing. Topical corticosteroids, either hydrocortisone pellets or triamcinolone in an adhesive base, are also useful. The problem with all these local treatments is that it is difficult to keep the drug in contact with the ulcer.

Behçet's syndrome (see Chapter 74)

Behçet's syndrome is a rare chronic relapsing disorder with ulceration of the mouth and genitalia, with uveitis [12]. There is a suggestion that it occurs more frequently in the Middle and Far East. Men are more commonly affected; it most frequently presents between the second and fourth decades.

The aetiology is unknown. There is a slightly increased familial incidence. Immunological studies have shown haemagglutinating antibodies against foetal oral mucosal extracts [14]. There is an increased incidence of HLA-B5 [13].

The pathology of the oral ulcers is similar to aphthous ulceration.

Clinically, the syndrome most frequently presents with painful oral ulceration of major or herpetiform type, which may precede the genital ulceration and uveitis by weeks or months (see Table 74.9). The central nervous system and lower gastrointestinal tract may be involved. The syndrome tends to run a chronic relapsing course. There is no effective treatment. The oral lesions are treated like recurrent aphthous ulcers.

Crohn's disease (see Chapter 52)

Oral lesions are not uncommon in Crohn's disease but are often missed by lack of observation [18]. Up to 20% of Crohn's patients have overt oral disease, but there is evidence that 70% of patients have minor histological abnormalities in macroscopically normal oral mucosa [2]. The lesions may occur at any age and are not sex related.

The aetiology of the oral lesions is ill-understood. It is likely that haematinic deficiency does not play a significant role as the oral lesions do not respond to treatment with haematinics [3, 19].

There are six major types of oral pathology in Crohn's disease:

1. Aphthous ulcers.
2. Areas of inflammatory hyperplasia and mucosal fissuring or cobble-stoning.
3. Indurated polypoid 'tag-like' lesions situated on the retro-molar and vestibular mucosa.
4. Persistent deep linear ulcers with hyperplastic margins.
5. Indurated fissures in the mid-line of the lower lip.
6. Diffuse swelling of the lips and cheek.

Microscopically, there is often evidence of surface fissuring with focal collections of lymphocytes in the submucosa and lamina propria. Secondary lymphoid follicles are less common. Initial thickening, perivascular mononuclear cell infiltration and neuronal hyperplasia are also seen.

Less commonly (in about 10% of lesions) typical Crohn's granulomata are present, together with a marked cellular infiltrate of lymphocytes, plasma cells and histiocytes in the lamina propria and submucosa [18]. Non-ulcerated areas of the epithelium may show a characteristic lymphocytic infiltration, together with a few neutrophils. Similar features may be seen in the fibrous stroma of the minor salivary glands.

The oral lesions are more frequent in patients with colonic disease, and in those with skin and joint involvement. The lesions may be asymptomatic and precede symptoms of bowel disease. They can be very painful and tend to run a chronic relapsing and remitting course.

There is no specific treatment, the management being symptomatic and similar in principle to the measures used for recurrent aphthous ulceration.

Ulcerative colitis (see Chapter 49)

Patients with ulcerative colitis, particularly those with active disease, have a variety of oral lesions of which the commonest is recurrent aphthous ulceration. Reports of the prevalence of oral lesions vary from 5 to 20%, but 30% of patients with ulcerative colitis may have minor histological abnormalities despite macroscopically normal oral mucosa [2].

Pyostomatis vegetans is almost specific to ulcerative colitis. Over six to eight weeks, the mucosa of the cheek and lips, and occasionally palate, swells and becomes inflamed with deep fissure-like ulcers and papillary projections of mucosa. Gingivitis may also occur with submandibular lymphadenopathy. Histology shows intra-epithelial abscesses with an eosinophilic infiltration and a few acantholytic cells. The epithelium may degenerate and the lamina propria becomes densely infiltrated with lymphocytes, eosinophils and histiocytes. Perivascular infiltration with eosinophils may be seen in the lamina propria.

Painful ulcerative lesions of the mouth, similar to pyoderma gangrenosum of the skin, are rare but may be associated with the skin lesions. The ulcers are irregular in shape, about 1.5–2 cm in diameter, with a grey base consisting of a fibrino-purulent membrane and rolled-out margins. They are associated with active colitis, develop over four to eight weeks, and may occur after panproctocolectomy in patients with stoma problems. Histologically, there is ulceration of the mucosa and a chronic inflammatory cell infiltrate in the lamina propria together with a few foreign body giant cells.

In a few patients with active ulcerative colitis, haemorrhagic irregularly-shaped ulcers can appear in the oral mucosa and skin of the cheeks, inner aspects of the thigh, buttocks and lower abdomen. The lesions commence as haemorrhagic bullae which ulcerate within three days. Histological features include cutaneous necrotizing vasculitis in the lamina propria and submucosa, fibrinoid necrosis of the venules and neutrophilic infiltration.

Glossitis occurs in both Crohn's patients and ulcerative colitics—it is related to haematinic deficiency, secondary candidiasis, or treatment with antibiotics or steroids.

Oral carcinoma

Oral carcinoma in western countries accounts for about 2% of all tumours, whereas in parts of India this figure rises to 50%. It is a disease found more commonly after the fourth decade. Its incidence is decreasing but it remains commoner in men than women. Causative factors include pipe smoking, tobacco chewing, alcohol consumption, chronic dental and oral infection (particularly infection with *Herpes simplex*, *Candida albicans* and *Treponema pallidum*), oral melanosis, submucous fibrosis and leukoplakia.

Both leukoplakia and submucous fibrosis have a high incidence of carcinomatous transformation. Submucous fibrosis, found in the Far East, is related to eating chillies. Five per cent of patients with leukoplakia, and 30% of cases showing epithelial atypia, undergo malignant change.

Pathology

Squamous carcinoma accounts for 90% of the tumours. Poorly differentiated and anaplastic lesions are rare on the lips. Spread is by local invasion, distant metastases being uncommon. Tumours of the lip and tongue account for 50% of the carcinomas, the remainder occur in about equal frequency in the mouth, cheek, palate and oropharynx. The lesions may be multiple.

Clinical features

Patients present with an ulcer or a lump, which gradually increases in size. Initially it is relatively painless but later may cause discomfort. Either a dry mouth or excessive salivary flow may be a feature. The lesions may bleed. Tumours of the tongue may cause local pain and referred earache when deeply invasive.

On inspection all lumps should arouse suspicion. Malignant ulcers tend to have everted edges and indurated bases. Biopsy of any chronic or indurated oral lesion is mandatory, particularly in middle-aged or elderly patients. Lesions from ill-fitting dentures may be confused clinically with carcinoma. The former tend to heal within a week or so of denture removal.

Recurrent aphthous ulcers, by their history of recurrence, should not cause too much confusion, but the oral lesions of inflammatory bowel disease may require biopsy to exclude malignancy.

Treatment

After establishing the diagnosis by biopsy, surgical excision of the lesion with block dissection of the regional lymph nodes is the treatment of choice. Extensive resections involving removal of the flow may be required for large invasive lesions.

Radiotherapy is a useful alternative for inoperable tumours and as a primary treatment for lip cancer. Occasionally a combined approach is required. Xerostomia is a common complication of radiotherapy.

Prognosis

The average five-year survival ranges from 20 to 50% depending on the site of the lesion and lymph node involvement. Lip cancer has a better prognosis with an 80% five-year survival.

Bullous and vesicular lesions

Pemphigus

The skin condition, pemphigus vulgaris, presents with oral manifestations in 50% of patients, but most patients develop oral involvement at some stage. The disease is rare; both sexes are affected, usually after the age of 30 years.

The aetiology is unknown. Serum antibodies of IgG class are found against interepithelial antigens of both skin and oral mucosa. The significance of this is uncertain. The oral pathology is of intra-epithelial bullae and acantholytic cells associated with diffuse leucocytic infiltration of the lamina propria.

The oral lesions consist of painful fluid-filled bullae, which burst after a few hours leaving shallow ulcers with ill-defined margins. These ulcers persist for weeks to months. The disease is chronic and associated with recurrent crops of new lesions. Routine investigations are valueless, but histology of direct scrapings from the lesions shows characteristic acantholytic cells.

The differential diagnosis includes the other oral bullous lesions of pemphigoid, erythema multiforme and lichen planus. All may be distinguished histologically. Recurrent aphthous ulcers are not characterized by bullae and have a well-defined margin.

Treatment is with systemic steroids, administered initially in a high dose, for example prednisolone 60–100 mg daily. Thereafter, the dosage is reduced to a level that will prevent formation of new lesions.

Azathioprine has been used for its steroid-sparing effect. Maintenance steroids and azathioprine are continued indefinitely.

Pemphigoid

Pemphigoid is another rare bullous lesion affecting the oral mucosa. It occurs a decade later than pemphigus and women are affected twice as commonly as men.

The aetiology is not known. Immunological factors may have a role as immunofluorescent studies demonstrate autoantibodies to the oral mucosal basement membrane. Pathological features are of subepithelial bullae with detachment of the epithelium from the lamina propria. In contrast to pemphigus, there are no acantholytic cells and the bullae are subepithelial, not suprabasilar.

Pemphigoid presents with bullous lesions affecting the mouth, genitalia and conjunctivae. The mouth alone may be involved but the mucous membranes of the upper gastrointestinal tract and vulva, vagina, penis and anus can be affected. The bullous lesions rupture within 48 hours leaving ulcerated areas which are relatively painless. Involvement of the gingiva leads to a raw, bleeding, painful gingivitis. The disease runs a chronic, relapsing course. Eye involvement may lead to blindness.

Treatment relies upon topical steroids if only the mouth is involved, or systemic prednisolone. Large doses are given initially but are then reduced to a maintenance dose sufficient to prevent the formation of new lesions.

Erythema multiforme

Erythema multiforme may occur at any age but is commoner in young males. It may be a drug reaction or be associated with infection. Many episodes are unexplained. In this condition, and its more severe form, the Stevens–Johnson syndrome, there are painful, extensive erosions and ulcers of the palate, tongue and cheek. Gingivitis is common with haemorrhagic crusting of the lips. These lesions may occur without the characteristic skin lesions making diagnosis difficult. A biopsy will exclude pemphigus, pemphigoid or lichen planus.

Treatment consists of stopping any causative drugs and symptomatic measures—topical tetracycline and topical or systemic steroids are useful.

Lichen planus

Lichen planus is often a symptomless oral disease which may also affect the skin. Its aetiology is uncertain. Pathological features include hyperkeratosis, hyperplasia, and degenerative liquefaction of the epithelial basal cell layer. There is a marked lymphocytic and monocytic infiltration of the lamina propria.

The lesions tend to occur after the third decade. There are three types: hypertrophic, erosive and bullous. The hypertrophic variety is often symptomless and may occur alone or with the other two types. It consists of tiny papillae and white striae affecting the posterior buccal mucosa, lips and dorsum of the tongue, although other areas may be involved. The striae give rise to a variety of patterned appearances that may fuse to form plaques, which can be particularly numerous on the dorsum of the tongue.

The bullous variety is rare, the bullae bursting to form ulcers. The erosive type is more common with large, shallow ulcers surrounded by striae and papules. The ulcers are painful. There is commonly an associated gingivitis. Systemic upset is rare unless secondary infection occurs.

The hypertrophic variety does not require treatment. The erosive variety tends to recur and local steroid therapy is needed until the lesions clear. The gingivitis is treated with saline mouth washes, salicy-late pastes and anaesthetic gels. Dental hygiene is important.

Gingivitis

Primary herpetic gingivostomatitis is caused by *Herpes simplex* infection; it occurs in young children more frequently than adults. It starts acutely with a sore mouth and throat, fever and gingivitis. Subsequently, vesicles and oral mucosal ulcers form. Initial crops of ulcers join producing large, shallow, irregular ulcers with surrounding erythema.

Infection starts with the entrance of the *Herpes* virus into the epithelial cell. Intranuclear viral replication takes place and vesicles form as more epithelial cells are affected and degenerate. Rupture of vesicles forms ulcers, which eventually heal without scarring. The disease may be distinguished from recurrent aphthous ulceration by the associated malaise, vesicle formation, sore throat and lymphadenopathy.

Treatment is symptomatic with soothing mouth washes, sedation and a light diet. Tetracycline mouth washes help combat secondary infection. Idoxuridine solution applied locally is beneficial in the early stages. Systemic acyclovir should be given to the immunodeficient.

Acute infective gingivitis (Vincent's infection) is characterized by acute ulceration of the inter-dental and marginal gingivae. It is fairly common and may affect any age group, although the prevalence is higher in younger adults and smokers.

Ill-health may be a predisposing factor—acute leukaemia, neutropenia or aplastic anaemia may be present with haemorrhagic gingivitis. The disease is probably caused by infection with oral commensals, Gram-negative anaerobes such as *Fusobacterium fusiformis*, *Borellia vincentii* or *Bacteroides melaninogenicus*. The precise role of micro-organisms is not established. Poor oral hygiene, pericoronitis and accumulation of dental plaque are important aetiological factors. Histological examination of the gums reveals acute inflammation with a marked polymorph infiltration and fibrinous exudate. There is necrosis of the epithelium and microvascular thrombosis.

Acute infective gingivitis is characterized by the acute onset of painful, bleeding gums, halitosis and a fever of up to 39°C. There is malaise, anorexia and regional lymphadenitis. Coincident with the gum inflammation there are necrotic ulcers affecting the inter-dental gingivae.

Primary herpetic patients are younger and have vesicles followed by ulceration over the whole oral mucosa, rather than a disease localized to the gingivae. Herpetic patients do not have such foul breath. Direct examination of smears from the lesions will also characterize the two diseases—organisms are found in gingivitis, but intranuclear inclusion bodies or giant cells in the herpetic patients.

Inadequate or no treatment leads to necrosed, chronically inflamed gingivae, with associated halitosis, gum bleeding and tooth decay. Antibiotics are the mainstay of treatment—oral penicillin is commonly used but, as Gram-negative anaerobes are involved, metronidazole orally (400 mg eight-hourly for 6 days) is appropriate. Attention to local hygiene is important, with repeated mouth washes using warm saline. Hydrogen peroxide mouth washes and sodium perborate have a cleansing action when in contact with oral debris. Teeth should be cleaned with a soft tooth brush. Recurrence of infection is prevented by strict oral hygiene using dental floss or tape, proper tooth-brushing, descaling and polishing of the teeth.

Bacterial infections

Cancrum oris is a rapidly spreading gangrene of the lips and cheek. It is rarely seen in Britain but may occur in association with terminal illness, particularly in immunodeficient patients. It is more commonly seen in tropical Africa.

Oral tuberculosis may be associated with pulmonary tuberculosis. It presents as a painful, persistent ulcer or plaque which exhibits a characteristic histological feature of the disease. The oral lesions respond to routine antituberculous therapy.

Primary **syphilis** presents as a chancre on the lip or tongue in the first four weeks of infection. The initial painless, firm nodule breaks down into an ulcer with indurated raised margins. There is regional lymphadenopathy. This stage is highly infective. Diagnosis rests on direct observation of *Treponema pallidum* by dark ground illumination. Serological tests are usually negative at this stage of the illness.

Secondary syphilis presents with a maculopapular rash and lymphadenitis 1–4 months after initial infection. Shallow 'snail track' ulcers affect the tonsils, tongue and lips. The saliva is still infectious and serological tests are positive.

Tertiary syphilis is seen 3–30 or more years after inadequately-treated or untreated infection. A gumma presents as a swelling which changes to a painless, punched-out ulcer on the palate, tongue or tonsil. It may heal or perforate. Leukoplakia is another manifestation presenting as an irregular white patch.

The treatment of oral syphilis is identical to that of syphilis in the rest of the body—an appropriately-administered antibiotic such as penicillin.

Candidiasis

Species of *Candida* are found as oral commensals in about half the normal population. Whether these commensals cause the infection is not known but predisposing factors include immunodeficiency, antibiotic therapy and systemic ill-health.

There are four clinical varieties of candidiasis [10].

Acute pseudomembranous candidiasis (thrush) is seen in young babies and debilitated adults. These are symptomless white papules or cotton-wool like exudates which, when rubbed off, leave an erythematous mucosa.

Acute atrophic candidiasis may follow thrush and is usually associated with antibiotic therapy. It is painful and is characterized by a smooth, red tongue, cheilitis and occasionally, sore red lips and cheek mucosa.

Chronic atrophic candidiasis only occurs in denture wearers. It consists of a diffuse erythema of the palate under the denture, with occasional white patches and angular cheilitis. Raised salivary IgA antibodies against *Candida albicans* are found, as are serum agglutinating and precipitating antibodies. These changes are not necessarily involved in pathogenesis, as they occur in a proportion of normal individuals [17]. Cell mediated immunity may be disturbed.

Chronic hyperplastic candidiasis presents as firm, diffuse white patches or papules with intervening erythema on the cheek, tongue or lips. The lesions persist for years and can be associated with chronic mucocutaneous candidiasis which in turn may be seen in immunodeficiency syndromes [8].

Oral antifungal agents are effective treatment for all forms of candidiasis except the chronic hyperplastic variety. Nystatin and amphotericin B suspension or lozenges are equally effective; patients should sleep without their dentures until the infection has cleared. Ketaconazole is reserved for use when other antifungal agents have failed. Chronic mucocutaneous candidiasis has to be treated with systemic antifungal agents, but the disease tends to recur when treatment is stopped.

Dental caries [9]

Dental caries or decay is caused by infection with micro-organisms aggregating on the tooth surface to form dental plaque. The disease is common in children and young adults. Dietary sugar, in combination with colonization by organisms (mainly *Streptococcus mutans*) produce acid that dissolves dental enamel. *Streptococcus mutans* also produces glucosyl transferase, an enzyme important in the synthesis of the extracellular polysaccharides that form the matrix of dental plaque.

Lack of dental and oral hygiene, plus excessive consumption of sucrose and dextrose in the form of sweets, play a leading role. Immunological features are probably largely irrelevant to the initial development of caries, although it has been postulated that relapse of caries follows a fall in serum antibodies against cariogenic bacteria and of salivary antibodies against *Streptococcus mutans* glucosyl transferase [4].

The bacterial plaque reacting with sucrose forms acid which demineralizes dental enamel. The bacteria penetrate further to reach dentine, which is destroyed by decalcification and proteolysis. The dental pulp becomes inflamed but cannot expand in the rigid walls of the tooth. Further spread of infection occurs through the root canal to the apical tissue, causing peri-apical inflammation and abscess formation or a chronic granuloma.

Patients complain of toothache worsened by food, hot or cold fluids. If early treatment is not given, the infection may cause death of the dental pulp, and abscess formation with cellulitis. There may be regional lymphadenopathy. Ludwig's angina is a more serious complication; it is a cellulitis caused by beta-haemolytic *Streptococci* which spreads along the fascial planes of the intra-maxillary and sub-lingual spaces to involve the glottis, causing respiratory obstruction and dysphagia.

Clearly, preventive treatment is most important. Measures include removal of plaque by regular tooth brushing, the use of dental tape, the avoidance of excessive sucrose and water fluoridation. With established caries conservative treatment by a dentist aims to remove the caries, to protect the pulp with suitable dressing and to restore the teeth with fillings. Abscesses are drained by intra-oral incision and appropriate antibiotic therapy.

Glossopyrosis and glossodynia

Complaints by patients of a sore tongue are common, but patients are often worried by normal appearances. Coating of the tongue caused by food particles and desquamation is normal. Smoking commonly causes a black staining, as may antibiotics.

Some patients complain of a burning sensation (glossopyrosis) or painful tongue (glossodynia). Usually, the tongue looks normal and an organic cause is unlikely. If iron, B_{12} and folate deficiencies have been excluded and reflux oesophagitis is not a problem, topical carbenoxolone, in the form of Bioral gel or Pyrogastrone tablets, may be helpful.

Glossitis

The tongue's appearance is abnormal, being either atrophic or reddened. Atrophic appearances are relatively common, particularly in older people. The aetiology is unknown, but it is wise to exclude iron, folate and B_{12} deficiency. A painful red tongue is commonly seen in association with oral thrush.

Erythema migrans or geographic tongue is characterized by an oval-shaped patch of erythema with well-defined edges affecting the dorsum of the tongue. It is often an incidental finding and the patient should be reassured.

Table 7.2. Disorders affecting taste (after Shiffman, [15].

Disorders	Taste
Nervous	
Bell's palsy	A/D
Damage to chorda tympani	A/D
Familial dysautonomia	A/D
Head trauma	A/D
Multiple sclerosis	A/D/D
Nutritional	
Cancer	A/D (sweet)
	Heightened (bitter in some cases)
Chronic renal failure	A/D/D (metallic taste)
Cirrhosis of the liver	A/D
Niacin (vitamin B_{12} deficiency)	A/D/D
Thermal burn	A/D/D
Zinc deficiency	A/D
Endocrine	
Adrenal cortical insufficiency	IDDR
Congenital adrenal hyperplasia	IDDR
Panhypopituitarism	IDDR
Cushing's syndrome	A/D
Cretinism	A/D
Hypothyroidism	A/D/D
Diabetes mellitus	A/D (glucose)
Gonadal dysgenesis (Turner's syndrome)	A/D
Pseudohypoparathyroidism	A/D (sour, bitter)
Local	
Facial hypoplasia	A/D
Sjogren's syndrome	A/D
Radiation therapy	A/D/D
Viral infectious	
Influenza-like infections	A/D/D
Other	
Cystic fibrosis	Individual variation
Hypertension	A/D (salt)
Laryngectomy	A/D/D

A/D denotes absent or diminished; A/D/D absent, diminished, or distorted; and IDDR, increased detection but decreased recognition.

Table 7.3. Drugs affecting taste (after Shiffman, [15]

Classification	Drug
Amoebicides and antihelmintics	Metronidazole; niridazole
Anaesthetics, local	Benzocaine; procaine hydrochloride, and others; cocaine hydrochloride; tetracaine hydrochloride
Anticholesteremic	Chlofibrate
Anticoagulants	Phenindione
Antihistamines	Chlorpheniramine maleate
Antimicrobial agents	Amphotericin B; ampicillin; cefamandole; Griseofulvin; ethambutol hydrochloride; lincomycin; sulphasalazine; streptomycin; tetracyclines; tyrothricin
Antiproliferative, including immunosuppressive agents	Doxorubicin and methotrexate; azathioprine; carmustine; vincristine sulfate
Antirheumatic, analgesic-antipyretic, anti-inflammatory agents	Allopurinol; cholchicine; gold; levamisole; D-penicillamine; phenylbutazone; 5-thiopyridoxine
Antiseptics	Hexetidine
Antithyroid agents	Carbimazole; methimazole; methylthiouracil; propylthiouracil; thiouracil
Agents for dental hygiene	Sodium lauryl sulfate (toothpaste)
Diuretics and antihypertensive agents	Captopril; diazoxide; ethacrynic acid
Hypoglycemic drugs	Glipizide; phenformin and derivatives
Muscle relaxants and drugs for treatment of Parkinson's disease	Baclofen; chlormezanone; levodopa
Opiates	Codeine; hydromorphone hydrochloride; morphine
Psychopharmacologic, including anti-epileptic, drugs	Carbamazepine; lithium carbonate; phenytoin; psilocybin; trifluoperazine
Sympathomimetic drugs	Amphetamines; phenmetrazine theoclate and fenbutrazate hydrochloride (combined)
Vasodilators	Oxyfedrine; bemifylline hydrochloride
Others	Germine monoacetate; idoxuridine; iron sorbitex; vitamin D; industrial chemicals, including insecticides

Actinomycosis

Infection with *Actinomycosis israeli* is rarely seen in Britain, but it is common in the tropics. Facio-cervical actinomycosis is the commonest clinical form and is generally associated with dental caries, infected gums, or periodontal disease.

The lower jaw is more frequently affected. The gums becoming indurated, nodules then appear on the jaw, submandibular tissues and lymph nodes. The swellings are painful. The overlying skin becomes indurated and cyanotic: abscesses point externally to form multiple sinuses. The pus contains visible granules which microscopically are Gram-positive mycelia. Secondary infection is common.

Treatment with antibiotics, preferably penicillin or cotrimoxazole, has to be prolonged and in high dosage until cure is obtained. Surgery is useful for extirpation of diseased tissue and to establish free drainage.

Disorders of taste

Patients frequently complain of abnormal taste sensation—a symptom that is difficult to assess objectively. The problem has been reviewed extensively [15]. Abnormal taste sensation has been attributed to nervous system, nutritional, or endocrine disease, as well as to trauma, virus infections, and local disease in the oropharynx (Table 7.2). A large range of commonly-used drugs are reported to alter taste sensation (Table 7.3).

References

1 Basu MK, Asquith P. Immunological aspects of the mouth. In: Asquith P, ed. *Immunology of the gastrointestinal tract.* Edinburgh: Churchill Livingstone, 1979:37–54.
2 Basu MK, Asquith P. Oral manifestation of inflammatory bowel disease. In: Farmer RG ed. *Clin Gastroenterol* 1980;9:307–321.
3 Basu MK, Asquith P, Thompson RA, Cooke WT.

Oral manifestation of Crohn's disease. *Gut* 1975;**16**:249–254.

4 CHALLACOMBE SJ, LEHNER T, GUGGENHEIM B. Serum and salivary antibodies to glucosyl transferase in dental caries. *Nature* 1972;**238**:219.

5 DONATSKY O, BENDIXEN G. In situ demonstration of hypersensitivity to Strep. 2. A in recurrent aphthous stomatitis by means of leucocyte migration test. *Acta Allergol* 1972;**29**:308–318.

6 FERGUSON R. (Univ. of Birmingham M.D. Thesis)

7 FERGUSON R, BASU MK, ASQUITH P, COOKE WT. Jejunal mucosal abnormalities in patients with recurrent aphthous ulceration. *Br Med J* 1976;**1**:11–13.

8 HIGGS JM, WELLS RS. Chronic mucocutaneous candidiasis: new approach to treatment. *Br J Dermatol* 1973;**89**:179–190.

9 JENKINS GN. Recent changes in dental caries. *Br Med J* 1985;**291**:1297–1298.

10 LEHNER T. Classification and clinico-pathological features of candida infection in the mouth. HI Winne, RE Hurley, eds *Symposium on candida infections.* Edinburgh 1966.

11 LEHNER T. Stimulation of lymphocyte transformation by tissue humogenates in recurrent oral ulceration. *Immunology* 1967;**13**:139–166.

12 LEHNER T. Oral ulceration and Behçet's syndrome. *Gut* 1977;**18**:491–511.

13 OHNO S, AOKI K, SUGUIRA S, NAKAYAMA E, ITAKURA K, AISAWA M. HLAs and Behçets syndrome. *Lancet* 1973;**ii**:1383–1384.

14 OSHIMA Y, SHIMUZU T, YOKOHARI R, MATSUMOTO T, KAMO K, KAAMI T, NAGAYA H. Clinical studies on Behçets syndrome. *Ann Rheum Dis* 1966;**22**:36–75.

15 SHIFFMAN SS. Taste and smell in disease. *New Engl J Med* 1983;**308**:1275–1279, 1337–1343.

16 TAYLOR KB, TRUELOVE SC, WRIGHT R. Serological reaction to gluten and cow's milk proteins in gastro-intestinal disease. *Gastroenterology* 1964;**46**:99–108.

17 WELLS RS. Chronic mucocutaneous candidiasis: a clinical classification. *Proc R Soc Med* 1973;**61**:801–802.

18 WIESENFELD D, FERGUSON MM, MITCHELL DN et al. Orofacial granulomatosis—a clinical and pathological analysis. *Q J Med* 1985;**54**:101–13.

19 WRAY, D, FERGUSON MM, MASON DK, HUTCHEN AW, DAGG JM. Recurrent apthae: treatment with vitamin B_{12}, folic acid and iron. *Br Med J* 1975;**2**:490–493.

Chapter 8
Diseases of the Salivary Glands

M. HOBSLEY

The salivary glands develop as outpouchings from the embryonic foregut and are therefore legitimately part of the gastrointestinal tract (Table 8.1). Salivary gland diseases are not common (Table 8.2).

Anatomy

The site and shape of a parotid gland is shown in Fig. 8.1. The normal gland is of the same consistency as its surroundings and is therefore impalpable. The facial nerve trunk enters the posterior aspect of the gland and then divides into six named branches which traverse the gland. The parotid duct runs forwards along the masseter muscle, 1 cm below the zygoma, to enter the mouth opposite the second molar

Table 8.2. Diseases of the salivary glands.

Trauma	External
	Surgical
Stones (strictures)	Submandibular; parotid
Infections	Bacterial
	Viral
Tumours	Benign
	Malignant
	Secondary
Connective tissue	Sjögren's disease
	Sicca syndrome
Sarcoidosis	
Other	Sialectasis
	Sialosis
	Non-specific enlargement

Table 8.1. The composition of saliva.

Volume	750 ml/day (70% submandibular, 25% parotid)
	Max. parotid flow 3–13 ml/5 min.
pH	6.2–7.4
Sp. Gr.	1002–1003
Inorganic constituents	Calcium
	Phosphorus
	Sodium
	Potassium
	Chloride
	Bicarbonate
Organic constituents	Amylase
	Glycoproteins
	Lysozyme
	Carbonic anhydrase
	Amino acids
	Urea
	Citrate
	Kallikrein

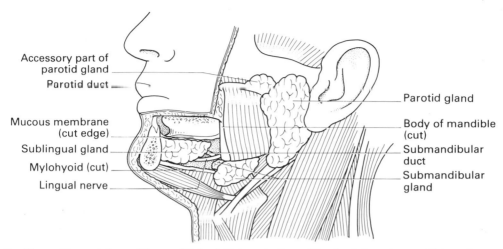

Fig. 8.1. The position and shape of the parotid gland. Note projections of the gland along the parotid duct, down into the neck behind the submandibular gland, and backwards over the mastoid process.

tooth. It is thick-walled with a lumen of less than 1 mm across.

Each submandibular gland has a deep portion in the floor of the mouth and a superficial portion that is usually firmer than its surroundings and therefore readily palpable in the neck. The lumen of the submandibular gland's duct is much larger than that of the parotid.

Diseases of the sublingual, and of the countless unnamed salivary glands in the mouth and pharynx are rare and will not be considered.

Clinical features and examination

Patients often complain of increased or decreased rates of salivary secretion but rarely can this be objectively confirmed (except in patients on tricyclic antidepressant drugs) [3]. Decreased salivation can occur early in the development of the sicca or Sjögren's syndrome and before palpable changes in the glands occur. It is unusual for studies of salivary function to be of any additional diagnostic value when a palpable abnormality is present.

Salivary gland swellings may be acute, chronic or recurrent, and either unilateral or bilateral (Table 8.3). Swelling may affect the whole gland (diffuse) or part of it (focal lump).

Table 8.3. A classification of salivary gland swellings.

Type		Diagnosis
Diffuse		
Bilateral	Acute	Mumps
		Ascending infection
	Chronic	Sjögren's
	or recurrent	Other (rare)
		including bilateral
		calculi
Unilateral	Acute	Mumps
		Ascending infection
	Chronic	Calculus
	or recurrent	Sjögren's
		Sicca syndrome
		Sarcoid
		Sialosis
		Other (rare)
Focal		
Bilateral	Acute	Lymph nodes
		(reactive;
		lymphoma)
	Chronic	Tumour, especially
		adenolymphoma
Unilateral	Acute	Abscess (calculi)
		'Inflammatory'
		tumour, e.g.
		adenolymphoma
	Chronic	Tumour (unless
		proved otherwise)

Each of the four major salivary glands should be assessed for enlargement, induration and the presence of a lump. An erroneous diagnosis of unilateral (or bilateral) chronic parotid enlargement is sometimes made when the enlarged structure is really the masseter muscle. This should be avoided by asking the patient to clench his teeth during the examination. The examination must include palpation of the submucosal (submandibular) and subcutaneous (parotid) ducts with inspection of their orifices into the mouth. In addition, one should test the functions of the facial, lingual and hypoglossal nerves, which may become involved by a disease of the salivary glands, and palpate the local drainage lymph node fields.

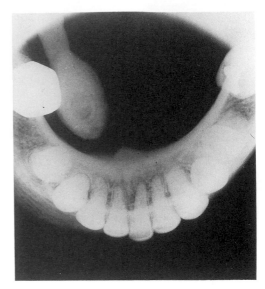

Fig. 8.3. Plain X-ray of the floor of the mouth (the occlusal view) showing a large submandibular calculus. Reproduced from [9].

Investigations

Radiology is particularly helpful in patients with recurrent swelling of a salivary gland [22]. Plain radiographs should include an intrabuccal 'dental' film to show the termination of the parotid duct (Fig. 8.2) or an occlusion film of the submandibular glands (Fig. 8.3). Water-soluble contrast media should be used for sialography [1] as oily agents stay in the ducts and can excite a foreign body reaction. Minimal force should be used for the injection to prevent extravasation from the ducts into the parenchyma of the gland which is likely if the ducts have been weakened by chronic inflammation. CT-sialography may be particularly helpful to identify small superficial parotid masses [4].

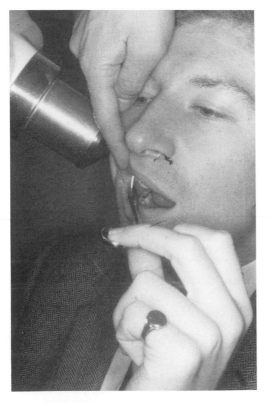

Fig. 8.2. Plain X-ray of the parotid region: intrabuccal view. The patient holds a small dental film in a pair of forceps between the cheek and the gum. Reproduced from [9].

Common diseases

Mumps

Mumps is caused by an RNA-virus of the influenza group. The parotitis is a non-specific, non-suppurative inflammation that starts after an incubation-period of 14–21 days. Orchitis, pancreatitis and rarely meningitis, or encephalitis may also occur [13]. A single attack (including approximately 30% of asymptomatic infections) confers life-long immunity. This makes mumps an unlikely cause of recurrent parotid swelling.

Mumps is the commonest cause of acute bilateral parotid enlargement. The submandibular glands may be involved as well as the parotid glands. Mumps can affect a single parotid gland although the other may later become involved. In a patient with circumstantial evidence favouring mumps, this is usually the correct diagnosis. When it occurs in a child or young adult and there is a history of a current epidemic or exposure to a known contact, there is little diagnostic doubt. If doubt exists, the specific mumps antibody should be measured at intervals to demonstrate a rising titre.

There is no specific treatment for mumps; rest is usually advised to reduce the risk of pancreatitis or orchitis, but there is no evidence of its efficacy. Simple analgesia should be given for relief of pain and fever.

Salivary calculi

Salivary calculi are more commonly encountered in the submandibular (rather than parotid) glands. The majority are found in the duct although some present while in the substance of the gland. The initial calculi are ovoid or cylindrical in shape and tend to block the duct system. The ducts proximal to the obstruction dilate and in the stagnant contents secondary stones can form (often spherical in shape). Both types of stone are composed of material similar to dental tartar with a variable concentration of calcium. Most calculi are radio-opaque. Recurrent or chronic unilateral enlargement of a salivary gland

is usually due to a salivary duct calculus [17, 23] Clinical features suggesting impaction of a calculus are a sudden onset of pain and swelling; a sensation of dryness in the ipsilateral half of the mouth during an attack; a relatively short duration of swelling or discomfort (from a few hours up to 10 days); and a fairly sudden end to the attack—sometimes with a gush of saliva into the mouth from the affected duct. As the submandibular duct is wider than the parotid duct, submandibular obstruction usually resolves in a few minutes or hours, whereas parotid obstruction lasts longer with a greater chance of ascending infection.

Submandibular duct stones are usually larger than those in the parotid duct and can often be palpated in the floor of the mouth. A parotid calculus is often more difficult to feel as it is smaller and less of the parotid duct is palpable in the cheek. However, there is often additional evidence supporting a parotid duct calculus such as oedema, swelling or deformity of the duct orifice or the fact that turbid saliva can be expressed from the duct. Plain X-rays and

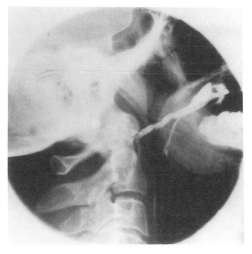

Fig. 8.4. Sialogram showing a stone in the parotid duct. The parotid duct is grossly distended apart from a few millimetres at its oral end.

sialography (Fig. 8.4) usually confirm the diagnosis.

Submandibular salivary stones are usually too large to pass spontaneously; if they are palpable in the floor of the mouth they can be removed by a local incision through the buccal mucosa and into the duct. The lingual nerve can be damaged if the stone is close to the deep part of the gland. Under these circumstances removal of the whole submandibular gland and its proximal duct (including the stone) should be undertaken through a cervical incision.

About 5% of patients with chronic submandibular swelling have no evidence of a stone—they should have the gland excised in case it harbours a tumour. A complaint that the gland is enlarged is common in depressed and anxious patients so one must

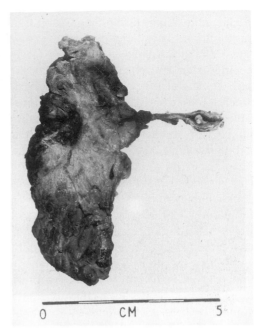

Fig. 8.6. Superficial parotidectomy specimen showing a parotid duct stone.

be convinced that it is abnormal before advising operation.

If a **parotid duct calculus** has impacted at the orifice of the duct it can be removed through the mouth (Fig. 8.5). If it lies further back the only way to remove it, without risking accidental damage to the facial nerve, is to perform a superficial conservative parotidectomy (Fig. 8.6). The risks of this operation have to be balanced against the severity of the patient's symptoms and the likelihood of the stone passing spontaneously.

Approximately 25% of patients with recurrent or chronic parotid swelling have no evidence of calculi—most show punctate sialectasis on sialography (Fig. 8.7).

Bacterial infection [16]

The oral cavity harbours many pathogenic bacteria. The risk of ascending infection is increased by any interference with the downward flow of sterile saliva. Thus, any

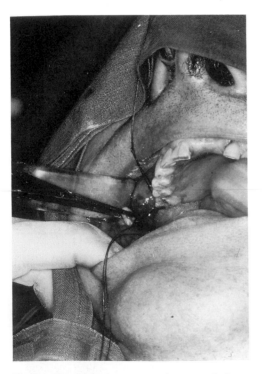

Fig. 8.5. Parotid duct meatotomy for removal of a calculus. The stay sutures in the buccal tissues above and below the duct steady the tissues while the orifice is slit open and the stone is extracted.

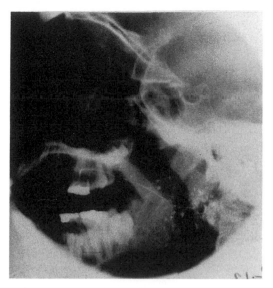

Fig. 8.7. Sialectasis: parotid sialogram showing a normal duct with blobs of contrast at the terminations of the finer ducts when dye has extravasated through the epithelium weakened by chronic inflammation.

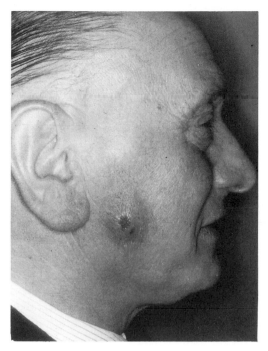

Fig. 8.8. Clinically diagnosable lump in the parotid region. This was an inflammatory mass situated in the parotid duct area. Inspection and palpation from within the mouth confirmed that this was a parotid duct calculus with a secondary abscess where the stone was penetrating into the cheek.

form of obstruction in the salivary duct (calculus, stricture or neighbouring lesion such as a dental abscess) or any reduction in the flow of saliva (dehydration or Sjögren's syndrome) can lead to secondary infection in the affected gland.

Ascending infection usually involves the whole salivary gland. The acute infection may resolve, produce an abscess or become chronic.

Localized inflammation, within an otherwise normal salivary gland, is usually due to a focal lesion; for example, a stone eroding through the wall of a duct to cause inflammation within the gland (Fig. 8.8), or a sterile inflammatory degeneration in a particular parotid neoplasm—the adenolymphoma.

The infected gland is usually inflamed, enlarged and tender. Pus discharging from the orifice of the parotid duct (Fig. 8.9) clinches the diagnosis of ascending parotitis. The patient should be treated with systemic broad-spectrum antibiotics such as amoxycillin and metronidazole. If the discharge stops, but parotid pain and tenderness grow worse or even fail to improve, a parotid abscess must be considered. There is no point in looking for fluctuation—the tense overlying parotid fascia masks this sign. Treatment is by drainage of the abscess through an incision at the point of maximal tenderness, under general anaesthesia. The incision should be made parallel to the direction of the nearest branch of the facial nerve to reduce the risk of damage to the nerve; once through the parotid fascia, blunt probing is used to locate and drain the abscess cavity.

Patients with **punctate sialectasis** appear to have a weak defence mechanism against ascending infections. The abnormality is not necessarily a reduction in the secretion

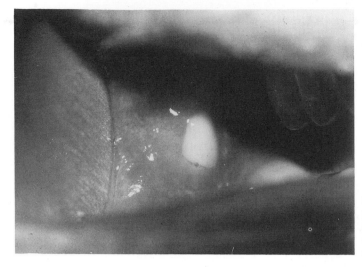

Fig. 8.9. Acute ascending parotitis. Thick, opaque pus is seen discharging from the orifice of the parotid duct, in the cheek opposite the second molar tooth.

rate of saliva, since many subjects have a normal secretion. Bouts of ascending infection occur—their onset is gradual, not related to eating and each episode usually lasts three to four weeks. Antibiotics usually help to cut short an attack but after several bouts of acute infection the parotid remains enlarged and indurated between attacks. Patients with severe symptoms due to recurrent infection may require a conservative parotidectomy.

Salivary gland neoplasms

Salivary gland neoplasms are rare—they account for only 2% of all neoplasms. They can present at any age, but most commonly in the fourth and fifth decades; the sexes are equally affected. The parotid is the commonest site [5]. In the parotid, 85% of tumours are benign adenomas, but in the submandibular glands malignant lesions account for 50% of the tumours seen [19]. There are no definite aetiological features, although half of all parotid carcinomas arise by malignant change in a benign tumour [18].

Table 8.4 gives a modification of the World Health Organization classification of salivary gland neoplasms [24].

Table 8.4. Histological classification of epithelial tumours salivary glands.

Benign	Pleomorphic adenoma
	Monomorphic adenoma, several
	varieties including adenolymphoma
Intermediate	Mucoepidermoid tumour
	Acinic cell tumour
Malignant	Adenoid cystic carcinoma
	Frank carcinoma

The **pleomorphic adenomas,** and much rarer **monomorphic adenomas,** are benign in that they do not infiltrate surrounding tissues but push them aside, and do not metastasize. However, unless excised with a clear margin of normal tissue, they show an unpleasant tendency to local recurrence, usually as multiple nodules (Fig. 8.10). The reason for this behaviour is that bosses of tumour project through an incomplete capsule and are likely to be shorn off and left in the bed of the tumour if enucleation is attempted (Fig. 8.11). Biopsy, either needle or surgical, is ill-advised because of the risk of tumour implantation and the fact that histological diagnosis of parotid tumours is difficult [24].

The **adenolymphoma** (not to be confused with lymphadenoma) is the second com-

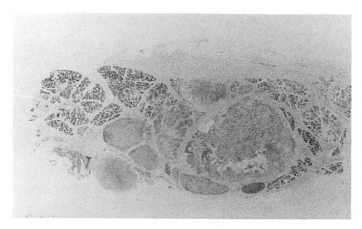

Fig. 8.10. Histological features of recurrent nodules of a pleomorphic salivary adenoma after previous enucleation of the tumour. The skin scar (top) has been excised to ensure clearance of nodules but as the tumour nodules extend to the deep aspect of the specimen some neoplastic tissue has probably been left behind.

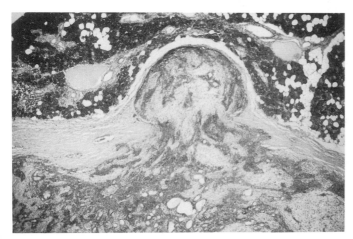

Fig. 8.11. A pleomorphic salivary adenoma showing the tumour (below) separated from the normal parotid tissue (above) by a capsule of compressed tissue with a 'boss' of tumour projecting through this capsule. Such bosses account for the strong tendency to recurrence after enucleation.

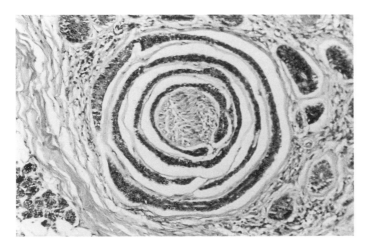

Fig. 8.12. The adenoid cystic carcinoma: this tumour infiltrates along the nerve sheath producing an onion-skin appearance around the central axon.

monest parotid tumour. It tends to be soft as it contains cystic spaces. It usually occurs in middle-aged men at the lower pole of the parotid. However, none of these features is sufficiently distinct to permit a confident clinical diagnosis. Adenolymphomas may be bilateral, or occur at multiple sites in the same gland. The latter may result in apparent recurrence after removal but, unlike the adenomas, it shows no potential for true implantation.

The **acinic cell tumour**, the **mucoepidermoid tumour**, the **adenoid cystic carcinoma** and **frank carcinomas** form an ascending scale of malignancy [17]. Locally, the tumours invade neighbouring structures such as skin, bone or facial nerve—the adenoid cystic carcinoma has a predilection for nerve-sheath (Fig. 8.12). The risk of widespread bloodborne metastases is greatest with a frank carcinoma.

Clinical presentation

About 90% of lumps in the parotid region are parotid neoplasms, of which 80% are pleomorphic salivary adenomas. The management strategy must therefore be designed to give good results should that be the case [6, 7].

In about 5% of patients there may be evidence of malignant invasion of skin, facial nerve or bone. Very rapid growth also suggests malignancy.

A lump in the submandibular region usually turns out to be a chronic swelling of the whole gland due to infection in association with a stone in the duct. If there is no evidence of a stone, it should be assumed that a tumour is present and the whole gland should be removed. The patient should be warned about possible damage to either the lingual, hypoglossal or the mandibular branch of the facial nerve.

Surgery

Unless a tumour is obviously malignant [2], the lump should be excised with a wide margin of normal tissue, if possible exposing and preserving the facial nerve and all its named branches **(conservative parotidectomy)**. The patient must be warned that dissection of the nerve often produces a temporary facial paresis and that, even in the absence of any clinical evidence of involvement of the facial nerve, it is occasionally found at operation that the lump is growing into the nerve instead of pushing it aside (Fig. 8.12), making it necessary to sacrifice a branch or some branches of the nerve **(semi-conservative parotidectomy)** or even the whole nerve **(radical parotidectomy)** [8, 12].

The results of surgery are good. For a patient with a pleomorphic (or monomorphic) adenoma operated on initially in this manner, where both surgeon and the pathologist agree that the tumour has been removed intact, the risk of recurrence appears to be zero [10, 11, 21].

Should the tumour prove on histological examination to be either an adenoid cystic or frank carcinoma, the patient should receive radiotherapy.

Complications of parotidectomy

Reactionary haemorrhage during the first 24 hours is common, despite suction drainage of the wound. The patient must return to theatre, the wound reopened under general anaesthesia and the clot evacuated with due deference the exposed facial nerve. Any bleeding point is secured and the wound again closed with suction drainage.

Postoperative facial paresis is common, although it is usually mild. After conservative parotidectomy it is always transient, although to a trained observer (as distinct from the patient) it may take several months to disappear completely.

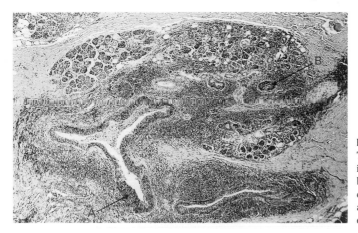

Fig. 8.13. Sjögren's syndrome. There is diffuse lymphocytic infiltration of the lobule. A branching duct shows hyperplasia of part of its epithelial lining (A) and there is a solid epimyoepithelial island (B).

A parotid fistula does not occur provided that most of the parotid duct is excised.

A late complication may be uncontrolled excessive sweating over the parotid area due to loss of normal sympathetic control.

Other conditions

Sjögren's syndrome

Sjögren described a combination of dry eyes, dry mouth, swellings of salivary glands and various connective tissue disorders such as rheumatoid arthritis [20]. The condition is commonest in middle-aged females and may be an autoimmune disease as 60% of patients have various autoantibodies present in their serum. Histologically there is a lymphocytic infiltration of the affected salivary glands with fibrinoid necrosis of the walls of the fine ducts. There is also an overgrowth of ductal cells—not only the columnar cells lining the ducts but also the contractile Purkinje or myoepithelial cells that lie on the outer aspect of the ducts —which can obliterate the lumen of the ducts (Fig. 8.13). Sialography shows punctuate sialectasis.

Some of the more severely affected patients respond favourably to steroids or immunosuppressive drugs, but most only require symptomatic measures [25].

Sarcoidosis

Enlargement of the parotid can be due to sarcoid infiltration of lymphatic tissue within the gland [15]. The Heerfordt's or Waldenstrom's syndrome of uveitis, fever, enlargement of the parotid and (sometimes) facial nerve palsy (uveoparotid fever) is very rare. Sarcoidosis usually responds to systemic steroids.

Branchial fistula

The rare first arch branchial fistula usually presents in children. The complete lesion is a fibrous track, lined with columnar epithelium, opening in the anterior wall of the cartilaginous external auditory meatus posteriorly and in the skin below the angle of the jaw anteriorly. In its course through the parotid gland it winds around the facial nerve [14].

References

1 ADAM EJ, WILLSON SA, CORCORAN MO, HOBSLEY M. The value of parotid sialography. *Br J Surg* 1983;**70**:108–110.

2 CORCORAN MO, COOK HP, HOBSLEY M. Radical surgery following radiotherapy for advanced carcinoma of the parotid. *Br J Surg* 1983;**71**:261–263.

3 CURRY TC, PATEY DH. A clinical test for parotid function. *Br J. Surg* 1964;**51**:891–892.

4 EYJOLFSSON O, NORDSHUS T., DAHL T. Sialography

and CT-Sialography. *Acta Radiol* [*Diagn*] (*Stockh*) 1984;**25:**361–367.

5 EVANS RW, CRUICKSHANK AH. *Epithelial Tumors of the Salivary Glands*. Philadelphia: Saunders, 1970.

6 HOBSLEY M. Salivary Tumours. *Br J Hosp Med* 1973;**10:**553–562.

7 HOBSLEY M. The management of a lump in the parotid region. In: MacFarland J, ed. *Postgraduate Surgery Lectures Vol. 1*. London: Butterworths, 1973:90–106.

8 HOBSLEY M. Head and Neck. In: Kirk RM, ed. *General Surgical Operations*. Edinburgh: Churchill Livingstone, 1978;342–365.

9 HOBSLEY, M. *Pathways in Surgical Management*. London: Edward Arnold, 1979.

10 HOBSLEY M. Sir Gordon Gordon-Taylor: two themes illustrated by the surgery of the parotid gland. *Ann Roy Coll Surg Engl* 1981;**63:**264–269.

11 HOBSLEY M. Surgery of the salivary glands. In: J Hadfield, M Hobsley, eds. *Current Surgical Practice Vol. 3*. London: Edward Arnold, 1981: 8–31.

12 HOBSLEY MM. *A Colour Atlas of Parotidectomy*. London: Wolfe Medical Publications, 1984.

13 JOHNSTONE JA, ROSS CAC, DUNN M. Meningitis and encephalitis associated with mumps infection. A 10-year survey. *Arch Dis Child* 1972;**47:**647–51.

14 MILLER PD, CORCORAN M, HOBSLEY M. Surgical excision of first cleft branchial fistulae. *Br J Surg.* 1984;**71:**696–697.

15 MITCHELL DN, SCADDING JG. Sarcoidosis. *Amer Rev Resp Dis* 1974; **110:**774–802.

16 PATEY DH. Inflammation of the salivary glands with particular reference to chronic and recurrent parotitis. *Ann Roy Coll Surg Engl* 1965;**36:**26–44.

17 PATEY DH. Recurrent swelling of the parotid gland (recurrent parotitis). In: WT Irvine, ed. *Modern Trends in Surgery Vol. 3*. London: Butterworths, 1971:261–283.

18 PATEY DH, THACKRAY AC, KEELING DH. Malignant disease of the parotid. *Br J Cancer* 1965;**19:**712–737.

19 RAFLA S. Submaxillary gland tumors. *Cancer* 1970;**26:**821–6.

20 SJÖGREN H. Zur kenntnis der Keratoconjunctivitis Sicca. *Acta Ophthalmol* (Kbh) 1933; suppl. **2:**1–151.

21 STEVENS LK, HOBSLEY M. The treatment of pleomorphic adenomas by formal parotidectomy. *Br J Surg* 1982;**69:**1–3.

22 SULEIMAN SI, HOBSLEY M. Radiological appearances of parotid duct calculi. *Br J Surg* 1980;**67:**879–80.

23 SULEIMAN SI, THOMSON JPS, HOBSLEY M. Recurrent unilateral swelling of the parotid gland. *Gut* 1979;**20:**1102–1108.

24 THACKRAY AC, LUCAS RB. *Tumors of the major salivary glands*. Washington DC: Armed Forces Institute of Pathology, 1974.

25 WHALEY K, WILLIAMSON J, CHISHOLM DM, WEBB J, MASON DK, BUCHANAN WW. Sjögren's syndrome. I. Sicca Components. *QJ Med* 1973;**42:**279–304.

SECTION III

DISEASES OF THE OESOPHAGUS

Chapter 9
Investigation of the Oesophagus

J. N. BLACKWELL & D.O. CASTELL

Most patients presenting with common oesophageal disorders will be diagnosed easily from the clinical history, supported by barium radiographic studies and upper gastrointestinal endoscopy with biopsy. Only in a minority of patients will more detailed investigation be required. However, diagnostic difficulties can occur when common oesophageal disorders present with atypical symptoms or manifestations. In addition we now recognize that disorders of oesophageal function occur more frequently than was previously thought.

Oesophageal Radiology

The barium-swallow has been the traditional initial investigation for assessing structural abnormalities, mucosal changes and motility disturbances. Although the technique draws its strength from being relatively straightforward, reliable information requires more than simple observation of the passage of the barium into the stomach with one or two 'spot' films. Effective radiological evaluation requires an understanding of the oesophageal anatomy and physiology and the use of a variety of examination techniques, tailored to the patient's symptoms or suspected diagnosis [11].

The full column technique is used to demonstrate strictures, carcinomas, large oesophageal ulcers, hiatal herniae, rings or pressure from extrinsic masses. Mucosal relief films are used to demonstrate early neoplasms, varices, small ulcers or erosions. Some lesions require both techniques for full definition. Double-contrast studies are possible but the sensitivity is not necessarily improved [19]. Dynamic recording using television, cine or rapid sequence spot films may be used to investigate motility. These techniques are especially useful for swallowing disorders arising from the tongue, pharynx or upper part of the oesophagus.

The clinical value of oesophagography depends upon the interest and experience of the radiologist. There are surprisingly few published evaluations of the accuracy and results of this technique. Reports from centres with a special interest in oesophageal disease serve more as an encouragement to other radiologists in what may be achieved, than as a help to the clinician in assessing the reliance he can place upon his own X-ray department. From a practical standpoint the best guidance is to 'know your radiologist'.

Reflux disease

Suspected gastro-oesophageal reflux disease is the most common indication for a barium swallow. Mucosal abnormalities can be detected in as many as 90% of patients with endoscopically-confirmed moderate or severe oesophagitis [19]. However, minor degrees of oesophagitis will be demonstrated in less than 16% of cases. Such results are, however, only achieved in a few radiology departments and most grossly underestimate the incidence of such changes.

Indirect evidence of reflux oesophagitis may be obtained by observing barium reflux into the gullet [20], but it should be remembered that occasional reflux occurs in normal individuals and can be provoked by a variety of manoeuvres. Only unprovoked free barium reflux can be regarded as a reliable indicator of an abnormality. Similarly, the presence of a hiatal hernia is not synonymous with reflux disease. Although hiatus herniae were demonstrable in 85% of patients with oesophagitis they were also seen in 40% of 'controls' [21]. The radiological detection of a hiatal hernia appears to relate more to the vigour of the technique used than to the presence of disease, reported incidences in control populations ranging from 1.3% to 100%. The incidence also increases with age and in the over 60s the demonstration of a small hiatal hernia seems usual.

Carcinoma

Radiology is effective in the diagnosis of oesophageal carcinoma. It should demonstrate all lesions causing narrowing of the lumen, which is usually present by the time most patients present. Difficulty can arise in differentiating peptic from malignant strictures and endoscopy with biopsy should always be performed before treatment is commenced. Barium studies are less effective in detecting early lesions that are less than 3.5 mm in diameter. Moss, Koehler and Margulis [16] reported that only 73% of carcinomas were detected by barium swallow, even with careful examination of the radiographs. The majority of mistakes were reporting a lesion benign when it was malignant, emphasizing the importance of endoscopy and biopsy.

Motility disorders

The best investigation for detecting motility disorders in the mouth, pharynx or oesophagus, is cine or video-fluoroscopy with the facility for slow replay. Motility disorders affecting the body or distal oesopha-

gus, other than achalasia, are poorly detected radiologically. Achalasia, when presenting late, is always diagnosable although caution is needed to exclude malignant disease at the cardia which may mimic achalasia. Early achalasia without oesophageal dilation may go unrecognized if the gastro-oesophageal junction is not thoroughly examined during routine radiology. In gross diffuse oesophageal spasm the radiological features have been given many colourful synonyms including 'rosary bead oesophagus' or 'corkscrew oesophagus'. However, these obvious changes are present only in a minority of patients with diffuse spasm. The majority are more likely to show less dramatic changes, such as tertiary contractions, which do not always correspond to any specific manometric abnormality. In other motility disorders oesophageal radiology is generally normal.

Endoscopy and oesophageal mucosal biopsy

Fibreoptic upper gastrointestinal endoscopy has become a simple and routine procedure. Modern instruments with their improved optics, controls and flexibility have resulted in markedly reduced discomfort and less hazard. None-the-less it should be remembered that complications can still occur—for example from the drugs used for sedation, from perforations and from haemorrhage. Perforation of the oesophagus or stomach from endoscopic damage has been reported in 0.14–0.65 per 1,000 procedures [24, 14].

Many gastroenterologists now use upper gastrointestinal endoscopy as the first diagnostic investigation without a preceding barium study. This approach seems correct where radiology is less reliable, such as in reflux oesophageal disease or diffuse mucosal disease, but is to be deprecated when dysphagia is the presenting symptom. When the patient has dysphagia, radiology should always precede endoscopy. Prior knowledge of the level of a stricture or other lesion may aid the safe passage of the endoscope, and should prevent the rare, but potentially dangerous, unwitting entry into a pharyngeal pouch or oesophageal diverticulum.

Reflux disease

The endoscopic diagnosis of moderate or severe oesophagitis presents no difficulty, the distal oesophagus showing erosions and haemorrhagic areas with exudate and friability. Mild oesophagitis is more difficult. However, erythematous longitudinal streaks extending upwards from the gastro-oesophageal mucosal junction, on the crest of the mucosal folds and with slight mucosal friability, correlate well with histological evidence of mild oesophagitis. It should be borne in mind that if the appearances are at all atypical, infective oesophagitis (*Candida* or *Herpes*) may be the cause.

The histological criteria for oesophagitis, initially described by Ismael-Beigi [12], have stood the test of time and clinical experience. A polymorphonuclear inflammatory cell infiltrate in the lamina propria indicates severe oesophagitis, while milder changes are identified by basal cell hyperplasia in the squamous epithelium and by an abnormal extension of the dermal papillae towards the mucosal surface. These changes are likely to represent a reparative response to mucosal injury and can be seen in mucosa that appears endoscopically normal. For this reason it is good practice to take mucosal biopsies from the lower oesophagus whenever reflux disease is suspected. These should not be taken within 2.5 cm of the gastro-oesophageal mucosal junction if they are to prove reliable [29]. There has been some dispute about the adequacy of biopsies using endoscopic 'pinch-forceps' as they are small and difficult to orientate, compared with those obtained using the Rubin tube or the Quinton suction biopsy machine. Nevertheless, several biopsies can be quickly and easily obtained at endoscopy and diagnostic difficulty is rarely encountered. The authors therefore do not recommend the routine use of suction biopsies in the diagnosis of reflux disease.

Strictures

When a stricture is present the clinical history and endoscopic appearance will usually indicate whether it is peptic or malignant in nature. None-the-less, exceptions do occur and malignancy is a recognized complication of long-standing oesophagitis associated with Barrett's oesophagus. It is, of course, mandatory to biopsy any potentially malignant oesophageal lesion with at least 4 biopsies from the upper margin and 2 from within the lumen of all strictures. Brush cytology samples from any suspected malignant lesion will increase the diagnostic pick-up rate. The only oesophageal lesions that should not be biopsied are the rare vascular malformations or varices. Fortunately these are usually easily recognizable.

Disorders of motility

Endoscopy is of no value in the diagnosis of these conditions, as the presence of the instrument and air insufflation makes interpretation of peristaltic activity impossible. Nevertheless, endoscopy should be undertaken in all cases of achalasia to exclude gastric fundal and lower oesophageal malignancy. In oesophageal spasm, and other motility disorders, endoscopy and biopsy should be considered in order to identify those patients whose motor disturbance is secondary to oesophagitis.

Bernstein acid-perfusion test
(Fig. 9.1)

This simple test, introduced by Bernstein and Baker [3], indicates sensitivity to acid of the distal oesophagus. A fine-gauge nasogastric tube is passed to the mid-oesophagus. Normal saline and subsequently, 0.1 N hydrochloric acid are then perfused at 7 ml/min for 30 minutes. If the patient experiences any symptoms with the acid, the perfusion is changed to sodium bicarbonate (0.1 N) and symptoms are reassessed. The changes in perfusate are made out of the patient's sight and without his knowledge. Reproduction of the patient's symptoms, relieved by the bicarbonate, indicates sensitivity of the oesophagus to acid and the probable cause of the patient's symptoms.

In patients with reflux disease pain usually occurs within 15 minutes of acid infusion—prolonged infusion can produce symptoms in normal individuals. This test is particularly useful when the patient's symptoms are atypical. A review of seven publications [22] found an overall sensitivity of 79% and specificity of 82% for the detection of oesophagitis. False positive tests can be reduced by only accepting pain occurring within 15 minutes of acid perfusion as positive.

Monitoring of oesophageal pH

This procedure measures the frequency and duration of episodes of gastro-oesophageal reflux over periods of time [18]. After the level of the lower oesophageal sphincter has been identified by manometry, a miniature pH electrode is passed until its tip lies 5 cm above this point. The electrode is connected to a pH meter and chart recorder. Record-

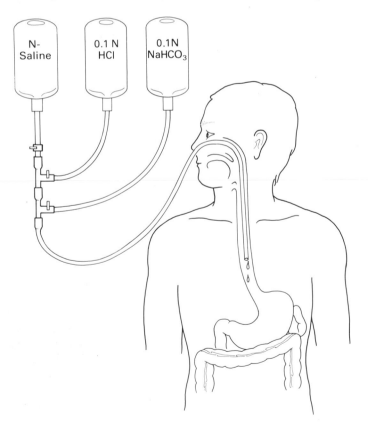

Fig. 9.1. Diagrammatical representation of a patient undergoing a Bernstein acid perfusion test.

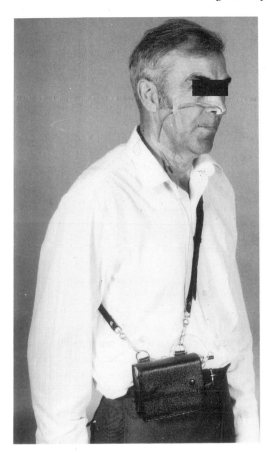

Fig. 9.2. Illustration of a patient undergoing a continuous 24 hour pH monitoring study using portable equipment.

ing the intraluminal pH identifies episodes of acid reflux occurrences and permits measurement of their duration [28]. Standard apparatus is not portable so the patient has to sit or recline in bed and therefore must be hospitalized. Recently a range of 24-hour portable monitoring systems have been developed that allow measurements to be made while the patient continues his daily activites (Fig. 9.2). Such systems provide precise measurements of the severity of reflux, its relationship to symptoms and to activities such as smoking, drinking, eating or sleeping [25].

Abnormal reflux is assessed by comparison with the range of reflux observed in healthy, asymptomatic subjects (Fig. 9.3). This technique has the highest sensitivity (88%) and specificity (98%) of any clinical test of gastro-oesophageal reflux. Early series [27] indicated that most reflux episodes occurred during the waking hours, particularly during the 2–3 hours after eating. Reflux at night, during quiet sleep was less pronounced. DeMeester [8] has reported variable reflux patterns, with some patients exhibiting reflux mainly when recumbent, others when upright and some with a mixed pattern. This technique has been used to document an association between reflux and nocturnal bronchospasm [13].

Clearly, prolonged monitoring of distal oesophageal pH is not needed in the assessment of most patients with oesophagitis. In those with typical symptoms and endoscopic features of oesophagitis, no further investigation is required. This test should be reserved for difficult cases of obscure chest pain, those with unusual symptomatology and the occasional patient with symptoms of reflux but with normal radiology, Bernstein test, and endoscopy with mucosal biopsy [9].

The pH probe is also used for the Standard Acid Reflux test [26]. In this test 300 ml of 0.1 N hydrochloric acid is placed within the stomach and reflux is induced by a variety of manoeuvres. In his review of this and other tests Richter [22] reports an overall sensitivity of 84% and specificity of 83% for this test. This is poorer than that seen with straightforward prolonged pH monitoring and it is therefore not a particularly useful test.

Gastro-oesophageal scintiscanning

This is a quantitative test of reflux [10], performed by filling the stomach with 300 ml of normal saline labelled with 99^m Tc-sulphur colloid. Gamma-camera scintiscanning over the stomach and lower oesophagus for sequential 30 second periods

Chapter 9

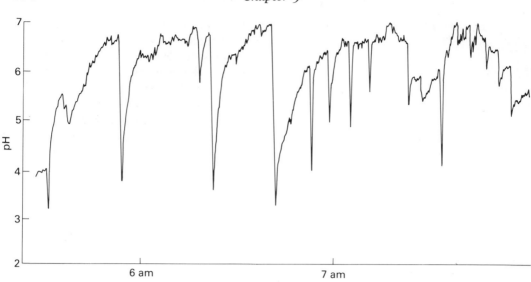

Fig. 9.3. Part of a 24-hour pH tracing showing prolonged episodes of gastroesophageal reflux.

indicates the frequency and duration of reflux. As intubation is not necessary the test is inherently attractive. Reports of its clinical value are variable and the authors' own experience in adults has not been encouraging. The test has, however, proved useful in children because of its non-invasive character [23].

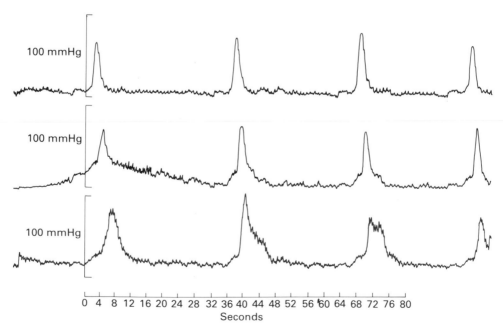

Fig. 9.4. A distal oesophageal manometric recording, in a normal subject, showing the peristaltic response to 4 'wet swallows'.

Oesophageal mucosal potential difference

Changes in potential difference can be measured across the gastro-oesophageal junction [17]. This can be used to accurately identify the level of the gastro-oesophageal junction and has been used to detect the presence of a Barrett's oesophagus. However, it is rarely indicated in routine patient assessment.

Studies of oesophageal motility

The limitation of radiology in assessing distal oesophageal motility led to the development of water-perfusion oesophageal manometry. The technique is now straightforward and reproducible, and equipment is available commercially [1, 6].

The basic equipment is illustrated in Fig. 9.5. A multi-lumen polyvinyl tube assembly is passed via the patient's nose or mouth into the oesophagus. Each lumen has side openings that are placed at intervals along the distal part of the tube so that intraluminal pressure may be measured at different levels. Water passes from the infusion pump, via a separate pressure transducer for each channel, to the multi-lumen catheter. The water exits through the distal side-openings in the catheter. The pressure transducers are linked to a multi-channel amplifier and chart recorder to obtain a permanent record. When a peristaltic wave or other pressure is exerted on the catheter assembly, the flow of water through the side holes is impeded and consequently the transducers register a rise of pressure.

To record the lower oesophageal sphincter pressure, the catheter assembly is passed until the lower three or four side-openings lie within the stomach. Gradual withdrawal then results in the side-openings passing upwards through the lower oesophageal sphincter and a rise of pressure is registered relative to intra-gastric pressure. The catheter is then held stationary within the oesophagus to record spontaneous and swallowing-induced motor activity. By convention the patient is given swallows of 5 ml of water to initiate primary peristalsis. (Fig. 9.4).

Using modern equipment and standardized techniques a spectrum of motility disorders has been described [2]. These include achalasia, diffuse oesophageal spasm, hypertensive lower oesophageal sphincter, high amplitude and prolonged duration peristalsis and non-specific motility disorders (see Chapter 10).

The major indications for manometry are unexplained dysphagia, obscure chest pain and before surgical treatment of reflux oesophagitis. Many patients with previously unexplained dysphagia have a motility dis-

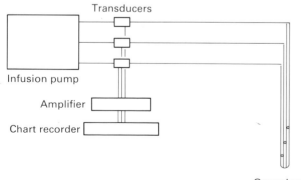

Transducers

Infusion pump

Amplifier

Chart recorder

Oesophageal catheter

Fig. 9.5. An illustration of the components of manometric equipment.

order detectable by manometric studies. Similarly, up to 50% of patients with obscure chest pain will show abnormal oesophageal motility on manometry. Prior investigation should exclude a cardiac cause and additional investigations may be required to detect unsuspected gastro-oesophageal reflux disease or unrelated gastrointestinal and musculo-skeletal disorders.

Provocation tests may be employed in patients with obscure chest pain. One example is the injection of the cholinergic drug edrophonium during a manometric study and a correlation is sought between the occurrence of the patient's typical chest pain and oesophageal contractions. The performance and interpretation of such provocation tests require considerable experience.

Oesophageal manometry should be per-formed before surgery is recommended for reflux oesophagitis. It may identify patients who are unlikely to benefit from, or who may develop other problems after the operation. Experience has shown that patients with significant abnormalities of peristalsis develop severe dysphagia or remain symptomatic after fundoplication. Alternatively, abnormal motility may be the cause of their symptoms [7]. Preoperative manometry would be expected to reduce the incidence of failures after fundoplication.

Radionuclide transit studies

In this technique [4] a gamma-camera with data processor is used to measure the transit time of a fluid bolus from mouth to stomach and to provide a qualitative assessment of the pattern of movement of the

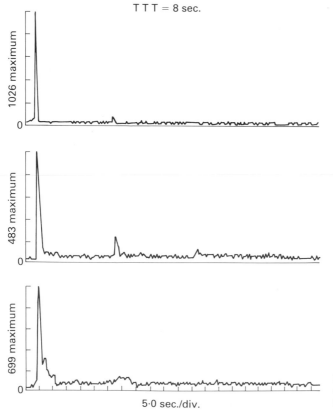

Fig. 9.6. A radionuclide transit test in a normal subject (total transit time = 8 secs.)

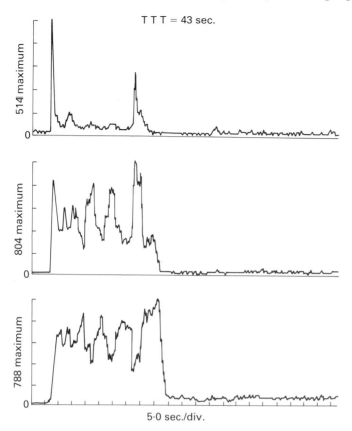

Fig. 9.7. A radionuclide transit test in a patient with diffuse oesophageal spasm (transit time = 43 secs. with 'to and fro' movements between mid- and lower oesophagus).

bolus within the oesophagus (Figs. 9.6 and 9.7). The test is simple, quick and non-invasive and causes little radiation exposure to the patient. For this reason it is attractive to patients and clinicians alike [15]. However, manometry still is required to further elucidate any motility disorder that is demonstrated.

Radionuclide tests appear to be particularly sensitive in detecting non-peristaltic spasm contractions and, in a prospective study, there was an 84% concordance with the results of manometric studies [5]. However, although sensitive in the detection of uncoordinated contractions, this test has provided normal results in some patients with hypertensive but normally relaxing lower oesophageal sphincters, and in some patients with abnormally high pressure or prolonged duration peristaltic waves (nutcracker oesophagus).

Conclusion

Most oesophageal disorders can be confidently diagnosed with the help of a careful history, good radiological assessment and endoscopy with biopsy and cytology. Prolonged pH monitoring, motility studies and radionuclide imaging are useful in the diagnosis of the difficult patient and in assessing the effects of treatment.

References

1 ARNDORFER RC, STEFF JJ, DODDS WJ, LINEHAN JH, HOGAN WJ. Improved infusion system for intraluminal esophageal manometry. *Gastroenterology* 1977;73:23–27.

2 BENJAMIN SB, CASTELL DO. Chest pain of esophageal origin. Arch Intern Med, 1982;**143**:772–776.
3 BERNSTEIN LM, BAKER LA. A clinical test for esophagitis. *Gastroenterology* 1958;**34**:760–781.
4 BLACKWELL JN, HANNAN WJ, ADAM RD, HEADING
RC. A radionuclide technique for assessing oesophageal function. *Nuclear Medicine Communication*
1982;**2**:291–296.
5 BLACKWELL JN, HANNAN WJ, ADAM RD, HEADING
RC. Radionuclide transit studies in the detection of
oesophageal dysmotility. *Gut* 1983;**24**:421–426.
6 BLACKWELL JN, CASTELL DO. Oesophageal motility:
recent advances and implications (Review). *Clin Sci*
1984;**67**:145–151.
7 BOMBECK CT, BATTLE WS, NYHUSS LM. Spasm in the
differential diagnosis of gastroesophageal reflux.
Arch Surg 1982;**104**:477–483.
8 DeMEESTER TR, JOHNSON LF, JOSEPH GJ, TOSCANO
MS, HALL AW, SKINNER DB. Patterns of gastro
esophageal reflux in health and disease. *Ann Surg.*
1976;**184**:459–470.
9 DeMEESTER TR, WANG CI. Technique, indications
and clinical use of 24 hr. oesophageal pH monitoring. *J Thorac Cardiovasc Surg* 1980;**79**:656–670.
10 FISHER RS, MALMUD LS, ROBERTS GS, LOBIS LF.
Gastroesophageal (GE) scintiscanning to detect
and quantitate GE reflux. *Gastroenterology*
1976;**70**:301–308.
11 GELFAND DW, OTT DJ. Anatomy and technique in
evaluating the oesophagus. *Semin Roentgenol*
16:168–181.
12 ISMAIL-BEIGI F, HORTON PF, POPE CE. Histological
consequences of gastroesophageal reflux in the distal esophagus of man. *Gastroenterology* 1970;**58**:
163–174.
13 JOLLEY SG, HEBST JJ, JOHNSON DG, MATTAK ME,
BOOK LS. Esophageal pH monitoring during sleep
identifies children with respiratory symptoms from
gastroesophageal reflux. *Gastroenterology* 1981;**80**:
501–506.
14 LANCET LEADER. Instrumental perforation of the
oesophagus. *Lancet* 1984;**i**:1279.
15 MALMUD LS, FISHER RS. Radionuclide studies of
esophageal transit and gastroesophageal reflux
(Review). *Sem Nucl Mec* 1982;**12**:104–115.
16 MOSS AA, KOEHLER RE, MARGULIS AR. Initial
accuracy of esophagograms in detection of small
esophageal carcinoma. *Am J Roentgenol* 1976;**127**:
909–913.
17 ORLANDO RC, POWELL DW, BRYSON JC, KINARD HB,
CARNEY CN, JONES JD, BOZYMSKI EM. Esophageal
potential difference measurements in esophageal
disease. *Gastroenterology* 1982;**83**:1026–1032.
18 ORR WC, JOHNSON LF, ROBINSON MG. Effect of sleep
on swallowing, esophageal peristalsis and acid
clearance. *Gastroenterology* 1984;**86**:814–819.
19 OTT DJ, GELFAND DW, WU WC. Sensitivity of
single-contrast radiology in esophageal disease: a
study of 240 patients with endoscopically verified
abnormality. *Gastrointest Radiol* 1983;**8**:105–110.
20 OTT DJ, DODDS WJ, WU WC, GELFAND DW, HOGAN
WJ, STEWART ET. Current status of radiology in
evaluating for gastroesophageal disease. *J. Clin
Gastroenterol* 1982;**4**:365–375.
21 OTT DJ, WU WJ, GELFAND DW. Reflux esophagitis
revisited: prospective analysis of radiologic accuracy. *Gastointest Radiol* 1981;**6**:1–7.
22 RICHTER JE, CASTELL DO. Gastroesophageal reflux
pathogenesis, diagnosis and therapy. *Ann Intern
Med* 1982;**99**:93–103.
23 RUDD TG, CHRISTIE PM. Demonstration of gastroesophageal reflux in children by radionuclide
gastroesophagography. *Radiology* 1979;**131**:483–
486.
24 SHAMIR M, SCHUMAN PM. Complications of fibreoptic endoscopy. *Gastrointes endos* 1980;**26**:86–
91.
25 SCHLESINGER PK, DONAHUE PE, SMID B, LAYDEN TJ.
Limitations of 24 hour intraesophageal pH monitoring in the hospital setting. *Gastroenterology*
1985;**89**:797–804.
26 SKINNER DB, BOOTH DJ. Assessment of distal esophageal function in patients with hiatal hernia
and/or gastroesophageal reflux. *Ann Surg* 1970;
172:627–637.
27 SPENCER J. Prolonged pH recording in the study of
gastroesophageal reflux. *Br J Surg* 1969;**56**:912–
914.
28 STANCIU C, HOARE RC, BENNETT JR. Correlation between manometric and pH tests for gastroesophageal reflux. *Gut* 1977;**18**:536–540.
29 WEINSTEIN WM, BOGOCH ER, BORVES KL. The normal human esophageal mucosa: a histological
reappraisal. *Gastroenterology* 1975;**68**:40–44.

Chapter 10
Disorders of Oesophageal Motility

G.N.J. TYTGAT & J.F.W.M. BARTELSMAN

Oesophageal motility is characterized by peristaltic waves that normally pass from the pharynx to the lower oesophageal sphincter (LOS) at a speed of 3–3.4 cm sec⁻¹. The resting lower oesophageal sphincter pressure is 15–25 mmHg (2.0 3.3 kPa) higher than intra-gastric pressure; this sphincter is approximately 3 cm long and may vary in position by 1–3 cm during respiration. Tonic contraction of the sphincter prevents reflux, while relaxation allows food and fluid to pass from the oesophagus into the stomach. Relaxation of the sphincter occurs during swallowing and when the oesophagus is distended. Peristalsis is provoked by swallowing (primary) or by distension of the oesophagus (secondary). The mechanisms controlling peristalsis and relaxation of the lower oesophageal sphincter are poorly understood [61].

Physiological control

There is convincing evidence for two neural mechanisms controlling peristalsis [26]. The first control unit lies in the swallowing centre of the brain stem nuclei and reticular formation. The second is an intrinsic mechanism situated in the smooth muscle of the oesophageal wall. Impulses arising in the brain stem are transmitted to the oesophagus via the vagal nerves. Relaxation of the lower oesophageal sphincter induced by swallowing is mediated through the vagal nerves, while relaxation following distension is through intrinsic pathways [40].

Normal oesophageal motility can be disturbed in several ways:

1. Loss of peristalsis, particularly when combined with impaired lower oesophageal sphincter relaxation, can cause dysphagia.
2. Defective peristalsis can prolong episodes of gastro-oesophageal reflux (defective clearing).
3. Peristaltic waves may be replaced by non-progressive, simultaneous or tertiary contractions, which can cause chest pain and dysphagia. This occurs particularly if the contractions have high amplitudes, long duration and are repetitive.
4. The lower oesophageal sphincter may have a high resting pressure or there may be absent or incomplete relaxation, resulting in dysphagia and retention of food in the oesophagus.
5. The lower oesophageal sphincter may have a low resting pressure or relax inappropriately (i.e. unprovoked by swallowing or distension), resulting in pathological gastro-oesophageal reflux.

Types of motility disorders

Oesophageal motility disorders may be either primary or secondary [85, 86, 88].

Primary motility disorders include achalasia, diffuse oesophageal spasm and non-specific, or intermediate-type motility disorders [14, 90]. The non-specific category includes vigorous achalasia and hypertensive lower oesophageal sphincter syndrome ('nutcracker' or 'super-squeezer') [7, 10]. Achalasia and diffuse oesophageal spasm share some clinical features and are thought to be two variants in a spectrum of primary disorders. In both, the smooth

muscle of the oesophagus is involved and
the methacholine test may be positive (see
Chapter 9). Transition from typical diffuse
oesophageal spasm to classical achalasia
has been described [90]. In such patients
the predominant symptoms change from
chest pain to dysphagia. In addition, some
patients may show manometric features of
a non-specific motility disorder, which subsequently progresses to that of achalasia.
Finally, it is not uncommon to find patients
that have clinical and manometric features
of both diffuse oesophageal spasm and
achalasia at the same time.

Secondary motility disorders are either
part of a systemic disease or of an inflammatory or malignant process involving the
oesophageal wall. This group includes conditions such as scleroderma and other connective tissue diseases, diabetes, amyloid,
alcoholic neuropathy, Chagas' disease and
chronic idiopathic pseudo-obstruction.

Primary motility disorders

Achalasia

This is a disease of unknown origin that
produces abnormal function of the lower
oesophageal sphincter and of the oesophageal body. The sphincteric defect includes basal hypertension and defective relaxation and the smooth muscle defect
includes increased resting pressure and abnormal peristaltic activity. These combined
defects lead to a severe dysfunction of the
gullet.

Incidence

This is not clearly established, but has been
estimated at 1:100,000 in Western countries [58, 85]. There are very few reports of
achalasia in tropical countries although in
Africa it is not uncommon [3]. Achalasia
can occur at any age, but is rare in children
(<5% in most series) and very uncommon

under 5 years of age [30]. The sex ratio is
equal in most reports [44]. In one study
from South Africa [78] it was three times
as common in black women, but equal between the sexes in whites.

Aetiology and pathophysiology

The cause of achalasia is not known. There
may be a genetic factor—familial achalasia
has been reported in siblings, but rarely in
parents and offspring [18, 70, 91].

Our understanding of the pathophysiological mechanisms involved remains fragmentary. Histological studies have shown
that there is a degeneration of, and a reduction in the numbers of neurons in the
myenteric nerve plexus of the lower oesophageal sphincter and oesophageal body
[12]. Abnormalities have also been seen in
the vagal dorsal motor nucleus, nucleus
ambiguous, and in the smooth muscle of
the oesophagus itself [12]. These findings
suggest that both vagal and intramural
pathways are involved in this disease [39].

Pharmacological studies in humans suggest that there is a defect in the intramural
inhibitory neurons of the lower oesophageal sphincter in most patients. The
sphincter and oesophageal wall have an increased sensitivity to cholinergic stimuli
such as methylcholine and carbachol [20,
50]. Edrophonium, a cholinesterase inhibitor, also increases the lower oesophageal
sphincter pressure [22] suggesting that
acetylcholine is still being released, presumably from intact post-ganglionic nerve
fibres. The site of denervation must therefore be at large pre-ganglionic nerve fibres.

In addition both the sphincter and oesophageal body display increased sensitivity
to stimulation by gastrin and pentagastrin
[21, 65]. In view of the hypersensitivity to
cholinergic stimuli this probably represents
a non-specific denervation hypersensitivity,
rather than implying a direct pathophysiological role for gastrin.

Cholecystokinin-octapeptide has been shown to induce relaxation of the lower oesophageal sphincter in normal individuals, but in achalasia it produces a paradoxical increase of sphincter pressure [28]. The normal response is explained by a direct excitatory effect upon the muscle followed by an indirect inhibitory effect through non-adrenergic inhibitory nerves. In achalasia, presumably, the latter pathway is impaired.

The causes of the neuron lesion in achalasia remain a mystery—a neurotoxic virus and an autoimmune process have been postulated [79].

Clinical features

The symptoms in the authors' patients are similar to those reported by others (Table 10.1). Symptoms are present for a variable period before diagnosis, ranging from a few weeks to many years. Usually they are gradual in onset, although occasionally the onset may be sudden.

The classical symptom is slowly progressive dysphagia for solids and liquids. In the early stages pain may accompany the dysphagia, but this gradually disappears while the dysphagia and regurgitation increase.

Regurgitation during and after meals is present in most patients. When it occurs at night it may lead to nocturnal drooling or aspiration into the airways, causing a nocturnal cough or aspiration pneumonia [44, 88]. In children recurrent respiratory symptoms due to aspiration often overshadow any symptoms of dysphagia and can lead to diagnostic difficulties [76, 91].

Pain is mostly perceived in the substernal area. Many patients have attacks of substernal cramps unrelated to meals, but frequently present at night. These attacks occur especially in patients with the vigorous or active type of achalasia and are caused by simultaneous high amplitude contractions of the oesophagus. In some patients these attacks are present only in the early phase of the illness. As a result of the dysphagia and regurgitation weight loss is not uncommon.

There is very little information about the natural history of this disease. Most patients are treated as soon as the diagnosis is made. However, in a few untreated patients, radiological and clinical findings are available from earlier assessments. These suggest that in some patients mega-oesophagus occurs within one year, but in others it may take over 20 years to develop (Fig. 10.1). Other patients' symptoms may remain virtually static for several years and then suddenly increase, with rapid weight loss and severe cachexia.

Carcinoma of the oesophagus is thought to occur with achalasia. The incidence

Table 10.1. Presenting symptoms.

	[43] (n = 75)	[87] (n = 133)	[4] (n = 200)
Dysphagia	80	97	100
Pain	52	58	60
Clinostatic regurgitation or vomiting	75	90	58
Weight loss	56	90	72
Nocturnal cough	—	30	—
Respiratory complications	—	7·5	14
Others	36	—	—

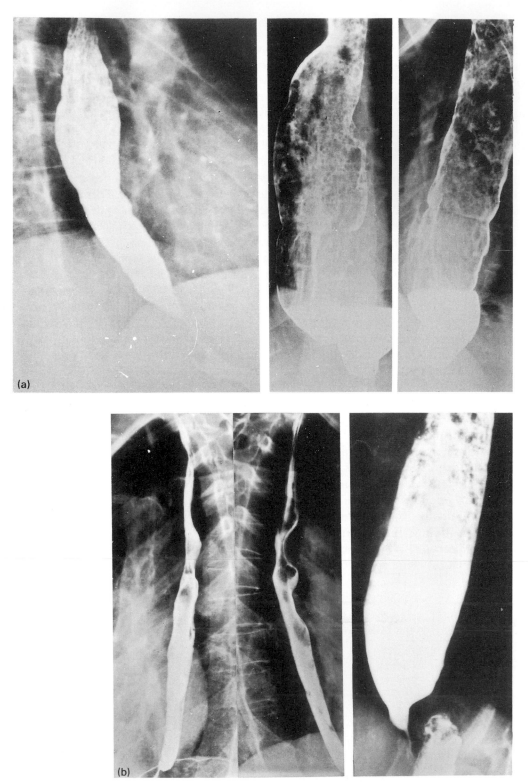

Fig. 10.1. (a) development of a mega-oesophagus over a 10-year period. (b) development of a mega-oesophagus over 1.5 years.

varies from nil to 20% in different series [19, 44]. It is thought to occur as a secondary complication of oesophagitis induced by food retention and stasis. If this assumption is correct early diagnosis and treatment should prevent the development of malignancy—but this remains unproven.

Diagnostic investigations

RADIOLOGY

Radiographic examination is usually the first investigation done in most cases. A chest X-ray may show the following features [80, 95]:
1. The right wall of the oesophagus may be seen as a shadow lying to the right of the mediastinum. A fluid/air level may be seen (Fig. 10.2).
2. On a lateral film the trachea may be displaced forward by the enlarged oesophagus.
3. The normal gas bubble in the stomach may be absent.
4. In some patients chronic pulmonary

changes from recurrent aspiration may be present.

Barium studies may show either absent or non-peristaltic contractions. It is essential to do this examination in both the upright and recumbent positions. In the latter position barium will be seen to move up and down the oesophagus with non-peristaltic contractions. When the patient is upright, some barium will pass into the stomach by gravity, even though the lower oesophageal sphincter opens poorly, but usually a column of barium and food debris remains in the oesophagus, retained by the poorly relaxing sphincter. Characteristically there is a smooth, tapered distal narrowing of the sphincter zone ('bird's beak') (Fig. 10.3). In about 20% of patients there is an asymmetrical, unilateral outpouching in the tapered segment, which may be mistaken easily for an ulcer niche (Fig. 10.4).

In the early stages the only abnormality may be simultaneous contraction waves, but later on the oesophagus becomes very dilated with food and fluid retention caus-

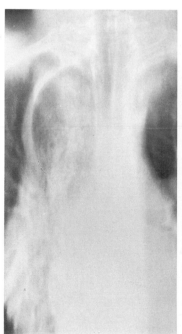
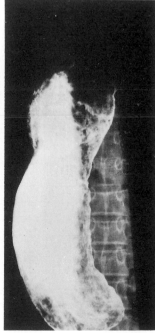

Fig. 10.2. The mega-oesophagus of achalasia shown as a visible fluid-filled shadow on the right side of the upper mediastinum.

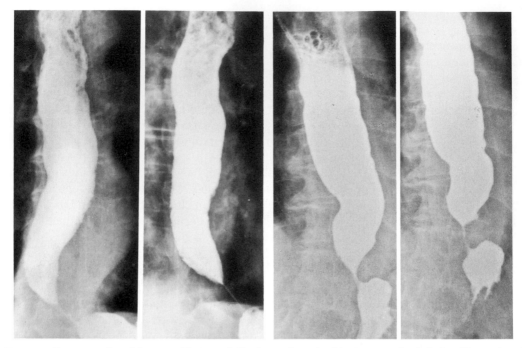

Fig. 10.3. Two examples of the smoothly-tapered distal oesophageal sphincter zone of achalasia with an absent gastric air bubble.

ing an air/fluid level. Finally the oesophagus becomes elongated, tortuous and sigmoid-shaped (mega-oesophagus) (Fig. 10.5).

Although cine-radiography may provide more refined information about motility it is rarely needed to make the diagnosis of achalasia in clinical practice [56].

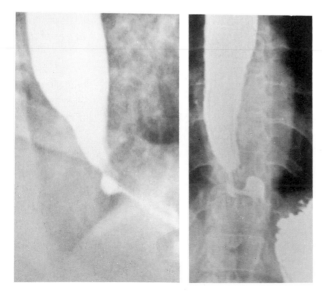

Fig. 10.4. Two examples of asymmetrical unilateral outpouchings in the area of the narrowed segment of achalasia.

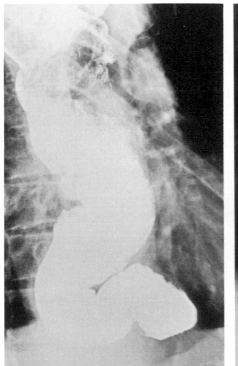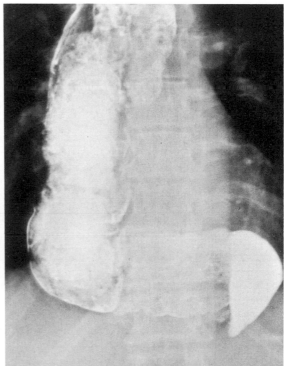

Fig. 10.5. Two examples of a tortuous sigmoid-shaped oesophagus, filled with food, in advanced achalasia.

ENDOSCOPY

Endoscopy has only a limited diagnostic role in achalasia. However, it must always be done to rule out an alternative cause for stenosis of the lower oesophagus. In true achalasia it should be possible to pass the endoscope through the sphincter into the stomach [72]. Usually there is a characteristic sensation of sudden yielding of the hypertensive sphincter as the endoscope passes into the stomach. Whenever the passage of a standard size endoscope (> 11 mm) is impossible, or very difficult, an organic cause for the stenosis should be suspected. The routine use of narrow calibre endoscopes can be misleading in this respect and should be avoided.

The cardia should always be inspected from the gastric side by using an inversion manoeuvre. Any suspicious lesion should be biopsied using large forceps, with further sampling of the deeper layers by repeat biopsy at the same site. Using this technique the authors have diagnosed submucosal carcinoma in a number of patients presenting with typical features of achalasia on manometry and radiology and with macroscopically normal fundic mucosa (Fig. 10.6). Carcinoma should be suspected in any patient whose symptoms are of short duration or are rapidly progressive, until proved otherwise.

MANOMETRY

In achalasia manometry shows non-peristaltic simultaneous contractions initiated by swallowing in the oesophageal body. These may be bi-, tri-, or multi-phasic (several waves after one swallow). This abnormality is often restricted to the distal two-thirds of

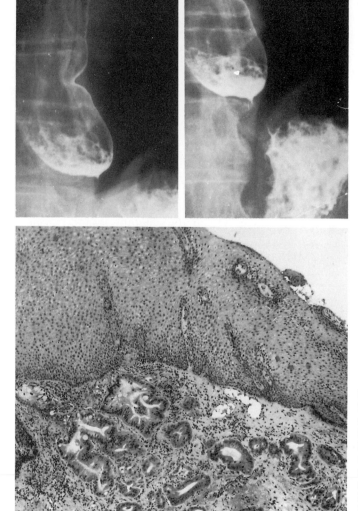

Fig. 10.6. A submucosal infiltrating adenocarcinoma of the cardia of the stomach mimicking the appearances of an achalasia. Note the nests of adenocarcinomatous glands lying deep to apparently normal surface squamous epithelium on the biopsy sample obtained using large forceps.

the oesophagus, with normal sequential waves in the upper third. In a dilated oesophagus these contractions are usually of low amplitude or even undetectable (Fig. 10.7). Subcutaneous methylcholine chloride (5–10 mg s.c.) causes a marked rise in resting oesophageal pressure which then gradually subsides.

The lower oesophageal sphincter resting pressure is high in most patients. Charac-teristically sphincter relaxation after swallowing is absent or incomplete, with the result that the lower oesophageal sphincter pressure fails to reach gastric fundal pressure, thus creating a constant barrier to oesophageal emptying (Fig. 10.7).

After adequate treatment the oesophageal diameter decreases and peristaltic contractions reappear in about one-third of patients [90] (Fig. 10.8), but a decrease of

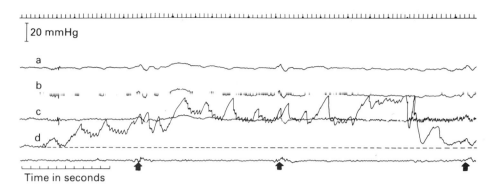

Fig. 10.7. Manometric pressure tracing from a patient with achalasia. (A = 33 cm; B = 38 cm; C = 43 cm; D = Sphincter Zone; Dashed line = end-expiratory pressure in the gastric fundus.) Note the simultaneous weak contractions within the oesophageal body and the absence of LOS-relaxation after swallowing (arrows).

lower oesophageal sphincter pressure of at least 60% would be expected after an adequate pneumatic dilatation.

OESOPHAGEAL SCINTIGRAPHY

This has been developed as a sensitive, quantitative, non-invasive test of oesophageal function [33, 37, 41, 73, 81] (see Chapter 9). It has proved particularly useful in evaluating the results of drug therapy [37], pneumatic dilatation, and surgical cardiomyotomy [41].

Differential diagnosis

Achalasia has to be differentiated from other primary and secondary motility disorders and from other conditions mimicking achalasia.

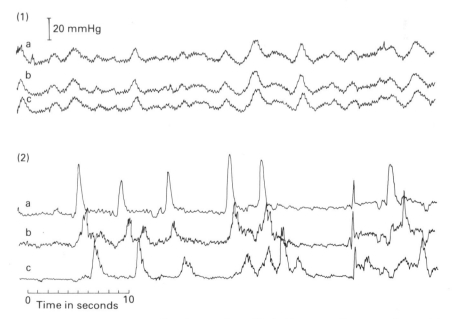

Fig. 10.8. Manometric pressure tracings, within the oesophageal body (A = 35 cm; B = 40 cm; C = 45 cm), obtained *before* (1) and 3 months *after* (2) pneumatic dilatation. Note the reappearance of peristaltic waves after treatment.

Amyloidosis [62] and idiopathic pseudo-obstruction [75] can cause oesophageal dilatation, loss of peristalsis and incomplete lower oesophageal sphincter relaxation.

Scleroderma can result in dilatation and aperistalsis with radiological features suggestive of achalasia due to peptic stricture at the cardia. However at manometry the resting sphincter pressure is low or absent [23, 93].

Malignant infiltration of the cardia by gastric, oesophageal [55], pancreatic or pulmonary carcinoma [82]; by gastric lymphoma [47]; or Hodgkin's disease [68] may all produce clinical and radiological features indistinguishable from primary achalasia. This 'secondary achalasia' should be suspected if the following triad of signs is present—symptoms for less than one year, age over 50 years and a weight loss of more than 7 kg.

Treatment

As the cause of achalasia is unknown, treatment is directed at lowering the lower oesophageal sphincter pressure to aid oesophageal emptying. At present this can be achieved in three ways: drug therapy; forceful dilatation; or cardiomyotomy.

DRUG THERAPY

There are several groups of drugs that lower the lower oesophageal pressure.

Anticholinergics

Oral and subcutaneous dicyclomine hydrochloride (10–20 mg) reduces LOS pressure and has produced symptomatic improvement in patients with achalasia [52].

Long-acting nitrates

Sublingual isosorbide dinitrate (5–10 mg) has been reported to relieve dysphagia and improve oesophageal emptying with apparently better results than those obtained with nifedipine [37].

Calcium antagonists

Sublingual nifedipine (10 mg) produced good or excellent results in most patients treated in a 6–18-month trial [9, 17]. While verapamil and sodium nitroprusside relax the lower oesophageal sphincter in the opossum [38], neither agent has been successful when used clinically [5].

At present the place of drug therapy in the long-term management of achalasia is not established. In the authors' experience unwanted effects (for example headaches) are common and limit the value of such treatments.

FORCEFUL DILATATION

There are many techniques for the forceful dilatation of the lower oesophageal sphincter, but all rely upon stretching the muscle layers causing weakening and rupture of the circular muscle fibres and connective tissue. Various types of pneumatic balloons are available commercially (Plummer-, Negus-, Mosher-, Browne-McHardy microvasive bag).

Correct positioning of the bag can be very difficult in the tortuous and dilated mega-oesophagus without the assistance of a guide-wire inserted under endoscopic control. The authors use either a commercially available balloon (Rider-Moeller cardia dilator 2.8, 3.8, and 4.8 cm in diameter) or balloons mounted on an Eder-Peustow guiding device [83, 84]. The authors prefer to use repeated dilatations with bags of progressively larger diameter, 3–4.5 cm [83, 84, 87, 88]. The bags are inflated to a pressure of 200 mmHg for 1 minute and then to 300 mmHg for a second minute under fluoroscopic control to check that the bag remains correctly positioned across the

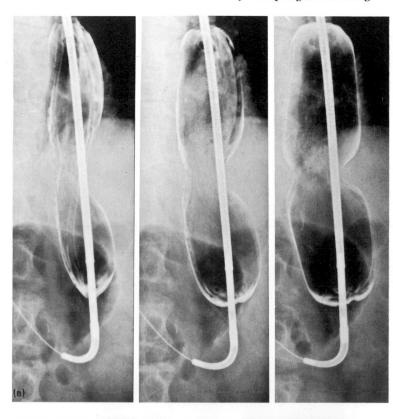

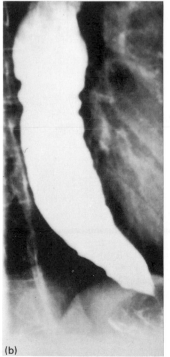

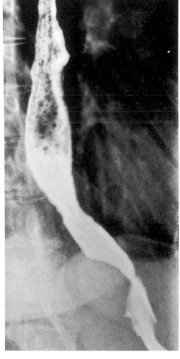

Fig. 10.9. (a) pneumatic balloon mounted upon a flexible guiding device (Eder-Peustow) and positioned using a guide-wire technique. Note the position of the sphincteric segment during the dilatation. (b) demonstration of the decrease in oesophageal luminal diameter *before* and 5 months *after* pneumatic dilatation. Note the widening of the sphincteric zone.

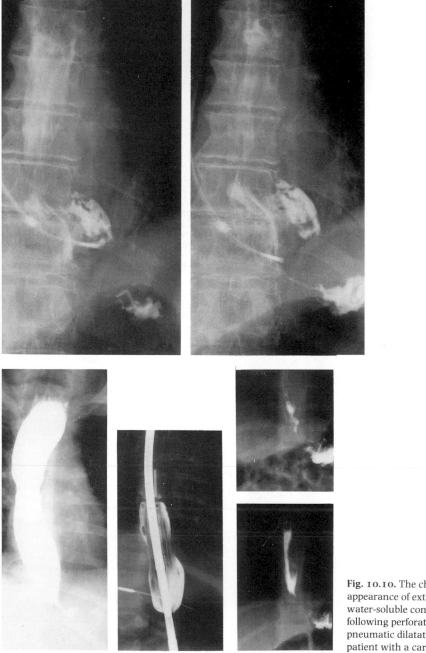

Fig. 10.10. The characteristic appearance of extravasation of water-soluble contrast medium following perforation after pneumatic dilatation in an elderly patient with a cardiac pacemaker.

sphincter zone (Fig. 10.9). These procedures can be performed on out-patients under mild or no sedation. Using a similar approach, with modified instruments, the authors have successfully treated a five-month-old infant.

An alternative to the guide-wire is to mount the balloon over a fine calibre endoscope [34, 96]. Forceful dilatation produces good to excellent results in over 70% of patients with achalasia [31, 87, 88].

The main acute complication is perforation—in less than 2% of patients. The perforation is usually a dorso-lateral tear just above the high pressure zone (Fig. 10.10). Surgical treatment is not always needed; if the perforation is small and contrast empties easily from the peri-oesophageal space into the stomach, conservative therapy can be successful [94]. Medical management consists of no intake by mouth, parenteral or intra-jejunal nutritional support and antibiotics [57].

The most important late complication is that of reflux oesophagitis. In all but one of our patients this was only moderately severe and responded to medical therapy.

Most gastroenterologists prefer pneumatic balloons to the semi-rigid Starck dilator, because of difficulties in insertion and positioning. However, a modified electro-mechanical Starck dilator has been introduced recently that allows continuous monitoring of the force applied and the diameter reached during dilatation. Experience with this new instrument is limited [35] so its place in management is not established.

CARDIOMYOTOMY

The operation most widely used in achalasia is Zayer's modification of Heller's operation—a single anterior cardiomyotomy incision. This approach produces good to excellent results in 65–88% of patients [88].

Controversy surrounds the length of my-otomy required (from 1–3 cm), the route of approach (whether thoracic, abdominal or combined), and the need for an anti-reflux operation at the same time [44, 87, 88]. Gastro-oesophageal reflux probably increases after myotomy and when it occurs clearance is impaired by the defective peristalsis of the oesophageal body. For this reason it seems reasonable to combine myotomy with an anti-reflux procedure but there is no agreement as to which operation is best. Many different procedures have been suggested—these include vagotomy and pyloroplasty [1], partial myotomy preserving some sphincter competence [78], a Nissen fundoplication [60], a partial fundoplication [36], a Belsey Mark IV repair [6, 92], or a hiatal repair [8]. According to the Chicago group [92] the best operation is a modified Belsey 270 degree fundoplication. This adds an effective anti-reflux valve mechanism without materially increasing the resistance to oesophageal emptying [6, 92].

A further controversial point is whether newly diagnosed achalasia should be treated immediately by surgery [89]. There has been one controlled trial in 38 patients which found in favour of cardiomyotomy as the primary treatment [24]. This trial has been criticized because of the method of forceful dilatation used. Most surgeons believe that myotomy should be used first. In justification they point to the results obtained in 899 patients treated at the Mayo clinic over a 27-year period with good-to-excellent results in 65% of the 431 patients treated by dilatation with 19% poor late results compared with 85% good-to-excellent results after myotomy, with only 6% poor results and a 3% incidence of late oesophagitis [63]. Others interpret these results as supporting the view that dilatation should be tried first and surgery should be reserved for those in whom it fails [88]. The authors also favour this approach as pneumatic dilatation is cheap, safe, easily repeatable and suitable for elderly or frail patients as an out-patient procedure. Dilatation has been shown to be effective if cardiomyotomy has failed [66].

PRACTICAL MANAGEMENT

We reserve operation for those in whom dilatation has failed, although we recognize that a major drawback is that surgery in these circumstances, is technically more difficult and hazardous because of scarring from the earlier dilatations. It has not yet been established that the results of myotomy under these circumstances are as good as those achieved when it is done as a primary treatment.

Surgery is indicated if there have been several unsuccessful attempts at forceful dilatation, if the patient's cooperation is poor, if malignancy is suspected, or if there are structural changes around the hiatus that make positioning of the balloon difficult or impossible.

Symptomatic diffuse oesophageal spasm

This disorder is characterized by chest pain and dysphagia caused by abnormal oesophageal contractions without a demonstrable organic lesion.

Aetiology and pathophysiology

The cause of this condition is unknown. It is associated with both neural and muscular abnormalities, but morphological studies have not identified the primary neural defect. Unlike achalasia, there are no histological changes in the neurons, or ganglion cells of the myenteric plexus, although chronic inflammatory cell infiltration may be present. Electron microscopic studies have shown diffuse degenerative changes in both myelinated and nonmyeli-

nated fibres of the vagus nerve [13]. At present the relationship between these changes and the abnormal contraction present in the oesophagus remains unexplained.

Clinical features

Symptomatic diffuse oesophageal spasm is recognized by a triad of clinical features: dysphagia with chest pain, abnormal oesophageal contractions on barium studies, and typical manometric abnormalities.

Pain is a prominent feature in 80–90% of patients. It may vary from mild substernal discomfort to very severe colic, often mimicking cardiac ischaemic pain [66]. Usually it is felt substernally but it may radiate into the jaw, neck, back, or down one or both arms. Duration can vary from a short attack to a persistent pain. Eating and emotional stress are commonly described as triggers for the pain and patients often avoid cold and carbonated drinks to reduce the frequency of attacks. Occasionally symptoms of odynophagia may be so severe that the patient avoids eating and loses weight [16].

Dysphagia is typically intermittent, occurs with solids and liquids and is often associated with the pain. Another typical feature, of diagnostic value, is that severe episodes are interspersed with periods of mild symptoms.

Patients are often referred to a cardiologist first as the pain mimics that of angina. When cardiac investigations are negative in a patient with chest pain, one should always consider an oesophageal motility disorder as the cause, even in the absence of dysphagia. Patterson [67] found diffuse oesophageal spasm and high-amplitude peristalsis in 18% of patients with unexplained chest pain but 77% of them had associated dysphagia for solids or liquids. Others have shown that as many as 65% of patients with chest pain and no coronary artery disease may have manometric oesophageal disorders [7, 10, 11, 31, 48, 53].

Diagnostic investigations

RADIOLOGY

The typical radiological features are 'segmental' or 'ladder' type spasm, described as a corkscrew, or rosary-bead oesophagus, or pseudo-diverticulosis. In addition there are tonic segmental contractions that lead to segmentation of the barium column [80] (Fig. 10.11).

In some patients the distal oesophagus may be narrowed (Fig. 10.12) or tightly contracted over a distance of several centimetres. With the patient recumbent, the barium is often trapped and pushed back into the proximal oesophagus. Usually there is no oesophageal dilatation, but the gullet wall may be thickened indicating hypertrophy. Food stasis is rare in diffuse spasm, but sometimes a retained food bolus may be seen with the sudden onset of dysphagia (Fig. 10.13).

It is important to realize that these changes are not seen in all patients with diffuse spasm on routine radiological assessment, while elderly patients may have the characteristic changes without symptoms [88].

MANOMETRY

Manometry is most helpful in diagnosis of this condition, although its manometric features have not always been clearly defined [88]. Usually these patients have various degrees of excessive motility with the following features: repetitive contraction waves; simultaneous non-peristaltic

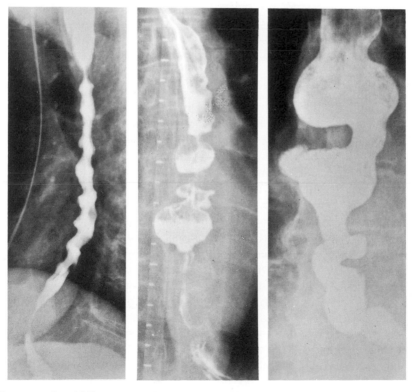

Fig. 10.11. Three examples of diffuse segmental oesophageal spasm of varying degrees of severity.

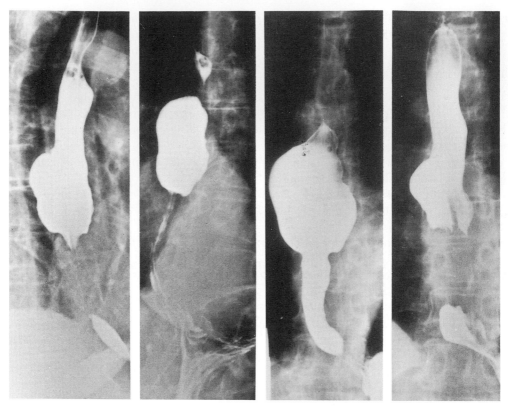

Fig. 10.12. An example of spasm in the distal oesophagus with segmental proximal dilatation. Various phases of contractile activity are shown.

contractions; long duration contractions; high amplitude waves and periods of normal peristalsis.

After a swallow the contraction waves are typically high in amplitude, increased in duration and repetitive (Fig. 10.14). The abnormal waves frequently occur simultaneously throughout the lower oesophagus, but this is not diagnostic. DiMarino and Cohen [27] have proposed that at least 30% of contractions must be abnormal to make the diagnosis. Others have suggested that contractions of a mean duration of 7.5 seconds are diagnostic [7]. A further feature is that of repetitive contractions—two or more in response to a single swallow [14].

It is more difficult to use the height of the pressure waves as this depends upon the compliance of the measuring system. Much higher amplitudes will be measured with low compliance systems, such as miniaturized intra-oesophageal pressure transducers.

Less common features are interrupted peristalsis (simultaneous pressure rise in proximal recording points and later pressure rise at a more distal site) and abnormally slow propagation of pressure waves in the distal oesophagus. Most patients have a normal lower oesophageal sphincter pressure and relaxation on swallowing [27], although in an occasional patient increased pressure and impaired relaxation can be detected. Some authors will not accept the diagnosis if the lower oesophageal sphincter function is impaired and it is our practice to categorize such patients under the titles 'vigorous' or 'active' achalasia. In a series

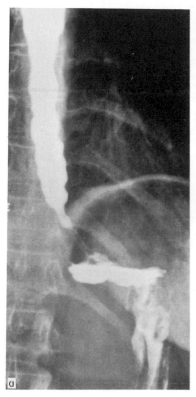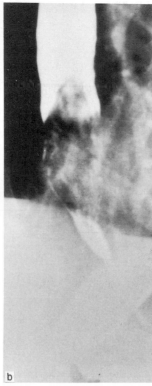

Fig. 10.13. An example of total dysphagia resulting from a food bolus obstruction (b) in a patient with diffuse oesophageal spasm (a).

reported by Van Trappen *et al.* [90] 24% of 156 patients, with oesophageal motility abnormalities and dysphagia, could not be classified as having achalasia, or diffuse oesophageal spasm.

PROVOCATION TESTS

Ergometrine and edrophonium provocation tests have been used to increase the diagnostic yield of manometry [3, 25, 53]. In a study of 42 patients, with suspected angina pectoris, 24 developed chest pain in association with abnormal motility after an ergometrine test, although six volunteers, known to have coronary artery stenosis, did not have such changes after this drug [3]. However, ergometrine can induce coronary artery spasm and is therefore not appropriate for routine clinical tests. Another stimulus that has been used is pentagastrin 6 μg/

kg body weight, but this has been disappointing in the diagnosis of diffuse oesophageal spasm [65].

Treatment

The therapy of diffuse oesophageal spasm is not clearly defined. Mild symptoms can be treated by reassurance and avoidance of known triggers. If emotional factors play a major role minor tranquillizers can help. Unfortunately the results of treating diffuse spasm are disappointing.

Anticholinergics, short and long-acting nitrates and nifedipine (30–40 mg/day) may produce moderate improvement in some patients [64, 88] and long-term oral hydralazine (25 mg b.d.) may help [59].

Pneumatic dilatation may be effective in some patients with severe dysphagia [29], but the benefit is much smaller than in

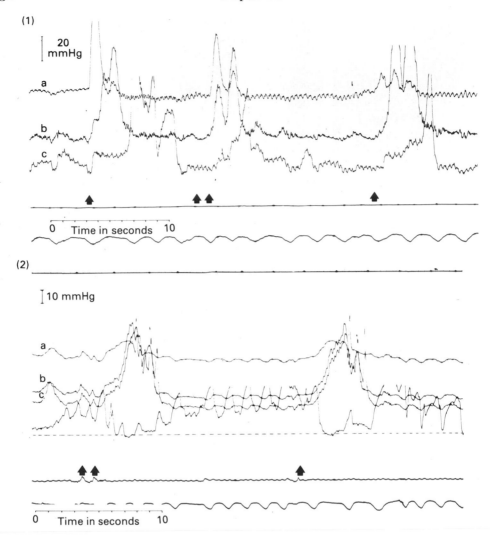

Fig. 10.14. Manometric pressure tracings in 2 patients with diffuse oesophageal spasm. (1) Tracings at A = 32 cm; B = 37 cm; C = 42 cm from nares in a patient presenting with chest pain. Note that contractions after swallowing (arrows) are sometimes peristaltic, sometimes simultaneous, biphasic or multiple. (2) Tracings at A = 40 cm; B = 45 cm; C = 50 cm; D = Sphincter zone in another patient with diffuse spasm. Note the simultaneous broad contractions and normal LOS-relaxation after swallowing (arrows).

achalasia with good results in only some 50% [87]. In addition the complication rate is higher, presumably because the oesophagus is not dilated and is contracting vigorously.

When symptoms are severe and unresponsive to medical therapy the patient should be considered for an extended oesophageal myotomy—up to the level of the aortic arch [51]. However, one should not embark upon this too easily, as the results can be poor and severe reflux oesophagitis, which can be difficult to control, may ensue.

Non-specific oesophageal motor disorders

Patients with chest pain and/or dysphagia often do not have typical manometric features of either achalasia or diffuse spasm. Such patients are classified under various headings, including vigorous achalasia, hypertensive lower oesophageal sphincter, or high-amplitude or vigorous peristalsis ('nutcracker' or 'supersqueezer') oesophagus.

Vigorous achalasia

In this condition the most striking abnormalities are high-amplitude, long-duration contractions. These are usually repetitive and have some features of diffuse oesophageal spasm [80, 83]. Such disordered contractility coincides with incomplete lower oesophageal sphincter relaxation. The spontaneous contractions are not initiated by swallowing and they are probably responsible for the severe chest pain. Otherwise the condition is very similar to classical achalasia.

The major difference lies in the response to treatment as pneumatic dilatation is of less benefit than in achalasia. In particular the attacks of retrosternal chest pain are difficult to relieve with medical therapy.

High amplitude or vigorous peristalsis

Recently attention has been focused on the motility disorder characterized by painful, hypertensive, broad, but peristaltic, contraction waves. This condition has a variety of additional names ('nutcracker' or 'supersqueezer' oesophagus). Patients with this condition have dysphagia and/or chest pain. Manometric features are contraction waves of high amplitude (greater than 200 mmHg) and long duration (greater than 7 seconds), but with normal peristaltic progression [7]. Ergometrine, acting via

alpha-adrenergic receptors, provokes pain in such patients. Therapy is similar to that used for diffuse oesophageal spasm [71].

Secondary oesophageal motility disorders

Scleroderma (systemic sclerosis)

Patients with scleroderma (or the syndrome associated with calcinosis, Raynaud's phenomenon, sclerodactyly and telangiectasia) frequently have severe abnormalities of oesophageal motility. These are due to smooth muscle atrophy with collagen replacement. Such abnormalities are found in 80% of patients with scleroderma, occurring usually in the third and fourth decades of life and twice as frequently in women as in men.

Oesophageal involvement is manifested by weak or absent smooth muscle contraction causing defective or absent distal peristalsis and diminished lower oesophageal sphincter pressure [74]. This combined defect leads to impaired oesophageal clearance causing severe reflux oesophagitis with stricture formation [45, 77]. The latter is usually the main cause of symptoms.

The diagnosis is suggested by the radiological finding of a peptic stricture with a non-contractile oesophagus. Typically the barium swallow shows a dilated oesophagus with a hiatus hernia and distal stricturing (Fig. 10.15). Manometry reveals weak or absent peristalsis [43], with a low or absent lower oesophageal sphincter pressure (Fig. 10.16).

These patients are notoriously difficult to treat and usually do not respond to standard anti-reflux measures. The H2-receptor antagonist cimetidine has been shown to be beneficial, but usually prolonged treatment at full dosage is necessary to maintain a remission [69]. As the results of medical therapy are so poor it is probably reasonable to consider anti-reflux surgery (i.e.

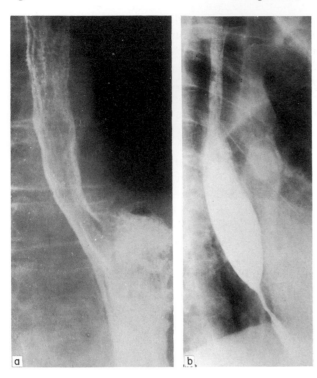

Fig. 10.15. Appearances of the oesophagus in advanced scleroderma. (a) Slightly dilated oesophagus with loss of contractile activity and the lower oesophageal sphincter. (b) Dilated oesophagus with loss of contractile activity but with distal narrowing secondary to reflux oesophagitis due to loss of the lower oesophageal sphincter.

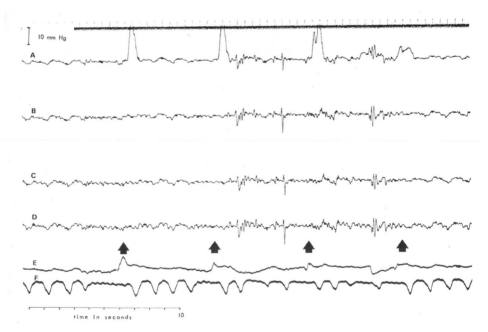

Fig. 10.16. Manometric pressure tracing (A = 18 cm; B = 23 cm; C = 28 cm; D = 33 cm; E = Swallowing record; F = respiratory record) in a patient with scleroderma. Note that contractions of the oesophagus after swallowing only occur in the proximal oesophagus.

Belsey repair). It is important not to use a Nissen 360° fundoplication, because this type of valve mechanism creates too much resistance to oesophageal emptying—in the presence of impaired peristalsis severe postoperative dysphagia will result [92].

Other causes of secondary oesophageal motility disorders

Patients with **mixed connective disease disorders** (including rheumatoid arthritis, systemic lupus erythematosus, dermatomyositis and polymyositis) may occasionally present with oesophageal problems similar to those found in scleroderma [42, 46].

Diabetes mellitus can occasionally be associated with motility disorders but rarely are these symptomatic. It is intriguing that the manometric pattern resembles that seen in diffuse oesophageal spasm, multipeaked pressure complexes have also been described [54]. **Amyloidosis** may cause similar changes when it involves the oesophageal neurones.

Chronic alcoholism may result in damage to the neurons of the myenteric plexus with the production of non-peristaltic contraction waves in the lower oesophagus, whereas the sphincter functions normally.

Myasthenia gravis can involve the pharynx and oesophagus leading to difficulties in swallowing. This dysfunction can be partially corrected by administration of edrophonium (2–8 mg).

Ageing can be associated with motility defects (segmentation and tertiary contractions) demonstrable on barium X-ray studies but manometric studies in such cases show only diminished pressure waves and symptoms are rare.

Chagas' disease

This is an important cause of abnormal oesophageal motility. The disease is caused by an infection with *Trypanosoma cruzi* which is transmitted by the bite of the *Triatoma megista* bug that lives in the thatched roofs and bedclothes of village huts in South America, Panama, Mexico and the southern United States. The oesophageal motility abnormalities are identical to those seen in achalasia and the mega-oesophagus develops about 30 years after the first attack.

References

1 ADAMS HD. A myenteric achalasia of the esophagus. *Surg Gynecol Obstet* 1964;**119**:215–256.
2 ALBAN-DAVIES H, KAYE MD, THADES J, DART AM, HENDERSON AH. Diagnosis of oesophageal spasm by ergometrine provocation. *Gut* 1982;**23**:89–97.
3 ANYANWU CH. Achalasia of the oesophagus in Nigeria. *J R Coll Surg Edinb* 1982;**27**:146–149.
4 BARTELSMAN JFWM, TYTGAT GNJ. *Amsterdam Series*. 1983.
5 BECKER BS, BURSKOFF R. Differential effect of verapamil on LES in normal subjects and those with achalasia. *Gastroenterology* 1981;**80**:1107.
6 BELSEY R. Recent progress in oesophageal surgery. *Acta Chir Belg* 1972;**71**:230–238.
7 BENJAMIN SB, GERHARDT DC, CASTELL DO. High amplitude, peristaltic esophageal contractions associated with chest pain and/or dysphagia. *Gastroenterology* 1979;**77**:478–483.
8 BLACK J, VORBACH AN, LEIGH-COLLIS J. Results of Heller's operation for achalasia. The importance of hiatal repair. *Br J Surg* 1976;**63**:949–953.
9 BORTOLOTTI M, LABO G. Clinical and manometric effects of Nifedipine in patients with esophageal achalasia. *Gastroenterology* 1981;**80**:39–44.
10 BRAND D, MARTIN D, POPE CE II. Esophageal manometrics in patients with angina-like chest pain. *Am J Dig Dis* 1977;**22**:300–304.
11 BRAND D, ILVES R, POPE CE II. Evaluation of esophageal function in patients with central chest pain. *Acta Med Scand [Suppl]* 1981;**644**:53–56.
12 CASSELLA RR, BROWN AL, SAYRE GP, ELLIS FH. Achalasia of the esophagus; pathologic and etiologic considerations. *Ann Surg* 1964;**160**:474–487.
13 CASSELLA RR, ELLIS FH JR, BROWN AL JR. Diffuse spasm of the lower part of the esophagus: Fine structure of esophageal smooth muscle and nerve. *JAMA* 1965;**191**:379–382.
14 CASTELL DO. The spectrum of esophageal motility disorders. *Gastroenterology* 1979;**70**:639–645.
15 CASTELL DO. Motor disorders of the esophagus. *N Eng J Med* 1979;**301**:1124.
16 CASTELL DO. Esophageal chest pain. *Am J Gastroenterol* 1984;**79**:969–971.
17 CASTELL DO. Calcium-channel blocking agents for

gastrointestinal disorders. *Am J Cardiol* 1985;
55:210B–213B.

18 CHAWLA K, CHAWLA SK, ALEXANDER LL. Familial achalasia of the esophagus in mother and son: a possible pathogenetic relationship. *J Am Geriatr Soc* 1979;**27**:519–520.

19 CHUONG JJM, DU BORIK S, McCALLUM RW. Achalasia as a risk factor for esophageal carcinoma; a reappraisal. *Dig Dis Sci* 1984;**29**:1105–1108.

20 COHEN BR, GUELRUD M. Cardiospasm in achalasia. Demonstration of supersensitivity of the lower esophageal sphincter. *Gastroenterology* 1971;**60**:769.

21 COHEN S, LIPSHUTZ W, HUGHES W. Role of gastrin hypersensitivity in the pathogenesis of lower esophageal sphincter hypertension in achalasia. *J Clin Invest* 1971;**50**:1241–1247.

22 COHEN S, FISHER R, TUCK A. The site of denervation in achalasia. *Gut* 1972;**13**:556–558.

23 COHEN S, FISHER R, LIPSHUTZ W, TURNER R, MYERS A, SCHUMACHER R. The pathogenesis of esophageal dysfunction in scleroderma and Raynaud's disease. *J Clin Invest* 1972;**51**:2663–2668.

24 CSENDES A, VELASCO N, BRAGHETTO I, HENRIQUEZ A. A prospective randomised study comparing forceful dilatation and esophagomyotomy in patients with achalasia of the esophagus. *Gastroenterology* 1981;**80**:789–795.

25 DALAL JJ, DART AM, ALBAN-DAVIES H, SHERIDAN DJ, RUTTLEY MST, HENDERSON AH. Coronary and peripheral arterial responses to ergometrine in patients susceptible to coronary and oesophageal spasm. *Br Heart J* 1981;**45**:181–185.

26 DIAMANT NE, El-SHARKAWY TY. Progress in gastroenterology. Neural control of esophageal peristalsis. A conceptual analysis. *Gastroenterology* 1977;**72**:546–556.

27 DiMARINO AJ JR, COHEN S. Characteristics of lower esophageal sphincter function in symptomatic diffuse esophageal spasm. *Gastroenterology* 1974;**66**:1–6.

28 DODDS WJ, DENT J, HOGAN WJ, PALEL GK, TOONLI J, ARNDORFER RC. Paradoxical lower esophageal sphincter contraction induced by cholecystokinin-octapeptide in patients with achalasia. *Gastroenterology* 1981;**80**:327–333.

29 EBERT EC, OUYANG A, WRIGHT SH, COHEN S, LIPSHUTZ WH. Pneumatic dilatation in patients with symptomatic diffuse esophageal spasm and lower esophageal sphincter dysfunction. *Dig Dis Sci* 1983;**28**:481–485.

30 ELDER JB. Achalasia of the cardia in childhood. *Digestion* 1970;**3**:90–96.

31 FELLOWS IW, OGILVIE AL, ATKINSON M. Pneumatic dilatation in achalasia. *Gut* 1983;**24**:1020–1023.

32 FERGUSON SC, HODGES K, HERSCH T, JINICH H. Esophageal manometry in patients with chest pain and normal coronary arteriogram. *Am J Gastroenterol* 1981;**75**:124–127.

33 FISHER RS, APPLEGATE LS, ROCK E, LORBER SH. Effect of bolus composition on esophageal transit: concise communication. *J Nucl Med* 1982;**23**:878–882.

34 FRIMBERGER E, KUHNER W, KUNERT H, OTTENJANN R. Results of treatment with the endoscope dilatator in 11 patients with achalasia of the esophagus. *Endoscopy* 1981;**13**:173–175.

35 FRIMBERGER E, KUHNER W, HAHN A, OTTENJANN R. Konservative behandlung der achalasia mit einem elektronisch-mechanischen dilatator. *Dtsch Med Wochenschr* 1982;**36**:1339–1342.

36 GALLONE L, PERI G, GALLIERA M. Proximal gastric vagotomy and anterior fundoplication as complementary procedures to Heller's operation for achalasia. *Surg Gynecol Obstet* 1982;**155**:337–341.

37 GELFOND M, ROZEN P, GILAT T. Isosorbide dinitrate and nifedipine treatment of achalasia: a clinical manometric and radionuclide evaluation. *Gastroenterology* 1982;**83**:963–969.

38 GOYAL RK, RATTAN S. Effects of sodium nitroprusside and verapamil on lower esophageal sphincter. *Am J Physiol* 1980;**238**:G40–G44.

39 GOYAL RK. Pathophysiology of achalasia and diffuse esophageal spasm. In: *Post-graduate course: the neuromuscular disorders of the gastrointestinal tract.* New York: AGA, 1981.

40 GOYAL RK, COBB BW. Motility of the pharynx; esophagus and the esophageal sphincters. In: Johnson, CR, ed. *Physiology of the Digestive System.* New York: Raven Press, 1981.

41 GROSS R, JOHNSON LF, KAMINSKI RJ. Esophageal emptying in achalasia, quantitated by a radioisotope technique. *Dig Dis Sci* 1979;**24**:945–949.

42 GUTIERREZ F, VALENZUELA JE, EHRESMANN GR, QUISMORIO FP, KITRIDOU RC. Esophageal dysfunction in patients with mixed connective tissue diseases and systemic lupus erythematosus. *Dig Dis Sci* 1982;**27**:592–597.

43 HAMEL-ROY J, DEVROEDE G, ARHAN P, TETREAULT L, DURANCEAU A, MENARD H-A. Comparative esophageal and anorectal motility in scleroderma. *Gastroenterology* 1985;**88**:1–7.

44 HARLEY HRS. *Achalasia of the cardia.* Bristol: John Wright & Sons Ltd, 1978.

45 HENDERSON RD, PEARSON FG. Surgical management of esophageal scleroderma. *J Thorac Cardiovasc Surg* 1973;**66**:686.

46 HOROWITZ M, McNEIL JD, MADDERN GJ, COLLINS PJ, SHEARMAN DJC. Abnormalities of gastric and esophageal emptying in polymyositis and dermatomyositis. *Gastroenterology* 1986;**90**:434–439.

47 KLINE MM. Successful treatment of vigorous achalasia with gastric lymphoma. *Dig Dis Sci* 1980;**25**:311–313.

48 KLINE M, CHESNE R, STURDEVENT RAL, McCALLUM RW. Esophageal disease in patients with angina-like chest pain. *Am J Gastroenterol* 1981;**75**:124–127.

49 KOTELES G, KEMENY P, REICH K. Familiare infantile achalasie. 3 Falle bei Geschwistern einer familie. *Mschr Klinderheilk* 1985;**123**:9–14.

50 KRAMER P, INGELFINGER FJ. Esophageal sensitivity to mecholyl in cardiospasm. *Gastroenterology* 1951;**19**:242–253.

51 LEONARDI IIK, SHEA JA, CROSIER RE, ELLIS FE JR. Diffuse spasm of the esophagus. Clinical, manometric and surgical considerations. *J Thorac Cardiovasc Surg* 1977;**74**:736–743.

52 LOBIS IF, FISHER PS. Anticholinergic therapy for achalasia. A controlled trial. *Gastroenterology* 1976;**70**:976.

53 LONDON RL, OUYANG A, SNAPE WJ, GOLDBERG S, HIRSCHFELD JW, COHEN S. Provocation of esophageal pain by ergonovine or edrophonium. *Gastroenterology* 1981;**81**:10–14.

54 LOO FD, DODDS WJ, SOERGEL KH, ARNDORFER RC, HELM JF, HOGAN WJ. Multipeaked esophageal peristaltic pressure waves in patients with diabetic neuropathy. *Gastroenterology* 1985;**88**:485–491.

55 McCALLUM RW. Esophageal achalasia secondary to gastric carcinoma. *Am J Gastroenterol* 1979;**71**:24–29.

56 MALMUD LS, FISHER RS. Scintigraphic evaluation of disorders of the esophagus, stomach and duodenum. *Med Clin North Am* 1981;**65**:1291–1310.

57 MATHUS-VLIEGEN EMH, TYTGAT GNJ. The role of endoscopy in correct and fast positioning of feeding tubes. *Endoscopy* 1983;**15**:78–84.

58 MAYBERRY JF, ATKINSON M. Studies of incidence and prevalence of achalasia in the Nottingham area. *Q J Med* 1985;**220**:451–456.

59 MELLOW MH. Effect of isosorbide and hydralazine in painful primary esophageal motility disorders. *Gastroenterology* 1982;**83**:364–370.

60 MENGUY R. Management of achalasia by transabdominal cardiomyotomy and fundoplication. *Surg Gynecol Obstet* 1971;**133**:482–484.

61 MEYER GW, CASTELL DO. Physiology of the esophagus. *Clin Gastroent* 1982;**11**:439–451.

62 MILLER RH. Amyloid disease, an unusual case of megalo-esophagus. *South African Medical J* 1969;**43**:1202–1203.

63 OKIKE N, PAYNE WS, NEUFELD DM, BERNATZ PE, PAIROLERO PC, SANDERSON DS. Esophagomyotomy vs. forceful dilatation for achalasia of the esophagus. *Ann Thorac Surg* 1979;**28**:100–102.

64 ORLANDO RC, BOZYMSKI EM. Clinical and manometric effects of nitroglycerin in diffuse esophageal spasm. *N Eng J Med* 1973;**289**:23–24.

65 ORLANDO RC, BOZYMSKI EM. The effect of pentagastrin in achalasia and diffuse esophageal spasm. *Gastroenterology* 1979;**77**:472–477.

66 PALMER ED. Treatment of achalasia when the Heller operation has failed. *Am J Gastroenterol* 1972;**57**:255–260.

67 PATTERSON DR. Diffuse esophageal spasm in patients with undiagnosed chest pain. *J Clin Gastroenterol* 1982;**4**:415–417.

68 PEEBLES WJ, ELMAHDI AM, ROSATA FE. Achalasia of the esophagus associated with Hodgkin's disease. *J Surg Oncol* 1979;**11**:213–216.

69 PETROKUBI RJ, JEFFRIES GH. Cimetidine versus antacid in scleroderma with reflux esophagitis: a randomised double-blind controlled study. *Gastroenterology* 1979;**71**:691–695.

70 POLONSKI L, GUTH PH. Familial achalasia. *Dig Diseases* 1970;**15**:291–295.

71 RICHTER JE, DALTON CB, BUICE RG, CASTELL DO. Nifedipine: A potent inhibitor of contractions in the body of the human esophagus. Studies in healthy volunteers and patients with the nutcracker esophagus. *Gastroenterology* 1985;**89**:549–554.

72 ROESCH W. Endoscopy in achalsia. *Postgrad Med J* 1974;**50**:211.

73 RUSSELL CVH, HILL LD, HOLMES ER III, HULL DA, GANNON R, POPE CE II. Radionuclide transit: A sensitive screening test for esophageal dysfunction. *Gastroenterology* 1982;**80**:887–892.

74 SALADIN TA, FRENCH AB, ZARAFONETIS CJD, POLLARD HJ. Esophageal motor abnormalities in scleroderma and related diseases. *Amer J Dig Dis* 1966;**11**:522–535.

75 SCHUFFLER MD, POPE CE. Esophageal motor dysfunction in idiopathic obstruction. *Gastroenterology* 1976;**70**:677–682.

76 SCHULTZ EH JR. Achalasia in children as a cause of recurrent pulmonary disease. *J Pediatr* 1961;**59**:522–528.

77 SEGEL MC, CAMPBELL WL, MEDOGER TA JR, ROUMM AD, Systemic sclerosis (scleroderma) and esophageal adenocarcinoma: Is increased patient screening necessary? *Gastroenterology* 1985;**89**:485–488.

78 SILBER W. Achalasia. *Lancet* 1965;**ii**:1287–1292.

79 SMITH B. The neurological lesion in achalasia of the cardia. *Gut* 1970;**11**:388–391.

80 STEWART ET. Radiographic evaluation of the esophagus and its motor disorders. *Med Clin North Am* 1981;**65**:1173–1194.

81 TOLIN RD, MALMUD LS, REILLEY J, FISHER RS. Esophageal scintigraphy to quantitate esophageal transit (quantitation of esophageal transit). *Gastroenterology* 1979;**76**:1402–1408.

82 TUCKER HJ, SNAPE WJ JR, COHEN S. Achalasia secondary to carcinoma: manometric and clinical features. *Ann Int Med* 1978;**89**:315–318.

83 TYTGAT GNJ. Endoscopic methods of treatment of gastrointestinal and biliary stenosis. *Endoscopy* (Suppl) 1980;**12**:57–68.

84 TYTGAT GNJ, DEN HARTOG JAGER FCA. Non-surgical treatment of cardio-esophageal obstruction. Role of endoscopy. *Endoscopy* 1977;**9**:211–215.

85 VAN TRAPPEN G, HELLEMANS J. In: *Diseases of the esophagus*. New York, Heidelberg: Springer Verlag, 1974.

86 VAN TRAPPEN G, HELLEMANS J. Esophageal motility disorders. *Front Gastrointest Res* 1978;**3**:49–75.

87 VAN TRAPPEN G, HELLEMANS J. Treatment of achalasia and related motor disorders. *Gastroenterology* 1980;**79**:144–154.

88 VAN TRAPPEN G, HELLEMANS J. Esophageal spasm and other muscular dysfunction. *Clinics Gastroenterol* 1982;**11**:453–477.

89 VAN TRAPPEN G, JANSSENS J. To dilate or to operate? That is the question. *Gut* 1983;**24**:1013–1019.

90 VAN TRAPPEN G, JANSSENS J, HELLEMANS J, COREMANS G. Achalasia, diffuse esophageal spasm and related motility disorders. *Gastroenterology* 1979;**76**:450–457.

91 VAUGHAN WH, WILLIAMS JL. Familial achalasia with pulmonary complications in children. *Radiology* 1973;**107**:407–409.

92 WATERS PF, DeMEESTER TR. Foregut motor disorders and their surgical management. *Med Clin North Am* 1981;**65**:1235–1268.

93 WEIHRAUCH TR, KORTING GW. Manometric assessment of oesophageal involvement in progressive systemic sclerosis, morphoea and Raynaud's disease. *Br J Dermatol* 1982;**107**:325–332.

94 WESDORP ICE, BARTELSMAN JFWM, DEN HARTOG JAGER FCA, TYTGAT GNJ. Treatment of instrumental esophageal perforation. *D Gut.* 1984;**25**:398–404.

95 WILLICH E. Achalasia of the cardia in children. Manometric, cinematographic and pharmacoradiographic studies. *Pediatr Radiol* 1973;**1**:229–236.

96 WITZEL L. Treatment of achalasia with a pneumatic dilator attached to a gastroscope. *Endoscopy* 1981;**13**:170–177.

Chapter 11
Oesophagitis and Hiatus Hernia

T. GLEDHILL & R. H. HUNT

In health the lower oesophageal sphincter lies below the diaphragm and is associated with the gastro-oesophageal mucosal junction. It is a physiological zone of high pressure that can prevent reflux, but it is not always effective, even in normal individuals. Reflux disease occurs when the frequency and volume of such regurgitation is excessive. The severity of oesophagitis that follows depends upon the balance between the frequency, content and volume of reflux on the one hand and the mucosal protective mechanisms on the other (Fig. 11.1).

Our understanding of reflux oesophagitis has been bedevilled by its association with hiatus hernia. Normal function of the lower oesophageal sphincter is partly dependent upon its anatomical position so that displacement into the thorax created by a hiatus hernia can predispose to reflux. Half of the patients with a radiologically demonstrated hernia have symptomatic reflux [86], yet over 30% of asymptomatic subjects have a hiatus hernia—a figure that rises to 50% in people over 50 years of age [26, 63].

A hiatus hernia can give rise to problems that are not caused by reflux. The sliding type of hernia (Fig. 11.2) may occupy a part of the thoracic cavity, causing cardiac or pulmonary embarassment. Peptic ulceration may occasionally occur within the hernia and is often resistant to treatment. If the hernia is of a paraoesophageal or

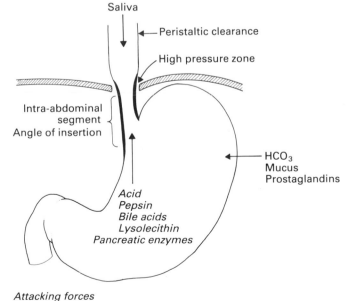

Saliva

Peristaltic clearance

High pressure zone

Intra-abdominal segment
Angle of insertion

HCO3
Mucus
Prostaglandins

Acid
Pepsin
Bile acids
Lysolecithin
Pancreatic enzymes

Attacking forces
Defending forces

Fig. 11.1. The aetiological factors in reflux oesophagitis—attack vs. defence.

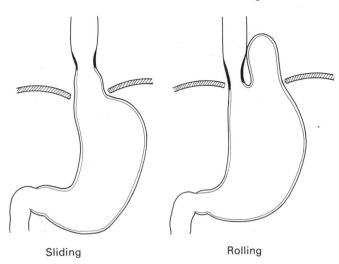

Sliding   Rolling

Fig. 11.2. Diagrammatic representation of a sliding and a para-oesophageal (rolling) hiatus hernia.

'rolling' type (Fig. 11.2) there is a substantial risk of obstruction and strangulation. Paraoesophageal herniae have a complete peritoneal covering and lie lateral to the gastro-oesophageal junction; usually they contain the gastric fundus. They probably arise because of failed closure of the medial pleuro-peritoneal canal or, more rarely, of the lateral pleuro-peritoneal canal (Bochdalek hernia). Classically paraoesophageal herniae cause dysphagia that is relieved by a change of posture.

Epidemiology

The incidence of heartburn in the general population is difficult to estimate. In a study of normal hospital personnel, 7% had daily and 36% had monthly episodes of heartburn [57]. The prevalence of this symptom in patients attending a gastroenterology clinic was found to be 15% [57]. Certainly reflux oesophagitis is a common cause of dyspepsia in the Western world.

Many factors associated with the aetiology of this condition are linked to a Western life-style—smoking, diet and obesity. Obesity and cigarette smoking are less common in African and Asian populations which may explain why this disease is rarely seen in such communities. Some believe that these differences can be explained by the low intake of dietary fibre in the Western diet.

Symptomatic reflux can occur at any age [79], but is most common at the extremes of life. Its presence in the infant may result from a poorly developed sphincter while in later life it may be caused by weakening of the sphincter with age. At other ages symptoms often begin after a sudden weight gain or during the last trimester of pregnancy.

Aetiology

Acid and pepsin

In animal experiments acid alone (even at low pH, 1.0–1.3) does not cause oesophagitis. At low acid concentrations oesophagitis occurs only when pepsin is also present—pepsin-induced changes are pH dependent—occurring maximally at pH 1.3, being absent at pH 2.5 [29]. Thus both acid and pepsin are involved in the production of mucosal damage.

Lower oesophageal sphincter incompetence

Oesophagitis results when incompetence of the lower oesophageal sphincter permits the reflux of acid and pepsin, which remains in the oesophagus for long enough to overcome the mucosal protective mechanisms [35]. Factors considered important in maintaining a high pressure zone in the lower oesophagus can be classified as anatomical or physiological (Table 11.1).

The **anatomical factors** include the presence of an intra-abdominal segment (compressed by abdominal pressure), the diaphragmatic hiatus, the angle between the stomach and oesophagus, the presence of mucosal folds and the circular muscle fibres of the lower oesophagus. **Physiological control** may be effected by 3 mechanisms—contraction in the basal state may be enhanced by cholinergic stimuli and, possibly, circulating gastrin [42]; relaxation occurs through adrenergic stimuli initiated during the pharyngeal phase of swallowing—in addition reflex relaxation of the lower oesophageal sphincter, initiated by food entering the upper oesophagus, persists until the peristaltic wave has passed distally; finally, a brief period of contraction occurs after the peristaltic wave has passed and this is mediated through cholinergic receptors. There is also evidence that dopaminergic receptors play a part in lower oesophageal function.

Although there have been reports showing an inverse correlation between lower oesophageal sphincter pressure and reflux [3], 25% of patients with reflux have 'normal' sphincter pressures. It is also recognized that reflux can occur in the presence of a raised lower oesophageal sphincter pressure [83]. This paradox has been clarified by the demonstration that sphincter pressure varies with time in normal and in refluxing patients [25]. Patients with oesophagitis fall into two groups, both having significantly more episodes of reflux during a 12-hour period than normal individuals. In one group reflux occurs spontaneously because of a low resting sphincter pressure, while in the other group reflux results from an increased frequency of lower oesophageal sphincter relaxation.

Diet

In addition to these physiological mechanisms, dietary factors also play a role. Ingestion of protein increases and fat decreases the lower oesophageal sphincter pressure. Eating chocolate, drinking alcoholic beverages and, especially, smoking relax the sphincter.

Drugs

Anti-cholinergic agents produce a fall in the lower oesophageal sphincter pressure and decrease the volume and alkalinity of the saliva passing down the oesophagus. While anticholinergics may reduce the volume of

Table 11.1. Factors important in maintaining a high pressure zone in the lower oesophagus.

Anatomical	Physiological
Right crus of diaphragm	Increase tone in sphincter
Mucosal 'choke'	Cholinergic
Oblique muscle of stomach	Adrenergic
Intra-abdominal oesophagus	Dopaminergic
Acute angle between oesophagus and stomach	

gastric secretion, they have little effect on the concentration of acid and tend to slow gastric emptying, which also increases the risk of reflux. For these reasons they are contraindicated in the management of this problem.

Heller, *et al.* [33] reported that **non-steroidal antiflammatory drugs** were taken more frequently in patients with peptic oesophageal strictures than they were in a control group. However, this study has been criticized for its selection of controls and it is not known whether these drugs are of aetiological importance or not.

Bile reflux

The action of acid and pepsin cannot explain the development of severe oesophagitis after a previous total gastrectomy. Under these circumstances the damage is probably caused by the combination of bile, bile salts, pancreatic enzymes and lysolecithins.

It is a frequent endoscopic observation that large amounts of bile are present in the stomach and lower oesophagus of patients with severe oesophagitis. Whether bile reflux is aetiologically important for many patients with oesophagitis is still controversial. However, it has been shown that surgical procedures that redirect bile flow (Roux-en-Y bypass) can result in healing of severe oesophagitis [88].

Nocturnal reflux

Nocturnal episodes of reflux may be particularly important, as it is during the night that intra-gastric acidity is greatest. During the day food partially buffers gastric acid and the total 'acid contact time' is thereby reduced.

Motility

Disorders of oesophageal or gastric motility may also cause oesophagitis [11, 55]

(Chapter 10). Oesophagitis can be a complication of delayed gastric emptying (e.g. pyloric stenosis) or after gastric surgery where bile reflux and/or acid reflux is increased. As many as 50% of patients with reflux may have delayed gastric emptying [52, 85].

Pregnancy

Reflux occurring during pregnancy may be attributed both to mechanical factors and to hormonal changes—oestrogens decrease lower oesophageal sphincter pressure and, characteristically, reflux improves dramatically following delivery.

Pathology

The changes seen endoscopically in the early stages of oesophagitis are erythema and engorgement of the lower oesophageal mucosa. Later the mucosa becomes opalescent and erosions develop progressing to form linear ulcers along the mucosal folds. These ulcers then become confluent resulting in a circumferential loss of oesophageal epithelium with a membranous exudative covering.

Although macroscopic oesophagitis is evidence of reflux, symptoms do not always correlate with the presence or severity of these changes [76]. Biopsy may be helpful in symptomatic patients even without macroscopic changes [41]. Initial mucosal damage causes increased epithelial desquamation and a compensatory cellular proliferation. This is characterized by elongated rete papillae and increased thickness of the basal zone (Fig. 11.3a). Ismail-Beigi, *et al.* [41] believe that 85% of patients with heartburn show these changes, which are absent in healthy controls. It is a wise precaution to ensure that biopsies are taken from an area at least 5 cm proximal to the gastro-oesophageal junction as changes of

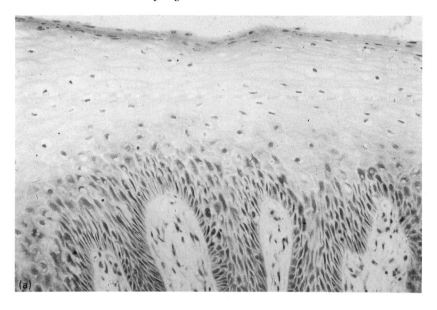

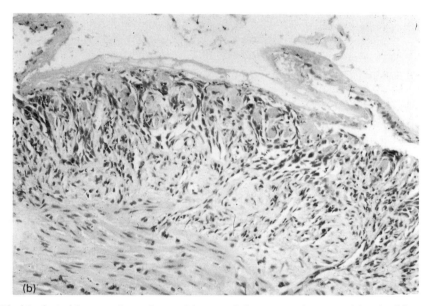

Fig. 11.3. The histological features of oesophagitis. (a) minimal change oesophagitis with basal cell hyperplasia and increase in the height of the papillae. (b) severe oesophagitis with ulceration of the surface epithelium, chronic inflammatory cell infiltrate and an inflammatory exudate on the surface.

oesophagitis may be found below this level in normal subjects [89].

More severe damage is reflected by loss of surface epithelium with inflammatory changes throughout all layers of the oeso-phageal wall (Fig. 11.3b). Healing is associated with fibrosis which may lead to stricture formation in 10–15% of patients at initial presentation [14]. The surface mucosa may be replaced by a metaplastic epithelium of antral, fundic, pyloric or intestinal cell types [62]. These changes result in a 'Barrett's oesophagus' in which the lower part of the oesophagus is lined by gastric rather than squamous epithelium [12, 35]. Barrett's oesophagus can also occur as a congenital condition (sometimes called congenital short oesophagus). It has been suggested that this metaplastic columnar epithelium reverts to a squamous epithelium after anti-reflux surgery [13], but this remains contentious. The gastric mucosa found in Barrett's oesophagus may undergo malignant transformation in approximately 10% of these patients [16, 36, 43, 56].

Presentation

The most common symptom of gastro-oesophageal reflux is **heartburn** [70]. This can be defined as a retrosternal discomfort or burning sensation that extends upwards to the throat, usually occuring after food and relieved by antacids. Heartburn is generally episodic and exacerbated by stooping or lying flat. It is usually relieved by antacids and made worse by swallowing citrus juice, spirits or hot drinks, or by any activity that increases intra-abdominal pressure. Heartburn provoked by exercise can be very difficult to distinguish from angina. Angina-like pain may be present in 10% of patients with reflux.

The impaired motility associated with inflammation of the oesophageal mucosa may result in **dysphagia** is almost 50% of patients, although stricture occurs in only 10%. Occasionally this dysphagia will be severe enough to result in loss of weight.

Another symptom of reflux is **waterbrash.** This is due to gastric fluid reaching the pharynx and causing a bitter or acid taste. This symptom must be distinguished from **regurgitation** which occurs when oesophageal contents return into the nasopharynx without producing a sensation of an acid or bitter taste. Regurgitation is often a symptom of obstruction and raises the suspicion of severe luminal narrowing due to a stricture, tumour or achalasia.

Other symptoms of oesophagitis include vomiting, nausea, back pain, epigastric (sub-xiphisternal) pain and odynophagia. Reflux can result in episodes of coughing and choking, and an association with nocturnal asthma is now recognized [4, 9, 46, 48].

Oesophagitis may present with **upper gastrointestinal bleeding** which is usually chronic in nature (presenting as iron-deficiency anaemia) rather than as a frank haematemesis. However, it is essential that a hiatus hernia seen on barium meal is not assumed to be the cause of chronic blood loss until other causes, particularly carcinoma of the colon, have been excluded.

The natural history of oesophagitis is variable—two-thirds of patients will be symptom-free 10 years after initiating medical treatment [2] while a few develop complications such as a stricture, bleeding and Barrett's oesophagus.

Differential diagnosis [21]

Heartburn can be difficult to distinguish from other causes of dyspepsia, notably duodenal and gastric ulceration. A useful distinguishing feature is that the pain of peptic ulcer tends to wake the patient from sleep, but heartburn occurs when lying flat and therefore prevents the patient from getting to sleep.

Difficulty may also be encountered in differentiating angina, cholelithiasis, pancreatic disease and the irritable bowel syndrome from reflux disease. Other clues in the history and physical examination will often help. Oesophagitis is supported by a clear history of reflux and the absence of physical signs. The importance of angina needs emphasizing as some reports suggest that almost half the patients with symptoms suggesting angina, but with normal cardiac studies, have gastro-oesophageal reflux as the cause of their pain [20, 22, 49, 68]. Appropriate medical or surgical therapy will abolish the chest pain in approximately 75% of patients.

Problems may also be encountered in differentiating oesophagitis from other causes of dysphagia. Achalasia is usually painless—pain, if present, occurs early in the disease, has a different distribution, or may be that of odynophagia due to **retention oesophagitis** (see Chapter 10). Carcinoma is suggested by the progressive nature of the dysphagia, absence of reflux, regurgitation, age and weight loss (see Chapter 13). Dysphagia may also be caused by a Schatzki ring, which has been described as a narrowing at the squamo-columnar junction demonstrated radiologically. It produces a notch, 19 mm or less in diameter, which is shown on distension of the oesophagus [71]. The ring has been blamed as a cause of the 'steakhouse syndrome' but it remains debatable as to whether it is a true entity or an annular peptic stricture.

Medical treatment

The aim of treatment is to break the cycle of reflux causing damage which impairs motility and causes further reflux [17, 47, 59].

General measures

General measures are recommended for mild symptoms. These include weight reduction in the obese patient, removal of tight clothing, avoidance of stooping or bending and smoking.

Cigarette smoking [23] and alcohol (when taken orally or intravenously [40]) decrease the lower oesophageal sphincter pressure and they should therefore be avoided. Coffee also lowers sphincter pressure while increasing gastric acid secretion

[19]—an undesirable combination. Other foods, notably chocolate and fats, have similar effects on the sphincter and certain beverages, such as orange and tomato juice, can increase symptoms and are best avoided [67].

Elevation of the head of the bed by 15 cm, which is better than simply increasing the number of pillows, will not prevent reflux but does tend to reduce the time that refluxed fluid remains in the oesophagus at night.

These simple, but important measures improve approximately 75% of patients with reflux symptoms. The remainder require more aggressive treatment with pharmacological agents, which act in three ways—neutralization of acid, inhibition of gastric secretion and elevation of the lower oesophageal sphincter pressure.

Antacids, alginates, carbenoxolone, anaesthetics and simethicone

Gastric alkalinization increases the lower oesophageal sphincter pressure [18, 37]. The aim of **antacids** is to increase intragastric pH, thereby decreasing the amount of refluxed acid. Antacids have, however, little effect upon intragastric acidity at night [44]. While many doctors regard antacids as the mainstay of therapy for reflux [44] objective proof of their benefit is lacking. Symptoms can be improved by taking antacids on an 'as required' basis, and regular use reduces the sensitivity of the lower oesophageal mucosa to acid.

Antacid-alginate mixtures produce a gel that floats on the gastric contents when the patient is erect decreasing the amount of acid refluxed into the lower oesophagus. The buffering capacity of these mixtures is minimal so presumably they work mainly as a physical barrier. Controlled trials have shown improvement of symptoms with an alginate/antacid mixture [5, 6]. One study, in which there was no symptomatic benefit, documented a reduction in episodes of reflux and acid contact time [80]. Three other trials have shown no benefit from combining antacid with alginates [31, 54, 73].

An alginate/antacid mixture has also been combined with a small dose of **carbenoxolone** (20 mg/tab. 'Pyrogastrone')—this is supposed to enhance healing of mucosal ulceration. It is reported that this preparation is significantly better than an antacid/alginate mixture alone [69]. However, its main drawback is that carbenoxolone can occasionally produce water retention and hypokalaemia, which in elderly people or patients with heart, liver or kidney disease, can be dangerous.

Antacids have also been combined with an acid stable **local anaesthetic agent** (oxethazine 10 mg/5 ml) in an attempt to increase pain relief. This is a popular combination ('Mucaine') in clinical practice but does not seem to have been subjected to a careful controlled trial.

The addition of a **simethicone derivative** to an antacid mixture ('Asilone') is claimed to reduce belching. Such defoaming agents should not be used with alginate mixtures as they destroy the gel.

Antacids are effective agents for symptom relief but they have not been shown to affect the inflammatory changes seen at endoscopy. Most gastroenterologists give the antacids after meals and at night but there is no good evidence concerning the best regime. Usually they are given for symptom relief and are continued for as long as they are required. Provided that they are not used in excessive doses, there are no serious side effects (with the exception of the carbenoxolone/alginate/antacid mixture). Antacids are often used in combination with other agents such as metoclopramide.

H$_2$-receptor antagonists

These agents have been extensively investigated in the management of reflux oesophagitis since **cimetidine** was first introduced in 1976. The rationale for their use is that they are capable of reducing acid secretion for a prolonged period, both during the day and the night. This acid reduction is accompanied by a decrease in peptic activity which could be of benefit. These drugs have no direct effect on the lower oesophageal sphincter but do reduce the number of reflux episodes [8]. Cimetidine has also been shown to reduce mucosal sensitivity to acid [7].

Early studies [53] showed that cimetidine (1.6 g/day) produced rapid symptom relief with an apparent improvement in the appearance of oesophagitis at endoscopy

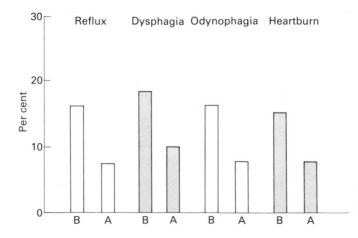

Fig. 11.4. Symptom relief achieved during treatment with cimetidine. (B) before treatment; (A) after four weeks of 400 mg q.d.s. (after [4]).

(Fig. 11.4). Subsequently a number of controlled trials of cimetide against placebo were reported. Tytgat [87] analysed the results of 11 controlled trials in 450 patients and showed that in nine of these cimetidine was significantly better than placebo in symptom relief. Over the last few years the second H_2-receptor antagonist **ranitidine** has also been tested in reflux oesophagitis. Controlled trials have shown that symptom relief is significantly better with ranitidine (150 mg twice daily) than with placebo, when given over a six week period [30, 39, 74, 91].

There is much more controversy over the effects of H_2-receptor antagonists on the healing of the mucosal ulceration seen endoscopically in this condition. Tytgat [84] concluded that cimetidine produced improvement in the endoscopic appearance of oesophagitis in around two-thirds of the patients treated. In addition Kothari, Mangla and Kalra [45] showed that cimetidine could heal the ulceration seen in Barrett's oesophagitis and Petrokubi and Jefferies [64, 65] demonstrated an improvement in symptoms and oesophagitis in patients with scleroderma. However, two studies failed to show any benefit from cimetidine in preventing recurrence of a peptic oesophageal stricture [28, 45] and one failed to reverse the metaplastic change seen in Barrett's oesophagus [91].

There are fewer reports on the use of ranitidine in oesophagitis. On theoretical grounds (if acid inhibition is the mode of action) then one might expect this drug to be more effective as a 150 mg dose of ranitidine is roughly equivalent to 800 mg of cimetidine in acid inhibitory terms. Certainly in the four controlled studies there was a significant improvement in the endoscopic appearance and histological grade of oesophagitis present at the end of the six week period, when compared with the pretreatment assessment and placebo response [10].

In conclusion, both cimetidine and ranitidine are effective agents for symptom relief in patients with reflux oesophagitis [55, 77] and both probably improve the mucosal inflammation/ulceration present. Unfortunately their use in long-term management remains controversial and there is little information on the value of 'maintenance' therapy in oesophagitis. Certainly symptoms tend to recur rapidly when these drugs are discontinued so some form of long-term treatment will be required in patients with severe oesophagitis.

Dopamine-receptor antagonists

Metoclopramide is a dopamine S_2-antagonist which causes an increase in lower oesophageal sphincter pressure and promotes gastric emptying [24, 80] without any effect upon gastric secretion. Two trials have shown a decrease in symptoms after this drug although neither showed an increase in lower oesophageal sphincter pressure or healing of the oesophagitis [15, 51]. Two further studies [61, 87] failed to show any significant effect in severe oesophagitis. It appears that any benefits achieved by metoclopramide depend upon the pre-existing weakness of the lower oesophageal sphincter—the weaker the sphincter, the smaller the rise in sphincter tone achieved by the drug. The major side-effect is that of extrapyramidal effects which can be serious and intractable in some elderly patients [60].

Domperidone is an alternative dopamine S_2-antagonist which appears to be more specific and potent than metoclopramide. It has the major advantage that it does not appear to produce extrapyramidal side-effects.

These agents have a relatively short duration of action so the timing of administration is probably quite critical. Reflux symptoms tend to occur after a meal so the usual recommendation is to give these drugs about 30 minutes before a meal (metoclopramide 10 mg and domperidone 10–20 mg three times daily). If reflux is most severe at night then a dose of these drugs may be given just before retiring.

Stable cholinergic agents

Bethanechol hydrochloride is a stable cholinergic agent that increases lower oesophageal sphincter tone, improves acid clearance from the lower oesophagus and speeds gastric emptying. Two trials have shown reduced symptoms and one, reduced oesophagitis after this drug, given in a dose of 25 mg 4 times daily [27, 82]. Bethanechol can, however, increase gastric secretion, produce acute retention and exacerbate glaucoma, so that its use is restricted.

Sucralfate

Aluminium sucrose sulphate has been shown to be of benefit in the management of peptic ulcer. In a recently reported placebo-controlled trial (using 1 g four times daily) complete healing of oesophagitis was achieved in 72% of those treated with sucralfate compared with only 40% of those treated with the placebo [90]. This is one of the first reported studies of this compound in this condition, so further information is required before it can be recommended for routine use.

Management strategy

It is important to take the time to provide patients with an adequate explanation of their problem. Reassurance, weight reduction, dietary advice and stopping smoking will alone control symptoms in many patients. Advice on correct posture when lifting and on elevating the head of the bed at night, may also be required.

Most patients will respond to an antacid/alginate preparation taken after meals and at bedtime. An antacid preparation can also be given 1–3 hours after meals if symptoms persist. If this fails, metoclopramide or domperidone should be used. At this stage more intensive investigation, such as endoscopy, should be considered. If endoscopy reveals severe inflammation, an ulcer or stricture then an H_2-receptor antagonist or carbenoxolone should be given.

When progress is good the treatment can be simplified by omitting the antacids between meals and lowering the bed head. It is wise to continue the antacid/alginate preparation while metoclopramide is gradually withdrawn.

If this approach to treatment fails it may be necessary to admit the patient for a period of intensive medical therapy, because in hospital the patient is more likely to comply with the doctor's advice and treatment. After relief experienced in hospital a patient is more likely to co-operate as an outpatient.

Surgical treatment should only be considered, in an uncomplicated patient, after all the above measures have failed and if severe symptoms persist that seriously interfere with the patient's life (see Chapter 12).

Treatment of complications

The complications of reflux oesophagitis include bleeding, stricture and Barrett's oesophagus. All are relative indications for surgery in the younger patient. In the elderly, bleeding and Barrett's epithelium should be treated with aggressive medical therapy using histamine H_2-receptor antagonists, metoclopramide or domperidone, and antacid or alginate/antacid preparations.

Strictures demand other measures. There is now little justification for rigid oesophagoscopy and bouginage. Modern fibreoptic instruments result in far fewer complications and allow dilatation to be done under sedation, with diazepam and pethidine, as

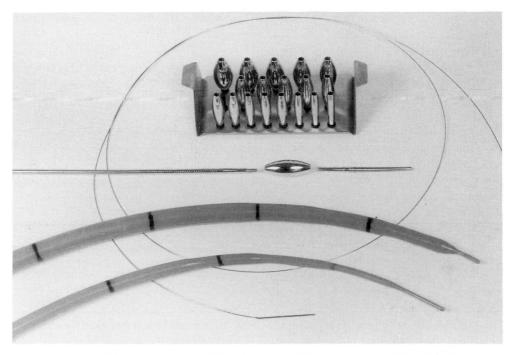

Fig. 11.5. Photograph of Eder-Peustow (top) and Celestin graduated dilators (bottom) with flexible guide-wire as used for endoscopic dilatation.

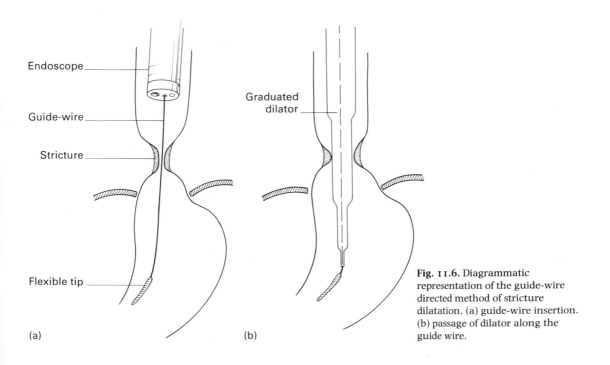

Endoscope

Guide-wire

Stricture

Flexible tip

(a)

Graduated dilator

(b)

Fig. 11.6. Diagrammatic representation of the guide-wire directed method of stricture dilatation. (a) guide-wire insertion. (b) passage of dilator along the guide wire.

an out-patient procedure in most patients.

Various dilators are available (Fig. 11.5) but two main techniques are in widespread use. The first, and most popular, is the use of a railroad technique for the insertion of graded dilators. A guide-wire is inserted at endoscopy and the dilator (Eder-Peustow: Celestin) is passed through the stricture using this 'rail' (Fig. 11.6). Perforation occurs in less than 1% of patients [58, 66, 75] and permanent relief of dysphagia is achieved in 50% of the patients who continue on medical treatment. This technique is easy to perform and is the preferred treatment for a newly diagnosed stricture. Which of these dilators is best remains controversial although two studies have suggested that the Celestin dilator is best for routine use [1, 38].

The second dilatation technique used is to get the patients to swallow a mercury-weighted, tapered rubber bougie after an initial endoscopic dilatation (Maloney bougie). Stoddard and Simms [66] have recently reported 534 dilatation performed in 109 patients using this dilator in the out-patients department without any sedation. There were no serious complications or perforations in this series. Another advantage of this technique is that, with suitable training, the patient can be taught to pass it on him or herself. This avoids the need for hospital admission completely and the patient can then continue this at home as long as is necessary. This method is probably the best one for a rapidly recurrent stricture.

References

1 ASTE H, MUNIZZI F, SACCOMANNO S, PUGLIESE V. Splitting and stretching dilatation of esophageal strictures. *Endoscopy* 1983;15:41–43.
2 ATKINSON M. Diseases of the digestive system. Hiatus hernia. *Br Med J* 1967;4:218–221.
3 ATKINSON M, EDWARDS DAW, HONOUR AJ. The oesophagogastric sphincter in hiatus hernia. *Lancet* 1957;2:1138–1142.
4 BARISH CF, WU WC, CASTELL DO. Respiratory complications of gastroesophageal reflux. *Arch Intern Med* 1985;145:1882–1888.
5 BARNADO DE, LANCASTER-SMITH M, STRICKLAND ID, WRIGHT JT. A double-blind controlled trial of Gaviscon in patients with symptomatic gastro-oesophageal reflux. *Curr Med Res Opin* 1975;3:388–391.
6 BEELEY M, WARNER JO. Medical treatment of symptomatic hiatus hernia with low density compounds. *Curr Med Res Opin* 1972;1:63–69.
7 BEHAR J, SHEANAN DC. Histologic abnormalities in reflux esophagitis, *Arch Pathol* 1975;99:387–391.
8 BENNET JR, MARTIN HD, BUCKTON G. Cimetidine in reflux oesophagitis. Hepatogastroenterology: *International Congress of Gastroenterology* 1980; 27 Suppl. Abstract XI: 30.
9 BERNSTEIN A, TEMPLE JG. Gastro-oesophageal reflux and bronchial asthma relationship? In: Baron JH, ed. *Cimetidine in the 80's*. Edinburgh: Churchill Livingstone, 1981:167–171.
10 BERSTAD A. Overview of ranitidine in reflux oesophagitis: its effect on symptoms, endoscopic appearance and histology. In: Misiewicz JJ, Wormsley, G eds. *The clinical use of Ranitidine*. Oxford: The Medicine Publishing Foundation, 1982: 297–304.
11 BOOTH DJ, KERNMERER WT, SKINNER DB. Acid clearing from the distal esophagus. *Arch Surg* 1968;96:731–734.
12 BOZYMSKI EM, HERLIHY KJ, ORLANDO RC. Barrett's esophagus. *Ann Intern Med* 1982;97:103–107.
13 BRAND DL, YLVISAKER JJ, GELFAND M, et al. Regression of columnar esophageal (Barrett's) epithelium after anti-reflux surgery. *N Engl J Med* 1980; 302:844–848.
14 BREMNER CG. Courses and prognosis. In: Truelove, SL, Ritchie, JA, eds. *Topics in Gastroenterology*. London: Blackwell Scientific Publications, 1976: 127–146.
15 BRIGHT-ASARE P, EL BASSOUSSI M. Cimetidine, metoclopramide or placebo in the treatment of symptomatic gastro-eosophageal reflux. *J Clin Gastroenterol* 1980;2:149–156.
16 CAMERON AJ, OTT BJ, PAYNE WS. The incidence of adenocarcinoma in columnar-lined (Barrett's) esophagus. *New Engl J Med* 1985;313:857–859.
17 CASTELL DO. Medical therapy for reflux esophagitis: 1986 and beyond. *Ann Intern Med* 1986;104: 112–114.
18 CASTELL DO, LEVINE SM. Lower esophageal sphincter response to gastric alkalinisation. A new mechanism for treatment of heartburn with antacids. *Ann Int Med* 1971;74:223–237.
19 COHEN S. Pathogenesis of coffee induced gastrointestinal symptoms. *N Engl J Med* 1980;303: 122–124.
20 DAVIES HA, JONES DB, RHODES J. 'Oesophageal angina' as the cause of chest pain. *JAMA* 1982; 248:2274–2278.

21 DE CAESTECKER JS, BLACKWELL JN, BROWN J, HEADING RC. The oesophagus as a cause of recurrent chest pain: which patients should be investigated and which tests should be used? *Lancet* 1985;ii:1143–1146.

22 DEMEESTER TR, SULLIVAN GO, BERMUDEZ G, MIDELL AI, CIMOCHOWSKI GE, O'DROBINAK J. Esophageal function in patients with angina type pain and normal coronary angiograms. *Ann Surg* 1982;196:488–498.

23 DENNISH HGW, CASTELL DO. Inhibitory effect of smoking on the lower esophageal sphincter. *N Engl J Med* 1971;284:1136–1137.

24 DILAWARI JB, MISIEWICZ JJ. Does oral metoclopramide increase cardiac sphincter pressure? *Gut* 1972;13:856.

25 DODDS WJ, DENT J, HODAN WJ et al. Mechanisms of gastro-esophageal reflux in patients with reflux esophagitis. *N Engl J Med* 1982;307:1547–1552.

26 DYER NH, PRIDIE RB. Incidence of hiatus hernia in asymptomatic subjects. *Gut* 1968;9:696–699.

27 FARRELL RL, ROLING GT, CASTELL DO. Cholinergic therapy of chronic heartburn. *Ann Intern Med* 1974;8:573–576.

28 FERGUSON R, DRONFIELD MW, ATKINSON M. Cimetidine in treatment of reflux oesophagitis with stricture. *Br Med J* 1979;2:472–474.

29 GOLDBERG HI, DODDS WJ, GEE S, MONTGOMERY C, ZBORALSKI FF. Role of acid and pepsin in acute experimental esophagitis. *Gastroenterology* 1969;56:223–230.

30 GOY JA, MAYNARD JH, MCNAUGHTON WM, O'SHEA A. Ranitidine and placebo in the treatment of reflux oesophagitis. *Med J Australia* 1983;2:558–561.

31 GRAHAM DY, LANZA F, DORSCH ER. Symptomatic reflux oesophagitis: a double blind comparison of antacids and alginate. *Curr Ther Res* 1977;22:653–658.

32 HAGUE AK, MERKEL M. Total columnar lined esophagus: a case for congenital origin. *Arch Pathol Lab Med* 1981;105:546–548.

33 HELLER SR, FELLOWS IW, OGILVIE AL, ATKINSON M. Non-steroidal anti-inflammatory drugs and benign oesophageal stricture. *Br Med J* 1982;285:167–168.

34 HELM JF, DODDS WJ, PELC LR, PALMER DW, HOGAN WJ, TEETER PC. Effect of esophageal emptying and saliva on clearance of acid from the esophagus. *New Engl J Med* 1984; 284–287.

35 HENNESSEY TPJ. Barrett's oesophagus. *Br J Surg* 1985;72:336–340.

36 HERLHY KJ, ORLANDO RC, BRYSON JC, BOZYMSKI EM, CARNEY N, POWELL DW. Barrett's esophagus: Clinical, endoscopic, histologic, manometric and electrical potential difference characteristics. *Gastroenterology* 1984:86:436–443.

37 HIGGS RH, SMITH RD, CASTELL DD. Gastric alkalinisation: effect on lower esophageal sphincter pressure and serum gastrin. *N Engl J Med* 1974;291:486–490.

38 HINE KR, HAWKEY CJ, ATKINSON M, HOLMES GKT. Comparison of the Eder-Peustow and Celestin techniques for dilating benign oesophageal strictures. *Gut* 1984;25:1100–1102.

39 HINE KR, HOLMES GKT, MELIKIAN V, LOUEI M, FAIRCLOUGH PD. Ranitidine in reflux oesophagitis. *Digestion* 1984;29:119–123.

40 HOGAN WJ, VIEGAS DE ANDRADE SR, WINSHIP DH. Ethanol induced acute oesophageal motor dysfunction. *J Appl Physiol* 1972;32:755–760.

41 ISMAIL-BEIGI F, HORTON PP, POPE CE. Histological consequences of gastro-esophageal reflux in man. *Gastroenterology* 1970;58:163–174.

42 JOELSSON PE, DEMEESTER TR, SKINNER DB, LAFONTAINE E, WATERS PE, O'SULLIVAN GC. The role of the esophageal body in the anti-reflux mechanism. *Surgery* 1982;92:417–424.

43 KALISH RJ, CLANCY PE, ORRINGER MB, APPLEMAN HD. Clinical, epidemiologic and morphologic comparisons between adenocarcinoma arising in Barrett's esophageal mucosa and in the gastric cardia. *Gastroenterology* 1984;86:461–467.

44 KEENAN RA, HUNT RH, VINCENT D, WRIGHT B, MILTON-THOMPSON GJ. The case for high dose antacid therapy in duodenal ulcer. *Gut* 1978; 19:A974.

45 KOTHARI T, MANGLA IC, KALRA TMS. Barrett's ulcer and treatment with cimetidine. *Arch Int Med* 1980;140:475–477.

46 LARRAIN A, CARRASCO J, GALLEQUILLOS J, POPE CE. Reflux treatment improves lung function in patients with intrinsic asthma. *Gastroenterology* 1981;80:1204.

47 LEADER. Management of gastro-oesophageal reflux. *Lancet* 1984;1054–1055.

48 LEADER. Gastric asthma? *Lancet* 1985;ii:1399–400.

49 LEADER. Angina and oesophageal disease. *Lancet* 1986;ii:191–192.

50 LIEBERMAN DA, KEEFFE EB. Treatment of severe reflux esophagitis with cimetidine and metoclopramide. *Ann Inter Med* 1986;104:21–26.

51 MCCALLUM RW, IPPOLITI AF, COONEY C, STURDEVANT RAL. A controlled trial of metoclopramide in symptomatic gastro-esophageal reflux. *N Engl J Med* 1977;296:354–357.

52 MCCALLUM RW, MENSH R, LANGE R. Definition of the gastric emptying abnormality present in gastro-esophageal reflux patients. *Gastroenterology* 1981;80:1226.

53 MCCLUSKIE RA, BARDHAN KD, SAUL DM, DUTHIE HL, GREANEY MB, IRVIN TP. Cimetidine in the treatment of oesophagitis. In: Burland, WL, Simkins, MA, eds. *Cimetidine.* Amsterdam Oxford: Excerpta Medica, 1977:297–304.

54 MCHARDY G. A multicentre randomised clinical trial of Gaviscon in reflux. *South Med J* 1978;71:16–21.

55 MADERN GJ, CHATTERTON BE, COLLINS PJ, HOROWITZ
    M, SHEARMAN DJC, JAMIESON GC. Solid and liquid
    gastric emptying in patients with gastro-oeso-
    phageal reflux. *Br J Surg* 1985;**72**:344–347.

56 NAFF AP, SAVERY M, OZZELLO L. Columnar-lined
    lower esophagus. An acquired lesion with malig-
    nant predisposition. Report on 140 cases of Bar-
    rett's esophagus with 12 adenocarcinomas.
    J Thor Cardiovasc Surg 1975;**70**:826–835.

57 NEBEL OT, FARNES MF, CASTELLO DO. Symptomatic
    gastro-esophageal reflux: Incidence and predispos-
    ing factors. *Dig Dis* 1972;**17**:993–996.

58 OGILVIE AL, FERGUSON R, ATKINSON M. Outlook
    with conservative treatment of peptic oesophageal
    stricture. *Gut* 1980;**21**:23–25.

59 OLSEN AM, SCHENGEL JF. Motility disturbances
    caused by esophagitis. *J Thor Cardiovasc Surg*
    1965;**50**:607–612.

60 ORME ME, TALLIS RC. Metoclopramide and tardive
    dyskinesia in the elderly. *Br Med J* 1984;**289**:
    397–398.

61 PAULL A, KERR GRANT A. A controlled trial of me-
    toclopramide in reflux oesophagitis. *Med J Aust*
    1974;**2**:627–629.

62 PAULL A, TRIER JS, DALTON MD, CAMP RC, LOEB P,
    GOYAL RK. The histologic spectrum of Barrett's
    esophagus. *N Engl J Med* 1976;**295**:476–480.

63 PETERMANS W, VANTRAPPEN G. Oesophageal dis-
    ease in the elderly. *Clin Gastroenterol* 1985;
    14:635–656.

64 PETROKUBI RJ, JEFFRIES GH. Cimetidine versus ant-
    acid in scleroderma with reflux oesophagitis. *Gas-
    troenterology* 1979;**77**:691–695.

65 PETROKUBI RJ, JEFFRIES EH. Chronic cimetidine
    therapy for reflux oesophagitis in scleroderma.
    Gastroenterology 1980;**78**:1236.

66 PRICE JD, STANCIU C, BENNETT JR. A safe method
    for dilating oesophageal strictures. *Lancet*
    1974;**1**:1141–1142.

67 PRICE SF, SMITHSON KW, CASTELL DO. Food sensi-
    tivity in reflux esophagitis. *Gastroenterology*
    1978;**2**:919–920.

68 RASMUSSEN K, RAVENSBAEK J, FUNCH-JENSEN P,
    BAGGER JP. Oesophageal spasm in patients with
    coronary artery spasm *Lancet* 1986;**i**:174–176.

69 REED PI, DAVIES WA. Controlled trial of a carben-
    oxolone/alginate antacid combination in reflux
    oesophagitis. *Curr Med Res Opin* 1978;**5**:637–644.

70 RICHTER JE, CASTELL DO. Gastroesophageal reflux.
    Pathogenesis, diagnosis and therapy. (Review)
    Ann Intern Med 1982;**97**:93–103.

71 SCHATZKI R, GARY JE. Lower oesophageal ring.
    Amer J Radiol 1956;**75**:246.

72 SCHWEITZER EJ, BASS BL, JOHNSON LF, HARMON JW.
    Sucralfate prevents experimental peptic esophagitis
    in rabbits. *Gastroenterology* 1985; **88**:611–619.

73 SCOBIE BA. Endoscopically controlled trial of algin-
    ate and antacid in reflux esophagitis. *Med J Austral*
    1976;**1**:627–628.

74 SHERBANIUK R, WENSEL R, BAILEY R *et al*. Raniti-
    dine in the treatment of symptomatic gastro-
    esophageal reflux disease. *J Clin Gastroenterol*
    1984;**6**:9–15.

75 SILVIS SE, NEBEL O, ROGERS G, SAGAURA C, MAN-
    DELSTORN. Endoscopic complications: Results of the
    1974 American Society for Gastrointestinal endos-
    copy survey. *JAMA* 1976;**235**:928–930.

76 SLADEN GE, RIDDELL RH, WILLOUGHBY JMT. Oeso-
    phagoscopy, biopsy and acid perfusion test in
    diagnosis of 'Reflux Oesophagitis'. *Br Med J* 1975;
    1:71.

77 SMOUT AJPM, BOGAARD JW, VAN HATTUM J, AKKER-
    MANS LMA. Effects of cimetidine and ranitidine on
    interdigestive and postprandial lower esophageal
    sphincter pressures and plasma gastrin levels
    in normal subjects. *Gastroenterology* 1985;**88**:
    557–63.

78 SONTAG SJ, SCHNELL TG, CHEJFAC G, *et al*. Barrett's
    oesophagus and colonic tumours. *Lancet* 1985;
    i:946–948.

79 SPENCE RAJ, COLLINS BJ, PARKS TG, LOVE AHG.
    Does age influence normal gastro-oesophageal
    reflux. *Gut* 1985;**26**:799–801.

80 STANCIU C, BENNETT JR. Alginate/anatacid in the
    reduction of gastro-oesophageal reflux. *Lancet*
    1974;**1**:109–111.

81 STODDART CJ, SIMMS JM. Dilatation of benign oeso-
    phageal strictures in the out-patient department.
    Br J Surg 1984;**71**:752–753.

82 THANIK KD, CHEY WY, SHAH AS. GUTIERREZ JG.
    Reflux esophagitis: effect of oral bethanecol on
    symptoms and endoscopic findings. *Ann Int Med*
    1980;**93**:805–808.

83 THURNER RL, DEMEESTER TF, JOHNSON LF. Distal
    esophageal sphincter and its relationship to
    gastro-esophageal reflux. *J Surg Res* 1974;**16**:
    418–426.

84 TYTGAT GMJ. Assessment and efficacy of cimetidine
    and other drugs in oesophageal reflux disease. In:
    Baron, JH, ed. *Cimetidine in the 80's*. Edinburgh:
    Churchill Livingstone, 1981:153–166.

85 VALENZUELA JE, MIRANDA M, ANSARI AN, LIM BR.
    Delayed gastric emptying in patients with reflux
    esophagitis. *Gastroenterology* 1981;**80**:1307.

86 VANSANT JH. Surgical management of hiatus her-
    nia with oesophageal reflux. *Am J Surg* 1978;
    44:179.

87 VENABLES CW, BELL D, ECCLESTON D. A double blind
    study of metoclopramide in symptomatic peptic
    oesophagitis. *Postgrad Med J [Suppl 4]* 1973:
    49:73–76.

88 WASHER GF, GEAR MWL, DOWLING BL, *et al*. Ran-
    domised prospective trial of Roux-en-Y duodenal
    diversion versus fundoplication for severe reflux
    oesophagitis. *Br J Surg* 1984;**71**:181–184.

89 WEINSTEIN WM, BOGOCH ER, BOWES FL. The normal
    human esophageal mucosa: a histological reap-
    praisal. *Gastroenterology* 1975;**68**:40–44.

90 WEISS W, BRUNNER H, BUTTNER GR *et al.* Treatment of reflux oesophagitis with sucralfate. *Dtsch Med Wochenschr* 1983;108:1706–1711.

91 WESDORP ICE, DEKKER W, KLINGENBERG-KNOL EC. Treatment of reflux oesophagitis with ranitidine. *Gut* 1983;24:921–924.

Chapter 12
Surgery for Gastro-Oesophageal Reflux

J.G. TEMPLE

There are two main indications for operation in gastro-oesophageal reflux—failure of medical treatment or a complication of oesophagitis (Table 12.1).

Table 12.1. Gastro-oesophageal reflux—indications for operation.

Failure of medical treatment	Intractability
Complications	Stricture
	Haemorrhage
	Respiratory problems

Indications

Failure of medical treatment

This is the commonest reason for operation, accounting for 85–92% of cases [32,55]. A strict and carefully supervised medical regimen should be tried initially; only when this has failed can intractability be accepted, that is to say when symptoms prevent an individual from leading a normal life [32]. This is therefore a very subjective decision depending upon the clinician's persistence and the patient's resilience [21]. Conventional medical treatment provides symptomatic relief in about 60% of cases [12], but has little objective effect on oesophageal function even after 12 months [5]. Recent experience with histamine H_2-receptor antagonists has not greatly increased the proportion of patients who remain free from serious symptoms [66]. A balance must therefore be struck between too early referral for operation and too prolonged perseverance with medical

treatment (see Chapter 11). This creates a strong case for joint management of the patient between physicians and surgeons.

Complications

Peptic stricture

A peptic stricture develops when reflux is inadequately controlled and is the indication for operation in 3–14% of those coming to surgery for reflux oesophagitis [31, 55].

Two types of stricture occur (Fig. 12.1)—either a short 'annular stricture' situated at the cardio-oesophageal mucosal junction, involving mainly mucosa and submucosa or a 'longitudinal stricture' extending from the cardio-oesophageal mucosal junction for a considerable distance up the oesophagus, sometimes as high as the aortic arch. The longitudinal stricture is often associated with a columnar lined Barrett's oesophagus (see Chapter 11).

Haemorrhage

Severe bleeding is a rare complication of reflux oesophagitis and usually occurs as a result of a penetrating ulcer in the oesophageal wall. Emergency surgery may rarely be needed to control this haemorrhage.

More often reflux oesophagitis leads to chronic blood loss and iron deficiency anaemia. This can continue even when good symptomatic control is achieved on medical therapy [67]. Persistent anaemia has been

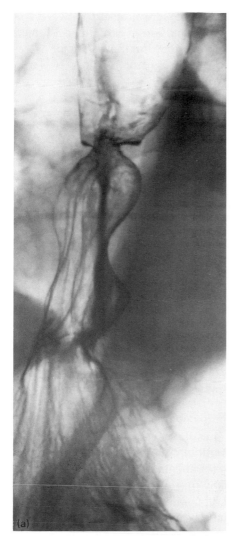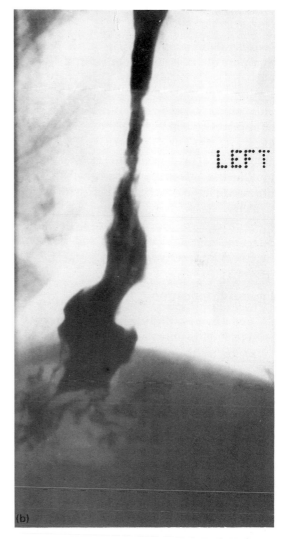

Fig. 12.1. Types of oesophageal stricture. (a) Short annular stricture; (b) Longitudinal stricture.

suggested as an indication for surgery, although many would disagree with this. All other causes of occult gastrointestinal bleeding must be excluded before recommending surgery for oesophagitis-induced anaemia (see Chapter 32).

Respiratory complications

Around 20–50% of patients with reflux may have significant respiratory problems [32, 67] due to repeated aspiration [41], sometimes leading to pulmonary fibrosis. A link between maturity onset asthma and gastro-oesophageal reflux has also been postulated [17, 50]. Although effective reflux control by medical [25] or surgical means [14, 67] improves asthmatic symptoms in such patients, improvement is not entirely explained by overspill into the bronchial tree.

Criteria for operation

Considerable variations occur in the interpretation of these indications for surgery, with operation rates varying from 10% [56] to 60% [1, 67] of all patients referred with reflux oesophagitis. Stricter criteria for operation can be defined by using additional objective evidence such as the endoscopic appearance of the oesophagitis, manometric findings, measurements of intra-oesophageal pH and Bernstein acid perfusion tests (see Chapter 9). Such selection criteria should ensure better and longer lasting surgical results and remove the risk of unnecessary surgery.

Types of operation

An effective operation for gastro-oesophageal reflux must correct any underlying cause, be technically simple and reproducible in different surgeons' hands and have a low morbidity, recurrence rate and mortality.

It is generally believed that the principal cause of reflux is incompetence of the lower oesophageal sphincter and that this does not depend on the position of the sphincter relative to the diaphragm (see Chapter 11). While a sliding hiatus hernia is often associated with reflux, it may be absent in 30% of patients with gastro-oesophageal reflux [12]. The aim of surgery, therefore, must be to create a high pressure zone which can maintain a pressure gradient between the intra-gastric and lower oesophageal lumen [5]. Whether tone in the sphincter is restored [32] or a predominantly one-way valve mechanism is created by the operation [14] remains unclear.

The operations used to correct reflux are listed in Table 12.2.

Anatomical repair

The Allison repair

Allison believed that restoration of a normal anatomical arrangement of the oesophago-gastric junction below the diaphragm would prevent reflux [1].

Using a thoracic approach the junction zone is mobilized, reducing any hiatus hernia that is present, and it is fixed in place by suturing the phreno-oesophageal ligament to the under surface of the diaphragm [1]. The crura are then sutured behind the oesophagus to narrow the hiatus (Fig. 12.2).

This operation corrects the hiatal hernia but ignores the physiological basis of reflux. Allison initially reported relief of symptoms in 82% of patients with a mortality of 0.3%, but follow-up results over a 20-year period were disappointing (Table 12.3) [2]. Similar data have been reported by other workers [43, 67] although their recurrence rates were lower because of shorter follow-up intervals.

Table 12.2. Operations for gastro-oesophageal reflux.

Anatomical repairs	Allison repair
	Boerema repair
Acid-decreasing operations	Truncal vagotomy and drainage
	Proximal gastric vagotomy
Anti-reflux operations	Nissen fundoplication
	Partial fundoplication
	Belsey mark IV operation
	Hill median arcuate repair
	Angelchik anti-reflux prosthesis

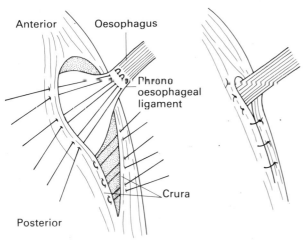

Anterior   Oesophagus

Phrono
oesophageal
ligament

Crura

Posterior

(a) Site of sutures   (b) After repair

Fig. 12.2. Technique of Allison repair, illustrated from above the diaphagm.

Table 12.3. Results of Allison repair. Twenty-year retrospective review; 374 patients.

	X-ray	No.	%
Symptom free	No hiatus hernia	47	12.6 } 24
	Hiatus hernia	43	11.4
Recurrent symptoms	No hiatus hernia	86	23 } 76
	Hiatus hernia	196	53

Gastropexy (Boerema's operation)

This operation differs fundamentally from most other procedures designed to prevent reflux as there is no attempt to create a valve mechanism.

An abdominal approach is used—any hiatus hernia present is reduced and the oesophagogastric junction is fixed by suturing 5 cm of the upper lesser curve of the stomach to the anterior abdominal wall under tension (Fig. 12.3). This is the crucial part of the operation [11] as it recreates a segment of intra-abdominal oesophagus. The crura are usually repaired posteriorly, although this is not essential [42].

Boerema reported a 1% mortality and 5% recurrence of hiatus hernia in 100 patients treated by this procedure. Others have not been able to confirm these good results (Table 12.4), and its use remains limited [20, 42].

Table 12.4. Results of gastropexy.

Reference	No.	Recurrent hiatus hernia %	Recurrent symptoms %
MAGAREY (1972) [42]	37	33	64
DE LAER & SPITZ (1983) [20]	50	42	62

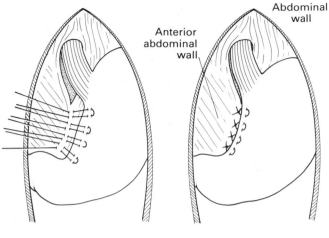

(a) Site of sutures   (b) After ligation   **Fig. 12.3.** Technique of Boerema's
   to anterior   of sutures   anterior gastropexy showing
   abdominal wall   suturing to inner surface of
                                                       anterior abdominal wall.

Acid-decreasing procedures

Berman and Berman [9] believed that a 'balanced procedure' for gastro-oesophageal reflux and hiatus hernia should include prevention of reflux (hiatal hernia repair), a decrease in gastric secretion (truncal vagotomy) and the promotion of gastric emptying (drainage procedure).

Pearson [52] has convincingly demonstrated that there is no place for this approach. In fact, those patients who underwent vagotomy and drainage with a hiatal hernia repair had more postoperative complications, related to the vagotomy,

than those who had an hiatal hernia repair alone (Table 12.5). Similar poor results have been reported by other groups [13, 23, 73].

Recently it has been suggested that proximal gastric vagotomy should be used as an adjunct in the control of gastro-oesophageal reflux [4, 34]. This type of selective vagotomy has the advantage of reducing the risk of dumping and diarrhoea but may increase the risk of lesser curve necrosis [36].

Vagotomy is only indicated, therefore, if there is a concurrent duodenal ulcer, if the nerves are damaged during mobilization of the oesophagus, or if it is required to help lengthen a shortened oesophagus [52].

Table 12.5. Results of acid-decreasing procedures [48].

	Hiatus hernia repair + Truncal vagotomy and drainage	Hiatus hernia repair
	No. = 87 %	No. = 50 %
Recurrent reflux	8	6
Post-vagotomy diarrhoea	27	2
Dumping	17.5	0

Anti-reflux procedures

The Nissen fundoplication

This operation is usually performed through an abdominal approach—the lower oesophagus is mobilized and any associated hiatus hernia is reduced. After mobilization of the upper part of the greater curve of the stomach the fundus is wrapped around the gastro-oesophageal junction and the lower 3–4 cm of oesophagus.

There are two ways in which this fundoplication may be constructed. In the classical method [48] the walls of the gastric fundus are anchored anteriorly with non-absorbable sutures passed through the muscle layer of the oesophagus (Fig. 12.4)—vagal nerve damage is a potential hazard of this technique. Rossetti's modification [57] avoids these anchoring stitches by simply wrapping the fundus loosely around the lower oesophagus (Fig. 12.5).

In the classical technique a 50 FG bougie is passed through the cardio-oesophageal junction to prevent excessive narrowing. This is also advisable when a 'floppy fundoplication' is fashioned. An important technical point is that tension on the repair must be avoided. This is achieved by adequate mobilization of the fundus. A plication 3–4 cm in length is generally sufficient and no crural narrowing is required as the bulky, loose, plication will remain '*in situ*' if adequate mobilization has been performed.

Fundoplication provides a substitute for an inadequate sphincter by compressing the lower oesophagus when intra-gastric pressure increases. This new high pressure zone maintains a pressure gradient against changing intra-gastric pressures sufficient to prevent gastro-oesophageal reflux under most physiological conditions [5]. The Nissen procedure is safe, with a mortality rate of less than 1% in experienced hands [52, 57]. It is the most certain procedure for preventing reflux, but has a higher incidence of unwanted effects than other anti-reflux operations [73]. A major advantage is that it can be done by either the abdominal or the trans-thoracic route [45].

Partial fundoplication

In this procedure the fundus is only wrapped around the anterior surface of the oesophagus. The rationale of a partial

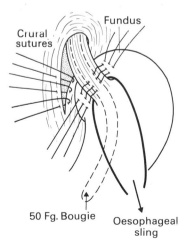

50 Fg. Bougie   Oesophageal sling

(a) Suture placement

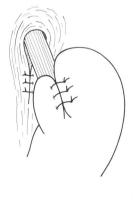

(b) After

Fig. 12.4. Technique for abdominal Nissen fundoplication showing sutures passing through the oesophageal wall and between the crura.

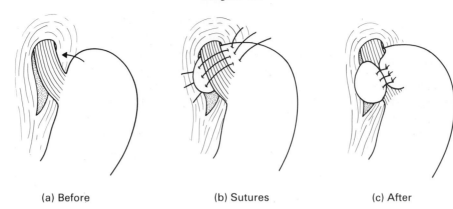

(a) Before   (b) Sutures   (c) After

Fig. 12.5. Demonstration of the 'floppy' type of Nissen fundoplication from below the diaphragm. Note the absence of crural sutures.

fundoplication is that it achieves as good control of reflux as does the full procedure, but the patient is still able to belch or vomit. It is usually recommended that it be combined with a crural repair and suturing of the stomach to the undersurface of the diaphragm—this suggests that partial fundoplication may not achieve complete control of reflux [27]. Long-term results of partial fundoplication are lacking, so full evaluation is impossible.

The Belsey mark IV repair

This is performed through a left thoracotomy. The distal oesophagus is mobilized with reduction of any associated hiatus hernia. A 240° fundoplication is then performed (Fig. 12.6) which creates a high pressure zone similar to that in the Nissen repair. This incomplete wrap allows belching and vomiting to occur normally, which Belsey believes is to be a fundamental prop-

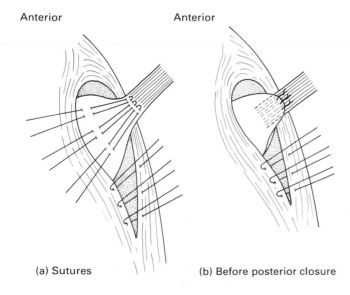

Anterior   Anterior

(a) Sutures   (b) Before posterior closure

Fig. 12.6. Technique for the transthoracic Belsey Mark IV repair, shown from above diaphragm.

erty of an acceptable anti-reflux operation [6]. An important part of the procedure is closure of the crura behind the oesophagus, which creates a posterior buttress. This should not be made too tight. The Belsey mark IV repair is a safe operation with a 1.2% mortality [19] but it does require a trans-thoracic approach.

The Hill posterior gastropexy repair

This was first described in 1961 [30]. It is based on the concept that symptoms are due entirely to the gastro-oesophageal reflux and that few hiatal herniae are incarcerated in the chest. The operation is performed using an abdominal approach. After mobilization of the oesophagus, the crura are approximated posteriorly and the oesophagogastric junction is then sutured to the medial arcuate ligament (Fig. 12.7). This can be difficult in an obese patient and minor modifications have been reported [39, 68]. The operation is, in effect, a posterior gastropexy creating a long segment of intra-abdominal oesophagus which is kept closed by positive intra-abdominal pressure. Inherent in the procedure is a reduction in the size of the cardiac opening, as a suture is passed through the anterior and posterior parts of the oesophago-gastric junction, where the phreno-oesophageal ligament is attached, and then through the medial arcuate ligament. Hill believes that this 'key suture' can only be inserted correctly using intra-operative manometry to create a pressure gradient of 50–55 mmHg across the junction zone. If this pressure is too high dysphagia results and if too low reflux can still occur. Several other imbrication sutures are then inserted from the oesophagogastric junction into the arcuate ligament, causing the anterior and posterior walls of the stomach to overlap the oesophagus. Butterfield [14] showed that both the Nissen and Hill repairs produced similar valvular effects suggesting that the Hill procedure is, in effect, a partial fundoplication [5, 63]. Its success probably depends more on the strong mechanical fixation of the junction zone to the medial arcuate ligament than to the creation of a partial fundoplication.

This procedure has a low mortality rate (0.4%) [32] and early and late complications are uncommon. While others have been unable to quite repeat the excellent results reported by Hill, they remain enthusiastic about it [19, 73].

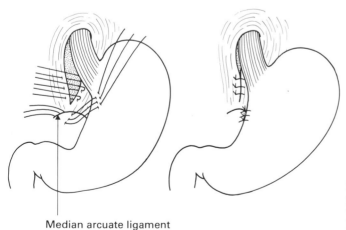

Median arcuate ligament

Fig. 12.7. Technique for the Hill posterior gastropexy with suture through the medial arcuate ligament.

The Angelchik anti-reflux procedure

This novel operation was first described in 1979 [3]. The Angelchik prosthesis is a 'C' shaped silicone elastomer shell filled with silicone gel which is held in place by a polyester reinforced Dacron tape [69]. The prosthesis is inserted through an abdominal approach, after mobilization of the oesophagus and any associated hiatus hernia (Fig. 12.8). Once inserted the prosthesis is tied loosely around the lower oesophagus, allowing space to insert a finger between it and the oesophageal wall. By contrast with other techniques the procedure is simple to perform and shows less variation between individual surgeons.

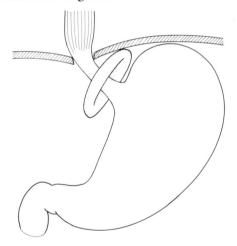

Fig. 12.8. Diagram of the Angelchik prosthesis in position.

The results are good in the short term with approximately 80% of patients relieved of their symptoms [3, 24, 64, 65, 72, 74]. The main problems have been erosion of the device into the gastrointestinal tract, disruption and migration of the prosthesis [8]. Exactly how it works is still unclear. It cannot function as a fundoplication, as it is too loose. In all probability its main action is as a posterior buttress, angulating and stretching the lower oesophagus (Fig. 12.9)

[7]. Much longer follow-up is needed before its place in the management of gastro-oesophageal reflux is established [37, 38, 46].

Results of anti-reflux procedures

It is difficult to compare the results of the various anti-reflux operations since there are very few prospective studies and different criteria and methods have been used to make objective assessments. Pearson *et al.* [53] believe that accurate and meaningful comparisons are virtually impossible. Therefore any operation for gastro-oesophageal reflux is most easily judged in terms of the complications associated with it (Table 12.6).

Table 12.6. Disorders after anti-reflux surgery.

1. Recurrence of gastro-oesophageal reflux

2. Complications of anti-reflux surgery
       perforation
       splenectomy
       transient dysphagia
       gas bloat syndrome
       vagal denervation
       gastric ulcer
       disruption of the repair

Recurrence of reflux

A relatively low incidence of recurrent symptomatic reflux occurs after a Nissen or Belsey repair (Table 12.7). Analysis of several series shows that overall recurrence occurs in 7% of patients after a Nissen and in 10% after a Belsey operation.

There are few long-term reports of the posterior gastropexy procedure. Hill reports a 5% anatomical and a 6% symptomatic recurrence rate in 511 patients. Other studies suggest an overall recurrence rate not dissimilar to that after fundoplication. A finding common to all these procedures is a tendency for recurrence to rise with the duration of follow-up, so long-term results are required when comparing different operations.

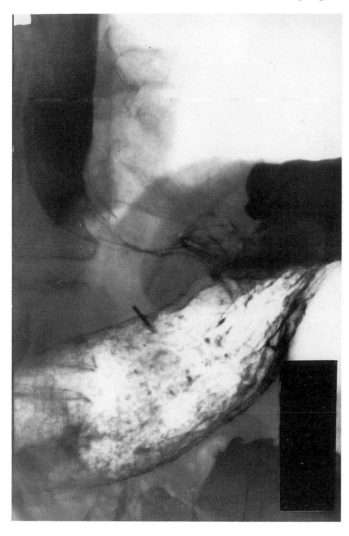

Fig. 12.9. Barium swallow showing the distortion of the lower oesophagus produced by the Angelchik prosthesis.

All the above procedures have lower recurrence rates than those found after anatomical repairs (Table 12.8), confirmed by direct comparison in the same centres [20, 43].

Perforation

This is more likely to occur during a second operation for recurrent gastro-oesophageal reflux, or when a stricture is present. A perforation occurring at the time of surgery is usually easy to recognize and repair. It is advisable to incorporate this repair in the subsequent plication as an added precaution. Late perforation is a rare and grave complication.

Damage to the spleen

During the Nissen and Belsey repairs, mobilization of the upper greater curve of the stomach is important. It is not unusual that during this the spleen may be damaged, resulting in an incidental splenectomy rate of around 7% [55]. As the damage is usually to the capsule, judicious packing should avoid splenectomy in many cases [59].

Table 12.7. Recurrence of gastro-oesophageal reflux.

Reference	*Nissen fundoplication* Symptomatic recurrences %
[73]	8
[70]	6
[57]	11.5
[55]	2
[44]	14
[43]	7.5
[26]	4
[20]	9.6
[27]	7
	Mean 7.7

Reference	*Belsey Mark IV* Symptomatic recurrences %
[62]	10
[67]	7
[49]	12.7
[63]	12
[29]	29.2
	Mean 13.1

Transient dysphagia

Transient dysphagia occurs in some 20% of patients after operations for gastro-oeso-phageal reflux [55]. It usually appears within two weeks of operation and resolves spontaneously within eight weeks. Many surgeons regard it as a feature of a success-ful operation. A dilatation may be required if it persists.

Gas bloat syndrome

Eructation is necessary for the normal relief of excess swallowed air [43]. After anti-reflux procedures the new pressure gradient may exceed the physiological mechanism for releasing air. This has been termed the 'gas bloat syndrome' [73]. Pooled data sug-gest that this occurs in some 12–16% of patients after any anti-reflux operation. For-tunately, it is usually mild and can be avoided by simple dietary measures. The length of the repair is probably crucial—if it exceeds 4 cm gas entrapment appears to be more likely.

Vagal denervation

The main vagal trunks can be damaged by division or stretching during the repair. This should be avoided by careful isolation of the nerves prior to the repair. In an un-complicated case this is usually straight-forward, but in the presence of severe peri-oesophagitis it can be difficult to identify the vagi. Damage will lead to gastric stasis. If this occurs a drainage procedure may be needed later, but the patient may recover normal gastric emptying during treatment with metoclopramide or domperidone (10 mg t.d.s. before meals).

Gastric ulcer

This may occur as a late complication of any operation for reflux, particularly if the vagal nerves are damaged. It occurs most commonly after a Nissen fundoplication—a 2.6–10% incidence [16, 61].

Table 12.8. Comparison of anatomical repair with anti-reflux operation.

	Anatomical repair	Recurrence %	anti-reflux operation	Rec %
[20]	Boerema	43	Nissen	9.6
[43]	Allison	⎰39 Anatomical ⎱18 Symptoms	Nissen	⎰6 Anatomical ⎱7.5 Symptoms

Dehiscence of the repair

The differences in success among various operations may reflect more the relative strengths of the tissues and of the suture materials used than any other factor. The Hill repair relies heavily on strong mechanical fixation of the gastro-oesophageal junction; the Nissen fundoplication depends on the mass of fundus wrapped around the lower oesophagus and the Belsey repair on fixation to the under-surface of the diaphragm. Both the latter operations should be performed without tension, or dehiscence is likely to occur—becoming apparent by the return of reflux symptoms.

Management of peptic strictures

A peptic stricture is a clear indication of severe reflux oesophagitis. It develops as a result of inadequate medical control, neglect by the patient or, rarely, for no apparent reason.

Two types of peptic stricture are recognized: firstly a short annular stricture, in which inflammation is confined to the mucosa and submucosa, usually close to the oesophagogastric junction; and secondly, the less common longitudinal ascending stricture, which signifies extensive transmural involvement and is often associated with a columnar lined, or Barrett's, oesophagus [28]. Malignancy must always be excluded in a stricture by adequate biopsies and brush cytology, as it occurs in up to 17% of patients [40].

The decision whether to treat by regular dilatation or operation is based upon the site and type of stricture, the ease of dilatation and the age and general health of the patient. Intermittent dilatation, using Eder-Peustow or Celestin dilators, is a safe and effective procedure in an elderly or frail patient (see Chapter 11, Fig. 11.5). Conversely, in a younger patient, re-stenosis may be rapid and surgery advisable as it

carries a low risk. Elective surgery becomes necessary in a number of such patients [51, 54], but whenever possible medical and surgical anti-reflux therapy should be aimed at preventing this complication. This is because the mortality of surgery for a stricture is some six times that for an uncomplicated anti-reflux operation [31].

The short (low) oesophageal stricture

Modern surgery for a stricture tends to be conservative in nature, as this has a lower risk. Radical surgery is reserved for those rare patients where dilatation of the stricture is impossible, or previous conservative procedures have failed [12]. In one series [11] these accounted for only 1% of all patients with a stricture. Even the initial tightness of the stricture is no guide to the likely long-term outcome of conservative surgery. Provided the stricture can be widely dilated (up to 50 Fg.), recurrence is less likely and resection is rarely required [51, 63].

The surgical alternatives are outlined in Table 12.9. Many series have demonstrated good results from anti-reflux surgery plus dilatation [11, 28, 33, 51]. Certainly the simplified approach of an anti-reflux operation, with dilatation at the time, is the

Table 12.9. Surgical alternatives for peptic oesophageal stricture.

Conservative
Belsey IV + dilatation
Nissen fundoplication + dilatation
Hill repair + dilatation
Thal stricturoplasty
Thal stricturoplasty + anti-reflux operation
Collis gastroplasty
Collis gastroplasty + anti-reflux operation

Radical
Resection of stricture + gastric replacement
Resection of stricture + jejunal replacement
Resection of stricture + colonic replacement

treatment of choice for all dilatable strictures requiring an operation. Good results with anti-reflux surgery alone for all, except trans-mural strictures, has been reported [45, 47].

The high stricture with a shortened oesophagus

For this type of stricture two different operative procedures are available.

The Thal stricturoplasty + intra-thoracic fundoplication

The Thal stricturoplasty (Fig. 12.10) can widen successfully a strictured oesophagus but, unless combined with an anti-reflux procedure, it increases gastro-oesophageal reflux. An intra-thoracic fundoplication should always be added to this procedure [33, 73]. There are, however, reservations about leaving a fundoplication within the thorax [27].

to be combined with either a Nissen fundoplication or Belsey Type IV repair in order to prevent further reflux—this can produce excellent results in selected patients [27, 53].

Radical surgery for oesophageal stricture

Resection of peptic strictures should be reserved for three indications: first, strictures which cannot be dilated—with the advent of modern flexible endoscopes and guidewire dilatation techniques such strictures are becoming rare (see Chapter 11); second, for strictures that are perforated during operative dilatation; third where conservative surgery fails.

Under these circumstances bowel interposition is preferable to oesophago-gastrectomy as it is associated with a lower operative mortality [6]. An alternative is a Roux-en-Y biliary bypass with antrectomy. This has been reported to give good results

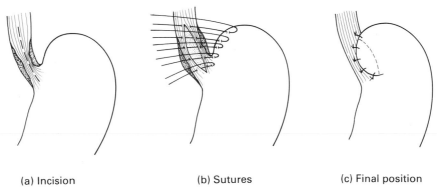

(a) Incision   (b) Sutures   (c) Final position

Fig. 12.10. Diagrammatic representation of the Thal stricturoplasty and fundoplication.

The Collis gastroplasty + anti-reflux operation

The Collis gastroplasty [18] creates a new lower oesophagus by fashioning the upper stomach into a tube (Fig. 12.11). This produces a new oesophago-gastric junction below the diaphragm, but without a sphincter mechanism. This procedure needs

[58, 71] particularly when bile reflux oesophagitis occurs after previous gastric surgery [22].

Management of surgical failures

There are several reasons for surgical failure [6], these include a failure to recognize chronic oesophagitis associated with oeso-

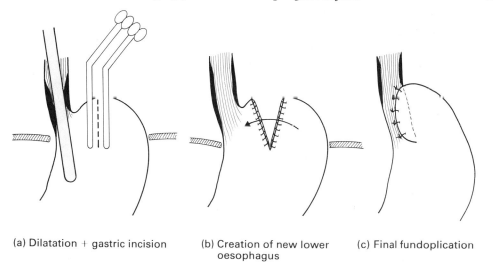

(a) Dilatation + gastric incision (b) Creation of new lower (c) Final fundoplication
oesophagus

Fig. 12.11. Diagram of the technique used to create a longer oesophagus when performing a gastroplasty with fundoplication.

phageal shortening, inexperience of the operator, technical error—the most common being inadequate mobilization and poor selection of patients.

Recurrence after operation for reflux is a difficult management problem. Most authorities recommend re-operation with greater attention to detail. Because mobilization may be difficult, the surgeon and patient must be prepared for a combined thoracoabdominal approach. Here again an antrectomy with Roux-en-Y can be a useful alternative [34, 60], but it should be combined with a truncal vagotomy to prevent stomal ulceration.

Choice of operative approach

Abdominal route

The oesophagogastric junction and lower oesophagus are intra-abdominal organs. The Hill posterior gastropexy can only be performed adequately through an abdominal approach, which is possible in most patients. The Nissen fundoplication seems to function best when it lies below the diaphragm—this is easiest to achieve from the

abdomen. The Angelchik procedure is only appropriate for the abdominal route.

Abdominal exploration also allows correction of any associated intra-abdominal pathology, for example gall stones or peptic ulcer, which can be present in 17–50% of patients [10].

Thoracic route

Mobilization of the lower oesophagus and hiatus hernia, particularly if there is associated peri-oesophagitis or oesophageal shortening, is easier through a thoracic approach. The disadvantage is that it usually precludes correction of any intra-abdominal pathology. The Belsey mark IV and Allison repairs were designed for a thoracic approach. Stricturoplasty and gastroplasty are also exclusively thoracic procedures, as they are only appropriate when oesophageal shortening is present.

The combined thoraco-abdominal approach should be reserved for recurrences, where wide exposure may be needed to guarantee adequate and safe mobilization of the lower oesophagus. It may also be required when a trans-thoracic operation is undertaken in the presence of coincidental biliary or gastric pathology.

Conclusion

For uncomplicated **gastro-oesophageal re-flux** the best operation is probably a Nissen fundoplication performed through an abdominal approach. It has a low mortality and is the most certain cure for reflux, although there is a higher incidence of troublesome sequelae than with other procedures [15, 35]. Many of these can be avoided by attention to technical details, such as adequate mobilization of the greater curve. The Hill posterior gastropexy repair is probably as effective, but is more difficult to do. The Belsey mark IV repair is technically the most exacting, but suffers the disadvantage that a trans-thoracic approach is essential.

When operation for an **oesophageal stric-ture** is necessary an anti-reflux procedure is the treatment of choice if the stricture can be dilated. However, if oesophageal shortening is also present, a Collis gastroplasty plus an anti-reflux procedure seems the best choice.

References

1 ALLISON PR. Reflux oesophagitis, sliding hiatal hernia, and the anatomy of repair. *Surg Gynecol Obstet* 1951;**92**:419–431.
2 ALLISON PR. Hiatus hernia (a 20 year retrospective review). *Ann Surg* 1973;**178**:273–276.
3 ANGELCHIK JP, COHEN R. A new surgical procedure for the treatment of gastro-oesophageal reflux and hiatal hernia. *Surg Gynecol Obstet* 1979;**148**:246–248.
4 BAHADORZADEH K, JORDON PH. Evaluation of the Nissen fundoplication for treatment of hiatal hernia; use of parietal cell vagotomy without drainage as an adjunctive procedure. *Ann Surg* 1975;**181**:402–408.
5 BEHAR J, BIANCANI P, SPIRO HM, STORER EH. Effect of an anterior fundoplication on lower oesophageal sphincter competence. *Gastroenterology* 1974;**67**:209–215.
6 BELSEY R. Mark IV repair of hiatal hernia by the trans-thoracic approach. *World J Surg* 1977;**1**:475–483.
7 BENJAMIN SB, KNUFF TK, FINK M, WOODS E, CASTELL DO. Angelchik anti-reflux prosthesis. Effects on the lower oesophageal sphincter of primates. *Ann Surg* 1983;**197**:63–67.
8 BENJAMIN SB, KERR R, COHEN D, MOTOPARTHY V, CASTELL DO. Complication of the Angelchik prosthesis. *Ann Intern Med* 1984;**100**:570–575.
9 BERMAN JK, BERMAN EJ. Balanced operations for esophagitis associated with esophageal hiatal hernia. *Arch Surg* 1959;**78**:889–896.
10 BIGHAM JA. Hiatus hernia repair combined with the construction of an anti-reflux valve in the stomach. *Br J Surg* 1977;**64**:460–465.
11 BOEREMA I. Repair by right-sided, subhepatic, anterior gastropexy. *Surgery* 1969;**65**:884–893.
12 BOMBECK CT. Invited commentary on gastro-oesophageal reflux without hiatal hernia. *World J Surg* 1977;**1**:450–451.
13 BREMNER CG. Hiatal hernia—Manometric and symptomatic assessment of failed surgical management in 60 patients. *S Afr Med J* 1977;**51**:924–926.
14 BUTTERFIELD WC. Current hiatal hernia repairs; similarities, mechanisms and extended indications—an autopsy study. *Surgery* 1971;**69**:910–916.
15 CARCASSONNE M, GUYS JM, DELARUE A, SARLES J. Surgery of gastroesophageal reflux. *World J Surg* 1985;**9**:269–276.
16 CAMPBELL R, KENNEDY T, JOHNSON GW. Gastric ulceration after Nissen fundoplication. *Br J Surg* 1983;**70**:406–407.
17 CLEMENCON GH, OSTERMAN PO. Hiatal hernia in bronchial asthma—the importance of concomitant pulmonary emphysema. *Gastroenterology* 1961;**95**:110–120.
18 COLLIS JL. Gastroplasty. *Thorax* 1961;**16**:197–206.
19 CSENDES AS, LARRAIN A. Effect of posterior gastropexy on gastroesophageal sphincter pressure and symptomatic reflux in patients with hiatal hernia. *Gastroenterology* 1972;**63**:19–24.
20 DELAET M, SPITZ L. A comparison of Nissen fundoplication and Boerema gastropexy in the surgical treatment of gastro-oesophageal reflux in children. *Br J Surg* 1983;**70**:125–127.
21 EARLAM RJ. Surgical procedures. In: *Clinical tests of oesophageal function*. London: Crosby, Lockwood and Staples, 1976.
22 EARLAM RJ. Bile reflux and the Roux-en-Y anastomosis. *Br J Surg* 1983;**70**:393–397.
23 FRANKLIN RH. Oesophageal surgery. *Ann Roy Coll Surg Engl* 1975;**57**:175–185.
24 GEAR MWL, GILLISON EW, DOWLING BL. Randomised prospective trial of the Angelchik anti-reflux prosthesis. *Br J Surg* 1984;**71**:681–683.
25 GOODALL RJR, EARIS JE, COOPER DN, BERNSTEIN A,

TEMPLE JG. The relationship between asthma and gastro-oesophageal reflux. *Thorax* 1983;**36**:2:116–121.

26 HAVIA T, INBERG MV, AALTO T, *et al.* Hiatal hernia. A follow-up study. *Acta Chir Scand* 1975;**141**:378–384.

27 HENDERSON RD. In: *The oesophagus; reflux and primary motor disorders.* London: Williams & Williams, 1980.

28 HERRINGTON JL JR, WRIGHT RS, EDWARDS WH, SAWYERS JL. Conservative surgical treatment for reflux esophagitis and esophageal stricture. *Ann Surg* 1975;**181**:552–566.

29 HIEBERT CA, O'MARA CS. The Belsey operation for hiatal hernia: a twenty year experience. *Am J Surg* 1979;**137**:532–535.

30 HILL LD, CHAPMAN KW, MORGAN EH. Objective evaluation of surgery for hiatus hernia and esophagitis. *J Thoracic Cardiovasc Surg* 1961;**41**:60–74.

31 HILL LD. Median arcuate repair for hiatus hernia and gastro-oesophageal reflux. In: *Controversy in surgery.* Philadelphia: W.B. Saunders Co., 1976.

32 HILL LD. Progress in the surgical management of hiatal hernia. *World J Surg* 1977;**1**:425–438.

33 HOLLENBECK JI, WOODWARD ER. Treatment of peptic oesophageal stricture with combined fundic patch fundoplication. *Ann Surg* 1975;**182**:472–476.

34 JOHNSON DG. Current thinking on the role of surgery in gastroesophageal reflux. *Pediatr Clin North Am* 1985;**32**:1165–79.

35 JONES NAG, ANDERS CJ. A new approach to the surgical treatment of reflux oesophagitis. *Ann Roy Coll Surg Engl* 1979;**61**:48–50.

36 KENNEDY T, MAGILL P, JOHNSTON GW, PARKES TG. Proximal gastric vagotomy, fundoplication and lesser curve necrosis. *Br Med J* 1979;**1975**.1:1455–1456.

37 KOZAREK RA, PHELPS JE, SANOWSKI RA, GROBE JL, FREDELL CH. An anti-reflux prosthesis in the treatment of gastroesophageal reflux. *Ann Intern Med* 1983;**98**:310–315.

38 LANCET LEADER. The angelchik anti-reflux prosthesis. *Lancet* 1985;**ii**:987.

39 LARRAIN A. Technical considerations in posterior gastropexy. *Surg Gynecol Obstet* 1971;**132**:299–300.

40 LORTAT-JACOB JL. Invited commentary. *World J Surg* 1977;**1**:473.

41 MAYS EE, DUBOIS JJ, HAMILTON GB. Pulmonary fibrosis associated with tracheo-bronchial aspiration. *Chest* 1976;**69**:512–515.

42 MAGAREY CJ. The results of 101 operations for symptomatic hiatus hernia. *Br J Surg* 1972;**59**:432–436.

43 McALHANY JC, THOMAS HF, WOODWARD ER. Gastroesophageal reflux after operative procedures for sliding hiatus hernia. *Am J Surg* 1972;**123**:657–663.

44 MOKKA RE, KAIRALUOMA MI, LARMI TK. Surgical treatment of peptic oesophageal stricture with Nissen fundoplication and intraoperative dilation. *Ann Chir Gynaecol* 1977;**66**:72–75.

45 MOGHISSI K. Intra-thoracic fundoplication for reflux stricture associated with short oesophagus. *Thorax* 1983;**38**:36–40.

46 MORRIS DL, JONES J, EVANS DF, *et al.* Reflux versus dysphagia: an objective evaluation of the Angelchick prosthesis. *Br J Surg* 1985;**72**:1017–1020.

47 NAEF AT, SAVARY M. Conservative operations for peptic oesophagitis with stenosis in columnar lined oesophaguses. *Ann Thorac Surg* 1972;**13**:543.

48 NISSEN R. Eine einfache operation zur benflussung der reflux oesophagitis. *Schweiz Med Wochenschr* 1956;**86**:590–592.

49 ORRINGER MB, SKINNER DB, BELSEY RH. Long-term results of the mark IV operation for hiatal hernia and analyses of recurrences and their treatment. *J Thorac Cardiovasc Surg* 1972;**63**:25–33.

50 OVERHOLT RR, ASHRAF MM. Esophageal reflux as a trigger in asthma. *NY State J Med* 1966;**66**:3030–3032.

51 PAYNE WS. Surgical management of reflux-induced oesophageal stenoses: results in 101 patients. *Br J Surg* 194;**71**:971–973.

52 PEARSON FE, STONE RM, PARRISH RM, FALK RE, DRUCKER WR. Role of vagotomy and pyloroplasty in the therapy of symptomatic hiatus hernia. *Am J Surg* 1969;**117**:132–137.

53 PEARSON FG, HENDERSON RD. Long-term follow-up of peptic strictures managed by dilatation, modified Collis gastroplasty and Belsey hiatus hernia repair. *Surgery* 1976;**80**:396–404.

54 PETERMANS W, VANTRAPPEN G. Oesophageal disease in the elderly. *Clin Gastroenterology* 1985;**14**:635–656.

55 POLK HC JR. Fundoplication for reflux oesophagitis: Misadventures with the operation of choice. *Ann Surg* 1976;**183**:645–652.

56 RAPHAEL HA, ELLIS FH, CARLSON HC, ANDERSON HA. Repair of sliding oesophageal hiatus hernia. *Arch Surg* 1965;**91**:228–232.

57 ROSETTI M, HELL K. Fundoplication for the treatment of gastro-oesophageal reflux in hiatal hernia. *World J Surg* 1977;**1**:439–444.

58 ROYSTON CMS, DOWLING BC, SPENCER J. Roux-en-Y anastomosis in the treatment of peptic oesophagitis with stricture. *Brit J Surg* 1975;**62**:605–607.

59 ROY D. The spleen preserved. *Br Med J* 1984;**289**:70–71.

60 SALO JA, LEMPINEN M, KIVILAAKSO E. Partial gastrectomy with Roux-en-Y reconstruction in the treatment of persistent or recurrent oesophagitis after Nissen fundoplication. *Br J Surg* 1985;**72**:623–625.

61 SIEFERS EC, TAYLOR TL, RICK GG, *et al.* The role of gastrin in the treatment of sliding hiatal hernia with reflux using the reefing method of

fundoplication. *Surg Gynecol Obstet* 1976;**143:**376–380.

62 SINGH SV. Present concept of the Belsey Mark IV procedure in gastro-oesophageal reflux and hiatal hernia. *Br J Surg* 1980;**67:**26–28.

63 SKINNER DB. Complications of surgery for gastro-oesophageal reflux. *World J Surg* 1977;**1:**485–492.

64 STARLING JR, REICHELDERFER MO, PELLET JR, BELZER FO. Treatment of symptomatic gastro-oeso-phageal reflux using the Angelchik prosthesis. *Ann Surg* 1982;**195:**686–691.

65 TEMPLE JG, TAYLOR TV, ALEXANDER-WILLIAMS J. A simple prosthetic treatment for gastro-oesophageal reflux. *J R Coll Surg Edinb* 1983;**26:**16–17.

66 TYTGAT GNJ. Assessment of the efficacy of cimeti-dine and other drugs in oesophageal reflux disease. In: Baron JH, ed. *Cimetidine in the 80's.* London: Churchill Livingstone, 1981.

67 URSCHEL HC, JR, PAULSON DL. Gastro-oesophageal reflux and hiatal hernia. Complications and ther-apy. *J Thorac Cardiovasc Surg* 1967;**53:**21–32.

68 VANSANT JH, BAKER JW, ROSS DG. Modification of the Hill technique for repair of hiatal hernia. *Surg Gynecol Obstet* 1976;**143:**637–642.

69 WALE RJ, ROYSTON CMS, BENNETT JR, BUCKTON GK. Prospective study of the Angelchik anti-reflux pros-thesis. *Br J Surg* 1985;**72:**520–524.

70 WALLS AD, GONZALES JG. The incidence of gas-bloat syndrome and dysphagia following fundopli-cation for hiatus hernia. *J R Coll Surg Edinb* 1977;**22:**391–394.

71 WASHER GF, GEAR MWL, DOWLING BL, GILLISON EW, ROYSTON CMS, SPENCER J. Randomised pro-spective trial of Roux-en-Y duodenal diversion versus fundoplication for severe reflux oesophagi-tis. *Br J Surg* 1984;**71:**181–184.

72 WEAVER KM, TEMPLE JG. The Angelchick prosthesis for gastro-oesophageal reflux: Symptomatic and ob-jective assessment. *Ann Roy Coll Surg Engl* 1985;**67:**299–302.

73 WOODWARD ER. Surgical treatment of gastro-oeso-phageal reflux and its complications. *World J Surg* 1977;**1:**453–461.

74 WYLLIE JH, EDWARDS DAW. A quantitative assess-ment of results with the Angelchick prosthesis. *Ann Roy Coll Surg Engl* 1985;**67:**216–221.

Chapter 13
Oesophageal Carcinoma: Features and Assessment

R.M. KIRK

Oesophageal carcinoma remains a dreaded disease because of its poor prognosis and its effect upon swallowing [2]. There has been an upsurge of interest in this disease over the last few years. An important stimulus has been the success of screening programmes in China and Japan to detect asymptomatic disease and effect surgical 'cures'. This has been achieved with much lower operative mortality rates than those achieved in Western countries. Another stimulus has come from new scanning techniques for assessing the extent of the disease and for monitoring the results of treatment.

Epidemiology

Considerable variation exists in the incidence of this disease in different parts of the world—it ranges from 5 per 100,000 in England and Wales, to 20 in the United States' black population, 25 in France [12, 13], 109 in the Taihang mountains of northern China [10], and 262 in the Caspian littoral of Iran [21]. Incidence also varies quite considerably in adjoining areas, for example the incidence of this tumour rises markedly between Gilan on the west to Mazandaran on the east of the Caspian sea [21]. In Africa there are considerable

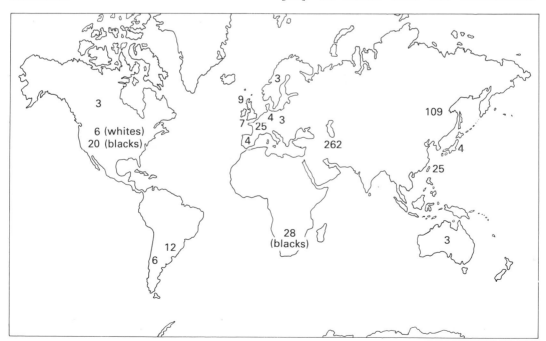

Fig. 13.1. Incidence of oesophageal cancer in different areas of the world recorded as deaths per 100,000 per year.

changes in incidence from one country to another, the highest being found in the Transkei and East Africa [7] where it is some 300 times commoner than in Nigeria [13].

These variations in incidence suggest that environmental factors play a major role in aetiology [9] (Fig. 13.1).

Aetiology

A number of aetiological factors of importance have been suggested [30].

Alcohol

Carcinoma of the oesophagus is commoner in publicans, waiters and brewery workers, and, with the exception of China, high incidence areas are associated with high alcohol intakes [32].

Tobacco

There is convincing evidence of an association between smoking and carcinoma of the oesophagus [34]. Very few patients are lifetime non-smokers.

Occupation

Norell *et al.* [27] have shown that Swedish vulcanization workers have a 10-fold increase in oesophageal cancer compared with matched controls.

Temperature of beverages

It has been suggested that there is a relationship between the temperature at which food and beverages are ingested and carcinoma of the oesophagus [11].

Diet

Considerable work has been undertaken looking at the association between diet and oesophageal carcinoma. A number of factors have been implicated including deficiencies in protein and vitamin intakes [14, 26]; mineral deficiencies in the soil [3]; the ingestion of certain cereal moulds (i.e. *Fusaria*) and the intake of nitrite and nitrosamines. In a recent study in China, in an area of high incidence, it was found that there were 10 times as many particles of silica in the oesophageal mucosa of patients residing in that area compared with the mucosa of controls from London [26]. It was suggested that this originated from dietary millet bran.

Other diseases

These include iron deficiency anaemia (Paterson-Kelly or Plummer-Vinson syndrome) [15] which is associated with cricopharyngeal carcinoma; achalasia of the cardia (see Chapter 10), caustic strictures [20], Barrett's oesophagus [4] (see Chapter 11) and long-standing oesophagitis. There is controversy as to whether the relationship between oesophagitis and carcinoma is a real or exaggerated one [23, 31].

Genetic factors

Genetic factors have been implicated in the carcinoma associated with sideropenic anaemia [23]. It has also been suggested that such factors play a part in the prevalence of carcinoma in certain localities and in familial tylosis.

Pathology

More than 90% of all oesophageal carcinomas are of the squamous type [24]; adenocarcinomas of the gastric fundus may invade the lower oesophagus and, rarely, an adenocarcinoma may arise within the oesophageal body. Presumably the latter

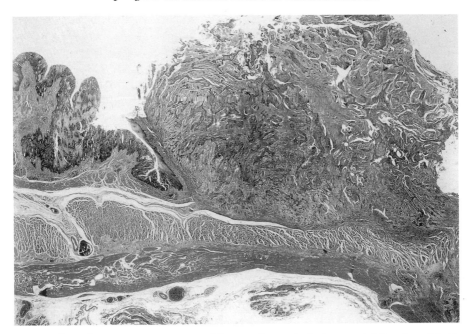

Fig. 13.2. Section through a squamous carcinoma of the oesophagus. At the bottom right is a deposit in the muscular wall of the oesophagus.

originates from ectopic areas of gastric mucosa and glands.

Recent endoscopic studies in China and Iran [8] have suggested that carcinoma is associated with an unusual form of oesophagitis in these areas. This oesophagitis is not like that seen in reflux oesophagitis, tends to involve the whole of the oesophagus and is associated with changes of leukoplakia in around 25% of cases. The carcinoma arises in the mucosa where, judging from experience in China [35], it remains localized for some time before invading the submucosa, muscularis mucosa and oesophageal wall.

Spread

When it becomes invasive the tumour spreads both longitudinally and circumferentially in the oesophageal wall. The gastric cardia offers no barrier so it can spread freely into the upper stomach. Tumour cells may enter the submucosal veins and lym-phatics giving rise to satellites at a distance from the site of origin. Local invasion may involve the pericardium, thoracic aorta, root of the lung, vagus nerves or trachea. If the trachea is involved, and tumour necrosis occurs, then a tracheo-oesophageal fistula may result. Alternatively, pulmonary tumours may invade the oesophagus leading to diagnostic difficulties.

For localization purposes the oesophagus is divided into four major areas: cervical and intrathoracic, upper-, middle- and lower-third. The distribution of tumours varies in different reports (Fig. 13.3) but the commonest sites are the lower- and middle-third.

Macroscopic appearance

Macroscopically an early tumour appears as a slight irregularity, depression or nodularity of the mucosa with some stiffness of the wall, sometimes accompanied by superficial ulceration. More advanced lesions

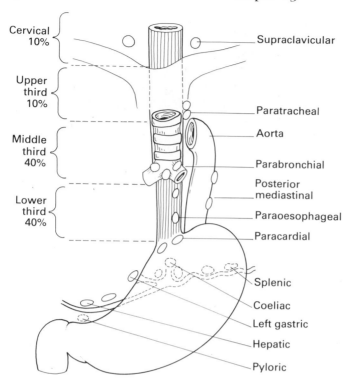

Fig. 13.3. The sites and occurrence of carcinoma of the oesophagus is shown on the left side. The glands that can be secondarily involved are illustrated. It is important to note that those closest to the tumour may not be those first involved.

produce thickening of the wall, ulceration or proliferative projections into the lumen. Circumferential lesions result in narrowing and irregularity of the lumen which can progress to partial or complete obstruction. Some oesophageal dilatation occurs above the obstruction but is rarely as marked as that seen with benign peptic strictures. Gross dilatation presumably does not occur because there is insufficient time.

Distant spread

Lymphatic spread occurs longitudinally within the posterior mediastinum. From here the spread is upwards to the supra-clavicular nodes (the right being involved as often as the left [29]), and downwards to the coeliac, upper gastric, hepatic and splenic lymph nodes within the abdomen [1]. It has been shown both radiologically [21] and pathologically [24] that this spread is not segmental and that lymph

node involvement may be extensive what-ever the site of the primary lesion. Blood borne spread occurs to the liver, lungs, and adrenal glands but this is seldom important clinically as the patient usually dies of the local effects of the tumour before wide-spread metastases become symptomatic.

Clinical features

The oesophagus produces a very limited range of symptoms. The most frequent is that of **dysphagia.** This may range from a slight sensation of hold up of food, the stick-ing of solid food, difficulty with fluids, to, finally, an inability to swallow anything, including saliva. The degree of dysphagia does not always represent the degree of luminal narrowing since a lump of meat, fruit stone, or fruit skin may impact and produce sudden total dysphagia in a pre-viously asymptomatic patient. It has been stated repeatedly in the past that the patient can easily localize the level of the obstruction but this has recently been challenged [14]—considerable discrepancies exist between the site of obstruction recorded by the patient and that of the actual lesion.

Whenever there is a severe degree of oesophageal narrowing food and fluid are retained above it. This leads to **regurgitation,** particularly when the patient lies down. Some of the contents will spill over into the larynx and trachea giving rise to coughing bouts or, at night, when the cough reflex is inhibited, to aspiration pneumonia. The cough can be productive and occasionally particles of food may be seen in the sputum. If a fistula develops respiratory symptoms and pulmonary damage are greatly increased.

Difficulty in swallowing leads to reduced nutritional intake and rapid **weight loss.** This is aggravated by the metabolic effects of the tumour itself.

Pain may be an important and distressing symptom of oesophageal carcinoma. Odynophagia (pain on swallowing) is caused by overdistension of the normal oesophagus above the obstruction; it goes when the swallowed food or fluid has passed the narrowing or has been regurgitated. Advanced tumours with extensive local infiltration (into aorta, spine or intercostal nerves) can produce a severe deep seated 'boring' pain.

Tumours in the cervical, upper- or middle-third can infiltrate the recurrent laryngeal nerves leading to **hoarseness of the voice. Severe haemorrhage** is unusual in oesophageal tumours although lower-third lesions may infiltrate the stomach and cause overt bleeding due to ulceration. Rarely the aorta may be invaded by a tumour at the level of the aortic arch and necrosis of this lesion can lead to sudden catastrophic haemorrhage. More commonly, bleeding is occult leading to iron deficiency anaemia.

Examination

Usually by the time that clinical signs develop the carcinoma is already far advanced. Supraclavicular glands should always be felt for on both sides. Extension of a primary cervical carcinoma or secondary glands may produce a palpable mass in the neck or produce tracheal displacement, or narrowing leading to stridor. Tumour, or glands, in the thoracic inlet or upper mediastinum may cause venous congestion. Superior venal caval compression or thrombosis presents as gross congestion of the veins in the neck, head and upper limbs with oedema of the arms. The liver may be enlarged and sometimes individual secondary nodules within it can be felt. Lower oesophageal tumours may produce an epigastric mass or ascites and trans-coelomic spread to the pelvis may lead to palpable nodules in the recto-vesical pouch on rectal examination. Occasionally blood borne metastases may result in distant skin nodules.

Investigations

Barium radiology

This is the recommended first line of investigation because of the difficulty in accurately localizing the level of the lesion on clinical grounds, which increases the risk of endoscopic perforation if the lesion is unexpectedly high. An early tumour may be detected by seeing a localized filling defect, thickening or distortion of the mucosal folds, superficial ulceration, spasm or stiffness of the affected segment of the oesophagus on the barium swallow [33]. Unfortunately it is rare for carcinoma to present at such an early stage and most are locally advanced at the time of presentation. In an advanced tumour the radiological features include luminal narrowing, filling defects, rigidity and irregularity of the lumen. A

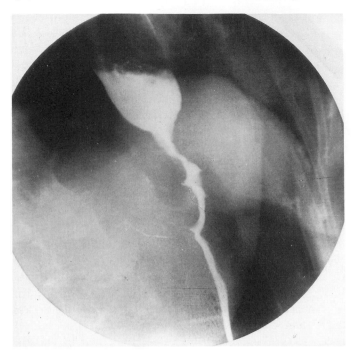

Fig. 13.4. Barium swallow showing typical irregular stricture of a carcinoma of the oesophagus.

malignant stricture is generally longer and more irregular than a benign one. Annular tumours may produce shouldering at their upper and lower ends producing a typical 'apple core' appearance. Food debris held up above a benign or malignant stricture may mimic the appearances of an intraluminal tumour.

The oesophagus may show some dilatation above the tumour but this is rarely of any magnitude. Barium may occasionally be seen to spill over into the larynx and trachea; this has to be distinguished from direct entry of barium from the oesophagus into the trachea through a fistula.

The films should be carefully examined to detect any surrounding soft tissue mass as this may provide evidence of the local extension of the carcinoma.

The stomach, particularly its upper half, should be carefully screened in order to detect filling defects or rigidity that might suggest extension of the tumour into the abdomen. Such changes may, of course, indicate that the carcinoma is arising primarily from the stomach with extension into the lower oesophagus.

Plain radiographs of the chest are also indicated. These may demonstrate evidence of lung collapse, pulmonary fibrosis, pleural effusion, pulmonary metastases, mediastinal widening and distortion or narrowing of the trachea or main bronchi—all features that suggest that the tumour is already far advanced.

Endoscopy

Endoscopy provides a valuable means of assessment and usually provides the conclusive diagnosis [18]. Modern fibreoptic instruments can be passed with little or no sedation and provide an excellent view of the lesion enabling biopsy and cytology specimens to be obtained and the level of the lesion to be recorded. Early carcinomas may be detected by careful brush cytology of any mucosal abnormality seen during inspection of the mucosa. Ulcerative or proliferative carcinomas are usually easily rec-

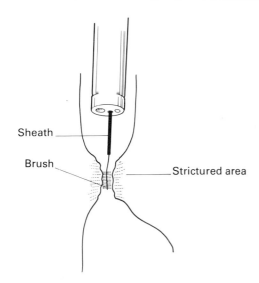

Fig. 13.5. Technique for obtaining cytological samples from a carcinoma of the oesophagus using a sheathed brush.

Sheath

Brush

Strictured area

ognized but infiltrating tumours may be more difficult as the mucosa can be intact over their surface. The small endoscopic biopsy forceps may not take a sufficiently deep bite for diagnostic purposes in such infiltrative lesions. It is essential therefore that multiple biopsies are taken using as large a biopsy forceps as possible, preferably with a central spike for more accurate positioning. The biopsies should be taken at several levels and at different quadrants, particularly when an infiltrative lesion is suspected. The biopsies should be adequately labelled as to their site of origin as the distance in centimetres from the incisor teeth.

The use of oesophageal cytological examination, in addition to biopsy, has proved extremely valuable. Specimens may be obtained by passing a sheathed cylindrical brush down the biopsy channel of the endoscope and brushing the area under suspicion (Fig. 13.5). The brush is then withdrawn and wiped on to clean, labelled, microscope slides which are dipped into fixative or sprayed with a fixative solution.

Finally the brush is agitated in a pot of fixative which is then spun down to look for malignant cells. A number of studies have shown that the use of both biopsy and cytological examination increases the diagnostic accuracy of endoscopy in malignant tumours to around 98%.

In the presence of a severe stricture it may be valuable to perform dilatation with Eder-Puestow or Celestin dilators. This procedure is not without risk as perforation is much commoner with malignant as opposed to benign strictures. However, it will allow a more adequate examination of the strictured area to be obtained with an assessment of the distal extent of the tumour. It has the added benefit of temporarily relieving the patient's dysphagia and improving the nutritional state prior to definitive treatment. Whenever possible the endoscope should be passed into the stomach—with the tip inverted it should be possible to examine the fundus, cardia and gastro-oesophageal junction to exclude a primary tumour or secondary invasion of these areas.

On rare occasions a positive diagnosis will not be made by fibreoptic endoscopy. As it is important not to submit a patient to what may be high risk treatment without a confirmed diagnosis rigid oesophagoscopy under general anaesthetic may be valuable. This will enable inspection under direct vision and deep biopsies using Brock's forceps can be obtained from all four quadrants at different levels. If necessary, a slim fibreoptic endoscope can then be passed through the rigid oesophagoscope to provide inspection of the stomach and oesophagus.

Bronchoscopy

Whenever the lesion is in the upper- or middle-third of the oesophagus a bronchoscopy should also be performed [5, 6]. This can be done either with a rigid or fibreoptic

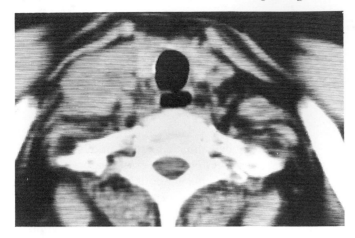

Fig. 13.6. Computerized tomographic scan (CT scan) through the cervical region of a patient with a squamous carcinoma of the mid-oesophagus. It shows extensive glandular involvement on the left side.

instrument. It is indicated to determine whether there has been any spread of the lesion into the trachea or main bronchi and to exclude a primary bronchial lesion secondarily invading the oesophagus. Occasionally a tracheo-oesophageal fistula can be detected by this examination.

Computerized axial tomography (CT)

Computerized axial tomography is of great value in assessing the extent of an oesophageal carcinoma. It should be performed from the root of the neck into the upper abdomen. When available it should be used routinely before submitting the patient to resection as it may show extensive invasion undetected by other means.

Other Investigations

Ultrasound examination of the liver can be useful in detecting metastatic deposits and in performing a guided needle biopsy/ cytology from suspicious areas.

Nuclear magnetic resonance has already been shown to detect oesophageal carcinoma and may, in the future, prove extremely useful in assessing the biological features of such tumours.

Recent Japanese work showing a high incidence of tumour deposits in the supraclav-

icular lymph nodes may make it reasonable to **biopsy** these before embarking on major resections, particularly if scanning techniques suggest involvement [19].

Differential diagnosis

Benign strictures

Various benign strictures including peptic, caustic, achalasic and post-cricoid webs can all give rise to diagnostic difficulty. Usually benign strictures are smooth and short, whereas malignant ones are long and irregular with shouldered edges. Generally the diagnosis is made on macroscopic inspection at endoscopy and confirmed by adequate biopsy and cytological examination. Occasionally histological and cytological examination fail to make the diagnosis (2–5% of cases) and the only clue to the malignant nature of the stricture is the rapid way in which symptoms recur after an apparently adequate dilatation. Under these circumstances there should be no hesitation in repeating the endoscopy and biopsies [19].

Benign ulcers

All ulcers, including those found above a columnar-lined oesophagus (Barrett's) should be regarded as malignant until multiple biopsies from several sites have shown no evidence of malignancy and brush cytology specimens are normal.

Benign tumours

These are relatively uncommon and rarely cause any major diagnostic difficulty. They include lipoma, leiomyoma, papilloma, and less common lesions such as pseudotumours, fibrovascular polyps and epithelial cysts.

Other malignant tumours

The commonest malignant tumour that causes diagnostic difficulty is that of an adenocarcinoma of the fundus of the stomach invading the lower oesophagus. Bronchial carcinomas can also involve the oesophagus by direct extension. Other, much rarer, malignant tumours include leiomyosarcoma, rhabdomyosarcoma, fibrosarcoma, lymphoma, pseudosarcoma and melanoma.

General assessment

The patient's general condition requires careful assessment before considering radical surgical treatment for carcinoma of the oesophagus (see Chapter 14). This should include estimation of the patient's haemoglobin, to exclude anaemia from chronic blood loss, and a full blood count including total lymphocyte count. A low lymphocyte count has been shown to correlate with a poor prognosis in many tumours.

Nutrition is often severely depleted with weight loss and reduced muscle bulk and power [17]. This can be further assessed by anthropometric measurements and by estimation of serum albumin and transferrin. If there is evidence of severe nutritional depletion this can be improved in a number of ways. If the patient can still swallow normally then a high protein, high calorie diet should be given as normal food, with or without supplementation with proprietary fluid preparations. Patients with dysphagia may have swallowing restored, for a period, by dilatation of the stricture but if this fails a fluid diet can be given either as regular drinks or continuously via a fine bore tube passed through the strictured area. Only if all these methods fail should intravenous or gastrosomy/jejunostomy feeding be considered. This is particularly valuable in the post-operative period.

References

1 AKIYAMA H, TSURUMARA M, KAWAMURA I, ONO Y. Principles of surgical treatment for carcinoma of the oesophagus. *Ann Surg* 1981;**194**:438–446.
2 BMJ LEADER. Cancer of the oesophagus. *Br Med J* 1976;**2**:135–136.
3 BURRELL RJW, ROACH WA, SHADWELL A. Oesophageal cancer in the Bantu of the Transkei associated with mineral deficiency in garden plants. *J Nat Cancer Inst* 1966;**36**:201–214.
4 CAMERON AJ, OTT BJ, PAYNE WS. The incidence of adenocarcinoma in columnar-lined (Barrett's) esophagus. *N Engl J Med* 1985;**313**:857–859.
5 CHOI TK, SIU KF, LAM KH, WONG J. Bronchoscopy and carcinoma of the esophagus I. Findings of bronchoscopy in carcinoma of the esophagus. *Am J Surg* 1984;**147**:757–759.
6 CHOI TK, SIU KF, LAM KH, WONG J. Bronchoscopy and carcinoma of the esophagus II. Carcinoma of the esophagus with tracheobronchial involvement. *Am J Surg* 1984;**147**:760–762.
7 COOK P. Cancer of the oesophagus in Africa. *Br J Cancer* 1971;**25**:853–880.
8 CRESPI M, GRASSI A, MUNOZ N, GUO-QUING W, GUANREI Y. Endoscopic features of suspected precancerous lesions in high-risk areas for esophageal cancer. *Endoscopy* 1984;**16**:85–91.
9 DAY NE. Cancer of the oesophagus. *Br Med J* 1984;**40**:329–334.
10 DAY NE. The geographic pathology of cancer of the oesophagus. *Br Med Bull* 1984;**40**:329–334.
11 DEJONG VW, BRESLOW N, GOHEWE-HONG J, SRIDHARRAN M, SHANMUGARATNAM K. Aetiological factors in oesophageal cancer in Singapore Chinese. *Int J Cancer* 1974;**13**:291–303.
12 DOLL R. Cancer in five continents. *Proc R Soc Med* 1972;**65**:49–55.
13 DOLL R. Strategy for the detection of cancer hazards in man. *Nature* 1977;**265**:589–596.
14 EDWARDS DAW, LOBELLO R. Site of referral of the sense of obstruction to swallowing. *Gut* 1982 **23**:A435.

15 Jacobs A, Kilpatrick GS. The Patterson-Kelly syndrome. *Br Med J* 1964;**2**:177–182.

16 Joint Iran-International Agency for Research on Cancer Study Group. Oesophageal cancer studies in the Caspian littoral of Iran: Results of population studies: a prodrome. *J Nat Cancer Inst* 1977;**59**:1127–1138.

17 Karran S. Who needs nutritional support? In: Lumley JSP, Craven JL, eds. *Surgical review.* London: Pitman, 1982:25–62.

18 Kirk RM. Oesophagoscopy. In: Dudley HAF, Pories W, eds. *Operative surgery.* 4th Ed. London: Butterworths, 1983.

19 Kirk RM, McLaughlin JE. In: Hadfield GJ, Hobsley M, Morson BC, eds. *Pathology in surgical practice.* London: Arnold, 1983.

20 Lansing PB, Ferrante WA, Oschner JL. Carcinoma of the oesophagus at the site of lye stricture. *Am J Surg* 1969;**118**:108–111.

21 Mahboubi E, Kmet J, Cook PJ, Day NE, Ghadirian P, Salmasizadeh S. Oesophageal cancer studies in the Caspian littoral of Iran: The Caspian Cancer Registry. *Br J Cancer* 1973;**28**:197–214.

22 McCourt JJ. Radiographic identification of lymph node metastases from carcinoma of the oesophagus. *Radiology* 1952;**59**:694–711.

23 Michel JO, Olsen AM, Docherty MB. The association of diaphragmatic hernia and gastro-oesophageal carcinoma. *Surg Gynecol Obstet* 1967;**124**:583–589.

24 Morson BC. The spread of carcinoma of the oesophagus. In: Tanner NC, Smithers DW, eds. *Tumours of the oesophagus.* Edinburgh: Livingstone, 1961:136–145.

25 Morson BC, Dawson IMP. *Gastrointestinal pathology.* 2nd ed. Oxford: Blackwell Scientific Publications, 1979.

26 Munoz N, Wahrendorf J, Bang LJ, et al. No effect of riboflavine, retinol, and zinc on prevalence of precancerous lesions of oesophagus. *Lancet* 1985;**ii**:111–114.

27 Norell S, Ahlbom A, Lipping H, Osterblom L. Oesophageal cancer and vulcanisation work. *Lancet* 1983;**i**:462–463.

28 O'Neill C, Pan Q-Q, Clarke G, et al. Silica fragments from millet bran in mucosa surrounding oesophageal tumours in patients in northern China. *Lancet* 1982;**i**:1202–1207.

29 Sannohe Y, Hiratsuka R, Doki K. Lymph node metastases in cancer of the thoracic oesophagus. *Am J Surg* 1981;**141**:216–218.

30 Silber W. Carcinoma of the oesophagus: aspects of epidemiology and aetiology. *Proc Nutr Soc* 1985;**44**:101–110.

31 Spechler SJ, Robbins AH, Rubins HB, et al. Adenocarcinoma and Barrett's esophagus. An over-rated risk? *Gastroenterology* 1984;**87**:927–933.

32 Tuyns AJ. Cancer of the oesophagus: further evidence of the relation to drinking habits in France. *Int J Cancer* 1970;**5**:152–156.

33 Wang Zheng-Yan. Radiological appearances in early oesophageal cancer. *J R Soc Med* 1980;**73**:849–851.

34 Weir JM, Dunn JE Jr. Smoking and mortality. A prospective study. *Cancer* 1970;**25**:105–112.

35 Wu K, Huang KC. Chinese experience in the surgical treatment of carcinoma of the oesophagus. *Ann Surg* 1979;**190**:361–365.

Chapter 14
Management of Carcinoma of the Oesophagus
A. WATSON

The incidence of oesophageal carcinoma appears to be increasing across the world. It remains one of the most depressing neoplasms to treat. In the West most tumours are advanced at the time of presentation, because approximately two-thirds of the circumference of the gullet is involved when dysphagia first occurs [17]. It is hardly surprising that inoperability rates of 65% are reported [36] and cure rates are poor. The magnitude of attempted curative surgery and the debilitated condition of many patients results in a cumulative operative mortality rate of 30% for squamous carcinoma [15]. As a consequence of this, and the advent of fibreoptic pulsion intubation as a relatively safe means of palliation, the role of resection in the United Kingdom is controversial.

In contrast, experience in Japan [3] shows that excellent long term results, with a low operative mortality, can be achieved when an early diagnosis is made. Perhaps it is in this direction that our efforts should be made. Newer diagnostic methods, including computerized axial tomography (CT) and magnetic resonance imaging (MRI), have enabled more accurate staging of the disease before operation. Concentration of effort on those whose chances of 'cure' are best can result in operative mortality rates comparable to those of palliative intubation [54], with the bonus of 'cure' in 10–20% [35]. Further help may come from accurate assessment of the relative merits of other treatments including mega-voltage radiotherapy and adjuvant chemotherapy.

Classification of oesophageal carcinoma

Oesophageal carcinoma may be classified by site, or tissue of origin (see Chapter 13)—each has therapeutic implications.

Tumours of the cervical and upper-third of the oesophagus are almost all squamous in type. They are usually radiosensitive and because of the magnitude of surgical excision, often involving pharyngo-laryngectomy, radiotherapy is the best treatment.

Carcinomas of the middle- and lower-third occur with approximately equal frequency. Most of middle-third tumours are squamous but adenocarcinomas can occur in this area. Many middle-third lesions are radiosensitive, but surgical excision is widely practised and is still considered the best treatment. The results of controlled trials are still awaited. Many lower-third lesions are adenocarcinomas, with a few arising from the stomach and extending upwards. The response to radiotherapy in these circumstances is disappointing and surgical treatment remains best.

Squamous carcinomas are associated with a better long-term survival than adenocarcinomas, which tend to be more advanced at the time of presentation [54]. The repeatedly reported association between gastro-oesophageal reflux, Barrett's oesophagus and adenocarcinoma is a cause for concern [26, 39]. Centres specializing in the surgical treatment of reflux oesophagitis and peptic strictures experience a higher proportion of adenocarcinomas than the oft-quoted incidence of 10%. While the incidence of adenocarcinoma complicating Barrett's oesophagus is only 2.5–10.0% [53] this is several hundred times that occurring in the general population, confirming the benefits of effective management of gastro-oesophageal reflux.

Objectives of treatment

The objectives of treatment are firstly to relieve dysphagia to prevent death from starvation, secondly to prolong survival, and thirdly to 'cure' the disease. In evaluating the success of therapy it is equally important that the chosen method of treatment has an acceptably low mortality.

The principal methods used are resection, intubation and radiotherapy, whilst palliative bypass, chemotherapy and laser therapy are less frequently employed. Each of these will be discussed in detail later, but in considering the objectives of treatment it is important to put them in perspective. Resection probably offers the best chance of 'cure', but mega-voltage radiotherapy may be considered potentially curative in a proportion of patients with squamous lesions.

Whilst resection has traditionally been associated with a high mortality rate [8, 15] some recent series report single figure mortalities [18, 35]. These show the impact of modern surgical and anaesthetic techniques together with improved nutritional and ventilatory support. Selection of patients is equally important and Wong (1981) has shown the dramatic influence of age and serious intercurrent disease on operative mortality. It is the opinion of most oesophageal surgeons that, with appropriate selection and attention to factors that influence survival, operative mortality should be less than 10%.

Radiotherapy has apparent advantages over surgery in avoiding operative mortality. However, this may be more apparent than real, if long-term survival figures are studied. It is fair to say that to date the full potential of radiotherapy has probably not been realized. This is because it has often been reserved for hopeless cases, which is reflected in overall one- and five-year survival rates of only 18% and 6% respectively [16].

In Lancaster the corresponding figures for surgically-treated patients, including operative mortality, are 51% one-year and 11.1% five-year survival. Only Pearson [44] reported prolonged survival after radiotherapy with a 20% five-year survival, but this series included relatively favourable lesions of the upper-third of the oesophagus. To date there has been no controlled trial of radiotherapy against radical surgery for localized lesions of the middle- and lower-thirds of the oesophagus.

Intubation is the mainstay of palliative surgery for advanced tumours or in patients unfit for resection. It is often viewed as a safer procedure than resection and, alone or combined with radiotherapy, as appropriate treatment for even those suitable for resection. Intubation, however, carries its own mortality and morbidity and, if used alone, denies any prospect of cure. Mortality rates range from 45% for surgical intubation [33] to 11–27% for endoscopic intubation [30, 40] if hospital, rather than procedure-related mortality is assessed. These figures are obviously more comparable to surgical results.

There is, therefore, no single ideal treatment for this disease. Each patient must be assessed from the standpoint of age, general health, site, type, and tumour stage, before any management decision is taken.

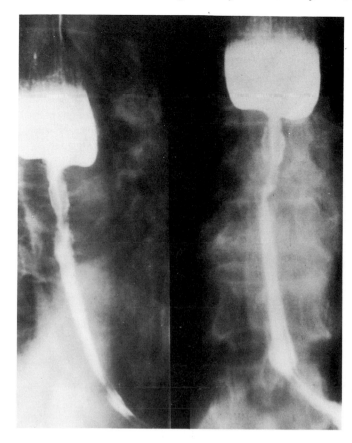

Fig. 14.1. Barium swallow showing 10 cm-long irregular stricture produced by a carcinoma. Inoperability can be inferred by the length of the lesion.

Pretreatment assessment
Diagnosis

Before any treatment programme is undertaken it is mandatory that a tissue diagnosis be made (see Chapter 13). Fibreoptic endoscopy is safer and provides better visualization than rigid oesophagoscopy. It is important that brush cytological samples be taken in addition to punch biopsies, in order to reduce the chance of false negative results and to increase the likelihood of determining the cell type. At endoscopy the opportunity should be taken to dilate the stricture or, if not possible, to insert a fine-bore feeding tube in order to improve the nutrition of the patient before therapy.

Table 14.1. Tumour staging and survival in histological types.

	Whole group	Adenocarcinoma	Squamous carcinoma
Localized to oesophageal wall (%)	9	0	23
Transgressed oesophageal wall (%)	19	15	23
Lymph node involvement (%)	72	85	44
Mean survival (months)	21.8	15.1	32.4

Tumour staging

Having confirmed the diagnosis, an attempt should be made to stage the tumour. This is more difficult than for some other tumours but advanced, and probably incurable, disease can be inferred from the presence of a recurrent nerve palsy, tracheal involvement with or without a fistula, or a tumour length greater than 7 cm [51]. Lateral spread of the tumour may be inferred from a large soft tissue shadow on a chest radiograph or with increased accuracy, by CT scanning [49]. Evidence of lymph node spread may also be sought by laparoscopy and mediastinoscopy [38], but correlation between lymph-node invasion and survival is poor. Postlethwait [46] has noted poor survival in node-negative cases and prolonged survival in some node-positive cases, which agrees with our experience in Lancaster. Distant spread invariably means incurable disease—hepatic deposits and supraclavicular or axillary nodes should be sought.

General health

Finally, if tumour assessment suggests a choice of treatments, the fitness of the patient to undergo thoraco-abdominal surgery needs to be investigated. Age is an important criterion, Wong [56] showed double the operative mortality in patients over 70 years, when compared to the 40–60 age group. The presence of serious intercurrent disease is also prognostically important. As most problems following resection are cardio-respiratory, pre-existing disease in these systems increases the risk. Cardiological and respiratory evaluation is therefore important, if there is any hint of a problem. Diabetes and chronic renal disease may also influence one against aggressive surgery.

On the basis of evaluation of the tumour and the patient, most clinical situations will resolve into 2 categories—a 'curative' or a 'palliative' approach. In Lancaster, with a high incidence of oesophageal carcinoma of 13.8 per 100,000 compared to 7.8 per 100,000 for the United Kingdom, the management policy during the last 10 years has used radical resection wherever appropriate, with 70 years as an arbitrary upper age limit, but relying more on biological than chronological age so that we have resected patients up to the age of 76 years. Using this approach, approximately 40% of our patients have undergone radical resection with an operative mortality of close to 9.7% [55].

Methods of treatment

These are best categorized according to their use in a curative or palliative capacity (Table 14.2).

Table 14.2. Methods of treatment

Curative therapy
(1) Radical surgery
(2) Radical radiotherapy

Palliative treatment
(1) Surgical by-pass
(2) Surgical intubation
(3) Endoscopic intubation
(4) Endoscopic dilatation
(5) Endoscopic laser therapy
(6) Palliative radiotherapy
(7) Chemotherapy

Radical surgery

This is the only treatment that has yielded long-term survival in a few patients. It is the best treatment for the relatively fit patient with a favourable tumour. It is important to appreciate that the success of such surgery depends on close teamwork involving anaesthetists, cardiologists, chest physicians and surgeons, with a skilled staff in the theatre and intensive care unit. The team must be dealing with enough patients to become familiar with the problems that follow and the best way to handle them. For this reason oesophageal cancer should be managed in centres with a special interest and expertise in oesophageal surgery. There is little place for the occasional oesophagectomist.

Preoperative preparation

Success with radical resection begins with careful selection and attention to preoperative preparation. It is important to spend a few days correcting pre-existing anaemia, fluid, electrolyte and nutritional deficiencies. The latter can be corrected either enterally, or parenterally (see Chapter 78). Enteral feeding is easier and safer to administer and can be done using high calorie, high protein feeds of known volume and composition either by mouth or via a fine-bore feeding tube if oral intake is poor. If this is impossible then parenteral feeding should be used. Whilst pre-operative nutritional support appears rational on general and immunological grounds [13], measurable benefit in such patients is controversial [7, 27].

In addition pre-operative physiotherapy is valuable and, in our experience, an explanatory visit from the intensive care unit team is psychologically beneficial. We also normally administer (unless contra-indicated) prophylactic sub-cutaneous low-dose heparin (5,000 units 8-hourly) and prophylactic antibiotics immediately before operation.

Operative technique

The principal factor governing surgical excision is the well-documented longitudinal submucosal spread of such tumours, beyond macroscopic disease [37]. Thus greater clearance is required than is normally practised in intestinal cancer surgery. This should be for at least 10 cm either side of the margin of the growth. In many series anastomotic dehiscence is the greatest cause of death [12]; it is significantly associated with residual tumour in the cut ends and for this reason wide exposure and adequate clearance is vitally important. The two-stage sub-total oesophagectomy (described by Ivor Lewis 1946), or the three-stage total oesophagectomy (described by McKeown 1972) are more likely to fulfil the objectives of radical surgery, than the more convenient left thoraco-abdominal approach. This is particularly true for tumours more than 5 cm above the cardia: we have observed frequent cardiac dysrhythmias in our limited use of the latter approach. There have been recent reports [23, 31] of resection without formal thoracotomy, the claimed advantage being a lower incidence of pulmonary problems, which has not always been borne out in practice.

The other major variable in surgical technique is the choice of organ to replace the resected oesophagus and its route of placement. Jejunum and colon have been used, but their use demands a more extensive operation with multiple anastomoses, and is accompanied by more complications [42]. For these reasons a tube constructed from the distal stomach has been the most popular replacement organ. This is generally placed trans-thoracically in the bed of the oesophagus, being the shortest and most natural route. Pre-sternal and retrosternal routes have been used by some workers to obviate the risk of mediastinitis if anastomotic leakage occurs [4, 28], but technical problems are common and fistulae may occur, causing some surgeons to abandon such techniques [34].

During the past 10 years we have used the Ivor Lewis approach in over 80% of our patients, reserving a left thoraco-abdominal approach for tumours of the cardia involving the lower oesophagus. As there has been no instance of residual tumour at the

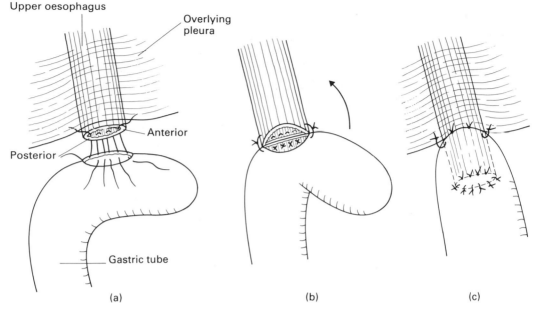

Upper oesophagus

Overlying pleura

Anterior

Posterior

Gastric tube

(a)   (b)   (c)

Fig. 14.2. Technical steps in making the gastro-oesophageal anastomosis using the apex of the gastric tube to seal the anastomosis. (a), placement of posterior layer of sutures; (b), posterior layer completed with start of anterior layer sutures; (c), overlapping of apex of stomach tube to seal the anastomosis.

resected margin and only one clinically important anastomotic leak using this method, we have used the three-stage total oesophagectomy in only three patients [55].

Practical surgical management

We employ the standard Ivor Lewis [32] technique starting with the abdominal procedure and then opening the chest through the bed of the right 5th or 6th rib. Pyloroplasty is not performed, except where pyloric or duodenal ulcer disease exists, as we have found it to be unnecessary; this avoids the problems of late biliary reflux oesophagitis. Adequate mobilization of the oesophagus is assisted by division of the azygous vein; we try to remove at least 10 cm of oesophagus on either side of the palpable tumour. The oesophago-gastric anastomosis is made, using non-absorbable sutures, on the posterior wall of the gastric remnant (after closure of the lesser curve)

with a large oesophageal tube across the anastomosis to prevent stricture formation. The anterior flap of stomach is sutured to the mediastinal pleura above the anastomosis to relieve tension on the suture line and act as a seal. Finally a fine-bore tube is passed through the anastomosis and pylorus to assist in post-operative nutritional support.

Postoperative management

Ventilatory support is maintained for 24 hours in the intensive care unit. Epidural analgesia is given via a thoracic catheter, to avoid respiratory depression induced by systemic analgesics and to assist cooperation with physiotherapy. Oral fluids are withheld for seven days and are only begun after a gastrografin swallow has confirmed anastomotic patency. Fluid and nutritional requirements are met by intravenous fluids and enteral feeding when bowel sounds have returned.

Results

There is a considerable variation in the published results of radical resection. In a review of 122 series Earlam & Cunha-Melo [15] reported a mean operative mortality of 29% (range 1–83%) and a five-year survival of 4% (range 1–13%). Whilst this review has attracted considerable attention it should be appreciated that many of the analysed series were published over 30 years ago, with operations presumably, being performed up to 10 years earlier.

There are, in contrast, several recently reported United Kingdom series with operative mortalities of around 10% [14, 35, 54], and American and Japanese series with mortalities of only 2–3% [3, 8]. Con-

Table 14.3. Death and morbidity following resection [55].

Causes of death	
Intractable cardiac arrhythmia	2
Cardiac failure	2
Pulmonary embolus	1
Mediastinitis	1
Bronchopneumonia	2
Morbidity (overall 35%)	
Chest infection	18
Cardiac arrhythmia	7
Cardiac failure	4
Thrombo-embolism	2
Empyema	1
Wound dehiscence	1
Mediastinitis	1

temporary five-year survival rates, corrected for operative mortality, are 8–18%, with 34.6% in Akiyama's highly selected patients with early oesophageal lesions.

In Lancaster of 82 patients undergoing resection for oesophageal carcinoma, over the last 10 years, the hospital mortality was 9.7%. The main causes of death and transitory morbidity were cardiorespiratory (Table 14.3). The current five-year survival rate is 11.1%. The quality of postoperative swallowing was excellent, normal swallowing being restored in 90% with only four

patients requiring dilatation for anastomotic narrowing. In the few instances of local recurrence it was a late feature, coinciding with rapid progression of the disease and widespread metastases, usually to liver but occasionally to chest, brain or bone.

Radical radiotherapy

Although radiotherapy has been used in the management of squamous carcinoma for a long time, evidence for its efficacy as a primary treatment is lacking. One problem is that it is frequently used where surgery is contra-indicated, by virtue of advanced disease or poor general condition. This may explain the poor results reported by Earlam and Cunha-Melo [16] in an analysis of 49 series: a one-year mean survival of 18% and a 5-year of only 6%. Only Pearson [44,45] has shown encouraging results with mega-voltage radiotherapy, reporting a 16% overall five-year survival in 288 patients treated for middle-third squamous carcinoma. Cederquist, *et al.* [10] using a similar tumour dose of 5,000 rads, could report only a 4% five-year survival.

The limitations of radiotherapy as a primary curative procedure presumably relate to the inability to irradiate more than 5 cm beyond the tumour margin because of an unacceptable reduction in tumour dose [45]. This has led others to attempt a combined approach of surgery with radiotherapy, the latter being given either pre- or post-operatively. In most series a pre-operative dose of 4–5,000 rads was given followed by surgery 2–4 weeks later [2, 43]. These reports suggest that increased resectability and five-year survival can be achieved, but at the expense of increased surgical mortality and morbidity.

The main theoretical advantage of radiotherapy is avoidance of operative mortality, but it is not without risk in its own right, particularly in elderly debilitated patients and many 'curative' courses are probably converted to 'palliative' ones for this reason [16]. In the report by Cederquist, et al. [10] 9% of patients died during therapy and most series report complications such as skin burns, pneumonitis, leucopenia, nausea or vomiting in a substantial number of patients. In addition, continuing dysphagia occurs in a high proportion of patients, because of either failure to eradicate the tumour or fibrosis. In Pearson's series [44] 3 out of his 20 five-year survivors never regained normal swallowing, and 50% needed regular dilatations.

The full potential of mega-voltage radiotherapy is unlikely to be realized until the results of prospective controlled trials have established how it should best be used. Fortunately such trials are now in progress and their results are awaited with interest.

Palliative treatment

This is required by approximately 60% of patients. The objectives are to relieve dysphagia by the least invasive technique, with as low a mortality as possible. In addition the aim is to avoid a prolonged period in hospital for someone whose life span is limited.

Surgical by-pass

Many authors have described a variety of palliative by-pass procedures, including anastomosing the gastric fundus above the tumour or using gastric tubes, or jejunal or colonic loops as a by-pass organ [41, 46]. Whilst excellent palliation is reported, this appears to be at the expense of a high operative mortality (up to 40%) and morbidity [1]. In the author's opinion the only justification for palliative by-pass is when inoperability is established at attempted resection, but this should be rare with adequate pre-operative assessment. There is no place for gastrotomy or oesophagotomy in modern practice.

Surgical intubation

Until the development of fibreoptic endoscopic intubation the insertion of a Celestin or Mousseau-Barbin prosthetic tube was the commonest palliative procedure for relief of dysphagia due to an inoperable tumour. Whilst the operative procedure is relatively minor and quickly performed, it carries a mortality of around 40% [33, 54]. This is probably partly due to the immunodepressive effect of surgery on an already debilitated patient but it also suggests that perforation, due to splitting of the tumour, occurs more frequently than is often realized. In our hands the quality of swallowing is less effective than after endoscopic intubation, with normal swallowing in only 15.4% of patients. This may reflect differences in internal diameter of the tubes that are used. It is suggested that surgical intubation should be reserved for those cases where endoscopic insertion is impossible, or when inoperability is only found at surgery [56].

Endoscopic intubation

Whilst endoscopic intubation has been practised for over a century using rigid oesophagoscopy, it is only with the advent of fibreoptic endoscopy that it has become an established technique [5, 11].

The principle of the technique is the pulsion passage of a prosthetic tube mounted on an introducer guided by a flexible wire through the tumour. Two tubes are in regular use in the United Kingdom, the Atkinson silicone-rubber tube and the Celestin latex rubber tube incorporating a nylon spiral to retain rigidity. Both have a funnel upper end and flange distally to prevent proximal displacement. There are two introducer systems: the semi-rigid Nottingham introducer with expandable olive at its end, to hold on to the tube, and the Celestin flexible introducer using a balloon to hold

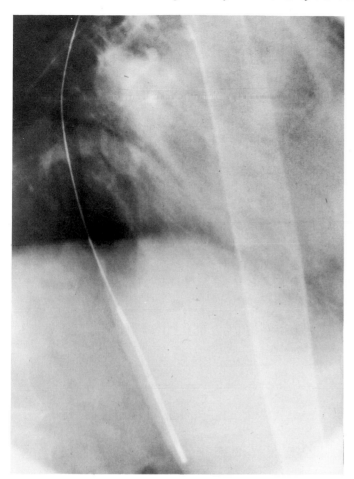

Fig. 14.3. Fluoroscopic view of guide-wire passed through an oesophageal tumour using endoscopic control.

Table 14.4. Quality of swallowing following resection, endoscopic intubation and surgical intubation [55].

Visick grade	Endoscopic intubation %	Surgical intubation %	Resection %
I (Normal swallowing)	33.3	15.4	90.3
II (Dysphagia for solids)	63.0	69.2	8.7
III (Dysphagia for semi-solids)	3.7	15.4	—
IV (Dysphagia for liquids)	—	—	—

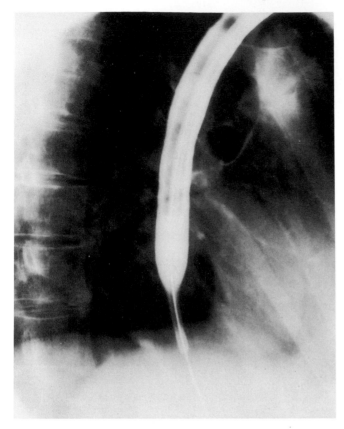

Fig. 14.4. Fluoroscopic appearance of Celestin dilator bougie passing through oesophageal tumour.

(a) Nottingham introducer

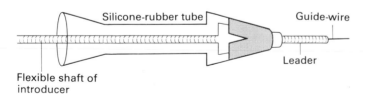

(b) Celestin insertion technique
(using fine calibre endoscope)

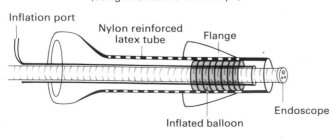

Fig. 14.5. Principle of the endoscopic insertion techniques for placement of oesophageal prostheses.

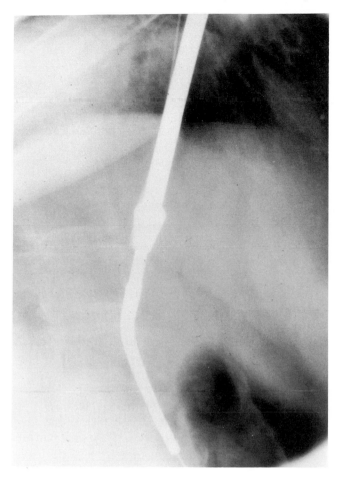

Fig. 14.6. Fluoroscopic appearance of Nottingham introducer passed through oesophageal tumour.

on to the tube; one version of the latter system allows a narrow calibre endoscope to be passed down its lumen to allow positioning of the tube under direct vision.

Technique

Dilatation is performed under sedation with diazepam plus pentazocine or pethidine, however, many prefer a general anaesthetic [6]. Once the diagnosis has been established and palliative intubation has been decided as the correct treatment, a guide-wire is inserted and the tumour is dilated with either an Eder-Peustow dilator or Celestin dilator (Chapter 11). Intubation is performed with an appropriately-sized tube and its position is checked by post-intubation endoscopy or fluoroscopy. Prophylactic broad-spectrum antibiotics should be given and oral fluids withheld until a post-intubation chest radiograph has excluded perforation. Food can then be given, advising the patient to chew thoroughly and to use a gaseous drink after each meal in order to reduce the risk of blockage.

The immediate results of endoscopic intubation are generally much better than those of surgical intubation. In order to evaluate the procedure it is important to compare 'hospital mortality' rather than that immediately following the procedure. In the Nottingham series [40] hospital mortality was 11% and in the Lancaster study

[55] it was 11.4%. Our mean hospital stay was 7.6 days compared to 13.0 days for operative insertion in a similar group of patients. Survival was not significantly different with a mean of 10.8 months for endoscopic, and 8.1 months for surgical, intubation. Studies of the quality of swallowing using a modified Visick grading system showed that 60% of patients in both groups were in grade 2 (dysphagia for solids). Neither group could match the 90.3% grade 1 (no dysphagia) found after resection, although 33.3% after endoscopic insertion were in this grade, compared with only 15.4% after surgical insertion (Table 14.4).

The main complications are perforation, tube migration and tube blockage. Early perforation occurred in 11% of patients in the Nottingham series and in 9% of our own. Late perforation has also been reported in patients who have received later radiotherapy. Tube migration is less of a problem now that tubes have a distal flange. Tumour extension may block above the tube, although the cause of a blocked tube is more commonly a food bolus. *In vivo* destruction of the latex Celestin tube has been reported [47].

Another use of endoscopic intubation is in the management of a **tracheo-bronchial fistula.** Several groups have reported patients in whom an endoscopically inserted tube has been used successfully to occlude such a fistula.

Endoscopic dilatation

Whilst this has been recommended as a palliative procedure [25] recurrent dysphagia usually occurs so rapidly that it is only useful as a temporary measure and as an aid to intubation.

Endoscopic laser photocoagulation

Laser photocoagulation (YAG laser) has recently been used as a palliative treatment [9, 20, 21, 22]. Reduction of tumour bulk and improved swallowing has been reported, but the procedure is time consuming, needing multiple applications each lasting up to 30 minutes. An additional disadvantage is the high cost of the equipment. Doubtless further improvements in this technique will be made, but currently endoscopic intubation remains the most feasible technique in most centres.

Palliative radiotherapy

Palliative radiotherapy is difficult to define, although frequently referred to in the literature [50]. There would appear to be little merit in offering radiotherapy in very advanced tumours, particularly those with widespread deposits, or tracheo-bronchial fistula, as there are alternative methods of rapid palliation. Palliative radiotherapy is ineffective in long tumours, and short ones should be treated with a curative dose. In most published series patients have undergone palliative radiotherapy because they could not tolerate a full therapeutic dose [19]. It is felt by some [36] that patients receiving palliative therapy fare no better than those who receive no radiation at all.

Chemotherapy

Although chemotherapy has been used intermittently over the last 15 years there are conflicting reports of its efficacy [24, 29, 48]. The most commonly used drug is **bleomycin** either alone, or in combination with other drugs or radiotherapy [52]. Despite several favourable reports no striking effect has been demonstrated with any agent. Whilst adjuvant chemotherapy is an attractive concept it appears unlikely, on present data, that it has any place in the management of oesophageal carcinoma.

Conclusion

Carcinoma of the oesophagus remains a formidable disease and only a palliative approach is possible in around 60% of patients at presentation. A curative approach is justified in the remaining 40% and, on the available evidence, radical resection surgery offers the best chance of restoring normal swallowing with a chance of long term survival. In units specializing in this condition an operative mortality of about 10% is attainable and normal swallowing should be restored in over 90%, with a 10–20% chance of long term 'cure'.

Of the many available palliative procedures endoscopic intubation using a flexible endoscope appears the safest and most effective.

The role of radiotherapy is as yet undefined and we must await the outcome of controlled trials to clarify its usefulness. Chemotherapy would not appear to have a role at present, but the results of studies with new agents are awaited with interest.

At present efforts must be directed at earlier diagnosis; more accurate staging before surgery and to further reducing the mortality associated with resection.

References

1 ANGORN IB, HAFFEJEE AA. Pulsion intubation v. retrosternal gastric bypass for palliation of unresectable carcinoma of the upper thoracic oesophagus. *Br J Surg* 1983;**70**:335–338.

2 AKAKURA I, NAKAMURA Y, KAKEGAWA T, NAKAKYAMA R, WATANABE H, YAMASHITA H. Surgery of carcinoma of the esophagus with pre-operative radiation. *Chest* 1970;**57**:47–57.

3 AKIYAMA H, TSURAMUARU M, KAWAMURA T, ONO Y. Principles of surgical treatment of carcinoma of the esophagus: Analysis of lymph node involvement. *Ann Surg* 1981;**194**:438–446.

4 ALLISON PR, DASILVA LT. The Roux loop. *Br J Surg* 1953;**41**:173–180.

5 ATKINSON M, FERGUSON R. Fibreoptic endoscopic palliative intubation of inoperable oesophagogastric neoplasms. *Br Med J* 1977;i:266–267.

6 ATKINSON M, FERGUSON R, OGILVIE AL. Management of malignant dysphagia by intubation at endoscopy. *J Roy Soc Med* 1979;**72**:894–897.

7 BELGHITI J, LANGONNET F, BOURSTYN E, FEKETE F. Surgical implications of malnutrition and immunodeficiency in patients with carcinoma of the oesophagus. *Br J Surg* 1983;70.339–341.

8 BERTELSEN S, AASTED A, VEJLSTED H. Surgical treatment for malignant lesions of the distal part of the esophagus and the esophagogastric junction. *World J Surg* 1985;**9**:633–638.

9 BUSET M, DUNHAM F, BAIZE M, deTOEUF J, CROMER M. Nd-YAG laser, a new palliative alternative in the management of esophageal cancer. *Endoscopy* 1983;**15**:353–356.

10 CEDERQUIST C, NIELSEN J. BERTHELSEN A, HANSEN HS. Cancer of the oesophagus. II Theory and outcome. *Acta Chir Scand* 1978;**144**:233–240.

11 CELESTIN LR. New techniques of intubation. *Proc World Congr of Dig Endoscopy* 1978;97.

12 CHASSIN JL. Oesophago-gastrectomy: data favouring end-to-side anastomosis. *Ann Surg* 1978;**188**:22–26.

13 DALY JM, DUDRICK SJ, COPELAND EM. The intravenous hyperalimentation: Effect on delayed cutaneous hypersensitivity in cancer patients. *Ann Surg* 1980;**192**:587–592.

14 DARK JS, MOUSALLI H, VAUGHAN R. Surgical treatment of carcinoma of the oesophagus. *Thorax* 1981;**36**:891–895.

15 EARLAM R, CUNHA-MELO JR. Oesophageal squamous cell carcinoma. I. A critical review of surgery. *Br J Surg* 1980;**67**:381–390.

16 EARLAM R, CUNHA-MELO JR. Oesophageal squamous cell carcinoma. II. A critical review of radiotherapy. *Br J Surg* 1980;**67**:457–460.

17 EDWARDS DAW. Carcinoma of the oesophagus and fundus. *Postgrad Med J* 1974;**50**:223–227.

18 ELLIS FH JR, GIBB SP. Esophago-gastrectomy for carcinoma. *Ann Surg* 1979;**190**:699–705.

19 ELLIS FH, SALZMAN FA. Carcinoma of the esophagus. Surgery v. radiotherapy. *Postgrad Med J* 1977;**61**:167–171.

20 FLEISCHER D. Palliative therapy for esophageal carcinoma by endoscopic Nd-YAG laser. *Laser Endosc* 1981;**2**:17–20.

21 FLEISCHER D, SIVAK MV. Endoscopic Nd-YAG laser therapy as palliative treatment for advanced adenocarcinoma of the gastric cardia. *Gastroenterology* 1984;815–820.

22 FLEISCHER D, SIVAK MV. Endoscopic Nd: YAG laser therapy as palliation for esophagogastric cancer. *Gastroenterology* 1985;**89**:827–831.

23 GARVIN PJ, KAMINSKI DL. Extra-thoracic esophagectomy in the treatment of esophageal cancer. *Am J Surg* 1980;**140**:772–778.

24 GISSELBRECHT C, CALVO F, MIGNOT L, *et al*. Treatment of advanced epidermoid carcinoma of the oesophagus with combined 5-fluorouracil and cis-

platinum (FAP). *Nouv Presse Med* 1982;11:1859–1862.

25 GRAHAM DY, DODDS SM, ZUBLER M. What is the role of prosthesis insertion in esophageal carcinoma? *Gastrointest Endosc* 1983;29:1–5.

26 HAGGITT RC, TRYZELAAR J, ELLIS FH, COLCHER H. Adenocarcinoma complicating columnar epithelium-lined (Barrett's) esophagus. *Am J Clin Path* 1978;70:1–5.

27 HEATLEY RV, WILLIAMS RHP, LEWIS MH. Pre-operative intravenous feeding—a controlled trial. *Postgrad Med J* 1979;55:541–545.

28 HEIMLICH HJ. Esophagoplasty with reversed gastric tube. *Am J Surg* 1972;123:80–92.

29 ICHIKAWA T. The clinical effect of Bleomycin against squamous cell carcinoma and further developments. *Prog Antimicrob Anticancer Chemother* (Proc Sixth Int Cong Chemother) 1970;2:288.

30 JONES DB, DAVIES PS, SMITH PM. Endoscopic insertion of palliative oesophageal tubes in oesophago-gastric neoplasms. *Br J Surg* 1981;68:197–198.

31 KIRK RM. A trial of total gastrectomy combined with total thoracic oesophagectomy without formal thoracotomy for carcinoma at or near the cardia of the stomach. *Br J Surg* 1981;68:577–579.

32 LEWIS I. The surgical treatment of carcinoma of the oesophagus with special reference to a new operation for growths of the middle-third. *Br J Surg* 1946;34:8–20.

33 LISHMAN AH, DELLIPIANI AW, DEVLIN HB. The insertion of oesophagogastric tubes in malignant oesophageal strictures: endoscopy or surgery? *Br J Surg* 1980;80:257–259.

34 MCKEOWN KC. Trends in oesophageal resection for carcinoma. *Ann R Coll Surg Engl* 1972;51:213–238.

35 MCKEOWN KC. Carcinoma of the oesophagus. *J R Coll Surg Edinb* 1979;24:253–274.

36 MILLER C. Carcinoma of the thoracic oesophagus and cardia. *Br J Surg* 1962;49:507–522.

37 MORSON BC. The spread of carcinoma of the oesophagus. In: Tanner NC, Smithers DW, eds. *Tumours of the oesophagus.* Edinburgh: Churchill Livingstone, 1961;136–145.

38 MURRAY GF, WILLCOX BR, STAREK PJK. The assessment of operability of oesophageal carcinoma. *Ann Thorac Surg* 1977;23:393–399.

39 NAEF AP, OZELLO L. Columnar-lined lower esophagus: an acquired lesion with malignant pre-disposition. *J Thorac Cardiovasc Surg* 1975;70:826–835.

40 OGILVIE AL, DRONFIELD MW, FERGUSON R, ATKINSON M. Palliative intubation of oesophagogastric neoplasms at fibreoptic endoscopy. *Gut* 1982;23:1060–1067.

41 ORRINGER MB, SLOAN H. Substernal gastric bypass of the excluded thoracic esophagus for palliation of esophageal carcinoma. *J Thorac Cardiovasc Surg* 1975;70:836–839.

42 PARKER EF, BALLENGER JF, SHULL KC. Esophageal resection and replacement for carcinoma. *Ann Surg* 1978;187:629–633.

43 PARKER EF, GREGORIE HB. Carcinoma of the esophagus long-term results. *JAMA* 1976;235:1018–1020.

44 PEARSON JG. The value of radiotherapy in the management of esophageal cancer. *Am J Roentgenol* 1969;105:500–513.

45 PEARSON JG. The present status and future potential of radiotherapy in the management of esophageal cancer. *Cancer* 1977;39:882–890.

46 POSTLETHWAIT RW. *Surgery of the oesophagus.* Hemel Hempstead: Appleton-Century-Crofts, 1979;341–395.

47 RANSEN MB, JOHN HT. Complications associated with the use of the Celestin tube for benign oesophageal obstruction. *Br J Surg* 1979;66:110–112.

48 RAVRY M, MOERTEL CG, SCHUTT AJ, HAHN RG, REITEMEIER RJ. Treatment of advanced squamous cell carcinoma of the gastro-intestinal tract with Bleomycin. *Cancer Chemother Rep* 1973;57:493–496.

49 ROBBINS AH, PUGATCH RD, GERZOF SG. Observations on the medical efficacy of computed tomography of the chest and abdomen. *Am J Roentgenol* 1978;131:15–19.

50 ROWLAND CG, PAGLIERO KM. Intracavitary irradiation in palliation of carcinoma of oesophagus and cardia. *Lancet* 1985;981–982.

51 RUBIN P. Cancer of the gastro-intestinal tract: II oesophagus. Treatment—localised and advanced. Pre-treatment laparotomy. *JAMA* 1974;227:184–185.

52 SOGA J, FUJIMAKI M, TNAKA O, SASAKI K, KAWAGUCHI M, MUTO T. Analysis of preoperative combined Bleomycin and radiation therapy for esophageal carcinoma. *World J Surg* 1983;7:230–235.

53 SPECHLER SJ, ROBBINS AH, RUBINS HB, *et al.* Adenocarcinoma and Barrett's esophagus. An over-rated risk. *Gastroenterology* 1984;87:927–933.

54 WATSON A. Resection or palliation in oesophageal carcinoma? *Proc World Cong Gastroenterol* 1982:9.

55 WATSON A. A study in the quality and duration of survival following resection, endoscopic intubation and surgical intubation in oesophageal carcinoma. *Br J Surg* 1982;69:585–588.

56 WONG J. Management of carcinoma of oesophagus: art or science? *J R Coll Surg Edinb* 1981;26:138–148.

Chapter 15
Other Diseases of the Oesophagus

A. W. DELLIPIANI

Congenital anomalies

These are dealt with in greater detail in Chapter 68, however a few remarks about how these affect the oesophagus are clearly required.

Oesophageal atresia and tracheo-oesophageal fistula

During embryonic development there may be a partial or complete failure of cannulation of the developing oesophagus [27]. In addition the cannulated part may become attached to the trachea leading to a tracheo-oesophageal fistula. This fistula may connect either to the upper or lower blind oesophageal pouch.

The clinical presentation is that of excessive salivation, choking, regurgitation and vomiting provoked by feeding. There may also be features of pulmonary aspiration. Early diagnosis, usually within a few hours of birth, should be made and investigation and treatment is generally undertaken by a highly specialized paediatric surgical team. A survival rate of over 70% can be expected if correctly managed [45].

Congenital cysts and reduplication

These are rarer abnormalities. Most occur in the lower oesophagus and may be associated with vertebral abnormalities including Klippel-Feil syndrome (congenital short neck) and spina bifida [1]. They are often asymptomatic but dysphagia may occur. Treatment is surgical.

Vascular abnormalities

Vascular abnormalities within the thorax may affect the oesophagus. The commonest is an aberrant right subclavian artery arising as a fourth branch from the thoracic aortic arch. The condition is usually asymptomatic but may give symptoms in older patients—'dysphagia lusoria'—presumably as a result of increased tortuosity or dilatation producing compression of an ageing oesophagus associated with a diminished propulsive activity.

Oesophageal perforation

Perforation may be either spontaneous or traumatic and is one of the most serious perforations affecting the gastrointestinal tract [15].

Spontaneous perforation is relatively uncommon [46]. It is usually seen in men and often occurs after a heavy meal followed by vomiting or straining. The mechanism is thought to be sudden and rapid overdistension of the oesophagus against a closed cricopharyngeal sphincter.

Traumatic perforation is more common. Chest injuries after a car crash can cause considerable diagnostic difficulties. Perforation may follow ingestion of a foreign body, or caustic fluid, but the commonest cause is instrumentation within the oesophagus [22]. This is much commoner after rigid oesophagoscopy than fibreoptic endoscopy, where the incidence is between 0.14–0.65/1000 [35, 50]. Other manipulative procedures, such as pneumatic dilatation, dilatation of benign and malignant strictures and insertion of prosthetic tubes, are all associated with the risk of perforation (see Chapters 10, 12 and 14). More subtle, and therefore more dangerous, are the perfora- tions that rarely occur after simple intubation during anaesthesia, or in the ward with, for example, the passage of a naso-gastric tube.

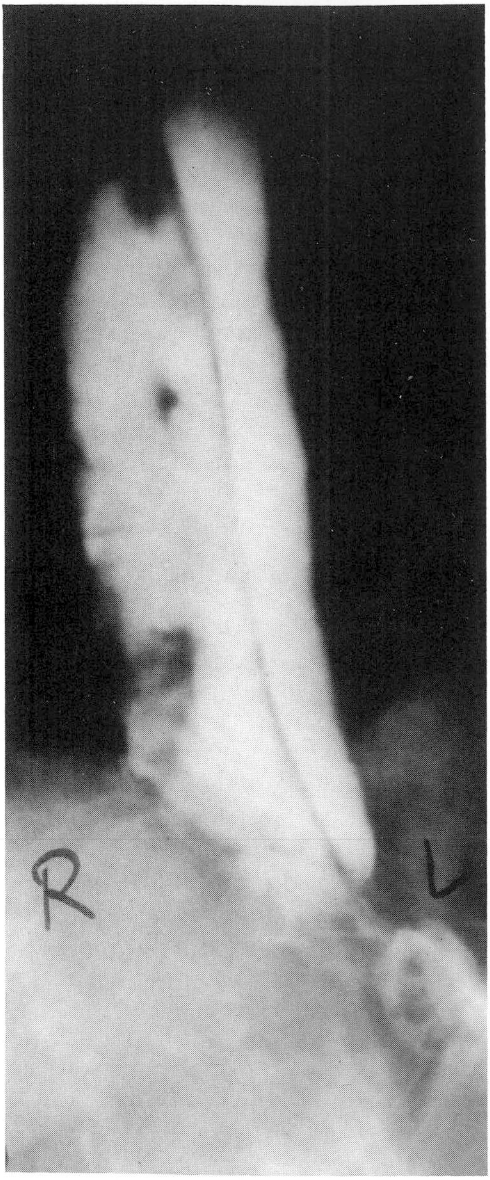

Clinical features

Perforations can occur in the cervical, intrathoracic or intra-abdominal segments of the oesophagus. Presenting symptoms depend on the site and size of the perforation and the persistence of leakage. Patients

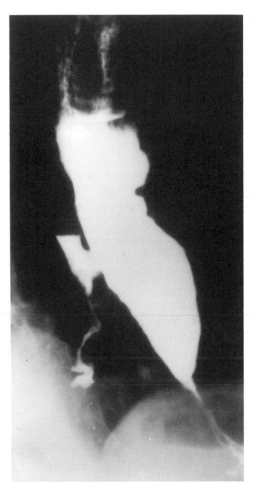

Fig. 15.1. The appearances shown on barium swallow in a 67-year-old man who presented with the sudden onset of severe chest pain, with pain on swallowing, due to a spontaneous perforation of the lower oesophagus.

Fig. 15.2. Instrumental (Hurst Bougie) perforation of the oesophagus in a patient with achalasia of the cardia. *Note* the typical dilatation of oesophageal body with tapered cardio-oesophageal junction.

with large perforations characteristically become very ill rapidly with severe pain in the chest, neck, or upper abdomen. Pain in the back is also common. Dysphagia, odynophagia, respiratory distress, cyanosis and pyrexia, also occur and the patient may be profoundly shocked.

Signs of mediastinal air are usually found—palpable crepitus in the neck due to surgical emphysema, or 'crackling' on auscultation of the chest is often present. A chest X-ray will usually confirm the diagnosis and may show a pleural effusion. However, the radiological features of a perforation may be delayed or absent with smaller perforations. Where there is doubt, especially in a patient with minimal symptoms, radiological assessment using a water soluble medium (e.g. Gastrografin) should confirm the diagnosis and locate the site of perforation (Figs 15.1, 15.2).

Management

Early diagnosis is the most important aspect of management. As spontaneous perforation is rare, and its features often mimic those of other intrathoracic and intra-abdominal emergencies, the initial diagnosis may be overlooked. In the most common type of perforation (that following oesophageal instrumentation), there is no excuse for missing the diagnosis and careful clinical and radiological assessment of a patient is mandatory if symptoms develop after such a procedure.

The treatment of large perforations is by surgical repair. Ideally this should be done within 24 hours, as after this period it becomes more difficult and some form of drainage and diversion procedure becomes necessary [35]. The mortality is high, especially after intrathoracic perforations [15, 39].

There is a small, but important role for non-operative management in this condition [36]. Where instrumental perforations occur in a 'clean oesophagus', such as at pneumatic dilatation, symptoms are often minimal and radiological assessment shows no leakage of contrast medium. Such perforations seal quickly and can be managed with analgesia, sedation, nasogastric aspiration and antibiotic therapy. Parenteral nutrition may be necessary but, in the author's experience, the nasogastric tube can usually be withdrawn within two to three days and light feeding resumed.

Foreign bodies

Oesophageal foreign bodies are most common in children, the mentally handicapped and the elderly. Many objects will impact in the cricopharyngeal region and are amenable to removal by laryngoscopy. Common foreign bodies include food boluses (Fig. 15.3), coins, needles and safety pins. In the absence of oesophageal disease most objects impact at the lower end of the oesophagus, though impaction in the mid-oesophagus occasionally occurs.

Clinical features

The patients complain of dysphagia and are, almost always, able to relate its onset to the ingestion of a particular object. In children and the mentally handicapped this history is not always present, and the symptoms may be refusal to eat, excessive salivation or regurgitation, or pain and discomfort in the chest. Localization requires postero-anterior and lateral X-ray views of the chest and cervical region. The features of a perforation should also be looked for on these radiographs. If the object is radiolucent, or there is doubt about the diagnosis—especially when the history is unreliable—a Gastrografin swallow may be needed (Fig. 15.4).

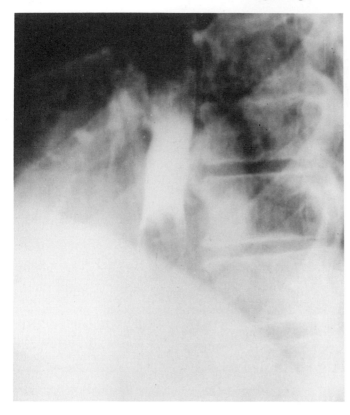

Fig. 15.3. Food bolus obstruction of the oesophagus in a patient presenting with acute onset dysphagia.

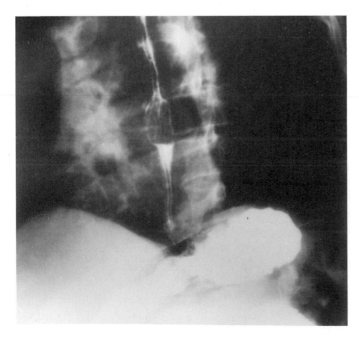

Fig. 15.4. Foreign body impacted in lower third of oesophagus (potato chip). Note normal mucosal appearance below this.

Management

If there is no undue distress, sedation may permit passage of a foreign body, such as an impacted meat bolus, into the stomach within a few hours. If the object does not move on, particularly if it is sharp, removal is necessary. This is not an area for the occasional endoscopist as considerable experience may be required. Fibreoptic endoscopy is now usually used, and is preferable to rigid oesophagoscopy because of the better view and lower risk of perforation. It may be possible to push the foreign body (for example food bolus) into the stomach ahead of the endoscope; otherwise it should be removed using an appropriate snare, or grasping forceps passed down the biopsy channel of the instrument. During withdrawal one must always be aware of the hazard of dropping the object into the larynx. Sharp or pointed objects may damage the oesophagus and pharynx during retrieval—this may be averted by passage of a flexible tube over the endoscope. This tube needs to be 50 cm long and, in an emergency, may be made out of garden hose. This tube is lubricated and passed over the proximal part of the endoscope before passage of the instrument. When the foreign body is found the tube is advanced beyond the end of the endoscope and the object is drawn into the tube before both are withdrawn. Though most endoscopists do these procedures using sedation, expert anaesthetic help should be readily available. When a foreign body has been pushed into the stomach it will almost always pass through the intestine without further problems but, if passage is delayed or the object is sharp, it should be removed from the stomach endoscopically.

Corrosive injuries

The ingestion of strongly acidic or, more commonly, alkaline solutions can severely damage the oesophagus [40]. This may be with suicidal intent or by accident, especially in children. Many corrosive substances are found amongst the ordinary household cleaning agents (for example household bleach). Swallowing alkaline solutions causes coagulative tissue necrosis with a variable penetration through the muscle layers depending upon contact time and strength. After a few days there is healing with granulation tissue and variable re-epithelialization and scarring.

Clinical features

The patient complains of pain in the mouth and chest. There is distress with dysphagia, odynophagia, excessive salivation, retching and vomiting. Features of a perforation should be looked for. Examination of the mouth will usually, but not invariably, show evidence of mucosal damage [14].

Management

Immediate management includes ingestion of a buffer to neutralize the toxic agent, potent analgesia and fluid replacement. Evidence of a perforation demands urgent surgical intervention. Otherwise it is important to assess the extent of the lesion within 12 hours of the injury using a flexible fibreoptic endoscope [9]. This assessment is important in planning early management, the length of hospitalization and the need to use a variety of therapeutic agents which, in themselves, are not without hazard. The objectives of treatment are to encourage healing and to anticipate, and attempt to diminish, the severity of stricture formation.

The traditional approach included analgesia, antibiotics, corticosteroids, sedation and intubation to keep the oesophagus open. Steroids were given in large doses for a period of three to six weeks (for example hydrocortisone 200 mg six hourly). Nutritional support by parenteral or intrajejunal feeding was needed.

This management approach has been challenged by Di Constanza *et al.* [10], who dispensed with intubation, routine antibiotics and corticosteroids. Precise advice is difficult to formulate because few have extensive experience of severely ill patients and there have been no controlled trials. In those where endoscopy shows only inflammation (Stage I) light feeding can be started immediately and prolonged hospitalization is not required. Where there is necrosis of the upper oesophageal mucosa only and/or the stomach (Stage II), or necrosis of the whole of the oesophageal mucosa (Stage III), parenteral feeding should be given for about 15 days. The author does not believe that antibiotics or intubation are required routinely but only in response to specific indications.

In the present state of uncertainty it would seem reasonable to give parenteral corticosteroids for Stage III cases. Radiological and endoscopic surveillance for stricture formation should begin after two to three weeks. The most popular way of managing strictures is by endoscopy and dilatation (Eder-Peustow or Celestin dilator). Intractable strictures may require surgical treatment using a by-pass procedure. This can be extremely difficult, particularly if the stricture starts in the pharynx and the stomach has been involved. Carcinoma is a recognized long term hazard in such patients [2].

Non-peptic oesophagitis

Monilial oesophagitis

This occurs in patients who are immunologically compromised, suffering from diabetes or hypoparathyroidism and after prolonged treatment with wide spectrum antibiotics or corticosteroids. Another pre-

disposing factor is impaired oesophageal emptying as occurs with carcinoma, strictures or motility disorders. Occasionally moniliasis occurs spontaneously [20].

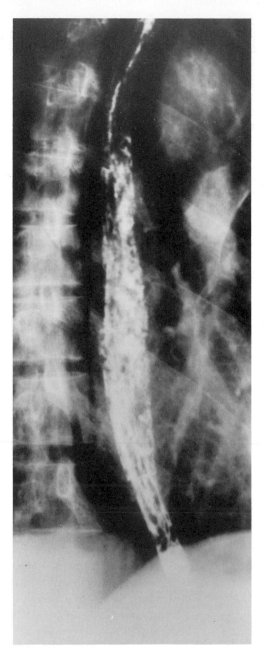

Fig. 15.5. Appearance of the oesophagus on a barium swallow in a patient with severe candidiasis.

Clinical features

Most patients are asymptomatic but there may be dysphagia or odynophagia. *Candida* can usually be seen as white plaques on the hard and soft palate, occasionally these typical oral lesions are absent (Chapter 7) [43]. A barium swallow may be normal, but it may show a ragged or nodular mucosal margin or ulceration with (occasionally) segmental narrowing (Fig. 15.5). The diagnosis is often made at endoscopy when white plaques are seen lying on the mucosa. In more advanced cases these plaques may be confluent with hyperaemia and frank ulceration of the mucosa. The yeast can be demonstrated microscopically on biopsies or brush cytology smears. The main differential diagnoses are severe reflux oesophagitis or an herpetic infection.

Treatment

Nystatin suspension (200,000 units in 2 ml) is swallowed two to four hourly for several weeks. Resistant or chronic cases may require more aggressive treatment— miconazole, which can be given either orally (250mg 6-hourly) or parenterally, has proved successful in this situation [37]. Ketoconazole is a systemic antifungal agent that can be given by mouth and this may be the treatment of choice in severely ill patients [12]. However there is recent evidence that an occasional patient may develop chronic liver damage on this agent so it must not be used as initial treatment. General management should include the identification and treatment of fungal infections in other parts of the body.

Herpes oesophagitis

Herpes simplex infection may also occur in the immuno-compromised [28] and the severely debilitated or terminally ill patient [3, 19]. It has also been described occasionally in normal individuals [32].

Clinical features

These may range from no symptoms to dysphagia, odynophagia, or rarely major bleeding [8, 42]. There are no distinctive radiological features. Endoscopy will show discrete, or confluent superficial ulceration that may mimic moniliasis. Typical eosinophilic inclusion bodies in biopsies, and a rise in complement fixing antibodies against herpes simplex in the serum, will confirm the diagnosis. The endoscopist must be aware of the danger of viral transfer when taking biopsies, particularly to the eyes, and precautions should be taken to avoid this.

Treatment

The traditional treatment for this condition was to use the same mode of management as one would use for peptic oesophagitis (see Chapter 11). However specific antiviral therapy for this condition is now available and should be used for any cases where the condition is severe. This is acyclovir (Zovirax) which should be given for at least five days (5 mg/kg i.v. 8 hrly, or 200 mg 4 hrly by mouth) [21].

Drug-induced oesophagitis

Several drugs have been implicated as a cause of oesophageal ulceration or stricture formation. These include emepronium bromide, potassium salts, iron preparations, some analgesics and antibiotics and even beta-adrenergic blockers. It has also been suggested that there is a higher incidence of benign oesophageal stricture in association with non-steroidal anti-inflammatory drugs [7, 16].

Drug induced oesophagitis is particularly likely to occur in old and debilitated patients whose oesophageal clearance may be impaired. Under these circumstances tablets and capsules may remain in the oesophagus for longer than normal producing local tissue damage. This is even more likely if there is an organic cause for hold-up. For these reasons patients should always be encouraged to take all their medications in the upright position with plenty of water to wash them down [18].

Radiation induced oesophagitis

Thoracic irradiation (as for bronchial carcinoma) may be followed by oesophagitis. Symptoms usually occur some weeks or months after the treatment has started. Symptoms may range from mild to severe and can include an achalasia-like disturbance of motility [44].

Treatment

Steroids have been recommended in the treatment of this condition [29] and recent animal work suggests that indomethacin may prevent severe oesophageal involvement, if it is given before the irradiation [30]. However, usually the symptoms are quite mild and it is difficult to justify routine prophylaxis.

Other non-peptic causes of oesophagitis

Infective causes, such as tuberculosis and syphilis, are now extremely uncommon but a giant oesophageal ulcer, associated with cytomegalovirus, has been described in a homosexual drug abuser [38]. Mucosal lesions have also been observed in Behçet's syndrome [23] and in Crohn's disease [25]. Pemphigoid and epidermolysis bullosa may also rarely affect the oesophageal mucosa [11, 31].

Webs and rings

Webs are formed from squamous epithelium whilst **rings** are lined by squamous epithelium on their upper surface and columnar on their lower. Unlike a ring, which tends to be circumferential, a web occupies only part of the oesophageal wall.

The **Paterson–Kelly or Plummer–Vinson syndrome** was originally described in 1919. The syndrome includes intermittent dysphagia, glossitis, koilonychia and iron-deficiency anaemia. It commonly presents in post-menopausal women although younger women and men may also be affected. In recent years its incidence has fallen, presumably as a result of better nutrition. Occasionally the dysphagia may occur in the absence of the complete syndrome and with a normal serum iron. The aetiology is obscure, though an auto-immune background has been suggested [6].

The pathological changes include degeneration of the epithelium over the upper oesophageal sphincter with fibrosis and lymphocytic infiltration. There may be web formation anteriorly in the post-cricoid region. Demonstration of this web requires a very careful radiological technique which is helped by cine-radiography (Fig. 15.6).

Management

This includes oral iron and the careful endoscopic examination of the post-cricoid area to exclude carcinoma. The passage of the endoscope itself is often sufficient to relieve the symptoms. As the condition is thought to be pre-malignant, regular follow-up with endoscopic surveillance is recommended [5].

Other webs and rings

It has been suggested that a 'ring' can also occur in the post-cricoid area, at the junction between ectopic gastric mucosa

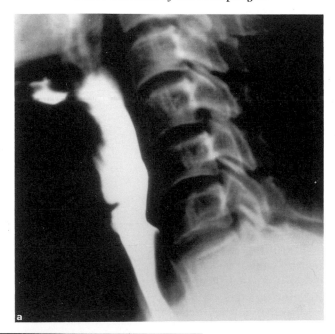

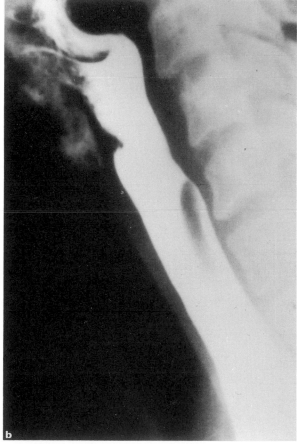

Fig. 15.6. (a) and (b): Two examples of post-cricoid webs demonstrated on barium swallows.

and the squamous epithelium of the upper oesophagus. This will mimic the Paterson–Kelly syndrome [47]. Rings may also occur at other sites within the oesophagus through a similar mechanism.

Webs can also rarely occur in the middle and lower part of the oesophagus. Their aetiology remains obscure [26, 41]. True webs are usually congenital and asymptomatic. In adults they may present with intermittent dysphagia or sudden food bolus obstruction. Treatment is by dilatation.

Schatzki rings occur in the lower oesophagus. Their aetiology is unknown and inflammation is usually absent. There is controversy as to their significance and whether they represent the site of the gastro-oesophageal mucosal junction or the presence of a hiatus hernia [17]. They are usually asymptomatic being found on barium swallow during the investigation of reflux or ulcer symptoms. Occasionally they present as intermittent dysphagia or bolus obstruction, particularly when eating under stressful circumstances (such as eating in public or at a banquet).

The diagnosis is made by a careful radiological technique and usually the ring can be seen endoscopically. Treatment is by dilatation which, in difficult cases, may have to be pneumatic in type, as for achalasia (see Chapter 10).

Oesophageal diverticula

Oesophageal diverticula are most often mucosal pouches protruding through the wall of the oesophagus (Fig. 15.7). True diverticula, where all the layers of the oesophagus are found, are rare and probably variants of a duplication of the alimentary tract. Most consist of the epithelium alone and are typically found in the pharynx, mid- and lower-oesophagus.

Pharyngeal pouch (Zenker's diverticulum) is the most important diverticulum of the oesophagus. It occurs (Fig. 15.8) just

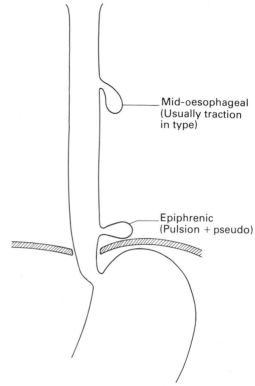

Fig. 15.7. Diagrammatic illustration of the sites of diverticula in the oesophagus.

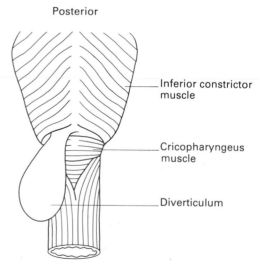

Fig. 15.8. Diagrammatic illustration of the anatomical site at which a pharyngeal pouch occurs.

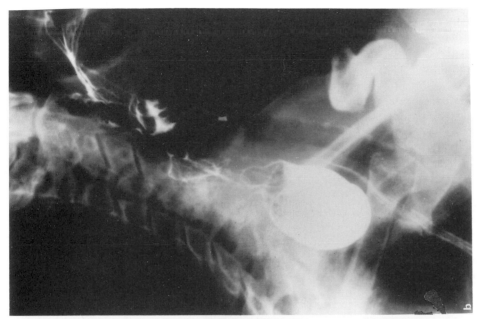

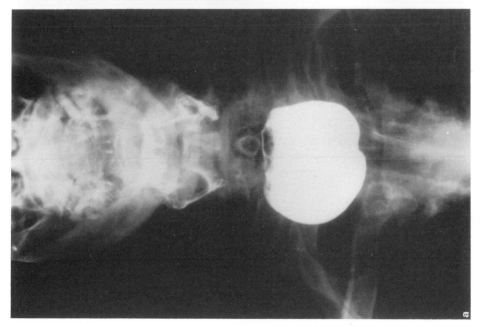

Fig. 15.9. (a) and (b): Anterior-posterior and lateral views of a pharyngeal pouch (Zenker's diverticulum).

above the crico-pharyngeal sphincter in the weak area between this and the superior constrictor muscle. Muscular incoordination of the crico-pharyngeal sphincter has been implicated in its aetiology [24]. Other pharyngeal diverticula can occur in particular occupations, such as glass blowers and wind instrument players, but these are rare.

A pharyngeal pouch usually presents with intermittent dysphagia, food regurgitation and occasional pulmonary aspiration. The patient is generally in the older age group and sometimes the dysphagia can become very severe with weight loss. Rarely a swelling may be palpable in the neck, after food, and some patients recognize the need to regurgitate or empty food from the pouch if normal swallowing is to be achieved. The diagnosis is made by a barium swallow with careful views of the neck area (Fig. 15.9). Endoscopy is not indicated and is dangerous in such patients.

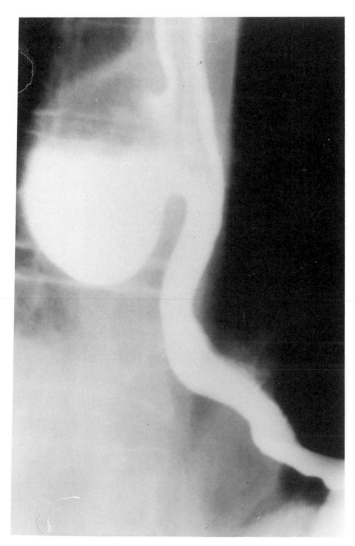

Fig. 15.10. Large diverticulum in the lower-third of the oesophagus shown on barium swallow—the patient was asymptomatic.

Treatment

Management is surgical, usually involving excision of the pouch with primary closure of the mucosa. Controversy reigns as to whether recurrence is prevented by a crico-pharyngeal myotomy at the same time as the excision. Elderly, debilitated patients, with a small pouch, may be helped by an endoscopic crico-pharyngeal myotomy alone [34, 49].

Other oesophageal diverticula

Diverticula in the mid-oesophagus are usually traction in type and are most often secondary to mediastinal inflammation, such as tuberculosis involving the peribronchial lymph nodes.

Epiphrenic or lower oesophageal diverticula are commonly associated with some motility defect (see Chapter 10). Most are wide necked (Fig. 15.10). Occasionally pseudo-diverticula occur in this area from the healing of an oesophageal ulcer. Treatment is conservative.

Intramural diverticulosis

This is an extremely rare condition in which collar-stud out-pouchings can be seen radiologically along the oesophageal wall. These are due to the dilatation of the oesophageal submucosal glands of unknown aetiology. It usually occurs in elderly patients whose complaint is of dysphagia. Motility disturbances are often present and may be severe [4, 13].

Benign oesophageal tumours

Leiomyoma

A leiomyoma is often detected incidentally at the time of a barium meal performed for another reason. Occasionally it may present with dysphagia or gastrointestinal bleeding.

The tumour is typically intramural and dumb-bell in shape. The radiological appearances are usually characteristic and, if the tumour is very large, it may be visible on a plain X-ray of the chest. On barium swallow the classical appearance is of a smooth filling-defect with a clearly defined edge—sometimes there is ulceration at its apex. Encirclement and obstruction of the lumen can occur. At endoscopy the lesion is covered by a healthy normal oesophageal mucosa, unless ulceration has occurred. Endoscopic biopsy is seldom helpful because it is impossible to take a deep enough bite for representative tissue. Treatment is surgical—usually local enucleation is possible but a local resection is sometimes required.

Other benign tumours

There are several other benign tumours that can occur in the oesophagus. These can be either mucosal or submucosal in origin. They include squamous papillomas, benign epithelial cysts, inflammatory fibrous polyp, haemangiomas, lymphangiomas, fibromas, lipomas and hamartomas [33].

Such tumours may be large or pedunculated, causing dysphagia. Occasionally a pedunculated tumour of the upper oesophagus may result in airways obstruction. The diagnosis is made on radiology and confirmed by endoscopy and biopsy, when appropriate. Treatment may be either surgical, with resection, or endoscopic by snare removal of a small pedunculated lesion.

References

1 ANDERSON HA, PLUTH JR. Chapter 11. In: Payne WS, Olsen AM, eds. *The esophagus*. Philadelphia: Lea and Febiger, 1974.
2 APPELQUIST P, SALMO N. Lye corrosive strictures of the esophagus—a review of 63 cases. *Cancer* 1980;**45**:2655–2658.
3 BUSS H, SCHARYJ M. Herpes virus infection of the esophagus and other visceral organs in adults. In-

cidence and clinical significance. *Am J Med* 1979;**66**:457–462.

4 CASTILLO S, ABURASHED A, KIMMELMAN J, ALEXANDER LC. Diffuse intramural esophageal pseudodiverticulosis. *Gastroenterology* 1977;**72**:541–545.

5 CHISHOLM M. The association between webs, iron deficiency and post-cricoid carcinoma. *Postgrad Med J* 1974;**50**:215–219.

6 CHISHOLM M, ARDRAN GM, CALLENDER ST, WRIGHT R. A follow-up study of patients with postcricoid webs. *Q J Med* 1971;**40**:409–420.

7 COLLINS FJ, MATHEWS HR, BAKER SE, STRAKOVA JM. Drug induced oesophageal injury. *Br Med J* 1979;**i**:1673–1676.

8 DENT J. What's new in the esophagus. *Dig Dis Sci* 1981;**26**:161–173.

9 DILAWARI JB, SURJIT SINGH, RAO PN, ANAND BS. Corrosive acid ingestion in man—a clinical and endoscopic study. *Gut* 1984;**25**:183–187.

10 DI CONSTANZA J, NOIRCLERC M, JOUGLARD J, *et al.* New therapeutic approach to corrosive burns of the upper gastrointestinal tract. *Gut* 1980;**21**:370–375.

11 ENG TY, HOGAN WJ, JORDAN RE. Oesophageal involvement in bullous pemphigoid. A possible cause of gastrointestinal haemorrhage. *Br J Dermatol* 1978;**99**:207–210.

12 FAZIO RA, WICKREMESINGHE PC, ARSURA EL. Ketoconazole treatment of candida esophagitis. *Am J Gastroenterol* 1983;**78**:261–264.

13 FROMKES J, THOMAS FB, MEKHJIAN H, CARDWELL JH, JOHNSON JC. Esophageal intramural pseudodiverticulosis. *Dig Dis Sci* 1971;**22**:690–700.

14 GAUDREAULT P, PARENT M, MCGUIGAN MA, CHICOINE L, LOVEJOY FH. Predictability of esophageal injury from signs and symptoms: a study of caustic ingestion in 378 children. *Pediatrics* 1983;**71**:767–770.

15 GOLDSTEIN LA, THOMPSON WR. Esophageal perforations—a fifteen year experience. *Am J Surg* 1982;**143**:495–503.

16 HELLER SR, FELLOWS IW, OGILVIE AL, ATKINSON M. Nonsteroidal anti-inflammatory drugs and benign oesophageal stricture. *Br Med J* 1982;**285**:167–168.

17 HENDRIX TR. Schatzki ring, epithelial junction and hiatus hernia. *Gastroenterology* 1980;**79**:584–585.

18 HEY H, JORGENSEN F, SORENSEN K, HASSELBLACH H, WAMBERG T. Oesophageal transit of six commonly used tablets and capsules. *Br Med J* 1982;**285**:1717–1719.

19 HOWILER W, GOLDBERG HI. Gastroesophageal involvement in Herpes Simplex. *Gastroenterology* 1976;**70**:775–778.

20 KODSI BE, WICKREMSINGHE PC, KOZINN PJ, ISWARA K, GOLDBERG PK. Candida esophagitis—A prospective study of 27 cases. *Gastroenterology* 1976;**71**:715–719.

21 JEFFRIES DJ. Clinical use of Acyclovir. *Br Med J* 1985;**290**:177–178.

22 LEADER ARTICLE. Instrumental perforation of the oesophagus. *Lancet* 1984;**ii**:1279–1280.

23 LEVACK B, HANSON D. Bechets disease of the oesophagus. *J Laryngol Otol* 1979;**93**:99–101.

24 LICHTER I. Motor disorders in the pharyngoesophageal pouch. *J Thorac Cardiovasc Surg* 1978;**76**:272–275.

25 LIVOLSI VA, JARETZKI A, III. Granulomatous oesophagitis. *Gastroenterology* 1973;**64**:313–319.

26 LONGSTRETH GF, WOLOCHOW DA, TU RT. Double congenital mid-esophageal webs in adults. *Dig Dis Sci* 1979;**24**:162–165.

27 DE LORIMIER AA, HARRISON MR. Esophageal atresia: embryogenesis and management. *World J Surg* 1985;**9**:250–257.

28 MCDONALD GB, SHARMA P, HACKMAN RC, MEYERS JD, DONNALL THOMAS Esophageal infections in immunosuppressed patients after marrow transplantation. *Gastroenterology* 1985;**88**:1111–1117.

29 NELSON RS, HERNANDEZ AJ, GOLDSTEIN HM, SACA A. Treatment of irradiation esophagitis. Value of hydrocortisone injection. *Am J Gastroenterol* 1979;**71**:17–23.

30 NORTHWAY MG, LIBSHITZ HI, OSBORNE BM, *et al.* *Gastroenterology* 1980;**78**:883–892.

31 ORLANDO RC, BOZYMSKI EM, BRIGGAMAN RA, BREAM CA. Epidermolysis bullosa: Gastrointestinal manifestations. *Ann Intern Med* 1974;**81**:203–206.

32 OSWENSBY LC, STAMMER JL. Oesophagitis associated with Herpes Simplex infection in an immunocompetent host. *Gastroenterology* 1978;**74**:1305–1306.

33 PATEL J, KIEFFER RW, MARTIN M, AVANT GR. Giant fibrovascular polyp of the esophagus. *Gastroenterology* 1984;**87**:953–956.

34 PAYNE WS. In: Payne WS, Olsen AM, eds. *The esophagus.* Philadelphia: Lea & Febiger, 1974.

35 PAYNE WS, BROWN PW, FONTANA RS. Chapter 9. In: Payne WS, Olsen AM, eds. *The esophagus.* Philadelphia: Lea & Febiger, 1974.

36 QUAYLE AR, MOORE PJ, JACOB G, GRIFFITHS CDM, ROGERS K. Treatment of oesophageal perforation by intubation. *Ann R Coll Surg Engl* 1985;**67**:101–102.

37 RUTGEERTS L, VERHAEGEN H. Intravenous miconazole in the treatment of chronic esophageal candidiasis. *Gastroenterology* 1977;**72**:316–318.

38 ST ONGE G, BEZAHLER GH. Giant esophageal ulcer associated with Cytomegalovirus. *Gastroenterology* 1982;**33**:127–130.

39 SANDRASAGRA FA, ENGLISH TAH, MILSTEIN BB. The management and prognosis of oesophageal perforations. *Br J Surg* 1978;**65**:629–632.

40 SCAPA E, ESHCHAR J. Chemical burns of the upper gastrointestinal tract. *Burns Incl Therm Inj* 1985;**11**:269–273.

41 SHIFLETT DW, GILLIAM JH, WU WC, AUSTIN WE,

OTT DJ. Multiple esophageal webs. *Gastroenterology* 1979;77:556–559.

42 SPRINGER DJ, DACOSTA LR, BECK IT. A syndrome of acute self limiting ulcerative esophagitis in young adults probably due to Herpes Simplex virus. *Dig Dis Sci* 1979;24:535–539.

43 TAVITIAN A, RAUFMAN J-P, ROSENTHAL E. Oral candidiasis as a marker for esophageal candidiasis in the acquired immunodeficiency syndrome. *Ann Int Med* 1986;104:54–57.

44 THORPE JAC, OAKLAND C, ADAMS IP, MATHEWS HR. Irradiation induced motor disorders of the oesophagus. *Gut* 1982;23:710–711.

45 TOCCALINO H, LICASTRO R, GUASTAVINO E, *et al.* Vomiting and regurgitation. *Clin Gastroenterol* 1977;6:267–297.

46 WALKER WS, CAMERON EWJ, WALBAUM PR. Diagnosis and management of spontaneous transmural rupture of the oesophagus (Boerhaave's syndrome). *Br J Surg* 1985;72:204–207.

47 WEAVER GA. Upper esophageal web due to a ring formed by a squamocolumnar junction with ectopic gastric mucosa (another explanation of the Paterson–Kelly syndrome). *Dig Dis Sci* 1979;24:959–963.

48 WESDORP ICE, BARTELSMAN JFWM, HUIBREGTSE K, DEN HARTOG JAGER FCA, TYTGAT GN. Treatment of instrumental oesophageal perforation. *Gut* 1984;25:398–404.

49 WORMAN LW. Pharyngo-oesophageal diverticulum—excision or incision. *Surgery* 1980;87:236–237.

50 WRIGHT RA. Upper esophageal perforation with a flexible endoscope secondary to cervical osteophytes. *Dig Dis Sci* 1981;25:66–68.

SECTION IV

DISEASES OF
THE STOMACH AND
DUODENUM

Chapter 16
Radiology and Endoscopy of the Stomach and Duodenum

T. G. GIRDWOOD & R. H. SALTER

For many years the conventional barium meal examination was the most important diagnostic technique for acute upper gastrointestinal disorders. The poor diagnostic accuracy of this procedure—approximately 70%—[3, 20] was not generally appreciated, because verification could only be made at laparotomy, or necropsy. Gastroscopy was done with rigid instruments and was unpleasant, potentially dangerous and of limited usefulness.

The introduction of fibreoptic endoscopy rapidly exposed the inadequacies of the conventional barium meal examination and prompted the development of more sophisticated radiological methods. The subsequent comparative studies of the two techniques led to realization that each has advantages and limitations.

Double-contrast radiology

Double-contrast radiology of the upper gastrointestinal tract was pioneered by Japanese radiologists and was simplified in the United Kingdom by Scott-Harden [26, 28].

Unlike the lumen-imaging approach of the conventional barium meal, double-contrast radiology is a technique of mucosal imaging, the mucosa being coated with a fine layer of barium and the lumen of the viscus distended with gas—usually CO_2. The double-contrast barium meal is quick, well tolerated by the patient and does not need premedication. The morbidity and mortality of the technique is negligible. The better diagnostic accuracy of the double-

contrast over the conventional technique is beyond doubt, the diagnostic sensitivity and specificity being approximately 92% and 85% respectively [14, 20, 22].

The main disadvantage is that although the double-contrast technique is comparatively easy to learn, interpretation of the radiographs needs considerable experience and diagnostic errors usually arise because of misinterpretation, rather than because of failure to show the lesion.

In the double-contrast barium meal the stomach and the duodenum are distended with gas (carbon dioxide, CO_2) and the entire mucosal surface is repeatedly coated with barium (Fig. 16.1). Fluoroscopy is used mainly for positioning and timing of the radiographs and to monitor gastric and duodenal distension by the gas. Duodenal and gastric contractions, the rate of gastric emptying and the presence or absence of sliding hiatus hernia and of gastro-oesophageal reflux are also detected by fluoroscopy. The diagnosis can be made from radiographs, if these are of high quality, so that the risk of observer error during screening is decreased.

The barium suspension used should be a compromise between high density and low viscosity and the volume given to the fasting patient varies between 50–200 ml. Distension is produced by the administration of gas-releasing tablets, or granules, or by getting the patient to swallow a drink with a high CO_2 content—these can be given either before, during, or after the barium. The volume of gas should be sufficient to distend the lumen, separating the walls and

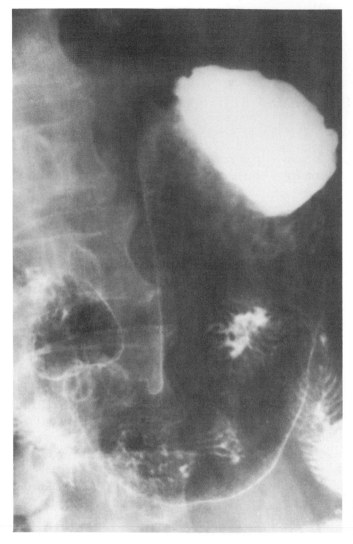

Fig. 16.1. Normal stomach and duodenum as demonstrated by double contrast barium meal.

stretching the mucosal folds, but without obliterating them (Fig. 16.1).

Many different modifications of the original double-contrast technique have been introduced, each with claimed advantages. However, the overall diagnostic sensitivity and specificity remain remarkably constant [16]. Particularly controversial is the routine use of smooth muscle relaxing agents during the examination. Despite the claimed improvement in diagnostic accuracy, the routine use of these agents such as intravenous hyoscine butylbromide (Bus-copan), or glucagon, advocated by Kreel, Herlinger and Glanville [19], has not led to any important improvement in the sensitivity and specificity of the method. A more selective approach, using parenteral smooth muscle inhibitors only when the stomach and duodenum are over-active, seems better practice.

Fibreoptic endoscopy

Fibreoptic endoscopy with modern instruments allows complete inspection of the lumen of the stomach and proximal duodenum. The technique is not difficult to learn and adequate interpretation skills can be acquired after 80–100 examinations, although higher numbers may be needed to establish reliability [18]. Apart from diagnostic accuracy, one important advantage of endoscopy is the facility of acquiring specimens for cytological and histopathological examination, which is particularly important when there is any suspicion of malignant disease. An expanding range of therapeutic procedures is being developed. Relative disadvantages are that endoscopy is invasive, time-consuming, usually needs the administration of sedatives and carries small, but definite morbidity and even mortality.

Some radiologists define the endoscopist's role as that of a sophisticated trouble-shooter [31], the need for this investigation being prompted by the result of good quality double-contrast radiography of the stomach and duodenum which, it can be argued, is a more cost-effective screening procedure. On the other hand most clinical gastroenterologists use endoscopy as the first diagnostic procedure in the investigation of symptoms thought to originate in the stomach or duodenum. During the last few years the number of endoscopies has increased enormously. The proportion of patients referred for either type of examination will be thus determined by local preferences and availability of facilities. The usefulness of open-access endoscopy for general practitioners remains to be determined [17].

The technique of fibreoptic endoscopy of the stomach and duodenum is detailed in many endoscopy texts [6, 7, 10, 36]. These also discuss choice, maintenance and cleaning of instruments, requirements for efficient endoscopy units, supporting staff and normal and abnormal appearances. The reader is directed to them for details.

The basic requirements are that after fasting for 6–8 hours, the patient is given a minimal intravenous dose of a drug such as diazepam, necessary to achieve sedation: usually between 10 and 20 mg. Many endoscopists combine this with a smooth muscle relaxant such as hyoscine butylbromide (Buscopan), 20–40 mg—there are many minor variations concerning premedication. With the patient reclining on the left side the selected endoscope (usually end-viewing) is introduced through a guarding mouthpiece held between the patient's teeth into the pharynx and the patient encouraged to swallow. When the instrument passes into the upper oesophagus it is guided down the oesophageal lumen under direct vision and through the lower oesophageal sphincter into the stomach. The endoscope is then passed down the stomach to the antrum and through the pylorus where the duodenal bulb and the second part of the duodenum are inspected. The instrument is then gradually withdrawn into the stomach with any abnormalities being recorded—some endoscopists photograph any abnormality encountered. The lumen of the stomach is thoroughly examined as the instrument is withdrawn towards the cardia. It is particularly important to inspect the fundus and cardia from below by retroverting the endoscope. Cytological exfoliative brushings and multiple targeted biopsies are taken as necessary for histopathological examination. In uncomplicated cases endoscopy usually takes 10–15 minutes in experienced hands. Premedication with diazepam induces a useful amnesia for the procedure. After endoscopy the patients must be told not to take anything by mouth for one hour if a local anaesthetic (Xylocaine 2%) spray to the fauces was used; it is usual to advise patients not to drive, or operate dangerous machinery for 24 hours, if intravenous diazepam was administered.

Closed circuit colour television or videotape recording allows the procedure to be

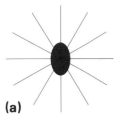

(a)

Fig. 16.2. (a) mucosal guideline pattern indicating a benign gastric ulcer. (b) arrow shows benign gastric ulcer indicated by characteristic guideline pattern.

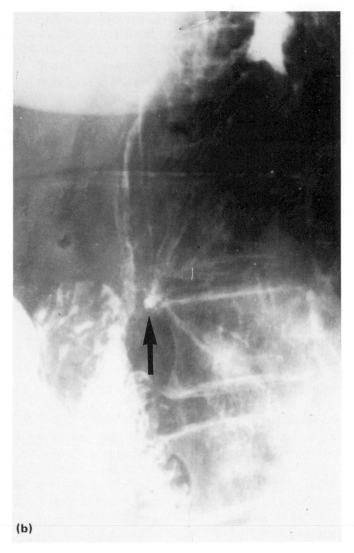

(b)

followed by interested observers; this is a valuable teaching aid, but it is not likely to be widely available.

The relative advantages and limitations of radiology and endoscopy in commonly encountered clinical situations are as follows.

X-ray negative dyspepsia

Further investigation of X-ray negative dyspepsia when the barium meal has been of the conventional type accounts for an ap-preciable fraction of an endoscopist's work-load. However, the endoscopic yield from the investigation of dyspeptic patients after a negative double-contrast barium meal is small (sensitivity approximately 96%) [23]. The practical implications of this are that if a good quality double-contrast barium meal done by an experienced radiologist does not show any abnormality, an alternative ex-planation should be sought for the patient's complaints, unless there are clinical poin-ters that strongly suggest upper gastro-intestinal disease. The role of endoscopy as

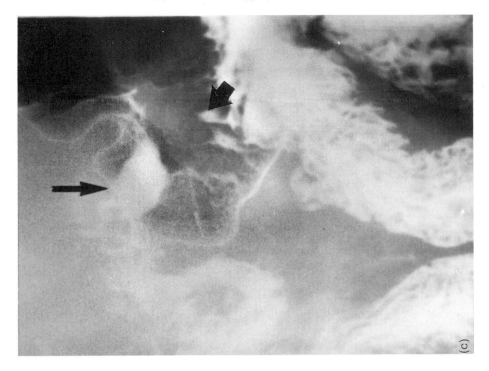

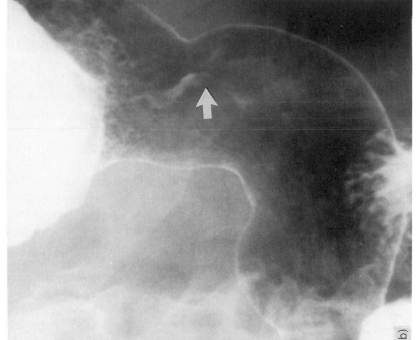

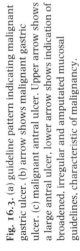

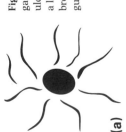

Fig. 16.3. (a) guideline pattern indicating malignant gastric ulcer. (b) arrow shows malignant gastric ulcer. (c) malignant antral ulcer. Upper arrow shows a large antral ulcer, lower arrow shows indication of broadened, irregular and amputated mucosal guidelines, characteristic of malignancy.

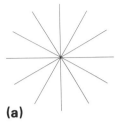

(a)

Fig. 16.4. (a) Mucosal guideline pattern indicating ulcer scar. (b) healed gastric ulcer. Ulcer crater no longer present, mucosal guidelines converge on the scar.

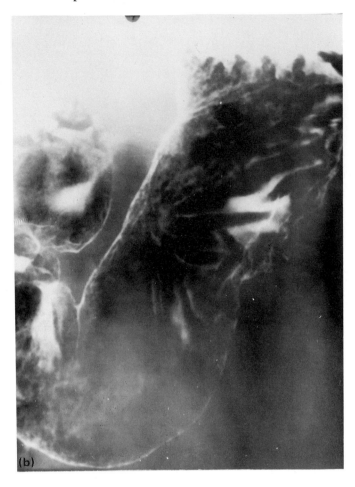

(b)

the first investigation of dyspepsia has been reviewed recently, with recommendations to minimize costs by reserving endoscopy for those whose symptoms persist despite treatment for six to eight weeks, while those who show no response, develop complications, have recurrent symptoms, or have a systemic illness should be endoscoped earlier [12].

Gastric ulcer

Unlike the conventional examination, the double-contrast barium meal is a reliable method for diagnosing gastric ulcer. The main radiological features of gastric ulceration demonstrated by the double-contrast technique are a barium niche of varying shape or, if the ulcer is on the anterior gastric wall, a ring shadow. The characteristics of the surrounding mucosal pattern are particularly important.

As it is impossible to distinguish with certainty between a benign lesion and an ulcerating gastric malignancy, endoscopy is mandatory in gastric ulcer, so that multiple targeted biopsies and exfoliative cytological brushings can be obtained. However, appearances of the mucosal pattern around the ulcer crater displayed by double-contrast radiology allow accurate differentiation between benign or malignant ulcers, regardless of the site, size, or shape of the crater [24]. The characteristic mucosal

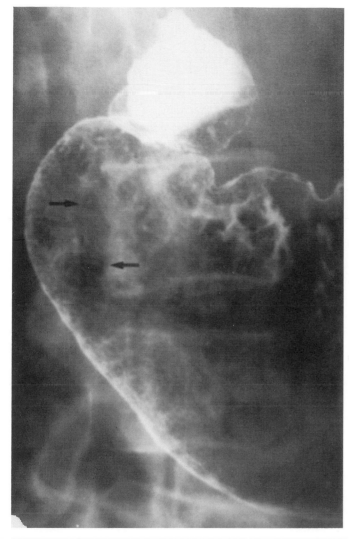

Fig. 16.5. Arrows show multiple gastric erosions in the antrum.

guidelines indicating a benign lesion are thin, straight and run directly into the rim of the ulcer crater, as shown in Fig. 16.2. [29]. In contrast, the mucosal guidelines indicating malignancy are thick, distorted and stop short of the crater rim [34, 35] (Fig. 16.3).

Even when radiological and endoscopic examinations indicate that a gastric ulcer is benign, careful follow-up is essential until the ulcer has healed to a scar. This is indicated radiologically by the guidelines converging on a central point [29] (Fig. 16.4), or endoscopically by scarring and complete epithelialization of the ulcer crater.

Small gastric erosions are clearly visible at endoscopy and can also be shown by the double-contrast technique, when they appear as translucent rings or ovoids of oedema with a small, central fleck of barium (Fig. 16.5).

Gastric polyps

The double-contrast barium meal and endoscopy have shown that gastric mucosal

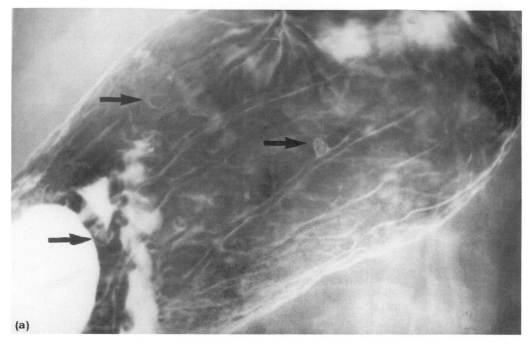

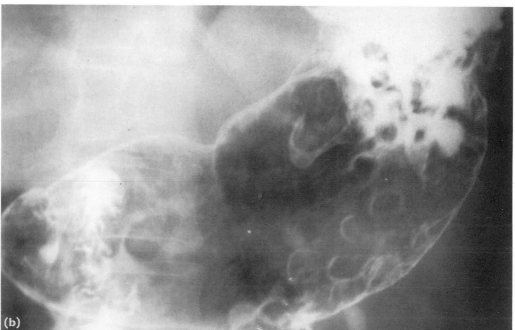

Fig. 16.6. (a) and (b) multiple gastric polyps.

polyps occur more often than previously realized [13]. The characteristic radiological pattern consists of filling defects with a sharply defined outer border, which is frequently slightly irregular (Fig. 16.6). The stalk of a pedunculated polyp may be visible. Gas bubbles can mimic gastric polyps, but they do not have a sharply defined border, or the slightly irregular outline. Moreover, gas bubbles tend to change location or disappear if several radiographs are taken and the area washed with barium between exposures [21].

The commonest variety is the hyperplastic gastric polyp, which tends to be small and multiple and carries no malignant potential. However, hyperplastic polyps may be found in association with carcinoma elsewhere in the stomach [4]. The adenomatous polyps that are premalignant tend to be single and larger than the hyperplastic variety and should be removed, preferably by endoscopic snare polypectomy.

Endoscopy of the patient with gastric polyps is mandatory in order to establish the

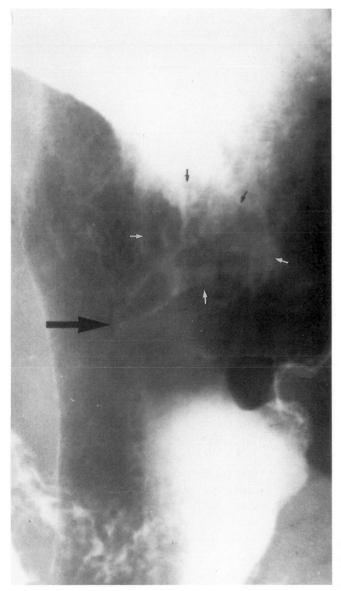

Fig. 16.7. Small arrows show early gastric carcinoma adjacent to benign gastric ulcer (large arrow).

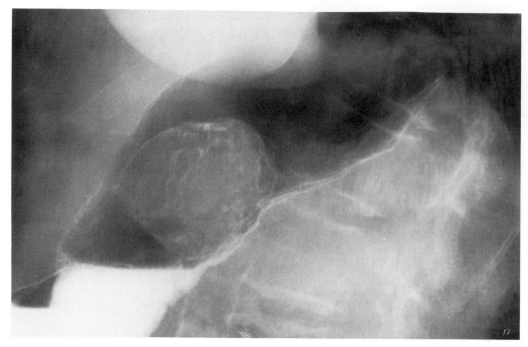

Fig. 16.8. Encephaloid gastric carcinoma.

diagnosis and to biopsy representative lesions to establish the type of polyp (see Chapter 27).

Gastric carcinoma

In addition to showing advanced lesions, the double-contrast barium meal is sufficiently sensitive to suggest the diagnosis of early gastric cancer, where the growth is confined to the mucosa and submucosa. The characteristic radiological features of early gastric cancer include an area of slightly elevated mucosal irregularity, or the presence of mucosal folds ending abruptly at some distance from a shallow ulcer, or a raised plaque [4, 34, 35] (Fig. 16.7).

The radiological features of advanced malignancy vary depending on the type of neoplasm. The encephaloid type is indicated by a mass projecting into the gastric lumen (Fig. 16.8) and sessile tumours show up as plaques or protrusions associated with an irregular guideline pattern and punctate mottling over the surface (Fig. 16.9) [32]. Submucosal infiltration produces decreased distensibility, or contraction—if diffuse, the condition is recognized as linitis plastica, or the 'leather bottle stomach' (Fig. 16.10) [26].

If radiology was the initial diagnostic investigation, the slightest suspicion of malignancy demands subsequent endoscopy and multiple biopsies and brushings for histological and cytological studies. The highest diagnostic yield is obtained when radiology and endoscopy are regarded as complementary. Early gastric cancer can only be diagnosed if an aggressive investigational approach is adopted using sophisticated radiological techniques together with endoscopy, in patients of middle age or older, presenting for the first time with persistent dyspepsia [4] (see Chapter 28).

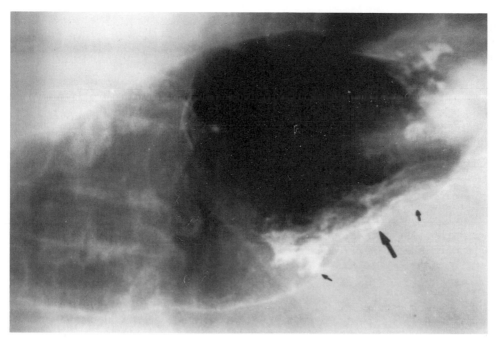

Fig. 16.9. Carcinomatous plaque with central ulceration (large arrow) on the greater curve of the stomach (small arrows).

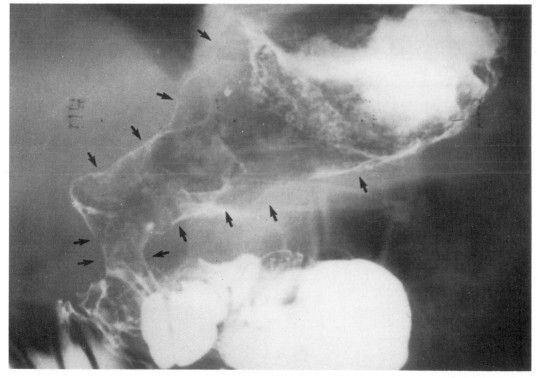

Fig. 16.10. Infiltrating gastric carcinoma; previous gastroenterostomy.

Gastric outlet obstruction

The commonest causes of gastric outlet obstruction in adults are a chronic stenosing duodenal ulcer and carcinoma of the distal stomach. Adult hypertrophic pyloric stenosis is rare.

The radiologist and the endoscopist may have to deal with retained gastric contents which should be aspirated before starting either procedure. It is usually possible to determine radiologically whether the obstructing lesion is on the gastric or the duodenal side of the pylorus and whether it is benign or malignant. Surgical intervention is usually indicated whatever the cause, but preoperative confirmation of carcinoma of the gastric outlet by endoscopic biopsy is helpful and usually possible despite the residue of fluid and food. It may be feasible to make a radiological diagnosis of a chronic stenosing duodenal ulcer causing pyloric obstruction, where it is impossible to pass the tip of the endoscope through the pylorus.

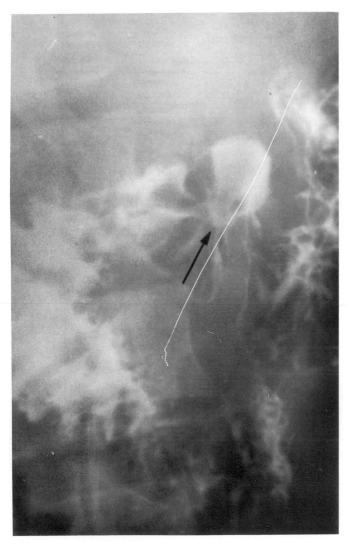

Fig. 16.11. Chronic duodenal ulcer.

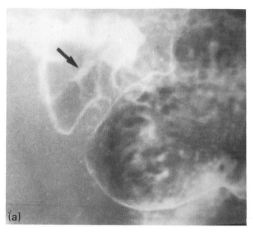 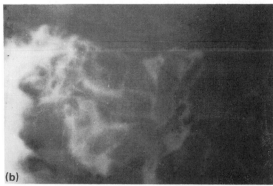

Fig. 16.12 (a) linear duodenal ulcer. (b) same ulcer healed to a scar.

Duodenal ulcer

Providing the duodenal cap can be adequately distended, the double-contrast barium meal can be used to show the presence or absence of duodenal ulcer, but deformity of the proximal duodenum in chronic ulceration may make it difficult to know if an ulcer crater is present. Failure to distend the duodenal bulb (irritable cap) is not a reliable pointer to the presence of an ulcer crater within it. Post-bulbar ulcers are infrequent but should be remembered as a possible diagnosis.

The main radiological features of duodenal ulcer are a barium niche situated in the posterior wall and a ring shadow if the ulcer is on the anterior wall of the duodenal cap. The ulcer may or may not be surrounded by converging guidelines (Figs. 16.11, 16.12(a)), or a surrounding mound of oedema appearing radiologically as a zone of translucency encircling the ulcer crater. Scarring is indicated by the convergence of guidelines on a central point with or without distortion of duodenal cap (Fig. 16.12(b)) [29].

Endoscopic confirmation is not essential when the classical picture of a duodenal ulcer is obtained radiologically. However, when the diagnosis is uncertain, or when it is not clear from radiology whether a duodenal ulcer is present, endoscopy is essential and must be combined with thorough visualization of the whole of the upper gastrointestinal tract. Endoscopy is particularly important if there is any doubt about the diagnosis and surgery is being considered. Routine biopsy of ulcers in the duodenum is not necessary, but if the lesion looks atypical, tissue should be collected for histopathological examination for the differential diagnosis of Crohn's disease or malignancy.

Occasionally it may be difficult at endoscopy to confirm or exclude the presence of an active ulcer crater in a grossly distorted duodenal bulb. Lesions in the duodenal fornix may be difficult to visualize and narrowing of the pyloric canal associated with a juxtapyloric duodenal ulcer may prevent duodenal intubation. A slim side-viewing endoscope should be used when adequate visualization has not been possible with an end- or oblique-viewing instrument. Duodenal ulcer is further discussed in Chapters 20–24.

The post-surgical stomach

The conventional barium meal was notoriously inaccurate in the post-operative sto-

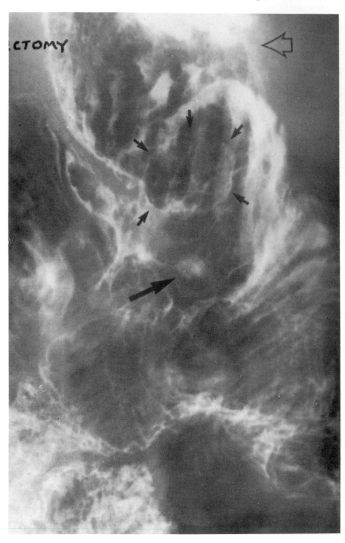

Fig. 16.13. Jejunal ulcer (solid large arrow) adjacent to stoma (solid small arrows) after Polya gastrectomy (gastric remnant indicated by open arrow).

mach [33] and fibreoptic endoscopy is the best procedure for the investigation of dyspepsia after ulcer surgery [5]. Bile reflux, difficulty of adequately distending the stomach and anatomical distortion may all contribute to the endoscopist's difficulties in this situation [25]. Double-contrast radiology is of some value in these patients, the technique being modified to overcome the problem of the rapid escape of the distending gas through a stoma or a freely open pylorus after pyloroplasty [11]. The best diagnostic accuracy stems from comple-

mentary use of endoscopy and double-contrast radiology. Using radiology and/or endoscopy, conditions such as gastro-oesophageal reflux of gastric juice, or bile, gastric or gastric remnant ulceration or malignancy, ulceration associated with gastroenterostomy, gastrointestinal anastomosis, or with pyloroplasty (Fig. 16.13), or recurrence of duodenal ulcer can all be diagnosed [25]. Ulceration recurrent after gastric operations is further discussed in Chapter 24.

Acute upper gastrointestinal bleeding

Endoscopy is the most accurate method of establishing the source of acute bleeding from the upper gastrointestinal tract and should be done as soon as practicable after the patient's admission to the hospital. In many units with limited staff trained in endoscopy this is difficult; in any case several studies have suggested that early endoscopy has not affected the outcome of acute gastrointestinal haemorrhage. Emergency endoscopy can be difficult, particularly when the patient is bleeding at the time of the examination and the diagnostic yield is smaller than under optimal circumstances [15, 37]. Detailed interpretation of endoscopic appearances in acute upper alimentary bleeding is discussed in Chapter 30.

Double-contrast radiology performed as soon as possible after admission [3] is claimed to have a diagnostic yield only slightly smaller than emergency endoscopy [9] and the modified technique is well tolerated by the patient [30]. The radiological features of recent or active bleeding are the presence of blood clot on an ulcer (Fig. 16.14) or an artery in the base of an ulcer (Fig. 16.15). Active bleeding at the time of examination appears as a central translucency due to blood oozing from the ulcer crater surrounded by a half-density barium-halo (Fig. 16.16) [30].

Arteriography should be considered if endoscopy fails to define the source of haemorrhage, but diagnostic success depends on presence of bleeding at the time of the examination and is precluded by previous barium studies. Arteriography may locate the bleeding site, but is rarely informative about its pathological basis. The angiographic catheter can be used for selective infusion of vasopressor agents, or injection of embolic material to stop the bleeding [1].

Therapeutic endoscopy

Although the main use of fibreoptic endoscopy of the stomach and duodenum is diagnostic, it can also be used for treatment [2]. Endoscopic polypectomy and using the diathermy snare for the endoscopic removal of

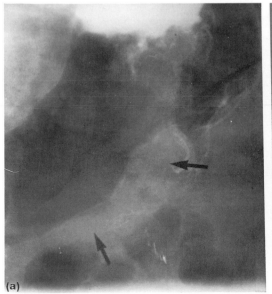 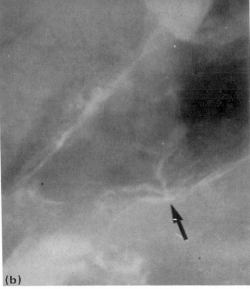

(a) (b)

Fig. 16.14. (a) blood clot adherent to greater curve. (b) clot moved to reveal underlying malignant ulcer indicated by bent broadened guidelines.

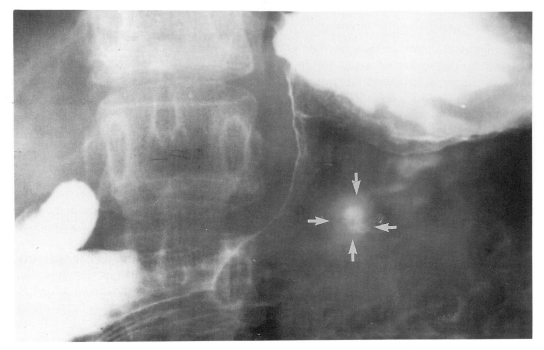

Fig. 16.15. Artery in the base of a bleeding gastric ulcer.

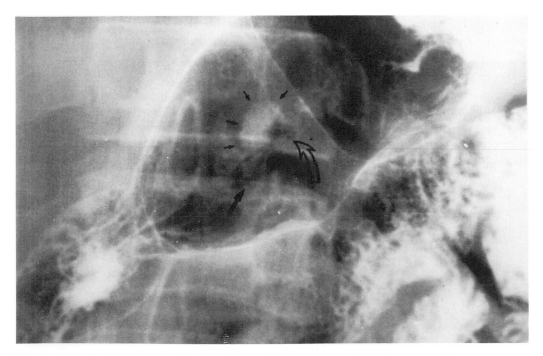

Fig. 16.16. Bleeding from a gastric ulcer. Curved arrow demonstrates central translucency, small arrows indicate halo and large solid arrow indicates ulcer guidelines.

foreign bodies which fail to leave the stomach are examples. The usefulness of endoscopic control of arterial bleeding using a laser beam, or electrocoagulation is at present being studied (see Chapter 30).

Conclusions

Double-contrast radiology of the upper gastrointestinal tract has high diagnostic sensitivity for the initial assessment of patients with upper gastrointestinal symptoms. The conventional single-contrast barium meal should be regarded as obsolete. Fibreoptic endoscopy improves diagnostic specificity and has the important advantage of direct visualization of lesions and the capability of establishing a histopathological diagnosis. Endoscopy is the investigation of first choice in the diagnosis of recurrent duodenal ulcer in the presence of deformity of the duodenal cap, in post-surgical problems and in acute gastrointestinal bleeding. It is mandatory whenever the presence of cancer is suspected and in the evaluation and follow up of gastric ulcer.

The choice of initial investigational technique depends on clinical circumstances and the availability of resources. The number of endoscopies done has increased enormously in recent years and in many units the demand for barium meal examinations has greatly decreased. Where available, endoscopy is generally preferred to radiology [8], but best results are obtained when both techniques are used in a complementary fashion.

References

1 ALLISON DJ. Gastrointestinal bleeding—radiological diagnosis. *Br J Hosp Med* 1980;**23**:358–365.
2 BENNETT JR, ed. *Therapeutic endoscopy and radiology of the gut.* London: Chapman and Hall, 1981.
3 COTTON PB. Fibreoptic endoscopy and the barium meal—results and implications. *Br Med J* 1973;ii:161–165.
4 COTTON PB, ed. *Early gastric cancer, proceedings of the second B.S.G., S.K. & F. International Workshop.* Smith Kline & French, 1981.
5 COTTON PB, ROSENBERG MT, AXON ATR, *et al.* Diagnostic yield of fibre-optic endoscopy in the operated stomach. *Br J Surg* 1973;**60**:629–632.
6 COTTON PB, WILLIAMS CB. *Practical gastrointestinal endoscopy.* 2nd ed. Oxford: Blackwell Scientific Publications, 1982.
7 DEMLING I, ELSTER K, KOCH H, RÖSCH W. *Endoscopy and biopsy of the oesophagus, stomach and duodenum.* 2nd ed. Philadelphia: W.B. Saunders Co., 1982.
8 DOOLEY CP, LARSON AW, STACE NH, *et al.* Double-contrast barium meal and upper gastrointestinal endoscopy. A comparative study. *Ann Intern Med* 1984;**101**:538–545.
9 FRASER GM. The double contrast barium meal in patients with acute upper gastrointestinal bleeding. *Clin Radiol* 1978;**29**:625–634.
10 FRÜHMORGEN P, CLASSEN M, eds. *Endoscopy and biopsy in gastroenterology.* Berlin: Springer-Verlag, 1980.
11 GIRDWOOD TG. In: James WB, ed. *The Double Contrast Barium Meal. Proceedings of a Symposium. Glasgow.* Rickmansworth: Concept Pharmaceuticals, 1976:24.
12 HEALTH AND PUBLIC POLICY COMMITTEE. American College of Physicians. Endoscopy in the evaluation of dyspepsia. *Ann Intern Med* 1985;**102**:266–269.
13 HERLINGER H. Double contrast radiology of gastric polyps. In: Nolan DJ, ed. *Double contrast barium techniques of the upper gastrointestinal tract. Proceedings of a Seminar, Oxford.* Rickmansworth: Concept Pharmaceuticals, 1979:28–29.
14 HERLINGER H, GLANVILLE JN, KREEL L. An evaluation of the double contrast barium meal (D.C.B.M.) against endoscopy. *Clin Radiol* 1977; **28**:307–314.
15 HOARE AM. Gastrointestinal bleeding—endoscopic diagnosis. *Br J Hosp Med* 1980;**23**:347–356.
16 JAMES WB, ed. *The double contrast barium meal. Proceedings of a symposium, Glasgow.* Rickmansworth: Concept Pharmaceuticals, 1976.
17 JONES R. Open access endoscopy. *Br Med J* 1985;**231**:424–426.
18 KLING PA, EDIN K, DOMELÖFF L. Observer variability in upper gastrointestinal fiber-endoscopy. *Scand J Gastroenterol* 1985;**20**:462–465.
19 KREEL L, HERLINGER H, GLANVILLE J. Technique of the double contrast barium meal with examples of correlation with endoscopy. *Clin Radiol* 1973;**24**:307–314.
20 LAUFER I, MULLENS JE, HAMILTON J. The diagnostic accuracy of barium studies of the stomach and duodenum. *Radiology* 1975;**115**:559–573.
21 NOLAN DJ, ANAND BS. In: Nolan DJ, ed. *The double contrast barium meal: a radiological atlas.* Chicago: Year Book Medical Pubs., Inc., 1980:57–67.
22 SALTER RH. Upper gastrointestinal endoscopy in perspective. *Lancet* 1975;ii:863–864.

23 Salter RH. X-ray negative dyspepsia. *Br Med J* 1977;ii:235–236.

24 Salter RH, Gill DK, Girdwood TG, McNeill RH, Athey G. Gastric ulcer—is endoscopy always necessary? *Br Med J* 1981;282:2097.

25 Salter RH, Girdwood TG, Scott-Harden WG, Cole TP. The radiological and endoscopic assessment of recurrent ulceration after peptic ulcer surgery. *Br J Radiol* 1978;51:257–259.

26 Samuel E, Laws JW, Whiteside CG, Sutton D. In: Sutton D, ed. *The gastrointestinal tract and abdomen: a textbook of radiology and imaging.* Edinburgh: Churchill Livingstone, 1980:681–712.

27 Scott-Harden WG. Double contrast (air-contrast) radiology of the stomach and duodenum. *Gut* 1972;13:850.

28 Scott-Harden WG. Evaluation of double contrast gastro-duodenal radiology. *Br J Radiol* 1973;46:153.

29 Scott-Harden WG. Radiological investigation of peptic ulcers. *Br J Hosp Med* 1973;10:149–153.

30 Scott-Harden WG. Radiology of acute upper digestive tract bleeding. *J R Coll Physicians Lond* 1974;8:365–374.

31 Scott-Harden WG. Radiology now—upper digestive tract radiology today. *Br J Radiol* 1976;49:658–659.

32 Scott-Harden WG. The stomach and duodenum. In: Lodge T, Steiner R E, eds. *Recent advances in radiology and medical imaging. Number 6.* Edinburgh: Churchill Livingstone, 1979:65–77.

33 Schulman A. Anastomotic gastro-jejunal ulcer: accuracy of radiological diagnosis in surgically proven cases. *Br J Radiol* 1971;44:422–433.

34 Shirakabe H. *Atlas of X-ray diagnosis of early gastric cancer.* Philadelphia: Lippincott, 1966.

35 Shirakabe H. *Double contrast studies of the stomach.* Stuttgart: George Thieme Verlag, 1972.

36 Sugawa C, Schuman BM. *Primer of gastrointestinal fibreoptic endoscopy.* Boston: Little, Brown, 1981.

37 Zambartas C, Cregeen RJ, Forrest JAH, Finlayson NDC. Accuracy of early endoscopy in acute upper gastrointestinal bleeding. *Br Med J* 1982;285:1540.

Chapter 17
Gastric Secretion

J. H. BARON

Physiology

The mucosa of the gastric body and fundus has different secretory functions from the antrum. The antrum does not secrete acid or pepsin, but contains cells that synthesize and release alimentary polypeptide hormones, such as gastrin.

The parietal cells in the body of the stomach secrete acid and intrinsic factor and the zymogen chief cells secrete pepsinogens which are converted by acid into pepsins. Alkaline mucus is secreted by the surface epithelial and mucous neck cells of the body and by the pyloric cells of the antrum. Microscopical anatomy of the gastric mucosa is described in Chapter 18. Acid and intrinsic factor are secreted by the same parietal cell. The number of parietal cells is correlated with the number of chief cells, so that measurement of acid alone is an expression of gastric secretory capacity with but few exceptions.

There are three interconnected phases of gastric secretion—cephalic, gastric and intestinal. These three phases overlap in time and are also mutually interrelated in a complicated nervous and hormonal system (Fig. 17.1). Not all the complexities have been unravelled, nor can it be certain that each of the separate mechanisms has a role in normal physiology.

The **cephalic phase** begins with the expectation, thought, sight and smell and perhaps chewing and swallowing of food stimulating vagal centres via the hypothalamus. The vagus nerves send preganglionic cholinergic efferent fibres to the nerve plexuses of many parts of the alimentary system. Postganglionic nerves from these plexuses stimulate the stomach and intestines directly, as well as potentiating indirectly their response to other stimuli. Thus the vagi excite the exocrine cells of the body of the stomach by direct cholinergic stimulation and by cholinergic potentiation of other stimuli, such as gastrin. The vagi affect the endocrine cells of the antrum of the stomach by direct cholinergic stimulation of gastrin release and by cholinergic potentiation of gastrin release by other stimuli, including distension and the chemicals in food.

The **gastric phase** begins when food enters the stomach. Food stimulates stretch receptors and possibly chemoreceptors in the body of the stomach eliciting local and vagovagal distension reflexes, which evoke acid secretion. When food reaches the antrum of the stomach its bulk stimulates stretch receptors and its peptides and amino acids stimulate chemoreceptors in the pyloric gland area. Specialized G cells in the mucosa of the antrum then release their gastrin hormones. Gastrins are carried by the blood stream and stimulate the parietal cells of the body of the stomach to secrete acid. The antrum has an important pH-dependent negative feedback system, by which acid in contact with the mucosa inhibits further release of gastrin.

The **intestinal phase** of gastric secretion begins when food and its digestive products enter the intestine. Neuroreceptors are stimulated and intestinal gastrins and other hormones released. Acid and fat entering

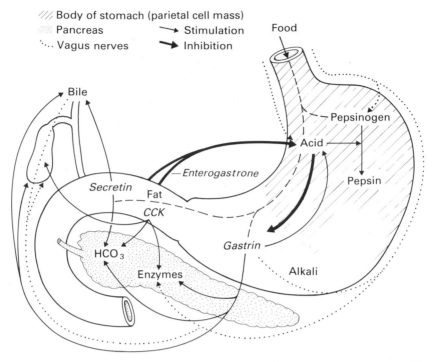

Fig. 17.1. The regulation of gastric acid secretion. Names in italics are hormones. Names in upper and lower case are alimentary secretions. The body of the stomach (parietal cell mass) is represented by oblique shading, and pancreas by stippling. The vagus nerves are shown as dotted lines. Stimulation is indicated by thin arrows, and inhibition by thick arrows ([1] adapted with permission of the editors of *Proc R Soc Med*).

the duodenum and intestine inhibit gastric acid secretion, another feedback system [1].

Summary

A meal entering the stomach elicits, by neural and endocrine mechanisms, secretion of acid and pepsins, which acidify, sterilize and initiate the digestion of the meal. When the resultant chyme reaches the antrum and duodenum it is partly neutralized by the alkaline secretion of the pyloric glands; duodenum, pancreas and by bile and it also causes inhibition of further acid secretion. The now liquefied meal is at the correct pH for intestinal digestion and absorption. The rate of entry of the chyme into the small intestine is closely controlled by a separate set of reflexes, discussed in Chapter 26.

Measurement of acid

Gastric secretion is measured to try to answer three questions: How many parietal (or chief) cells are there in the stomach of this patient? Are all, some or none of these cells innervated by branches of the vagus nerves? Are there excess gastrins stimulating these parietal cells [2, 4]?

Technique

The three important tests are measurements of basal, maximal and cephalic-stimulated secretion. Procedures are best standardized to generally accepted standards for reliability and for comparisons with tests performed elsewhere. Our 1968 protocol in the Department of Surgery, Royal Postgraduate Medical School, Hammersmith Hospital, London, can be summarized:

1. Tests are best performed early in the morning and can comprise basal secretion alone, or basal followed by maximal, or basal and cephalic, or basal-cephalic-maximal. The combined tests spare the patient from having to attend on subsequent occasions.

2. The patient should be fasting from the previous night and should not have taken antacids that morning, or any drugs affecting gastric secretion during the preceding 24 hours.

3. The test is explained to the patient.

4. The patient's weight (kg) and height (cm) are measured and recorded.

5. The patient lies comfortably on a couch and a nostril (preferably the right) and throat are sprayed with a solution of 3% lignocaine in isotonic saline. The gastric tube is plastic, radio-opaque throughout, 14–16 mm in circumference, 125 cm long, and of the Levin type with holes close to the tip. The tube, well lubricated with liquid paraffin, is passed through the nose. The patient is asked to swallow repeatedly while the tube is being pushed steadily and rapidly down through the pharynx and oesophagus into the stomach. Gagging and retching are minimized by instructing the patient to take deep breaths.

6. A 20–50 ml syringe is attached to the end of the tube, using an adaptor if necessary and the stomach emptied of the **resting juice** and air by repeated syringe suction. If there is food retained in the stomach of a fasting patient, it should be washed out and the test repeated after a day on a fluid diet.

7. The tube can be positioned fluoroscopically in the body of the stomach. The **water recovery** test is an alternative to fluoroscopy. The patient drinks 20 ml of water and this is recovered by aspiration. The tube is then withdrawn 2–5 cm at a time and the water recovery test repeated after each withdrawal until the shortest possible tube

position is achieved with satisfactory recovery. The tube is taped to the face and the stomach is again emptied.

8. The tube is connected to a pump with continuous suction at a subatmospheric pressure of 30 to 50 mmHg. The pump suction is interrupted frequently (e.g. every 5 minutes) by manual syringe suction followed by injection of 10 ml air down the tube from a syringe, or side-arm bulb, to clear aspirated mucus, or mucosa blocking the holes in the tube. Minor adjustments of tube position may be necessary to allow satisfactory aspiration.

9. For **basal secretion** one 60-minute, or four 15-minute aspirates are collected and labelled with the times of the collection periods.

10. **Pentagastrin** (Peptavlon, ICI), 6 μg/kg, is injected intramuscularly (i.m.), the time recorded, and four consecutive 15-minute, or six 10-minute aspirates are collected and labelled with the exact times. This test is preceded by the basal hour and may also be preceded by a cephalic test (sham feeding).

11. A **pentagastrin infusion** test may be done as an alternative to the single parenteral injection. An intravenous (i.v.) infusion of 0.9% NaCl is started and after the basal period pentagastrin 6 μg/kg/h is infused for 90 minutes with six consecutive 15-minute, or nine 10-minute, aspirates.

12. **Cephalic** tests

a. With **sham feeding** the patient chews and spits out a tasty meal, such as steak and salad, or a toasted sandwich. A mouthful of food is well chewed and then spat out, and the mouth washed out with a small amount of water to ensure that no food particles are swallowed. The chew, spit and rinse is repeated for several cycles for ten minutes, during which gastric secretion is aspirated continually, with further aspirations for further five 10-minute periods. Peak, or maximum, acid output is calculated as for pentagastrin-stimulated acid.

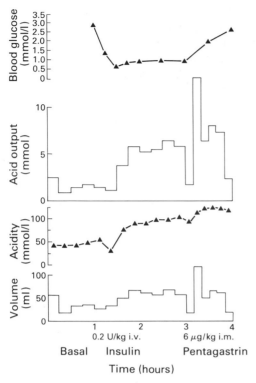

Fig. 17.2. Blood glucose and gastric secretory volume, acidity and acid output one hour before, and two hours after a single intravenous injection of insulin 0.2 U/kg, and one hour after an intramuscular injection of pentagastrin 6 μg/kg ([5] adapted with permission of Macmillan Publishers Ltd).

b. For the **single intravenous injection of insulin** test 2 ml of venous blood for estimation of glucose is taken at 0 minutes, and soluble insulin B.P. (20 U/ml) 0.2–1.0 U/kg is injected intravenously through the same needle. Eight 15-minute aspirates are collected and labelled. Venous blood, 2 ml for glucose estimation, is taken at 30 and 45 minutes after the insulin injection.

c. The **insulin infusion** test is an alternative to the test with a single intravenous injection of insulin. An intravenous infusion of 0.9% NaCl is started and after the basal period soluble Insulin B.P. in a dose of 0.15 u/kg/h is infused for 150 minutes during which ten 15-minute collec-

tions of gastric juice are made. Venous blood, 2 ml for glucose estimation is taken at 0, 45, 60, 75, 90 and 120 minutes. These insulin tests are always preceded by the basal hour test. A cephalic test sham feeding, single intravenous injection of insulin or insulin infusion may be followed by either of the pentagastrin tests—that is a basal-cephalic-maximal test either by single injection (Fig. 17.2) or by intravenous infusion (Fig. 17.3). During an insulin test, the patient's comments and appearance are recorded. Glucose, 50 ml of 50%, is kept immediately available and is injected intravenously if the patient has symptoms of hypoglycaemia. At the end of any test a drink of glucose, or sweetened tea is given and the patient is not allowed to leave the laboratory until recovered from the hypoglycaemia.

13. The volume (ml), pH (units) and titratable acidity (mmol/l) are measured and the amount of acid (mmol) in each specimen calculated: Volume (l) × Titratable acidity = Acid output (mmol).

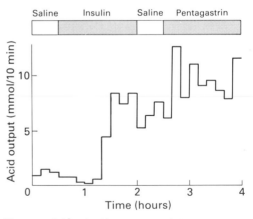

Fig. 17.3. Acid output in response to intravenous infusion of soluble insulin 0.15 U/kg-h for 90 minutes followed after 30 minutes of infusion with 0.9% saline, by infusion of pentagastrin 6 U/kg-h for 90 minutes. Blood glucoses were: basal 72 mg/100 ml (4.0 mmol/h); at 60 minutes 25 mg/100 ml (1.4 mmol/h); at 90 minutes, 43 mg/100 ml (2.4 mmol/h) ([5] adapted with permission of Macmillan Publishers Ltd).

14. Basal acid output (BAO) and peak acid output after pentagastrin (PAO$_{Pg}$) and after insulin (PAO$_I$) or sham feeding (PAO$_{SF}$) are expressed as mmol/h [9].

Agonists

Maximal secretion is evoked by a dose of agonist sufficient to stimulate all the parietal cells of the stomach. The natural secretagogue, pure gastrin I or II has been used as a maximal stimulus, but is not available for routine tests because of expense. The active C-terminal tetrapeptide sequence Try. Met. Asp. Phe-NH₂ has the entire range of physiological activities of the natural gastrin hormone. This sequence

has been synthesized as **tetragastrin** which also can produce maximal gastric acid output. The synthetic peptide mostly in use is pentagastrin (Peptavlon, ICI).

Pentagastrin stimulates acid similarly to gastrin and the highest peak acid is achieved by a dose of 6 μg/kg given subcutaneously, or intramuscularly—the usual routine. Pentagastrin given intravenously, or even subcutaneously, may rarely produce severe unwanted effects such as fainting, bradycardia and hypovolaemia, all rapidly responding to intravenous antihistamine, or hydrocortisone and suggesting an idiosyncratic or a hypersensitivity response.

Histamine was the first gastric stimulant commonly used. It is only in the last 30

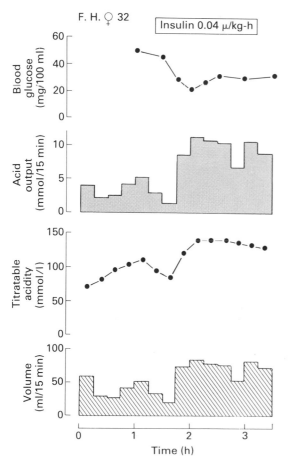

Fig. 17.4. Blood glucose and gastric secretory volume, acidity and acid in 1 hour before and 2½ hours after an intravenous infusion of insulin 0.04 u/kg/h ([8] adapted with permission of the editors of *Am J Dig Dis*).

Chapter 17

years that the development of antihistamines to block the H_1 effects of histamine elsewhere in the body allowed augmented doses of histamine sufficient to provide maximal acid secretion by stimulation of H_2 receptors to be used. Histamine is the cheapest gastric stimulant, either when given subcutaneously, or by intravenous infusion, but in most centres pentagastrin is used for reasons of safety and comfort. The histamine analogue Histalog (also known as betazole, or ametazole) is rarely used today.

Peak acid output after **insulin** is correlated with hypoglycaemia, measured either as the lowest blood glucose, or the fall, or the rate of fall of blood glucose. Hypoglycaemia provides a quantitative glycopaenic stimulus which produces a quantitative vagal secretory response. The optimal dose

of insulin for single intravenous injection is 0.2 u/kg because in most subjects this dose lowers blood glucose sufficiently to elicit a maximal vagal acid response (Fig. 17.2). The pathway of this response is through the hypoglycaemia-sensitive cephalic centres in the lateral hypothalamus. The 0.2 u/kg dose acts without decreasing blood glucose to excessively low concentrations, at which gastric secretion is depressed. An intravenous infusion of insulin decreases blood glucose concentration less severely than a standard insulin test and has milder unwanted effects, yet it achieves comparable acidity and acid output (Figs. 17.3 and 17.4). Nevertheless insulin tests should not be done in patients with heart disease or abnormal electrocardiograms and should be avoided in patients over 65 years of age.

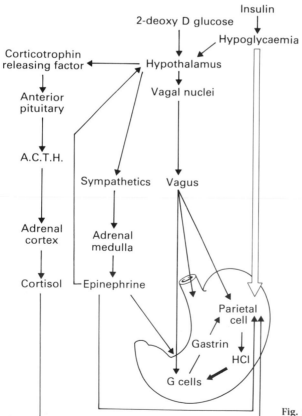

Fig. 17.5. Glycopaenia and the stomach (see text) ([4] adapted with permission of Little, Brown & Co.).

Continuous medical supervision during the test is essential even in the young and healthy.

Unfortunately glycopaenic stimulation of the hypothalamus produces para-sympathetic and sympathetic responses and hypoglycaemia may affect gastric parietal and antral G-cells, as well as adrenals. The adrenal-sympathetic system may be a neural non-vagal pathway. Beta-blockers decrease insulin-stimulated acidity and acid output in patients with duodenal ulcer before and after vagotomy, so that part of the acid response after vagotomy is probably due to sympathetic pathways rather than to inadequate vagal section (Fig. 17.5).

Sham feeding by chew-and-spit evokes acid secretion from the stomach similar to that resulting from adequate sham feeding where the thought, sight, smell, ingestion and swallowing of the food is followed by expulsion of the food through an oesophagostomy, without it having entered the stomach. The chew-and-spit sham feeding vagal stimulus is highly reproducible and evokes acid output comparable to the insulin test, that is about half the maximal. Sham feeding has replaced the insulin test in many centres for two reasons. Firstly, it is simpler, safer and less unpleasant for the patient. Secondly, sham feeding does not have the same stimulatory effect as insulin does on non-vagal pathways, either on those inhibiting gastric acid leading to a falsely low acid output, or on those stimulating the adrenal-adrenaline-gastrin cells, giving a falsely high acid output.

Expression of results

After a single injection of an agonist by any route acid output rises from a basal level to its highest rate—i.e. peak—and then declines to basal levels again. Acid output was once expressed as all that collected during the total period of stimulation following the agonist, such as 1 hour after histamine,

gastrin, tetragastrin and pentagastrin, or $1\frac{1}{2}$–2 hours after histalog and about 2–4 hours after insulin. Today acid output is commonly expressed as a collection made during the peak period of secretion, but this peak period may have variable timing (Fig. 17.6). **Peak acid output** is the sum of the two consecutive highest collection periods (conveniently expressed in mmol/h), and this peak acid output after a single injection of agonist approximates to the plateau acid output after intravenous infusion, which is not commonly used routinely because it is more complicated and less convenient than a single injection. The term **maximal acid output** is generally used to denote the highest observed acid output, whether peak acid output after a single injection or plateau acid output after an intravenous infusion. The term maximum acid output (MAO) is sometimes used for the output in the whole hour (0–60 minutes) after a stimulant.

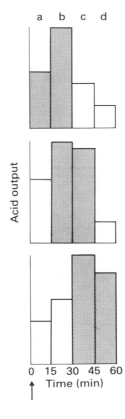

Fig. 17.6. Patterns of acid response during the hour after a single parenteral injection of histamine or pentagastrin. The shaded columns represent the three possible positions of peak acid output (PAO)— the sum of the two highest consecutive periods. (i) the first half-hour, a+b, (ii) the middle half-hour, b+c, (iii) the last half-hour c+d. PAO is calculated in mmol/h as output 2 × (a+b), or 2 × (b+c), or 2 × (c+d). Maximum acid output MAO, is often used for the whole 60 minute period after the injection of histamine or pentagastrin:MAO mmol/h=(a+b+c+d) ([2] adapted with permission of Butterworths).

Biological factors

Maximal acid output is an expression of the secretion of every parietal cell, the **parietal cell mass.** The size of the stomach is related constitutionally to bodily habitus and it is obviously important to express acid output of children in terms of body weight. This calculation can be done for adults, or acid can be related to lean body mass, surface area or, simplest of all, height. Such corrections largely eliminate the apparently lower acid outputs in women (Table 17.1), but for

Table 17.1. The mean (range) of basal and peak acid output (mmol/h).

	Basal	Peak acid output
Healthy men	1 (0–5+)	22 (<1–45)
Healthy women	1 (0–5+)	12 (<1–30)

routine purposes most data are still presented uncorrected for body build. There are also ethnic variations, so that short lean populations may need higher doses of agonists for maximal secretion and may also have small parietal cell masses.

Corrections for loss and reflux

The gastric aspirate is a mixture of the acid secreted by parietal cells, alkali secreted by non-parietal cells, and contamination of these gastric components by reflux of pancreatic, biliary and intestinal secretions from the duodenum, and swallowed saliva. Some gastric contents are lost through the pylorus. Saliva is inevitably secreted and swallowed, even though the patient is asked to spit it out.

About 10–20% of the secreted gastric acid may be lost through the pylorus rather than aspirated. This loss is probably not a constant proportion of the rate of secretion, so that the effect may be lower at higher rates of secretion. This loss can be corrected for by constantly infusing an inert non-

absorbable marker, such as phenol red, through a separate gastric tube. By measuring the concentration of marker in the gastric aspirates it is possible to calculate, and correct for, gastroduodenal loss. This calculation is usually not done in routine tests.

Reflux of alkali from the duodenum, neutralizing and diluting gastric acid, is variable. It can be prevented by a separate duodenal intubation, which makes the test much more difficult to do. It can also be estimated from measurements of the sodium concentration in gastric aspirates, but again this refinement is rarely used in routine clinical practice. Finally, acid may diffuse back from the lumen through the gastric mucosa, but there is no certainty of the magnitude of this factor in reducing observed gastric acidity (Fig. 17.7).

Alkaline secretion and mucus

The mucosal resistance to attack by acid-pepsin is commonly divided into two

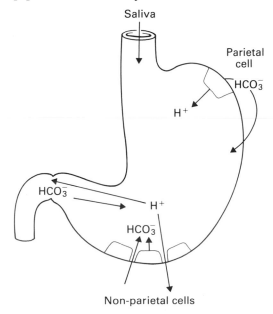

Fig. 17.7. Five possible causes of hypoacidity ([3] adapted with permission of the editors of *Rendiconti di Gastroenterologia*).

barriers, superficial mucus and the layer of mucosal cells. Mucus is a viscous secretion of the mucous glands of the stomach, together with cell fragments, leucocytes and various salts. By volume more than 90% of mucus is water with a matrix of glycoprotein, and mucus is a partial barrier to the passage of acid and pepsin from the gastric lumen attacking the cells of the gastric mucosa. These cells form the second barrier because of the rapid turnover of 4–6 days of the mucosal cell layer.

Mucus also allows the passage from mucosa to lumen of bicarbonate secreted by the surface mucous cells. The maximal alkaline output of the mucous cells is probably no more than 10% of the maximal acid output secreted by the parietal cell mass. However, this bicarbonate may be confined in the unstirred layer of mucus to form a high concentration barrier to acid—if that amount of alkali had merely been released into the lumen generally it would be relatively ineffective against the greater mass of acid (Fig. 17.8). Physical and chemical methodology of mucus is inadequate for routine testing [3, 8, 10].

Pepsins

The chief cells secrete pepsinogens. Virtually all are released into the gastric lumen where they are split by acid into their respective pepsins. Gastric pepsins are not measured routinely because, in general, acid and pepsin secretion are closely correlated.

A mere 1% of pepsinogens pass from the chief cells into the blood where they can be measured as total serum pepsinogens. Fundic serum pepsinogen I (PGI) is correlated with basal and peak acid output and shows encouraging prospects of becoming a tubeless test of gastric secretory capacity suitable for routine use. This fundic (I), but not the antro-duodenal (II), pepsinogen is excreted as urine pepsinogen (uropepsin), another approximate indicator of chief cell mass. Measurements of pepsinogen concentrations are not used routinely at present [6].

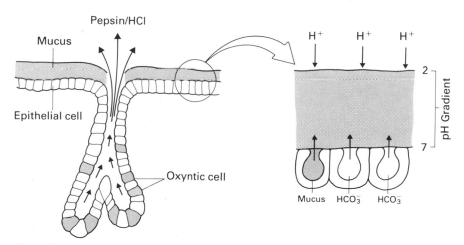

Fig. 17.8. 'Mucus-bicarbonate' barrier. Diagrammatic representation of the gastric epithelium illustrating the interaction between hydrogen and bicarbonate ions within the mucus gel layer. Hydrogen ions diffusing from the lumen are neutralized by bicarbonate ions secreted by the surface cells, thus creating a pH gradient across the mucus interface ([9] adapted with permission of the editors of *Clin Sci*).

Indications for tests

Clinical practice

Clinical tests of gastric acid are occasionally helpful in patients with X-ray or endoscopy negative ulcer-like dyspepsia, in that they might suggest that a particular patient probably has, or probably does not have duodenal ulcer disease. There seems little place for routine acid tests on patients with gastric ulcer or carcinoma, or duodenal ulcer disease.

Basal secretion and pentagastrin-stimulated acid output should ideally be measured in all patients before all operations for duodenal ulcer, as well as in patients with recurrent dyspepsia after gastrectomy. These tests should be done, together with a cephalic test such as sham feeding or insulin, in all patients after vagotomy as part of the assessment of the operation. These tests, and measurements of serum gastrin should be performed in patients with recurrence of dyspepsia after vagotomy to seek a cause for recurrent ulceration and to help in planning revision operations.

Measurement of basal and maximal secretion may be needed in patients taking acid-lowering drugs, especially if they are not responding clinically, so that the dose may be adjusted, or the anti-secretory drug changed if suitably low acid outputs are not being achieved with a particular drug in the particular dose used. They are essential in monitoring effective medical treatment in the very rare cases of gastrinoma [5].

Research

Gastric secretion tests are widely used in research on the pathophysiology of gastric and duodenal ulcer, oesophagitis and duodenitis, and in diseases in other organs affecting gastric secretion, for example, liver, kidneys, endocrine, or intestinal. The tests are commonly used for the assessment of anti-secretory drugs to determine dose and frequency of drug to produce satisfactorily low acid output to allow ulcer healing and sustained remission [7].

References

1 BARON JH. Physiological control of gastric acid secretion. *Proc R Soc Med* 1971;**64**:739–741.
2 BARON JH. Gastric function tests. In: Wastell C, ed. *Chronic duodenal ulcer.* London: Butterworths, 1972:82–114.
3 BARON JH. Gastric secretion and diseases of mucosal barrier. *Rendiconti di Gastroenterologia* 1977;**9**:41–46.
4 BARON JH. Gastric secretion tests. In: Nyhus LM, Wastell C, eds. *Surgery of the stomach and duodenum.* Boston: Little, Brown & Co, 1977:133–147.
5 BARON JH. *Clinical tests of gastric secretion: history, methodology and interpretation.* London: Macmillan, 1978.
6 BARON JH. Pathophysiology of gastric acid and pepsin secretion. In: Domschke W, Wormsley KG, eds. *Magen und Magenkrankheiten.* Stuttgart: Thieme Verlag, 1981:131–149.
7 BARON JH. Current views on the pathogenesis of peptic ulcer. *Scand J Gastroenterol* 1982;**17**:1–10.
8 CROMPTON J, REES WDW. Gastroduodenal bicarbonate secretion: its role in protecting the stomach and duodenum. In: Pounder RE, ed. *Recent advances in gastroenterology*, 6. Edinburgh: Churchill Livingstone, 1986:35–50.
9 GIRVAN DP, HANSKY J, SPENCER J, BARON JH. The response of gastric secretion and serum gastrin to insulin infusion in patients with duodenal ulcer. *Am J Dig Dis* 1974;**6**:103–133.
10 REES WDW, TURNBERG LA. Mechanisms of gastric mucosal protection: a role for the mucus bicarbonate barrier. *Clin Sci* 1982;**62**:343–348.

Chapter 18
Gastritis

S.J. LA BROOY

Gastritis is associated with the aetiology of certain well-defined diseases such as pernicious anaemia and Ménétrièr's disease. Its association with other more common diseases, such as gastric ulceration and carcinoma of the stomach is less well understood at present, but may ultimately prove more important. The study of gastritis is difficult because even severe mucosal changes may be asymptomatic or have no specific radiological, gastroscopic, secretory or serologic features [35]. Gastritis is therefore an essentially histopathological diagnosis.

Classification

The normal mucosa of the stomach is divided into that of the body and the pylorus. Body mucosa consists of a single layer of epithelial cells which dips to form shallow gastric pits into which open the gastric glands. The upper part of the glands consist of parietal and mucin-secreting neck cells, and the lower part of chief cells (Fig. 18.1). Antral mucosa lines approximately the lower-third of the stomach; on the lesser curve it extends proximally for a variable distance. In pyloric mucosa the gastric pits are longer and may branch. The glands here are usually mucin-producing with only occasional parietal cells (Fig. 18.2). Small numbers of round inflammatory cells may occur in the lamina propria in normal mucosa. Inflammatory changes in the gastric mucosa may be divided into acute or chronic gastritis.

Acute gastritis

Acute gastritis occurs as a result of direct injury to the gastric mucosa by many agents and is discussed in Chapter 19.

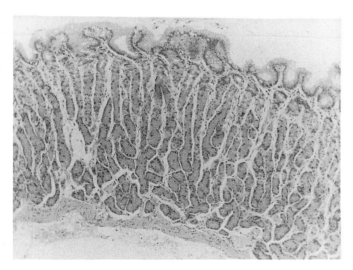

Fig. 18.1. Normal body mucosa. Short gastric pits, regular surface epithelium.

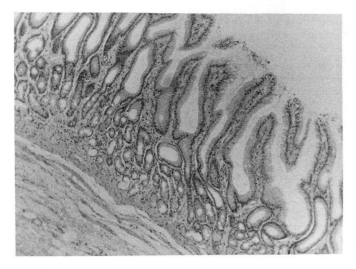

Fig. 18.2. Normal antral mucosa. The pits are slightly longer.

Chronic gastritis

Classification of chronic gastritis is complex. The most widely accepted classification is that proposed by Whitehead [63] and a simplified version of this is used here based on three factors: the type of mucosa involved; the grade of gastritis; and the presence and type of metaplasia. (Table 18.1)

tritis is different and they are associated with different diseases—peptic ulcer with the former and pernicious anaemia with the latter. Though the terms type A and type B gastritis are still used, the definition of gastritis by the site of involvement and severity is more precise.

Table 18.1. Modification of the generally accepted classification of gastritis [63].

Mucosal type	Chronic gastritis	Metaplasia
Pyloric (type B)	Superficial	Pseudopyloric
Body (type A)	Atrophic	Intestinal

Type of mucosa

Strickland and Mackay [54] first postulated the division of chronic gastritis into two broad categories. Type A gastritis involves the body of the stomach, is associated with hypo- or anacidity, antibodies to gastric parietal cells in the serum and impaired absorption of vitamin B_{12}. Type B gastritis involves the antrum alone and is associated with normal acid secretion. The distinction between the two types of gastritis is important. The aetiology of antral and fundal gas-

Grade of gastritis

Superficial gastritis and gastric atrophy are probably extremes of the same disease process [49]. In superficial gastritis there is increased infiltration of the lamina propria by lymphocytes and plasma cells. This alone is insufficient for diagnosis, as there is no agreement on what constitutes a normal degree of round-cell infiltration. Polymorphonuclear leucocyte infiltration of surface epithelium and formation of aggregates in the gastric pits (crypt abscesses) are there-

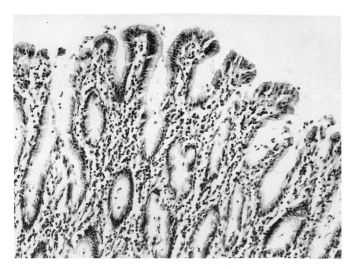

Fig. 18.3. Superficial gastritis. Gastric mucosa with inflammatory cells in the surface epithelium and in the lumen of the glands.

fore helpful. Epithelial cells may show degenerative or regenerative changes with irregularities in the size, shape and nuclear characteristics. Regeneration may result in an epithelium several layers thick (Fig. 18.3). The presence of normal glands and reticulin pattern distinguishes superficial from atrophic gastritis (Fig. 18.4). In atrophic gastritis there is distortion of reticulin pattern, dilatation and tortuosity of the gastric pits with atrophy of the gland tubules and disappearance of the parietal and chief cells (Figs 18.5 and 18.6). There are increased numbers of plasma cells and lymph-

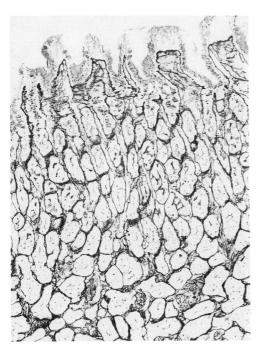

Fig. 18.4. Normal reticulin stain of gastric body mucosa.

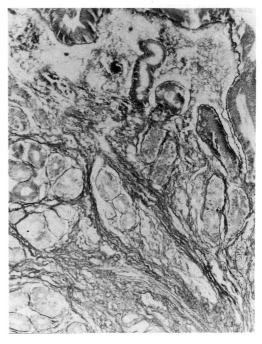

Fig. 18.5. Reticulin stain in atrophic gastritis. In contrast to Fig. 18.4, the reticulin network is condensed and irregular.

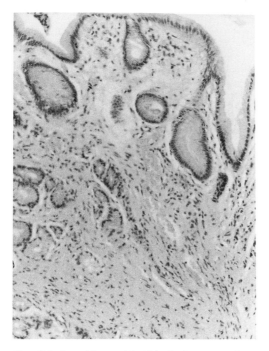

Fig. 18.6. Atrophic gastritis. The glands are atrophic.

ocytes in the epithelium. Gastric atrophy is characterized by a complete disappearance of fundic glands, absence of regenerative changes and inflammatory cell infiltration and mucosal thinning. Metaplastic changes occur.

Metaplasia

Pseudopyloric metaplasia generally occurs in atrophic gastric mucosa and has no clinical significance. It consists of increased mucin-secreting cells in the gastric glands, so that eventually the appearance mimics normal pyloric mucosa within the body of the stomach.

Intestinal metaplasia also occurs only in the presence of atrophic gastritis, more commonly in the pyloric mucosa. The cells are morphologically and functionally identical with small bowel cells. Villous formation may occur (Fig. 18.7). In a small proportion of intestinal metaplasia cells resemble colonic more than small bowel mucosa. It is uncertain whether small bowel metaplastic changes progress to colonic type. Recent evidence suggests that metaplastic cells with colon-like appearances may be more specifically linked with gastric carcinoma [46].

Hypertrophic gastropathy (Ménétrièr's disease)

The term gastropathy is used because histopathological evidence of mucosal inflammation may be absent in Ménétrièr's disease. Although it is invariably classified as a form

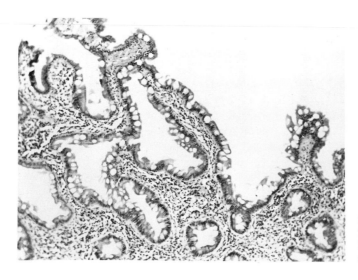

Fig. 18.7. Intestinal metaplasia. The normal gastric epithelium has been replaced by villiform structures containing goblet cells.

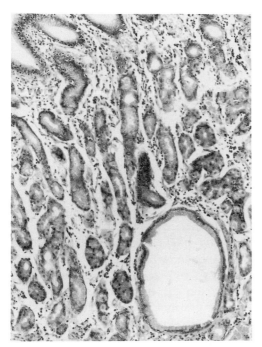

Fig. 18.8. Ménétrièr's disease. Gastric body mucosa with characteristic cyst formation.

of gastritis, it is no longer considered such in the strictest sense of the word.

The most characteristic features are the enlarged convoluted gastric folds in the body of the fundus of the stomach which rarely involve the antrum. The mucosa is thickened and the gastric pits elongated. The surface epithelium is hyperplastic and mucin-secreting cells of the surface and neck type line the gastric pits and extend into the basal part of the glands. Mucin-containing cysts occur deep in the mucosa and may extend through the muscularis mucosa. The glands are elongated with reduced numbers of parietal and chief cells. The muscularis mucosa is thickened and spikes of it may extend up between the glands. Inflammatory cell infiltrates may be present, but this is thought to be a local reaction to rupture of the mucin cysts. Pseudopyloric metaplasia may occur (Fig. 18.8).

Granulomatous gastritis

Granulomas can occur in the gastric mucosa in Crohn's disease, sarcoidosis, tuberculosis, syphilis and histoplasmosis. They may be associated with severe or mild mucosal inflammation. This form of gastritis is rare and it is impossible to distinguish the different causes on histopathological grounds alone unless caseation (indicative of tuberculosis) is present. Diagnosis is dependent on systemic manifestations of the individual diseases. Granulomas can also be caused by food particles and foreign bodies which are thought to enter through breaks in the gastric mucosa.

Eosinophilic gastritis

This diffuse lesion usually involves only the antral mucosa and is characterized by oedema of the lamina propria and submucosal layers, with an infiltrate of eosinophils and polymorphonuclear leucocytes, which is usually heaviest in the submucosa, but may extend through to the serosa.

Epidemiology

Most of the epidemiological data pertains to diseases associated with chronic gastritis, such as pernicious anaemia and gastric cancer, rather than to gastritis itself. This is understandable as the condition is so often asymptomatic. The incidence of pernicious anaemia is estimated at 0.13% in individuals of Scandinavian, English and Irish descent. It occurs less frequently in Mediterranean races and is rare in Arabs, Orientals and Bantu South Africans. Gastric cancer has a high incidence in Japan, South America and Finland [25]. It is not known whether gastritis occurs more commonly in these areas. Prevalence rates of gastritis in random population samples vary from 27–78%, with only a small proportion of severe atrophic gastritis (Table 18.2). However,

Table 18.2. Prevalence of chronic gastritis in the normal population.

Country	Type of sample	Number of subjects	Distribution			
			Normal	Superficial	Atrophic	Severe atrophy
Finland [48]	Random rural population	142	47%	25%	25%	3%
Estonia, USSR [61]	Random rural population	155	22%	72%		6%
Australia [21]	Hospital patients without gastrointestinal symptoms and normal volunteers	336	16.4%	36.6%	36.6%	10.4%
Finland [16]	Random rural and urban population	431	36%	62%		2%

these figures may not be universally applicable.

Age

Gastritis of the body and antrum is more common with increasing age (Fig. 18.9).

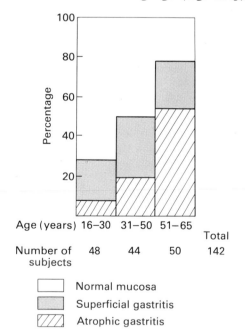

Age (years) 16–30   31–50   51–65   Total

Number of   48   44   50   142
subjects

☐ Normal mucosa
▨ Superficial gastritis
▨ Atrophic gastritis

Fig. 18.9. The distribution by age of superficial and atrophic gastritis in a randomly selected group of normal subjects from a rural Finnish population. Superficial gastritis occurred with the same frequency in all age groups but there was a significant increase of atrophic gastritis in subjects older than 50 years of age [44].

Pernicious anaemia is also most common in the sixth to eighth decades. If, however, atrophic gastritis precedes pernicious anaemia by ten or more years [47], then atrophic gastritis must occur earlier in these patients than in the general population. Evidence that this does indeed happen in first-degree relatives of patients with pernicious anaemia supports this theory (Fig. 18.10). Juvenile pernicious anaemia is due to a congenital absence of intrinsic factor and is not associated with gastritis [17, 33].

Sex

Atrophic gastritis is more common in women [60]. This is consistent with the female preponderance of 2:1 in pernicious anaemia in the United Kingdom and Scandinavia [7].

Aetiology

The aetiology of gastritis is multifactorial. Chronic atrophic gastritis of the body (type A) and antral gastritis (type B) have different causes and clinical features and should therefore be considered separately.

Chronic atrophic gastritis (type A)

A 27-year follow-up study of subjects with normal gastric mucosa or superficial gastritis has shown that the latter eventually progress to atrophic gastritis [49]. The cause of the initial insult to the gastritic mucosa is unknown, though genetic, environmental and immunological mechanisms are all believed to be involved in the development of atrophic gastritis and pernicious anaemia.

Genetics

Chronic atrophic gastritis occurs more commonly and at an earlier age in first-degree relatives of patients with pernicious anaemia (Fig. 18.10) and the familial incidence of the disease is 20 times greater than in the normal population [29]. Pernicious anaemia is also associated with other genetically determined features such as blue eyes, prematurely grey hair and blood group A, though this last association is weak [5]. Attempts to associate atrophic gastritis with specific HL-A types have not been successful [30, 59, 64]. The mode of inheritance in pernicious anaemia is unknown.

Environmental factors

Many agents have been shown to cause acute injury to the gastric mucosa, but their role in the development of chronic gastritis is not clear. Alcohol, tobacco, drugs such as aspirin, and hot food and beverages have all been suggested as causes of chronic gastritis, but the evidence from clinical studies is either weak or contradictory.

Chronic gastritis is more common in the lower socio-economic classes [9], but this is not related to increased consumption of alcohol and tobacco in these groups. The role of diet in chronic gastritis has never been assessed. Iron deficiency anaemia is also associated with chronic atrophic gastritis, but whether this is a primary aetiological factor or a secondary effect of gastritis is uncertain.

Immunology

The presence of humoral and cell-mediated specific immunological factors in patients

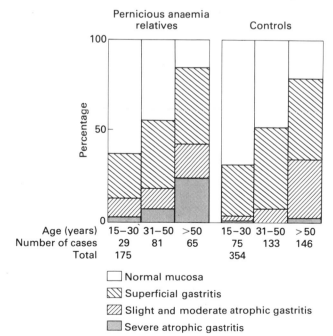

Fig. 18.10. The occurrence of superficial and atrophic gastritis of the gastric body in first-degree relatives of pernicious anaemia probands and computer-matched control subjects. Superficial gastritis is as common in both groups, but severe atrophic gastritis is significantly more common ($p < 0.01$) in relatives of patients with pernicious anaemia and occurs earlier [57].

Table 18.3. Auto-antibodies in patients with pernicious anaemia and thyroid disease compared with the normal population [65].

Subjects		Age (yrs)	With antibodies		
			to Parietal cells	to Intrinsic factor	to Thyroid cytoplasm
Normal	Men	under 55	5.6%	very rare	5.2%
		over 55	9.2%	1%	
	Women	under 55	14.7%	very rare	12.2%
		over 55	22.3%	1%	17.8%
Patients with pernicious anaemia			84%	56%	55%
Relatives of patients with pernicious anaemia			36%	6%	50%
Patients with gastritis			47%	rare	rare
Patients with myxoedema			32%	4%	47%
Relatives of patients with myxoedema			20%	–	46%

with chronic atrophic gastritis and pernicious anaemia suggests that immune mechanisms may be important in the pathogenesis of the disease. The most common is an antibody specific for the smooth cytoplasmic membrane of the gastric parietal cell (parietal cell antibody) which can be found in the serum, gastric juice and gastric mucosa [19]. Circulating parietal cell antibodies are found in most patients with pernicious anaemia and a high proportion of their relatives. They occur in the normal population, but incidence in individuals with chronic atrophic gastritis is significantly higher (Table 18.3). Parietal cell antibodies are also more common in other autoimmune diseases, in particular thyroid disease [64], and in diabetes mellitus, vitiligo and Addison's disease.

Antibodies to intrinsic factor occur less frequently than parietal cell antibodies in patients with pernicious anaemia, but are more specific for the disease. They are rare in relatives of patients with pernicious anaemia and those with atrophic gastritis (Table 18.3). Two types of intrinsic factor antibody have been identified. Type I (blocking antibody) prevents formation of the intrinsic factor-vitamin B_{12} complex by attaching itself to the intrinsic factor receptor site. Type II (binding antibody) reacts with the already formed intrinsic factor-vitamin B_{12} complex at a different site to prevent absorption [41]. These antibodies occur in the serum and gastric juice. The latter is a potent inhibitor of vitamin B_{12} absorption and may be found in the absence of circulating antibodies [39]. Type I antibody is usually the one measured in the serum as type II antibody is less common and rarely occurs in the absence of type I. Circulating intrinsic factor antibodies are more likely to be found in younger patients with pernicious anaemia [41].

Circulating thyroid antibodies are found in 50% of patients with pernicious anaemia and their relatives (Table 18.3) and lymphocytotoxic antibodies in 30%.

The presence of altered cell-mediated immunity is shown by lymphocyte transformation and migration inhibition to gastric juice, intrinsic factor concentrate and other antigens in patients with pernicious anaemia [55]. Similar observations have been recorded in patients with chronic atrophic gastritis [13].

Bacteriology

Gastric spiral bacteria have been repeatedly reported and then forgotten during the past half century. Endoscopic antral biopsies showed curved bacilli to be present in 80% of patients with gastric ulcer [52], but the observation remained dormant until Warren and Marshall [62] described them again and since then the subject has been intensively investigated. These organisms, now provisionally termed *Campylobacter pyloridis*, are S-shaped or curved Gram-negative flagellate rods and are strongly associated with active antral gastritis and also with gastric, or duodenal ulceration [27, 28, 36]. A complement-fixing antibody has been found in 90% of patients with gastritis and 13% of those with normal mucosa [11]. The organisms reside deep to the layer of gastric mucus covering the antral epithelium. It is possible that these bacilli may be an important factor in gastritis and also perhaps in some forms of peptic ulcer.

Pathophysiology

The initiating mechanism in the development of chronic atrophic gastritis is unknown and there is no evidence that acute mucosal injury leads to chronic gastritis. Autoimmune phenomena are important, especially in the development of pernicious anaemia, but aetiology cannot be explained on this alone, as pernicious anaemia has been described in patients with coexistent immunoglobulin deficiency [56]. Humoral antibodies are therefore not necessary for the development of pernicious anaemia. It is possible that some initial damage to the gastric mucosa causes antibody formation at the cellular level. This may either initiate or perpetuate chronic inflammatory changes in genetically predisposed individuals, which finally lead to the production of circulating antibodies. It would explain why humoral antibodies are less common in chronic atrophic gastritis than in pernicious anaemia.

Antral gastritis (type B)

Much less is known about the aetiology of antral gastritis. Duodenogastric reflux is thought to be important—bile salts damage the gastric mucosa and duodenogastric reflux is an important factor in gastric ulcer, which is invariably associated with antral gastritis [38].

Clinical features

Gastritis presents in a number of ways—the main problem for the clinician is deciding if symptoms are due to gastritis or whether it is incidental.

Gastrointestinal haemorrhage

Bleeding can occur in patients with acute mucosal injury where it takes the erosive form. Haemorrhage is of varying degree of severity and may be life-threatening. This subject is dealt with in Chapters 19 and 30.

Dyspepsia

Gastritis may be the only lesion found in patients with dyspeptic symptoms. However, many patients with dyspepsia have a normal gastric mucosa, so it is unlikely that gastritis itself is responsible for these symptoms [10, 35]. It is important, therefore, to exclude other causes of dyspepsia in these patients.

Anaemia

Anaemia may be of the iron-deficiency, or megaloblastic type. Though iron-deficiency anaemia is associated with atrophic gastritis the relationship is not causal and evidence of dietary deficiency or blood loss must be sought. The clinical features of pernicious anaemia are more clearly defined.

In **pernicious anaemia** the onset of symptoms is often insidious and non-specific, thus delaying diagnosis. Most patients have symptoms of anaemia, vague dyspepsia, anorexia and soreness of the tongue, as well as paraesthesiae and cerebral disturbances, such as depression and impaired memory. In more severe cases cardiac failure due to anaemia may be present. Sub-acute combined degeneration of the spinal cord is less common now (7% of patients), but symptoms may antedate the anaemia. Rarer neurological manifestations include psychosis, ophthalmoplegia, impotence, bladder atony and retrobulbar neuritis. Examination may show anaemia more severe than the symptoms indicate and mild icterus. There may be brownish pigmentation of the skin and patches of vitiligo. Glossitis occurs in about 50% of patients. The spleen may be palpable, but is not grossly enlarged. Neurological signs consistent with damage to the dorsal and lateral columns of the spinal cord may be present.

Other associated diseases

Chronic gastritis has been associated with dermatitis herpetiformis, polycythaemia rubra vera, Sjögren's disease, scleroderma, rheumatoid arthritis, systemic lupus erythematosus and hookworm infestations. There is no evidence that gastritis is of any clinical significance in these diseases.

Diagnosis

The diagnosis of gastritis can only be established by gastric mucosal biopsy. A normal barium meal does not exclude the diagnosis of atrophic gastritis and mild gastritis has no specific radiological features. Gastroscopy allows visualization of the mucosa of the stomach and duodenum and permits multiple tissue sampling with accurate localization of biopsies. Unfortunately correlation between endoscopic and histological appearances of the gastric mucosa is poor, especially in superficial gastritis where reddening and oedema of the mucosa with exudates may not reflect the degree of mucosal inflammation. Correlation with atrophic gastritis is better, the mucosa being paler with increased prominence of submucosal vessels and a paucity of rugae on the greater curve. Gastric juice may be scanty.

Investigation

The presence of superficial gastritis is not likely to be of clinical significance and further investigation should be directed to other causes for the symptoms.

When chronic atrophic gastritis is diagnosed, especially if it is severe and the patient is not elderly, the line of investigation should be:

1. to establish the diagnosis of pernicious anaemia if macrocytic anaemia is present;
2. to exclude subclinical vitamin B_{12} deficiency where the haemoglobin is normal;
3. to establish the risk factors for the patient developing pernicious anaemia.

Haematology

Haemoglobin concentration may be normal even in severe atrophic gastritis. Macrocytosis may occur before the onset of anaemia. Iron deficiency anaemia may also be present. In some patients with pernicious anaemia haemoglobin concentration may be extremely low and is usually less than 7–8 g/ml if the patient has symptoms. Oval macrocytes with a wide variety of cell-body inclusions are characteristic and erythrocyte survival is shortened. Leucocytes are normal, or low in number and the ratio of hypersegmented neutrophils is increased (<0.17). Thrombocytopaenia may occur. The bone marrow in pernicious anaemia is characterized by the presence of megaloblasts. Giant metamyelocytes may also be found. Megakaryocytes may be normal or reduced.

Biochemistry

The main biochemical investigation is the measurement of serum vitamin B_{12} and of its absorption. Serum vitamin B_{12} is low ($<100 \mu g/ml$) due to decreased absorption, which can be demonstrated by measuring the urinary excretion of ingested [58]Co-labelled B_{12} (Schilling test). Less than 10% of the ingested dose is excreted by patients with pernicious anaemia.

Abnormally low absorption of vitamin B_{12} also occurs in severe atrophic gastritis without pernicious anaemia and there is evidence of progressive deterioration with time in these patients, to levels found in pernicious anaemia [66]. As the abnormal vitamin B_{12} absorption is due to a lack of intrinsic factor secretion, a more sensitive measurement is of intrinsic factor in gastric juice. Only very small amounts of intrinsic factor are necessary for vitamin B_{12} absorption. The normal range of secretion is 1,000–10,000 u/h with less than 200 u/h being secreted in pernicious anaemia [6]. Patients with atrophic gastritis have intrinsic factor secretion in the pernicious anaemia range long before abnormalities in serum vitamin B_{12} and B_{12} absorption occur [18]. The Schilling test is, however, much simpler to do, does not involve intubation and is sensitive enough for diagnosis, especially where an improvement of vitamin B_{12} absorption can be shown by the addition of intrinsic factor to the ingested B_{12}.

In patients with anacidity and atrophic gastritis fasting serum gastrin is raised to 100–1,000 pmol/l, being highest in patients with pernicious anaemia [53]. This is due to response to the removal of the inhibitory effect of gastric acid [23]. In some patients with severe atrophic gastritis with antral involvement, serum gastrin may be normal. Serum pepsinogen I concentrations are related to gastric acid secretion, being significantly lower in anacidic patients [40]. It has been suggested that the measurement of serum gastrin and pepsinogen I may prove to be a non-invasive screening procedure for severe atrophic gastritis and pernicious anaemia as they are a specific and sensitive indicator of mucosal disease [58]. It must be remembered, however, that the radioimmunoassay may not be readily available and screening may not be important except in areas with a high incidence of atrophic gastritis and gastric cancer.

Immunology

Measurement of parietal cell and intrinsic factor antibodies is moderately helpful in the diagnosis of pernicious anaemia. Parietal cell antibodies may occur very commonly (70–90%), but unfortunately are not specific. Where they occur in relatives and in patients with atrophic gastritis they may be useful in determining the likelihood of developing the disease. Intrinsic factor antibodies are specific for pernicious anaemia but as they are absent in 30–40% of patients, they are, at best, only an aid to diagnosis. Measurement of cell-mediated immune responses will remain unhelpful in practical terms until their role in the aetiology of the disease has been more clearly defined.

Gastric acid secretion is related to the degree of chronic gastritis, anacidity being associated with severe atrophic gastritis. Patients with pernicious anaemia, unless of the juvenile type, are anacidic and unresponsive to stimulation with histamine or pentagastrin.

Treatment

As no specific symptoms are associated with gastritis, management of these patients is directed towards such symptoms as they have.

Antral gastritis

As reflux of bile may be an aetiological factor, cholestyramine and aluminium hydroxide, which bind bile salts, may be tried. There is no evidence that they relieve symptoms, however, even in the operated stomach, where bile reflux is greater [31].

Atrophic gastritis

Treatment here is as for non-specific dyspepsia. Antacids, anticholinergics and antiflatulents may be used. Avoidance of foods that aggravate symptoms is probably sound advice. Iron-deficiency anaemia may be corrected. None of these measures will improve or change the progress of gastritis.

Pernicious anaemia

Vitamin B_{12} therapy has significantly lowered the mortality in this disease. Most deaths tend to occur soon after diagnosis and are usually due to effects of prolonged severe anaemia [26]. The main problem in treating the disease is the reluctance of some patients to continue therapy for life. Even in these cases relapses may take up to two years to occur. The maintenance dose of vitamin B_{12} is 1,000 μg of cyanocoba-

lamin by intramuscular injection every two months.

Prognosis

Long-term studies show that patients with normal gastric mucosa may develop superficial and even atrophic gastritis over a 20-year period, though in more than 50% the mucosa remains normal. In patients with superficial gastritis the inflammation either persists or develops into atrophic gastritis (50%) in the same period [49]. The most important factor in the prognosis is the development of atrophic gastritis, because in these patients the risk of gastric carcinoma may be higher than in the general population. In pernicious anaemia gastric cancer occurs three to four times more commonly [2]. A similar risk probably operates in patients with atrophic gastritis, though this is not so well documented [50]. Rarely, patients with anacidity as a result of autoimmune atrophic gastritis, most of whom will have pernicious anaemia, develop enterochromaffin-like (ECL) cell hyperplasia which leads to multiple polypoidal carcinoid tumours of the stomach; these tumours probably grow very slowly [15]. They are interesting because uninterrupted, long-term anacidity produced by potent inhibitors of acid secretion gives rise to hypergastrihaemia, which is thought to be the cause of ECL cell hyperplasia.

Whether atrophic gastritis is a precancerous condition, or whether both diseases share some common genetic factor is uncertain. It is postulated that the tumour arises in areas of intestinal metaplasia [32] and there is some evidence that intestinal metaplasia is more common in patients with gastric carcinoma [34]. On the other hand, the specificity of metaplasia as an indicator of gastric cancer is poor, as it may occur in up to 20% of the population [16]. The specificity of intestinal metaplasia as a precancerous condition may be enhanced by recognizing different sub-types. The colonic-type of metaplasia has been reported to have a much stronger association with carcinoma [46] and further differentiation may help in defining the group of patients with atrophic gastritis at greatest risk. There is an increased risk of gastric argyrophil cell carcinoid tumours, which could be potentially malignant, in patients with pernicious anaemia [4, 15].

Hypertrophic gastropathy (Ménétrièr's disease)

The original description of this disease by Ménétrièr in 1888 was of gastric rugal hypertrophy with hypoproteinaemia and a normal or decreased acid secretion. Since then a variant of this disorder associated with hypersecretion of gastric acid has been recognized [43, 45]. The condition is rare and can occur at any age. Men are more often affected than women. The cause is unknown.

Clinical features

Symptoms may persist for up to 20 years before diagnosis. The commonest presentation is that of ulcer-like dyspepsia relieved by antacids. Anorexia, nausea and vomiting may also occur, the latter sometimes being due to intermittent obstruction by the enlarged gastric folds. Gastrointestinal haemorrhage is another feature of the disease and may be due to peptic ulceration or diffuse haemorrhagic gastritis. Some patients have weight loss and hypoproteinaemia with ascites or oedema.

Investigations

Presenting symptoms determine the initial line of investigation. Diagnosis is not always easy. The classical radiological features of enlarged tortuous rugae, particularly on the greater curve, with sluggish peristalsis can be found in the Zollinger-Ellison syndrome or carcinoma and may be mistaken for the latter [37]. Gastroscopic findings are probably even less reliable, as the appearance of the mucosal folds depends heavily on the degree of air insufflation. Classical gastroscopic features are tortuous, oedematous and nodular folds which may look inflamed and are covered in mucus; erosions may be present. In one large series less than a third of the patients were correctly diagnosed by gastroscopy [12], but increasing experience with fibreoptic endoscopy may well improve this. Gastroscopic biopsies are usually of inadequate depth for diagnosis of Ménétrièr's disease, as are *per oral* suction biopsies. The definitive diagnosis has been made by full thickness surgical biopsies of the gastric mucosa in the past, though electrosurgical snare biopsy through the endoscope may provide an alternative [3]. Basal and stimulated gastric acid secretion varies from anacidity to hypersecretion. In the latter, measurements of serum gastrin are helpful in distinguishing this condition from the Zollinger-Ellison syndrome [1].

Hypoproteinaemia is one of the most important features of Ménétrièr's disease. This is due to protein loss from the gastric mucosa which can be determined by the retrieval of intravenously administered radiolabelled albumin (^{131}I or ^{51}Cr) in the gastric aspirate [6]. There is evidence that this protein loss is non-selective [20] and may occur through abnormality of epithelial cell 'tight' junctions [22]. There is also increased breakdown of proteins, even when serum protein concentrations are normal [20].

Differential diagnosis

Gastric carcinoma may have similar radiological features and be associated with gastric protein loss. The diagnosis can usually be excluded by gastroscopy and multiple biopsies.

Granulomatous gastritis is usually associated with systemic disease and granulomas may be present in mucosal biopsies.

Zollinger-Ellison syndrome is difficult to distinguish from the hypersecretory form of Ménétrièr's disease. The definitive difference is the presence of grossly elevated serum gastrin levels, and their response to provocative tests in the former.

Treatment

Prolonged treatment with anticholinergics, such as propantheline bromide 15 mg four times a day improves symptoms and hypoproteinaemia [51]. The mechanism of this is uncertain. Cimetidine 1 g/day gives similar improvement [24] and an initial trial of medical treatment is reasonable in all patients before surgery as it carries a high mortality. Correction of hypoproteinaemia and electrolyte balance is essential before surgery. Vagotomy and/or partial gastrectomy has proved effective [42, 44]. In most patients symptoms abate and protein concentrations return to normal with treatment. Where hypoproteinaemia persists, or severe haemorrhage occurs after surgery, total gastrectomy may have to be done.

Prognosis

Spontaneous remission of the disease has been reported [14]. Most patients, if they survive surgery, do well, but carcinoma has been reported in patients with Ménétrièr's disease [8]. In such a rare condition this association may be significant.

Granulomatous gastritis

This is a rare condition, associated with various systemic illnesses such as Crohn's disease, tuberculosis, sarcoidosis and syphilis. Patients may have dyspepsia, symptoms of gastric outlet obstruction, or haemorrhage. Radiological appearances may mimic gastric ulceration, pyloric stenosis, duodenal ulcer, linitis plastica, or be normal. Diagnosis is made on the presence of granulomas in gastric mucosal biopsies and the presence of systemic disease elsewhere, for example small bowel involvement in Crohn's disease. There are no specific gastroscopic features (except perhaps a cobble-stone appearance in Crohn's disease) and isolation of the infecting organism in tuberculosis and syphilis is not common. In the latter this is because gastric involvement usually manifests in the tertiary stage of the disease. In tuberculosis and syphilis treatment of the disease invariably results in improvement of the gastric lesion, though surgery may be indicated where fibrosis has occurred. In Crohn's disease and sarcoidosis surgery is avoided unless absolutely necessary.

Eosinophilic gastritis

There are two forms of this. A localized eosinophilic lesion is more properly termed **eosinophilic granuloma**. Eosinophilic granulomas generally occur in the antrum, are well localized and present with ulceration, or pyloric obstruction. There is no peripheral eosinophilia or associated allergic phenomena and the condition responds best to local resection.

Diffuse eosinophilic gastritis is usually associated with marked peripheral eosinophilia. About half the patients suffer from asthma or other allergies. Patients present with fever, abdominal pain, diarrhoea and pyloric obstruction; haemorrhage (from ulcers) and peritonitis may occur. The response to corticosteroid therapy is good, though exacerbations may occur.

References

1 BERENSON MM, SANNELLA J, FRESTON JW. Ménétrièr's disease: Serial morphological, secretory and serological observations. *Gastroenterology* 1976;**70**: 257–263.

2 BLACKBURN EK, CALLENDER ST, DACIE JV, *et al.* Possible association between pernicious anaemia and leukaemia; a prospective study of 1625 patients with a note on the very high incidence of stomach cancer. *Int J Cancer* 1968;3:163–170.

3 BJORK JT, GREENEN FJ KOMOROWSKI RA, SOERGEL KH. Ménétrièr's disease diagnosed by electrosurgical snare biopsy. *JAMA* 1979;238:755–1756.

4 BORCH K, RENVALL H, LIEDBERG G. Gastric endocrine cell hyperplasia and carcinoid tumours in pernicious anaemia *Gastroenterology* 1985;88:638–648.

5 CALLENDER ST, DENBOROUGH MA, SNEATH J. Blood groups and other inherited characters in pernicious anaemia. *Br J Haematol* 1957;3:107–114.

6 CITRIN Y, STERLING K, HALSTED JA. The mechanism of hypoproteinaemia associated with giant hypertrophy of the gastric mucosa. *N Eng Jl Med* 1957;257:906–912.

7 CHANARIN I. *The megaloblastic anaemias.* London: Blackwell Scientific Publications Ltd, 1969.

8 CHUSID LR, HIRSCH I, COLCHER H. Spectrum of hypertrophic gastropathy. *Arch Intern Med* 1964;114:621–628.

9 EDWARDS FC, COGHILL NF. Aetiological factors in chronic atrophic gastritis. *Br Med J* 1966;2:1409–1415.

10 EDWARDS FC, COGHILL NF. Clinical manifestations in patients with chronic atrophic gastritis, gastric ulcer and duodenal ulcer. *Q J Med* 1968;37:337–360.

11 ELDRIDGE J, LESSELLS AM, JONES DM. Antibody to spiral organisms on gastric mucosa *Lancet* 1984;1:1237–1239.

12 FEIBER SS. Hypertrophic gastritis, report of two cases and analysis of fifty pathologically verified cases from the literature. *Gastroenterology* 1955;28:39–42.

13 FIXA B, KOMÁRKOVÁ O, NOŽIČKA Z. Leucocyte migration inhibition test with two gastric antigens in pernicious anaemia and in simple atrophic gastritis. *Acta Hepato-gastroenterol (Stuttg)* 1979;26:43–45.

14 FRANK B, KERN F. Ménétrièr's disease: spontaneous metamorphosis of giant hypertrophy of the gastric mucosa to atrophic gastritis. *Gastroenterology* 1967;53:953–960.

15 HARVEY RF, BRADSHAW MJ, DAVIDSON CM, WILKINSON SP, DAVIES PS. Multifocal gastric carcinoid tumours, achlorhydria and hypergastrinaemia. *Lancet* 1985;i:951–954.

16 IHÁMAKI T, VARIS K, SIURALA M. Morphological, functional and immunological state of the gastric mucosa in gastric carcinoma families. *Scand J Gastroenterol* 1979;14:801–812.

17 IMMERSLUND O. Idiopathic chronic megaloblastic anaemia in children. *Acta Paediatr Scand* [Suppl 119] 1960;40:1–115.

18 IRVINE W, DAVIES SH, HAYNES RC, SCARTH L. Secretion of intrinsic factor in response to histamine and to gastrin in the diagnosis of Addisonian pernicious anaemia. *Lancet* 1965;i:736–737.

19 IRVINE WJ, DAVIES SH, TERTELBAUM S, DELAMORE IW, WYNN-WILLIAMS A. The clinical and pathological significance of gastric parietal cell antibody. *Ann NY Acad Sci* 1965;124:657–691.

20 JARNUM S, JENSEN KBN. Plasma protein turnover (albumin, transferrin, IgG, IgM) in Ménétrièr's disease (giant hypertrophic gastritis): evidence of non-selective protein loss. *Gut* 1972;13:128–137.

21 JOSKE RA, FINCKH ES, WOOD IJ. Gastric biopsy. A study of 1,000 consecutive successful gastric biopsies. *Q J Med* 1955;24:269–294.

22 KELLY DG, MILLER LJ, MALAGALEDA JR, HURZENGA KA, MARKOWITZ H. Giant hypertrophic gastropathy (Ménétrièr's disease): Pharmacologic effects of protein leakage and mucosal ultrastructure. *Gastroenterology* 1982;83:581–589.

23 KORMAN MG, STRICKLAND RG, HANSKY J. The functional 'G' cell mass in atrophic gastritis. *Gut* 1972;13:349–351.

24 KRAG E, FREDERIKSEN H-J, OLSEN N, HENRIKSEN JH. Cimetidine treatment of protein-losing gastropathy (Ménétrièr's disease) *Scand J Gastroenterol* 1978;13:635–639.

25 LANGMAN MJS. *The epidemiology of chronic digestive disease.* London: Edward Arnold, 1979.

26 LAWSON DH, MURRAY RM, PARKER HLW. Early mortality in the megaloblastic anaemias. *Q J Med* 1972;41:1–14.

27 MARSHALL BJ, ARMSTRONG JA, MCGRECKIE DB, GLAUCY RJ. Attempt to fulfill Koch's postulates for pyloric camopylobacter. *Med J Aust* 1985;142:436–439.

28 MARSHALL BJ, WARREN JR. Unidentified curved bacilli in the stomach of patients with gastritis and peptic ulceration. *Lancet* 1984;1:1311–1314.

29 MCINTYRE PA, HAHN R, COULEY CL, GLASS B. Genetic factors in predisposition to pernicious anaemia. *Bull Johns Hopkins Hospital* 1959;104:309–314.

30 MAWHINNEY H, LAWTON JWM, WHITE AG, IRVINE WJ, HL-A3 and HL-A7 in pernicious anaemia and autoimmune atrophic gastritis. *Clin Exp Immunol* 1975;22:47–53.

31 MESHKINPOUR H, ELASHOFF H, STEWART H. Effect of cholestyramine on the symptoms of reflux gastritis. A randomised double blind crossover study. *Gastroenterology* 1977;73:441–443.

32 MING SC, GOLDMAN H, FREIMAN DG. Intestinal metaplasia and histogenesis in carcinoma in human stomach. *Cancer* 1967;20:1418–1429.

33 MOLLIN DI, BAKER SJ, DONIACH I. Addisonian pernicious anaemia without gastric atrophy in a young man. *B J Haematol* 1955;1:278–289.

34 MORSON BC, DAWSON IMP. *Gastrointestinal pathology.* London. Blackwell Scientific Publications, 1979.

35 PALMER ED. Gastritis: a revaluation. *Medicine (Balt)* 1954;**33**:199–290.

36 PRICE AB, LEVI J, DOLBY JM, DUNSCOMBE PL, SMITH A, CLARK J, STEPHENSON ML, *Campylobacter pyloridis* in peptic ulcer disease: microbiology pathology, and scanning electron microscopy. *Gut* 1985;**26**:1138–88.

37 REESE DF, HODGSON JR, DOCKERTY MB. Giant hypertrophy of the gastric mucosa (Ménétrièr's disease): a correlation of the roentgenographic, pathologic and clinical findings. *Am J Roentgenol* 1962;**88**:619.

38 RHODES J. Etiology of gastric ulcer. *Gastroenterology* 1972;**63**:171–182.

39 ROSE MS, CHANARIN I. Intrinsic factor antibody and absorption of Vitamin B12 in pernicious anaemia. *Br Med J* 1971;**i**:25–26.

40 SAMLOFF IM. A study of the relationship between serum group I pepsinogen levels and gastric acid secretion. *Gastroenterology* 1975;**69**:1196–1200.

41 SAMLOFF IM, KLEINMAN MS, TURNER MD, SOBEL MV, JEFFIRES GH. Blocking and binding antibody to intrinsic factor and parietal cell antibody in pernicious anaemia. *Gastroenterology* 1968;**55**:575–583.

42 SCOTT HW, SHULL HJ, LAW DH. Surgical management of Ménétrièr's disease with protein-losing gastropathy. *Ann Surg* 1975;**181**:765–777.

43 SCHINDLER R. On hypertrophic glandular gastritis, hypertrophic gastropathy and parietal cell mass. *Gastroenterology* 1963;**45**:77–83.

44 SEARCY RM, MALAGELADA J-R. Ménétrièr's disease and ideopathic hypertrophic gastropathy. *Ann Intern Med* 1984;**100**:565–570.

45 SIMSON JNL. Hyperplastic gastropathy. *Brit Med J* 1985;**291**:1298–1299.

46 SIPPONEN P. Intestinal metaplasia and gastric carcinoma. *Ann Clin Res* 1981;**13**:139–143.

47 SIURALA M, ERÄMMA E, NYBERG W. Pernicious anaemia and atrophic gastritis. *Acta Med Scand* 1960;**166**:213–223.

48 SIURALA M, ISOKOSKI I, VARIS K, KEKKI M. Prevalence of gastritis in a rural population. *Scand J Gastroenterol* 1968;**3**:211–223.

49 SIURALA M, SALMI HJ. Long-term follow-up of subjects with superficial gastritis or a normal gastric mucosa. *Scand J Gastroenterol* 1971;**6**:459–463.

50 SIURALA M, VARIS K, WILJASALO M. Studies of patients with atrophic gastritis: a 10–15 year follow-up. *Scand J Gastroenterol* 1966;**1**:40–48.

51 SMITH RL, POWELL DW. Prolonged treatment of Ménétrièr's disease with an oral anticholinergic drug. *Gastroenterology* 1978;**74**:903–906.

52 STEER HW, COLIN-JONES DG. Mucosal changes in gastric ulceration and their response to carbenoxolone sodium. *Gut* 1975;**16**:590–597.

53 STOCKBRÜGGER R, ANGERVALL I, LUNDQVIST G. Serum gastrin and atrophic gastritis in achlorhydric patients with and without pernicious anaemia. *Scand J Gastroenterol* 1976;**11**:713–719.

54 STRICKLAND RG, MACKAY I. A reappraisal of the nature and significance of chronic atrophic gastritis. *Am J Dig Dis* 1973;**18**:426–440.

55 TAYLOR KB. Pernicious anaemia. In: Truelove SC, Willoughby CP, eds. *Topics in Gastroenterology*, Vol 7, Oxford: Blackwell Scientific Publications, 1979.

56 TWOMEY JJ, JORDAN PH, LAUGHTER AH. The gastric disorder in immunoglobulin deficient patients. *Ann Intern Med* 1970;**72**:499–504.

57 VARIS K, IHÄMAKI T, HARKONEN M, SAMLOFF IM, SIURALA M. Gastric morphology, function and immunology in first-degree relatives of probands with pernicious anaemia. *Scand J Gastroenterol* 1979;**14**:129–139.

58 VARIS K, ISOKOSKI M. Screening of Type A gastritis. *Ann Clin Res* 1981;**13**:133–138.

59 VARIS K, SAMLOFF IM, TIILIKAINERN A, *et al. Gastritis in first-degree relatives of pernicious anaemia, gastric cancer patients and controls in the genetics and heterogeneity of common gastrointestinal diseases.* New York, London, Toronto, Sydney, San Francisco: Academic Press, 1980.

60 VILLAKO K, SIURALA M. Behaviour of gastritis and related conditions in different population samples. *Ann Clin Res* 1981;**13**:114–118.

61 VILLAKO K, TAMM A, SAVISAAR E, RUTTAS H. Prevalence of antral and fundal gastritis in a randomly selected group of an Estonian rural population. *Scand J Gastroenterol* 1976;**11**:817–822.

62 WARREN JR, MARSHALL B. Unidentified curved bacilli on gastric epithelium in active chronic gastritis. *Lancet* 1983;**1**:1273–1275.

63 WHITEHEAD R. Mucosal biopsy of the gastrointestinal tract. *Major problems in pathology* (vol. 3). Philadelphia, London, Toronto: W. B. Saunders Co, 1979.

64 WHITTINGHAM S, YOUNGCHAIND U, MACKAY IR, BUCKLEY JD, MORRIS PJ. Thyrogastric autoimmune disease, studies on the cell-mediated immune system and histocompatibility antigens. *Clin Exp Immunol* 1975;**19**:289–299.

65 WINTROBE MM. *Clinical haematology.* Philadelphia: Lea and Febiger, 1981.

66 WOOD IJ, RALSTON M, COWLING DC. Vitamin B12 deficiency in chronic gastritis. *Gut* 1964;**5**:27–37.

Chapter 19
Gastric Mucosal Injury

M. M. COHEN

Introduction

Gastric mucosal damage occurs in a bewildering array of circumstances. It is not surprising that it has a number of synonyms depending on the perceived aetiology, for example, acute stress erosions, stress ulceration, acute gastritis, erosive gastritis, Curling's ulcer, Cushing's ulcer and acute gastric mucosal lesions. Of these, the last is probably the most useful because it does not attribute a specific cause and clearly distinguishes the condition from inflammatory gastritis and chronic peptic ulceration. The salient features of gastric mucosal injury are rapid onset (sometimes within minutes) and lack of inflammatory component. It is focal, multiple, superficial, and heals rapidly when the damaging agent is withdrawn. The lesion is histologically the same no matter how induced, but the depth varies with the severity and duration of the injury. A simple classification based on aetiology is: drugs, e.g., aspirin and ethanol; physical agents, e.g., corrosives and freezing; injury and illness; psychological.

Silen [56] has stressed that in situations such as critical illness or extensive burns, a pre-existing peptic ulcer diathesis can be reactivated and that this complication, occurring later in the course of the illness, must be distinguished from the early development of multiple acute erosions. Certain drugs also can induce or reactivate a peptic ulcer. The stress of confinement causes mucosal damage in the rat but there is little data to support the widely held view that psychological stress can cause gastric injury in man [61].

The clinical features of gastric mucosal injury are variable. There may be no symptoms whatsoever, or there may be exsanguinating haemorrhage from multiple erosions developing in a desperately ill patient in the intensive care unit.

Ulceration of the gastroduodenal mucosa has been viewed as a disease of too much acid. Schwartz's dictum 'no acid ... no ulcer' certainly holds true, in that mucosal ulceration will not occur in the complete absence of acid, but very little acid is required for mucosal injury to occur. Gastric ulcer and particularly acute gastric mucosal lesions are due more to a defect in mucosal defence (and thus, an impaired ability to deal with whatever acid is present), than to hyperacidity.

This chapter will consider acute gastric mucosal damage and its pathogenesis and will deal with the various agents which have been incriminated in the aetiology of acute gastric mucosal damage and the possible mechanisms by which this damage might occur.

Epidemiology

It is difficult to measure the prevalence of gastric mucosal injury. Damage is present in many asymptomatic individuals. Most of those challenged have a significant increase in faecal blood loss after oral non-steroid anti-inflammatory drugs (NSAID) (Fig. 19.1), presumably due to the development of acute gastric mucosal lesions [30]. Most normal subjects develop endoscopically obvious lesions of the stomach (less commonly of the duodenum) after a short course of

Chapter 19

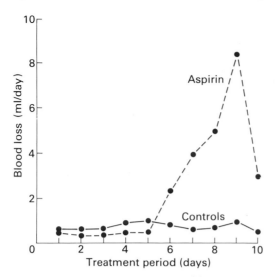

Fig. 19.1. Daily faecal blood loss in healthy young men who received either aspirin 600 mg or placebo four times daily for three days. Blood loss measured with the 51 Cr labelled red cell technique [5, 29].

NSAID [38]. Endoscopy shows that acute mucosal lesions occur in most patients who have sustained injury, severe burns, or critical illness [13, 40]. Yet, few of these individuals actually develop frank gastro-intestinal bleeding. Langman [37] reviewed the epidemiological evidence for the association between aspirin and acute bleeding and found a history of aspirin ingestion within 48 hours of hospital admission twice as frequently in patients with gastrointestinal bleeding than in control patients. Between 20 and 30 thousand million aspirin tablets are taken annually in the United States alone and there are over 300 proprietary preparations that contain aspirin. Despite this vast consumption, gastrointestinal bleeding has not reached epidemic proportions and indeed, Levy [39] pointed out that aspirin cannot be a common cause of major bleeding because the hospital admission rate for haemorrhage (excluding patients with peptic ulcer) is only 15 per 100,000 heavy aspirin users per annum and the use of aspirin for 1 to 3 days per week is not associated with risk

of significant bleeding. Grossman and his colleagues summarized the problem succinctly, 'If you are an aspirin salesman, you can say that taking aspirin is safe because so few aspirin users get ulcers, or bleeding. But, if you are an ulcer doctor, you will say that these drugs are important causes of ulcers and bleeding because up to 30% of persons with these diseases are regular users of aspirin. Both statements are correct … it depends on your point of view' [35].

The prevalence of acute gastric mucosal injury induced by alcohol is even more difficult to determine. Every endoscopist has seen severe erosive gastritis following a bout of drinking, but in relation to the quantities of alcohol consumed the problem is relatively rare. Gastritis was seen in 88% of non-alcoholic men endoscoped within six hours of an alcoholic binge [46]. Endoscopic examination of the mucosa three hours after a single dose of 1 g/kg ethanol, showed an obvious mucosal lesion in every subject [23]. Mucosal adaptation to aspirin and alcohol must occur, as only a minority of chronic aspirin users, or chronic alcoholics have visible endoscopic damage of the mucosa. Aspirin adaptation has also been shown in normal subjects [24].

Clearly, while mucosal damage is common, its clinical significance is uncertain. Frank haemorrhage in intensive care unit patients has shown a marked decline in the past two decades. This decline preceded the introduction of vigorous prophylaxis with antacids or histamine H_2 receptor antagonists and may simply reflect a general improvement in the care of these patients [42].

Pathology

Acute mucosal lesions are usually multiple and widely distributed. They are more prominent in the proximal stomach than in the antrum and the duodenum is often spared. The typical lesion is a discrete

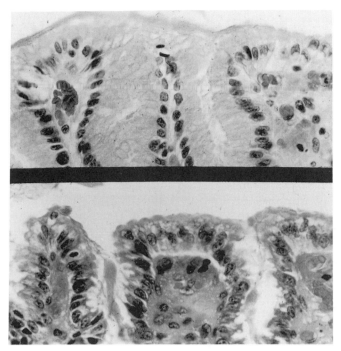

Fig. 19.2. The upper biopsy of gastric mucosa is normal and shows pits lined by mucus filled cells with regular basal nuclei. The lower biopsy is from the same subject after five days aspirin 650 mg q.i.d. The biopsy was taken from an area of mucosa which appeared macroscopically normal. The pits are distorted. The cells are depleted of mucus and their nuclei are of variable size and shape. Both sections stained by H&E [11].

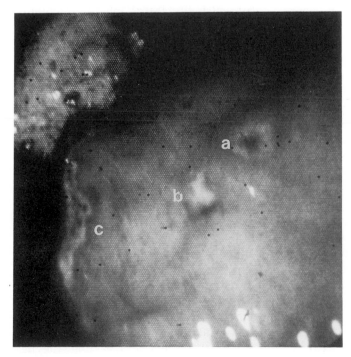

Fig. 19.3. Endoscopic appearance of the gastric mucosa of a healthy volunteer after five days of regular aspirin (two tablets four times daily). (a) discrete circular submucosal haemorrhage. (b) 3 mm erosion. (c) serpiginous erosion on the crest of a gastric ruga. This is an unusually severe injury with this dose of aspirin but illustrates well the variety of acute mucosal lesions visualized endoscopically.

circular shallow erosion which is due to cellular necrosis to a depth limited by the muscularis mucosae. Extravasation of blood causes submucosal haemorrhage and bleeding into the gastric lumen. Infrequently the erosions penetrate through the muscularis mucosae into the submucosa, where a small artery may be eroded leading to brisk haemorrhage. The mucosa between the erosions is not entirely normal, but a loss of surface mucus and irregularity of the nuclei within somewhat flattened cells is present [11] (Fig. 19.2). There are no histological features to characterize lesions due to different agents, although erosions in patients with aspirin injury and intracranial disease occur more often in the antrum and duodenum.

At endoscopy (Fig. 19.3) the typical lesions appear as discrete, circular or linear brown/black, submucosal haemorrhages which are most prominent on the tops of the gastric rugae. The remainder of the mucosa may look normal, or may be diffusely oedematous and erythematous and in severe drug induced injury may be 'beefy' red and friable and bleed at the touch of the endoscope. The loss of surface cells cannot be detected by the naked eye and only in the most severe case is the endoscopist able to visualize erosions which appear as white areas surrounded by submucosal haemorrhage. The depth of these erosions cannot be accurately assessed but it is likely that these are the lesions which extend into the submucosa. Because of their very small size, the erosions cannot usually be visualized radiologically [53] without special techniques (see Chapter 16). Endoscopy is the key to diagnosis and must be done within 12 to 24 hours of admission to hospital, or the opportunity to make the diagnosis may be lost.

Aetiology and pathogenesis

The precise mechanism by which drugs and different stresses cause mucosal erosions is not yet fully understood. Nor is it clear why these lesions are focal, rather than diffuse. Hypersecretion of gastric acid is an obvious possible cause, but gastric injury is usually not associated with hypersecretion of acid. Most ulcerogenic drugs have no marked effect on acid secretion. Caffeine stimulates acid and pepsin [9], but is not ulcerogenic. Acid hypersecretion does not occur in thermal injury, nor in the critically ill. Only in neurosurgical cases is there convincing evidence of increased acid secretion [45]. The more likely explanation is a defect in mucosal defence. Mucosal resistance has been extensively investigated and several possible mechanisms are worth considering in some detail.

The gastric mucosal barrier

This term denotes the powerful barrier to acid which the gastric mucosa maintains. At times, the pH on the luminal side of the mucosal cell will be as low as 1.0 and on its other side 7.4. It is this concentration gradient across a single layer of cells which has been termed the gastric mucosal barrier. It is a biochemical not a structural barrier. Its precise location is unknown. The barrier concept was developed by Davenport during the 1960s in a series of simple but elegant studies in dogs with Heidenhain pouches [16] based on the original observations made by Teorell [57]. Davenport showed that the normal mucosa allowed a small trickle of hydrogen ion to diffuse back from the lumen to the interstitial tissue and that this passive transport was markedly increased by the presence of many agents (e.g., aspirin, ethanol, bile salts) in contact with the mucosa. He called this phenomenon 'disruption of the mucosal barrier' and showed that the dis-

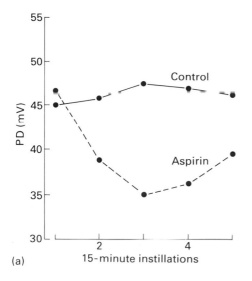

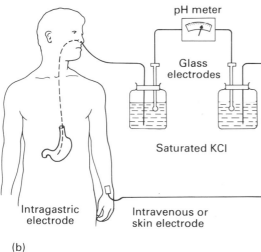

Fig. 19.4. (a) typical fall in human gastric mucosal potential difference (PD) in response to aspirin: 20 mM acetylsalicylic acid was placed in the stomach during instillations 2 and 3. (b) diagram of the apparatus for measurement of PD in man.

appearance of hydrogen ion from the gastric pouch was accompanied by the efflux into the pouch lumen of a large amount of sodium ion, a small amount of potassium ion and some fluid. It is not known whether this ionic flux occurs across, or between the surface mucosal cells. Increased back-diffusion of hydrogen ion is accompanied by a

decrease in gastric transmucosal potential difference (PD) which is normally around 40–60 mV with the surface of the mucosa negative relative to the interstitium (Fig. 19.4). In humans it is impossible to make accurate determinations of ionic flux and the correlation between mucosal permeability and PD has been used to study the mucosal barrier [21]. The generation of PD is multi-factorial and changes in secretory activity have profound effects upon it. The mucosal barrier is difficult to measure in humans [20].

It has been postulated that increased interstitial hydrogen ion concentrations cause local histamine release which, in turn, increases acid damage of submucosal vessels which is followed by extravasation of a protein-rich fluid into the gastric lumen and bleeding culminating in cell necrosis (Fig. 19.5). This attractive hypothesis is consistent with the obligatory role of acid in the pathogenesis of mucosal injury. The effect of aspirin on the mucosal barrier has been extensively studied and it has been shown to disrupt the barrier in a dose related and pH dependent manner [14]. The abnormal mucosal permeability is associated with intracellular changes detectable with electron-microscopy and characterized by condensation of the nuclear chromatin, cytoplasmic oedema and vacuolation [28].

Aspirin, indomethacin and ethanol disrupt the mucosal barrier but some ulcero-

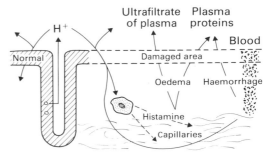

Fig. 19.5. Diagram of the gastric mucosal barrier (adapted from Davenport [15]).

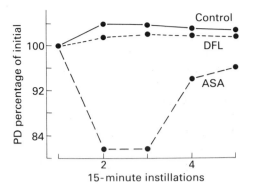

Fig. 19.6. Potential difference study in normal human subjects demonstrates that diflunisal (DFL), a recent addition to the list of NSAID, does not 'break' the gastric mucosal barrier. ASA and diflunisal in equimolar concentration were added during instillations 2 and 3 only.

genic drugs, e.g., ibuprofen, naproxen, phenylbutazone and steroids, have no demonstrable effect on the barrier (Fig. 19.6). Prednisone potentiates the barrier damaging effect of aspirin, and aspirin and ethanol potentiate each other. Bile salts increase back-diffusion of hydrogen ion and bile reflux is common in patients with gastric ulcer, gastritis and also in the critically ill. The hypothesis that bile reflux could be the cause of acute mucosal lesions in these situations [25] is attractive but unproven. Intensive care unit patients [55] and patients with thermal injury [48] have increased back-diffusion of hydrogen ion, but recent animal experiments suggest that visible mucosal damage can occur in haemorrhagic and septic shock without any preceding alteration in permeability. Even a profound fall of mucosal blood flow does not by itself disrupt the mucosal barrier [32]. This has led to the suggestion that it is the ratio of hydrogen ion back-diffusion to mucosal blood flow that is important. Despite its elegance, the hypothesis of mucosal barrier disruption does not provide a unifying explanation for gastric mucosal injury.

Tissue perfusion

Mersereau and Hinchey [44] suggested that there is a direct relationship between the degree of ischaemia and the severity of mucosal injury, but decreased mucosal perfusion does not cause the typical gastric mucosal lesions. There are few functional arterio-venous shunts in the gastric mucosa, so it is unlikely that focal shunting of blood is an important mechanism of damage [1]. The focal lesions are characterized microscopically by congestion and haemorrhage, rather than by ischaemia. Agents such as isoprenaline, which increase blood flow, protect against damage by 'barrier breakers' such as bile salts and indomethacin [50]. This may be due to the more rapid removal of hydrogen ion which has back-diffused, or perhaps to a more efficient intramucosal buffering of it.

Another view of the role of tissue perfusion in acute mucosal lesions has been developed by Menguy [43] who showed that haemorrhagic shock is followed rapidly by a profound decrease in mucosal ATP. He proposed that the mucosal lesions seen in shock are the result of a focal mucosal energy deficit. A deficiency of energy substrate can also be caused by drugs without major changes in perfusion (e.g. aspirin uncouples oxidative phosphorylation and reduces mucosal ATP).

Cell turnover

Epithelial cell turnover is fast in the stomach (within one to three days) and constitutes an important defence mechanism against chronic irritation. It is not an important factor in the defence against acute gastric mucosal lesions, which can arise within minutes of the administration of aspirin or ethanol. However, the resistance which develops to these drugs (many chronic alcoholics and long-term aspirin users have entirely normal gastric mucosa at endoscopy) may be due to a more rapid cell turnover [18]. The increased susceptibility to mucosal damage observed in patients on corticosteroids, or after irradiation could be due to some impairment of epithelial renewal.

Mucus–bicarbonate barrier

Hollander [29] suggested that the two key factors in mucosal resistance are epithelial renewal and the layer of mucus which clings tenaciously to the surface of the gastric mucosa. Mucus was believed to provide an impermeable barrier to acid, but modern analysis of the composition of mucus has shown that it consists of more than 95% water and, as expected from this observation, does not impede the passage of hydrogen ion. Human gastric mucus forms a layer 0.5 mm thick [2] of a viscoelastic gel consisting of a complex glycoprotein with a molecular weight of around 2 million [47]. This coating not only protects the delicate mucosa from mechanical trauma by food, etc., but also maintains an aqueous environment for the mucosal surface.

In the past few years, the long suspected [54] alkaline non-parietal secretion into the gastric lumen has been conclusively de-

monstrated. Bicarbonate is secreted by the fundal and antral mucosa, is carbonic anhydrase-dependent and possibly regulated through cholinergic mechanisms in response to changes in pH. Prostaglandins may regulate bicarbonate and mucus secretion [3]. About 10 times more hydrogen ion than bicarbonate ion is secreted by the gastric mucosa, but much of the acid is lost due to buffering by food, neutralization by refluxed bile and by gastric emptying. The amount of hydrogen ion reaching the surface of the mucosa may not exceed the amount of bicarbonate secreted and retained close to the mucosa by the mucus gel. Experiments using microelectrodes confirm that there is a pH gradient across the mucus layer and that the pH at the surface of the mucosa is close to seven [62]. Bicarbonate trapped within the unstirred layer of mucus seems to act as an efficient neutralizer of luminal acid (Fig. 19.7).

If this theory concerning the mucus-bicarbonate barrier is true, the main obstacle preventing the diffusion of hydrogen ion into the mucosa may be present within the unstirred layer of mucus rather than at the apical membrane, or tight junctions as suggested by the gastric mucosal barrier theory. Anything that damages, or prevents

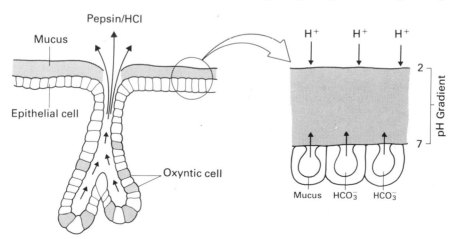

Fig. 19.7. Diagram of the 'mucus-bicarbonate' barrier. Hydrogen ion diffusing towards the epithelium is neutralized by bicarbonate ions trapped in the mucus. A pH gradient is created across the mucus unstirred layer [49].

the formation of this mucus layer is potentially ulcerogenic.

Aspirin, indomethacin and ethanol inhibit bicarbonate secretion, interfere with mucus formation and change its composition [22]. In certain diseases mucus secretion is decreased but we do not know what happens to gastric mucus in the clinical conditions associated with the development of acute mucosal injury. This will be a fruitful area for future investigation.

Prostaglandins

Prostaglandins (prostacylin and PGE_2) are found in high concentrations in the gastric mucosa. Both are products of the cyclooxygenase pathway of arachidonic acid metabolism (Fig. 19.8). The function of mucosal prostaglandins is unknown. They are rapidly metabolized locally and by the liver and lung, so that virtually none reach the systemic arterial circulation. They probably act as local modulators of cell function. The prostaglandins are vasoactive, affect motility, inhibit gastric acid and stimulate bicarbonate and mucus secretion. All of these actions are potentially useful for mucosal defence. The most striking property of prostaglandins so far identified is their ability, in minute amounts applied topically, to prevent damage to the gastric mucosa by

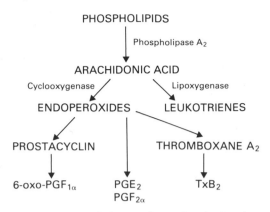

Fig. 19.8. The arachidonic acid cascade. NSAID such as aspirin and indomethacin are powerful inhibitors of cyclooxygenase. Corticosteroids inhibit phospholipase A_2.

many necrosing substances [5, 51] (Fig. 19.9). This 'cytoprotective' effect is independent of any action on acid secretion. In the rat, the protective dose of most prostaglandins is 100 times smaller than the antisecretory dose [52]. Similar protection has been demonstrated in humans using faecal blood loss [6, 8] (Fig. 19.10), mucosal potential difference [7, 10] (Fig. 19.11) or endoscopy to assess mucosal damage (Fig. 19.12).

This evidence does not prove that endogenous prostaglandins defend the mucosa, [27], but additional support for this view is available. Mild irritants [4] and stress [59,

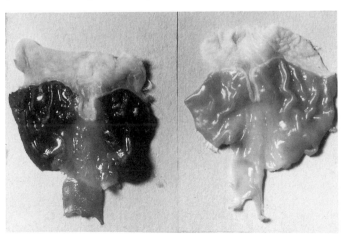

Fig. 19.9. Cytoprotection. The rat on the left was given 1 ml 100% ethanol 1 hour before it was killed. There is extensive damage (black area) to the glandular corpus. The forestomach and the antrum are spared. The rat on the right received, in addition, 10 μg 16,16-dimethyl PGE_2 topically 20 minutes earlier. The ethanol damage has been completely prevented.

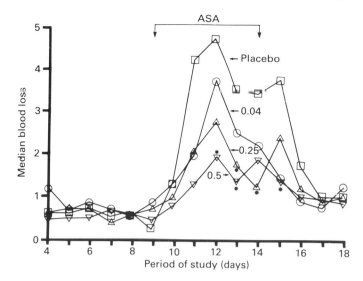

Fig. 19.10. A study of faecal blood loss measured by 51 Cr PGE₂ provides a dose-related protection against ASA injury. The doses of PGE₂ are in mg given q.i.d. The dose of ASA was 650 mg q.i.d. Even at the lowest dose of PGE₂ there is some reduction in the ASA damage. None of the doses provided total protection. Asterisks indicate values significantly lower than placebo [6].

60] can protect rats against the subsequent application of strong irritants and stress. This protection is abolished by pre-treatment with indomethacin—an inhibitor of prostaglandin synthesis and the protected animal has a higher than normal rate of endogenous prostaglandin production and release [34]. This is strong evidence that endogenous prostaglandins are involved in

mucosal defence. How prostaglandins provide this protection is not yet understood, but perhaps they act by stimulating mucus or bicarbonate secretion, mucosal blood flow, the sodium pump, or are in some way essential for the maintenance of cell membrane integrity.

Ever since Vane showed that aspirin and indomethacin are potent inhibitors of the cyclooxygenase system [58], it has been assumed that their ulcerogenic action is due to inhibition of prostaglandin synthesis. Not all non-steroid anti-inflammatory drugs disrupt the gastric mucosal barrier, but all to varying degrees inhibit prostaglandin synthesis. A clear relationship between prostaglandin inhibition and mucosal damage cannot be shown [11] and it is likely that NSAID have more than one mechanism of action as gastric irritants [19] (Fig. 19.13). Smoking may decrease gastric luminal prostaglandins [41]. Agents such as bile salts and ethanol are not known to inhibit prostaglandin synthesis, so this does not explain their ulcerogenic action [31]. The effects on gastric mucosal prostaglandin synthesis of thermal injury, increased intracranial pressure and critical illness have not been studied. Chronic gastric ulcer may possibly be a local prostaglandin de-

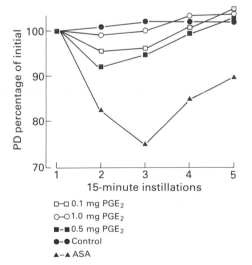

□—□ 0.1 mg PGE₂
○—○ 1.0 mg PGE₂
■—■ 0.5 mg PGE₂
●—● Control
▲—▲ ASA

Fig. 19.11. The effect of three different doses of PGE₂ on human PD. ASA and PGE₂ were added to the stomach during instillations 2 and 3 only. All doses of PGE₂ prevented the ASA induced fall in PD.

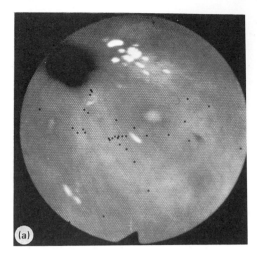
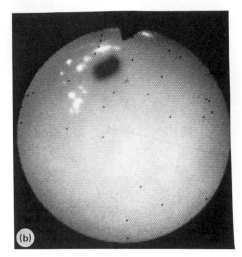

Fig. 19.12. In a double-blind study a synthetic analogue of PGE₂ (enprostil) significantly reduced mucosal damage induced by ASA 650 mg q.i.d. for five days. (a) appearance of antral mucosa after ASA and placebo. Note the presence of several discrete white erosions. (b) appearance of antral mucosa after ASA and 7 μg enprostil b.i.d. The mucosa shows only minimal erythema.

ficiency disease [63] and it is not inconceivable that stress ulceration could be the result of a prostaglandin deficiency, or perhaps exhaustion of local synthesizing capacity. Synthetic prostaglandins are being intensively investigated as possible prophylactic agents in drug and stress-induced erosive gastritis [8, 10] and for treatment of chronic peptic ulceration.

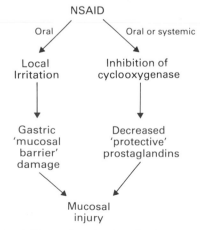

Fig. 19.13. Proposed mechanism of gastric mucosal damage by non-steroid anti-inflammatory drugs (NSAID).

Clinical aspects

The four clinical categories of acute gastric mucosal injury were listed in the introduction to this chapter. We indicated that there was little or no data to support the view that psychological stress causes acute injury. Damage by corrosive agents and freezing is not common and while the patient suffering such an injury can present formidable difficulty in management, the pathogenesis is clearly understood.

The remaining two categories of acute mucosal injury are probably best viewed as separate clinical entities, namely: injury induced by drugs; and injury induced by critical illness and/or trauma. Of these two clinical problems, the second is by far the more difficult to manage and presents the greater therapeutic challenge. The reason, of course, is that the cause cannot be removed.

Prophylaxis

The prevention of drug-induced injury is largely a matter of education. The public needs to be informed of the potential hazard of aspirin, the numerous guises in which it is found and that for most ailments paracetamol is safer [36]. The doctor should know that all NSAID, despite the vigorous claims of the pharmaceutical industry to the contrary, cause gastric mucosal irritation. Alcoholic binges are particularly likely to damage the mucosa.

Prevention of 'stress erosions' is much more contentious. Meticulous attention to the intensive care of the critically ill is probably the single most important factor. Early mechanical ventilation for respiratory failure, gastric decompression and the urgent drainage of pus are crucial. Inhibition of gastric acid secretion is important, especially in the neurosurgical patients. Antacids are of proven value if used vigorously, to keep the gastric pH above 3.5 [26]. Inhibitors of acid secretion, such as cimetidine or ranitidine are much easier to use but are not of proven value and may conceivably do more harm than good, as it has been shown experimentally that the inhibited mucosa is more susceptible to injury [33]. Prostaglandins have yet to be tested. No one has shown that prophylaxis against stress bleeding saves lives.

Treatment

The management of patients with acute gastric mucosal injury due to aspirin, alcohol, etc., depends entirely on the severity of the symptoms. Minor upset without significant blood loss needs no more than general supportive care. Major haemorrhage demands endoscopy to establish the diagnosis. Treatment is with liberal doses of antacid (e.g. 60 ml Mylanta every hour) after washing the stomach free of blood clot with ice-cold tap water, or saline, through a wide-bore double lumen nasogastric tube. These patients virtually never need surgery.

The treatment of patients who develop major bleeding while in the intensive care unit is essentially similar. The mainstay of treatment is vigorous administration of antacids. Histamine H_2 receptor antagonists are of no proven value. The infusion of vasopressin directly into the left gastric artery has been tested [12], but as this drug also causes mucosal ischaemia, its use may be harmful. Occasionally a patient will not respond to medical therapy and surgery becomes necessary. The most appropriate surgical treatment has not been established, but probably the safest course in these desperately ill patients is to suture the bleeding lesions and carry out a truncal vagotomy and sub-total gastrectomy [17]. Either the operative mortality, or the rebleed rate is unacceptable with any other operation.

References

1 Archibald LH, Moody FG, Simons M. Measurement of gastric blood flow with radioactive microspheres. *J Appl Physiol* 1975;38:1051–1056.

2 Bickel M, Kauffman GL. Gastric gel mucus thickness: effect of distension, 16,16-dimethyl prostaglandin E_2 and carbenoxolone. *Gastroenterology* 1981;80:770–775.

3 Bolton JP, Palmer D, Cohen MM. Stimulation of mucus and non-parietal cell secretion by the E_2 prostaglandins. *Am J Dig Dis* 1978;23:359–364.

4 Chaudhury TK, Robert A. Prevention by mild irritants of gastric necrosis produced in rats by sodium taurocholate. *Dig Dis Sci* 1980;25:830–836.

5 Cohen MM, ed. *Biological protection with prostaglandins (Vol II)*. Boca Ratou, Florida: CRC Press, 1986.

6 Cohen MM, Cheung G, Lyster DM. Prevention of aspirin-induced faecal blood loss by prostaglandin E_2. *Gut* 1980;21:602–606.

7 Cohen MM, Clark L. Prevention of aspirin damage to human gastric mucosa with simultaneous administration of prostaglandin E_2. *Can J Surg* 1983;26:116–118.

8 Cohen MM, Clark L, Armstrong L, D'Souza J. Reduction of aspirin-induced fecal blood loss with low dose misoprostol tablets in man. *Dig Dis Sci* 1985;30:605–611.

9 Cohen MM, Debas HT, Holubitsky IB, Harrison RC. Caffeine and pentagastrin stimulation of human gastric secretion. *Gastroenterology* 1971;61:440–444.

10 Cohen MM, McReady DR, Clark L, Sevelius H. Protection against aspirin-indured antral and duo-

denal damage with enprostil: a double-blind endoscopic study. *Gastroenterology* 1985;**88**:382–386.

11 COHEN MM, MACDONALD WC. Mechanism of aspirin injury to human gastroduodenal mucosa. *Prostagl Leukotr Med* 1982;**9**:241–255.

12 CONN HO, RAMSBY GR, STORER EH, *et al.* Intra arterial vasopressin in the treatment of upper gastrointestinal hemorrhage: a prospective, controlled clinical trial. *Gastroenterology* 1975;**68**:211–221.

13 CZAJA AJ, MCALHANY JC, PRUITT BAJ. Acute gastroduodenal disease after thermal injury: an endoscopic evaluation of incidence and natural history. *N Engl J Med* 1974;**291**:925–929.

14 DAVENPORT HW. Damage to the gastric mucosa: effects of salicylate and stimulation. *Gastroenterology* 1965;**49**:189–196.

15 DAVENPORT HW. Salicylate damage to the gastric mucosal barrier. *N Engl J Med* 1967;**226**:1307–1312.

16 DAVENPORT HW. Backdiffusion of acid through the gastric mucosa and its physiological consequences. In: Glass GBJ, ed. *Progress in Gastroenterology*. New York: Grune and Stratton, 1970;48.

17 DELANEY JP, MICHEL HM. Hemorrhagic gastritis following operation. In: Najarian JS, Delaney JP, eds. *Critical surgical care*. Miami, Florida: Symposia Specialists, 1977:357–379.

18 EASTWOOD GL. Epithelial renewal in gastroduodenal mucosal injury. In: Harmon JW, ed. *Basic mechanisms of gastrointestinal mucosal cell injury and protection*. Baltimore/London: Williams and Wilkins, 1981:49–63.

19 EASTWOOD GL. Ultrastructural effects of ulcerogens. *Dig Dis Sci* 1985;**30**:95S–104S

20 FROMM D. Gastric mucosal 'Barrier'. *Gastroenterology* 1979;**77**:396–398.

21 GEALL MG, PHILLIPS SF, SUMMERSKILL DM. Profile of gastric potential difference in man. *Gastroenterology* 1970;**58**:437–443.

22 GLASS GBJ, SLOMIANY BL. Derangement of biosynthesis, production and secretion of mucus in gastrointestinal injury and disease. In: *Mucus in health and disease*. Elstein M, Parke DV, eds. New York/London: Plenum Press, 1977;311–347.

23 GOTTFRIED EB, KORSTEN MA, LIEBER CS. Alcohol-induced gastric and duodenal lesions in man. *Am J Gastroenterol* 1978;**70**:587–592.

24 GRAHAM DY, SMITH JL, DOBBS SM. Gastric adaptation occurs with aspirin administration in man. *Dig Dis Sci* 1983;**28**:1–6.

25 GUILBERT J, BOUNOUS G, GURD FN. Role of intestinal chyme in the pathogenesis of gastric ulceration following experimental hemorrhagic shock. *J Trauma* 1969;**9**:723–743.

26 HASTINGS PR, SKILLMAN JJ, BUSHNELL LS, SILEN W. Antacid titration in the prevention of acute gastrointestinal bleeding. A controlled, randomised trial in 100 critically ill patients. *N Engl J Med* 1978;**298**:1041–1045.

27 HAWKEY CJ, RAMPTON DS. Prostaglandins and the gastrointestinal mucosa: are they important in its function, disease or treatment? *Gastroenterology* 1985;**89**:1162–1188.

28 HINGSON DJ, ITO S. Effect of aspirin and related compounds on the fine structure of mouse gastric mucosa. *Gastroenterology* 1971;**61**:156–177.

29 HOLLANDER F. Gastric secretion of electrolytes. *Fed Proc* 1952;**11**:706–714.

30 HOLT PR. Measurement of gastrointestinal blood loss in subjects taking aspirin. *J Lab Clin Med* 1960;**56**:717–726.

31 ITO S, LACEY ER. Morphology of rat gastric mucosal damage, defense and restitution in the presence of luminal ethanol. *Gastroenterology* 1985;**88**:250–260.

32 KIVILAAKSO E, FROMM D, SILEN W. Relationship between ulceration and intramural pH of gastric mucosa during haemorrhagic shock. *Surgery* 1978;**84**:70–78.

33 KIVILAAKSO E, SILEN W. Pathogenesis of experimental gastric mucosal injury. *N Engl J Med* 1979;**301**:364–369.

34 KONTUREK SJ, BRZOZOWSKI T, PIASTUCKI I, RADECKI T, DEMBINSKI A, DEMBINSKI-KIEC A. Role of locally generated prostaglandins in adaptive gastric cytoprotection. *Dig Dis Sci* 1982;**27**:967–971.

35 KURATA JH, ELASHOFF JD, GROSSMAN MI. Inadequacy of the literature on the relationship between drugs, ulcers, and gastrointestinal bleeding. *Gastroenterology* 1982;**82**:373–376.

36 LANCET. Aspirin or paracetamol (editorial). *Lancet* 1981;**ii**:287–289.

37 LANGMAN MJS. Epidemiological evidence for the association of aspirin and acute gastrointestinal bleeding. *Gut* 1970;**11**:627–634.

38 LANZA FL, ROYER GL, NELSON RS, *et al.* The effects of motrin, indocin, aspirin, naprosyn and placebo on the gastric mucosa of normal volunteers. A gastroscopic and photographic study. *Dig Dis Sci* 1979;**24**:823–828.

39 LEVY M. Aspirin use in patients with major upper gastrointestinal bleeding and peptic ulcer disease. *N Engl J Med* 1974;**290**:1158–1162.

40 LUCAS CE, SUGAWA C, RIDDLE J, *et al.* Natural history and surgical dilemma of 'stress' gastric bleeding. *Arch Surg* 1971;**102**:266–273.

41 MCREADY DR, CLARK A, COHEN MM, Cigarette smoking reduces human gastric luminal prostaglandin E_2. *Gut* 1985;**26**:1192–1196.

42 MENGUY R. The prophylaxis of stress ulceration. *N Engl J Med* 1980;**302**:461–462.

43 MENGUY R, DESBAILLETS L, MASTERS YF. Mechanism of stress ulcer: influence of hypovolemic shock on energy metabolism in the gastric mucosa. *Gastroenterology* 1974;**66**:46–55.

44 MERSEREAU WM, HINCHEY EJ. Effect of gastric acid-

ity on gastric ulceration induced by haemorrhage in the rat utilising a gastric chamber technique. *Gastroenterology* 1973;**64**:1130–1135.

45 NORTON L, GREER J, EISEMAN B. Gastric secretory response to head injury. *Arch Surg* 1970;**101**:200-204.

46 PALMER ED. Gastritis: a re-evaluation. *Medicine* 1954;**33**:199–290.

47 PEARSON J, ALLEN A, VENABLES C. Gastric mucus: isolation and polymeric structure of the undegraded glycoprotein: its breakdown by pepsin. *Gastroenterology* 1980;**78**:709–715.

48 RAI K, COURTEMANCHE AD, COHEN MM. Gastric mucosal permeability in burned patients: correlation with endoscopy. *J Surg Res* 1976;**20**:71–75.

49 REES WDW TURNBERG LA. Biochemical aspects of gastric secretion. *Clin Gastroenterol* 1981; **10**: 521–554.

50 RITCHIE WP JR, SHEARBURN EW III. Influence of isoproterenol and cholestyramine on acute gastric mucosal ulcerogenesis. *Gastroenterology* 1977; **73**:62–65.

51 ROBERT A, NEZAMIS JE, LANCASTER C, HANCHAR AJ. Cytoprotection by prostaglandins in rats: prevention of gastric necrosis produced by alcohol, HCl, NaOH, hypertonic NaCl, and thermal injury. *Gastroenterology* 1979;**77**:433–443.

52 ROBERT A, SCHULTZ JR, NEZAMIS JE, LANCASTER C. Gastric antisecretory and antiulcer properties of PGE_2, 15-methyl PGE_2, and 16,16-dimethyl PGE_2. Intravenous, oral and intrajejunal administration. *Gastroenterology* 1976;**70**:359–370.

53 ROESCH W. Erosions of the upper gastrointestinal tract. *Clin Gastroenterol* 1978;**7**:623–634.

54 SCHIERBECK NP. Ueber Kohlensaure im Ventrikel. *Scand Arch Physiol* 1892;**8**:437–474.

55 SKILLMAN JJ, GOULD SA, CHUNG RSK, SILEN W. The gastric mucosal barrier: clinical and experimental studies in critically ill and normal man, and in the rabbit. *Ann Surg* 1970;**172**:564–584.

56 SKILLMAN JJ, SILEN W. Stress ulcers. *Lancet* 1972;ii:1303–1306.

57 TEORELL T. Untersuchungen über die magensaftsekretion. *Scand Arch Physiol* 1933;**66**:225–230.

58 VANE JR. Inhibition of prostaglandin synthesis as a mechanism of action for aspirin-like drugs. *Nature (New Biol)* 1971;**231**:232–235.

59 WALLACE JL, COHEN MM. Gastric mucosal protection with chronic mild restraint: role of endogenous prostaglandins. *Am J Physiol* 1984;G127–132.

60 WALLACE JL, TRACK NS, COHEN MM. Chronic mild restraint protects the rat gastric mucosa from injury by ethanol or cold-restraint. *Gastroenterology* 1983;**85**:370–375.

61 WEINER H. Stress and ulcers—the continuing association. *Gastroenterology* 1983;**84**:189–190.

62 WILLIAMS SE, TURNBERG LA. Demonstration of a pH gradient across mucus adherent to rabbit gastric mucosa: evidence for a 'mucus-bicarbonate' barrier. *Gut* 1981;**22**:94–96.

63 WRIGHT JP, YOUNG GO, KLAFF LJ, WEER LA, PRICE SK, MARKS IN. Gastric mucosal prostaglandin E levels in patients with gastric ulcer disease and carcinoma. *Gastroenterology*. 1982;**82**:263–267.

Chapter 20
Aetiology of Peptic Ulcer

M. J. S. LANGMAN

Epidemiology

Peptic ulceration is a major cause of ill health in Western communities and in many other areas, although the reasons why it develops are poorly understood. This indifferent appreciation arises in three important ways. Firstly, we are hindered in drawing epidemiological maps because frequency figures derived in one area can seldom be directly compared with those obtained in another, as no standard method of ascertainment can be applied. Secondly, ulcer disease is not a single entity, but many early analyses have failed to make the distinction between gastric and duodenal ulcers. It is now becoming clear that there are differential trends in frequency distribution between ulcer diseases in, for instance, the elderly and in young adults, which suggest that multiple environmental as well as genetic factors influence incidence patterns. Thirdly, testing aetiological hypotheses is impeded by inability to derive reliable methods of examining the importance of likely candidates, such as dietary items.

Descriptive data

Mortality rates

Deaths ascribed to peptic ulcers arise primarily through complications of bleeding and perforation and following operations. It follows that ulcer mortality data essentially describe patterns of complications of ulcer

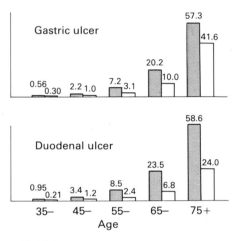

Fig. 20.1. Age specific death rates from peptic ulcer in England and Wales as rates per 100,000 *per annum* in 1973–77 [11].

disease in the elderly. Thus the chances of dying from peptic ulceration rise several hundredfold in later adult life in the United Kingdom and similar patterns can be discerned in other countries with a Western culture [9] (Fig. 20.1). Those who examine death rates from peptic ulceration in different communities have to consider whether the fluctuating patterns should be ascribed to differences in standards of clinical practice, to varying methods of coding the cause of death (thus post-operative deaths might be ascribed primarily to the underlying ulcer in some places and to complicating post-operative conditions in another), or to differences in the age structure of the population under review.

Whatever the variations may be that

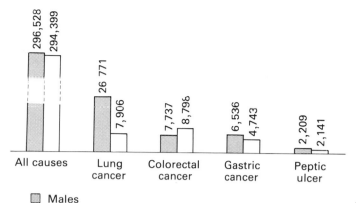

Males
Females

Fig. 20.2. Selected causes of death in England and Wales, 1979 [38].

occur as a result of such difficulties, deaths from peptic ulcer still constitute a minor proportion of all deaths in Western communities. This is illustrated in Fig. 20.2, which compares peptic ulcer mortality rates with those for other causes of death in the United Kingdom [38].

Autopsy surveys

Autopsy surveys show that more than a fifth of all men and a tenth of all women have been found to have evidence of present, or past ulcer disease. Table 20.1 contrasts figures obtained in Leeds, England and Rotterdam, the Netherlands [1, 6, 28, 58].

At least four factors hinder interpretation of these figures. Firstly the likelihood of de-

tecting active ulcers, or ulcer scars, will depend upon the care with which they are sought. Ulcers may heal completely without scarring, so that prevalence data will be underestimated. The autopsy rate in many Western countries has fallen progressively in recent years. The group now selected for examination may be unrepresentative of the larger group formerly considered, whilst in its turn this group is likely to contain individuals with different characteristics from the living population. Thus a group of people dying in accidents may contain a higher proportion of drinkers. Despite such difficulties, the figures emphasize the general frequency of ulcer in Western communities, and the relative importance of gastric or duodenal ulcers.

Table 20.1. Percentage prevalence of gastric and duodenal ulcer at selected ages in Leeds, England and Rotterdam, the Netherlands.

Gastric ulcer				
Age	Leeds		Rotterdam	
20–29	2.7	2.0	0.7	0.4
40–49	7.0	3.2	9.8	1.4
60–69	4.1	6.0	9.3	6.4
Duodenal ulcer				
Age	Leeds		Rotterdam	
20–29	11.0	3.5	4.9	1.2
40–49	16.8	8.0	10.4	5.7
60–69	12.0	8.0	10.1	4.6

Hospital admission rates

In many countries such as the United Kingdom and the United States the reasons for hospital admission are noted in a sample population. Changes in admission rates may indicate that the frequency of ulcer disease is altering, but they may result from differences in treatment fashions. Kurata [24] has suggested that recent declines in overall hospital admission rates for ulcer in the United States mainly reflect such changes. Perforated ulcer is coded as a specific subset and as it is a mandatory cause of hospital admission, changes in perforation rates may be better guides to changes in ulcer frequency. Perforation rates have in general fallen in the United Kingdom [11].

Special surveys

The criteria used in conducting such surveys have varied greatly. Thus they may depend on simple questionnaires designed to elicit dyspepsia, or they have concentrated upon previously diagnosed ulcer, supplemented by selected examination of individuals who admit to symptoms. Matters are further complicated by the radical change in diagnostic method now in progress, as radiology is supplemented and later replaced by endoscopy.

Geographical and temporal patterns of ulcer frequency in populations of European origin

Temporal variations

During the last hundred years the frequency pattern of peptic ulceration has changed greatly. The changes have been particularly well documented in the United Kingdom and Scandinavia, but it is likely that the same general trends have occurred in most, if not all, European population groups. Two, and possibly three phases can be discerned, covering periods from about the mid-nineteenth century to the early twentieth century, from then until the mid-twentieth century, and a recent phase.

1850–1900

Before this period peptic ulceration was poorly described, but then there were increasingly frequent descriptions of gastric ulceration, especially as a disease of younger women. Duodenal ulcer was rarely mentioned before the last decade. Since this period antedated the introduction of diagnostic methods, the cases described were essentially those dying from bleeding, or perforated ulcer. The paucity of descriptions of duodenal ulcer seems likely to reflect lack of occurrence, rather than misclassification,

Table 20.2. Proportions of men and women with gastric ulcers in four one-year surveys [26].

	Perforated ulcer	Ulcer deaths		
	1867	1912	1918	1924
Aged less than 35 years:				
Men	18	182	167	151
Women	96	338	214	109
M:F ratio	0.2 : 1	0.5 : 1	0.8 : 1	1.4 : 1
Aged 35 years or more:				
Men	42	691	900	1219
Women	43	635	713	620
M:F ratio	1.0 : 1	1.1 : 1	1.3 : 1	2.0 : 1

or failure of detection. Table 20.2 compares the figures collected by William Brinton [6] in London for gastric ulcer frequency according to age, with the distribution of deaths from gastric ulcer recorded 50 years later in the United Kingdom. Even allowing for the introduction of successful treatment methods and for the increased proportion of elderly people in the population, there has been an obvious change. Exact timing is difficult, but descriptions of duodenal ulcer seem to have become common between 1890 and 1910 throughout western Europe and North America.

1900–1960

Duodenal ulcer prevalence rose to several times that of gastric ulceration and gastric ulcer became a disease of the elderly. Initial changes seem to have been rapid, but in the latter 20 years duodenal ulcer frequency seems to have climbed slowly to a peak.

1960 and later

Alternative views have been that ulcer frequency, in particular, of duodenal ulcer has fallen, or that no material change has occurred. The former view is supported by consideration of figures from the United Kingdom and the latter by data from Denmark and the United States [24, 5]. In the United Kingdom there is clear evidence that the ulcer perforation rate has fallen greatly in younger people, but no change, or even an increase, has been detected in the elderly—especially in women (Fig. 20.3), while in the United States it seems likely that decreases in admission and disability rates arise at least in part due to changes in patterns of medical practice, rather than in disease behaviour [19, 24, 36, 56]. We do not know why ulcer frequency has varied in the last hundred years. Analysis of individual sets of figures suggests that

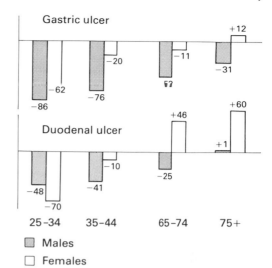

Fig. 20.3. Percentage change in admission rates for ulcer perforation in England and Wales as average rates for 1958–62 related to those for 1973–77 [11].

changes, particularly in the late nineteenth and early twentieth century occurred rapidly, suggesting that factors responsible may have only operated for a short time beforehand. Susser and Stein [52] proposed that the rising frequency of duodenal ulcer after the 1930s was a cohort phenomenon, those born in the period of financial depression being unduly susceptible to late ulcer disease by reason of exposure to, or deprivation of some factor, or factors.

Geographical variations

It is difficult to compare data collected in different places at different times and in different ways. Furthermore, little information has been obtained in European populations, except in north western areas. In places such as Australia and North America the lack of a uniform system of health care has hindered those seeking to collect figures. Table 20.3 outlines some of the major variations in ulcer frequency in different populations [26]. A common feature is the generally greater prevalence of duodenal than of gastric ulcer. There have been rare

Table 20.3. Ulcer frequency in some different parts of the world [26].

Area	Type	Distribution
Africa	Almost all duodenal, stenosis and obstruction relatively frequent. Almost all men.	Common on W. Coast, Nile Congo watershed, N. Tanzania, N. Ethiopia. Rare in north savannah of W. Coast, S. Ethiopia, N. Nigeria, most of Zaire and Zambia.
India	Almost all duodenal. Stenosis and obstruction relatively frequent. Almost all men.	Common in south and in Assam; rarer in north.
Europe	Duodenal and gastric both generally common (DU two to four times as frequent as GU).	No recognized areas of rarity, but some regional variations, e.g. DU two to three times as frequent in Scotland as in S. England.
N. America	Duodenal ulcer fairly common. Gastric ulcer probably less frequent than in Europe.	Probably fairly even.
Australia	Mainly duodenal ulcer, but relatively high frequency of gastric ulcer in younger women.	Gastric ulcer may be especially common in New South Wales and Queensland.

exceptions—in the north Norwegian population of Drammen and in a Peruvian Andean group. An increased frequency of gastric ulcer was recorded in younger women in Australia in the late 1940s and attributed to heavy intake of compound analgesics.

Ulcer frequency can vary distinctly within population groups. Thus in the United Kingdom duodenal ulcer frequency,

Table 20.4. Regional admission rates per 1,000 population with perforated peptic ulcer in the United Kingdom.

	Duodenal	Gastric
South		
East Anglia	0.07	0.08
Wessex	0.08	0.08
Oxford	0.13	0.04
South-west	0.14	0.02
North		
Leeds	0.22	0.07
Liverpool	0.23	0.03
Manchester	0.23	0.10
Newcastle	0.31	0.10
Scotland	0.45	0.07

measured by the perforation rate, rises progressively from South to North, whereas gastric ulcer frequency does not seem to change particularly [7] (Table 20.4).

Socio-economic variation

Classical textbook descriptions distinguish between duodenal ulcer as a disease of the affluent and gastric ulcer as an illness of the poor. The limited data available suggest that this may have been so 50 years ago, but that gastric and duodenal ulcer are now relatively more common in poorer people, as measured by mortality rates and frequency data (Table 20.5) [21, 30, 45]. There do not seem to be special occupations that confer special risks. The differential liability to peptic ulcer of college-educated and non-college-educated individuals in the United States is almost certainly attributable to the same socio-economic class factors (Table 20.6) [21]. Searches for background of significant stressful life events have generally been disappointing [32].

Table 20.5. Ulcer mortality (standardized mortality ratios) [45] and morbidity [30] by socio-economic class.

		Socio-economic class				
		I	II	III	IV	V
Mortality						
1959–63						
Gastric		46	58	94	106	109
Duodenal		70	84	113	102	136
Morbidity						
Gastric	Observed	6	11	12	13	28
	Expected	2	11	30	14	7
Duodenal	Observed	13	41	125	136	158
	Expected	14	80	218	108	52

Table 20.6. Smoking habits, ulcer frequency and educational attainment in men [21].

	Percentage with ulcers		
	Elementary school only	High or trade school	College
Smokers	15.1	13.3	10.7
Non-smokers	7.7	6.2	6.1

Ulcer frequency in non-European populations

Any difference in ulcer prevalence between European and non-European populations could be due to inherent variations in susceptibility conferred by racial characteristics, or to changes in the pressure of predisposing factors. Distinguishing between these can be difficult. In the black and white populations living in the United States ulcer frequency and death rates do not seem to differ greatly [23], although judgement is impeded by difficulty in standardizing for social factors and in being sure that both racial groups have the same standards of medical care and hence the same chances of ulcer diagnosis.

The liability of underdeveloped tropical populations to ulcer disease is illustrated by experience in Africa and India [53, 54].

Africa

Frequency of duodenal ulcer seems to vary very widely from extremely rare to comparatively common, but gastric ulcer outside the Republic of South Africa seems to be generally uncommon. Areas of high ulcer frequency seem to have no standard characteristics; they include areas on the West coast, in the Nile–Congo watershed, North Tanzania and Northern Ethiopia.

India

Again, virtually all ulcer is duodenal and as in Africa most disease is described in men where stenosis and obstruction seem to be frequent features. Contrasts have been drawn between the high prevalence of ulcer in the South and in Assam and its relative rarity in the North, such as in the Punjab.

Other areas

Although it is difficult to define simple comparative figures, it is clear that ulcer is a common problem in South America, in Chinese and Japanese populations and elsewhere.

Predisposing factors

Diet

Despite the great attraction of hypotheses linking dietary factors to liability to peptic ulceration, supportive evidence is fragmentary. Two alterations of dietary balance that have been thought could influence liability to peptic ulceration are changes in the proportions of protein, or carbohydrate and changes in dietary fibre content [53]. Epidemiological study of these, or any other dietary factors, are hindered in several ways. No one knows for what period any noxious influence must operate for peptic ulcer to develop, nor if there is any incubation period between exposure and occurrence of ulceration. No retrospective dietary questionnaires have been devised which measure reliably the patterns of food eaten in an antecedent period. We have therefore depended on three other sources of evidence. The geographical distribution of ulcer disease has been compared with the general diet patterns of those areas, the physiological qualities of foods as buffering agents have been related to their potential as predisposing or preventive agents and the influence of foods upon the development of ulcers in experimental animals has been examined. None of these forms of inquiry satisfies. Broad comparisons of ulcer frequency with composition of the diet are hindered by the poor knowledge of the distribution of ulcer disease, the time interval which it may take before ulcer develops and the impossibility of knowing whether an association with a specific dietary compo-

nent represents a direct, or an indirect phenomenon. Matters are further complicated because controlling for one factor can transform from positive to negative an apparent association with another. If foods such as proteins are found to have high buffering capacities, then such properties may well become valueless if they are more potent stimuli to secretion. The relevance of experimental animal models to human peptic ulcer is doubtful.

Dietary protein content

If duodenal and gastric ulcer are now diseases of the poor then associations with reduced dietary protein intake might be detected simply because poorer people are less able to buy expensive protein-containing foods. Examination of patterns of ulcer prevalence in tropical Africa do not necessarily suggest a correlation with protein intake.

Dietary fibre

Like many other diseases, peptic ulceration has been attributed to diminished dietary fibre intake. Fibre is a heterogeneous commodity and it may therefore be unreasonable to regard it as a unity; nevertheless a correlation can be detected between fibre deficient diets and an increased frequency of ulcer in parts of Southern India. The consistency of such an association elsewhere needs closer examination.

Beverage intake

An examination of the later frequency of peptic ulcer in Harvard and Pennsylvania students [39] who completed questionnaires as students about (inter alia) their tea, coffee, alcohol, milk and cola-type soft drink intake showed that coffee and cola drink consumption tended to be associated with an increased frequency of later ulcer, whereas milk intake seemed to be associated with protection, and tea and alcohol intake had negligible associations. We do not know if these were direct influences, but additive effects were noted between coffee and cola intake and cigarette smoking.

Acid and pepsin secretion

Basal and pharmacologically, or physiologically stimulated acid (and pepsin) secretion has been extensively studied in relation to the pathogenesis of duodenal and gastric ulcer, (see Chapter 17) but no general conclusions have been reached. Most studies reporting differences between ulcer and control populations show an overlap between the study groups, while others report observations on small numbers of intensively studied subjects, so that results may be affected by selection. Although a lot is known about factors controlling acid and pepsin secretion, in most patients the development of an ulcer probably results from an imbalance between those factors and mucosal resistance, and very little is known about the latter. The importance of various attack and defence mechanisms may be different in different patients.

Duodenal ulcer

As a group, patients with duodenal ulcer have higher acid outputs than controls. About 30% have higher basal acid secretion probably because of a larger parietal cell mass. Nocturnal rates of acid secretion are elevated and there is a higher peak secretion of acid. Acid output in patients with duodenal ulcers may also be higher than in normals during the day, but only a few patients have been thus studied [20]. The sensitivity of the parietal cells to secretagogues may be greater and more gastrin may be released from the antral G cells in patients with duodenal ulcer than in controls; the number of G cells is probably greater than normal. Inhibition of gastrin release by antral reflexes may be impaired in duodenal ulcer patients. These factors may lead to an increased acid and pepsin load entering the duodenum, especially as some (but not all) studies of gastric emptying in duodenal ulcer have reported it to be faster than in controls [34]. Increased basal and nocturnal rates of acid secretion and enhanced release of gastrin in response to a meal has led to postulation of an increased vagal drive, or tone in duodenal ulcer disease, but direct evidence for this idea is lacking. It has been pointed out that peak secretion of at least 15 mmol/h is needed for a duodenal ulcer to develop and that duodenal ulcer hardly ever occurs in individuals whose peak secretory capacity is below that level [4].

Whatever the distribution of secretory capacity in patients with duodenal ulcers, 70–80% of them heal after a short course of drugs that do not inhibit acid output, thus indicating the importance of other factors [10].

Acid and pepsin secretion usually move in parallel but may become dissociated, for example during administration of secretin which inhibits acid but stimulates pepsin. Precursors of pepsin—the pepsinogens—are found in the gastric fundal and body mucosa and can be measured by radioimmunoassay in the serum, where they have been divided into pepsinogen I (PgI), II (PgII) and a slow migrating protease (SMP): PgI has been most studied. PgI is above the normal range (50–175 ng/ml) in 50–60% of patients with duodenal ulcer, is higher in severe ulcer disease, correlates with secretory capacity of the stomach and is inherited as an autosomal dominant trait; it can be used as a marker of ulcer disease in some families. PgI contains at least five electrophoretically discrete bands which convert into four enzyme species, pepsins 1 to 4. It is possible that duodenal ulcer may be associated with increased secretion of pepsin I. The rate of breakdown of gastric mucus by pepsin I may be higher than that due to the other pepsin species; mucus acts as a barrier to the entry of pepsin into the epithelial cells, while being continuously eroded on its luminal surface by the enzyme. The interplay of these genetic and biochemical factors in duodenal ulcer needs to be worked out [55].

Gastric ulcer

Basal and peak acid secretion in patients with gastric ulcer falls within the normal range. Patients with ulcers in the body of the stomach tend to have lower acid outputs than those with prepyloric, or those with duodenal ulcer. Low acid secretion in patients with gastric body ulcers is probably a consequence of chronic atrophic gastritis which invariably accompanies this disease; back-diffusion of acid through the pathological mucosa may also play a part [4].

Thus in a multifactorial disease, abnormalities of control of gastric secretion may also be multifactorial and involve increased basal acid output, excessive cephalic acid response, abnormally high maximal acid secretion, hyper-sensitivity to gastrin, postprandial hypergastrinaemia and faulty regulation of gastrin release. The most frequent abnormalities are probably abnormally high nocturnal and postprandial secretion, possibly present in some 60% of patients with duodenal ulcer [25].

Mucosal resistance

This is a much invoked, but ill-understood factor in the aetiology of mucosal injury and of peptic ulcer. Viscous mucus [2] forming an adherent layer covering the epithelium may entrap bicarbonate secreted by the mucosa in an unstirred layer, creating a steep pH gradient from the lumen at pH of about 1.5, to the mucosal surface where it approaches neutrality [44]. Rapid turnover of epithelial cells would also tend to increase mucosal resistance. Mucosal resistance may be lowered by ulcerogenic drugs, or by reflux of bile into the stomach—duodenogastric reflux is more prominent in patients with gastric ulcer than in controls.

Prostaglandin E_2 (PGE_2) is synthesized by the gastric mucosa. Sub-antisecretory doses of various prostaglandins protect experimental animals against ulcerogenic agents, while prostanoid synthetase inhibitors increase the incidence of ulceration. This phenomenon has been called cytoprotection [46]. Its mechanism is poorly understood, but it may depend on maintenance of epithelial haemoperfusion.

Smoking

An association between smoking and peptic ulceration is now well-proven. Smokers are more likely to die from ulcers than nonsmokers, and those who have been smokers in earlier life are more liable to later ulceration. It seems unlikely that the association between smoking and peptic ulceration simply reflects a tendency for poorer people to smoke heavily. The association between smoking and peptic ulceration seems to hold independently of educational level and amongst doctors smoking was associated with an increased prevalence of ulceration [21, 37]. Smoking also decreases intraluminal PGE_2 concentrations in the stomach [33] and habitual smoking may increase acid secretory capacity [40], although the evidence for this is not entirely convincing.

Drug intake

There is considerable difficulty in determining whether corticosteroids, aspirin and other non-steroidal anti-rheumatoid agents are important precipitants of ulcer complications and/or cause ulcers to develop *de novo.* Anecdotal evidence describing the proportions of individuals with ulcer who have taken specific agents are valueless without comparative controls and when controlled studies are conducted those which consider prescription drugs must take into account the vagaries of prescribing habits from one individual to another, whilst analyses of the consumption of non-prescription agents must allow for drug taking which is consequential upon the presence of symptoms of an established lesion in considering what additional proportion may be causal.

Corticosteroids

Any increase in ulcer frequency in long term takers of corticosteroid drugs could be attributed to ulcer developing in debilitated people. Conn and Blitzer [13] took account of this possibility by comparing the frequency of ulcer in corticosteroid takers and non-takers in 42 controlled trials of therapy for a variety of conditions. They concluded that no significant risk was attached to such treatment, but the frequency of ulcer did in fact double over control levels when dosage was the equivalent of, or more than 20 mg of prednisolone.

Non-aspirin, non-steroidal anti-inflammatory drugs (NSAIDs)

Despite the widespread belief that drugs like phenylbutazone and indomethacin are common and perhaps important causes of ulcer and ulcer complications, supportive evidence is not abundant. An early suggestion that they were prone to cause antral greater curve ulceration has not been supported and it remains unclear whether any increase, which has inevitably been attributed to inhibition of prostaglandin synthesis in the mucosa, is in the frequency of gastric or duodenal ulcer. Medication with NSAIDs is, however, strongly correlated with admission to hospital because of

intestinal bleeding, or perforation, and the risk in elderly people of bleeding gastric or duodenal ulcer is increased by two to four times. A rising frequency of ulcer perforation in the United Kingdom in elderly people may also, in part, be related to NSAID intake [9, 51, 57].

Aspirin

The extent of any risk of haematemesis or melaena as a consequence of aspirin intake is difficult to determine. Studies, which have uniformly shown there to be a higher proportion of aspirin takers amongst those with haematemesis or melaena compared with hospital patients without bleeding, have usually failed to take account of the possibility that patients took aspirin because of symptoms associated with the presence of the bleeding lesion. When this has been done then in broad terms about one-third of all aspirin intake could be equated with that of control individuals without bleeding, one-third could, by reference to a parallel increase in paracetamol intake, be attributed to intake consequential upon the presence of the bleeding lesion (it being assumed that paracetamol does not cause acute upper gastrointestinal bleeding), but a remaining third was unaccounted for, and could be causal [12]. Levy [29] in analysing data from the Boston Collaborative Drug Surveillance Program concluded that occasional intake was not a risk factor, but that chronic regular use might be associated with a risk of the order of 15 per 100,000 regular users per year. Our own figures suggest that some risk may attach to occasional use perhaps of the order of one episode for every quarter million doses, as well as a risk associated with regular use. Data obtained in controlled trials of aspirin prophylaxis for cardiovascular disease confirm that treatment is associated with an increased risk of upper gastrointestinal bleeding (Table 20.7).

Table 20.7. Episodes of haematemesis or melaena recorded during controlled trials of therapy for thromboembolic diseases.

	AMIS [3]	CDPR [15]	PARIS [41]
Aspirin	8.2	6.2	6.4
Placebo	4.9	4.6	2.5

Figures record the percentage of individuals reporting such events. Each trial lasted approximately three years, and aspirin dosage was in the range 900–1000 mg daily.

AMIS —Aspirin, myocardial infarction study research group.
CDPR —Coronary drug project research group.
PARIS —Persantin-aspirin reinfarction study research group.

The risk of developing ulcers as opposed to the complications of ulcers has also been disputed. In Australia, and to a lesser extent in North America, long term use has been thought to cause chronic gastric ulceration. Consumption chronically of compound aspirin-phenacetin-based analgesic mixtures has been blamed for a high frequency of chronic gastric ulcer in middle-aged women in Eastern Australia, although lately the thesis has been disputed by the finding that a parallel increase in paracetamol-based analgesic intake is also detectable [42].

Associated disease

Many other illnesses have been claimed to increase the chances of chronic peptic ulceration developing in the same individual. Assessment is complicated because inevitably the chances of having a second disease diagnosed are enhanced by being under medical surveillance already. Furthermore, disease clustering might occur because of common associations with social factors or with characteristics such as smoking habits. Problems of assessment are discussed in detail elsewhere [14, 17].

Once all figures have been taken into account it seems likely that cirrhotic liver disease, hyperparathyroidism and chronic renal disease after transplantation or during dialysis are associated with an increase in liability to peptic (usually duodenal) ul-

ceration. Another factor which seems to be related to heightened liability to peptic ulcer is low blood pressure within the normal range. At least two sets of data support this surprising conclusion; the basis is unclear [35, 39].

Patients with diabetes mellitus seem by contrast to be relatively protected from developing peptic ulceration, either probably, because atrophic gastritis reduces acid secretory potential, or because of a high frequency of autovagotomy [18, 22]. The role of *Campylobacter* infection in predisposing to gastritis or duodenitis is, at present, unclear [43].

Genetic factors

Any increase in the frequency of peptic ulceration within families may imply the working of common environmental or genetic factors, or both.

It has been known for nearly forty years that peptic ulceration follows a familial pattern, that within such families one type of ulceration tends to prevail, and that the increased ulcer frequency is observed both across and within generations. Although these patterns are consistent with the operation of inherited factors they could also result from environmental influences [16].

The existence of racial influences upon liability to peptic ulceration has long been postulated, but it has been difficult to decide if observed differences in ulcer prevalence or mortality between, say, coloured and white populations are due to differing inherent susceptibility to varying exposure to environmental predisposing factors, or to greater or lesser chances of disease diagnosis. Kurata and Haile [23] in analysing United States data noted that crude death rates from ulcer, hospitalization rates and ulcer prevalence as judged by responses to questionnaires were all higher in white than in non-white populations, but whether these differences were real or whether they arose through, for instance, a lesser tendency for non-whites to ascribe symptoms to ulcer or to gain access to diagnostic facilities, is questionable.

Genetic markers

The finding that people of blood group A [1] have a slightly increased liability to develop gastric cancer was followed quickly by the discovery that duodenal ulcer was more common in those of blood group O than in those of groups A, B or AB, and that AB (O) H non-secretors (those incapable of secreting these blood group substances in water soluble form) are also more prone to ulceration than secretors [8].

The effects of secretor status and of ABO blood group are exerted independently and the effects of both upon the chances of developing ulcers are modest—in general terms those of blood group O are about 25% more liable and those who are non-secretors about 30% more liable to duodenal ulceration than the remainder.

Further analysis has shown that the blood group association is most marked for complicated ulcer, especially bleeding ulcer [27], and once this has been taken into account any overall association of blood group with duodenal ulcer may be slight or non-existent. The pattern in gastric ulceration is less clear. Although some data suggest a broadly similar picture to that seen in duodenal ulcer, other results indicate that gastric ulcers above the angulus are associated with blood group A, and those below with group O.

The basis for the observed associations is uncertain but no correlation has been detected between acid or pepsinogen secretory potential and blood group or secretor status.

Pepsinogens are separable electrophoretically into five fast moving bands (group I) and two slower moving bands (group II). Two patterns, of hyperpepsinogenaemia or normopepsinogenaemia, are detectable within group I. Hyperpepsinogenaemia I seems to be inherited as an autosomal dominant characteristic, and is associated with liability to duodenal ulcer. The risk is somewhat greater than that associated with ABO blood group or secretor status, though not markedly so, and normopepsinogenaemic individuals remain at risk of duodenal ulceration [49, 50].

The case has been pressed [47] for suggesting that other features, which include an increased gastrin response to a protein meal, and rapid gastric emptying are heritable and predispose to duodenal ulcer but could do with more support. Taken overall it seems likely that the frequency of duodenal ulcer and the changes in distribution patterns are explained by the interplay of environmental influences with genetic variation contributing to background susceptibility.

Examination of HLA groups in ulcer patients have revealed no consistent trends.

References

1 Aird I, Bentall HH, Mehigan JA, Roberts JAF. The blood groups in relation to peptic ulceration and carcinoma of colon, rectum, breast and bronchus. *Br Med J* 1954;ii:315–321.

2 Allen A. Structure and function of gastrointestinal mucus. In: Johnson LR, ed. *Physiology of the gastrointestinal tract.* New York: Raven, 617–639.

3 Aspirin. Myocardial Infarction Study Research Group. A randomized controlled trial of aspirin in

persons recovered from myocardial infarction. *JAMA* 1980;243:661–669.

4 BARON JH. Current views on the pathogenesis of peptic ulcer. *Scand J Gastroenterol [Suppl 80]* 1982;17:1–10.

5 BONNEVIE O. Peptic ulcer in Denmark. *Scand J Gastroenterol [Suppl 63]* 1980;15:163–174.

6 BRINTON W. *On the pathology, symptoms and treatment of ulcer of the stomach.* London: Churchill, 1867.

7 BROWN RC, LANGMAN MJS, LAMBERT PM. Hospital admissions for peptic ulcer during 1968–72. *Br Med J* 1976;1:35–37.

8 CLARKE CA, EDWARDS JW, HADDOCK DRW, HOWEL EVANS AW, McCONNELL PB, SHEPPARD PM. ABO blood groups and secretor character in duodenal ulcer. *Br Med J* 1956;ii:725–731.

9 COLLIER DStJ, PAIN JA. Non-steroidal anti-inflammatory drugs and peptic ulcer perforation. *Gut* 1985;26:359–363.

10 COLIN-JONES D.G. There is more to healing ulcers than suppressing acid. *Gut* 1986;27,475–480.

11 COGGON D, LAMBERT P, LANGMAN MJS. Twenty years of hospital admissions for peptic ulcer in England and Wales. *Lancet* 1981,i:1302–1304.

12 COGGON D, LANGMAN MJS, SPIEGELHALTER D. Aspirin, paracetamol, and haematemesis and melaena. *Gut* 1982;23:340–344.

13 CONN HD, BLITZER BL. Non-association of adrenocorticosteroid therapy and peptic ulcer. *N Engl J Med* 1976;294:473–479.

14 COOKE AR, LANGMAN MJS. Gastric and duodenal ulcer and their associated diseases. *Lancet* 1976;i:680–683.

15 CORONARY DRUG PROJECT RESEARCH GROUP. Aspirin in coronary heart disease. *J Chronic Dis* 1976;29:625–642.

16 DOLL R, KELLOCK TD. The separate inheritance of gastric and duodenal ulcers. *Ann Eugenics* 1951;16:231–240.

17 DONALDSON RM. Factors complicating observed associations between peptic ulcer and other diseases. *Gastroenterology* 1975;68:1608–1614.

18 DOTEVALL G. Incidence of peptic ulcer in diabetes mellitus. *Acta Med Scand* 1959;164:463–477.

19 ELASHOFF JD, GROSSMAN MI. Trends in hospital admissions and death rates for peptic ulcer in the United States, from 1970 to 1978. *Gastroenterology* 1980;78:280–285.

20 FELDMAN M, RICHARDSON DT. Total 24-hour gastric acid secretion in patients with duodenal ulcer. Comparison with normal subjects and effects of cimetidine and parietal cell vagotomy. *Gastroenterology* 1986;90:540–544.

21 FREIDMAN GD, SIEGELAAB AB, SELTZER CC. Cigarettes, alcohol, coffee and peptic ulcer. *New Engl J Med* 1974;290:469–473.

22 HOSKING DJ, MOODY F, STEWART IM, ATKINSON M. Vagal impairment of gastric secretion in diabetic autonomic neuropathy. *Br Med J* 1975;2:588–590.

23 KURATA JH, HAILE BM. Racial differences in peptic ulcer disease: fact or myth? *Gastroenterology* 1982;83:166–172.

24 KURATA JH, HONDA GD, FRANKL H. Hospitalization and mortality rates for peptic ulcers: a comparison of a large health maintenance organisation and United States data. *Gastroenterology* 1982;83:1008–1016.

25 LAM SK. Pathogenesis and pathophysiology of the duodenal ulcer. In: Isenberg JI, Johanssen C, eds. *Clin Gastroenterol* 1984;13:447–471.

26 LANGMAN MJS. *The epidemiology of chronic digestive disease.* London: Arnold, 1979.

27 LANGMAN MJS, DOLL R. ABO blood groups and secretor status in relation to clinical characteristics of peptic ulcer. *Gut* 1965;6:270–273.

28 LEVI IS, DE LA FUENTE AA. A post mortem study of gastric and duodenal peptic lesions. *Gut* 1963; 4: 349–359.

29 LEVY M. Aspirin use in patients with major upper gastrointestinal bleeding and peptic ulcer disease. *New Engl J Med* 1974;290:1158–1162.

30 LITTON A, MURDOCH WR. Peptic ulcer in South West Scotland. *Gut* 1963;4:360–366.

31 McCONNELL RB, LINAKER BD, GEORGE J. Genetic markers and severity of duodenal ulcer. *Prog Clin Biol Res* 1983;173:245–254.

32 McINTOSH JH, NASIRY RW, COATES C, MITCHELL H, PIPER DW. Perception of life event stress in patients with chronic duodenal ulcer. A comparison of the rating of life event by duodenal ulcer patients and community controls. *Scand J Gastroenterol* 1985;20:563–568.

33 McREADY DR, CLARK I, COHEN MM. Cigarette smoking reduces gastric luminal prostaglandin E_2. *Gut* 1985;26:1192–1196.

34 MADDERN GH, HOROWITZ M, HETZEL DJ, JAMIESON GG. Altered solid and liquid gastric emptying in patients with duodenal ulcer disease. *Gut* 1985;26:689–693.

35 MEDALIE JH, NEUFELD HN, GOLDBOURT U, KAHN HA, RISS E, ORON D. Association between blood pressure and peptic ulcer incidence. *Lancet* 1970;ii:1225–1226.

36 MENDELOFF AI. What has been happening to duodenal ulcer? *Gastroenterology* 1974;67:1020–1022.

37 MONSON RR. Cigarette smoking and body form in peptic ulcer. *Gastroenterology* 1970;58:337–344.

38 OFFICE OF POPULATION, CENSUSES AND SURVEYS. *Mortality Statistics in England and Wales,* 1979; O.P.C.S.

39 PAFFENBARGER PS, WING PL, HYDE RT. Chronic disease in former college students. XIII Early precursors of peptic ulcer. *Am J Epidemiol* 1974;199:307–315.

40 PARENTE P, LAZZARONI M, SANGALETTI O, BARONI S, BIANCHI PORRO G. Cigarette smoking, gastric

acid secretion and serum pepsinogen I concentrations in duodenal ulcer patients. *Gut* 1985;**26**:1327–1332.

41 PERSANTIN-ASPIRIN REINFARCTION STUDY RESEARCH GROUP. Persantin and aspirin in coronary heart disease. *Circulation* 1980;**62**:449–468.

42 PIPER DW, McINTOSH JH, ARIOTTI DE, FENTON BH, MacLENNAN R. Analgesic ingestion and chronic peptic ulcer. *Gastroenterology* 1981;**80**:427–432.

43 PRICE AB, LEVI J, DOLBY JM, *et al. Campylobacter pyloridis* in peptic ulcer disease: microbiology, pathology, and scanning electron microscopy. *Gut* 1985;**26**:1183–1188.

44 REES WDW, TURNBERG LA. Mechanism of gastric mucosal protection: a role for the mucus-bicarbonate barrier. *Clin Sci* 1982;**62**:343–348.

45 REGISTRAR GENERAL'S DECENNIAL SUPPLEMENT. *Occupational mortality tables for 1959–63.* London: HMSO, 1971.

46 ROBERT A. Current history of cytoprotection. *Prostaglandins [suppl]* 1981;**21**:89–96.

47 ROTTER JI. The genetics of gastritis and peptic ulcer. *J Clin Gastroenterol [Suppl 2]* 1981;**3**:36–43.

48 ROTTER JI, PETERSEN GM, SAMLOFF IM, *et al.* Genetic heterogeneity of hyperpepsinogenemic I and normopepsinogenemic I duodenal ulcer disease. *Ann Intern Med* 1979;**91**:372–377.

49 ROTTER JI, SONES JQ, SAMLOFF IM, *et al.* Duodenal ulcer disease associated with elevated serum pepsinogen I. *N Engl J Med* 1979;**300**:63–66.

50 SAMLOFF IM, LIEBMAN WM, PANITCH NM. Serum group I pepsinogen by radioimmunoassay in control subjects and patients with peptic ulcer. *Gastroenterology* 1975;**69**:83–90.

51 SOMERVILLE K, FAULKNER G, LANGMAN M. Non-steroidal anti-inflammatory drugs and bleeding peptic ulcer. *Lancet* 1986;**i**:462–466.

52 SUSSER S, STEIN Z. Civilisation and peptic ulcer. *Lancet* 1962;**i**:115–118.

53 TOVEY F. Duodenal ulcer and diet. In: Burkitt, DP, Trowell, HC, eds *Refined carbohydrate foods and disease.* London: Academic Press, 1973.

54 TOVEY FI, TUNSTALL M. Duodenal ulcer in black populations in Africa south of the Sahara. *Gut* 1975;**16**:564–576.

55 VENABLES CW. Mucus, pepsin and peptic ulcer. *Gut* 1986;**27**:233–238.

56 VOGT TM, JOHNSON RE. Recent changes in the incidence of duodenal and gastric ulcer. *Am J Epidemiol* 1980;**111**:713–720.

57 WALT R, KATSCHINSKI B, LOGAN R, ASHLEY J, LANGMAN M. Rising frequency of ulcer perforation in elderly people in the United Kingdom. *Lancet* 1986;**i**:489–492.

58 WATKINSON G. The incidence of chronic peptic ulcer found at necropsy. *Gut* 1960;**i**:14–31.

Chapter 21
The Presentation of Peptic Ulcer

K. D. BARDHAN

The presentation of ulcer disease

Clinical features

The cardinal symptom of patients with ulcer disease is epigastric pain, usually recurrent, often long-standing, related to meals and relieved by antacids. Many ancillary symptoms, such as heartburn, or distension, may also be present. Much less often patients present as an emergency with haemorrhage or bleeding.

The pain or discomfort is mainly epigastric or in the upper right quadrant and may radiate to the back. The relapses generally last 1–4 weeks, but troublesome pain may last only a few days. The remissions are of varying length, commonly 1–6 months and 1–4 relapses a year are usual. During the attacks the pain fluctuates in intensity and there are pain-free intervals. Food may relieve or worsen the pain, or may have no effect. Nocturnal pain is common and wakes the patient between 1 and 3 a.m. Vomiting may be present, usually relieves the pain and may thus be self-induced. There are various other dyspeptic symptoms, the commonest being heartburn. The disease runs a long course [1].

There are wide variations from this average picture, nor is the pattern unique to peptic ulcer and the features of duodenal and of gastric ulcer are virtually indistinguishable clinically [8, 10, 11, 19]. This means that the differentiation of gastric from duodenal ulcer has to be established by endoscopy or by radiology.

Age and sex

Duodenal ulcer used to be a disease of the young and gastric ulcer a disorder of the middle aged, but an older population is now affected. However, the disease affects people of any age. Duodenal ulcer is 3–5 times more common in men than in women, though the ratio varies in different parts of the world; the difference is much less marked in gastric ulcer. Thus, a young man with ulcer symptoms is far more likely to have a duodenal than a gastric ulcer, while in an old woman the chances can be almost equal [20].

Characteristics of ulcer pain (see Chapter 3)

Patients use various descriptions of the pain such as pressure, or burning, or hunger, but these are not discriminatory. The pain is not uniformly severe throughout a relapse. It is often severe for 1–4 days (or longer) and the patient may therefore describe the length of the relapse in those terms, but milder symptoms commonly precede or follow the severe pain for several days. The relapses also vary in severity. Even when severe and continuous, the pain fluctuates in intensity. During the 24 hours the pain is episodic, attacks lasting $\frac{1}{2}$ to 2 hours, although the duration is difficult to measure accurately as patients seek relief from food or drugs. This pattern is different from biliary colic, where the intense pain lasts for a few hours only and is followed by gradually fading discomfort. Fleeting pain lasting seconds or minutes is not acteristic of ulcer disease. Nocturnal pain that wakes the patient affects more than half the subjects with severe symptoms; its relief by antacids is strongly indicative of duodenal ulcer.

The diagnostic importance of the relation between food and pain is exaggerated. It is said that food relieves pain of duodenal ulcer which rarely occurs soon after meals, but 1–2 hours later; in gastric ulcer food only rarely relieves and pain develops soon after. But this is frequently not so; the results vary from centre to centre and the relation is not unique to ulcer disease.

The pain is usually epigastric. Less commonly it is in the right hypochondrium. Ulcer pain can occur in other sites but if it is perceived in the lower abdomen, it is very unlikely to be due to ulcer disease. Ulcer pain may be felt over a wide area, but the patients are usually (but not invariably) able to localize the area of pain with one finger—the 'pointing sign'. In contrast, patients with functional disorders are seldom able to localize their pain and may use the flat of the hand to indicate the area of pain.

The pain may radiate at some stage in 60% of patients—generally to the back or to other areas of the abdomen. As a result of gastro-oesophageal reflux, retrosternal pain or heartburn is common.

An abrupt increase in the severity of pain, or a change from its previous pattern was thought to be indicative of ulcer penetration. These changes include: colicky intense pain instead of a burning discomfort, location in the right upper quadrant instead of the epigastrium, radiation to the back, the loss of diurnal rhythm, or failure of antacids and/or food to relieve the symptoms. However, increasing severity and radiation are a part of the natural history of the disease and these changes are also found in patients whose ulcers have not involved other tissues.

Relieving factors

Food, antacids, vomiting and rest are usually considered to relieve ulcer pain, but the pattern is variable. Vomiting may be self-induced if the patient has discovered that this relieves the pain. Spontaneous vomiting does not necessarily mean that irreversible pyloric stenosis is present and it usually settles with medical treatment. It is rarely severe enough to produce serious dehydration and metabolic alkalosis.

Mechanism of pain

Not much is known about the mechanism of pain which presumably arises from the ulcer crater; irritation of the lower oesophagus by acid may contribute to duodenal ulcer pain [9]. The afferent pathway mediating the sensation of pain has not been worked out, and although most vagal fibres are said to be afferent, it is not known whether the vagus is the main nerve conducting painful stimuli from the stomach and the first part of the duodenum. Acid is generally accepted as an important factor provoking the pain and quick relief of it by antacids or milk, supports this hypothesis. The situation must be more complex, as recent close surveillance of patients with duodenal ulcer during trials of maintenance treatment has shown that a proportion of ulcers relapse without any symptoms being perceived by the patients. The apparent paradox of relief of ulcer pain by food (which stimulates acid secretion) can be explained by the considerable buffering capacity of foodstuffs, especially protein, so that despite maximal or near maximal secretion of acid postprandially, the intragastric pH rises after meals. The return of pain some two hours after meals signifies that gastric emptying has depleted the intraluminal reserves of buffer, but gastric secretion of acid continues, presumably providing the trigger for pain. Nocturnal pain may be related to night-time hypersecretion of acid, often present in patients with duodenal ulcer. The role of locally released products of inflammation, or of histamine, kinins and prostanoids in the mediation of pain is unknown. Gastric or duodenal motility has been invoked as a factor in causation of pain, but its importance is doubtful.

Course

Ulcer disease is characterized by relapses and remissions often over many years, but with the exception of carcinoma of the stomach, other conditions mimicking ulcer disease, such as the irritable bowel syndrome, have a similar course. Relapses lasting more than two weeks followed by clear-cut and complete remissions of at least one and often several months, are more characteristic of ulcer disease than of functional disorder. The reasons for the cyclical nature of ulcer disease and its seasonal variations are unknown (see Chapter 20) [3, 17].

Gastric carcinoma

Relentless anorexia, weight loss and pain may strongly suggest the diagnosis, but in some it can only be made by endoscopy, biopsy and cytological brushings of the gastric lesion.

Examination

The diagnosis of duodenal, or gastric ulcer cannot be made at physical examination, but some useful clinical points can be gathered. Epigastric tenderness is often present, but is not diagnostic. It is usually absent in ulcer disease during remissions and it can be elicited in functional disorders [26]. Physical examination determines the site of pain and excludes the presence of abdominal masses or organomegaly. The general nutrition of the patient and his or her abil-

ity to localize the site of pain with precision are worth noting. In patients with vomiting as a prominent symptom it is useful to look for visible gastric peristalsis and a succussion splash—their presence denotes severe organic pyloric channel obstruction, which may be due to fibrosis and scarring associated with long-standing duodenal ulcer, but also to antral carcinoma.

Special categories of peptic ulcer

Ulcers in children and the elderly

Ulcer disease in childhood is rare and as the picture may be atypical, the diagnosis may be missed. The main features may be poor feeding, vomiting, and failure to grow. Under the age of seven the pain may be generalized or at the umbilicus, right hypochondrium, or right iliac fossa, with or without vomiting. Symptoms in the teenager resemble those in adults [15, 16, 23, 24, 31].

In **ulcer disease in the elderly** difficulties in diagnosis may arise because the patient is unable to give a clear history or the symptoms are vague or misleading. Pain may be wrongly attributed to other co-existing conditions, such as gallstones, or constipation. The patient may be receiving drugs causing abdominal pain, such as non-steroidal anti-inflammatory compounds. The history may be short, complications occur more frequently and mortality from them is high [2, 4, 25, 33, 36].

Pyloric channel ulcers

Less than 5% of peptic ulcers occur at the pylorus. Some studies indicate that the clinical picture is the same as in duodenal ulcer, but in other reports unusually high incidence of nausea and vomiting (55%–83% versus 10% in duodenal ulcer), atypical pain (33%–79% versus 10%), weight loss (33%–54% versus 9%) have been emphasized. Vomiting may or may not be related to meals or may be nocturnal, or painless. The pain, though epigastric, may be colicky, severe, almost constant, with little or no remission, unrelated to food or worsened by it [14, 29, 35].

Post-bulbar duodenal ulcers

Fewer than 5% of duodenal ulcers are post-bulbar. Their presence raises the possibility of a gastrinoma. Most have the usual pattern of ulcer pain, but if the ulcer penetrates surrounding tissues, the pain is mainly in the right upper quadrant, or in the back. There is an unusually high incidence of haemorrhage (38%) and duodenal obstruction is common (10%) [27].

Giant ulcers

Giant ulcers are rare. Patients with giant duodenal ulcers (larger than 2 cm diameter) usually have an atypical acute illness: severe and intractable pain spread diffusely in the epigastrium and right upper quadrant, unrelated to meals and unrelieved by antacids, vomiting, weight loss and an unusually high incidence of bleeding (86%), pancreatic penetration (71%), or obstruction (36%) are the clinical features. Multiple complications are uncommon in duodenal ulceration, but occur in those with giant lesions. Hypoalbuminaemia can also be present [21]. Patients with giant gastric ulcers may have similar symptoms, but in addition occasionally present with weight loss and the clinical picture may resemble carcinoma of the stomach. However, giant gastric ulcers carry no special risk of malignancy.

Bleeding and obstruction are said to occur more frequently in combined gastric and duodenal ulcers [28].

Complications

About 25% of ulcer patients bleed and 10% perforate at some time during the course of their disease. These complications can also be the first indication of ulcer disease—38% of 513 peptic ulcer patients presenting with bleeding and approximately 33% of 198 patients presenting with perforation, did not have antecedent symptoms of ulcer [6, 22].

Pyloric obstruction

Most patients have an associated duodenal ulcer. Vomiting is a prominent symptom. The pattern varies—frequent but of small volume and containing recently eaten food, the more classic voluminous vomits which contain old food, or nocturnal vomiting only—in some it is absent [7].

The differential diagnosis of the symptoms of ulcer disease

The range of conditions

Only some 25% of patients referred to gastrointestinal units with a suspected peptic ulceration have this diagnosis confirmed on investigation. Most of the remainder will be diagnosed as suffering from functional alimentary disorders, such as the irritable bowel syndrome. Oesophagitis, gastro-oesophageal reflux, gallstones are the next most numerous group, followed by gastric cancer and a wide range of conditions affecting the gut [10, 13, 18, 19, 30, 32, 34]. It follows that functional disease of the gut can closely resemble ulcer disease.

There are several problems in making the diagnosis. First, several conditions produce upper gastrointestinal symptoms, but as the variety of symptoms is limited, there is inevitably a similarity in their clinical picture. Second, two (or more) conditions may co-exist of which one causes the symptoms or

both cause symptoms, either simultaneously or at different times. Third, in most
instances, there are no physical signs except
for the location of pain.

A correct clinical diagnosis is commonly
made in less than half the patients presenting with upper gastrointestinal symptoms,
but when a more detailed history is taken,
the accuracy rises [5, 11, 12]. The reasons
for the poor performance include:

1. The symptoms traditionally recorded,
though interesting, may not have much
value in distinguishing one disease from another, for example nausea.

2. The questions may not elicit the important attributes of the symptoms. For example, questions concerning pain in the
evening, or at night, should elicit the
information whether the pain actually
wakes the patient from sleep.

3. The questions may be insufficient in detail—for example, was the night pain relieved by antacids, or a milky drink?

4. The answer may be vague, or it may be
wrongly assessed, for example the episodes
of pain lasted for two weeks and not just
for the 2–3 days of severe pain, of which
the patient complains.

5. Some features have great discriminant
value, but only when present, for example
jaundice.

6. All the features in the history are not
considered.

For further details concerning the discriminant value of symptoms see Chapter 3.

It must be clearly understood that a definite diagnosis of all those conditions affecting the upper alimentary tract that can be
subsumed under the label 'acid/pepsin disease' and which include duodenal and gastric ulceration, cannot be made without
investigation—preferably by endoscopy, or
by double contrast radiology (see Chapter
16). However, the need for investigation
does not exempt the clinician from taking
an accurate history and doing a careful and
thorough physical examination of the

patient. It is an essential preliminary to ar-
ranging the tests in such a way that a definite diagnosis is reached with the least in-
convenience to the patient and lowest
expenditure of time and money. It need
hardly be said that in areas where investigations are not readily available and if
the doctor wishes to try a period of treatment before referring the patient for tests,
the careful clinical appraisal is paramount.

References

1 BOCKUS HL. Diagnosis of peptic ulcer. In: Bockus HL, ed. *Gastroenterology*. 3rd ed. Philadelphia, London, Toronto: W. B. Saunders Company, 1974.

2 COLIN-JONES DG. Problems of peptic ulceration in the elderly. *Postgrad Med J* [Suppl 5] 1975;51:41–45.

3 CREAN GP, CARD WI, BEATTIE AD, *et al.* 'Ulcer-like dyspepsia'. *Scand J Gastroenterol* 1982;17:Suppl 79; 9–15.

4 CUTLER CW. Clinical patterns of peptic ulcer after sixty. *Surg Gynec Obs* 1958;107:23–30.

5 DE DOMBAL FT. Analysis of foregut symptoms. In: Baron JH, Moody FG, eds. *Gastroenterology: Foregut, Vol. 1.* London, Boston, Sydney, Wellington, Durban, Toronto: Butterworths, 1981.

6 DE DOMBAL FT. Surgery for acute abdominal pain. 1982 OMGE progress report. *Scand J Gastroenterol* 1984;19: Suppl 95:28–40.

7 DWORKEN HJ, ROTH HP. Pyloric obstruction associated with peptic ulcer. *JAMA* 1962;180:1007–1010.

8 EARLAM R. A computerised questionnaire analysis of duodenal ulcer symptoms. *Gastroenterology* 1976;71:314–317.

9 EARLAM R. On the origins of duodenal ulcer pain. *Lancet* 1985;i:973–974.

10 EDWARDS FC, COGHILL NF. Clinical manifestations in patients with chronic atrophic gastritis, gastric ulcer, and duodenal ulcer. *Q J Med* 1968; New series 37:337–360.

11 FOX J, BARBER D, BARDHAN KD. Effects of on-line symptom-processing on history-taking and diagnosis—a simulation study. *Int J Biomed Comput* 1979;10:151–163.

12 FOX J, BARBER D, BARDHAN KD. Alternative to Bayes? A quantitative comparison with rate-based diagnostic inference. *Methods Inf Med* 1980;19:210–215.

13 GEAR MWL, ORMISTON MC, BARNES RJ, ROCYN-JONES J, VOSS GC. Endoscopic studies of dyspepsia in the community: an 'open-access' service. *Br Med J* 1980;ii:1135.

14 GLICKMAN MG, SZEMES G, LOEB P, MARGULIS AR.

Peptic ulcer of the pyloric region. *Am J Roentgenol Radium Ther Nucl Med* 1971;**113**:147–158.

15 GOLDBERG HM. Duodenal ulcers in children. *Br Med J* 1957;**i**:1500–1502.

16 GROSSMAN MI. *Peptic ulcer: A guide for the practicing physician.* Chicago, London: Year Book Medical Publishers, 1981.

17 HALL WH, READ RC, MESARD L, LEE LE, ROBINETTE CD. The calendar and duodenal ulcer. *Gastroenterology* 1972;**62**:1120–1124.

18 HOLDSTOCK G, WISEMAN M, LOEHRY CA. Open-access endoscopy service for general practitioners. *Br Med J* 1979;**1**:457–459.

19 HORROCKS JC, DE DOMBAL FT. Clinical presentation of patients with 'dyspepsia'. *Gut* 1978;**19**:19–26.

20 KURATA JH, HAILE BM, ELASHOFF JD. Sex differences in peptic ulcer disease. *Gastroenterology* 1985;**88**:96–100.

21 MISTILIS SP, WIOT JF, NEDELMAN SH. Giant duodenal ulcer. *Ann Intern Med* 1963;**59**:155–164.

22 MORGAN AG, CLAMP S. OMGE International upper gastro-intestinal bleeding survey 1978–1982. *Scand J Gastroenterol* 1984;**19**: Supplement 95; 41–58.

23 NORD KS, LEBENTHAL E. Peptic ulcer in children. *Am J Gastroenterol* 1980;**73**:75–80.

24 NORD KS, ROSSI TM, LEBENTHAL E. Peptic ulcer in children. *Am J Gastroenterol* 1981;**75**:153–157.

25 PERMUTT RP, CELLO JP. Duodenal ulcer disease in the hospitalised elderly patient. *Dig Dis Sci* 1982;**27**:1–6.

26 PRIEBE WM, DA COSTA LR, BECK IT. Is epigastric tenderness a sign of peptic ulcer disease? *Gastroenterology* 1982;**82**:16–19.

27 RAMSDELL JA, BARTHOLOMEW LG, CAIN JC, DAVIS GD. Postbulbar duodenal ulcer. *Ann Intern Med* 1957;**47**:700–710.

28 RICHARDSON CT. Gastric ulcer. In: Sleisenger MH, Fordtran JS, eds. *Gastrointestinal disease.* Philadelphia, London, Toronto: WB Saunders Company, 1978.

29 RUFFIN JM, JOHNSTON DH, CARTER DD, BAYLIN GJ. Clinical picture of pyloric channel ulcer. *JAMA* 1955;**159**:668–671.

30 SAUNDERS JHB, OLIVER RJ, HIGSON DL. Dyspepsia: incidence of non-ulcer disease in a controlled trial of ranitidine in general practice. *Br Med J* 1986;**292**:665–669.

31 SEAGRAM CGF, STEPHENS CA, CUMMING WA. Peptic ulceration at the Hospital for Sick Children, Toronto, during the 20 year period 1949–1969. *J Pediatr Surg* 1973;**8**:407–413.

32 SJUDIN I, SVEDLUND J, DOTEVALL G, GILLBERG R. Symptom profiles in chronic peptic ulcer disease. A detailed study of abdominal and mental symptoms. *Scand J Gastroenterol* 1985;**20**:419–427.

33 STAFFORD CE, JOERGENSON EJ, MURRAY GC. Complications of peptic ulcer in the aged. *California Medicine* 1956;**84**:92–94.

34 TALLEY NJ, PIPER DW. The association between non-ulcer dyspepsia and other gastrointestinal disorders. *Scand J Gastroenterol* 1985;**20**:896–900.

35 TEXTER EC, SMITH HW, BUNDESEN WE, BARBORKA CJ. The syndrome pylorique. *Gastroenterology* 1959;**36**:573–579.

36 WHORWELL PJ, CLOUTER C, SMITH CL. Oesophageal motility in the irritable bowel syndrome. *Br Med J* 1981;**282**:1101–1102.

Chapter 22
Medical Treatment of Peptic Ulcer

D.G. COLIN-JONES

There are many causes for upper abdominal pain that may mimic peptic disease. Before embarking on any specific treatment for peptic ulceration it is important to confirm the diagnosis, with either a double-contrast barium meal or endoscopy. This is particularly important when long-term maintenance treatment or surgery are being considered. With gastric ulceration there is an appreciable incidence of unexpected malignancy, which in the United Kingdom is approximately 6–10% of ulcers examined. This emphasizes the need to investigate first.

The natural history of a patient's ulcer

Any medical treatment should be given with the knowledge of the natural history of the ulcer diathesis, with its tendency to spontaneous relapse and healing, and the variability of symptoms. In general practice, Fry [50] found that 16% of his patients had surgical treatment for ulcer because of symptoms, 23% because of complications, while most patients (61%) were treated medically with symptomatic relief in many. He postulated that symptoms reached a peak about 10 years after the ulcer started, and then gradually subsided. This view is supported by a Scandinavian study [58], which reviewed 154 duodenal ulcer (DU) patients diagnosed 13 years previously. Thirty-seven per cent had been treated medically and had virtually no symptoms, 29% had only mild symptoms, while 12% had severe symptoms and 22% had surgery. Thus nearly two-thirds of Scandinavian patients had little trouble from their peptic ulcer 13 years after diagnosis. Another review of over 300 patients [81] produced similar data, with the severity of ulcer symptoms reaching a plateau after about 15 years. The reasonable hope that a patient will have long periods of remission, and possibly that the ulcer disease will tend to burn itself out rather than increase in severity, forms an important basis for medical treatment.

It is often difficult to predict the future course of the ulcer in individual patients (Table 22.1). An interesting study by Massarrat and Eisenmann [110] has given some information on this point. These workers treated DU patients with low dose antacids and analysed a large number of clinical, endoscopic and secretory factors. Four factors were considered to be adverse—long duration of the present ulcer pain, smoking, stenosis of the duodenal bulb, and a high peak acid output. If only one of these was present, the spontaneous healing rate was 80%; this fell to 28% in the presence of three adverse factors. These observations have been supported by other work, which suggests that smoking is an important adverse factor that will materially influence the response to medical treatment [80, 138]. The prognosis in patients whose ulcers healed with low dose antacids seemed to be very good, since in the experience of Frederiksen, et al. [48] 61% had two recurrences or fewer over a two year observation period. By the same token, a DU which took longer to heal than

288

Table 22.1. Adverse factors for duodenal ulcer healing.

Symptoms	Frequent relapses
	Prolonged severe pain in last attack
Complications	Previous haemorrhage or perforation
	Stenosis
Endoscopy	Deep and large DU
	Stenosis of the duodenal bulb
	Associated very severe duodenitis
Strong family history	
Smoking	
Long history, young when symptoms began	
High peak acid output	

average tended to run a more refractory course [5].

Much can be learned about the natural history of ulcer disease from the patients who were given a placebo while taking part in controlled trials of ulcer treatments. From these studies it soon became clear that there was a wide variation in the spontaneous healing rate of ulcers in different countries, with the United Kingdom having a low spontaneous healing rate of about 25–30%, while a high spontaneous healing rate was recorded in the United States (Fig. 22.6) and Switzerland [118]. Various explanations have been offered. The self-administration of antacids is probably important (a common practice in the United States), but so too is delay in seeking and obtaining medical help, which might select ulcers that are slow to heal.

General management

Reduction of adverse factors

Non-steroidal anti-inflammatory drugs

It is well known that non-steroidal anti-inflammatory drugs (NSAIDs) damage the gastric mucosa producing inflammation, erosions and ulcers [29]. About 25% of dyspeptic patients on NSAIDs do not have an ulcer when investigated— they only need symptomatic measures. Clearly NSAIDs

should be avoided by any patient who has an ulcer. However, this poses real problems in the management of rheumatoid arthritis, for which they are so useful. Buffered or slow-release preparations have been developed with the aim of decreasing the irritant effect, but with only limited success. Some patients need continuous anti-ulcer treatment in the hope of diminishing the damaging effect of NSAIDs on the gastric and duodenal mucosa. NSAIDs have recently been shown substantially to increase the risk of haemorrhage from peptic ulceration [135]. The risk is highest in the elderly, who consume increasing quantities of these drugs [149].

Smoking

Smoking is strongly associated with peptic ulceration, with a poorer prognosis for spontaneous healing [110, 137] and a worse response to medical treatment [60, 80]. So should we advise our patients to stop smoking? An endoscopic survey has shown that the association between peptic ulceration and smoking is lost when ex-smokers are compared with smokers [2], which suggests that giving smoking up is beneficial. On the other hand, the relapse rate of gastric ulcer (GU) was not diminished by stopping smoking in one study [123]. It has been suggested that smoking diminishes the overnight acid-inhibiting effect of H_2-antagonists [18]. This is a most interesting hypothesis, but it has not been confirmed [38].

Alcohol

Not only is ingested alcohol a stimulus to acid secretion, but it is also a gastric irritant. However, the importance of these actions in the development and the treatment of peptic ulcers is uncertain—indeed a moderate intake of alcohol was found to be an advantage by one group [137]. Most gastroenterologists advise avoidance of excessive spirits, while allowing a moderate intake of other alcoholic drinks.

Bed rest

For many years physicians advised bed rest in order to relieve symptoms and heal the ulcer. This has been subjected to only one clinical trial in GU [40], and an advantage was gained with rest and consumption of milk and alkali. However, with modern drug treatment there is no additional benefit from hospitalization [44].

Diet

For many years a bland diet was routinely advised for ulcer patients, with small fre-

quent meals of soft consistency and bland taste. So established did these regimens become, that many patients still expect to receive dietary advice in great detail. There is no evidence to support the use of these so-called 'gastric diets'. The most important influence on intragastric pH is the buffering effect of the food and this is smaller with a milk diet, than with normal meals. When a 'gastric diet' was compared with a normal and with a convalescent diet (halfway between the entirely bland and the normal), no difference was found in 24-hour intragastric acidity (Fig. 22.1). The scientific basis for using these diets, therefore, does not exist.

At the other end of the dietary spectrum it is thought that a high fibre diet may be beneficial [104]—in India the frequency of duodenal ulcers in a population eating food requiring much chewing, is lower than in an area where the diet needs much less chewing. This study suggested that the chewing produced a good flow of saliva, postulating that salivary mucus acts as a buffer for intragastric acidity. Malhotra then went on to compare duodenal ulcer patients put onto an uncooked high fibre diet, or a cooked rice diet [104]. Over a five-year period the patients on the rice diet experienced a relapse rate of 81%, compared with a 14% relapse rate in those on

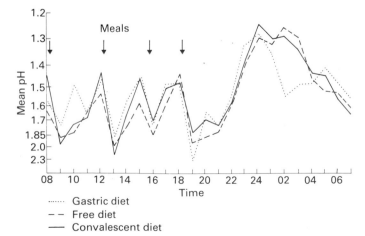

Fig. 22.1. Mean acidity of gastric contents in 12 DU patients on three separate days when each took one of the three diets. The acidity of the gastric contents was not altered by the type of diet taken [94].

the unrefined wheat diet. Rydning, Berstad, Aadland, *et al.* [131] randomly allocated their patients after ulcer healing to either a high or a low fibre diet; 80% relapsed on the low fibre, and 45% on the high fibre diet—this was significantly different. The study, however, can be interpreted by stating that a low fibre diet increased the relapse rate, rather than that a high fibre diet decreased it. The effect of different diets on intragastric acidity has been studied in some detail [94, 103]. However, some foods appear to confer protection against experimental ulcers by a method other than buffering of gastric acid [39] with certain foods containing a lipid-soluble protective agent [67, 74]. This is a most interesting area, which requires further study. At present it would seem sensible to advise patients to eat a normal diet, with a good roughage content, to avoid foods which they find upset them, and to take three balanced meals each day.

Clinical trials

Placebo-controlled trials monitored with endoscopy have shown that symptoms do not always correlate with ulcer activity, so that relief of pain and, particularly in the case of duodenal ulcer, radiological control, are inadequate for an accurate assessment of the efficacy of a particular drug. It is also important to ensure that the groups compared are similar in terms of age, duration of symptoms, smoking habits etc. Peterson and Elashoff [119] have shown that very large numbers are necessary in each treatment group if small differences are expected between the efficacy of the treatments under investigation. For example, if there is a chance of a 10% difference between two treatments, 375 patients would be needed in each arm of the trial to demonstrate it. One way to recruit such numbers is to involve many centres, but this poses its own problems because of differing populations and standards of practice. Results of controlled trials therefore are vital, but they should be treated as guidelines to the best treatment. Other factors, such as unwanted effects, cost, acceptability, or speed of symptom relief also need to be considered before making a decision on which drug to use.

Drug treatment

As discussed in Chapter 20, the rational basis for treatment is the attempt to restore equilibrium between the aggressive action of acid pepsin and perhaps bile, and the defensive mechanisms of the mucosa. Although acid output is stimulated physiologically by eating, because of the buffering effect of food the pH of the stomach is at its lowest, not after eating, but during the night and shortly before meals (Fig. 22.1). The DU patient's acid secretion differs most from the normal overnight, as spontaneous basal secretion falls to very low levels in the normal person in the sleeping hours—an effect that is much less pronounced in the DU patient [41].

Antacids

Antacids have been the mainstay of ulcer therapy and have been used to relieve the symptoms for many centuries. A recent review of studies comparing different antacids with placebo showed that in less than half the studies was antacid significantly better than placebo, and that there was poor correlation between relief of symptoms and the dose of antacid used [73]. Thus, although antacids are firmly established in the patient's (and the doctor's) mind as giving symptom relief, they have only a limited capacity to do so. Many patients testify to the very temporary relief of ulcer pain by antacids. Further critical assessment of antacids compares the neutralizing capacity of the various available products. A review of some antacids available in North America showed that the neutralizing capacity varied from 4.2 to 70.4 mmol H^+/10 ml of antacid; most antacids were in the range 22 to 28 mmol [47].

In addition to this variability in neutralizing capacity, other differences must be considered. For example, the sodium content of many antacids is high—Mist. Mag. Trisil. B.P.C. has Na^+ 6.3 mmol/10 ml, whereas Maalox has only 0.1 mmol/10ml. The buffering capacity is not the only consideration—aluminium salts will bind bile salts, thereby decreasing their irritant properties to the gastric epithelium which might be important. Finally, recent studies suggest that aluminium salts increase prostaglandin production in the gastroduodenal mucosa.

Ulcer healing

Although antacids may not be of striking value in the relief of ulcer symptoms, controlled clinical trials do point to their effectiveness in healing ulcers. However, the dose of antacid required is high, with frequent administration usually one and three hours after a meal, and has varied from 200 to 1008 mmol per 24 hours [65]. With these regimens healing rates comparable to those with cimetidine have been obtained. The rationale for their use is shown by 24-hour studies, using doses of antacid during the day (Fig. 22.2). The effect on the intragastric acidity was very similar to that produced by cimetidine, except during the night. A high dose regimen tends to produce unwanted effects, such as diarrhoea in 30% of patients [120], and requires a high degree of patient compliance because of the volume of medication which needs to be carried about during the day, and the sheer feat of memory that is required. More recently a trial from India showed that healing of DUs reached 85% with 207 mmol/day antacid, while healing rates were 46% with 103.5 mmol/day and 88% with 414 mmol/day [82]. Thus a moderate dose of antacid taken six times during the day can heal DU without appreciable side-effects. There is less information available regarding antacids in gastric ulcer. A large study [44] investigated healing rates in 206 patients given cimetidine and antacid (Mylanta), cimetidine and dummy antacid, or dummy cimetidine and Mylanta. There was a slight, but not significant advantage for cimetidine and antacid and benefits were similar in the three groups.

Antacids have been used in combination

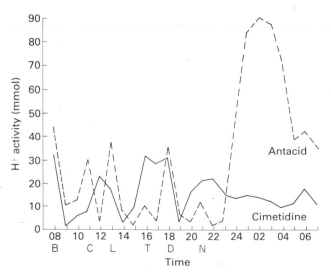

Fig. 22.2. Intragastric H^+ activity in 24 h in six patients given antacid 30 ml after each meal (B = breakfast; L = lunch; D = dinner), or cimetidine 200 mg three times daily and 400 mg at night (N) [113]. C = coffee; T = tea.

with other treatments, such as cimetidine or trimipramine— healing rates were 86–100%. They have also been used in combination with the anticholinergic hyoscyamine [140]. After six weeks placebo had healed 33%, cimetidine 83% and antacid plus hyoscyamine 96%. There is therefore quite a good case for the use of antacids, either alone in high dosage, or in lower doses, but in combination with another treatment that inhibits secretion of acid.

Antacids (Maalox, 3 tablets twice daily) have been reported to be as effective as cimetidine 400 mg at night in the prevention of DU relapse; Maalox 3 tablets daily was ineffective [6].

Unwanted effects of antacids

The most common side-effects are diarrhoea, common with magnesium salts, or constipation with aluminium salts.

Calcium-containing antacids

The use of calcium antacids has substantially diminished in recent years, because it is thought that they produce a rebound of acid secretion. This is because following a rise in gastric pH, calcium stimulates the release of gastrin from the antral G cells. Calcium is also an aggravating factor in the rare milk-alkali syndrome, which may follow prolonged ingestion of large amounts of antacids, especially with milk, leading to hypercalcaemia, hypercalcuria and eventually nephrocalcinosis with renal failure. The ingested alkali causes an alkaline urine, which tends to precipitate calcium phosphate within the kidney, resulting in renal damage. Potassium loss is also increased. Treatment should be prompt, stopping milk and antacids and rehydrating vigorously. Recovery is variable, but always limited once nephrocalcinosis has developed. Fortunately nowadays this syndrome is uncommon.

Aluminium-containing antacids

Aluminium combines with phosphate in the intestine decreasing its absorption and may therefore cause hypophosphataemia with weakness, anorexia and tiredness. Increased calcium loss through the kidney may also result, leading to osteomalacia.

Sodium and fluid retention

This may occur as a result of inadvertent administration of sodium-containing antacids to patients in developed, or incipient cardiac failure. With a high sodium-containing antacid such as liquid Gaviscon (6.3 mmol in 10 ml), oedema, hypertension and heart failure may be a problem.

Interference with drug absorption

Antacids influence the absorption of other drugs either by adsorption, particularly onto the aluminium moiety of the antacid, or by raising the intragastric pH. Absorption of tetracycline and digoxin is decreased. Absorption of cimetidine and ranitidine is decreased by about one-third with the use of Mylanta—a mixture of aluminium and magnesium hydroxide [112].

Histamine H_2-receptor antagonists

These drugs have revolutionized the medical management of peptic ulcer. For many years histamine has been known to be a powerful stimulant of gastric acid secretion, yet this effect is not blocked by conventional antihistamines. This led Black and his colleagues to develop the concept of a second histamine receptor (H_2) which was found chiefly in the gastric mucosa [14]. They were able to demonstrate H_2-receptors, initially using burimamide, and later the more potent and specific competitive antagonist, metiamide. Their investigations demonstrated that H_2-receptors were

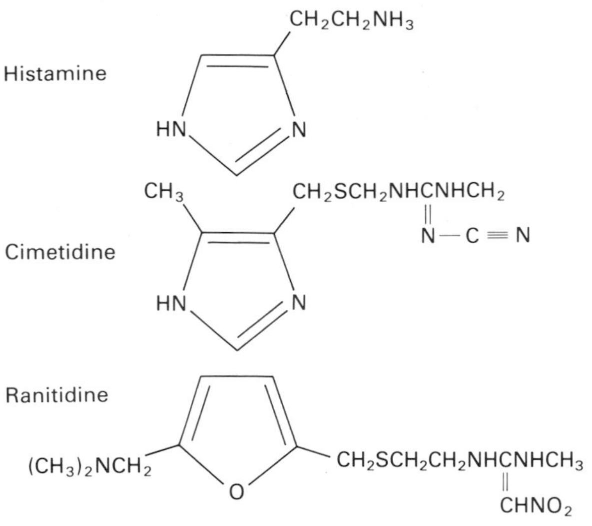

Histamine

$CH_2CH_2NH_3$

Cimetidine

CH_3 $CH_2SCH_2NHCNHCH_2$
                                    $\|$
                            $N-C\equiv N$

Ranitidine

$(CH_3)_2NCH_2$ $CH_2SCH_2CH_2NHCNHCH_3$
                                    $\|$
                            $CHNO_2$

Fig. 22.3. Structures of histamine, cimetidine and ranitidine.

also located in other parts of the body, notably in the atrium of the heart, the blood vessels and the uterus. Nonetheless, the main effect of these drugs in humans is powerful inhibition of gastric secretion. Histamine is a messenger involved in the final pathway leading to stimulation of gastric secretion by the parietal cell, so that H_2-receptor antagonists inhibit acid secretion in response not only to histamine, but also to vagal stimulation and food.

Metiamide was the first potent H_2-antagonist given to patients. It contained a thiourea group on the side chain which was responsible for the occurrence of reversible marrow depression and neutropenia in nearly 1% of patients treated with this drug. It has therefore been withdrawn. Its successor, cimetidine, contains a cyanoguanidine group instead of the thiourea (Fig. 22.3). Patients who had marrow depression with metiamide have subsequently recovered while treated with cimetidine. A few instances of marrow depression with cimetidine have been reported, but these are extremely rare.

The next available H_2-antagonist was ranitidine which differed from its predecessors in having a furan, instead of the imidazole ring. Further drugs in this class have

been developed and are being evaluated at present.

H_2-antagonists are a most effective group of compounds substantially inhibiting acid secretion, enabling most ulcers to heal [126, 144].

Cimetidine

Cimetidine is well absorbed from the gastrointestinal tract and is excreted largely unchanged in the urine. Its half-life is of the order of 110 minutes. Initially it was therefore recommended that it should be given with each meal, 200 mg three times a day and 400 mg at night, in order to obtain good control of gastric acidity (Fig. 22.4). However, later trials [79] have shown that cimetidine is as effective in a dose of 400 mg twice daily. The evening dose is effective in inhibiting nocturnal gastric secretion and more recently 800 mg nightly has been shown to be as effective as the more conventional 400 mg twice daily [25].

Efficacy—short-term healing

Many double-blind, controlled trials of cimetidine and placebo in DU have now been done. The end-point in all these trials is

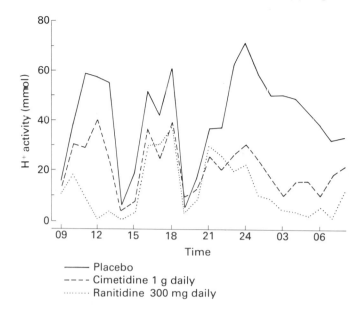

Placebo
- - - - Cimetidine 1 g daily
.... Ranitidine 300 mg daily

Fig. 22.4. Intragastric H+ activity during 24 h in 10 DU patients given either cimetidine (1 g/day) or ranitidine (150 mg twice daily) [150].

endoscopically confirmed healing of the DU. Wormsley [154] reviewed 46 trials, which gave an average healing rate of 73% on cimetidine compared with 42% on placebo, after four to six weeks of treatment. The evidence is overwhelming that cimetidine is highly effective for healing ulcers in the short term. Prolonged treatment will increase the number of ulcers healed, up to as much as 90% after three months [98]. In gastric ulcer (GU) the results are similar [31], with about 75% healing on cimetidine—better than placebo [56].

Relapse rate

Unfortunately, the relapse rate is high, highest in the first six months, with most recurrences occurring during the first three months. The figures vary from country to country, but about two-thirds of the patients appear to relapse in six months, and about 80% in a year. Controlled trials have shown that about 15–30% of ulcers relapse asymptomatically, the patients being unaware that their ulcer has recurred [4]. Is it possible to decrease the incidence of recurrence by prolonging treatment? Gudmand-Hoyer, *et al.* [59] and Bardhan [7], have shown that there is no difference in the relapse rate when the drug is stopped, irrespective of whether the treatment was given for one, three, six months, or a year. It would appear then, that cimetidine has made no difference to the natural history of the disease. However, preliminary results from a large maintenance trial over three years suggests that DUs that do not relapse during two years on cimetidine 400 mg at night have a lower relapse rate in the third year, when changed to placebo [148]. Prolonged maintenance, can, therefore, be used to select the patient with a less severe course for his DU. Of some interest is the finding from placebo-controlled trials that ulcers that healed on placebo have a lower relapse rate when subsequently receiving placebo as maintenance therapy [24], again presumably reflecting a benign type of DU which tends to heal spontaneously.

Maintenance

Intragastric acidity is greatest in the early hours of the morning. All H_2-antagonists inhibit nocturnal secretion (Fig. 22.4) and thus a night-time maintenance dose to keep the ulcer healed seems sensible. Cimetidine 400 mg at night is effective, and the relapse rate of DU during one year declines to about 25%, as long as treatment is taken; relapse rate on placebo is about 75% (Fig. 22.5). Maintenance treatment is therefore a very useful means of keeping the patient free of symptoms and of diminishing the potential risk of complications from the ulcer (Table 22.2).

Maintenance treatment may raise difficult problems of patient management, however. Questions such as: 'How long?', 'What dose?', 'Should ulcer healing be checked by regular endoscopy?', 'How should patients be selected for maintenance therapy?', 'Is it safe?', need to be considered and answered.

The optimal dose for cimetidine maintenance therapy appears to be 400 mg at night; there is little advantage in increasing the dose to 800 mg (Fig. 22.5). Relapse rates vary from centre to centre, but the dose can be increased to 400 mg twice daily (or 800 mg at night) if relapse occurs whilst on maintenance therapy [124]. Repeated endoscopy is probably not justified in DU. It is an invasive investigation, which cannot ensure that the DU will remain healed, even if it is at the time of the examination. Symptoms are not always correlated with ulcer recurrence, as about 15% of recurrences are silent. Nonetheless, symptomatic assessment seems to be the most practical way of managing the patients on maintenance therapy, once the initial diagnosis has been established by endoscopy. Length of treatment and selection of patients will be discussed later under general management.

For GU there is much less information on maintenance therapy than there is for DU, but cimetidine can lower the relapse rate (Table 22.3). Since the recurrence rate of GU is about 50% over two years [61], there is a real need for an effective maintenance

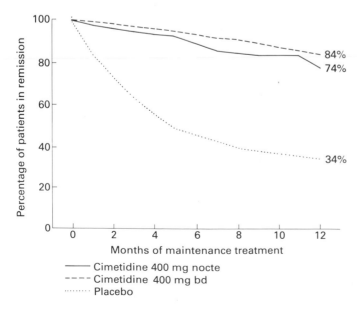

Fig. 22.5. Percentage of patients in clinical remission during treatment with cimetidine 400 mg twice daily (n = 184); cimetidine 400 mg nocte (n = 179), or placebo (n = 333) [23].

Table 22.2. Results of selected long-term trials of maintenance treatment with cimetidine.

| | No. of patients | | | | Relapse rate | | | |
| | | | | | Cimetidine | | Placebo | |
Reference	Cimetidine	Placebo	Cimetidine dosage	Duration of treatment	with symptoms %	without symptoms %	with symptoms %	without symptoms %
[8]	29	31	400 mg × 2	6 months	14	7	58	10
[10]	23	24	400 mg at night	12 months	9	0	58	8
[15]	21	24	800 mg at night	6 months	14	10	50	38
[16]	19	23	400 mg × 2	12 months	16	0	61	17
[57]	26	30	400 mg at night	6 months	27	0	80	0
[62]	20	20	400 mg × 2	12 months	5	0	80	20

therapy [100]. There is much more justification for serial endoscopy with multiple biopsy and exfoliative brush cytology in the follow-up of GU, because of the risk of missing a malignant ulcer, or early gastric cancer [87].

Resistant ulcers

There are a number of ulcers that do not heal on cimetidine—in the trials 10–25%. The reasons for this are not clear [125]. Non-compliance is a possibility and most likely to be important in patients asked to take treatment for a prolonged period [19]. Symptomatic ulcers tend to be associated with non-compliance, while compliant patients tend to get asymptomatic recurrences. Compliance has not been much studied, but plays only a small part in the re-

sistant ulcer. It is possible that some ulcers simply heal at a slower rate—this is difficult to investigate. Another suggestion has been that there is failure to absorb the drug. Gledhill, *et al.* [54] have shown that the serum concentrations after a dose of cimetidine are much as expected, both in those who heal swiftly and in those who do not. The same workers found that the inhibition of overnight acid secretion was much greater in the responders than in the non-responders, and that this was independent of concentrations of cimetidine in the blood. They postulated a reduced sensitivity of the parietal cell to cimetidine, but the mechanism is unknown. A further idea has been that inhibition of pepsin secretion is variable. Pepsin secretion is decreased somewhat less than acid by H_2-antagonists, but Cargill, *et al.* [28] could find no correlation be-

Table 22.3. Results of maintenance trials of cimetidine in gastric ulceration.

| Author | No. patients | Duration of treatment | Daily dosage | Percentage remaining healed | | Significance |
				Cimetidine	Placebo	
[13]	19	12 months	800 mg	100	44	$P < 0.025$
[101]	24	11 months	1000 mg	82	14	$P < 0.002$
[78]	31	12 months	800 mg	100	56	$P < 0.02$

tween relapse and pepsin concentrations. Switching treatment from an acid-inhibiting to a different drug may be useful. Thus 10 of 13 patients in whom the DU did not heal after cimetidine 1 g for four weeks, healed on tripotassium dicitrato bismuthate [84, 125].

Adverse effects

The adverse effects of cimetidine can be grouped into those related to the drug itself, and those related to blockade of histamine H_2-receptors (Table 22.4).

The most important group of unwanted effects are those resulting from the **altered metabolism of other drugs** which also use the hepatic cytochrome P450 enzyme system. Since cimetidine is partially metabolized by the P450 enzyme system, there is competition between drugs at this enzyme site, and therefore prolongation of their action. The most important of these

Table 22.4. Adverse effects of cimetidine.

Related to its action
  Diarrhoea (possible bacterial colonization of small bowel)
  Possible increase in gastric nitrosamine formation (theoretical risk of gastric cancer in the long term)
Related to its metabolism
  Anti-androgenic effects
    Impotence
    Gynaecomastia
  Elevation of liver enzymes
    Hepatitis (rare)
  Interstitial nephritis (rare)
  Confusion in very sick or elderly
  Neutropenia (rare)
  Arthralgia
  Interference with metabolism of other drugs, notably warfarin, diazepam, propranolol, phenytoin, theophylline, chlormethiazole
  Pancreatitis (rare)
Unlikely to be clinically significant
  Elevation of serum creatinine
  Alteration of immune responsiveness
  Possibility of bradycardia
  Skin rash (usually transient)

interactions are with warfarin, diazepam, phenytoin and propranolol. Other drugs involved are chlordiazepoxide, theophylline, chlormethiazole, and caffeine. These important interactions must be borne in mind when prescribing.

Confusion has been reported in elderly patients suffering from severe liver or renal disease; it is suggested that blood concentrations of cimetidine rise and the drug penetrates the blood-brain barrier where it acts on some unspecified receptor site in the CNS. A smaller dose should avoid this uncommon problem [35].

There is no experimental evidence suggesting **bone marrow toxicity** with cimetidine, but a review [129] collected 25 cases of neutropenia, of which five were likely to be related to cimetidine. Neutropenia, therefore, is a rare complication.

Cimetidine has a weak **anti-androgenic action.** Gynaecomastia seems to occur more commonly in the Zollinger-Ellison syndrome, than in simple peptic ulcer. It is probably mediated by displacement of testosterone from its receptor binding sites in peripheral tissues. Cimetidine has been reported to lower the libido and sperm count, but more recent evidence suggests that there is no effect on the latter [45]. Seven cases of **pancreatitis** in patients treated with cimetidine have been reported in the United Kingdom, two of which recurred on rechallenge [153].

The other group of unwanted effects that may arise from the use of cimetidine stems from its **inhibitory effects on gastric acidity.** Lowered secretion of intrinsic factor occurs with cimetidine and ranitidine, but is unlikely to be clinically important unless very long-term treatment is given [156]. Rebound hypersecretion of acid after stopping treatment does not occur in humans. Of more concern is the postulate put forward by Elder, *et al.* [43], that cimetidine could cause gastric cancer. There are two strands to this hypothesis. Firstly, raising the intragastric pH causes an increase in the number of bacteria in the stomach capable of converting dietary nitrates to nitrites and to nitrosamines, which are carcinogenic. Secondly, cimetidine itself could be nitrosated to the potentially carcinogenic N-nitrosocimetidine. These ideas have been investigated by a number of workers with differing conclusions. However, N-nitrosocimetidine has only been produced in the laboratory, it requires a neutral or alkaline pH for the process to occur, and has not been shown to occur *in vivo* in man. The subject has been discussed by Colin-Jones, *et al.* [34], who concluded that in most patients developing gastric cancer after treatment with cimetidine a diagnosis of a pre-existing cancer was missed. It is difficult to imagine that cimetidine would cause gastric cancer in the short-term treatment of peptic ulcer.

This is, however, an important area, and the need to monitor carefully the effects of long-term therapy remains. The hypothesis that nitrates and nitrites in the diet are converted to nitrosamines by bacteria is based on circumstantial evidence. In the long-term it is possible that elevation of intragastric pH could increase the concentration of carcinogens in the stomach. At present, however, there is not sufficient evidence, although this hypothesis cannot be dismissed. Nonetheless, very long-term treatment with drugs that powerfully inhibit acid secretion should not be given without an adequate clinical reason [90].

Despite these adverse effects of cimetidine, in practice it is a very well-tolerated and remarkably safe drug [99]—some 25 million patients had received it between 1976 and 1982.

Ranitidine

Ranitidine was the second H_2-antagonist to become commercially available [126]. It has a different structure from cimetidine,

being a furan with a different side chain (Fig. 22.3). It is well absorbed from the gastrointestinal tract, with a bioavailability of about 50%. Approximately half the oral dose is excreted unchanged in the urine, with most of the remainder excreted in the faeces. The half-life is 130 minutes. It is a highly effective, specific, competitive H_2-antagonist, some five times more potent than cimetidine on a mol for mol basis [117]. The usual dose advised was 150 mg twice daily, but now 300 mg at night has been found to be equally effective. Ranitidine 150 mg twice a day results in a 69% inhibition of intragastric acidity during 24 hours compared with 49% inhibition using cimetidine 1 g in divided doses (Fig. 22.4) [150].

Healing rates

Assessed against placebo in the short-term treatment of DU, ranitidine 150 mg twice daily (Fig. 22.6), produces a highly significant increase in ulcer healing rate, with 80% healing compared with 31% in the placebo group. Trials comparing ranitidine with cimetidine involving some 1200 patients have been reviewed by Colin-Jones [32] (Fig. 22.7). The healing rate of DU with ranitidine 150 mg twice daily was 76%, and with cimetidine 1 g daily 70%. Despite the problems of comparing results from different units and countries, this advantage in favour of ranitidine is probably significant [77]. Most assessments of ranitidine in the short-term management of DU are based on the 150 mg twice daily regimen. However, a single 300 mg dose of ranitidine given at night results in similar healing rates—96% after four weeks of treatment [72]. Once daily medication is convenient and may improve compliance. As with cimetidine, prolonging treatment with ranitidine increases the DU healing rate.

Ranitidine also increases the healing rate of GU. An open Japanese study [142] assessed the response of more than 400

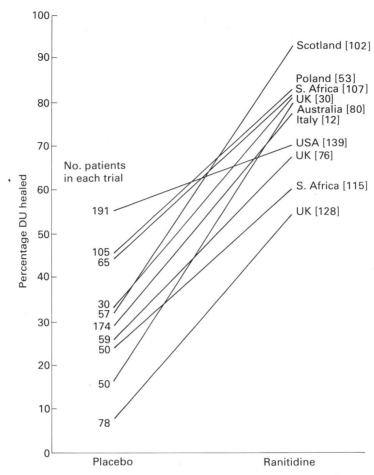

Fig. 22.6. Differences in healing rates of DU on placebo, or ranitidine 150 mg twice daily. Results of ten endoscopically-controlled trials.

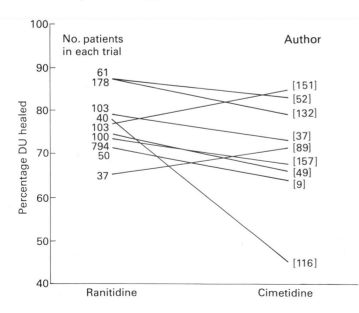

Fig. 22.7. Healing rates of DU on cimetidine 1g in divided doses, or ranitidine 150 mg twice daily. Results of endoscopically-controlled trials.

Table **22.5**. Ranitidine and cimetidine in the acute treatment of gastric ulcers (controlled trials).

	No. patients	Dropped out	Cimetidine in 4	8 weeks	Percentage healed on Ranitidine in 4	8 weeks
Cape Town, South Africa [155]	65	9	57	79	58	91
Belgium [3]	260	63	62	87	66	78
Netherlands [95]	70	8	66	84	63	90

patients treated with ranitidine using endoscopies at two week intervals, measuring acid secretion and ulcer size, thus evaluating a number of factors that might affect healing. The healing rate was unaffected by the site of the GU or by the size of the ulcer, but the large ulcers healed more slowly. Nor did acid secretion affect the healing rate. In a small controlled trial against gefarnate, ranitidine was clearly superior. Other studies from the United Kingdom, Poland, Canada and Norway have all shown ranitidine to be superior to placebo with increased healing rate with longer treatment [130]. Comparisons of ranitidine with cimetidine in GU have shown them to be similarly effective (Table 22.5).

Maintenance treatment

Prevention of recurrence of DU by ranitidine has been reviewed by Boyd, *et al.* [17]. Cumulative data indicate that the annual recurrence rate of healed duodenal ulcers was 31% on ranitidine 150 mg at night, compared with 79% recurrence during a year's treatment with placebo. In the ranitidine group 11% of the relapses were asymptomatic and 20% symptomatic—emphasizing the need for regular check endoscopy in clinical trials, if not in clinical practice. The choice of an H_2-antagonist may be important in determining the outcome of maintenance therapy. In a trial of ranitidine 150 mg, or cimetidine 400 mg given at night to 484 patients with healed DU, the relapse rate was significantly lower in those

receiving ranitidine—8% vs. 21% at four, 14% vs. 34% at eight and 23% vs. 37% at 12 months. Similar results were obtained in another independent trial using an identical protocol [55, 134]. These results, obtained using the recommended maintenance doses of the two H_2-antagonists, may reflect the five-fold greater potency of ranitidine over cimetidine. As with cimetidine, prolonging treatment with ranitidine increases the DU healing rate.

There is less information pertaining to GU. In 150 patients studied the relapse rate during one year's treatment with ranitidine 150 mg at night was 22%—significantly less than the 56% recurrence rate on placebo [17].

Resistant ulcers

Open and uncontrolled studies of patients who have failed to respond to treatment with cimetidine and then have been given ranitidine show a 74% to 94% healing rate after four weeks on ranitidine [22]. Several studies have shown that prolonging treatment with cimetidine or ranitidine beyond the customary four or six weeks to 12 weeks markedly diminishes the number of unhealed ulcers [5]. There is, as yet, no convincing evidence that changing the H_2-antagonist will improve the healing rate [86, 125]. Smoking is an adverse factor [18, 69, 80].

Adverse effects

Ranitidine is remarkably well tolerated, with rare adverse effects. Unlike cimetidine, it does not affect the cytochrome P450 enzyme system, and so has no interactions with other drugs.

It is therefore the best treatment for patients who require concomitant use of anticonvulsants or anticoagulants. Ranitidine has no anti-androgenic activity. Two cases of ranitidine-induced bradycardia have been reported, but it is doubtful whether they are clinically relevant. In clinical trials trivial adverse effects have occurred in less than 5% of patients, of which headache, tiredness, diarrhoea and skin rash are the most common. However, a similar incidence of these symptoms has been recorded in the patients given placebo. There appears to be no adverse effect on the bone marrow, but hepatitis has been reported [62]. Ranitidine cannot be nitrosated so there is no risk of a carcinogenic nitrosoranitidine. However, the same comments apply to all powerful inhibitors of acid secretion. Theoretically there could be long-term risk through alteration of the intragastric environment—a predisposition to gastric cancer could conceivably result. This was discussed under cimetidine above.

Other H₂-receptor antagonists

Numerous other H$_2$-antagonists have been developed and are being evaluated clinically, but the most potent may produce cellular changes with long-term use in the rat [90] and some have been withdrawn.

Other H$_2$-antagonists include famotidine which, in preliminary studies, appears very similar to ranitidine but on a molar basis even more potent [69]. Whether the next group of H$_2$-antagonists will prove to have any advantage will have to be demonstrated, since experience with cimetidine and ranitidine is vast (more than 50 million patients treated).

Carbenoxolone

Carbenoxolone was the first drug to show a significant advantage over placebo in the healing of GU, but its place in the treatment of peptic ulcer is now mainly historical. Carbenoxolone is a synthetic compound derived from glycyrrhizinic acid, which is extracted from liquorice root. It is an interesting compound, claimed to increase the production of gastric mucus thus strengthening the mucosal barrier. It has a minor action in decreasing intragastric peptic activity, but little effect on gastric acid secretion. Studies in GU showed carbenoxolone to be more effective than placebo in most trials, but the percentage of ulcers that healed was low, usually in the 50–60% region [152]. Marketed in a delayed-release capsule as Duogastrone, it was meant to release the carbenoxolone in the gastric antrum and therefore in high concentrations in the antrum and proximal duodenum. Endoscopically controlled trials show that this position-release capsule is significantly more potent than placebo in healing DU, with 60–81% of ulcers healed. Comparative trials of cimetidine and carbenoxolone in GU show a trend in favour of cimetidine, which is not always significant [83, 121].

Adverse effects

Unfortunately carbenoxolone has a mineralocorticoid action, causing sodium and water retention with hypertension, sometimes with resulting peripheral and pulmonary oedema. It also causes hypokalaemia. This is particularly a problem in the elderly, or in patients with renal or cardiopulmonary disease, in whom it is contraindicated. Up to 50% of patients may have symptomatic or biochemical abnormalities on treatment with carbenoxolone. Administration of an aldosterone antagonist, spironolactone, will abolish these unwanted effects, but seems also to diminish its effectiveness in healing GU. These unwanted effects seriously degrade the usefulness of carbenoxolone in treating peptic ulcer disease.

Anticholinergic drugs

Anticholinergic drugs inhibit acid output—basal secretion by 40–50% and food-stimulated secretion by about 30%. Unfortunately, the dose needed for suppression of acid will produce adverse effects. Cholinergic blockade gives rise to blurred vision, dry mouth, difficulty with micturition in men, constipation and delay in gastric emptying. Clinical trials have not given consistent results and most studies were done before endoscopic assessment of ulcer healing became established. A recent assessment suggests that propantheline 120 mg daily, although slower, produces healing similar to cimetidine after eight weeks' treatment—86% with propantheline and 94% with cimetidine [1].

The adverse effects and lack of a clear-cut advantage decreases the usefulness of anticholinergic drugs in peptic ulcer disease.

Pirenzepine

Pirenzepine is a selective anticholinergic that appears to be relatively specific for the muscarinic receptors in the gastric mucosa [46]. It inhibits acid and pepsin secretion by about 50%. It has little effect on gastric emptying and because of its selectivity has fewer unwanted effects than conventional anticholinergic drugs. It has an interesting pharmacological profile, inhibiting insulin-stimulated (through the vagus) pepsin secretion, but not that stimulated by pentagastrin [133]. Pirenzepine has a synergistic action with cimetidine, the latter depressed acid response by 60%, pirenzepine by 58%, but both drugs by 89% [96].

Adverse effects

Although much more selective than the conventional anticholinergic drugs, unwanted effects do occur in some 50% of patients—the commonest is a dry mouth. Most patients reporting a dry mouth did not stop the treatment and at the end of the trial had grown accustomed to this symptom. Adverse effects are therefore minor and can be tolerated, in contrast with other anticholinergics. Experience with pirenzepine has been smaller than with the H_2-antagonists, so the possibility of other adverse effects cannot be entirely excluded.

Efficacy

Clinical trials have shown pirenzepine to be superior to placebo and of similar efficacy to cimetidine. Thus 70–80% of DUs and GUs will heal during four to six weeks of pirenzepine 50 mg twice daily [66, 122, 145]. Maintenance studies are still in an early phase, but suggest broadly similar relapse rates compared with cimetidine—for example, 15% relapse rate over 24 weeks on cimetidine compared with 29% (not significant) on pirenzepine [27, 71].

Treatment with pirenzepine combined with an H_2-antagonist is theoretically attractive, but has been little exploited. However, the combination with cimetidine did appear to diminish the incidence of rebleeding from peptic ulcers on comparison with either drug alone, but did not expedite ulcer healing [96].

Trimipramine

Trimipramine is a tricyclic antidepressant which has anticholinergic effects. It could work centrally through its antidepressant action, or through antisecretory activity, or through another mechanism. The number of trials with this drug is limited and it has chiefly been studied in Scandinavia. About

80% of DUs will heal on trimipramine, but further work is needed [11].

Adverse effects

These include those due to cholinergic blockade—dry mouth and constipation. Drowsiness and lethargy are more prominent.

Tripotassium dicitrato bismuthate (TDB)

Tripotassium dicitrato bismuthate has been available for a number of years as a liquid with a strong ammoniacal smell. It is now also available as tablets that have to be chewed and are more acceptable. TDB may work by chelating with protein and granulation tissue at the base of the ulcer crater to form a protective layer, the reaction occurring at an acid pH. It therefore may prevent peptic digestion at the base of the ulcer. Trials have consistently given favourable results, with up to 86% healing rates reported for DU [147] and GU [141]. Although similar rates of healing are achieved, symptom relief may not be as swift as with H_2-antagonists [108]. Of particular interest is the possibility that the relapse rate may be lower after healing of the ulcer with TDB. Thus in one trial DU recurrence was 85% one year after cimetidine and 39% after TDB [108]. In another trial 120 patients with DU healed 97% of their

DUs after eight weeks treatment with either TDB, or ranitidine, but 12 months afterwards the relapse rate was 89% in those who were treated with ranitidine and 62% in those who had had TDB for eight weeks—a significant difference [93] (Fig. 22.8). This effect of TDB on the relapse rate is most intriguing. The explanation is quite unknown but the recently discovered *Campylobacter pyloridis* which is associated with gastritis [88] is susceptible to bismuth salts—further investigation is clearly needed [33].

Adverse effects

These are minor and include darkening of the stool, and an unpleasant ammoniacal taste which many patients find disagreeable. There is a theoretical risk of bismuth toxicity, but when the drug is used for one or two courses it is unlikely to be a problem, unless there is renal failure [125].

Sucralfate

Sucralfate is an aluminium sulphated sucrose and was thought to work similarly to TDB by binding to the base of the ulcer and protecting from acid and pepsin digestion of the granulation tissue [21]. Additionally it has been shown that sucralfate increases local prostaglandins [33, 68]. As TDB, it has to be taken before meals and is not absorbed. A number of clinical trials point

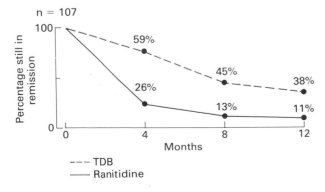

Fig. 22.8. Duodenal ulcer recurrence after ulcer healing with either ranitidine or tripotassium dicitrato bismuthate (TDB) [93].

to its efficacy, with similar rates of healing of DU after four weeks of sucralfate (80%) or cimetidine (76%) [109]. Sixty-three per cent of GUs healed on sucralfate, compared with 75% on cimetidine [106]. The suggestion that the relapse rate of GU after a course of sucralfate is lower than that after cimetidine [105] is not convincing, but further studies are needed.

Liquorice extract (Caved-S)

This is an impure extract of liquorice to which antacid and frangula are added. It is incxpensive and has few side-effects because glycyrrhizinic acid (which has aldosterone-like activity) has been removed. It is claimed that Caved-S acts through a mucosal protecting effect. Initial results with Caved-S were not consistent, but the trend suggests its superiority to placebo. One study shows Caved-S to be as effective as cimetidine in the short-term treatment of GU. It also decreases the relapse rate during one year's maintenance treatment [114].

Adverse effects

Caved-S contains frangula, which may occasionally produce diarrhoea. It is well tolerated, if the patient does not object to the strong taste of liquorice.

Prostaglandins

There is an intense interest in prostaglandins, because of their cytoprotective properties. Prostaglandins may heal ulcers either through inhibition of acid secretion or, in sub-inhibitory doses, through their putative cytoprotective activity. Small doses of synthetic prostaglandins appear to protect the mucosa, inhibit acid secretion and, apart from diarrhoea, to have only minor unwanted effects. Experimentally these substances prevent ulcers in animals, speed the rate of healing of artificially induced ulcers,

and appear to protect the mucosa against non-steroidal anti-inflammatory drugs. In one large multi-centre study, 67% of DUs healed on a synthetic PGE_2 analogue, arbaprostil 100 μg four times daily compared with 39% of DUs healing on placebo [143, 146]. Smoking retarded healing in the placebo, but not in the prostaglandin treated patients, in contrast to experience with H_2-antagonists. Misoprostil and enprostil are the most advanced synthetic prostaglandin analogues and preliminary trials suggest efficacy similar, or slightly inferior to that obtained with H_2-antagonists [91].

Adverse effects

Adverse effects are due to changes in motility or fluid handling by the small intestine, with loose stools and diarrhoea occurring in one-third of the patients, although only a few had to discontinue treatment. Prostaglandins have also been shown to protect the upper gastrointestinal tract in patients taking indomethacin for rheumatic diseases [75]. Their relative importance in anti-ulcer therapy is not clearly established at the time of writing.

Omeprazole

Omeprazole is a substituted benzimidazole that specifically blocks the H^+K^+ATP-ase in the parietal cell. Thus it suppresses acid secretion by direct action on the gastric proton pump. It seems to be remarkably specific. The inhibition of acid secretion lasts more than 72 hours. Complete inhibition of acid secretion may be achieved with doses of 40 mg daily [26, 111]. Omeprazole is susceptible to an acid environment and therefore has to be taken in an enteric-coated form. A preliminary study showed no difference in healing rates of DU in patients treated with omeprazole 20, 30, 40 or 60 mg daily [36]. In a trial involving 132 DU patients, at two weeks 73% of ulcers treated on omeprazole 30 mg daily healed, while 46% healed on cimetidine 1 g daily. After four weeks treatment the healing rate was 92% and 74% respectively. There was no difference in the relapse rate in the two groups during a six month follow-up [92].

Adverse effects

Because of its powerful inhibitory properties with consequent anacidity, omeprazole produces marked hypergastrinaemia. Long-term administration of omeprazole to rats produced marked hyperplasia of enterochromaffin-like cells (ECL cells), with the formation of ECL tumours in the gastric mucosa, especially in the female animals [90, 42]. Antrectomy appears to prevent the hypergastrinaemia and the ECL cell hyperplasia. Because of this, the place of omeprazole in routine clinical practice is at the moment uncertain. It has however, a definite, if limited, usefulness in the management of the hypersecretion in the Zollinger-Ellison syndrome. Multifocal gastric carcinoid tumours are rare, but have been described in patients with pernicious anaemia [64].

Other compounds

In a remarkable trial of **acetazolamide** in Romania, over 2000 patients with gastric ulcer were treated with either acetazolamide, or a placebo. The basal acid output was strikingly decreased, almost to zero, and at the end of one month 98.8% of ulcers had completely healed. In contrast, healing occurred in only 47% of patients on placebo [127]. This drug has also been shown by the same group to heal 91% of over 8400 duodenal ulcers in only two weeks. Such figures are unsurpassed, but the work clearly needs repeating by other units. **Proglumide** is claimed to interact with gastrin and by its antigastrin effects to reduce acid secretion. Trials of this drug are too sparse and too small for a useful opinion to be given of its role in treating ulcers. **Trithiozine** is an anti-secretory compound whose mechanism of action is not known. Nonetheless it inhibits acid secretion, is more effective than placebo, and in studies in Spain and Italy has been shown to be comparable to cimetidine. Further studies are needed. **Gefarnate** is derived from cabbage and has been shown to be inferior to the H_2-antagonists [142]. For a brief period, **hormonal therapy** was tried, using oestrogens, secretin and urogastrone (an extract derived from urine), but all had disadvantages. **Somatostatin** greatly inhibits acid secretion and may be useful in gastrointestinal bleeding, but has to be given parenterally.

Practical management of patients with peptic ulcers

The number and effectiveness of available treatments is almost bewildering. It is therefore important to use these powerful drugs appropriately. Firstly, the diagnosis has to be established with air-contrast barium radiology, or endoscopy. It is particularly important to perform biopsy and cytology in GU in order to detect possible malignancy [87]. It is sensible to check endoscopically on complete healing of the GU at six or eight weeks, to make sure that malignancy has not been missed and also because an ulcer is less likely to recur and cause complications if it is completely epithelialized, rather than just smaller and asymptomatic [123]. Repeat endoscopy to check on healing of DU is unnecessary, because the ulcer may recur at any time and be asymptomatic. Repeat endoscopy in DU becomes necessary if symptoms change, complications occur, or if pain persists despite an adequate period of medical treatment with apparently good compliance.

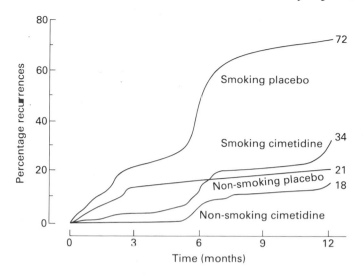

Fig. 22.9. Duodenal ulcer recurrence during maintenance treatment with either cimetidine 400 mg nocte or placebo, related to smoking habit [138].

General management

Patients should stop smoking, as smoking adversely affects the response to treatment with H_2-antagonists and the relapse rate in smokers is probably higher [80, 138] (Fig. 22.9). Salicylates should be avoided and other non-steroidal anti-inflammatory drugs reduced to a minimum and given in a form least likely to irritate the gastric mucosa. Alcohol is not prohibited, but should be taken in moderation and with meals, rather than on an empty stomach.

Diet is a subject dear to the hearts of our patients. Advise the patients to avoid foods which upset them, but to eat a normal balanced diet with small, frequent meals. A good fibre content would also seem desirable. Now that we have powerful drugs, hospitalization, long periods off work and psychiatric assistance are rarely needed.

Principles of treatment

Until diagnosis, antacids provide symptomatic relief. After the diagnosis has been confirmed, definitive treatment should be given. In short-term management the healing rates are remarkably similar with the wide range of available drugs, despite their dissimilar pharmacological attributes. However, the H_2-antagonists have advantages. Firstly, they give swift and reliable symptomatic relief, especially if they are combined with antacids for the first week—the pain usually clears within three to five days. This symptomatic relief is probably swifter than with other treatments. Secondly, they have been assessed in great detail and in many countries, so that much is known of their mode of action and adverse effects. Thirdly, and probably most importantly, maintenance therapy with cimetidine and ranitidine has been far more thoroughly assessed than with any other drugs. A short course of most treatments will heal about 80% of DU, but most ulcers recur within six months. The physician should tailor maintenance therapy to the needs of the individual, finding the best method of keeping the ulcer healed, either by continuous maintenance treatment, or by intermittent short courses of therapy whenever symptoms recur, or (increasingly seldom) by surgery.

Which H_2-antagonist? As cimetidine interacts with some drugs, ranitidine is preferred if the patient is receiving concomitant treatment. Either ranitidine

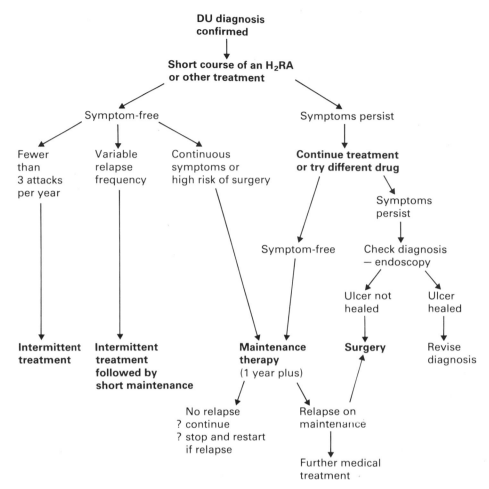

Fig. 22.10. Suggested management of uncomplicated duodenal ulceration.

or cimetidine may be used in most patients as first line treatment, as their healing rates are similar. The greater experience with cimetidine and its lower cost are offset by fewer adverse reactions with ranitidine and probably slightly greater efficacy. The clinician must choose.

Drug management

The patients should be given a four to six week course of the preferred drug. The course should be repeated when symptoms recur, as it is impracticable to endoscope all patients routinely to see if the ulcer remains

healed. There is a suggestion from one very small study that treatment should be given only until symptoms are relieved [85], but this approach is novel and needs further support before being recommended as routine. Patients who still have symptoms may continue on H_2-antagonist for a further six weeks, when fewer than 10% of ulcers will still be present [5]. If the patient is still symptomatic, surgery should be considered (Fig. 22.10) or one of the alternative drugs tried.

After a single course most patients are better—how do we keep them that way? The choice is between continuous maintenance therapy or intermittent treatment with a full dose for four to six weeks when symptoms recur. Maintenance therapy reduces not only the relapse rate but also the risk of complications [20]. Using data from the literature, Sonnenberg [136] has developed a model concluding that maintenance therapy is the most efficacious and safe compared with surgery or intermittent therapy. But not every ulcer patient needs continuous therapy. Thus medical practice ranges from a brief course for each symptomatic relapse to life-long maintenance with an H_2-antagonist to diminish the risk of complications. The management should be tailored to the individual patient.

Table 22.1 sets out factors that carry a poor prognosis and so point to the need for surgery or long-term maintenance therapy. The patient with good features, especially if he or she experiences only two or three attacks annually, needs only intermittent therapy. The patient with a history of frequent severe attacks of pain needs maintenance therapy. There seems to be no tachyphylaxis, so that each course is usually as effective as the first. A previous complication such as haemorrhage, would point towards long-term maintenance or surgery. Relapses occur while on maintenance therapy but are normally infrequent (Fig. 22.5). However, the refractory ulcer (one which is slow to heal and swiftly recurs on stopping treatment) has a much higher relapse rate even while on maintenance therapy [4]. These patients may be offered surgery [51, 63].

How long should maintenance treatment last?

The patient with persistent ulcer faces the prospect of continous medication. In the elderly patients or in the presence of high operative risk (especially if there have been previous complications of the ulcer) maintenance should be for life. For younger patients, two years of maintenance treatment is suggested [148]; it should then be stopped to assess the speed with which the ulcer recurs. Depending upon the swiftness and severity of recurrence, the patient can be offered either a further full dose short course followed by maintenance therapy, or surgery.

In the patient with variable frequency of relapses, maintenance need not be so prolonged. Thus maintenance will probably be needed for only three to four months in some, and a prolonged remission may follow.

When a full dose course is completed, should we stop treatment abruptly, or tail off with a night dose for a few weeks? At present we have no information on this point, but many physicians consider that a gradual tapering of treatment makes sense. After, say, six weeks on a full dose of the H_2-antagonist, they advise a further four to six weeks on maintenance. This is a reasonable practice. It must be stressed that a careful clinical assessment is needed for each individual to give some indication of the course of that patient's ulcer. The most appropriate regimen can then be advised.

References

1 ADAMI H-O, BJORKLUND O, ENANDER L-K, *et al.* Cimetidine or propantheline combined with antacid therapy for short-term treatment of duodenal ulcer. *Dig Dis Sci* 1982;27:388–393.
2 AINLEY CC, FORGACS LC, KEELING PWN, THOMPSON RPH. Smoking and peptic ulceration: an outpatient endoscopic survey. *Gut* 1982;23:904.
3 BARBIER P. Belgian peptic ulcer study group. Single blind comparative study of ranitidine and cimetidine in patients with gastric ulcer. *Gut* 1984;25:991–1002.
4 BARDHAN KD. Long-term management of duodenal ulcer: a physician's view. In: Baron JH, ed. *Cimetidine in the 80s.* Edinburgh: Churchill Livingstone, 1981.
5 BARDHAN KD. Refractory duodenal ulcer. *Gut* 1984;25:711–717.
6 BARDHAN KD. Can antacids prevent duodenal ulcer relapse? *Gut* 1986;27:A612.

7 BARDHAN KD, COLE DS, HAWKINS BW, FRANKS C. Does treatment with cimetidine extended beyond initial healing of duodenal ulcer reduce the subsequent relapse rate? *Br Med J* 1982;**284**:621–623.

8 BARDHAN KD, SAUL DM, EDWARDS JL. Double-blind comparison of cimetidine and placebo in the maintenance of healing of chronic duodenal ulceration. *Gut* 1979;**20**:158–162.

9 BARR GD, PARIS CH, MIDDLETON WRJ, PIPER DW. Comparison of ranitidine and cimetidine in duodenal ulcer healing. In: Misiewicz JJ, Wormsley KG, eds. *The clinical use of ranitidine. Proceedings of the Second International Symposium on Ranitidine.* Oxford: Medicine Publishing Foundation, 1982.

10 BERSTAD A, AADLAND E, CARLSEN E. Maintenance treatment of duodenal ulcer patients with a single bedtime dose of cimetidine. *Scand J Gastroenterol* 1979;**14**:827.

11 BERSTAD A, BJERKE K, CARLSEN E, AADLAND E. Treatment of duodenal ulcer with antacids in combination with trimipramine or cimetidine. *Scand J Gastroenterol* 1979;**13**:44–50.

12 BIANCHI PORRO G, PETRILLO M, LAZZARONI M. Ranitidine in the short-term treatment of duodenal ulcer: a multi-centre endoscopic double-blind trial. In: Misiewicz JJ, Wormsley KG, eds. *The clinical use of ranitidine. Proceedings of the Second International Symposium on Ranitidine.* Oxford: Medicine Publishing Foundation, 1982.

13 BIRGER JENSEN K, MOLLMANN KM, RAHBEK I, et al. Prophylactic effect of cimetidine in gastric ulcer patients. *Scand J Gastroenterol* 1979;**14**:175–176.

14 BLACK JW, DUNCAN WAM, DURANT CJ, GANELLIN CR, PARSONS EM. Definition and antagonism of histamine H$_2$-receptors. *Nature* 1972;**236**:385–340.

15 BLACKWOOD WS, MAUDGAL DP, NORTHFIELD TC. Prevention by bedtime cimetidine of duodenal ulcer relapse. *Lancet* 1978;**i**:626–627.

16 BODEMAR G, WALAN A. Maintenance treatment of recurrent peptic ulcer by cimetidine. *Lancet* 1978;**ii**:403–407.

17 BOYD EJS, WILSON JA, WORMSLEY KG. Maintenance treatment of duodenal and gastric ulcer with ranitidine. In: Riley AJ, Salmon PR, eds. *Ranitidine. Proceedings of an International Symposium held in the context of the Seventh World Congress of Gastroenterology.* Amsterdam: Excerpta Medica, 1982.

18 BOYD EJS, WILSON JA, WORMSLEY KG. Smoking impairs therapeutic gastric inhibition. *Lancet* 1983;**i**:95–97.

19 BOYD EJS, WILSON JA, WORMSLEY KG. Effects of treatment compliance and overnight gastric secretion on outcome of maintenance therapy of duodenal ulcer with ranitidine. *Scand J Gastroenterol* 1983;**18**:193–200.

20 BOYD EJS, WILSON JA, WORMSLEY KG. Safety of ranitidine maintenance treatment of duodenal ulcer. *Scand J Gastroenterol* 1984;**19**:394–400.

21 BROGDEN RN, HILL RC, SPEIGHT TM, AVERY GS. Sucralfate. A review of its pharmacodynamic properties and therapeutic use in peptic ulcer disease. *Drugs* 1984;**27**:194–209.

22 BRUNNER G, LOSGEN H, HARKE U. Ranitidine in the treatment of cimetidine resistant ulceration of the upper gastrointestinal tract (German). *Therapiewoche* 1982;**32**:4154–4158.

23 BURLAND WJ, HAWKINS BW, BERESFORD J. Cimetidine treatment for the prevention of duodenal ulcer: an international collaborative study. *Postgrad Med J* 1980;**56**:173–176.

24 BURLAND WJ, HAWKINS BW, HORTON RJ, BERESFORD J. The long-term treatment of duodenal ulcer with cimetidine. In: Wastell C, Lance P, eds. *Cimetidine: The Westminster Hospital symposium.* Edinburgh: Churchill Livingstone, 1978.

25 CAPURSO L, DALMONTE PR, MAZZEO F, et al. Comparison of cimetidine 800 mg once daily and 400 mg twice daily in acute duodenal ulceration. *Br Med J* 1984;**289**:1418–1420.

26 CARLSSON E, WALLMARK B, POUNDER E. Biochemical, pharmacology and clinical properties of omeprazole, an inhibitor of hydrogen potassium ATPase. In: Pounder RE, ed. *Recent advances in gastroenterology-6.* Edinburgh: Churchill Livingstone, 1986:17–35.

27 CARMINE AA, BROGDEN RN. Pirenzepine. A review of its pharmacodynamic and pharmacokinetic properties and therapeutic efficacy in peptic ulcer disease and other allied diseases. *Drugs* 1985;**30**:85–126.

28 CARGILL JM, PEDEN N, SAUNDERS JHB, WORMSLEY KG. Very long-term treatment of peptic ulcer with cimetidine. *Lancet* 1978;**ii**:1113–1115.

29 CARUSO I, BIANCHI PORRO G. Gastroscopic evaluation of anti-inflammatory agents. *Br Med J* 1980;**280**:75–78.

30 CHATTERJI AN. A double-blind and randomised placebo-controlled study of ranitidine in duodenal ulcer patients. *Hepatogastroenterology [Suppl 299]* 1980.

31 COLIN-JONES DG. Gastric ulcer—short-term healing with cimetidine and other drugs. In: Baron JH, ed. *Cimetidine in the 80s.* Edinburgh: Churchill Livingstone, 1981.

32 COLIN-JONES DG. Ranitidine in the treatment of peptic ulceration. In: Riley AJ, Salmon PR, eds. *Ranitidine. Proceedings of an International Symposium held in the context of the Seventh World Congress of Gastroenterology.* Amsterdam: Excerpta Medica, 1982.

33 COLIN-JONES DG. There's more to healing ulcers than suppressing acid. *Gut* 1986;**27**:475–480.

34 COLIN-JONES DG, LANGMAN MJS, LAWSON DH, VESSEY MP. Cimetidine and gastric cancer: prelimi-

nary report from post-marketing surveillance. *Br Med J* 1982;**285**:1311–1313.

35 COLIN-JONES DG, LANGMAN MJS, LAWSON DH, VESSEY MP. Post-marketing surveillance of the safety of cimetidine: twelve-month morbidity report. *Q J Med* 1985;**215**:253–268.

36 COOPERATIVE STUDY. Omeprazole in duodenal ulceration: acid inhibition, symptom relief, endoscopic healing, and recurrence. *Br Med J* 1984;**289**:525–528.

37 COSTELLO FT, FIELDING JD, LEE FI. Comparison of ranitidine and cimetidine in short-term healing of duodenal ulcer. *Gastroenterology* 1982;**82**:1037.

38 DEAKIN M, RAMAGE JK, COLIN-JONES DG, *et al*. Does smoking affect the response to cimetidine in duodenal ulcer disease? *Gut* 1985;**26**:A546.

39 DIAL EJ, LICHTENBERGER LM. A role for milk phospholipids in protection against gastric acid. Studies in adult and suckling rats. *Gastroenterology* 1984;**87**:379–385.

40 DOLL R, PYGOTT F. Factors influencing the rate of healing of gastric ulcers: admission to hospital, phenobarbitone and ascorbic acid. *Lancet* 1952;**i**:171–175.

41 DRAGSTEDT LR. Peptic ulcer. An abnormality in gastric secretion. *Am J Surg* 1969;**117**:143–156.

42 ELDER JB. Inhibition of acid and gastric carcinoma. *Gut* 1985;**26**:1279–1283.

43 ELDER JB, GANGULI PC, GILLESPIE IE. Cimetidine and gastric cancer. *Lancet* 1979;**i**:1005.

44 ENGLERT E, FRESTON JW, GRAHAM DY, *et al*. Cimetidine, antacid and hospitalisation in the treatment of benign gastric ulcer. A multicentre double blind study. *Gastroenterology* 1978;**74**:416–425.

45 ENZMANN GD, LEONARD JM, PAULSEN CA, ROGERS J. Effect of cimetidine on reproductive function in men. *Clin Res* 1981;**29**:26A.

46 FELDMAN M. Inhibition of gastric acid secretion in selection and non-selective anticholinergics *Gastroenterology* 1984;**84**:361–366.

47 FORDTRAN JS, MORAWSKI BA, RICHARDSON CT. In vivo and in vitro evaluation of liquid antacids. *N Engl J Med* 1973;**288**:923–928.

48 FREDERIKSEN H-JB, MATZEN P, MADSEN P, *et al*. Spontaneous healing of duodenal ulcers. *Scand J Gastroenterol* 1984;**19**:417–421.

49 FREITAS D, PONTES F, PINHO C, *et al*. Clinical trial of ranitidine in duodenal ulcer in Portugal. *Scand J Gastroenterol* 1982;**17**:366A.

50 FRY J. Peptic ulcer: a profile. *Br Med J* 1964;**2**:809–812.

51 GEAR MWL. Proximal gastric vagotomy versus long-term maintenance treatment with cimetidine for chronic ulcer disease. *Br Med J* 1983;**286**:98–99.

52 GIACOSA A, CHELI R, MOLINARI F, PARODI MC. Comparison between ranitidine, cimetidine, pirenzepine and placebo in the short-term treat-

ment of duodenal ulcer. *Scand J Gastroenterol* 1982;**17**:215–219.

53 GIBINSKI K, NOWAK A, GABRYELEWICZ A, *et al*. Multicentre double-blind trial of ranitidine for duodenal ulcer. *Hepatogastroenterology* 1981;**28**:216.

54 GLEDHILL T, BUCK M, McEWAN J, PAUL A, HUNT RH. Effect of cimetidine 1 g per day on nocturnal intragastric acidity and acid secretion in cimetidine non-responders. *Gut* 1982;**23**:454 A.

55 GOUGH KR, BARDHAN KD, CROWE JP, *et al*. Ranitidine and cimetidine in prevention of duodenal ulcer relapse. *Lancet* 1984;**ii**:659–662.

56 GRAHAM DY, AKDAMAR K, DYCK WP, *et al*. Healing of benign gastric ulcer; comparison of cimetidine and placebo in the United States. *Ann Intern Med* 1985;**102**:573–576.

57 GRAY GR, SMITH JS, MACKENZIE J, GILLESPIE G. Long-term cimetidine in the management of severe duodenal ulcer dyspepsia. *Gastroenterology* 1978;**74**:397–401.

58 GREIBE J, BUGGE P, GJORUP T, LAURITZEN T, BONNEVIE O, WULFF HR. Long-term prognosis of duodenal ulcer: follow-up study and survey of doctors' estimates. *Br Med J* 1977;**2**:1572–1574.

59 GUDMAND-HOYER E, BIRGER JENSEN K, KRAG E, RASK-MADSEN J, RAHBEK J. Prophylactic effect of cimetidine in duodenal ulcer disease. *Br Med J* 1978;**1**:1095–1097.

60 GUGLER R, ROHNER H-G, KRATOCHVIL P, BRANDSTATTER G, SCHMITZ H. Effect of smoking on duodenal ulcer healing with cimetidine and oxmetidine. *Gut* 1982;**23**:866–871.

61 HANSCOM DH, BUCHMAN E. The follow-up period from the Veterans Administration co-operative study on gastric ulcer. *Gastroenterology* 1978;**61**:585–591.

62 HANSKY J, KORMAN MG, HETZEL DJ, SHEARMAN DJC. Relapse rate after cessation of 12 months cimetidine in duodenal ulcer. *Gastroenterology* 1979;**76**:1179 A.

63 HARLING H, BALSEV I, BENTZEN E. Parietal cell vagotomy or cimetidine maintenance therapy for duodenal ulcer? A prospective controlled trial. *Scand J Gastroenterol* 1985;**20**:747–750.

64 HARVEY RF, BRADSHAW MJ, DAVIDSON CM, WILKINSON SP, DAVIES PS. Multifocal gastric carcinoid tumours, achlorhydria and pernicious anaemia. *Lancet* 1985;**i**:951–953.

65 HEADING RC. Antacids and duodenal ulcer. *Gut* 1984;**25**:1195–1198.

66 HENRY DA, HAWKEY C, SOMERVILLE K, BURNHAM WR, BELL GD, LANGMAN MJS. Pirenzepine and cimetidine in duodenal ulcer: a comparative study. In: Dotevall G, ed. *Advances in gastroenterology with the selective antimuscarinic compound, pirenzepine.* Amsterdam: Excerpta Medica, 1982.

67 HOLLANDER D, TARNAWSKI A. Dietary essential

fatty acids and decline in peptic disease—a hypothesis. *Gut* 1986;27:239–242.

68 HOLLANDER D, TARNAWSKI A, KRAUSE WJ, GERGELY H. Protective effect of sucralfate against ethanol-induced gastric mucosal injury in the rat. *Gastroenterology* 1985;88:366–374.

69 HOWARD JM, CHREMOS AN, COLLEN MJ, *et al.* Famotidine, a new, potent, long-acting histamine H2-receptor antagonist: comparison with cimetidine and ranitidine in the treatment of Zollinger-Ellison syndrome. *Gastroenterology* 1985;88:1026–1033.

70 HULL DH, BEALE PJ. Cigarette smoking and duodenal ulcer. *Gut* 1985;26:1333–1337.

71 IRELAND A. Pirenzepine and cimetidine in the prevention of duodenal ulcer relapse. In: *Pirenzepine: new aspects in research and therapy.* Excerpta Medica, Amsterdam, 1984.

72 IRELAND A, GEAR P, COLIN-JONES DG, *et al.* Ranitidine 150 mg twice daily vs 300 mg nightly in treatment of duodenal ulcers. *Lancet* 1984;ii:274–275.

73 ISENBERG WI. Effect of antacids on dyspeptic symptoms. In: Halter F, ed. *Antacids in the Eighties.* Munich: Urban and Schwarzenberg, 1982.

74 JAYARAJ AP, TOVEY FI, CLARK CG. Possible dietary protective factors in relation to the distribution of duodenal ulcer in India and Bangladesh. *Gut* 1980;21:1068–1076.

75 JOHANSSON C, KOLLBERG B, NORDEMAR R, SAMUELSSON K, BERGSTROM S. Protective effect of prostaglandin E2 in the gastrointestinal tract during indomethacin treatment of rheumatic disease. *Gastroenterology* 1980;78:479–483.

76 JONES DB, ROSE JDR, SMITH PM, CALCRAFT BJ. Treatment of peptic ulcer with ranitidine—a clinical trial. In: Misiewicz JJ, Wormsley KG, eds. *The clinical use of ranitidine.* Oxford Medicine Publishing Foundation, 1982.

77 JONES DB, YEOMANS ND. Cimetidine versus ranitidine in short term healing of duodenal ulcers. *Gut* 1985;26:642.

78 KANG JY, CANALESE J, PIPER DW. The use of long-term cimetidine in the prevention of gastric ulcer relapse—double blind trial. In: *Proceedings of the Annual Scientific Meeting of the Gastroenterology Society of Australia,* 1979: A9.

79 KERR GD. Cimetidine: twice daily administration in duodenal ulcer—results of a U.K. and Ireland multicentre study. In: Baron JH, ed. *Cimetidine in the 80s.* Edinburgh: Churchill Livingstone, 1981.

80 KORMAN MG, HANSKY J, MERRETT AC, SCHMIDT GT. Ranitidine in duodenal ulcer: incidence of healing and effect of smoking. *Dig Dis Sci* 1982;27:712–725.

81 KRAG E. Long-term prognosis in medically treated peptic ulcer. A clinical, radiographical and statistical follow-up study. *Acta Med Scand* 1966;180:657–670.

82 KUMAR N, VIJ JC, KAROL A, ANAND BS. Controlled therapeutic trial to determine the optimum dose of antacids in duodenal ulcer. *Gut* 1984; 25:1199–1202.

83 LABROOY SJ, TAYLOR RH, HUNT RH, *et al.* Controlled comparison of cimetidine and carbenoxolone sodium in gastric ulcer. *Br Med J* 1979;1:1308–1309.

84 LAM SK, LEE NW, KOO J, HIN WM, FOK KH, NG M. Randomised crossover trial of tripotassium dicitrato bismuthate versus high dose cimetidine for duodenal ulcers resistant to standard doses of cimetidine. *Gut* 1984;25:703–706.

85 LANCE P, GAZZARD BG. Controlled trial of cimetidine for symptomatic treatment of duodenal ulcers. *Br Med J* 1983;286:937–938.

86 LANCET (Editorial). Cimetidine-resistant duodenal ulcers. *Lancet* 1985;i:23–24.

87 LANCET (Editorial). Gastric ulcer or cancer? *Lancet* 1985;ii:202.

88 LANCET (Editorial). Pyloric Campylobacter finds a volunteer. *Lancet* 1985;iii:1021–1022.

89 LANGMAN MJS, HENRY DA, BELL GD, BURNHAM WR, OGILVY A. Cimetidine and ranitidine in duodenal ulcer. *Br Med J* 1980;2:473–474.

90 LANGMAN MJS. Antisecretory drugs and gastric cancer. *Br Med J* 1985;290:1850–1852.

91 LAURITSEN K, LAURSEN LS, HAVELUND T, BYTZER P, SVENDSEN LB, RASK-MADESEN J. Enprostil and ranitidine in duodenal ulcer healing: double blind comparative trial. *Br Med J* 1986;292:864–866.

92 LAURITSEN K, RUNE S, BYTZER P, *et al.* Effect of omeprazole and cimetidine on duodenal ulcer. *N Engl J Med* 1985; 312:958–961.

93 LEE FI, SAMLOFF IM, HARDMANN M. Comparison of tripotassium dicitrato bismuthate tablets with ranitidine in healing and relapse of duodenal ulcers. *Lancet* 1985;i:1299–1301.

94 LENNARD-JONES JE, BARBOURIS N. Effect of different foods on acidity of the gastric contents in patients with duodenal ulcer. *Gut* 1965;6:113–117.

95 LOCKEFEER JHM, POP P, SCHENK Y, STUIFBERGEN WNHM, DEJONG MJ. A multicentre comparison of ranitidine and cimetidine in the treatment of gastric ulcer. In: Wesdorp ICE, ed. *The clinical use of ranitidine. Proceedings of a symposium held in Amsterdam 14–15 May 1982.* Guildford: Theracom, 1982.

96 LONDONG W, HASFORD J, SANDER R, *et al.* Prevention of recurrent bleeding from gastro-duodenal ulcers by combined application of cimetidine and pirenzepine: a double-blind randomised and multicentre trial. In: Dotevall G, ed. *Advances in Gastroenterology with the selective antimuscarinic compound, pirenzepine.* Amsterdam, Excerpta Medica, 1982.

97 LONDONG W, LONDONG V, PRECHTL R, WEBER TH, VONWERDER K. Interactions of cimetidine and pirenzepine on peptone-stimulated gastric

acid secretion in man. *Scand J Gastroenterol* 1980;**15**:103–112.

98 McCarthy DM. Peptic ulcer: antacids or cimetidine? *Hosp Pract* 1979;**14**:52–87.

99 McGuigan J. A consideration of the adverse effects of cimetidine. *Gastroenterology* 1981; **80**:181–192.

100 Machell RJ. Gastric ulcer: long-term treatment with cimetidine. In: Baron JH, ed. *Cimetidine in the 80s*. Edinburgh: Churchill Livingstone, 1981.

101 Machell RJ, Ciclitira PJ, Farthing MJG, Dick AP, Hunter JO. Cimetidine in the prevention of gastric ulcer relapse. *Postgrad Med J* 1979;**55**:393–395.

102 MacKay C, Mohammed R, Lee FI, Fielding JD, Holmes GKT, Hine K. The effect of ranitidine, a new histamine H_2-receptor antagonist, on healing rate of duodenal ulceration. *Gastroenterology* 1981;**80**:1219 A.

103 Malhotra SL. New approaches to pathogenesis of peptic ulcer. *Am J Dig Dis*; 1970;**15**:489–496.

104 Malhotra SL. A comparison of unrefined wheat and rice diets in the management of duodenal ulcer. *Postgrad Med J* 1978;**54**:6–9.

105 Marks IN, Lucke W, Wright JP, Girdwood AH. Ulcer healing and relapse rates after initial healing with cimetidine or sucralfate. *J Clin Gastroenterol* 1981;**3**:163–165.

106 Marks IN, Wright JP, Denyer M, Ganisch JAM, Lucke W. Comparison of sucralfate with cimetidine in the short-term treatment of chronic peptic ulcers. *S Afr Med J* 1980;**57**:567–573.

107 Marks IN, Wright JP, Denyer M, Hatfield A, Girdwood AH, Lucke W. Ranitidine heals duodenal ulcers. *S Afr Med J* 1982;**61**:152.

108 Martin DF, Hollander D, May SJ, Ravenscroft M, Tweedle DEF, Miller JP. Difference in relapse rates of duodenal ulcer after healing with cimetidine or tripotassium dicitrato bismuthate. *Lancet* 1981;i:7–10.

109 Martin F, Farley A, Gagnon M, Bensemana D. Comparison of the healing capacities of sucralfate and cimetidine in the short-term treatment of duodenal ulcer: a double-blind randomised trial. *Gastroenterology* 1982;**82**:401–405.

110 Massarrat S, Eisenmann A. Factors affecting the healing rate of duodenal and pyloric ulcers with low-dose antacid treatment. *Gut* 1981;**22**:97–102.

111 McArthur KE, Collen MJ, Maton PN, *et al*. Omeprazole: effective, convenient therapy for Zollinger–Ellison syndrome. *Gastroenterology* 1985;**88**:939–944.

112 Mihaly GW, Marino AT, Webster LK, Jones DB, Louis WJ, Smallwood RA. High dose of antacid (Mylanta II), reduces bioavailability of ranitidine. *Br Med J* 1982;**285**:998–999.

113 Milton-Thompson GJ. Monitoring of 24 hours acid secretion during antacid treatment. In: Halter F, ed. *Antacids in the eighties*. Munich: Urban and Schwarzenberg, 1982.

114 Morgan AG, McAdam WAF, Pacsoo C, Darnborough A. Comparison between cimetidine and Caved-S in the treatment of gastric ulceration and subsequent maintenance therapy. *Gut* 1982;**23**:545–551.

115 Moshal MG, Spitaels JM, Khan F. A double-blind endoscopically controlled trial of ranitidine in a high incidence area. *Scand J Gastroenterol* 1980;**16**:129.

116 Peden NR, Boyd EJS, Saunders JHB, Wormsley KG. Ranitidine in the treatment of duodenal ulceration. *Scand J Gastroenterol* 1981;**16**:325–329.

117 Peden NR, Saunders JHB, Wormsley KG. Inhibition of pentagastrin-stimulated and nocturnal gastric secretion by ranitidine. *Lancet* 1979;i:690–692.

118 Peter P, Gonvers JJ, Pelloni S, *et al*. Cimetidine in the treatment of duodenal ulcer. In: Creutzfeldt W, ed. *Cimetidine. Proceedings of an International symposium on histamine H_2-receptor antagonists*. Amsterdam: Excerpta Medica, 1978.

119 Peterson WL, Elashoff J. Placebo in clinical trials of duodenal ulcer: the end of an era? *Gastroenterology* 1980;**79**:585–587.

120 Peterson WL, Sturdevant RAL, Frankl HD, *et al*. Healing of duodenal ulcer with an antacid regimen. *N Engl J Med* 1977;**297**:341–345.

121 Petrillo M, Bianchi Porro G, Valentini M. Cimetidine and carbenoxolone sodium in the treatment of gastric ulcer: an open pilot study. *Curr Ther Res* 1982;**26**:990.

122 Petrillo M, Lazzaroni M, Prada A, Daniotti S, Bianchi Porro G. A controlled trial of pirenzepine versus carbenoxolone in the treatment of gastric ulcer: preliminary results. In: Dotevall, G., ed. *Advances in gastroenterology with the selective antimuscarinic compound, pirenzepine*. Amsterdam: Excerpta Medica, 1982.

123 Piper DW, Greig M, Coupland GAE, Hobbin E, Shinners J. Factors relevant to the prognosis of chronic gastric ulcer. *Gut* 1975;**16**:714–718.

124 Pounder RE. Model of medical treatment for duodenal ulcer. *Lancet* 1981;i:29–30.

125 Pounder RE. Duodenal ulcers that will not heal. *Gut* 1984;**25**:697–702.

126 Pounder RE. Histamine H_2-receptor antagonists and gastric acid secretion. *Parmac Therap* 1984;**26**:221–234.

127 Puscas I, Dindelegan D, Contrasiu P. Carbonic anhydrase inhibitors in the treatment of gastric ulcer. *Scand J Gastroenterol* 1982;**17**:371 A.

128 Roberts DM, Wilson JA, Ratcliffe GE, Waring AJ, Reilly MJ, Lloyd JS. Clinical trial of ranitidine in the treatment of peptic ulcer. *Br J Clin Pract* 1982;**36**:9–12.

129 Rowley-Jones D, Flind AC. Continuing evaluation of the safety of cimetidine. In: Baron JH, ed.

Cimetidine in the 80s. Edinburgh: Churchill Livingstone, 1981.

130 RYAN FP. A comparison of ranitidine and placebo in the acute treatment of gastric ulcer. In: Misiewicz JJ, Wormsley KG, eds. *The clinical use of ranitidine. Proceedings of the second international symposium on ranitidine.* Oxford: Medicine Publishing Foundation, 1982.

131 RYDNING A, BERSTAD A, AADLAND E, ODEGAARD B. Prophylactic effect of dietary fibre in duodenal ulcer disease. *Lancet* 1982;2:736–738.

132 SCHILLER KFR. Short-term treatment of duodenal ulcer: comparison of ranitidine with cimetidine, U.K. data. In: Misiewicz JJ, Wormsley KG, eds. *The clinical use of ranitidine. Proceedings of the second international symposium on ranitidine.* Oxford: Medicine Publishing Foundation, 1982.

133 SHEERS R, ROBERTS NB. The effects of pirenzepine and ranitidine on pepsin secretion. In: Dotevall G, ed. *Advances in gastroenterology with the selective antimuscarinic compound pirenzepine.* Amsterdam: Excerpta Medica, 1982.

134 SILVIS SE. Results of the USA ranitidine maintenance trials. *Am J Med* 1984;77:33–38.

135 SOMERVILLE K, FAULKNER G, LANGMAN MJS. Nonsteroidal anti-inflammatory drugs and bleeding peptic ulcer. *Lancet* 1986;i:462–464.

136 SONNENBERG A. Comparison of different strategies for treatment of duodenal ulcer. *Br Med J* 1985;290:1185–1187.

137 SONNENBERG A, MULLER-LISSNER SA, VOGEL E, et al. Predictors of duodenal ulcer healing and relapse. *Gastroenterology* 1981;81:1061–1067.

138 SONTAG S, GRAHAM DY, BELSITO A, et al. Cimetidine, cigarette smoking, and recurrence of duodenal ulcer. – *Engl J Med* 1984;311:689–693.

139 SPIRO HM. United States multicentre studies of ranitidine. In: Misiewicz JJ, Wornesley KG, eds. *The clinical use of ranitidine. Proceedings of the Second International symposium on ranitidine.* Oxford: Medicine Publishing Foundation, 1982.

140 STROM M, GOTTHARD R, BODEMAR G, WALAN A. Antacid/anticholinergic, cimetidine and placebo in treatment of active peptic ulcers. *Scand J Gastroenterol* 1981;16:593–602.

141 SUTTON DR. Gastric ulcer healing with tripotassium dicitrato bismuthate and subsequent relapse. *Gut* 1982;23:621–624.

142 TAKEMOTO T, OKITA K, NAMIKI M, ISHIKAWA M, TSUNEOKA K, OSHIBA S. Clinical evaluation of H_2-receptor antagonists in the therapy of gastric ulcer in Japan. In: Riley AJ, Salmon PR, eds. *Ranitidine. Proceedings of an international symposium held in the context of the Seventh World congress of Gastroenterology.* Amsterdam: Excerpta Medica, 1982.

143 TARNAWSKI A, HOLLANDER D, STACHURA J, KRAUSE WJ, GERGELY H. Prostaglandin protection of the gastric mucosa against alcohol injury—a dynamic time-related process. *Gastroenterology* 1985;88:334–352.

144 THOMAS JM, MISIEWICZ JJ. Histamine H_2-receptor antagonists in the short- and long-term treatment of duodenal ulcer. *Clin Gastroenterol* 1984;13:501–541.

145 TROTMAN I, COLLEY S, HOWARD O, et al. A controlled trial of pirenzepine and cimetidine in the treatment of duodenal ulcer. In: *Advances in gastroenterology with the selective antimuscarinic compound, pirenzepine.* Amsterdam, Excerpta Medica, 1982.

146 VANTRAPPEN G, JANSSENS J, POPIELA T, et al. Effect of 15(R)-15-methyl prostaglandin (Arbaprostil) on the healing of duodenal ulcer: a double-blind multicenter study. *Gastroenterology* 1982;83:357–363.

147 VANTRAPPEN G, RUTGEERTS P, BROECKAERT L, JANSSENS J. Randomised open controlled trial of colloidal bismuth subcitrate tablets and cimetidine in the treatment of duodenal ulcer. *Gut* 1980;21:329–333.

148 WALAN A, BIANCHI PORRO G, HENTSCHEL E. Maintenance cimetidine for up to 3 years. *Lancet* 1985;i:115–116.

149 WALT R, KALSCHINSKI B, LOGAN R, ASHLEY J, LANGMAN MJS. Frequency of ulcer perforation in elderly people in the United Kingdom. *Lancet* 1986;i:489–492.

150 WALT RP, MALE PJ, RAWLINGS J, HUNT RH, MILTON-THOMPSON GJ, MISIEWICZ JJ. Comparison of the effects of ranitidine, cimetidine and placebo on the 24 hour intragastric acidity and nocturnal acid secretion in patients with duodenal ulcer. *Gut* 1981;22:49–54.

151 WALT RP, TROTMAN IF, FROST R, et al. Comparison of twice-daily ranitidine with standard cimetidine treatment of duodenal ulcer. *Gut* 1981;22:319.

152 WATKINSON G. Closing remarks: 'Ten years later'. In: Avery-Jones F, Langman MJS, Mann RD, eds. *Peptic ulcer healing: recent studies on carbenoxolone.* Lancaster: MTP Press Ltd, 1978.

153 WILKINSON ML, O'DRISCOLL R, KIERNAN TJ. Cimetidine and pancreatitis. *Lancet* 1981;i:610–611.

154 WORMSLEY KG. Short-term treatment of duodenal ulceration. In: Baron JH, ed. *Cimetidine in the 80s.* Edinburgh: Churchill Livingstone, 1981: 3–8.

155 WRIGHT JP, MARKS IN, MEE AS, et al. Ranitidine in the treatment of gastric ulcer disease. In: Misiewicz JJ, Wormsley KG, eds. *The clinical use of ranitidine. Proceedings of the Second International symposium on ranitidine.* Oxford: Medicine Publishing Foundation, 1982.

156 YEOMANS ND, HANSON RG, SMALLWOOD RA, MIHALY GW, LOUIS WJ. Effect of chronic ranitidine treatment on secretion of intrinsic factor. *Br Med J* 1982;285:264.

157 ZEITOUN P, D'AZEMAR P. International multicentre clinical trial of ranitidine in duodenal ulcer. Comparison with cimetidine. In: Misiewicz JJ, Wormsley KG, eds. *The clinical use of ranitidine. Proceedings of the Second International symposium on ranitidine*. Oxford: Medicine Publishing Foundation, 1982.

Chapter 23
Surgical Management of Peptic Ulcer

D.C. CARTER

Elective operation for peptic ulceration

The decision to recommend surgery for peptic ulceration is taken by balancing the risks and potential benefits of operation against those of continued medical therapy. In general, surgery gives worst results if an operation is done when it is not indicated, if the operation chosen is not appropriate, or if the operation selected is carried out badly. Great judgement is often needed to determine the need for surgery. At the extremes it is obviously incorrect to submit a young patient with a duodenal ulcer to operation when he or she has only a short history of mild dyspepsia, while it is equally incorrect to deny surgery to an otherwise healthy patient with a long history of intractable and incapacitating ulcer pain. It is in the area between these extremes that decisions may be difficult. Hard and fast rules are not practicable. The decision must be based on detailed consideration of the particular circumstances of each individual, and it is most likely to be correct when the views of the clinician responsible for past medical management are taken into account. The patient may have been managed from the time of referral to hospital by a medical gastroenterologist who has decreed the timing of surgical consultation. Alternatively, he or she may have been managed from the outset by a surgeon with a declared interest in gastroenterology. The best approach probably lies in a clinic run jointly by a physician and surgeon who have evolved a tried and tested policy of treatment. The approach offers the best prospect for a rational and informed decision about the need for surgery and, perhaps equally important, allows objective evaluation of the results of operation.

Duodenal ulcer

Indications for elective operation

It is only the minority of duodenal ulcer patients who have symptoms severe enough to warrant attendance at hospital and eventual consideration for surgical management. In assessing the need for operation the following factors are taken into account.

Unequivocal diagnosis

Given the ready availability of endoscopy as a means of complementing barium meal examination, there should be no doubt regarding the diagnosis of duodenal ulceration. It is inexcusable to carry out ulcer surgery on the basis of 'non-ulcer dyspepsia', equivocal radiological deformity of the duodenum, or slight stippling of the pyloroduodenal area at operation.

Intractability

Some two-thirds of patients coming to surgery do so because medical treatment has failed to heal their ulcer or keep it healed. Surgery should not be recommended until the patient has had at least one full course of a potent ulcer-healing drug. The advent

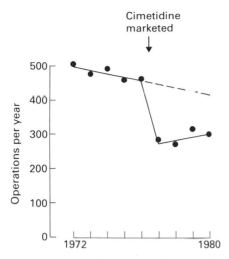

Fig. 23.1. Number of patients with duodenal ulcer coming to operation in six UK centres before and after the introduction of cimetidine [52].

of the H_2-receptor antagonists has markedly reduced the number of patients coming to ulcer operation (Fig. 23.1), but the number of operations may rise to some extent as patients fail on long-term medical management.

The duration and severity of symptoms are the accepted means of defining the need for operation. Care must be taken in interpretation. For example, a patient with a 10-year history of pain may seem a good candidate for surgery, but closer questioning may reveal that he or she has only experienced a few bouts of mild discomfort readily controlled by antacid therapy. On the other hand, surgery may be indicated strongly in a patient with 18 months of intractable dyspepsia which has made considerable inroads into his or her enjoyment of life and ability to work. Night pain can be particularly distressing and merits extra weighting, while loss of time from work and number of hospital admissions are other important indices of severity.

'Earning' was the term coined to denote the practice of postponing surgery in favour of prolonged medical therapy in the hope of reducing the incidence of poor results of surgery. Small *et al.* [46] could find no evidence linking the outcome of operation to the length of history or age of the patient and the 'earning' policy has fallen into disrepute. At the same time, many surgeons still consider that young patients fare less well after operation and submit them to surgery only after prolonged trial of medical treatment.

Natural history of duodenal ulcer

Duodenal ulceration is characterized by episodes of relapse interspersed with periods of remission. In one study from the south of England [12] symptoms increased progressively to peak after five to 10 years. Thereafter the tendency to remission increased and the disease gradually became quiescent. During the cycle some 16% of patients came to surgery to control symptoms, while a further 16% experienced bleeding, 7% perforated and 1% developed pyloric stenosis. In a more recent long-term study from Denmark involving 154 patients, 34 had come to operation while of the 120 treated conservatively, 19 continued to experience symptoms of some severity [18]. It is clear that surgery is not needed for many patients with duodenal ulcer and our ability to control symptoms by effective medical therapy now allows many patients to avoid operation who might have come to surgery in the past.

Ulcer complications

A history of ulcer bleeding or perforation strengthens the case for operation if symptoms return or persist. Pyloric stenosis is an absolute indication for surgery, although incomplete obstruction due to oedema and spasm may resolve once medical treatment has healed the ulcer. Stenosis may develop for the first time in patients receiving H_2-receptor antagonists and it is conceivable that accelerated healing with these agents may favour the development of stenosis [17].

Personality

As Small *et al.* [46] have shown, patients with psychiatric disability are less likely to achieve good results following surgery, particularly when suffering from less severe forms of ulcer disease. However, 70% of their patients with psychiatric problems did obtain good results and there was no evidence that operation exacerbated mental disability. Neurotic and emotionally unstable patients must not be denied operation on the grounds that 'they need their ulcer' as a focal point for their distress. The relief of physical symptoms is usually associated with improvement in psychological symptoms. At the same time, ulcer surgery must not be advocated as a panacea for anxious neurotic individuals. Those who drink and smoke to excess are also less likely to have good results from operation, but once again, should not be denied surgery on these grounds alone.

Long-term medical treatment or operation

Very few patients fail to derive some benefit from modern medical treatment and ulcer healing can be expected while on H_2-re-ceptor antagonists in 70–90% of patients (see Chapter 24). While maintenance therapy can prolong remission there is no evidence that it affects the natural history of the ulcer, or decreases the high relapse rate when therapy is stopped [1, 22] (Fig. 23.2). Gray *et al.* [17] studied the effect of long-term cimetidine in 50 patients originally accepted for elective ulcer surgery. At five-year assessment 20 had undergone surgery because of inadequate control of symptoms (13 patients) or complications of ulcer disease (7 patients). Twelve patients remained well on continuous therapy, while 18 who had discontinued treatment experienced recurrence of symptoms until cimetidine was restarted.

Gear [13] randomized patients with long-standing duodenal ulceration to long-term cimetidine, or highly selective vagotomy. With follow-up for one to four years the rate of ulcer recurrence was 54% in the medically treated group and 10% in those treated by operation. There can be no doubt that ranitidine and cimetidine have a valuable place in initial treatment and surgery is avoided in those patients whose ulcers heal rapidly and remain healed. Ulcers that recur on maintenance therapy can be treated by a return to full dose therapy, but after one to two years of medical management it is reasonable to discuss surgery. Just as there is no evidence that surgery is less

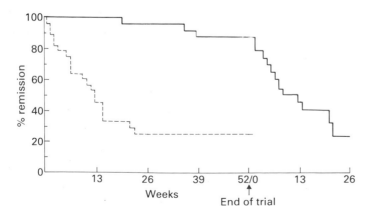

Fig. 23.2. Relapse rate in duodenal ulcer patients after healing had been achieved with a short course of cimetidine. The first group of patients (dotted line) received no further medical treatment; the second group (solid line) went on to a 12-month course of maintenance cimetidine before stopping treatment [22].

likely to be successful in those patients with severe ulcer disease [51], so there are no substantial grounds for believing that surgical cure is less likely in patients who have failed to respond to agents such as cimetidine.

Risks of surgery and post-operative sequelae

All clinicians concerned with the decision to recommend operation must be fully conversant with its risks and the likelihood of post-operative sequelae. Furthermore, they

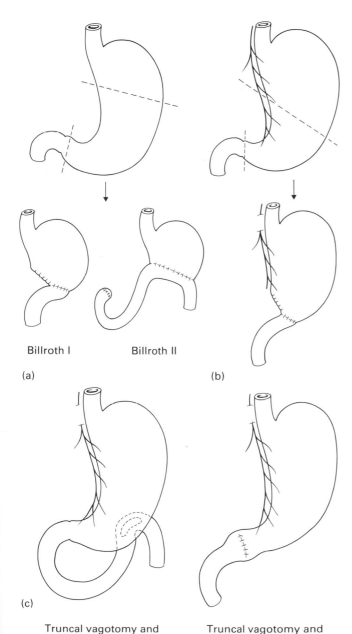

Billroth I   Billroth II

(a)   (b)

(c)

Truncal vagotomy and   Truncal vagotomy and
gastroenterostomy   pyloroplasty

Fig. 23.3. Operations available for duodenal ulcer. (a) partial gastrectomy with gastroduodenal (Billroth I) or gastrojejunal (Billroth II) anastomosis; (b) truncal vagotomy and antrectomy using a gastroduodenal anastomosis; (c) truncal vagotomy and gastrojejunostomy or pyloroplasty.

must discuss them fully so that the patient takes an active part in the decision. The risks are influenced by the type of operation to be undertaken, but in some patients, notably those with cardiorespiratory insufficiency, the risks of surgery patently outweigh its potential benefits and long-term medical treatment is the answer. Informed patient participation is essential if undue disappointment and recrimination are to be minimized when the results of surgery are sub-optimal.

Elective operation for duodenal ulcer

The ideal operation for duodenal ulcer is one that is safe, cures the ulcer and is free from undesirable effects due to altered gastrointestinal anatomy and physiology. None of the operations available are ideal and in assessing their relative worth, safety is the overriding consideration. In the past great emphasis was laid on a low incidence of recurrent ulcer but it is now apparent that severe dumping and diarrhoea may be more incapacitating and more difficult to treat.

Operations available

Partial gastrectomy without vagotomy (Fig. 23.3) reduces acid-pepsin secretion by removing the antrum which is the major source of gastrin production, and a variable amount of the oxyntic region of the stomach. This means removal of two-thirds to three-quarters of the distal stomach. Continuity is restored by gastroduodenal (Billroth I) or gastrojejunal (Billroth II) anastomosis. Resection can be confined to antrectomy if truncal vagotomy is added; partial gastrectomy without vagotomy is now seldom used in the treatment of duodenal ulcer.

Truncal vagotomy with antrectomy inhibits gastric secretion by removing the

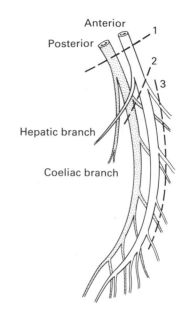

Fig. 23.4. Diagram of the abdominal vagi showing the level of nerve section in (1) truncal vagotomy, (2) selective vagotomy and (3) highly selective vagotomy.

major source of gastrin production, while abolishing the direct vagal drive to acid-pepsin secretion. Although popular in the United States, there are anxieties regarding its safety and incidence of unwanted effects, which have restricted its use in Europe as a primary ulcer operation.

Truncal vagotomy and drainage by gastrojejunostomy or pyloroplasty is safer than resection, but has a high incidence of recurrent ulceration and is by no means free from undesirable effects. Selective vagotomy and drainage was introduced to overcome these deficiencies; it was hoped that the risk of recurrence would be diminished by the more meticulous dissection required to divide only those vagal fibres destined for the stomach (Fig. 23.4). At the same time, it was anticipated that preserving the vagal supply to extragastric structures would lower the incidence of side-effects. Neither expectation has been fulfilled and the operation is not universally accepted.

Highly selective vagotomy is the safest of

all ulcer operations, in that the gut is not opened. The operation denervates only the acid-pepsin secreting part of the stomach but preserves the vagal supply to the antrum and pylorus (thus obviating the need for a drainage procedure), and to extragastric structures (Fig. 23.4). The operation demands meticulous technique to ensure adequate reduction of acid-pepsin secretion [14]. A number of variations have been described such as lesser curve myotomy [50] and anterior highly selective/posterior truncal vagotomy [23], but none seems likely to replace the standard operation.

Comparison of available operations

Operative mortality

Operations entailing resection with anastomosis are inherently more likely to produce life-threatening complications than those that avoid resection or do not even open the gastrointestinal tract. Although many trials apparently fail to show a higher operative mortality following resection, it must be remembered that patients were not included in many studies if extensive inflammation in and around the duodenum precluded resection, or the surgeon considered that all trial operations could not have been performed with equal safety. In the Leeds-York trial [15], partial gastrectomy, truncal vagotomy and antrectomy, and truncal vagotomy and gastrojejunostomy were all done without mortality, but these results achieved by skilled specialists may not represent those obtained in general surgical practice. While there were no significant differences between the four operations studied in the Veterans Administration trial [38], partial gastrectomy carried the highest mortality rate of 1.8%, a figure which may be more representative of the general experience.

Truncal vagotomy and drainage was at one time the safest ulcer operation with an operative mortality of just under 1% [3]. It has now been displaced by highly selective vagotomy with its mortality rate of only 0.3% [25].

Nature of perioperative complications

Following Billroth II gastrectomy the major complications include mechanical obstruction (at the stoma, afferent or efferent limb), leakage from the duodenal stump or stoma, haemorrhage from the suture lines, or traumatic pancreatitis or bile duct injury. After Billroth I gastrectomy the major complications are obstruction at the stoma, or leakage and bleeding at the suture line. The complications of truncal vagotomy and antrectomy are essentially those of partial gastrectomy without vagotomy.

Complications after truncal vagotomy and drainage include obstruction at the gastrojejunostomy or pyloroplasty, and bleeding or leakage from the suture lines. All of these problems are relatively uncommon as are oesophageal perforation and splenic damage in the course of vagotomy.

Necrosis of the lesser curve is a rare specific complication of highly selective vagotomy. Its pathogenesis is not clear, but the submucosal blood supply in the lesser curve is relatively poor and the risk of necrosis may be increased if the short gastric vessels are also divided, as in splenectomy or in preparation for fundoplication. The complication presents as perforation or bleeding in the post-operative period. Severe pain is the warning symptom and urgent re-operation is required as the complication has a mortality rate of 50%. Gastric stasis is a rare complication of highly selective vagotomy and necessitates early re-operation in 0.1% of patients [25].

Recurrent ulceration

Truncal vagotomy and antrectomy usually has a recurrence rate of less than 1% [3,

Table 23.1. Incidence of recurrent ulceration in trials of highly selective vagotomy in the treatment of duodenal ulceration*.

| | Trial operation | | | | | |
| | Highly selective vagotomy | | Vagotomy drainage | | Vagotomy antrectomy | |
Reference	n.	% Recurrence	n.	% Recurrence	n.	% Recurrence
[48]	64	5	62	5		
[30]	77	8	76	3		
[34]	50	26	50	14		
[2]	83	16	176	12		
[44]	86	3	37	3	50	0
[28]	45	2			47	0
[4]	116	3			106	1

*The incidence of recurrence may well rise with further follow-up; standard definition of ulcer recurrence not employed for all trials.

44], whereas partial gastrectomy without vagotomy is followed by recurrence in 1–13% of patients according to the amount of stomach resected.

The incidence of recurrent ulceration after truncal vagotomy and drainage ranges from 2–27% [46] with a mean value of about 10%. Information is still accruing regarding recurrence after highly selective vagotomy. Early reports of a rate of 22% [31] probably reflect inadequate technique, rather than failure of the operation itself and in most recent reports the operation has a recurrence rate at least equal to that of truncal vagotomy and drainage (Table 23.1).

Recurrent ulceration in most patients is due to failure to achieve complete vagal denervation of the acid-pepsin secreting area of the stomach. In only a small handful of patients can other explanations be invoked, such as the presence of a gastrinoma or a retained antrum after Billroth II gastrectomy. Some surgeons are better vagotomists than others, but this ability is not necessarily the prerogative of consultants [26]. It has been suggested that known hypersecretors should have antrectomy added to vagotomy, but as Johnston *et al.* [27] showed, patients with preoperative peak acid outputs in excess of 50 mmol/h fared

no worse than those with lower levels of secretion after highly selective vagotomy (see Chapter 24).

So-called 'selective' nerve stains do not help to achieve complete vagotomy, but some surgeons employ intragastric pH mapping (the Grassi test) to ensure denervation of the entire acid-secreting area. The test can also be used to define the boundary between antrum and corpus during highly selective vagotomy, but most surgeons rely on anatomical landmarks and avoid opening the stomach. When carrying out highly selective vagotomy it is particularly important to clear at least 5 cm of the oesophagus of all vagal fibres. Regardless of the type of vagotomy being performed, the key to avoiding ulcer recurrence is a meticulous and unhurried search for undivided vagal fibres.

Unwanted effects of gastric surgery

One of the main reasons for the move away from partial gastrectomy was the recognition of its long-term sequelae—weight loss, malabsorption, metabolic bone disease and anaemia and post-cibal symptoms such as dumping, diarrhoea and reactive hypoglycaemia (see Chapter 25). It was hoped that truncal vagotomy and drainage would avoid these troublesome and often incapacitating problems, but this hope has been unfulfilled. For example, in the Leeds-York trial only 70% of patients were placed in the satisfactory Visick grades I or II after truncal vagotomy and gastroenterostomy, compared with 78% after truncal vagotomy and antrectomy and 77% after Polya partial gastrectomy [15, 16]. Independent assessment of patients in the Veterans Administration trial showed that 83% achieved excellent or good results after vagotomy and drainage, as opposed to 89% after truncal vagotomy and antrectomy [38].

Interpretation of all trial results is hampered by varying definitions of unwanted effects and of their severity and in some cases by a lack of objective independent assessment. It is now clear that operations incorporating truncal vagotomy are not free of metabolic side-effects and that dumping and diarrhoea affect between 10% and 30% of patients and are severe in 2–5%. In the past these sequelae have been attributed to the vagotomy, but dumping and diarrhoea may well be attributable to gastric incontinence following gastric resection, or a drainage procedure.

Insufficient time has elapsed to assess the long term effects of highly selective vagotomy, but in that the operation avoids resection or gross disturbances of gastric emptying, there are good grounds for optimism. Dumping and diarrhoea affect only 2–3% of patients and are hardly ever classed as severe. It is of interest that in a study of post-surgery symptoms, only 84% of hernia repair patients were classified as Visick I or II compared to 90% of patients after highly selective vagotomy [41]. In the same context, Kennedy *et al.* [29] found no difference in Visick classification between patients after highly selective vagotomy and a group of patients without gastrointestinal disease who had not undergone surgery.

Risk of developing gastric cancer

It now seems likely that gastric resection favours the development of cancer in the gastric remnant. It is hypothesised that reflux of bile and pancreatic juice leads to chronic irritation, while hypochlorhydria favours bacterial proliferation with increased generation of carcinogenic nitrosamines from nitrites in food. Significant dysplasia is observed in the gastric remnant in some 20% of patients examined 20 years after gastrectomy [43, 45]. Some 5% of patients presenting with gastric cancer will have had previous resection for benign disease, whereas stump cancer develops in approximately 3% of all patients having resection for peptic ulcer. It is not yet certain whether the risk after truncal vagotomy and drainage is the same as that after resection, but the operation causes hypochlorhydria, allows reflux and may increase the nitrosamine content of the stomach. No information is available about the risks, if any, of developing gastric cancer after highly selective vagotomy but the presence of an innervated intact pylorus might be expected to decrease the reflux factor postulated as important in the genesis of cancer after gastrectomy. Acid secretion may partly recover after selective, or highly selective vagotomy [37].

Recommendations

Operations that avoid resection are safer than those which do not and highly selective vagotomy is the safest operation of all. Although truncal vagotomy and antrectomy offers the best guarantee of freedom from recurrence, highly selective vagotomy offers the best prospect of avoiding the undesirable side-effects of gastric surgery. In that ulcer recurrence is easier to treat (medically and surgically) than severe dumping and diarrhoea, highly selective vagotomy must be regarded as the operation of choice. For patients with pyloric stenosis, truncal vagotomy and gastrojejunostomy is indicated.

Gastric ulcer

Gastric ulcers are conveniently classified into three types: single ulcers located most often on the lesser curvature (type I), ulcers found in association with duodenal ulcers (type II), and prepyloric ulcers (type III). Type II gastric ulcers are usually regarded as secondary to the duodenal ulcer to which treatment is directed, while type III ulcers are regarded as a variant of duodenal ulceration for treatment purposes, once malignancy has been excluded. Unless stated otherwise, the remainder of this section is devoted to the treatment of type I ulcers.

Indications for elective operation

While duodenal ulceration is usually regarded primarily as a medical disorder that sometimes needs surgery, gastric ulcer is seen by many clinicians as a surgical disorder which in some cases can be treated medically. Protagonists of surgical treatment offer the following argument against conservative management:

1. It exposes the patient to the hazards of ulcer complications, notably bleeding and perforation and may deny surgery to patients with occult cancer at a stage when it can still be cured.

2. It is expensive and needs frequent hospital attendance with admission for further investigation and treatment.

3. Gastric ulcer has a recurrence rate of 50% when patients are followed for five years.

The counter-argument may be summarized as:

1. Most gastric ulcers are benign and modern diagnostic techniques greatly reduce the risk of overlooking malignancy.

2. Surgery carries a risk of mortality and subsequent unwanted effects.

3. Recurrent gastric ulcers respond just as well to therapy as the initial ulcer and drugs are available for safe, effective, long-term therapy.

In practice, the decision to recommend surgery still rests on evaluation of the balance between the risks and potential benefits of medical and surgical treatment for the individual. The considerations are similar to those outlined for duodenal ulcer, but with two important differences—gastric ulcer patients are often older and frailer and the risk of overlooking malignancy cannot be ignored.

Evaluation of the risk of malignancy

Malignant degeneration in a previously benign gastric ulcer is probably an extremely rare event. The difficulty lies in distinguishing between benign and malignant ulceration. Some 4–14% of gastric ulcers thought initially to be benign turn out to be malignant [21, 36]. Age, symptoms and ulcer location are not particularly useful in differentiation. Duodenal deformity, or coexistent duodenal ulceration suggest that the gastric ulcer is benign, although this premise has been questioned [36]. Endoscopic inspection is more reliable than radiology, but must be accompanied by multiple biopsies of the inside margin of the ulcer and its base, with additional brush cytological examination if possible.

Given that an ulcer is diagnosed as benign, medical treatment is usually recommended, particularly if the patient is elderly, frail, or suffering from cardiorespiratory insufficiency. However, vigilance must not be relaxed and healing must be assessed, preferably by repeat endoscopy and multiple biopsy after six to eight weeks. Surgery should be considered if the ulcer has not healed. Failure to heal is suspicious, as many malignant ulcers show some healing with medical therapy [40]. When the risks of surgery are high, a case can be made for persisting with medical treatment provided repeat biopsies exclude malignancy. Failure of ulcer healing after 12 weeks on medical treatment is an indication for surgery, unless the risks of operation are great, or the ulcer was originally larger than 2.5 cm in diameter and sufficient healing has occurred to justify a further month of treatment to complete the healing process.

Elective operation for gastric ulcer

As in duodenal ulceration, the ideal operation for gastric ulcer should be safe, free from ulcer recurrence and not attended by undesirable effects. A fourth consideration can never be ignored, namely the risk of overlooking gastric cancer at a potentially curable stage. The aim of surgery is to cure ulceration by decreasing the levels of acid and pepsin secretion, although it is accepted that failure of gastric mucosal defences may have primary importance in pathogenesis.

Comparison of operations available

Partial gastrectomy

Billroth I partial gastrectomy is the standard operation for gastric ulcer and is generally preferred to Billroth II partial gastrectomy and pylorus-preserving partial gastrectomy [35]. While Billroth I gastrectomy has been without operative mortality in some studies [6, 7], its overall operative mortality is probably 1–2%. The reported ulcer recurrence rate varies greatly, but may be as high as 20% [39, 42], while the unwanted effects are the same as those of resection for duodenal ulcer. Resection of more than 50–60% of the stomach is unnecessary. When the ulcer is high on the lesser curve, extensive resection can be avoided by leaving the ulcer in place after multiple biopsies to exclude malignancy, or by resecting the distal half of the stomach plus a tongue of lesser curve including the ulcer.

Truncal vagotomy and drainage

This approach avoids gastric resection, but does not remove the ulcer-bearing area of the stomach. Unless the ulcer is excised, multiple biopsies are imperative to exclude malignancy. The early results of vagotomy and drainage were very encouraging, with a low recurrence rate and up to 90% of patients achieving satisfactory results [10], but later studies reported a recurrence rate of 22% at five years [8]. When vagotomy and drainage was compared to Billroth I gastrectomy in a controlled trial there were no operative deaths after either operation, but morbidity was twice as high after resection [5]. There were no significant differences between the operations in terms of functional results; the recurrence rate was 3% after gastrectomy and 11% after vagotomy and drainage, but this difference was not statistically significant.

Highly selective vagotomy with ulcer excision

Duthie and Bransom [6] have reported a controlled trial of this operation versus Billroth I gastrectomy in 56 patients followed for an average of four years. There were no operative deaths but significantly more morbidity was observed after resection. The ulcer recurrence rate was 15% after highly selective vagotomy and 7% after gastrectomy. Follow-up of this series has now been extended for an average of eight years [39]. The recurrence rate has risen to 23% after vagotomy and to 17% after gastrectomy. If patients with ulcer recurrence are excluded, all highly selective vagotomy patients are in Visick grades I and II as opposed to only 62% of the gastrectomy patients.

Although these results from highly selective vagotomy are encouraging, the recurrence rate is disquieting and the operation may not be possible if there is marked inflammation and fibrosis extending into the lesser omentum from the ulcer.

Recommendations

Billroth I gastrectomy is still the standard operation for gastric ulcer. In skilled hands it carries an acceptable mortality rate and probably the lowest rate of ulcer recurrence. Resection removes the ulcer and avoids the risk of overlooking malignancy. Vagotomy may be preferred to resection in patients with high lesser curve ulcers, particularly when the patient is underweight, or is a relatively poor operative risk. Highly selective vagotomy with ulcer excision requires further evaluation, but the excellent functional results have to be balanced against a high recurrence rate. Finally it must not be forgotten that there is a long-term cancer risk following gastric resection. While this risk may not be high enough to affect the choice of operation in all patients, it seems reasonable to try to avoid resection in young subjects.

Emergency operation for peptic ulceration

Haemorrhage

Approximately 90% of patients admitted with upper gastrointestinal bleeding settle on conservative management. Further haemorrhage increases mortality by a factor of 4–12 and is more likely in patients with a large index bleed who are shocked on admission and in gastric rather than duodenal ulceration. Early endoscopy has increased the accuracy of diagnosis of the source of bleeding, but has not influenced prognosis [9], although endoscopic stigmata of recent haemorrhage have been shown to have prognostic importance in

predicting rebleeding. Lesions showing fresh bleeding, fresh or altered adherent blood clot or slough, or a protruding vessel are all associated with significantly greater risk of further haemorrhage [11, 20].

The decision to abandon conservative management in favour of surgery is often difficult and should be taken by experienced surgeons. In general, operation is indicated if overt bleeding continues or recurs. The indications are strengthened if the patient is older than 55 years and has any of the endoscopic stigmata mentioned above.

Truncal vagotomy and pyloroplasty is probably the standard operation for bleeding duodenal ulcer and the bleeding point is undersewn at the start of the pyloroplasty. Rebleeding is less likely after truncal vagotomy and antrectomy, but this gain has to be balanced against an increased mortality and morbidity after resection in ill patients. In gastric ulceration fear that the ulcer may be malignant means that resection is favoured, unless the patient is a poor surgical risk and the ulcer is high on the lesser curve. Under these circumstances it is safer to carry out vagotomy and drainage with excision of the ulcer or multiple biopsy. Although some centres have managed to reduce the mortality of bleeding peptic ulcer to as low as 2% [24], overall mortality is probably still between 5% and 10% and mainly affects the older patients. Non-surgical means of arresting haemorrhage, notably endoscopic laser photocoagulation have given encouraging early results [33, 49] and merit further evaluation as an alternative to surgery.

Perforation

In one large survey from the west of Scotland, the mortality rate in perforated duodenal ulcer was 11% and of perforated gastric ulcer 27% [32]. While these figures are higher than those reported from some hospitals, the overall experience of a region may be more representative. A large proportion of patients are elderly and it is clear that perforation remains a potentially lethal condition.

Although perforation can be managed conservatively, operation is normally preferred and the decision lies between simple closure and definitive surgery such as truncal vagotomy and drainage. Simple closure is followed by recurrent dyspepsia in most patients. Griffin and Organ [19] found on long-term follow-up that 78% of their patients had either come to reoperation, died from ulcer complications, or were under active treatment for ulcer symptoms. On the other hand, definitive emergency surgery is not needed in all cases, as 20–50% of patients with perforation of acute ulcers experience no further dyspepsia after simple closure.

Some surgeons advocate simple closure routinely for perforated duodenal ulcer, while others employ definitive surgery unless the patient's general condition is poor, there is established peritonitis, or the surgeon is inexperienced. A third approach consists of simple closure of ulcers judged to be acute, with definitive surgery only in patients who have had dyspepsia for more than three months or chronic scarring at operation and when none of the criteria mentioned above are present. Admittedly some 50–80% of the patients with so-called acute ulcers may still come to definitive operation, but this approach avoids unnecessary ulcer surgery in the remainder. Truncal vagotomy and drainage is generally preferred as the definitive operation, as the perforation can be incorporated in the pyloroplasty. Truncal vagotomy and antrectomy is best avoided on grounds of safety, but there is current interest in closure of the perforation plus highly selective vagotomy.

In perforated gastric ulcer there is a stronger case for definitive surgery with ulcer resection. About 10% of perforated gastric ulcers prove to be malignant and even when the ulcer is benign, simple closure is followed by a higher incidence of reoperation than is the case in perforated duodenal ulcer. Although truncal vagotomy and gastric resection is preferred, a lesser procedure may be safer in elderly, unfit patients with an ulcer high on the lesser curve.

References

1 BARDHAN KD. Long-term management of duodenal ulcer—a physician's view. In: Baron JH, ed. *Cimetidine in the 80s*. Edinburgh: Churchill Livingstone, 1981: 95–112.

2 CHRISTIANSEN J, JENSEN HE, EJBY-POULDEN P, BARDRAM L, HENRIKSON FW. Prospective controlled vagotomy trial for duodenal ulcer. Primary results, sequelae, acid secretion and recurrence rates two to five years after operation. *Ann Surg* 1981;**193**:49–55.

3 COX DJ, SPENCER J, TINKER J. Clinical results reviewed. In: Williams JA, Cox AG, eds. *After vagotomy*. London: Butterworths: 1969; 119–130.

4 DORRICOTT NJ, MCNEISH AR, ALEXANDER-WILLIAMS J, et al. Prospective randomized multicentre trial of proximal gastric vagotomy or truncal vagotomy and antrectomy for chronic duodenal ulcer: interim results. *Br J Surg* 1978;**65**:152–154.

5 DUTHIE HL. Surgery for gastric ulcer. *World J Surg* 1977;**1**:29–34.

6 DUTHIE HL, BRANSOM CJ. Highly selective vagotomy with excision of the ulcer compared with gastrectomy for gastric ulcer in a randomised trial. *Br J Surg* 1979;**66**:43–45.

7 DUTHIE HL, KWONG NK. Vagotomy or gastrectomy for gastric ulcer? *Br Med J* 1973;**4**:79–81.

8 EASTMAN MC, GEAR MW. Vagotomy and pyloroplasty for gastric ulcers. *Br J Surg* 1979;**66(4)**:238–241.

9 EASTWOOD GL. Does the patient with upper gastro-intestinal bleeding benefit from endoscopy? Reflections and discussion of recent literature. *Dig Dis Sci* 1981;**26(7)**:22–26.

10 FARRIS JM, SMITH GK. Long-term appraisal of the treatment of gastric ulcer in situ by vagotomy and pyloroplasty with a note on the Jaboulay procedure. *Am J Surg* 1973;**126(2)**:292–299.

11 FOSTER DN, MILOSZEWSKI KJA, LOSOWSKY MS. Stigmata of recent haemorrhage in diagnosis and prognosis of upper gastrointestinal bleeding. *Br Med J* 1978;**1**:1173–1177.

12 FRY J. Peptic ulcer—a profile. *Br Med J* 1964;**2**:809–812.

13 GEAR MWL. Proximal gastric vagotomy versus

long-term maintenance treatment with cimetidine for chronic duodenal ulcer: a prospective randomised trial. *Br Med J* 1983;286:98–99.

14 GOLIGHER JC. A technique for highly selective (parietal cell or proximal gastric) vagotomy for duodenal ulcer. *Br J Surg* 1974;61:337–345.

15 GOLIGHER JC, DE DOMBAL FT, DUTHIE HL, et al. Five to eight year results of Leeds-York controlled trials of elective surgery for duodenal ulcer. *Br Med J* 1968;2:781–787.

16 GOLIGHER JC, PULVERAFT CN, IRVIN TT, et al. Five to eight-year results of truncal vagotomy and pyloroplasty for duodenal ulcer. *Br Med J* 1972;1:7–13.

17 GRAY GR, McWHINNIE D, SMITH IS, GILLESPIE G. Five-year study of cimetidine or surgery for severe duodenal ulcer dyspepsia. *Lancet* 1982;i:787–788.

18 GRIEBE J, BUGGE P, GJORUP T, LAURITZEN T, BONNEVIE O, WULFF HR. Long-term prognosis of duodenal ulcer: follow-up study and survey of doctors estimation. *Br Med J* 1977;2:1572–1574.

19 GRIFFIN GE, ORGAN CH JR. The natural history of the perforated duodenal ulcer treated by suture plication. *Ann Surg* 1976;183:382–385.

20 GRIFFITHS WJ, NEUMANN DA, WELSH JD. The visible vessel as an indicator of uncontrolled or recurrent gastrointestinal haemorrhage. *N Engl J Med* 1979;300(25):1411–1413.

21 GROSSMAN MI. Resumé and comment (Veterans Administrative Cooperative Study on Gastric Ulcer). *Gastroenterology* 1971;61:635–640.

22 GUDMAND-HOYER E, BIRGER JK, KRAG E. Prophylactic effect of cimetidine in duodenal ulcer disease. *Br Med J* 1978;1:1095–1097.

23 HILL GL, BARKER MCJ. Anterior highly selective vagotomy with posterior truncal vagotomy: a simple technique for denervating the parietal cell mass. *Br J Surg* 1978;65:702–705.

24 HUNT PS, KORMAN MG, MARSHALL RD, PECK GS, McCANN WJ. Bleeding duodenal ulcer: reduction in mortality with a planned approach. *Br J Surg* 1979;66:633–635.

25 JOHNSTON D. Operative mortality and postoperative morbidity of highly selective vagotomy. *Br Med J* 1975; 545–547.

26 JOHNSTON D, GOLIGHER JC. The influence of the individual surgeon and of the type of vagotomy upon the insulin test after vagotomy. *Gut* 1971;12:963–967.

27 JOHNSTON D, PICKFORD IR, WALKER BE, GOLIGHER JC. Highly selective vagotomy for duodenal ulcer: do hypersecretors need antrectomy? *Br Med J* 1975;1:716–718.

28 JORDAN PH. A prospective study of parietal cell vagotomy and selective vagotomy-antrectomy for treatment of duodenal ulcer. *Ann Surg* 1976;183:619–628.

29 KENNEDY T, JOHNSTON GW, MACRAE KD, SPENCER EF Anne. Proximal gastric vagotomy: interim

30 KOFFMAN CG, ELDER JB, GILLESPIE IE, et al. A prospective randomized trial of vagotomy in chronic duodenal ulceration. *Br J Surg* 1979;66:145–148.

31 KRONBORG O, MADSEN P. A controlled, randomized trial of highly selective vagotomy versus selective vagotomy and pyloroplasty in the treatment of duodenal ulcer. *Gut* 1975;16:268–271.

32 MACKAY C, MACKAY HP. Perforated peptic ulcer in the West of Scotland 1964–1973. *Br J Surg* 1976;63:157–158.

33 MACLEOD IA, MILLS PR, MACKENZIE JF, JOFFE SN, RUSSELL RI, CARTER DC. Neodymium yttrium aluminium garnet laser photocoagulation for major haemorrhage from peptic ulcers and single vessels: a single blind controlled study. *Br Med J* 1983;286:345–348.

34 MADSEN P, KRONBORG O. Recurrent ulcer $5\frac{1}{2}$–8 years after highly selective vagotomy without drainage and selective vagotomy with pyloroplasty. *Scand J Gastroenterol* 1980;15:193–198

35 MAKI T, SHIRATORI T, HATAFUKU T, SUGAWARA K. Pylorus-preserving gastrectomy as an improved operation for gastric ulcer. *Surgery* 1967;61:838–845.

36 MOUNTFORD RA, BROWN P, SALMON PR, ALVARENGA C, NEUMANN CS, READ AE. Gastric cancer detection in gastric ulcer disease. *Gut* 1980;21:9–17.

37 ØRNSHOLT J, AMDRUPE, ANDERSEN D, HØSTRUP H. Århus County vagotomy trial: gastric secretory alterations during the first year after selective vagotomy. *Scand J Gastroent* 1985;18:455–463.

38 POSTLETHWAIT RW. Five year follow-up results of operations for duodenal ulcer. *Surg Gynecol Obstet* 1973;137(3):387–392.

39 REID DA, DUTHIE HL, BRANSOM CJ, JOHNSON AG. Late follow-up of highly selective vagotomy with excision of ulcer compared with Billroth I gastrectomy for benign gastric ulcer. *Br J Surg* 1982;69:605–607.

40 SAKITA T, OGURON Y, TAKASU S, FUKUTOMI H, MIWA T, YOSHIMORI M. Observations on the healing of ulcerations in early gastric cancer. The life cycle of the malignant ulcer. *Gastroenterology* 1971;60:835–844.

41 SALAMAN JR, HARVEY J, DUTHIE HL. Importance of symptoms after highly selective vagotomy. *Br Med J* 1981;283:1438.

42 SAPALA JA, PONKA JL. Operative treatment of benign gastric ulcers. *Am J Surg* 1973;125(1):19–28.

43 SAVAGE A, JONES S. Histological appearances of the gastric mucosa 15–27 years after partial gastrectomy. *J Clin Pathol* 1979;32:179–186.

44 SAWYERS JL, HERRINGTON JL, BURNEY DP. Proximal gastric vagotomy compared with vagotomy and antrectomy and selective gastric vagotomy and pyloroplasty. *Ann Surg* 1977;186:510–515.

45 SCHRUMPF E, STADAAS J, MYREN J, SERCK-HANSSEN

A, AUNE S, OSNES M. Mucosal changes in the gastric stump 20–25 years after partial gastrectomy. *Lancet* 1977;ii:467–469.

46 SMALL WP, CAY EL, DUGARD P, *et al*. Peptic ulcer surgery selection for operation by 'earning'. *Gut* 1969;10:996–1003.

47 STABILE BE, PASSARO E. Recurrent peptic ulcer. *Gastroenterology* 1976;70:124–135.

48 STODDARD CJ, VASSILAKIS JS, DUTHIE HL. Highly selective vagotomy or truncal vagotomy and pyloroplasty for chronic duodenal ulceration: a randomized, prospective clinical study. *Br J Surg* 1978;65:793–796.

49 SWAIN CP, BOWN SG, STOREY DW, KIRKHAM JS, NORTHFIELD TC, SALMON PR. Controlled trial of argon laser photocoagulation in bleeding peptic ulcers. *Lancet*, 1981;ii:1313–1316.

50 TAYLOR TV. Lesser curve vagotomy: an experimental study. *Ann Surg* 1980;191:414–418.

51 WEAVER RM, TEMPLE JG. Proximal gastric vagotomy in patients resistant to cimetidine. *Brit J. Surg*, 1985;72:177–178.

52 WYLLIE JH, ALEXANDER-WILLIAMS J, KENNEDY TL, *et al*. Effect of cimetidine on surgery for duodenal ulcer. *Lancet* 1981;ii:1307.

Chapter 24
Recurrent Ulceration After Surgery

O. KRONBORG

There are many causes of unsuccessful surgery for peptic ulcer. The aetiology of peptic ulcer is partly unknown and the decreased gastric acid secretion that follows ulcer surgery may not always cure the ulcer and prevent recurrence. Other factors, for example genetic, age, sex, race, diet, gastrin, or life-style may be important in ulcer recurrence or healing.

However, peptic ulcer almost never occurs in the presence of anacidity [4], and seldom in patients with a maximal acid secretion of a few mmol/h. This provides the rationale of acid-lowering surgery. However, inadequate gastric resection, incomplete vagotomy, gastrinomas and possibly antral G-cell hyperplasia may result in inadequate decrease of acid and pepsin secretion and surgical failure. Ulcer surgery may result in gastric stasis, but this is not a proven cause of recurrent ulcer in man. Defective protective mechanisms of the gastroduodenal mucosa have not been demonstrated as a cause of recurrence. Environmental factors for example, stress, coffee, tobacco, alcohol and drugs such as non-steroidal anti-inflammatory compounds and steroids may contribute to recurrence of ulcer after gastric surgery. Aetiology of recurrent ulceration after gastric surgery is therefore complex.

Definitions

Types of recurrent ulceration after surgery are in Table 24.1. Gastrojejunal ulcer is located near the anastomosis after a gastrojejunostomy, or a Pólya gastrectomy, while

Table 24.1. Recurrent ulceration and original surgery.

Type of recurrent ulcer	Original surgery
Gastrojejunal ulcer	Gastrojejunostomy $\pm$ vagotomy
	Billroth II
Gastroduodenal ulcer	Billroth I $\pm$ vagotomy
Duodenal ulcer	Vagotomy $\pm$ pyloroplasty
Gastric ulcer	Any
Pyloric ulcer	Vagotomy $\pm$ pyloroplasty
Prepyloric ulcer	Vagotomy $\pm$ pyloroplasty
Jejunal ulcer	Any
Suture ulcer	Any

a gastroduodenal ulcer is found near the anastomosis after a Billroth I resection. A pyloric ulcer is located in the pyloric ring and a prepyloric ulcer in the distal 2–3 cm of the antrum. The former is usually included among duodenal ulcers (DUs), while the latter is considered a gastric ulcer (GU). Suture ulcers are ulcers in relation to visible non-absorbable sutures, such as silk.

Billroth II is used as meaning a 2/3 Pólya gastrectomy with a gastrojejunal anastomosis. Billroth I covers antrectomy and hemigastrectomy with a gastroduodenal anastomosis. An antrectomy may be associated with a gastroduodenostomy or a gastrojejunostomy.

Vagotomy means all types of vagotomy including truncal, selective and highly selective, while drainage may be a pyloroplasty or a gastrojejunostomy.

Incidence

Recurrent ulcer rates (Table 24.2) are generally lower in women than in men after surgery for DU [26, 32], they are similar after surgery for GU. Most recurrences after DU are in the duodenum after vagotomy and drainage procedures and in the anastomosis after partial resection. Recurrences after surgery for GU are located in the stomach, but may be at the anastomosis after resection. GU amounts to 10–20% of all recurrences and is most frequent after vagotomy.

Recurrence rates are significantly lower after Billroth II or antrectomy and vagotomy than after any type of vagotomy, regardless of whether the original ulcer was duodenal [45] or gastric [56]. Ten- to 20-year follow-up studies suggest a figure of

Table 24.2. Average incidence of recurrent ulceration.

Original operation		Recurrence rate %
		%
for *duodenal ulcer*	Gastrojejunostomy	40
	Truncal vagotomy	20
	Truncal vagotomy and drainage	10
	Selective vagotomy and drainage	10
	Highly selective vagotomy	15
	Billroth II resection	5
	Vagotomy and antrectomy	3
for *gastric ulcer*	Wedge resection	20
	Vagotomy and drainage	15
	Highly selective vagotomy ± excision	15
	Billroth I	2
	Billroth II	1
for *prepyloric ulcer*	Highly selective vagotomy	25
	Vagotomy and drainage	10
	Billroth II	5

25% recurrence after vagotomy and drainage [67, 87]. This high incidence of reulceration is only exceeded by those after gastrojejunostomy alone for DU [15]. Recurrence rates after highly selective vagotomy without drainage for DU appear to be higher than after other types of vagotomy with drainage [10, 60, 89] and are much higher when the operation is done for pre-pyloric, or pyloric ulcer [3]. Recurrence rates after surgery for DU + GU may not be higher than after surgery for DU [48]—antrectomy alone for combined ulcers results in 10% recurrences within 1 to 4 years [16].

Aetiology

Aetiology is complex, perhaps because of the heterogeneity of possible causes of the primary peptic ulcer. However, most recurrent ulcers are due to inadequately performed surgery or to the wrong operation being done.

Length of history before surgery and activity of ulcer may adversely influence the risk of recurrent ulcer after surgery [60, 93]. Discriminant function analysis of possible factors influencing risk of recurrence after highly selective and total vagotomy and drainage has demonstrated acid secretion to be the most important variable, accounting for 50% of the total variance, while other factors contributed less [39].

Gastrojejunostomy

Gastrojejunostomy does not diminish secretion of acid and pepsin and the risk of recurrence is very high if it is used for DU. One series [11] demonstrated a low recurrence rate in patients with pyloric stenosis, but acid secretion measurements before surgery had no prognostic value. In another large series recurrence rate was very low (3/139) in patients with a maximal acid secretion before surgery of less than 30 mmol/h [82]. Diversion of acid from the duodenum and regurgitation of bile and pancreatic juice through the stoma neutralizing low, or low normal acid secretion may be effective in preventing recurrence. Unfortunately, this will account for only 25% of the men and 50% of the women with DU. It is unknown why recurrence after gastrojejunostomy happens later than after other types of surgery.

Gastric resection

Inadequate resections of the parietal cell mass and retained antral tissue in the duodenal stump after Billroth II operations increase the risk of recurrence. Hemigastrectomy, or a lesser procedure results in a higher recurrence rate than a 2/3 gastrectomy [25]. Maximal acid secretion is significantly higher in patients with recurrent gastrojejunal ulcer after Billroth II and gastroduodenal ulcer after Billroth I than in those without recurrence [79]. There is no threshold of acid secretion, except anacidity [4], that will protect from recurrence. Peak acid output above 15 mmol/h is found in 50% of recurrences and 10% of non-recurrences after Billroth I and II.

High plasma gastrin concentrations in patients with retained antral tissue in the duodenal stump after Billroth II are the rule, but normal values have also been described. Retained antral tissue after Billroth II is associated with a very high recurrence rate [62]. Retained tissue has been reported in one-third of patients after Billroth II, but is usually less common [14]. The diagnosis can be made by a technetium pertechnetate radioisotope scan [9], but may also be apparent at endoscopy of the afferent loop, or more rarely on a barium meal. Decrease in plasma gastrin concentration during the administration of iv secretin favours the diagnosis of retained antral tissue, rather than the Zollinger-Ellison syndrome [33].

Retained antral tissue after Billroth I may be harmless. The higher risk of recurrent ulcer after Billroth I than after Billroth II procedure for DU may be due to inadequate resection of the parietal cell mass in the former, because the surgeon may be afraid of tension at the gastroduodenal anastomosis after resection [6]. Anatomically determined antrectomy for GU [2], has not been shown to influence the very low recurrence rate after 'blind' antrectomy, but smaller wedge resections with, or without drainage carry high recurrence rates [7]. On the other hand, larger pylorus-preserving resections for GU have resulted in no recurrent ulcers in the hands of the originators [80]; recurrence after surgery for GU may have less to do with acid than DU, but so far studies of mucosal defence and gastric emptying have not shown any factors being responsible for it.

Gastric vagotomy

Incomplete vagotomy, as defined by an acid response to insulin hypoglycaemia, is strongly related to increased risk of recurrent ulcer, regardless of type of vagotomy or location of the original ulcer [47, 48]. At reoperation often one or more major, intact vagal trunks are apparent, suggesting incomplete vagotomy. Regeneration of large vagal nerves does not occur in humans. An acid response of a few mmol/h may indicate small intact nerve fibres, but larger responses mean intact major trunks or several small fibres after selective, or highly selective vagotomy [43, 91]. Re-vagotomy after total vagotomy usually results in a substantial inhibition of acid response to insulin [42]. Incomplete highly selective vagotomy is usually due to incomplete division of the nerves in the cardiac region and at the junction between gastric body and the antrum. More extensive oesophageal dissection results in more complete vagotomies and fewer recurrent ulcers [29, 50]. The use of anatomical landmarks of Latarjet's nerves for preservation of antral innervation after highly selective vagotomy results in incomplete denervation of the lower part of the parietal cell mass in 25% of the patients [70] and these have a higher acid response to sham-feeding than the remaining 75% [66]. However, leaving six instead of 10 cm of the antral lesser curve innervated seems not to influence the recurrence rate [59].

Sham-feeding is a better and safer way of stimulating the vagal acid output than insulin [88], and should replace insulin hypoglycaemia as a test for completeness of vagotomy, despite the lower acid response [49]. Peak acid output to pentagastrin or histamine decreases by 50–60% after any type of vagotomy and remains stable during the next few years, unless there is a large response to insulin in the early post-vagotomy period, in which case a substantial increase of acid secretion and risk of recurrent ulcer will occur [32]. Measurement of peak acid output is, therefore, unsuitable for the evaluation of completeness of vagotomy in the early postoperative period.

It has been suggested that the ratio between insulin (or sham-feeding) and pentagastrin-stimulated secretion measures 'vagal drive' and has predictive value before, as well as after vagotomy in estimating the risk of recurrent ulcer. So far this has not been confirmed after vagotomy [65]. The acid response to insulin increases with time after vagotomy, but patients with no response, or only a small response in the early post-vagotomy period end up with an acid secretion of no more than 5 mmol/h after several years—this is only 20% of the pre-vagotomy response [41, 58]. Nerve regeneration by sprouting may take place, but an early increase of the acid response may be due to neuropraxia during the operation of otherwise intact nerves.

Basal and stimulated secretion of pepsin decreases after vagotomy [92], but is difficult to measure and not usually used in practice. The relation between pentagastrin- and insulin-stimulated acid and pepsin secretions in patients with recurrent ulcer after vagotomy is similar to that in patients with active ulcer (not a scar) before vagotomy [93]. Serum pepsinogen I is also related to acid secretion and risk of recurrent ulcer and the pepsinogen response to Histalog is related to the acid response to insulin [74].

Plasma gastrin concentrations are usually raised after any type of vagotomy. The response to hypoglycaemia is possibly related to the acid response after vagotomy, but does not depend on the vagus alone. High basal gastrins may indicate the existence of the Zollinger-Ellison syndrome, but may also be due to antral G-cell hyperplasia [24], which results in acid hypersecretion and increased risk of recurrent ulcer. The pancreatic polypeptide response to hypoglycaemia is abolished by truncal vagotomy [77], but the role of the peptide in pathogenesis of recurrent ulcer is unknown.

The number of parietal cells, expressed by pre-operative peak acid output, influences the risk of recurrence after vagotomy for DU, but the relationship is still controversial. The risk of recurrence after total vagotomy and pyloroplasty, or after selective vagotomy and pyloroplasty, increases with increasing pre- and post-operative peak acid output [44, 51]. Similar decreases in peak acid output in patients with and without recurrent ulcer suggest that it is the remaining acid output that is the important determinant of recurrence, and not the amount of the inhibition. Selection of surgery for DU, vagotomy in patients with low and normal acid secretion and adding an antrectomy in those with high acid secretion, has resulted in very few recurrences [72], lending support to the statement that only low and normal acid secretors have a small risk of recurrence after vagotomy. With only one exception [97], several series of patients given highly selective vagotomy have demonstrated no relation between pre-operative peak acid output and recurrent ulcer [3, 5]. Still, the risk of recurrence seems to be related to post-operative peak acid output as well as to basal acid secretion and insulin-stimulated secretion [54, 55, 65]. Drainage used with total or selective vagotomy, to avoid gastric stasis probably does not influence recurrence of ulcer; rates are similar with pyloroplasty, or gastrojejunostomy [38]. Highly selective vagotomy originally used with drainage [31] is now used without because of near normal gastric emptying, but it is followed by a high recurrence rate, especially in prepyloric ulcer [3]. The reason for this is not clear; there is a tendency to more recurrences after selective vagotomy and pyloroplasty done for prepyloric ulcer, than after DU, suggesting that decreased acid output is less important than in DU. Adding a pyloroplasty to a highly selective vagotomy does not change acid secretion and it is doubtful whether the risk of recurrence is affected [97]. Highly selective vagotomy has been used instead of total vagotomy and drainage for GU, in order to prevent increased biliary reflux which might predispose to recurrent ulcer, but this has not affected the 15% risk of recurrent GU [20]. Some recurrent GUs are due to incomplete vagotomy [61]. The role of gastric stasis and environmental factors is not clear.

Recurrences after vagotomy and drainage for DU + GU are less frequent than after this operation for GU alone [19, 48]—no recurrences were detected in these two small series despite pre-operative acid secretion being similar to that in DU patients.

Truncal and selective vagotomies carry similar rates of incomplete vagal section and recurrent ulcer [36, 73]. On the other hand, there is a higher risk of problems after highly selective vagotomy [1, 60, 71]. Moreover, follow-up after this procedure is less than 10 years and the recurrence rate may increase further with time [53].

Location of recurrent ulcers after V±P is similar to pre-operative location in most vagotomy and pyloroplasty. Recurrent gastric ulcers constitute some 10% of recurrences after vagotomy and pyloroplasty for DU—these recurrences may be associated with prolonged gastric emptying [1], but also with an incomplete vagotomy.

Vagotomy and antrectomy

Elimination of the vagal and antral stimulation of gastric secretion is the most effective way of preventing recurrence of duodenal and combined ulcers. Antrectomy implies resection of 30–40% of the stomach, including the pylorus. Acid secretion decreases more than after other types of surgery. Even so, an incomplete vagotomy may not always be compensated for by antrectomy (even if it is extended to a hemigastrectomy) and a recurrent ulcer may still follow [18, 68]. Antrectomy alone inhibits the peak acid output by 50%— this may be less than after a complete vagotomy. It is, therefore, not surprising that the recurrence rate after total vagotomy and antrectomy may rise to 10% or more, especially if some operations are done by inexperienced surgeons [90]. The type of vagotomy has no influence on recurrence rate. Billroth I and II reconstructions result in a similarly low recurrence rate [30].

Gastrinoma and hypercalcaemia

Gastrinomas have been found in less than 2% of patients with recurrent ulceration [85], but the increasing use of gastrin assays may increase this figure. Recurrent ulcers due to the Zollinger-Ellison syndrome may be in the jejunum and often perforate. Hyperparathyroidism with hypercalcaemia is an even rarer disease associated with recurrent ulcer. Peptic ulcer is 10 times more frequent in patients with hypercalcaemia.

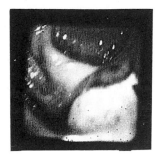

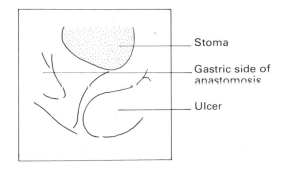

Stoma

Gastric side of anastomosis

Ulcer

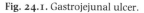

Fig. 24.1. Gastrojejunal ulcer.

Diagnosis

Diagnosis of recurrent ulceration is now usually obtained by endoscopy (Figs 24.1 and 24.2) but some ulcers may be diagnosed at surgery, or even at autopsy. Symptoms are not always helpful in the diagnosis of recurrence. Moderate or severe epigastric pain with no or little vomiting was diagnostic of recurrent ulcer in 14 of 17 patients [35]. However, recurrent ulceration may also be symptomless [21].

Most patients with endoscopically verified recurrence have pain similar to that of the original ulcer [43, 86], but the location may vary. Pain in the left hypochondrium is common in patients with gastric or jejunal ulcer [98]. Less than half of the patients have vomiting, which may indicate stomal obstruction, but not necessarily recurrence. Weight loss, diarrhoea, and faeculent eructations suggest a gastro-jejuno-colic fistula [63] (Fig. 24.3). Symptoms of acute pancreatitis may be present in patients with recurrent ulcers penetrating the pancreas.

Haematemesis, or melaena occurs in 15% and chronic bleeding in another 25% of recurrences [21]. Perforation affects 5–10% of the patients with recurrent problems. The clinical situation is made more complicated by the occurrence of dyspepsia without demonstrable recurrent ulcer in some 15% of patients after different types of

vagotomy [40]. Regurgitation of acid and heartburn may be associated with recurrent ulcer, but this is by no means invariable.

Symptoms of recurrent ulcer may occur from days to many years after surgery and GU may appear later than DU [69]. For example, gastrojejunal ulcer after Billroth II appears within the first two years in two-thirds of the patients, while after simple gastrojejunostomy it may take 10 years, or longer to develop. Recurrence after vagotomy for DU increases steadily with time, a rate of 10% being reached within 10 years. Most of the few recurrences after vagotomy and antrectomy occur within the first two years after the operation. Physical findings do not contribute to the diagnosis of recurrent ulcer, unless complications such as bleeding, perforation, or gastro-jejuno-colic fistulae are present.

Barium meal radiology may miss 50% of recurrent ulcers after resection as well as after vagotomy and drainage [21, 23, 94], and should now be replaced by endoscopy. Gastro-jejuno-colic fistulae are best demonstrated by barium enema (Fig. 24.3).

At endoscopy it is important to biopsy gastric and prepyloric ulcers, to exclude cancer. Tests of gastric acid secretion after pentagastrin stimulation are not useful for diagnostic purposes. However, insulin, or better sham-feeding, tests should be done to identify incomplete vagotomies. All patients with recurrent ulceration should have

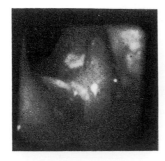

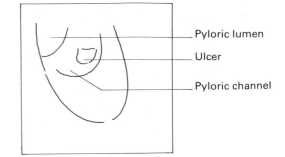

Pyloric lumen
Ulcer
Pyloric channel

Fig. 24.2. Ulcer in a pyloroplasty.

measurements of fasting plasma gastrin and serum calcium concentrations, to diagnose the Zollinger-Ellison syndrome or hyperparathyroidism, either of which may be responsible for recurrent ulcer.

Recurrent ulcers may not be in the same place as the original ulcer. Ulcers recurrent after vagotomy for DU are most frequently located in the duodenum, but may be in the stomach [81] or in the prepyloric region [31]. Gastrojejunal ulcers are usually in the jejunum and most often in the distal limb [98]. Multiple recurrent ulcers have been reported in some 10% of patients with recurrence [76].

Suture ulcers are detected by endoscopy (Fig. 24.4) [83]—relationships to clinical symptoms are not clear and sutures may be visible endoscopically without any ulcer. The increasing use of absorbable sutures may eliminate this problem.

Treatment

Medical treatment has gained proponents after the introduction of histamine H_2-receptor antagonists. On the other hand, conventional therapy with diet, antacids and anticholinergics carries an ulcer-related mortality of 11% and a further relapse rate of 40% [85] and is not to be recommended.

Anastomotic ulcers after Billroth I and II heal after 8 weeks treatment with cimetidine 1 g daily in 85–100% of the patients and most of these are symptom-free before healing is complete [17, 22, 28]. However, relapses occur rapidly after stopping the drug. During maintenance therapy with cimetidine 800 mg daily, 15% relapse within the first year [22].

Recurrent ulcers after vagotomy heal in 50–90% of the patients after 4–6 weeks' treatment with cimetidine [12, 39, 96], but relapse in most after stopping therapy. During maintenance therapy 15–30% relapse during the first one to two years and nearly all relapse after stopping cimetidine. Increasing the maintenance dose to 1 g daily has not resulted in a lower recurrence rate in the first year [75]. Recurrence rates during more than two years' maintenance therapy are not known yet, but patients will probably stop the treatment in increasing numbers and the risk of relapses will increase. Use of short courses of cimetidine or ranitidine during exacerbations may be attractive in otherwise fit patients. H_2-receptor antagonists have a place as a means of healing the recurrent ulcer to buy time in order to make subsequent surgery easier and less risky. Postponing surgery for years may increase the risk not only of surgery, but also because of ulcer complications such as haemorrhage, or perforation.

The final assessment of H_2-receptor antagonists in the treatment of ulcers recurrent after surgery must await the results of randomized trials, comparing these drugs with surgical treatment [39, 84].

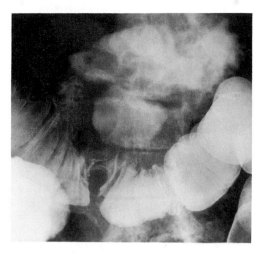 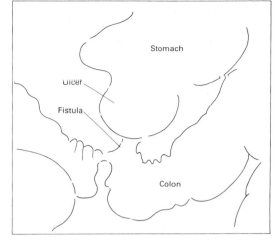

Fig. 24.3. Gastro-jejuno-colic fistula.

Surgical treatment

Surgical treatment (Table 24.3) of recurrent ulcer after surgery is more effective and is followed by a lower mortality than conventional medical therapy.

Gastrojejunal ulcer after gastrojejunostomy alone may be treated successfully by a 2/3 Pólya gastrectomy in 90% of the patients [6, 27, 98], but the operative mortality is 2–3% [85]. Vagotomy may result in more recurrences, but the mortality is low [95]. Closing the gastrojejunostomy and performing a highly selective vagotomy decreases the unwanted effects of vagotomy, but may carry a higher re-recurrence risk. Total and selective vagotomy should probably only be done in poor risk patients and not in those with acid hypersecretion. Vagotomy and antrectomy is followed by a very low risk of new recurrence (1–2%), but the mortality is 1–2%. A gastro-jejuno-colic fistula is treated with resection of the antrum and the fistula and vagotomy.

Vagotomy for gastrojejunal ulcer after Billroth II resection carries a risk of reulceration of 10% [14, 27], and a mortality of 0–1% [14, 98]. The vagotomy may be done through the chest with the same low mortality as abdominal vagotomy [52]. Re-re-

section with vagotomy may diminish the small risk of recurrence further, but the mortality can be 7%. Re-resection alone results in a recurrence rate of 20% [85]. Reports of excision of retained antral tissue in the duodenal stump are anecdotal but usually successful, vagotomy is probably an adequate treatment for these patients [14, 78].

The most effective treatment of recurrent ulcer after vagotomy and drainage or highly selective vagotomy is re-vagotomy and antrectomy, which inhibits acid secretion more than re-vagotomy alone and is followed by new recurrences in no more than 1–2% [37, 43], irrespective of whether Billroth I or II reconstruction is used. Both reconstructions are associated with severe dumping and bile regurgitation in at least 5–10% [64]. Re-vagotomy may be difficult to do because of dense adhesions. Omitting this part of the operation in patients with no acid response to insulin has resulted in 6% of new recurrences after antrectomy alone [39]. Re-vagotomy alone is followed by high recurrence rates in spite of the presence of acid response to insulin before re-vagotomy [21, 64] or apparently intact vagal trunks after previous total vagotomy in most patients [34]. Re-vagotomy

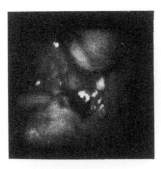

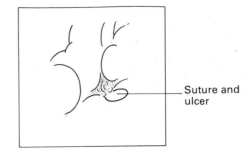

Suture and ulcer

Fig. 24.4. Suture ulcer.

alone in patients with incomplete vagotomy [91], which seems a logical procedure, has not been fully evaluated, but a large parietal cell mass increases the risk of recurrence after total or selective vagotomy regardless of the completeness of vagotomy [44, 51].

Repeating a highly selective vagotomy is not attractive in most patients having had this operation before [57].

Two-thirds gastrectomy for recurrence after vagotomy must be avoided, as it carries at least the same re-recurrence rate as

Table 24.3. Surgical treatment of recurrent ulceration.

Recurrent ulcer	Treatment
Gastrojejunal ulcer after gastrojejunostomy	Selective or truncal vagotomy ± antrectomy Billroth II
Gastrojejunal ulcer after gastrojejunostomy and vagotomy	Revagotomy + antrectomy Billroth II
Gastrojejunal ulcer after Billroth II	Selective or truncal vagotomy ± resection
Gastroduodenal ulcer after Billroth	Selective or truncal vagotomy ± resection
Gastroduodenal ulcer after Billroth II + vagotomy	Revagotomy ± re-resection
Duodenal ulcer after vagotomy ± pyloroplasty	Revagotomy ± antrectomy Antrectomy
GU after resection	Vagotomy ± Re-resection
GU after vagotomy ± drainage	Antrectomy
GU after excision	Antrectomy
Pyloric and prepyloric ulcer after vagotomy ± pyloroplasty	Revagotomy ± antrectomy Antrectomy
Suture ulcer	Removal of sutures

re-vagotomy and antrectomy; mortality and late untoward effects are more frequent [13, 14]. It seems rational to treat the few re-recurrences after vagotomy and antrectomy with re-vagotomy and/or re-resection, after exclusion of the Zollinger-Ellison syndrome which may demand a different approach.

Gastric recurrence after vagotomy for GU may be treated with antrectomy including the ulcer [20], while the very rare recurrent GU after antrectomy may be treated with further resection, with vagotomy. The results of these operations are only known from small series, but mortality and side-effects are similar to those reported after surgery for recurrent DU.

All recurrent ulcers carry a mortality because of risk of severe bleeding and perforation and this must be added to the mortality of one or more reoperations. The risk of recurrent ulcer should therefore be reduced to a minimum and vagotomy and antrectomy should be preferred after previous vagotomy or drainage alone, while vagotomy alone may be sufficient after previous resection, provided the resection was no less than a complete antrectomy.

Prevention

Vagotomy is used more often and gastrojejunal ulceration after Billroth II should, therefore, be rarer. However, Pólya gastrectomy is still used despite its well known untoward sequelae; the risk of recurrence may be diminished by a larger resection, but then the risk of unwanted effects also increases. Resection distal to the pylorus eliminates the risk of leaving antral tissue in the duodenal stump. The risk of gastrojejunal ulcer after gastrojejunostomy alone can be diminished by the use of this operation only in patients with low acid secretion and severe pyloric stenosis.

The largest problem is how to prevent an incomplete vagotomy. Several intra-operative tests have been designed [46], but none has shown a significant decrease of recurrence in randomized studies with a long follow-up. The main objection against intra-operative testing is that the trauma of the vagus caused by the dissection may account for false negative intra-operative tests [8]. An extensive dissection of the cardiac region results in more complete vagotomies and fewer recurrences [29, 50]. Vagotomy should be learned from an expert who has a known low recurrence rate and should not be done by a surgeon who is doing it only occasionally. Post-operative tests for completeness of vagotomy should be done during training of vagotomists, thus supplying a feedback and making the surgeons change their technique if faulty. The acid response to insulin is higher when highly selective vagotomy is done by surgeons inexperienced in this operation [46].

Total and selective vagotomy should be avoided in patients with hypersecretion, while it is still a matter of dispute whether this precaution is necessary for highly selective vagotomy. Some, but not all surgeons would advise pentagastrin tests before total and selective vagotomy, and they can be recommended as screening for the Zollinger-Ellison syndrome, if plasma gastrin measurements are not easily available. The latter should always be done in patients with recurrent ulcer. A low peak acid output (PAO) may allow a gastrojejunostomy to be done without a vagotomy.

The best way of preventing recurrence after surgery for peptic ulcer is to do a complete vagotomy and antrectomy, but adverse effects are more frequent and mortality is higher than after highly selective vagotomy alone.

Recurrence of GU is usually prevented by antrectomy alone, but because of the lower mortality, vagotomy may be preferred, in spite of a higher risk of recurrence. Excision alone, or wedge excision should be avoided. Prepyloric ulcer should not be treated with highly selective vagotomy without drainage.

It is customary to recommend complete or partial abstinence from alcohol, tobacco, coffee and anti-inflammatory drugs to decrease the risk of recurrent ulcer after gastric surgery. Some of these recommendations may be valid and some (smoking) are justified on general grounds, but there are no systematic data at the moment to support them.

References

1 AMDRUP E, BRANDSBORG M, BRANDSBORG O, LOEV-GREEN NA. Inter-relationship between serum gastrin concentration, gastric acid secretion and gastric emptying rate in recurrent peptic ulcer. *World J Surg* 1979;3:235–240.

2 AMDRUP E, KRAGELUND E, JENSEN HE. Precise antrectomy for gastric ulcer. *Acta Chir Scand* 1972; 138:517-520.

3 ANDERSEN D, AMDRUP E, HOESTRUP H, SOERENSEN FH. The Aarhus County vagotomy trial: Trends in the problem of recurrent ulcer after parietal cell vagotomy and selective gastric vagotomy with drainage. *World J Surg* 1982;6:86–92.

4 BARON JH. The clinical use of gastric function tests. *Scand J Gastroenterol* [Suppl 6] 1970;5:9–46.

5 BLACKETT RL, JOHNSTON D. Recurrent ulceration after highly selective vagotomy for duodenal ulcer. *Br J Surg* 1981;68:705–710.

6 BOLES RS, MARSHALL SF, BERSOUX RV. Follow-up study of 127 patients with stomal ulcer. *Gastroenterology* 1960;38:763–766.

7 BUHL O, CAMPBELL UD. Gastric ulcer treated with segmental resection without pyloroplasty. *Acta Chir Scand* 1974;140:528–530.

8 CARTER DC, WHITFIELD HN, MACLEOD IB. The effect of vagotomy on gastric adaptation. *Gut* 1972;13:874–879.

9 CHAUDHURI TK, SHIRAZI SS, CONDON RE. Radioisotope scan—a possible aid in differentiating retained gastric antrum from Zollinger-Ellison syndrome in patients with recurrent peptic ulcer. *Gastroenterology* 1973;65:697.

10 CHRISTIANSEN J, JENSEN HE, EJBY-POULSEN P, BARDRAM L, HENRIKSEN FW. Prospective controlled vagotomy trial for duodenal ulcer. *Ann Surg* 1981;193:49–55.

11 CLARK DH, KAY AW. The results of partial gastrectomy and selected gastrojejunostomy in treatment of duodenal ulcer. *Scot Med J* 1959;4:158–162.

12 CLARK CG, BOULOS PB. Cimetidine and the gastric surgeon. *World J Surg* 1979;3:745–752.

13 CLARK CG, WARD MWN. Polya gastrectomy for recurrent ulceration following vagotomy. *Br J Surg* 1982;69:259–260.

14 CLEATOR IGM, HOLUBITSKY IB, HARRISON RC. Anastomotic ulceration. *Ann Surg* 1974;179:339–351.

15 COOPER WA. End results in the treatment of peptic ulcer by posterior gastro-enterostomy. *Surgery* 1946;23:425.

16 DAVIS Z, VERHEYDEN CN, VAN HEERDEN JA, JUDD ES. The surgically treated chronic gastric ulcer: an extended follow-up. *Ann Surg* 1977;185:205–209.

17 DELLEFAVE GF, PAOLUZI P, BERGONZI L, DEMAGISTRIS L, SPARVOLI C, CARRATU R. Cimetidine and postgastrectomy recurrent ulcer. *Rend Gastroenterol* 1977;9:150.

18 DORRICOTT NJ, McNEISH AR, ALEXANDER-WILLIAMS J, *et al.* Prospective randomized multicentre trial of proximal gastric vagotomy or truncal vagotomy and antrectomy for chronic duodenal ulcer: interim results. *Br J Surg* 1978;65:152–154.

19 DOUGLAS MC, DUTHIE HL. Vagotomy for gastric ulcer combined with duodenal ulcer. *Br J Surg* 1971;58:721–724.

20 DUTHIE HL, BRANSOM CJ. Highly selective vagotomy with excision of the ulcer compared with gastrectomy for gastric ulcer in a randomized trial. *Br J Surg* 1979;66:43–45.

21 FAWCETT AN, JOHNSTON D, DUTHIE HL. Revagotomy for recurrent ulcer after vagotomy and drainage for duodenal ulcer. *Br J Surg* 1969;56:111–116.

22 FESTEN HPM, LAMERS CBH, DRIESSEN WMM, VAN-TONGEREN JHM. Cimetidine in anastomotic ulceration after partial gastrectomy. *Gastroenterology* 1979;77:83–85.

23 FREDENS M, KRONBORG O, MADSEN P, PALBOEL J. Radiography in the diagnosis of recurrent duodenal ulceration following vagotomy and pyloroplasty. *Scand J Gastroenterol* 1971;6:559–561.

24 GANGULI PC, POLAK JM, PEARSE AGE, ELDER JB, HEGARTY M. Antral gastrin-cell hyperplasia in peptic-ulcer disease. *Lancet* 1974;i:583–586.

25 GOBBEL WG, SHOULDERS HH. Gastric resection. In: Postlethwait RW, ed. *Results of surgery for peptic ulcer*. Philadelphia; WB Saunders: 142–168.

26 GOLIGHER JC, PULVERTAFT CN, DEDOMBAL FT, *et al.* 5–8 year result of Leeds/York controlled trial of elective surgery for duodenal ulceration. *Br J Surg* 1968;2:781–787.

27 GREEN WER, KENNEDY T, HASSARD T, SPENCER EFA. Management of recurrent peptic ulceration. *Br J Surg* 1978;65:422–426.

28 GUGLER R, ROHNER HG, KOLLMEIER J, MIEDERER S, MÖKEL W. Recurrent and stomal ulceration after partial gastrectomy. In: Baron JH, ed. *Cimetidine in the 80s*. Edinburgh: Churchill Livingstone, 1981;58–62.

29 HALLENBECK GA, GLEYSTEEN JJ, ALDRETE JS, SLAUGHTER RL. Proximal gastric vagotomy: effects of two

operative techniques on clinical and gastric secretory results. *Ann Surg* 1976;184:435–442.

30 HERRINGTON JL. Truncal vagotomy with antrectomy—1976.*Surg Clin North Am* 1976;56:1335–1347.

31 HOLLE F, HART W. Neue Wege der Chirurgie des Gastroduodenalulkus *Med Klin* 1967;62.441–450.

32 HOLST-CHRISTENSEN J, HANSEN OH, PEDERSEN T, KRONBORG O. Recurrent ulcer after proximal gastric vagotomy for duodenal and prepyloric ulcer. *Br J Surg* 1977;64:42–46.

33 INGRAM G, HERRING DW, VENABLES CW, et al. Plasma gastrin activity in patients with recurrent peptic ulceration. *Br J Surg* 1971;58:298–300.

34 JULER GL, DAGRADI AE, STEMPIEN SJ, COMBS RC. Evaluation of recurrent duodenal ulcer after vagotomy-pyloroplasty. *Am J Surg* 1976; 132:243–248.

35 KEIGHLEY MRB, HOARE AM, HORROCKS JC, DeDOMBAL FT, ALEXANDER-WILLIAMS J. A symptomatic discriminant to identify recurrent ulcer in patients with dyspepsia after gastric surgery. *Lancet* 1976;i:278–279.

36 KENNEDY T, CONNELL AM, LOVE AHG, MacRAE KD, SPENCER EFA. Selective or truncal vagotomy? Five-year results of a double-blind, randomized, controlled trial. *Br J Surg* 1973;60:944–948.

37 KENNEDY T, GREEN WER. Stomal and recurrent ulceration: medical or surgical management? *Am J Surg* 1980;139:18–21.

38 KENNEDY T, JOHNSTON GW, LOVE AHG, CONNELL AM, SPENCER EFA. Pyloroplasty versus gastrojejunostomy results of a double-blind, randomized, controlled trial. *Br J Surg* 1973;60:949–953.

39 KOO J, LAM SK, ONG GB. Cimetidine versus surgery for recurrent ulcer after gastric surgery. *Ann Surg* 1982;195:406–412.

40 KRONBORG P. Truncal vagotomy and drainage in 500 patients with duodenal ulcer. *Scand J Gastroenterol* 1971;6:501–509.

41 KRONBORG O. The stability of the insulin test result after truncal vagotomy and drainage for duodenal ulcer. *Scand J Gastroenterol* 1971;6:637–644.

42 KRONBORG O. *An evaluation of the insulin test.* Copenhagen: FADLs forlag, 1972.

43 KRONBORG O. A follow-up of patients operated upon for recurrence after vagotomy and drainage for duodenal ulcer. *Scand J Gastroenterol* 1973;8:123–128.

44 KRONBORG O. Gastric acid secretion and risk of recurrence of duodenal ulcer within 6–8 years after vagotomy and drainage. *Gut* 1974;15:714–719.

45 KRONBORG O. Surgical treatment of duodenal ulcer. *Acta Gastroenterol Belg* 1978;41:435–441.

46 KRONBORG O. Present status of tests of completeness of vagotomy. In: Pichlmaier H, Junginger T, eds. *Selektive proximale Vagotomie.* Stuttgart: Thieme, 1979:72–79.

47 KRONBORG O. Completeness of vagotomy: anatomy, pathophysiology and clinical consequences. *Scand J Gastroenterol* 1981;16:577–580.

48 KRONBORG O. Truncal vagotomy and drainage for gastric ulcer. In: Baron J, ed. *Vagotomy in modern surgical practice* London: Butterworths, 1982.

49 KRONBORG O, ANDERSEN D. Acid response to sham feeding as a test for completeness of vagotomy. *Scand J Gastroenterol* 1980;15:119–121.

50 KRONBORG O, JOERGENSEN PM, HOLST-CHRISTENSEN J. Influence of different techniques of proximal gastric vagotomy upon risk of recurrent duodenal ulcer and gastric acid secretion. *Acta Chir Scand* 1977;243:53–56.

51 KRONBORG O, MADSEN P. Relationships between gastric acid secretion and recurrent duodenal ulcer after selective vagotomy and pyloroplasty in men. *Scand J Gastroenterol* 1976;11:465–469.

52 LEHR L, PICHLMAYR R. Low-risk thoracic vagotomy for anastomotic ulceration *World J Surg* 1982;6:93–97.

53 LIAVAAG I, ROLAND M. A seven-year follow-up of proximal gastric vagotomy Clinical results. *Scand J Gastroenterol* 1979;14:49–56.

54 LIAVAAG I, ROLAND M. A seven-year follow-up of proximal gastric vagotomy: Secretory studies. *Scand J Gastroenterol* 1979;14:409–416.

55 LIEDBERG G, OSCARSON J. Selective proximal vagotomy: short-term follow-up of 80 patients. *Scand J Gastroenterol [Suppl 20]* 1973;8:12.

56 LIEDBERG G, OSCARSON J. Selective proximal vagotomy and gastric resection for gastric ulcer. In: Pichlmaier H, Junginger T, eds. *Selektive proximale Vagotomie.* Stuttgart: Thieme, 1979:61–63.

57 LIEDBERG G, QVARFORT P. Reoperation for recurrence after selective proximal vagotomy. In: Pichlmaier H, Junginger T, eds. *Selektive proximale Vagotomie.* Stuttgart: Thieme, 1979:27–28.

58 LYNDON PJ, GREENALL MJ, SMITH RB, GOLIGHER JC, JOHNSTON D. Serial insulin tests over a five-year period after highly selective vagotomy for duodenal ulcer. *Gastroenterology* 1975;69:1188–1195.

59 LYNDON PJ, JOHNSTON D, GREENALL MJ, BAKRAN A, GOLIGHER JC. Interim results of a prospective randomized trial of highly selective vagotomy versus a more proximal type of gastric vagotomy for duodenal ulcer: clinical and secretory findings. *Gut* 1975;16:829.

60 MADSEN P, KRONBORG O. Recurrent ulcer 5½–8 years after highly selective vagotomy without drainage and selective vagotomy with pyloroplasty. *Scand J Gastroenterol* 1980;15:193–199.

61 MADSEN P, KRONBORG O, HANSEN OH, PEDERSEN T. Billroth I gastric resection versus truncal vagotomy and pyloroplasty in the treatment of gastric ulcer. *Acta Chir Scand* 1976;142:151–153.

62 McKITTRICK LS, MOORE FD, WARREN R. Complications and mortality in subtotal gastric resection for

duodenal ulcer: report on two-stage procedure. *Ann Surg* 1944;**120**:531–561.

63 MEYER KA, STEIN IF. Management of recurrent peptic ulcer. *Surg Gynecol Obstet.* 1952;**94**:35–45.

64 MUSCROFT TJ, TAYLOR EW, DEANE SA, ALEXANDER-WILLIAMS J. Reoperation for recurrent peptic ulceration. *Br J Surg* 1981;**68**:75–76.

65 NIELSEN HO, BEKKER C, KRONBORG O, ANDERSEN D. Gastric acid response to sham feeding and pentagastrin before and after parietal cell vagotomy in patients with duodenal ulcer. *Scand J Gastroenterol* 1982;**17**:133–136.

66 NIELSEN HO, MUNOZ JD, KRONBORG O, ANDERSEN D. The antrum in duodenal ulcer patients. *Scand J Gastroenterol* 1981;**16**:491–495.

67 NOBLES ER. Vagotomy and gastroenterostomy 15-year follow-up of 175 patients. *Am Surg* 1966;**32**:177–182.

68 NYLAMO EI, INBERG MV, NELIMARKKA OI. The insulin test and recurrence of ulcer after vagotomy and antral resection or drainage. *Acta Chir Scand* 1980;**146**:127–132.

69 O'LEARY JP, WOODWARD ER, HOLLENBECK JI, DRAGSTEDT LR. Vagotomy and drainage procedure for duodenal ulcer: the results of seventeen years experience *Ann Surg* 1976;**183**:613–617.

70 POPPEN B. Parietal cell vagotomy. *Acta Chir Scand* [Suppl] 1978:484.

71 RAY DJ, KOFFMAN CG. Four-year results of prospective trial for duodenal ulcer (TVP v. HSV). *Br J Surg* 1981;**68**:889.

72 ROBBS JV. Prospective evaluation of selection for operation for duodenal ulcer based on acid secretory studies. *S Afr Med J* 1980;**58**:151–153.

73 ROBBS JV, BANK S, MARKS IN, LOUW JH. A comparison between selective and truncal vagotomy with drainage in duodenal ulceration. *S Afr Med J* 1973;**47**:1291–1396.

74 SAMLOFF IM, SECRIST DM, PASSARO E. The effect of betazole on serum group I pepsinogen levels: studies in symptomatic patients with and without recurrent ulcer after vagotomy and gastric resection or drainage. *Gastroenterology* 1976;**70**:1997–2013.

75 SAUNDERS JHB, CARGILL JM, PEDEN NR, et al. Cimetidine for ulcer recurring after surgery. *Br Med J* 1978;**1**:1619.

76 SCHIRMER BD, MEYERS WC, HANKS JB, KORTZ WJ, JONES RS, POSTLETHWAIT RW. Marginal ulcer: A difficult surgical problem. *Ann Surg* 1982;**195**:653–661.

77 SCHWARTZ TW, HOLST JJ, FAHRENKRUG J, et al. Vagal, Cholinergic regulation of pancreatic polypeptide secretion. *J Clin Invest* 1978;**61**:781–789.

78 SCOBIE BA, McGILL DB, PRIESTLEY JT, ROVELSTAD RA. Excluded gastric antrum stimulating the Zollinger-Ellison syndrome. *Gastroenterology* 1964;**47**:184–187.

79 SCOBIE BA, ROVELSTAD RA. Anastomotic ulcer: significance of the augmented histamine test. *Gastroenterology* 1965;**48**:318–325.

80 SEKINE T, SATO T, MAKI T, SHIRATORI T. Pylorus-preserving gastrectomy for gastric ulcer-one-to nine-year follow-up study. *Surgery* 1975;**77**:92–99.

81 SLANEY G, BEVAN PG, BROOKE BN. Vagotomy for chronic peptic ulcer. A five-year follow-up. *Lancet* 1956;**i**:221–224.

82 SMALL WP, BRUCE J, FALCONER CWA, SIRCUS V, SMITH AN. The results of a policy of selective surgical treatment of duodenal ulcer. *Br J Surg* 1967;**54**:838–841.

83 SMALL WP, SMITH AN, FALCONER CWA, SIRCUS W, BRUCE J. Suture line ulcer after gastric surgery. *Am J Surg* 1968;**115**:477–481.

84 SORGI M, ALEXANDER-WILLIAMS J, DONOVAN I, et al. Prospective trial of treatment of recurrent ulcer. *Gastroenterology* 1982;**82**:1186.

85 STABILE BE, PASSARO E. Recurrent peptic ulcer. *Gastroenterology* 1976;**70**:124–135.

86 STEINBERG DM, GREEN G, TOYE DKM, ALEXANDER-WILLIAMS J. The accuracy of methods of diagnosis in patients with suspected recurrent ulcer after vagotomy *Aust NZ J Surg* 1975;**45**:252–256.

87 STEMPIEN SJ, DAGRADI AE, LEE ER, et al. Status of duodenal ulcer patients 10 years or more after vagotomy-pyloroplasty. *Gastroenterology* 1970;**58**:997.

88 STENQUIST B, KNUTSON U, OLBE L. Gastric acid responses to adequate and modified sham feeding and to insulin hypoglycaemia in duodenal ulcer patients. *Scand J Gastroenterol* 1978;**13**:357–362.

89 STOREY DW, BOULOS PB, WARD MWN, CLARK CG. Proximal gastric vagotomy after five years. *Gut* 1981;**22**:702–704.

90 SVENSSON AA. Vagotomy with antrum resection. *Acta Chir Scand* 1974;**140**:50–56.

91 TAYLOR TV, PEARSON KW, TORRANCE B. Revagotomy for recurrent peptic ulceration. *Br J Surg* 1977;**64**:477–481.

92 VENABLES CW. The value of a combined pentagastrin/insulin test in studies of stomal ulceration. *Br J Surg* 1970;**57**:757–761.

93 VENABLES CW. The value of endoscopy and secretion studies in the management of recurrent symptoms after surgery for peptic ulceration. *J R Coll Surg Edinb* 1973;**18**:297.

94 WALTERS W, CHANCE DP, BERKSON J. A comparison of vagotomy and gastric resection for gastrojejunal ulceration: a follow-up study of 301 cases. *Surg Gynecol Obstet* 1955;**100**:1–10.

95 WALTERS W, PRIESTLEY JT, BELDING HH. Vagotomy in the treatment of gastrojejunal ulceration. *JAMA* 1952;**148**:803–808.

96 WASTELL C. The treatment of recurrent ulceration after vagotomy with cimetidine. 1978. In: *Cimetidine, The Westminster Hospital Symposium 1978.* Edinburgh: Churchill Livingstone, 84–90.

97 WASTELL C, COLIN J, WILSON T, WALKER E, GLEESON J, ZEEGEN R. Prospectively randomised trial of proximal gastric vagotomy either with or without pyloroplasty in treatment of uncomplicated duodenal ulcer. *Br Med J* 1977;2:851–853.

98 WYCHULIS AR, PRIESTLEY JT, FOULK WT. A study of 360 patients with gastrojejunal ulceration. *Surg Gynecol Obstet* 1966;122:89–99.

Chapter 25
Sequelae of Gastric Surgery

F. SABBATINI, J. R. SIEWERT AND A. L. BLUM

Sequelae of gastric surgery may occur even if the operation was performed correctly and for the correct indications. Every surgical intervention so far devised for the treatment of peptic ulcer deranges gastric function [1]. Nearly all patients experience some adverse effects during the first weeks or months following surgery but, in most patients, the symptoms decrease with time, with psychological and physiological adaptation. For these reasons results of gastric operations should be assessed six months, or longer, after surgery. If symptoms persist, a post-surgical syndrome is diagnosed. Attempts at prediction before surgery whether persisting symptoms will develop [43], have not been widely adopted.

Sequelae of gastric surgery are classified in Table 25.1. The occurrence of only one type of post-surgical syndrome is uncommon. The patient often presents with a combination of bilious vomiting in the fasting state, a small reservoir syndrome with epigastric fullness, early post-cibal dumping, and intermittent diarrhoea. A few syndromes are associated with a particular operation—the small reservoir syndrome occurs only after partial gastric resection, the afferent loop syndrome only after a Billroth II procedure. Most syndromes may occur after any type of surgery—diarrhoea, for example, may follow vagotomy or partial gastric resection.

The first and most important step in the assessment of a patient with post-surgical complaints is a detailed history. Table 25.2 shows how, using the symptoms of epigastric pain or discomfort, the sequelae may be classified. Many laboratory tests are often used, but in most cases they are of little practical value in the planning of treatment.

The incidence of persisting symptoms after gastric surgery is difficult to assess—their severity decreases with time. The diagnosis is mainly based on subjective criteria

Table 25.1. Classification of sequelae of gastric surgery.

Syndromes that may follow any type of gastric surgery.

Frequent

    Early dumping
    Bilious vomiting
    Gastric stasis
    Diarrhoea
    Weight loss
    Late metabolic sequelae

Rare

    Malabsorption
    Late dumping
    Reflux oesophagitis
    Phytobezoars
    Gastric mycosis

Controversial

    Postsurgical gastric cancer
    Postsurgical gastritis
    Postsurgical cholelithiasis

Syndromes that may follow particular operations.

After vagotomy

    Postoperative dysphagia
    Gastric necrosis

After partial gastric resection

    Small reservoir
    Stomal invagination
    Afferent loop syndrome
    Retained antrum

Table 25.2. Differential diagnosis of epigastric discomfort or pain.

Epigastric discomfort and/or pain experienced during			Bilious vomiting	Recurrent ulcer	Outlet obstruction	Small reservoir	Early dumping
Fasting	Relieved by	bile vomiting	+				
		food vomiting			+		
		eating		+			
		antacids		+			
	Worsened by	eating	+		+	+	
		antacids	+				
After meals	Relieved by	bile vomiting	+				
		food vomiting	+		+	+	
		antacids		+			
		lying down					+
	Worsened by	antacids	+				
		lying down	+				
Fasting and after meals	Relieved by	bile vomiting	+				
		eating		+			
		antacids		+			
	Worsened by	eating	+		+	+	

and therefore dependent on the questions asked and on the interpretation of the answers and, finally, on the way that an interviewer deals with a typical case of a mixed syndrome. The most often used assessment of the overall outcome of surgery is the grading system according to Visick.

Syndromes following any type of gastric surgery

Frequent syndromes

Early dumping

Early dumping is caused by very rapid gastric evacuation of food—the gastric contents are 'dumped' into the small bowel.

In the first weeks after any type of gastric surgery nearly all patients experience mild to severe dumping. The proportion of patients in whom dumping symptoms persist for more than six months varies between 15% to 50% after partial gastric resection, 10% to 30% after vagotomy and drainage procedures, and 2% to 7% after proximal gastric vagotomy respectively [4, 25, 61].

Pathophysiology (Fig. 25.1)

Accelerated gastric emptying after gastric surgery occurs because pyloric function is lost or impaired after partial gastric resection, gastroenterostomy, or pyloroplasty, or because denervation of the proximal stomach by vagotomy impairs receptive relaxation of the gastric body. Rapid gastric emptying of food leads to the formation of hypertonic chyme in the small intestine. This is particularly prominent when hypertonic solutions are ingested, or when food constituents such as carbohydrates are dissolved in small volumes of gastric and intestinal juice, or when starch is rapidly split into osmotically active fragments by amylase. Why hypertonic chyme produces dumping symptoms is not exactly clear. It has been postulated that intestinal distension triggers autonomic reflexes and then symptoms such as tachycardia and sweating. Dumping symptoms may be reproduced by balloon distension of the jejunum [41]. Another postulated mechanism is systemic hypovolaemia, following rapid equi-

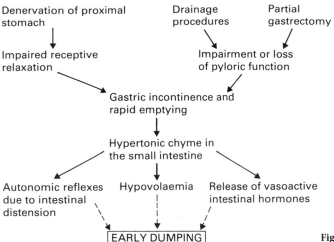

Fig. 25.1. Pathophysiology of early dumping.

libration between hypertonic intraluminal and isotonic extraluminal fluid compartments. However, hypovolaemia is not likely to be the principal cause of dumping, because the syndrome occurs even if blood volume is maintained by intravenous infusion [9]. Hypertonic chyme releases gut regulatory peptides such as enteroglucagon, neurotensin and vasoactive intestinal peptide from the small intestine and this may lead to symptoms of dumping [5, 6, 15, 30, 63].

Clinical features

Early dumping is characterized by abdominal and systemic symptoms (Table 25.3)

during the first 30 minutes after a meal. Most patients complain of abdominal and systemic symptoms, but abdominal symptoms may occur without systemic symptoms and vice versa.

The diagnosis of a dumping syndrome is suggested by a history of early post-cibal symptoms provoked mostly by sweets, improved by lying down and by the absence of symptoms while fasting. Symptoms beginning more than half an hour after a meal do not suggest early dumping. Epigastric fullness during a meal, followed by pain and relieved by vomiting suggests a small reservoir syndrome, rather than dumping. Vomiting may occur during dumping, but if vomiting is the main problem and occurs

Table 25.3. Symptoms of early dumping.

	Abdominal symptoms		Systemic symptoms	Relation to food intake
Main symptoms	Epigastric and/or abdominal fullness	and/or	Sweating Faintness Palpitations	Early post-cibal symptoms, provoked mostly by sweet food, improved by lying down
Additional symptoms	Nausea, vomiting, eructations, epigastric pain, abdominal cramps, diarrhoea	and/or	Headache Flushing Pallor	No symptoms in fasting state

also while fasting, or if the vomited material is heavily bile-stained, bilious vomiting, rather than dumping should be suspected.

Provocation tests have been used in the diagnosis of the dumping syndrome. Symptoms may be provoked by instillation of hypertonic glucose into the small bowel [22]. After the ingestion of a hypertonic solution of radiolabelled glucose, rapid gastric emptying, low plasma volume, and a rapid and abnormally high rise of serum glucose suggest dumping [59]. These tests are not always helpful in the diagnosis. It is often better to treat the patient and assess the response.

Medical treatment aims to alter the diet so that formation of hypertonic solutions in the small bowel will be prevented. The patients are advised to take small and frequent meals. Starchy and sweet foods must be avoided and liquids should be drunk before and not during or after meals. Solid food is preferred to semi-solid. Many patients profit from food with a high fibre content. These measures will substantially alleviate symptoms in most patients, but occasionally they persist. Oral pectin will decrease or abolish symptoms of dumping provoked by glucose—apparently by slowing down rapid gastric emptying—but is as yet to emerge as a practical treatment [4, 6]. Drug treatment has been suggested for these patients, but results are often disappointing. Theoretically glucoside-hydrolase inhibitors (for example acarbose before meals) should prevent the formation of hypertonic solutions by inhibiting the cleavage of starch [47]. However, despite decreased concentrations of plasma glucose and insulin it usually does not improve the symptoms. Insulin 10–20 units or tolbutamide 250–500 mg, 30 minutes before meals are given with the intention of accelerating glucose absorption and thus minimizing the exposure of the small bowel to hypertonic solutions, but again the clinical results are not satisfactory. Serotonin an-

tagonists, such as cyproheptadine 4 mg or ketanserin 10 mg, are given alone or in combination before meals in order to prevent systemic effects of vasoactive hormones; controlled studies with these compounds are not yet available. Intravenous somatostatin inhibits the secretion of gut regulatory peptides and decreases the symptoms of early dumping, it also prevents the reactive hypoglycaemia of late dumping by inhibiting the release of insulin and of gastric inhibitory polypeptide, but it has to be given parenterally [40].

Surgical treatment includes the conversion of a Billroth II to a Billroth I anastomosis in patients with a gastric resection, or the interposition of an isoperistaltic jejunal segment between the gastric remnant and the duodenum [21]; reconstruction of a pyloroplasty has also been tried.

In spite of enthusiastic reports of small series, the results of surgical treatment have not been convincing. It is therefore advisable to consider surgery only in those who have been incapacitated by symptoms for several years and who have not responded to medical treatment.

Bilious vomiting

Bilious vomiting is reported to occur in 10% to 20% of patients after partial gastric resection or vagotomy and drainage. After proximal gastric vagotomy the incidence varies between nil and 7% [4, 25, 61].

The main cause of symptoms is gastric irritation by bile refluxed from the small bowel into the stomach. The antro-pyloric anti-reflux barrier (Fig. 25.2) is lost after distal gastric resection or gastroenterostomy and is weakened by pyloroplasty, or antral denervation. Contact of bile with gastric mucosa is prolonged by slow gastric emptying, and it has been suggested that a vicious circle exists between gastric irritation by bile and slowed gastric emptying. Proximal gastric vagotomy possibly leads to

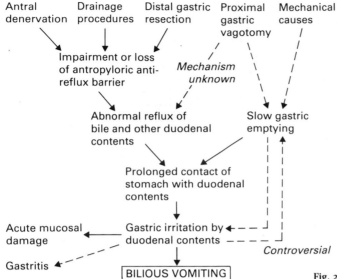

Antral   Drainage   Distal gastric   Proximal   Mechanical
denervation   procedures   resection   gastric   causes
                                               vagotomy

Impairment or loss   *Mechanism*   Slow gastric
of antropyloric anti-   *unknown*   emptying
reflux barrier

Abnormal reflux of   Slow gastric
bile and other duodenal   emptying
contents

Prolonged contact of
stomach with duodenal
contents

Acute mucosal   Gastric irritation by
damage   duodenal contents
                                              Controversial
Gastritis

BILIOUS VOMITING

Fig. 25.2. Pathophysiology of bilious vomiting.

bilious vomiting by this mechanism in patients with pre-existing high rates of duodenogastric reflux, but a direct effect of refluxed bile and other duodenal contents on gastric emptying has not been demonstrated consistently [72].

Bilious vomiting can be reproduced in symptomatic patients by gastric instillation of autologous intestinal contents, but apparently not by artificial bile acid solutions [50]. It is therefore unknown whether bile acids produce bilious vomiting only in the presence of additional substances (such as lysolecithin), or whether they are not responsible for bilious vomiting at all. Bile acid solutions produce acute mucosal damage in a dose-dependent manner [20], but do not lead to nausea and vomiting. Bile reflux has also been implicated in the production of chronic gastritis, and chronic gastritis is present in most patients with bilious vomiting. However, a causal relationship between bile reflux and chronic gastritis and between gastritis and nausea and vomiting, is uncertain. It is likely that gastritis in patients with bilious vomiting is an incidental finding, not specifically related to bile reflux or symptoms (see Chapter 18).

Most patients complain of epigastric pain or burning, typically before breakfast, relieved by vomiting of heavily bile-stained gastric contents. Nocturnal pain relieved by vomiting of bile, nocturnal heartburn and rarely, postprandial pain improved by vomiting of food mixed with bile-stained gastric juice may also occur. Food and antacids, or lying down usually worsen epigastric distress. Prolonged vomiting can lead to malnutrition and loss of weight. The occurrence of bile vomiting is related to the severity of reflux, but in an individual patient the likelihood of bile vomiting cannot be predicted on the basis of reflux tests. Most patients with marked postoperative reflux are asymptomatic. Additional factors, such as slow gastric emptying and poorly defined individual susceptibility determine whether reflux leads to bilious vomiting.

Differential diagnosis

The differential diagnosis of vomiting and epigastric pain is shown in Tables 25.2 and 25.4. None of the symptoms occurring in patients with bilious vomiting are specific,

Table 25.4. Differential diagnosis of vomiting.

Syndrome	Bile only	Vomiting Bile + food	Food only	Comment
Bilious vomiting	+ +	+ −	− −	Also in fasting state, repeatedly
Small reservoir	− −	+ −	+ +	Soon after meal
Outlet obstruction	− −	− −	+ +	Often late post-prandial
Early dumping	− −	− −	+ −	Vomiting not a main symptom
Afferent loop	+ +	+ −	− −	Very rare syndrome

but their combination leads to the diagnosis.

Formal reflux tests do not contribute much to the diagnosis, but can be useful to document reflux if surgical treatment of bilious vomiting is planned. The most reliable tests are the determination of bile acids in fasting gastric aspirates [28] and the assessment of the rate of reflux of a radiolabelled marker excreted in bile [54, 73, 78]. Gastric aspiration of marker solutions infused into the duodenum and the assay of bilirubin and trypsin in gastric juice are rarely done. Radiological evaluation of reflux following the intraduodenal infusion of contrast material [11], and endoscopical evaluation of reflux are unreliable. Endoscopy should be done in order to exclude recurrent ulceration and to assess whether oesophagitis is present. Gastric erythema is reported to occur more frequently in patients with bilious vomiting, whereas gastritis is common after any type of gastric surgery and cannot be used as a diagnostic criterion. Gastric secretory tests are unhelpful.

Medical treatment

Medical treatment aims to decrease the exposure of the gastric mucosa to intestinal contents. Cholestyramine 4 g three times daily [49], or hydrotalcite 1 g four times daily [26], or antacid gel containing aluminium hydroxide and magnesium hydroxide with a buffering capacity of 150 to 500

mmol daily can be used to inactivate bile salts in the stomach. Ursodeoxycholic acid 450 mg given in the evening replaces a fraction of bile salts toxic to the stomach; metoclopramide 10 mg or domperidone 10 mg half an hour before meals accelerate gastric emptying and decrease nausea. The results with any medical treatment are not very encouraging.

Surgical treatment

Surgical treatment is indicated for correction of severe bilious vomiting. Good results have been described with Roux-en-Y interposition of a jejunal 35 to 50 cm loop [2, 78] provided that the indications for the conversion are correct [42]. Hoare, *et al.* [27] suggest that the preoperative determination of fasting bile acids reflux should be more than 120 mmol/l, if surgery is to be performed. A disadvantage of Roux-en-Y conversion is an increased risk of ulcer recurrence.

Gastric stasis

Gastric stasis is caused by outlet obstruction or disordered gastric motility (Fig. 25.3). A frequent functional cause is antral denervation due to vagotomy [16], especially in patients with inadequate drainage procedures. Mechanical causes include outlet obstruction due to recurrent, or stomal ulcer. Rare causes include gastric or intestinal bezoars, an inadequately constructed, nar-

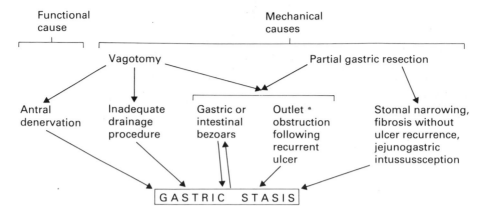

Fig. 25.3. Pathophysiology of gastric stasis.

row, or kinked stoma, stomal fibrosis without recurrent ulcer and jejunogastric intussusception. Sometimes gastric stasis due to diabetes or scleroderma becomes manifest after gastric surgery.

Symptoms

Symptoms consist of post-prandial epigastric fullness which is relieved by eructation and in severe cases by vomiting of food. Characteristically the vomited material is not bile stained.

Diagnosis

Epigastric fullness due to gastric stasis is a common postoperative symptom. If it persists, or newly arises after an interval of well-being, endoscopy is indicated and gives the best information on possible mechanical cause.

Medical treatment

Medical treatment for patients with antral denervation consists of metoclopramide or domperidone 10 mg before meals and at bedtime [51]. For treatment of bezoars of recurrent ulcer see Chapter 24. Surgical treatment is necessary for those with mechanical outlet obstruction.

Diarrhoea

Diarrhoea which may follow gastric surgery should be defined as the passage of 200 g or more of stool per day. Unfortunately, as diarrhoea is not uniformly defined in many studies, its incidence is difficult to assess. Incidence is higher after truncal vagotomy and drainage (approximately 30%) and selective vagotomy (approximately 20%) than after proximal gastric vagotomy or partial resection (<10%) [25, 35].

The two principal factors are gastric incontinence [44] and denervation of the small bowel with rapid intestinal transit [14]. Vagotomy appears to prevent the development of the normal feeding pattern of small intestinal motility. It is not clear whether vagotomy interferes with the gastric migrating myoelectric complexes [48, 58]. Rare causes of postoperative diarrhoea are shown in Fig. 25.4. For example, bacterial overgrowth of the small bowel has been described after gastric surgery as a consequence of low gastric acidity and disturbed intestinal motility, but appears to contribute little to the development of postoperative diarrhoea [17]. Denervation of the biliary tract was thought to produce increased volume of the gallbladder, increased concentration of bile acids in the small intestine and, in consequence, diar-

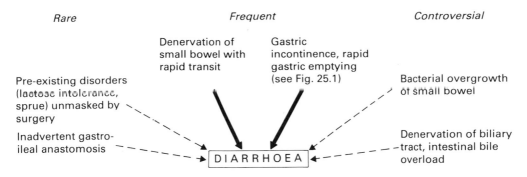

Rare   *Frequent*   *Controversial*

Denervation of small bowel with rapid transit

Gastric incontinence, rapid gastric emptying (see Fig. 25.1)

Pre-existing disorders (lactose intolerance, sprue) unmasked by surgery

Inadvertent gastro-ileal anastomosis

Bacterial overgrowth of small bowel

Denervation of biliary tract, intestinal bile overload

DIARRHOEA

Fig. 25.4. Pathophysiology of diarrhoea.

rhoea. This is unlikely, because cholecystectomy aggravates postoperative diarrhoea [71].

Clinical features and diagnosis

The diarrhoea appears most commonly within one or two hours of eating—less frequently it occurs also while fasting, or even at night. In a typical case of post-prandial diarrhoea no further tests are needed. In patients with continuous diarrhoea also occurring at night rare causes, such as bacterial overgrowth of the small intestine, or pre-existing disorders unmasked by surgery such as coeliac syndrome or IgA deficiency, should be looked for.

Treatment

The treatment of uncomplicated post-surgical diarrhoea is similar to that of the dumping syndrome. In addition, antidiarrhoeal drugs such as loperamide up to 8 capsules per day or codeine 30 mg up to four times daily, may be given. Cholestyramine 4 g three times per day has been shown to be helpful [3]. Surgical procedures, similar to those performed for dumping, have been done in severe diarrhoea. The results are not entirely satisfactory, and surgery should be regarded as a last resort measure in severe cases resistant to energetic medical treatment.

Weight loss

Postoperative weight loss is the most frequent consequence of gastric surgery. Although weight loss is easy to define and to measure, the data concerning the incidence of post-surgical weight loss are contradictory. In prospective studies weight loss has been claimed to occur rarely [45], occasionally [56], often [57], or mainly in patients who were initially overweight [76]. Postoperative body weight decreases in more than half of the patients with partial gastric resection, in one third of the patients with vagotomy and pyloroplasty, but those with proximal gastric vagotomy usually maintain their body weight.

Postoperative weight loss is usually due to malnutrition (Fig. 25.5). The two frequent causes are a diminished intake of food because of attempts to avoid food-related symptoms such as pain, dumping, diarrhoea or vomiting, and early satiety due to a small gastric reservoir, or gastric stasis. Malabsorption is a rare cause of weight loss after gastric operations.

For diagnosis it is very useful to keep accurate records of the patient's pre- and postoperative body weight.

A detailed evaluation of the diet, preferably done by a professional dietitian, is of central importance. Typically, the patients avoid eating because of the fear of food-related symptoms or because of early

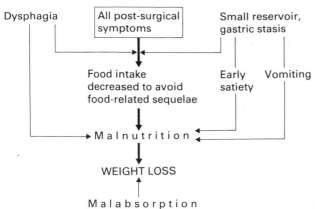

Fig. 25.5. Pathophysiology of weight loss.

satiety—in these circumstances, a metabolic evaluation of weight loss is not necessary. In patients with weight loss despite adequate nutrition, particularly in those with an increased faecal volume, diagnostic tests for malabsorption should be done (see Chapter 41). Provided there is no evidence of malabsorption and the patient's weight remains stable after the initial loss, no specific treatment is necessary apart from ensuring that the patient eats a nutritionally balanced diet. Often patients gain weight during hospitalization and lose it again after discharge from the hospital [8].

Late metabolic sequelae

Late metabolic sequelae consist of anaemia, or osteomalacia several years after surgery. These disorders are frequent but seldom severe.

Mild anaemia with haemoglobin values around 12 g/dl is present in most patients ten years after partial gastrectomy [75]; in menstruating women anaemia develops within five years. Severe anaemia with haemoglobin values below 10 g/dl leading to clinical symptoms is infrequent after partial gastric resection and especially rare after vagotomy. Disturbed calcium metabolism is observed in about 20% of the patients within 10 years after partial gastric resection, but rarely leads to symptoms.

Bone disease is mainly due to malnutrition with decreased intake of calcium and vitamin D [37]. Malabsorption of calcium and vitamin D is rare. Increased incidence of bone fractures [55] and symptomatic osteomalacia have been described after partial gastric resection. Increased serum alkaline phosphatase has been reported 10 years after truncal vagotomy, but it is unknown whether this is due to bone disease [76]. It is not clear whether neuropathy due to vitamin B_{12} deficiency is increased after gastric surgery.

The most important cause of anaemia is iron deficiency (Fig. 25.6) which may be due to decreased dietary intake of iron, or to chronic blood loss, for example in patients with erosive stomal gastritis. Contributing factors might be increased intragastric pH with impaired conversion of dietary (ferric) iron to ferrous state, faster small bowel transit time and duodenal bypass in partial gastric resection with Billroth II anastomosis. Conversion of dietary iron from ferric to ferrous is not a prerequisite for its absorption [77] and absorption is not restricted to the duodenum [18]. An additional cause contributing to anaemia is vitamin B_{12} deficiency. The intake of B_{12} may be too low in malnourished patients; rapid gastric emptying may prevent the formation of the B_{12}-intrinsic factor complex; ileal absorption of B_{12} may be impaired by

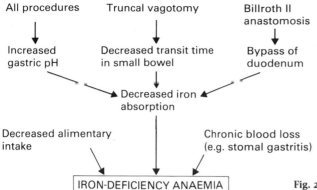

All procedures → Increased gastric pH

Truncal vagotomy → Decreased transit time in small bowel

Billroth II anastomosis → Bypass of duodenum

→ Decreased iron absorption ←

Decreased alimentary intake

Chronic blood loss (e.g. stomal gastritis)

IRON-DEFICIENCY ANAEMIA

Fig. 25.6. Pathophysiology of iron deficiency anaemia

rapid intestinal transit and bacterial overgrowth. Inadequate production of intrinsic factor is an unlikely cause except in patients with total gastric resection. Folic acid deficiency, another consequence of malnutrition, may also aggravate anaemia.

Diagnosis

The diagnosis of these disorders rests upon laboratory estimation of haemoglobin and haematological variables and the concentrations of B_{12}, folate, serum iron and iron binding capacity, calcium, phosphate and alkaline phosphatase. In cases of bone pain, radiological examination may show pseudofractures or Looser zones, while a trephine bone biopsy may help in the differentiation ·between osteoporosis and osteomalacia.

Treatment

Treatment depends on oral replacement. Oral iron 300 mg daily is usually successful in iron deficiency anaemia. Treatment should be continued even after correction of anaemia, because relapses frequently occur [75]. In cases of macrocytic anaemia associated with iron deficiency, parenteral vitamin B_{12}, 1000 mcg every two months and oral folate 10 or 15 mg daily should be given in addition.

Rare syndromes

Mild malabsorption

Mild malabsorption is often found after gastric surgery when appropriate tests (see Chapter 41) are performed. However, symptomatic malabsorption is rare [8]. Symptomatic malabsorption may be due to a pre-existing disorder, such as coeliac disease, which has been unmasked by surgery.

The pathophysiological factors that have been implicated in postoperative malabsorption include bacterial overgrowth secondary to denervation of the small intestine and low intragastric acidity. As a consequence, deconjugation of bile salts and utilization of dietary proteins [31], or vitamins (for example, B_{12}) by bacteria occurs. Due to dumping and intestinal denervation, the passage of food is rapid—there is poor mixing and inadequate time for absorption. In addition, rapidly emptied and propulsed food fails to mix with bile and pancreatic juice, increasing malabsorption.

Late dumping

Late dumping is rare and due to hypoglycaemia occurring two to three hours after a meal. The possible pathophysiological mechanisms are shown in Fig. 25.7. The symptoms are those of hypoglycaemia—

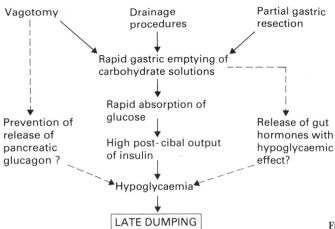

Fig. 25.7. Pathophysiology of late dumping.

sweating, palpitations, weakness, fatigue and mental confusion. Medical treatment consists in dietary adjustments. During an attack, ingestion of sugar usually promptly resolves the syndrome.

Reflux oesophagitis

Oesophagitis is rarely caused by partial gastric resection or vagotomy [7]. On the other hand, heartburn is quite frequent. Increased incidence of reflux oesophagitis has been reported in non-operated patients with duodenal ulcer [23]. Reports of reflux oesophagitis occurring as a consequence of surgery should be interpreted with care, unless the oesophagus has been examined before surgery. Partial gastric resection and vagotomy rarely cause oesophagitis. This is

in contrast to total gastrectomy where reflux oesophagitis is a major problem.

The two major causes of post-surgical oesophagitis are alkaline duodenogastric reflux with bilious vomiting and gastric stasis (Fig. 25.8). It has been speculated that duodenal exclusion in patients with a Billroth II anastomosis may interfere with postprandial closure of the lower oesophageal sphincter [33], but this is unproven. It has also been claimed that the sphincter is weakened by vagal denervation. However, vagotomy does not lower the resting sphincter pressure or the pressure response to pentagastrin. Proximal gastric vagotomy may even have a favourable effect on oesophagitis—it has been reported that pre-existing oesophagitis heals within one year after surgery [67]. Mechanical damage of

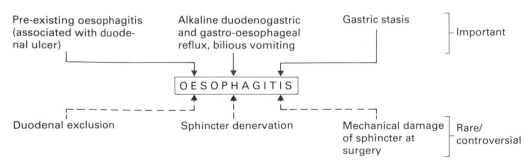

Fig. 25.8. Pathophysiology of reflux oesophagitis.

the sphincter region might occur during proximal gastric vagotomy but this has not been described as a cause of oesophagitis.

Oesophagitis is diagnosed by endoscopy (see Chapter 11 for details). Treatment of alkaline reflux is more difficult than the treatment of acid reflux. The same drugs as used for bilious vomiting may be given. In addition, reflux may be decreased by elevation of the head of the bed, frequent small meals, refraining from late meals, a low fat diet and abstinence from smoking. Drugs such as metoclopramide 10 mg three times daily or urecholine 25 mg four times daily may improve oesophageal clearance. When despite surgery gastric acidity is high, histamine H_2-antagonists are given (for example ranitidine 150 mg twice daily). Surgical treatment should only be resorted to if energetic medical therapy has not controlled the symptoms. The procedures recommended are identical to those described for the treatment of bilious vomiting. Fundoplication is rarely necessary—it should be avoided after partial gastric resection because it further decreases the size of the gastric reservoir.

Phytobezoars

Phytobezoars are rare, but ulcer surgery is a risk factor for their development. They are found in the stomach after vagotomy and in the small intestine after partial gastric resection. Phytobezoars are mainly composed of fruit fibres [53] and often overgrown by yeast and fungi; pure yeast and fungal bezoars are very rare (see also below). Phytobezoars develop in patients with high fibre consumption. Their formation is probably a consequence of slowed emptying of solids in general and fibre in particular: this may occur after gastric surgery despite the rapid emptying of fluids. An additional factor after distal gastric resection is the loss of the capacity of the antrum to fragment solid food residues.

A gastric bezoar may manifest itself with epigastric fullness or pain, nausea, and early satiety. Many gastric bezoars are asymptomatic. Small intestinal bezoars may lead to acute intestinal obstruction.

Conservative medical treatment of gastric bezoars is often successful. Administration of papain, a proteolytic enzyme, together with sodium bicarbonate may lead to dissolution of the bezoar [52]. Endoscopic fragmentation has also been tried. After removal of the bezoar patients should be advised to decrease their fibre intake and to avoid unripe fruit and uncooked vegetables. In cases of intestinal obstruction due to a bezoar, emergency surgery is usually performed (see Chapter 26).

Gastric mycosis

Gastric mycosis has been reported after antrectomy and vagotomy. It is very rare after other types of surgery. Candida and torulopsis are usually found. Predisposing factors are delayed gastric emptying, increased intragastric pH and mucosal damage due to duodenogastric reflux [34].

Most patients with fungal growth in the stomach are asymptomatic. Symptoms of epigastric fullness, pain, nausea, vomiting and foul-smelling eructations may occur with massive overgrowth. The stomach may be filled with fungal material, which may form bezoar-like structures. Medical management consists of repeated gastric lavage with acetylcysteine in order to break up the bezoars and flush out the viscous gastric contents. In addition, metoclopramide 10 mg three times daily and nystatin may be given orally. Unfortunately, the long-term results are not satisfactory.

Controversial syndromes

Post-surgical gastric cancer

It is not clear whether the incidence of gastric cancer increases after surgery for peptic ulcer. In experimental animals the incidence of gastric cancer increases when administration of an exogenous carcinogen is combined with a Billroth II anastomosis. The risk is smaller with a Billroth I. Increased concentrations of nitrites, precursors of carcinogenic N-nitroso compounds, have been found in gastric juice of patients with distal gastric resection with Billroth I and Billroth II anastomosis, but not after vagotomy. Elevated concentrations of N-nitroso compounds were found only after Billroth II procedures [64]. Gastritis, considered an essential step in carcinogenesis, develops after gastric surgery [58]. Other factors that may increase the risk of gastric cancer such as intestinal metaplasia, bile reflux, gastric stasis and bacterial overgrowth of the stomach are also present after surgery. A role for bile reflux is supported by the observation that after distal gastric resection carcinoma usually develops near the stoma.

Endoscopic surveys of populations apparently at high risk for the development of gastric cancer—such as patients after gastric resection—have reported an increased prevalence of gastric neoplasia, and a similar percentage of patients have been found to have severe dysplasia, which some consider to be equivalent to carcinoma *in situ*—the proportion of patients with gastric cancer or severe dysplasia ranges from 1.5% to 6.5%. Although the evidence is not conclusive, the risk of malignancy is probably confined to patients who have had a partial gastrectomy or a gastrojejunostomy. The risk is greater in patients who have had the operation for gastric rather than for duodenal ulcer and it becomes manifest 20 or more years after the surgery. A recent study suggested that the risk of cancer 20 years after gastric surgery increases 3.7-fold in those who have had the operation for duodenal ulcer and 5.5-fold in those who had it for gastric ulcer [12]. It also has to be remembered that only a small proportion

of late deaths after gastric resection will be caused by neoplasm of the gastric stump [13]. Interestingly, one study showed an increased risk for carcinoma of the lung, the colon and the pancreas after gastric surgery. The high incidence of extra-alimentary carcinomas was probably due to smoking [46]. Those who believe in an increased risk of gastric stump cancer advocate screening programmes with serial endoscopies in patients who survive for more than 10 years after partial gastric resection. Others have shown that in areas with a relatively low incidence of gastric cancer, the yield of these screening programmes is low [68] and poorly justified [39]. Exception could be made for selected patients who had a partial gastrectomy at an early age and who therefore remain at risk for a long time.

Cancer after partial gastric resection has a similar age distribution as primary gastric cancer. The symptoms of stump cancer are usually vague and often mimic symptoms of the original peptic ulcer, or of benign post-gastrectomy syndromes. They tend to be ignored by patients and physicians. The prognosis of cancer after gastric resection is even worse than for primary cancer—the overall five-year survival rate is below 1%.

Postoperative gastritis

Postoperative gastritis may or may not be an undesirable post-surgical syndrome, or 'a consequence of any successful operation for peptic ulcer' [2]. Gastritis is relatively uncommon in duodenal ulcer patients. In patients with gastric ulcer, gastritis is almost always found in the distal stomach [24], except in patients with the ulcer in the proximal part of the gastric body.

Gastritis in the antrum and in the body is found in almost all patients after partial resection for gastric and duodenal ulcer. The question whether athropic gastritis develops after vagotomy, and in particular after proximal gastric vagotomy, is not settled. In the distal stomach the incidence is reported to be more than 80%, while in the proximal stomach it is apparently low [2, 65]. Postoperative gastritis is thought to be asymptomatic. There is no convincing evidence for a causative role of gastritis in the symptoms of bilious vomiting [20]. Treatment is therefore not indicated.

Postoperative cholelithiasis

Postoperative cholelithiasis may, or may not be a complication of gastric surgery. Gallstones may coexist with duodenal ulcer and in about 10% of the patients the gallbladder is removed when the ulcer is treated surgically. The following pathophysiological mechanisms have been proposed: after vagotomy stasis in a dilated gallbladder and an accumulation of biliary sludge occur [74]. Cholecystokinin release may be low due to duodenal exclusion. It has also been claimed that after surgery the bile acid pool decreases and the cholesterol saturation index increases, but this has not been confirmed in recent studies [66, 70]. Most importantly, an increased risk of gallstones has not been demonstrated in prospective studies.

Syndromes following particular operations

After vagotomy

Post-vagotomy dysphagia

After vagotomy one fifth of patients complain of transient dysphagia. The pathophysiology is poorly understood, but the dysphagia is probably mostly due to surgical trauma, with the formation of oedema or haematoma around the distal oesophagus [20]. In cases with persisting symptoms a fibrous mass may surround and compress the oesophagus [69]. It is unlikely that dysphagia is due to the denervation of the lower oesophageal sphincter, or of the distal oesophagus, because truncal, selective and proximal gastric vagotomy would not be expected to interfere with oesophageal function. Experimentally, high-thoracic bilateral vagotomy interferes with distal oesophageal motility, while distal forms of vagotomy have no effect [36]. Dysphagia may occur in alkaline oesophagitis as a consequence of a stenosis.

Diagnostic assessment depends on radiology or endoscopy. The radiological picture may mimic achalasia, or even fundic carcinoma. Endoscopy usually shows concentric narrowing of the lumen with a normal mucosa, but reflux oesophagitis may be present. As the symptoms usually disappear spontaneously within a few weeks after the operation, no treatment is necessary. If the dysphagia persists, dilatation is the first line of treatment, but the results are not always satisfactory. Surgical treatment consists of excision of the scar tissue surrounding the distal oesophagus.

Gastric necrosis after vagotomy

Necrosis of the lesser curvature is a rare complication of selective or proximal gastric vagotomy [32]. The injury to the gastric wall is due to devascularization. Uraemia appears to be a risk factor. The patients develop acute peritonitis a few days after the operation. Prophylactic reperitonealization of the lesser curvature is performed by many surgeons during the operation.

After partial resection

Small reservoir

Extensive (80–90%) resection of the stomach decreases the gastric reservoir to a point where the patient experiences epigastric fullness, early satiety, pain, nausea and vomiting even with small meals. Most of these patients also have additional complications such as dumping and bilious vomiting. They finally suffer from severe malnutrition.

Medical management is difficult. In some patients, surgical treatment consisting of transformation of a sub-total into a total gastrectomy and the construction of a jejunal pouch has been done—the results are variable.

Stomal invagination

Stomal invagination is a rare consequence of a Billroth II anastomosis. Stomal invagination may lead to recurrent attacks of gastric outlet obstruction and, when the invaginate becomes ischaemic and necrotic, to an acute abdomen [29].

The diagnosis is made at endoscopy. It is possible to perform a reposition by means of the endoscope. Subsequent surgery, with abdominal fixation of the loop is necessary.

Afferent loop syndrome

The afferent loop syndrome is a very rare consequence of partial gastric resection with Billroth II anastomosis. The afferent loop syndrome reported in older publications was probably bilious vomiting [72].

The syndrome is caused by a kinked afferent loop. When bile and pancreatic juice are secreted into it in response to a meal, emptying of the loop does not occur and distension of the loop with epigastric pain results. Symptoms are relieved by explosive vomiting of intestinal contents. An acute afferent loop syndrome in the early postoperative period may lead to leakage from the blind end of the loop and to biliary peritonitis. Treatment is surgical.

Retained antrum

Retained antrum is another very rare syndrome. It may occur when during distal gastric resection with Billroth II anastomosis a part of the antrum is left at the duodenal stump. This part of the antrum continuously secretes gastrin, because inhibition of gastrin release by gastric acid does not occur. This leads to acid hypersecretion by the gastric remnant and to severe recurrent ulceration. The treatment consists of resection of the retained antrum.

References

1 ALEXANDER-WILLIAMS J, DONOVAN IA. Effects of gastric operations. In: Booth CC, Neale G. eds. *Disorders of the small intestine.* Oxford: Blackwell Scientific Publications, 1986:93–100.
2 ALEXANDER-WILLIAMS J, HOARE AM. Partial gastric resection. In: Blum AL, Siewert JR, eds. *Postsurgical syndromes.* London: WB Saunders Co., 1979:321–353.
3 ALLAN JG, RUSSELL, RI. Cholestyramine in treatment of postvagotomy diarrhoea—double-blind controlled trial. *Br Med J* 1977;1:674–676.
4 AMDRUP E, ANDERSEN D, HOSTRUP H. The Aarhus county vagotomy trial. I. An interim report on primary results and incidence of sequelae following parietal cell vagotomy and selective vagotomy in 748 patients. *World J Surg* 1978;2:85–90.
5 BLACKBURN AM, CRISTOPHIDES ND, GHATEI MA, *et al.* Elevation of plasma neurotensin in the dumping syndrome. *Clin Sci* 1980;59:237–243.
6 BLOOM SR, ROYSTOM CMS, THOMPSON JPS. Enteroglucagon release in the dumping syndrome. *Lancet* 1972;ii:789–791.
7 BLUM AL, SIEWERT JR. *Reflux-Therapie.* Berlin: Springer-Verlag.
8 BRADLEY EL, ISAACS J, HERSH T, DAVIDSON ED, MILLIKAN W. Nutritional consequences of total gastrectomy. *Ann Surg* 1975;182:415–428.
9 BUDD DC, MCREARY ML. Gastric phytobezoar: still another postgastrectomy syndrome. *Am Surg* 1978; 44:104–107.
10 BUTZ R. Dumping syndrome studied during maintenance of blood volume. *Ann Surg* 1961;154:225–234.
11 CAPPER WM, AIRTH GR, KILBY JO. A test for pyloric regurgitation. *Lancet* 1966;ii:621–623.
12 CAYGILL C, HILL MJ, KIRKHAM JS, NORTHFIELD TC. Mortality from gastric cancer following gastric surgery for peptic ulcer. *Lancet* 1986;i:929–931.
13 CLARK CG, FRESINI A, GLEDHILL T. Cancer following gastric surgery. *Br J Surg* 1985;72:591–594.
14 CONDON JR, ROBINSON V, SULEMAN MI, FAN VS, MCKEOWN MD. The cause and treatment of postvagotomy diarrhoea. *Br J Surg* 1975;62:309–312.

15 CUSCHIERI A, ONABANJO OA. Kinin release after gastric surgery. *Br Med J* 1971;**3**:565–566.

16 DOZOIS RR, KELLY KA, CODE CF. Effect of distal antrectomy on gastric emptying of liquids and solids. *Gastroenterology* 1971;**61**:675–681.

17 DRASAR BS, SHINER M. Studies on the intestinal flora. *Gut* 1969;**10**:812–819.

18 DUTHIE HL. The relative importance of the duodenum in the intestinal absorption of iron. *Br J Haematol* 1964;**10**:59–68.

19 EBEID FH, RALPHS DNL, HOBSLEY M, LEQUESNE LP. Dumping symptoms after vagotomy treated by reversal of pyloroplasty. *Br J Surg* 1982;**69**:527–528.

20 EDWARDS DAW. Post-vagotomy dysphagia. *Lancet* 1970;**ii**:90–92.

21 ELDH J, KEWENTER J, KOCK NG, OLSON P. Long-term results of surgical treatment for dumping after partial gastrectomy. *Br J Surg* 1974;**61**:90–93.

22 FENGER HJ, ANDREASSEN M, GOSTA DAVIDSEN H. The dumping syndrome and its experimental provocation. *Acta Chir Scand* 1961;**121**:142–150.

23 GAUMANN N, VOGEL E, JOST L, et al. Koinzidenz peptischer Läsionen im oberen Gastrointestinaltrakt. *Schweiz Med Wschr* 1983;**113**:351–357.

24 GEAR MWL, TRUELOVE SC, WHITEHEAD R. Gastric ulcer and gastritis. *Gut* 1971;**12**:639–645.

25 GOLIGHER JC, PULVERTAFT CN, IRVIN TT, et al. Five to eight years results of truncal vagotomy and pyloroplasty for duodenal ulcer. *Br Med J* 1972;**i**:7–13.

26 HOARE AM, MCLEISH A, THOMPSON H, ALEXANDER-WILLIAMS J. Hydrotalcite in the treatment of bile vomiting. *Br J Surg* 1977;**64**:849–850.

27 HOARE AM, MCLEISH A, THOMPSON H, ALEXANDER-WILLIAMS J. Selection of patients for bile diversion surgery: use of bile acid measurement in fasting gastric aspirates. *Gut* 1978;**19**:163–165.

28 HOARE AM, KEIGHLEY MRB, STARKEY B, ALEXANDER-WILLIAMS J. Measurement of bile acids in fasting gastric aspirates: an objective test for bile reflux after gastric surgery. *Gut* 1978;**19**:166–169.

29 HOVELIUS L. Jejunogastric intussusception after gastric resection. Report of two cases. *Acta Chir Scand* 1971;**137**:491–494.

30 JOHNSON LP, JESSEPH JE. Evidence for a humoral etiology of the dumping syndrome. *Surgical Forum* 1961;**12**:316–317.

31 JONES EA, CRAIGIE A, TAVILL AS, FRANGLEN G, ROSENOER VM. Protein metabolism in the intestinal stagnant loop syndrome. *Gut* 1968;**9**:466–469.

32 KALAJA E, CLEMMESEN I, BANKE L, KRAGELUND E, CHRISTIANSEN PM. Accidents and complications in selective and proximal gastric vagotomy. *Surgery* 1975;**77**:140–143.

33 KOELZ HR, LEPSIEN G, HOLLINGER AP, et al. Effect of intraduodenal peptone on the lower esophageal pressure in the dog. *Gastroenterology* 1978;**75**:283–285.

34 KONOK G, HADDAD H. Postoperative gastric mycosis. *Surg Gynecol Obstet* 1980;**150**:337–341.

35 KOO J, LAM SK, CHAN P, et al. Proximal gastric vagotomy, truncal vagotomy with drainage, and truncal vagotomy with antrectomy for chronic duodenal ulcer. A prospective, randomized controlled trial. *Ann Surg* 1983;**197**:265–271.

36 KRAVITZ JJ, SNAPE WJ, COHEN S. Effect of thoracic vagotomy and vagal stimulation on esophageal function. *Am J Physiol* 1978;**234**:E359–E364.

37 LEADING ARTICLE. Osteomalacia after gastrectomy. *Lancet* 1986;**i**,77–78.

38 LEEDS AR, EBIED F, RALPHS DNL, METZ G, DILAWARI JB. Pectin in the dumping syndrome: reduction of symptoms and plasma volume changes. *Lancet* 1981;**1**:1075.

39 LOGAN RF, LANGMAN MJS. Screening for gastric cancer after gastric surgery. *Lancet* 1983;**ii**:667–669.

40 LONG RG, ADRIAN TE, BLOOM SR. Somatostatin and the dumping syndrome. *Br Med J* 1985;**290**:886–888.

41 MACHELLA TE. Mechanism of the post-gastrectomy dumping syndrome. *Gastroenterology* 1950;**14**:237–252.

42 MALAGELADA J-B, PHILLIPS SF, SHORTER RG, et al. Postoperative reflux gastritis: pathophysiology and long-term outcome after Roux-en-Y diversion. *Ann Intern Med* 1985;**103**:178–183.

43 MCCOLL I, DRINKWATER JE, HULME-MOIR I, DONNAN SPB. Prediction of success or failure of gastric surgery. *Br J Surg* 1971;**58**:768–771.

44 MCKELVEY STD. Gastric incontinence and postvagotomy diarrhoea. *Br J Surg* 1970;**57**:741–747.

45 MCKEOWN KC. A prospective study of the immediate and long-term results of Pólya gastrectomy for duodenal ulcer. *Br J Surg* 1972;**59**:849–868.

46 MCLEAN ROSS AH, SMITH MA, ANDERSON JR, SMALL WP. Late mortality after ulcer surgery for peptic ulcer. *N Engl J Med* 1982;**307**:519–522.

47 MCLOUGHLIN JC, BUCHANAN KD, ALAM MJ. A Glycoside–hydrolase inhibitor in treatment of dumping syndrome. *Lancet* 1979;**ii**:603–605.

48 MARIK F, CODE CF. Control of the interdigestive myoelectric activity in dogs by the vagus nerves and pentagastrin. *Gastroenterology* 1975;**69**:387–395.

49 MESHKINPOUR H, ELASHOFF J, STEWART H, III, PHARM D, STURDEVANT AL. Effect of cholestyramine on the symptoms of reflux gastritis. *Gastroenterology* 1977;**73**:441–443.

50 MESHKINPOUR H, MARKS JW, SCHOENFIELD LJ, BONNORIS GG, CARTER S. Reflux gastritis syndrome: mechanism of symptoms. *Gastroenterology* 1980;**79**:1283–1287.

51 METZGER WH, CANO R, STURDEVANT RAL. Effect of

metoclopramide in chronic gastric retention after gastric surgery. *Gastroenterology* 1976;71:30–32.

52 MIR AM, MIR MA. Phytobezoar after vagotomy with drainage or resection. *Br J Surg* 1973; 60:846–849.

53 MORIEL EZ, AYALON A, EID A, RACHMILEWITZ D, KRAUSZ MM, DURST AL. An unusually high incidence of gastrointestinal obstruction by persimmon bezoars in Israeli patients after ulcer surgery. *Gastroenterology* 1983;84:752–755.

54 MULLER-LISSNER SA, SONNENBERG A, MULLER-DUYSING W, WILL N, HEINZEL F, BLUM AL. Quantitative measurement of duodenogastric reflux in man. *Scand J Gastroenterol [Suppl 67]* 1981;16:43–46.

55 NILSSON BE, WESTLIN NE. The fracture incidence after gastrectomy. *Acta Chir Scand* 1971; 137:533–534.

56 POSTLETHWAIT RW. Five year follow-up results of operations for duodenal ulcer. *Surg Gynecol Obstet* 1973;137:387–392.

57 PRICE WE, GRIZZLE JE, POSTLETHWAIT RW, JOHNSON WD, GRABICKI P. Results of operation for duodenal ulcer. *Surg Gynecol Obstet* 1970;131:233–244.

58 PULIMOOD BM, KNUDSEN A, COGHILL NF. Gastric mucosa after partial gastrectomy. *Gut* 1976;17:463–470.

59 RALPHS DNL, THOMPSON JPS, HOBSLEY M, LE QUESNE LP. A dumping provocation test. In: Baron JH, Alexander-Williams J, Allgower M, Muller C, Spencer J, eds. *Vagotomy in modern surgical practice.* London: Butterworths, 1982:263–264.

60 REHNBERG O, FAXEN A, HAGLUND U, KEWENTER J, STENQUIST B, OLBE L. Gastric mycosis following gastric resection and vagotomy. *Ann Surg* 1982; 196:21–25.

61 REID DA, DUTHIE HL, BRANSOM CJ, JOHNSON AG. Late follow-up of highly selective vagotomy with excision of the ulcer compared with Billroth I gastrectomy for treatment of benign gastric ulcer. *Br J Surg* 1982;69:605–607.

62 REVERDIN N, HUTTON MR, LING A, *et al.* Vagotomy and the motor response to feeding. In: Christensen J, ed. *Gastrointestinal motility.* New York: Raven Press, 1980;359–364.

63 SAGOR GR, BRYANT MG, GHATEI MA, KIRK RM, BLOOM SR. Release of vasoactive intestinal peptide in the dumping syndrome. *Br Med J* 1981; 282:507–510.

64 SCHLAG P, BOCKLER R, ULRICH H, PETER M, MERKLE P, HERFARTH C. Are nitrite and N-nitroso compounds in gastric juice risk factors for carcinoma in the operated stomach? *Lancet* 1980;i:727–729.

65 SCHUMPELICK V, GARBRECHT A, BEGEMANN F. Pyloric reflux and gastritis. In: Baron JH, Alexander-Williams J, Allgower M, Muller C, Spencer J, eds. *Vagotomy in modern surgical practice.* London: Butterworths, 1982: 275–283.

66 SHAFFER EA. The effect of vagotomy on gallbladder function and bile composition in man. *Ann Surg* 1982;195:413–418.

67 SIEWERT R. Dysphagia, achalasia and gastro-oesophageal reflux. In: Baron JH, Alexander-Williams J, Allgower M, Muller C, Spencer J, eds. *Vagotomy in modern surgical practice.* London: Butterworths, 1982:267–274.

68 SONNENBERG A. Endoscopic screening for cancer of the gastric stump. *Gastroenterology* 1983;84: 1316.

69 SPENCER JD. Postvagotomy dysphagia. *Br J Surg* 1975;62:354–355.

70 STEMPEL JM, DUANE WC. Biliary lipids and bile acid pool size after vagotomy in man. Evidence against a predisposition to gallstones. *Gastroenterology* 1978;75:608–611.

71 TAYLOR TV, LAMBERT ME, QURESHI S, TORRANCE B. Should cholecystectomy be combined with vagotomy and pyloroplasty? *Lancet* 1978;i:295–298.

72 TOYE DKM, ALEXANDER-WILLIAMS J. Post-gastrectomy bile vomiting. *Lancet* 1965;ii:524–526.

73 TOLIN RD, MALMUD LS, STELZER F, *et al.* Enterogastric reflux in normal subjects and patients with Billroth II gastroenterostomy. *Gastroenterology* 1979;77:1027–1033.

74 TOMPKINS RK, KRAFT AR, ZIMMERMAN E, LICHTENSTEIN JE, ZOLLINGER RM. Clinical and biochemical evidence of increased gallstone formation after complete vagotomy. *Surgery* 1972;71:196–200.

75 TOVEY FI, CLARK CG. Anaemia after partial gastrectomy: a neglected curable condition. *Lancet* 1980;i:956–958.

76 VENABLES CW, WHELDON EJ, JOHNSTON IDA. The long-term metabolic sequelae of truncal vagotomy and drainage. In: Baron JH, Alexander-Williams J, Allgower M, Muller C, Spencer J, eds. *Vagotomy in modern surgical practice.* London: Butterworths, 1982:288–294.

77 WALKER RJ, WILLIAMS R. Abnormalities of the gastrointestinal transport of iron. *Semin Nucl Med* 1972;2:235–250.

78 WICKREMESINGHE PC, DAYRIT PQ, MANFREDI OL, FAZIO RA, FAGEL VL. Quantitative evaluation of bile diversion surgery utilizing 99mTc HIDA scintigraphy. *Gastroenterology* 1983;84:354–363.

Chapter 26
Disorders of Gastric Motility

R. C. HEADING

After ingestion food is subjected in the stomach to grinding and mixing with gastric secretions before being delivered to the duodenum in a controlled fashion. In the normal stomach accommodation of ingested food is accompanied by relaxation of the gastric fundus, while peristaltic contractions of the distal stomach fulfil grinding, mixing and propulsive functions. Relaxation of the proximal and the peristaltic contractions of the distal stomach are mediated by vagal reflexes, but they are also affected by local reflexes within the stomach wall, by sympathetic innervation and by hormonal influences. Disorders of gastric motility comprise disorders of the accommodation mechanism as well as disorders of peristalsis—both may be responsible for abnormalities of gastric emptying. Impaired accommodation accelerates emptying, especially of liquids, during the first few minutes after consumption, while impairment of peristalsis results in delayed gastric emptying, especially of solids. These abnormalities may coexist, notably in the post-vagotomy stomach.

For practical purposes previous gastric surgery is the only important cause of abnormally rapid gastric emptying, while the differential diagnosis of delayed gastric emptying is more complex. Here only major disorders of direct clinical significance are considered, but it should be noted that minor abnormalities of gastric emptying may also be clinically relevant. For example accelerated gastric emptying may contribute to duodenal ulceration [14] and impaired gastric emptying may contribute to gastro-oesophageal reflux [16].

Recognition of abnormal gastric motility

When abnormal gastric motility is suspected, objective confirmation is often desirable. The physician should therefore be aware of the use and limitations of the relevant investigations. Suspected gastric retention (impaired gastric emptying) and abnormally rapid gastric emptying are considered separately.

Suspected gastric retention

Passage of a **nasogastric tube** and aspiration of the gastric contents is usually the simplest way to confirm gross gastric retention. Recovery of food residue, or of a volume of gastric secretion exceeding 150 ml may be considered abnormal, if aspiration is done after an overnight fast. A grossly distended stomach can sometimes be recognized on a plain abdominal X-ray (Fig. 26.1).

A **barium meal** after an overnight fast will immediately identify abnormal food and fluid residue in the stomach. This may be the only information gained, because peristalsis is often absent in a pathologically distended stomach and the retained food and fluid usually prevent satisfactory display of the distal antrum, pylorus and duodenum (Fig. 26.2). Endoscopy, or further radiological examination should therefore

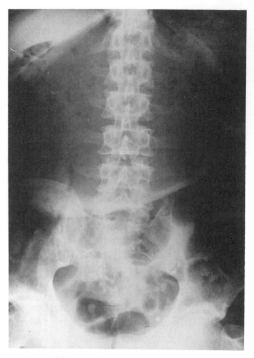

Fig. 26.1. Abdominal X-ray showing gross gastric distension.

be undertaken after 48 hours of nasogastric aspiration, with gastric lavage if necessary. It should then be possible to identify any mechanical obstruction (for example pyloric stenosis, gastric carcinoma) responsible for the gastric retention.

The use of a **gamma camera** to measure gastric emptying after ingestion of a test meal labelled with a gamma emitting radionuclide is a sensitive method of identifying delayed gastric emptying. Impaired emptying of a solid, or of a mixed solid-liquid meal may sometimes be demonstrable when radiology with liquid barium has shown no abnormality. However, gamma camera measurements of gastric emptying are not widely available at present and are not for routine use. They may be helpful when there is persistent clinical suspicion of delayed gastric emptying and other investigations have proved inconclusive [7, 16, 18, 21].

Measurements of intragastric pressure

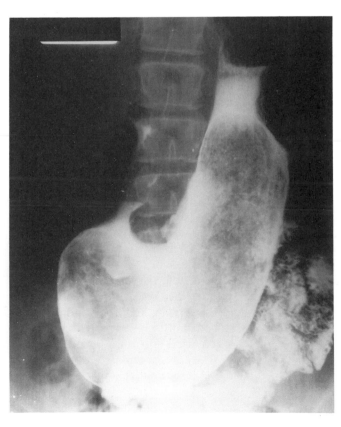

Fig. 26.2. Gastric distension and retention of food demonstrated by barium meal. The gastric contents prevent satisfactory display of the distal antrum and pylorus.

using techniques similar to those in oesophageal manometry and **electrophysiological recording** from the stomach are performed in a few research laboratories, but do not at present have a role in clinical practice.

Suspected rapid gastric emptying

Measurement of gastric emptying may very occasionally be helpful in the assessment of patients with symptoms thought to be a consequence of previous gastric surgery, particularly if revisional surgery is being considered. However, it must be recognized that all the commonly employed gastric operations result in an early phase of increased gastric emptying and that this is therefore an expected finding in such patients (Fig. 26.3). **Intubation methods** can be used to measure gastric emptying rate and are used in research but are seldom applied to the clinical assessment of individual patients [4, 10, 17].

Contrast radiology using barium suspen-sion will often show rapid gastric emptying in patients who have undergone partial gastrectomy, or vagotomy and drainage. However, radiological assessment is at best semi-quantitative and only an extreme degree of abnormality (for example, complete emptying of the stomach in five minutes) may be taken as a hint that clinical problems of dumping or diarrhoea may be anticipated.

Radionuclide methods measure gastric emptying rate and thus define abnormalities quantitatively. A greater acceleration of early gastric emptying usually occurs in patients with dumping or diarrhoea after gastric surgery, than in post-operative patients without these symptoms (Fig. 26.4). Gastric emptying measurements may therefore sometimes contribute to the assessment of patients with troublesome postoperative symptoms of uncertain significance. However, there is no standard technique for such measurements and their clinical value has not yet been clearly defined.

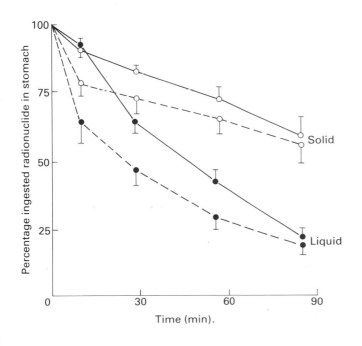

Fig. 26.3. Gastric emptying of radionuclide-labelled solid and liquid components of a meal in 12 normal subjects (solid lines) and 12 patients with truncal vagotomy and Heineke-Mikulicz pyloroplasty (broken lines). Note the acceleration of early (10 minute) emptying in the postoperative group.

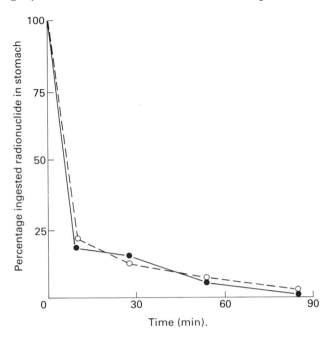

Fig. 26.4. Gastric emptying of radionuclide-labelled solid (solid circles) and liquid (open circles) components of a meal in a patient with severe dumping and diarrhoea after vagotomy and pyloroplasty. Compare with Fig. 26.3.

Clinical features of abnormal gastric motility

Impaired gastric accommodation resulting from vagotomy, or partial gastrectomy renders many patients unable to consume large meals and leads them to complain of early satiety or post-prandial epigastric fullness.

Rapid early gastric emptying resulting from gastric surgery predisposes to the early dumping syndrome and to postoperative diarrhoea. These disorders are described in Chapter 25.

Impaired gastric emptying may cause epigastric discomfort, fullness, nausea or vomiting. The vomiting may be projectile and contain food eaten many hours previously. Left-sided lower abdominal discomfort and severe heartburn of recent onset are less common complaints. Not all patients with gastric retention suffer these classical symptoms and sometimes gross retention may be associated with non-specific complaints, or symptoms not obviously

originating from the upper gastrointestinal tract. Persistent gastric retention usually causes decreased food intake and loss of weight; recurrent vomiting causes dehydration and electrolyte disturbance. Physical findings may include abdominal distension and occasionally an outline of the distended stomach may be visible through the abdominal wall. A succussion splash may be present.

Gastric retention due to mechanical obstruction

Common causes of gastric retention due to upper gastrointestinal obstruction include pyloric stenosis due to chronic peptic ulceration (Chapter 28) and gastric carcinoma (Chapter 28). The latter may also cause gastric retention without mechanically obstructing the lumen if extensive malignant infiltration of the antrum interferes with gastric peristalsis. Less common causes include inflammatory and neoplastic disorders of the duodenum, duodenal diverti culum and pancreatic pseudocyst (Chapter 29).

Hypertrophic pyloric stenosis, which usually presents in infancy, may occasionally become manifest in adult life, as adult hypertrophic pyloric stenosis. The pyloric channel is elongated and narrow, as a consequence of hypertrophy of the pyloric muscle. The clinical features are those of gastric retention. An epigastric mass often palpable in infants with this condition, is not a feature of the adult form. Treatment is surgical. Because carcinoma of the pyloric region is the main differential diagnosis, resection of the abnormal area is usually necessary to make the correct diagnosis with certainty.

Intragastric bezoars

Trichobezoars—tangled masses of hair—sometimes form in the stomachs of women who habitually chew their hair. The accumulation forms a loose mass in which food residue becomes trapped and eventually the bezoar may grow to a size sufficient to cause mechanical obstruction of the gastric outlet. **Phytobezoars** are similar, but are composed of dietary vegetable matter. It is said that they may develop in normal individuals who consume a vegetarian diet with an unusually large component of indigestible fibrous foods, but phytobezoars are most often encountered in patients whose gastric peristalsis is impaired, such as those who have undergone surgical vagotomy. Impairment of the normal crushing and grinding actions of gastric peristalsis permits an accumulation of fibrous vegetable material within the stomach, which may eventually form a discrete mass sufficient to obstruct the gastric outlet.

Management of both types of bezoar consists of attempting to break up the mass through an endoscope, with the intention of reducing it to fragments which might pass through the pylorus. In addition drugs promoting gastric peristalsis, such as metoclopramide 10 mg three times daily before meals, are usually prescribed. Surgery is occasionally necessary to remove large bezoars, notably the rare trichobezoars that extend through the pylorus into the duodenum.

Positional duodenal obstruction

Mechanical obstruction of the third part duodenum at the root of the mesentery may occasionally be encountered in very ill patients who are immobile. The following case history is illustrative.

Case report

A 20 year old woman suffered a septicaemia complicated by acute renal failure and endocarditis. Three thoracotomies were necessary within eight weeks, to insert an aortic and then a mitral valve prosthesis and to deal with a haemopericardium. She required assisted ventilation, haemodialysis and intravenous nutrition but eventually improved. Normal feeding was considered. She was 15 kg below her normal weight, was profoundly weak, and was constrained to a semi-recumbent supine position partly by physical weakness and partly by positioning of two intravenous cannulae. Twenty-four hours after beginning oral fluids *ad lib*, she complained of nausea. Abdominal examination revealed the outline of a grossly distended stomach with visible antral peristalsis—1900 ml of fluid were removed by nasogastric aspiration. A second attempt at oral fluids produced a similar result within 24 hours. Fluoroscopic examination with barium demonstrated gastric and duodenal dilatation with complete

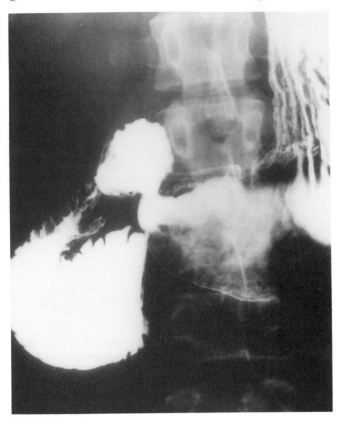

Fig. 26.5. (See case report). Complete obstruction of the third part of the duodenum was relieved when the patient was turned to the left lateral position. The stomach had been emptied by nasogastric aspiration before the radiological examination was undertaken.

obstruction of the third part duodenum when the patient was supine (Fig. 26.5), but no obstruction was apparent with the patient in the left lateral position. Oral fluids were recommenced and the patient assisted to a left lateral position every two hours. There was no recurrence of gastric retention. She gradually improved and ordinary diet was successfully resumed when she was able to sit. She eventually recovered completely.

This positional duodenal obstruction is not well described in the medical literature, perhaps because the survival of such profoundly weak and immobile patients is rare. Major gastric retention as in this case is uncommon, but it is obviously important to recognize its benign nature and the simple treatment. Very rarely, a similar chronic obstruction of the duodenum may occur [2].

Gastric retention without mechanical obstruction

Nausea due to any cause will inhibit gastric motility. Vomiting prevents the development of gross gastric retention and distension.

Acute gastric dilatation

Various acute conditions partly or completely inhibit gastric motility predisposing to gastric retention and distension, which in this context is sometimes termed acute gastric dilatation. It is now seen infrequently, simply because fasting and naso-gastric aspiration, or early surgery constitute part of the conventional management of the disorders predisposing to it, and acute gastric dilatation is usually prevented. Well recognized causes include severe pain of any origin, major trauma, inflammatory conditions, such as acute cholecystitis, appendicitis, pancreatitis and septicaemia, and metabolic disorders including diabetic ketoacidosis, hepatic encephalopathy, severe hypothyroidism and hypo- and hypercalcaemia. **Post-surgical gastric stasis** is described in Chapter 25.

Gastric retention in diabetes

Severe hyperglycaemia and diabetic ketoacidosis cause a reversible inhibition of gastric motility.

Chronic gastric retention (sometimes called diabetic gastroparesis or diabetic gastric atony) may occur in diabetic patients with autonomic neuropathy. Gastric peristalsis is impaired due to damage to vagal nerve fibres and perhaps also to myenteric neurones, leading to gastric retention and distension. The clinical features are those of gastric retention together with problems of diabetic control, resulting from the erratic delivery of ingested food to the small intestine. Symptoms characteristically vary in severity from week to week and the degree of gastric stasis may also vary. Diagnosis rests on the demonstration of autonomic neuropathy and on the exclusion of other causes of gastric retention. The symptoms of diabetic gastroparesis are invariably relieved when the stomach is emptied by nasogastric aspiration and the persistence of symptoms on completion of this procedure is an indication to seek some other explanation for the patient's complaints. Treatment consists of optimizing control of the diabetes, together with the prescription of metoclopramide 10 mg, or domperidone 10 or 20 mg before meals to promote gastric peristalsis and minimize nausea [25]. It may be helpful to give these drugs parenterally in the first instance. Treatment should be continued until improvement occurs; long-term therapy is not always necessary. Surgery (pyloroplasty or antrectomy) is rarely helpful. These patients have a poor prognosis, because diabetic gastroparesis is a manifestation of severe autonomic neuropathy, co-existing with other serious complications of diabetes. Approximately half of the patients are dead within three years of the gastroparesis being recognized.

Other causes

Drug induced gastric retention by narcotic analgesics, ganglion blocking drugs and drugs with anti-cholinergic activity may cause clinically important gastric stasis. Review of the treatment and stopping the drugs or decreasing the dose will cure the condition.

Impaired gastric peristalsis with gastric retention may occur in several **diseases which affect muscle**, including dermatomyositis, scleroderma and myotonic muscular dystrophy. Delayed gastric emptying is often part of the chronic intestinal pseudo-obstruction syndrome (Chapter 47).

Gastric emptying is delayed in some patients with unexplained upper gastrointestinal symptoms (**'functional' dyspepsia**) [11, 13]. Some of these cases are apparently due to abnormalities of antral peristalsis, while others may follow a viral illness. Most remain unexplained [22, 24, 27]. Contrary to the expectation of many clinicians, recent research has failed to indentify abnormalities of gastric emptying in patients with irritable bowel syndrome [3]. Experimental severe stress inhibits gastric motility, but the relevance of this observation to the psychological disorders encountered clinically is uncertain. Gastric emptying is impaired in anorexia nervosa [9].

Duodenogastric reflux

Reflux of duodenal fluid containing bile and pancreatic secretions into the stomach occurs to some extent in normal individuals, but it is controlled by co-ordination of pyloric and proximal duodenal contractions, such that the pylorus is usually closed when the duodenum contracts. Moreover, any fluid refluxed into the antrum during emptying of a meal from the stomach will almost immediately be returned to the duodenum before mixing with the more proximal gastric contents. In the fasting state duodenal contents refluxed into the stomach are returned to the duodenum by the intermittent powerful gastric contractions which constitute phase 3 of the interdigestive migrating motor complex [11].

Increased duodenogastric reflux has been identified in patients with peptic ulcer of the stomach or duodenum [5, 6, 23]. In some cases it seems likely that this reflux occurs because deformity of the pylorus prevents its adequate closure when the duodenum contracts, while in other instances the normal co-ordination between pyloric and duodenal contractions may be lost. Major duodenogastric reflux occurs when the distal antrum and pylorus are resected or bypassed, as in Billroth I gastrectomy or gastroenterostomy.

The injurious effects of bile on the gastric mucosa are discussed in detail in Chapter 19; the possible relevance of duodenogastric reflux to the genesis, or maintenance of peptic ulcer in the stomach should be noted.

Measurement of duodenogastric reflux

Although the measurement of duodenogastric reflux is a procedure more appropriate to research than to everyday clinical practice, a brief description of the techniques employed is given below. It is worth emphasizing that while direct observation of duodenal contents flowing into the stomach at upper gastrointestinal endoscopy should not be regarded as clinically important because of the unnatural circumstances of endoscopy, the recovery of heavily bile stained fluid from a fasting stomach is suggestive of an abnormal degree of reflux.

X-ray fluoroscopy after injection of contrast down a fine bore nasoduodenal tube can be used to identify duodenogastric reflux [5, 6]. In normal subjects, reflux of contrast into the stomach is exceptional. **Intraduodenal infusion** of markers such as polyethylene glycol, may be used to quantify duodenogastric reflux by relating the amount infused into the duodenum to the amount recovered by nasogastric aspiration [12]. **Bile acid concentrations** in fluid aspirated from the fasting stomach have been shown to correlate with fluoroscopic evidence of reflux and with the severity of symptoms attributed to duodenogastric reflux in patients who have previously undergone gastric surgery [8].

Radionuclide methods are a relatively recent development [19, 26]. A derivative of amino diacetic acid labelled with technetium 99m (^{99m}Tc HIDA) is given intravenously and becomes concentrated in the bile. Gamma camera images of the subject's abdomen taken up to 60 minutes after injection will show isotope in the liver, in the duodenum and the small bowel; an outline of the stomach is obtained only in individuals with duodenogastric reflux. The radioactivity in the stomach area on the image can be measured and provides an index of the amount of duodenogastric reflux.

Drugs used to treat gastric motility disorders

Metoclopramide chemically a derivative of procainamide, is an anti-emetic which in addition stimulates gastric peristalsis. Its pharmacology is still controversial, but the drug is a dopamine antagonist which apparently also enhances acetylcholine release from myenteric cholinergic neurones [1]. Metoclopramide has been shown to increase the gastric emptying rate and to improve symptoms in patients with delayed gastric emptying not due to mechanical obstruction. The usual dose is 10 mg three times daily. Recognized adverse reactions include a dystonia resembling that seen with phenothiazines, hyperprolactinaemia and gynaecomastia. Agitation and claustrophobia may be provoked by intravenous administration.

Domperidone a dopamine antagonist, is an anti-emetic acting on the chemoreceptor trigger zone, but crosses the blood brain barrier to a very limited extent. The drug has been shown to increase gastric peristalsis and emptying when these are impaired and to improve symptoms attributed to gastric hypomotility. It is assumed that these effects result from dopamine antagonism, but overall the drug has not been studied as fully as metoclopramide. The usual dose is 10 mg four times daily. Hyperprolactinaemia and gynaecomastia are rare adverse reactions.

References

1 ALBIBI R, MCCALLUM RW. Metoclopramide: pharmacology and clinical application. *Ann Intern Med* 1983;98:86–95.
2 ANDERSON JR, EARNSHAW PM, FRASER GM. Extrinsic compression of the third part of the duodenum. *Clin Radiol* 1982;33:75–81.
3 CANN PA, READ NW, BROWN C, HOBSON N, HOLDSWORTH CD. Irritable bowel syndrome: relationship of disorders in the transit of a single solid meal to symptom patterns. *Gut* 1983;24:405–411.
4 CLARKE RJ, ALEXANDER-WILLIAMS J. The effect of preserving antral innervation and of a pyloroplasty on gastric emptying after vagotomy in man. *Gut* 1973;14:300–307.
5 COCKING JB, GRECH P. Pyloric reflux and the healing of gastric ulcer. *Gut* 1973;14:555–557.
6 FLINT FJ, GRECH P. Pyloric regurgitation and gastric ulcer. *Gut* 1970;11:735–737.
7 HEADING RC, TOTHILL P, MCLOUGHLIN GP, SHEARMAN DJC. Gastric emptying rate measurement in

man. A double isotope scanning technique for simultaneous study of liquid and solid components of a meal. *Gastroenterology* 1976;71:45–50.
8 HOARE AM, KEIGHLEY MRB, STARKEY B, ALEXANDER-WILLIAMS J. Measurement of bile acids in fasting gastric aspirates: an objective test for bile reflux after gastric surgery. *Gut* 1978;19:166–169.
9 HOLT S, FORD MJ, GRANT S, HEADING RC. Abnormal gastric emptying in primary anorexia nervosa. *Br J Psychiatry* 1981;139:550–552.
10 HURWITZ A. Measuring gastric volumes by dye dilution. *Gut* 1981;22:85–93.
11 JIAN R, DUCROT F, PIEDELOUP C, MARY JY, NAJEAN Y, BERNIER JJ. Measurement of gastric emptying in dyspeptic patients: effect of a new gastrokinetic agent (cisapride). *Gut* 1985;26:352–358.
12 KEANE FB, DIMAGNO EP, MALAGELADA JR. Duodenogastric reflux in humans: its relationship to fasting antroduodenal motility and gastric pancreatic and biliary secretion. *Gastroenterology* 1981;81:726–731.
13 LABO G, BORTOLOTTI M, VEZZADINI P, BONORA G, BERSANI G. Interdigestive gastroduodenal motility and serum motilin levels in patients with idiopathic delay in gastric emptying. *Gastroenterology* 1986;90:20–26.
14 LAM SK, ISENBERG JI, GROSSMAN MI, LANE WH, HOGAN DL. Rapid gastric emptying in duodenal ulcer patients. *Dig Dis Sci* 1981;27:598–604.
15 MADDERN GJ, HOROWITZ M, HETZEL DJ, JAMIESON GG. Altered solid and liquid gastric emptying in patients with duodenal ulcer disease. *Gut* 1985;26:689–693.
16 MCCALLUM RW, BERKOWITZ DM, LERNER E. Gastric emptying in patients with gastroesophageal reflux. *Gastroenterology* 1981;80:285–291.
17 MALAGELADA JR, LONGSTRETH GF, SUMMERSKILL WHJ, GO VLW. Measurement of gastric functions during digestion of ordinary solid meals in man. *Gastroenterology* 1976;70:203–210.
18 MEYER JH, MACGREGOR IL, GUELLER R, MARTIN P, CAVALIERI R. ^{99m}Tc tagged chicken liver as a marker of solid food in the human stomach. *Dig Dis Sci* 1976;21:296–304.
19 MUHAMMED I, HOLT S, MCLOUGHLIN GP, TAYLOR TV. Non invasive estimation of duodenogastric reflux using technetium 99m p-butyl iminodiacetic acid. *Lancet* 1980;ii:1162–1165.
20 MULLER-LISSNER SA. Measurements of bile salt reflux are influenced by the method of collecting gastric juice. *Gastroenterology* 1985;89:1338–1341.
21 OSTICK DG, GREEN G, HOWE K, DYMOCK IW, COWLEY DJ. Simple clinical method of measuring gastric emptying of solid meals. *Gut* 1976;17:189–191.
22 PERKEL MS, MOORE C, HERSH T, DAVIDSON ED. Metoclopramide therapy in patients with delayed gastric emptying. *Dig Dis Sci* 1979;24:662–666.
23 RHODES J, BARNARDO DE, PHILLIPS SF, ROVELSTAD

RA, HOFFMAN AF. Increased reflux of bile into the stomach in patients with gastric ulcer. *Gastroenterology* 1969;57:241–252.

24 RHODES JB. ROBINSON RG, McBRIDE N. Sudden onset of slow gastric emptying of food. *Gastroenterology* 1979;77:569–571.

25 SNAPE WJ, BATTLE WM, SCHWARZ SS, BRAUNSTEIN SN, GOLDSTEIN HA, ALAVI A. Metoclopramide to treat gastroparesis due to diabetes mellitus. *Ann Intern Med* 1982;96:444–446.

26 TOLIN RD, MALMUD LS, STELZER F, *et al.* Enterogastric reflux in normal subjects and patients with Billroth II gastroenterostomy. *Gastroenterology* 1979;77:1027–1033.

27 YOU CH, LEE KY, CHEY WY, MENGUY R. Electrogastrographic study of patients with unexplained nausea bloating and vomiting. *Gastroenterology* 1980;79:311–314.

Chapter 27
Benign Gastric Tumours

J. B. ELDER

Benign gastric tumours are considered rare, but are not all that uncommon in gastrointestinal practice. They are sometimes asymptomatic, quite small and are often only discovered at gastroscopy. The term benign may be misleading, as some may show foci of malignant or premalignant change. Some are not tumours in the true sense, but represent a gastric mucosal inflammatory response [22] (Fig. 27.1).

Prevalence and aetiology

The incidence of benign gastric tumours is equal in men and women and has a peak between the fifth and seventh decade of life, [31]. In routine post-mortem studies the incidence of benign gastric tumours is low, ranging from 0.33% in one series of 20,000 autopsies [52] to 0.9% in another of 14,620 autopsies [41]. Gastric polyps account for most such lesions, estimated at 0.4% in a large pooled series of 80,000 autopsies

reported by Bentivegna and Panagopoulos [3]. The advent of upper gastrointestinal fibre-endoscopy has revealed a greater incidence of benign tumours in patients undergoing this procedure—a review of 13,200 consecutive endoscopies uncovered an incidence of 2.7% of benign gastric tumours [30], while in a consecutive series of 2420 patients investigated by double contrast barium meal examination benign tumours were found in 38 patients—an incidence of 1.6%, four times the average rate noticed at autopsy in the general population [19]. Polyp-like lesions of a purely inflammatory type were present in just under 1% in the series of 13,200 consecutive gastroscopies reported by Laxen, *et al.* [30], in 1982. Clearly those examined for upper gastrointestinal symptoms have an increased chance of having a benign gastric tumour.

In most cases the aetiology of benign gastric tumours is unknown, but there is a relationship between atrophic gastritis and

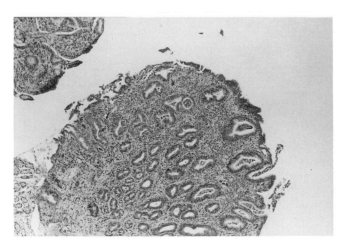

Fig. 27.1. Inflammatory polyp showing dense infiltrate of inflammatory cells separating the glandular elements (H & E × 35) (Histopathology Figs by courtesy of Dr A Ahmed, University of Manchester).

inflammatory benign polyps of the stomach [37]. Some are genetic as in association with familial polyposis coli [43]; some are associated with small bowel polyps in the Peutz-Jeghers syndrome and are very different from true adenomas. The gastric polyps found in cases of Peutz-Jeghers syndrome are formed from clearly differentiated proliferations of all cell types in the antrum and fundus including smooth muscle elements [12]. Other genetically determined conditions in which gastric polyps may occur include Gardner's syndrome [17], the Cronkhite-Canada syndrome [10] and familial adenomatosis coli [27], in which there is an association with polyps and benign tumours of the large and small intestine. The incidence of benign gastric tumours is high in pernicious anaemia, ranging from 6% to 20% of patients [14, 24, 34].

Pathology

The pathology of benign gastric tumours covers a wide range of distinct histological entities [8, 35, 37, 40, 50, 56]. They may be classified into four groups: epithelial tumours, mesenchymal tumours, developmental lesions (hamartomas and heterotopies) and fibroinflammatory pseudotu-

mours. The mean relative percentages of benign gastric tumours in 2,725 cases is illustrated in Fig. 27.2 [11]. Histological criteria are crucial to such distinctions; not surprisingly there are some tumours that are difficult to classify, lying between inflammatory lesions and benign tumours, or between the latter and malignant tumours. Several authors have reviewed this problem [23, 26, 33, 38, 53].

Epithelial lesions

Epithelial lesions are often referred to as polyps. Gastric polyps may be pedunculated, villous, sessile or smooth and broad based. Hyperplastic polyps [37] sometimes known as regenerative polyps [35] or as the hyperplasiogenous polyp of Elster [16], make up the majority (70%) of the polypoid lesions seen (Fig. 27.3). There is still no agreement in the classification of polypoid adenomas, Morson and Dawson [38] contending that true gastric adenomas are uncommon. Often repeated biopsy evidence is required for precise definition of a differentiated or hyperplastic polyp (Fig. 27.3) from a true adenomatous polyp or other lesion. Such a distinction is important as the hyperplastic lesion is of weak malignant potential, while

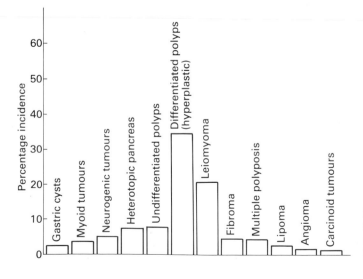

Fig. 27.2. Relative percentage incidence of benign gastric tumours from 2725 pooled cases (after [11]).

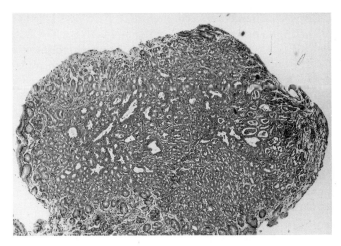

Fig. 27.3. Hyperplastic (regenerative) polyp showing superficial ulceration of the surface. Note the marked increase in the gastric glandular tissue and the absence of inflammatory infiltrate (H & E × 35) (courtesy of Dr A. Ahmed).

the adenomatous polyp (Fig. 27.4) is more closely associated with gastric malignancy. Even repeated biopsies may miss foci of carcinoma. Ming and Goldman [35] studied 90 cases of gastric polyps and found the ratio of hyperplastic to adenomatous polyps of 4:1. Almost 70% of those with adenomatous polyps also had gastric cancer, while only 4% of those with hyperplastic polyps were considered to have gastric carcinoma. In a more recent study Laxen, *et al.* [30] found that carcinoma of the stomach was associated in 38% of patients with true adenomas. On the other hand Morson and Dawson [38] state that hyperplastic regenerative polyps have no significant cancer potential.

Benign adenomatous gastric polyps originate in the glandular structures of the gastric wall and may be single or multiple, commonly presenting between 50 and 60 years of age with a similar age distribution in both sexes. Most of the lesions are in the antrum [31] and often have a tubulo-villous pattern. Lesions referred to as adenomatous polyps of Ming, Goldman [35] and Morson [37], commonly have a papillary appearance and are often bigger than the hyperplastic or differentiated polyps. The rate of malignant transformation is uncertain. It may be as high as 38% in adenomatous polyps, but others report an incidence as low as 3.7% [31]. The more extreme view of Monaco, *et al.* [36], that there is

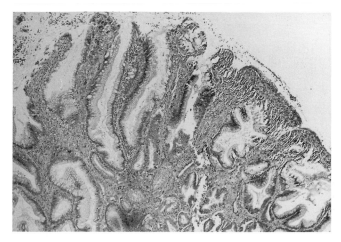

Fig. 27.4. Adenomatous polyps with tubulo-villous pattern and focal intestinal metaplasia (H & E × 100) (courtesy of Dr A. Ahmed).

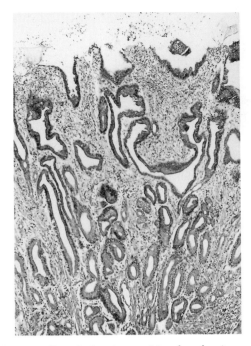

Fig. 27.5. Peutz-Jeghers type gastric polyp, showing branching glands and interglandular smooth muscle elements arising from muscularis mucosae (H & E × 40) (courtesy of Dr A. Ahmed).

no evidence that a stomach with multiple polyps runs a greater risk of cancer than any other, is not the view of most authors. De-differentiated adenomas and papillomas are sometimes associated with chronic atrophic gastritis and intestinal metaplasia. Lesions larger than 2 cm diameter are prone to un-

dergo cancerous change [9, 26, 58]. Other polypoid lesions of the stomach such as sessile or pedunculated villous tumours are rarer, but have been associated with intestinal metaplasia. Diffuse gastric polyposis accounts for less than 5% of all gastric polyps [7]. Gastric polyps occur in multiple familial polyposis, in multiple neurofibromatosis and in the Peutz-Jeghers syndrome (Fig. 27.5). Ranzi, *et al.* [4] found adenomatous polyps in the stomach in seven of nine patients with familial polyposis coli, and gastric and/or duodenal polyps were found in 28 of 34 such patients by Jarvinen, *et al.* [27], indicating that the incidence of neoplastic polyps in the upper gastrointestinal tract of these patients may be much higher than previously suspected. While the histology of these lesions is not an entirely settled matter and grey areas may exist in separating the different groups, it is clear that large (> 2 cm diameter), multiple adenomatous and villous polyps have an incidence of malignancy of the order of 20–40% [21, 26, 30, 35, 46], a situation reminiscent of that in the colon.

Developmental lesions

Developmental lesions include many malformations or ectopic tissues. The commonest is a gastric pancreatic heterotopic

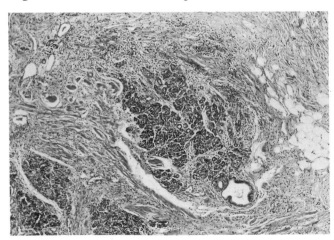

Fig. 27.6. Ectopic submucosal pancreatic tissue surrounded by bundles of smooth muscle (H & E × 35) (courtesy of Dr A. Ahmed).

rest (Fig. 27.6), which accounted for 7% of all benign gastric lesions in a large series [11]—it is usually close to the pylorus [28, 40].

The heterotopic pancreas occurs twice as often in men, is often less than 3 cm in diameter and need not breach the mucosa, but simply present as a thickening in the pre-pyloric region. Ectopic pancreatic tissue can undergo inflammatory, and rarely, malignant change, and is seldom related to the patient's symptoms [13].

Other developmental lesions, such as ectopic Brunner's glands and myoepithelial hamartoma, polypoid eosinophilic granuloma, gastric teratoma and dermoids, are all very rare [38]. Gastric xanthelasmata are endoscopically seen as small, yellow, plaque-like lesions, due to large numbers of foamy macrophages in the submucosa [29]. Their cause is unknown, but they are not associated with hypercholesteraemia. Benign gastric cysts are extremely rare, as are duplications of the stomach [1, 42].

Mesenchymal tumours

Mesenchymal tumours arise from any of the connective tissue elements of the stomach—the most common are spindle cell tumours, or leiomyomas. Arising from either the longitudinal or circular muscle coats, they make up approximately 50% of all benign gastric tumours [51]. They can be clinically troublesome, largely because of acute or chronic haemorrhage from vessels lying just under the mucosa covering the tumours (Fig. 27.7) producing iron-deficiency anaemia, with or without abdominal pain. Many varieties of histological patterns are found and it can be difficult, or sometimes impossible to say whether a leiomyoma will be benign or malignant from the histological appearances alone, which may be bizarre (Fig. 27.8) [38]. More often than not the appearance is benign, with no evidence of metastases.

Mixtures of different cellular components can occur and composite names such as angiofibroleiomyoma arise (Fig. 27.9). The incidence of malignancy in smooth muscle tumours of the stomach may be as high as 1 in 10 [5, 48]. The sex incidence is said to be equal and there are no known predisposing factors. Their growth usually directs the projection of the bulk of the tumour into the lumen. Rather more rarely the serosal surface is involved, giving a 'dumbbell' appearance. The differential diagnosis must include glomus tumours [2, 55], true fibromas (a rare tumour) or neurilemmoma-Schwannoma [47, 50]. While such

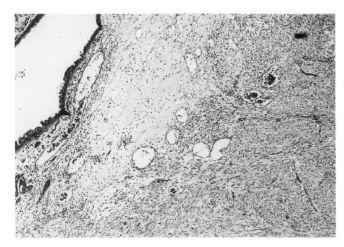

Fig. 27.7 Leiomyoma. Note the attenuated gastric mucosa and underlying large vascular channels (H & E × 35) (courtesy of Dr. A. Ahmed).

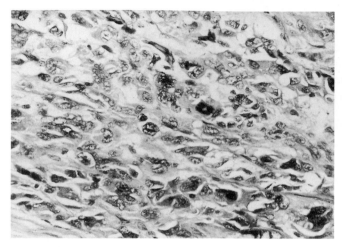

Fig. 27.8. Leiomyoma with bizarre pleomorphic cells.

tumours are seldom palpable, they are often ulcerated as can be easily seen at endoscopy.

Surgical treatment of leiomyomas is usually a wedge resection originating as they do in the muscle cells of the gastric wall.

Leiomyoblastoma

Leiomyoblastoma, characterized by Martin, *et al.* [32], has been given a variety of names, including reticulohistiocytoma and histiocytofibroma—over 200 cases are now documented. These appear as lesions of well demarcated antral tumours and present with pyloric obstruction in many instances.

Histologically, there are typical cells with a round, central and regular nucleus, surrounded by a peripheral clear halo in the cytoplasm giving the cell the characteristic appearance of an 'Owl's eye' [49] (Fig. 27.10). These appearances are sometimes focal, being part of a leiomyoma of varied cell type. At least 10% of these tumours undergo malignant change [5].

Gastric lipomas

Gastric lipomas are often large lobulated swellings in the submucosa of the antrum; they project into the lumen of the stomach sometimes undergoing necrosis and haemorrhage. These rare tumours [54] are

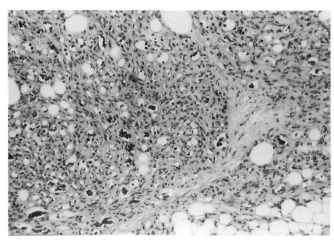

Fig. 27.9. Mixed leiomyoma. Note the prominent vascular channels scattered among the smooth muscle cells and rim of fibrous tissue (H & E × 100) (courtesy of Dr A. Ahmed).

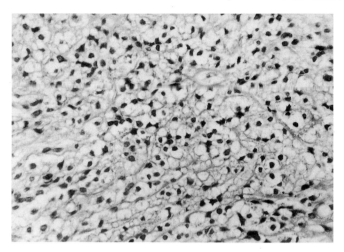

Fig. 27.10. Leiomyoblastoma showing dark nuclei surrounded by a clear cytoplasmic halo (H & E × 250) (courtesy of Dr A. Ahmed).

sometimes regarded as hamartomas, rather than essentially benign neoplasms [38].

Fibroinflammatory pseudotumours

Fibroinflammatory pseudotumours are small lesions, usually < 1 cm in diameter, often associated with gastritis (Fig. 27.1) and composed of fibrous stomach elements with inflammatory cells and sometimes plasma cells and lymphocytes. They usually lie in the antral submucosa, are whitish in colour at endoscopy and may extend to the muscularis mucosa. The aetiology is controversial and they are believed to be part of an inflammatory response, perhaps modified by a local allergic reaction. Others have suggested that these inflammatory fibroid lesions may have a neurogenic origin [18].

Pseudolymphoma or benign lymphoid hyperplasia of the stomach

Pseudolymphoma or benign lymphoid hyperplasia of the stomach [57] consists usually of a fibrotic, flat, ulcerated lesion on the lesser curvature which is radiologically similar to a carcinoma. On biopsy it consists of lymph follicles and fibrosis with or without ulceration of the mucosa. The lesion has clearly demarcated margin and often

involves only the mucosa and submucosa. The differential diagnosis is from gastric carcinoma and lymphoma. Similar lesions have been found in the duodenum and rectum. Essentially benign, it carries a good prognosis [33] (see Chapter 28).

Clinical features of benign epithclial gastric tumours

While benign epithelial gastric tumours are found in approximately 1–3% of patients undergoing upper GI endoscopy, they are found with greater frequency in selected groups—when patients with severe hypochlorydria or achlorhydria are screened, 2–5% are found to have benign adenomatous polyps of thc stomach [56]; in those with pernicious anaemia the incidence of hyperplastic polyps increases to 5–8% [14, 15, 24].

Patients with benign epithelial tumours often complain of epigastric pain [39], which is perhaps related to the almost invariable inflammatory changes, often with superficial ulceration of the polyp (Fig. 27.3). Thirty per cent have nausea and vomiting and as most lesions are in the antrum, it is not uncommon for pedunculated polyps to prolapse through the pylorus or present at the gastric outlet causing intermittent obstruction. In other patients symptoms are vague and non-specific consisting of epigastric fullness, discomfort, tiredness, (iron-deficiency anaemia), wind and nausea. Haematemesis is surprisingly rare—probably in less than 10% of such patients. Melaena is more common. Eighty per cent to 90% of patients have anacidity or severe hypoacidity (MAO < 1 mmol hr^{-1}). Weight loss may be present in up to a third of patients.

After the history, family history and examination, investigations should include proctoscopy and sigmoidoscopy, a blood count and film, gastroscopy and multiple biopsies, including the use of the diathermy snare loop if appropriate, and if available, cytological examination of gastric washing and a maximal gastric acid output test to pentagastrin 6 μg/kg body weight subcutaneously. Serum B_{12} estimation should also be routine [14]. A double-contrast barium meal and follow-through examination should also be performed [4].

Clinical management

Management depends on the histological nature of the gastric lesion. Small pedunculated polyps with a pedicle can be removed by endoscopic techniques, either at one or several sessions clearing the entire stomach of all the lesions for histological examination. Endoscopic snaring is replacing a more aggressive policy of partial or total gastric resection. Continued management on these lines would be justified only in the absence of malignant change at the tip of a polyp or elsewhere. Cautery of the base of any lesion resected is a sensible manœuvre, because of risk of bleeding—in a series of 48 endoscopic gastric polypectomies, two bleeding episodes requiring direct surgery were reported from the Mayo Clinic by ReMine, *et al.* [44]. No deaths resulted from these procedures, but of the 12 adenomatous polyps removed (25% of the total number), all less than 2 cm diameter, two contained foci of *in situ* malignancy.

Many patients with gastric polyps are in the older age group and may have other illnesses, making gastric resection risky. It is clear that regular endoscopic surveillance in this group is preferred.

Spontaneous disappearance of gastric polyps has been described in patients with pernicious anaemia [15, 25], but new polyps appeared in 20% of patients. The authors [15] commented that all the lesions were non-neoplastic, with the characteristics of regenerative polyps. They discounted the role of gastrin in polyp production [6]. This view may have to be revised in the light of reports of enterochromaffin-like cell (ECL) hyperplasia and multifocal gastric carcinoid tumours occurring in patients with pernicious anaemia [20] and in experimental animals treated with high doses of omeprazole and thus with hypergastrinaemia. Such studies emphasize the dynamic state of the gastric mucosa in atrophic gastritis with hyperplastic polyps and underline the need for regular endoscopic follow-up, perhaps at six, or 12 month intervals. There are no known means of prevention and apart from antacids there is little indication for any anti-ulcer preparations. Where polyps show severe intestinal metaplasia, or are frankly neoplastic, or are recurring rapidly, total gastrectomy must be considered if antrum and fundus are involved; in some patients antral resection alone will suffice. Such radical surgical treatment should become less necessary if vague upper gastrointestinal symptoms or unexplained anaemias are investigated promptly by endoscopy and dealt with by endoscopic snare-polypectomy and laser [44, 45].

References

1 ABRAMI G, DENNISON WM. Duplications of the stomach. *Surgery St. Louis* 1961;**49**:794–801.
2 APPELMAN HD, HELWIG EB. Glomus tumours of the stomach. *Cancer* 1969;**23**:203–213.
3 BENTIVEGNA S, PANAGOPOULOS AG. Adenomatous gastric polyps. *J Gastroenterol* 1965;**44**:138–148.

4 BONFIELD RE, MARTEL W, BATASKIS JG. The significance of small gastric filling defects. *Surg Gynecol Obstet* 1968;**127**:1231–1235.

5 BOSE B, CANDY J. Gastric leiomyosarcoma. *Gut* 1970;**11**:875–880.

6 BRANDBORG M, ELSBORG L, ANDERSEN D. Gastrin concentrations in serum and gastric mucosa in patients with pernicious anaemia. *Scand J Gastroenterol* 1977;**12**:537–541.

7 CARLSON E, WARD JG. Surgical considerations in gastric polyps, gastric polyposis and giant hypertrophic gastritis in 74 cases. *Surg Gynecol Obstet* 1958;**107**:727–738.

8 CONDON RE. Unusual disorders of the stomach and duodenum. In: Nyhus LM, Wastell C, eds. *Surgery of the Stomach and Duodenum.* 3rd Edition. Boston: Little, Brown & Co, 1977.

9 CORNET P, RENAULT P, CARNOT F. Polypes gastrique. Polypose et gastrite chronique. *Arch Fr Mal App Dig* 1971;**60**:507–524.

10 CRONKHITE LW, CANADA WJ. Generalised gastrointestinal polyposis. An unusual syndrome of polyposis, pigmentation, alopecia and onychoatrophia. *New Engl J Med* 1955;**252**:1011–1015.

11 DEBRAY CH, MARTIN E. Benign gastric tumours. In: Bockus H, ed. *Gastroenterology* Vol. 1. Philadelphia: Saunders, 1974.

12 DODDS WJ, SCHULTZE WJ, HENSLEY GT. Peutz-Jeghers syndrome and gastrointestinal malignancy. *Am J Roentgeno Radium Ther Nucl Med* 1972;**115**:374–377.

13 DOLAN RV, REMINE WH, DOCKERTY MB. The fate of heterotopic pancreatic tissue. *Arch Surg* 1974;**109**:762–765.

14 EKLOF O, ENGSTEDT L, REIZENSTEIN P. Intrinsic factor deficiency, achlorhydria and malignancy in polyps of the stomach and duodenum. *Acta Med Scand* 1962;**171**:601–612.

15 ELSBORG L, ANDERSEN D, MYHRE-JENSEN O, BASTRUP-MADSEN P. Gastric mucosal polyps in pernicious anaemia. *Scand J Gastroenterol* 1977;**12**:49–52.

16 ELSTER K. Histologic classification of gastric polyps. In: Morson BC, ed. *Current topics in pathology.* Heidelberg: Springe Verlag, 1977;**63**:77–93.

17 GARDNER EJ, RICHARDS RC. Multiple cutaneous and subcutaneous lesions occurring simultaneously with hereditary polyposis and osteomatosis. *Am J Hum Genet* 1953;**5**:139–147.

18 GOLDMAN, RL, FREIDMAN, NB. Neurogenic nature of so-called fibroid polyps of the stomach. *Cancer N.Y.* 1967;**20**:134–143.

19 GORDON R, LAUFER I, KRESSLER HY. Gastric polyps on routine double-contrast examination of the stomach. *Radiology* 1980;**134**:27–29.

20 HARVEY RF, BRADSHAW MJ, DAVIDSON CM, WILKISON SP, DAVIES PS. Multifocal gastric carcinoid tumours. Achlorhydria and hypergastrinaemia. *Lancet* 1985;**i**:951–954.

21 HAY LJ. Surgical management of gastric polyps and adenomas. *Surgery* 1956;**39**:114–119.

22 HELWIG EB, RANIER A. Inflammatory fibroid polyps of the stomach. *Surg Gynecol Obstet* 1953;**96**:355–367.

23 HOLMES FJ. Morphogenesis of gastric adenomatous polyps. Transformation to invasive carcinoma of intestinal type. *Cancer* 1966;**19**:794–802.

24 HUPPLER EG, PRIESTLEY JT, MARLOCK CG, GAGE RP. Diagnosis and results of treatment in gastricpolyps. *Surg Gynecol Obstet* 1960;**110**:309–313.

25 IIADA M, YAO T, WATANABE H. Spontaneous disappearance of fundic gland polyposis: report of the cases. *Gastroenterology* 1980;**79**:725–728.

26 JAMIESON GG, LUDBROOK J. The problem of 'benign' polypoid lesions of the stomach. *Aust NZ J Surg* 1971;**41**:123–130.

27 JARVINEN H, NYBERG M, PETTOKOALLIO P. Upper gastrointestinal tract polyps in familial adenomatosis coli. *Gut* 1983;**24**:333–339.

28 KILMAN WJ, BERK RN. The spectrum of radiographic features of aberrant pancreatic rests involving the stomach. *Radiology* 1977;**123**:291–296.

29 KIMURA K, HIRAMOTO T, BUNCHER CR. Gastric xanthelasma *Arch Pathol* 1969;**87**:110–117.

30 LAXEN F, SIPPONEN P, IHAMAKI T, HAKPILUOTO A, DORTSCHEVA Z. Gastric polyps; their morphological and endoscopical characteristics and relation to gastric carcinoma. *Acta Pathol Microbiol Immunol Scand [A]* 1982;**90**(3):221–228.

31 MARSHAK RH, FELDMAN F. Gastric polyps. *Am J Dig Dis* 1965;**10**:909–935.

32 MARTIN JF, BAZIN P, FEROLDI J, CABAUNE F. Tumours intra-murales de l'estomac; considerations microscopiques àpropos de 6 cas. *Ann Anat Path (Paris)* 1960;**5**:484–497.

33 MATTINGLY CS, CIBULL ML, RAM MD, HAGIHARA PF, GRIFFEN WO. Pseudolymphoma of the stomach. *Arch Surg* 1981;**116**:25–29.

34 MILN DC, HANNAH G. The single gastric polyp. *Br J Surg* 1968;**55**:599–602.

35 MING SC, GOLDMAN H. Gastric polyps: a histogenic classification and its relation to carcinoma. *Cancer* 1965;**18**:721–726.

36 MONACO AP, ROTH SI, CASTLEMAN B, WELCH CF. Adenomatous polyps of the stomach: A clinical and pathological study of 153 cases. *Cancer* 1962;**15**:456–467.

37 MORSON BC. Gastric polyps composed of intestinal epithelium. *Br J Cancer* 1959;**9**:550–557.

38 MORSON BC, DAWSON IMP. Benign Epithelial Tumours and 'Polyps'. In: *Gastrointestinal pathology.* Oxford: Blackwell Scientific Publications, 1979: 140–147.

39 NEIMARK S, ROGERS AI. Gastric polyps: A review. *Amer J Gastroenterol* 1982;**77**:585–587.

40 PALMER ED. Benign intramural tumours of the sto-

mach. A review with special reference to gross pathology. *Medicine* 1951;**30**:81–181.

41 PLACHTA A, SPEER FD. Gastric polyps and their relationship to carcinoma of the stomach. *Amer J Gastroenterol* 1957;**28**:160–175.

42 POTTER EL. *Pathology of the foetus and infant.* Chicago: Medical Publishers, 1961.

43 RANZI T, CASTAGNONE D, VELIO P, BIANCHI P, POLLI EE. Gastric and duodenal polyps in familial polyposis coli. *Gut* 1981;**22**:363–367.

44 REMINE SG, HUGHES RW Jr, WEILAND LH. Endoscopic gastric polypectomies. *Mayo Clinic Proceedings* 1981;**56**:371–375.

45 RICHEY GD, DIXON JA. Ablation of atypical gastric mucosa and recurrent polyps by endoscopic application of laser. *Gastrointestinal Endoscopy* 1981;**27**:224–225.

46 ROSATO FE, NOTO JA. Gastric polyps. *Am J Surg* 1966;**111**:647–650.

47 RUTTEN APM. Neurogenic tumours of the stomach. *Br J Surg* 1965;**52**:920–925.

48 SALMELA H. Smooth muscle tumours of the stomach: a clinical study of 112 cases. *Acta Clin Scand* 1968;**134**:384–391.

49 SCHOFIELD PF, FOX HH. Leiomyoblastoma of stomach. *Br J Surg* 1965;**52**:928–930.

40 SKANDALAKIS JE, GRAY SW, SHEPHARD D, BOURNE GH. Smooth muscle tumours of the alimentary tract. Springfield, Ill.: Springfield: Charles C Thomas, 1962.

51 STOUT AP. Bizarre smooth muscle tumours of the stomach. *Cancer* 1962;**15**:400–409.

52 THOMPSON HL, OYSTER JM. Neoplasm of the stomach other than carcinoma. *Gastroenterology* 1950;**15**:185–243.

53 TOMASULO J. Gastric polyps—Histologic types and their relationship to gastric carcinoma. *Cancer* 1971;**27**:1346–1355.

54 TURKINGTON RW. Gastric lipoma. Report of a case and revision of the literature. *Am J Dig Dis* 1965;**10**:719–726.

55 WEITZNER S. Glomus tumours of the stomach. *Am J Gastroenterol* 1969;**51**:322–328.

56 WELCH JP. *Polypoid lesions of the gastrointestinal tract.* Philadelphia: Saunders, 1964.

57 WRIGHT CJE. Pseudolymphoma of the stomach. *Human Pathol* 1973;**4**:305–318.

58 YAMADA T, ICHIKAWA H. X-ray diagnosis of elevated lesions of the stomach. *Radiology* 1974;**110**:79–83.

Chapter 28
Gastric Cancer and Lymphoma

I   GASTRIC CANCER *by* J. L. CRAVEN

II   GASTRIC LYMPHOMA *by* A. S. MEE

I   GASTRIC CANCER

Stomach cancer causes the death of more than 14,000 people per year in the United Kingdom, where a patient with stomach cancer has less than a 10% chance of surviving five years. Low rates of early diagnosis, operability and curative resection combine to produce this depressing prognosis. Though improved results of treatment have been reported from Japan during the past 25 years, these have not been attained in the West. The degree of fatalism which surrounds therapy of this disease [44] needs to be countered by reviewing research in epidemiology, aetiology, pathogenesis and pathology and by reconsidering the effect that screening, early diagnosis, radical surgery and adjuvant therapy can have at improving survival.

Epidemiology

Stomach cancer data [14] show a wide range in international age adjusted rates of incidence (Fig. 28.1) and wide regional differences occur within countries. Howe [29] has reported a three-fold range in the UK, Munoz, *et al.* [53] a four-fold range in Columbia and Craven, *et al.* [11] have shown that even within a high-incidence area of South Wales there is a five-fold range of incidence (Fig. 28.2). Incidence in Japanese and other migrant populations with high native rates shows that these fall until they approximate to those of the host country. In all countries the rate in women is much lower than in the men, but this difference

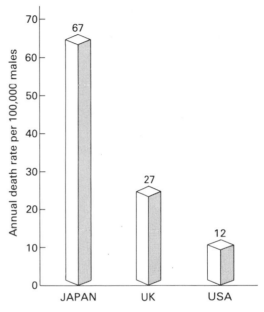

Fig. 28.1. Male death rates from stomach cancer in different countries.

is less pronounced before the age of 45. In the last 30 years the incidence of stomach cancer has been decreasing everywhere and in all age groups.

Aetiology

There is a slight excess of gastric cancer in first degree relatives and in those with blood group A, but it is likely that genetic factors are not very important. Studies of migrants and the universal declining incidence suggest a predominant role for environmental factors. The age-specific incidence rates suggest a gradual change in gastric mucosal cells due to exogenous carcinogens, though

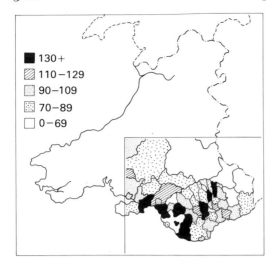

Fig. 28.2. Local variation in incidence of stomach cancer in South Wales, 1969–73. Standardized by age and sex for the whole of South Wales cancer registry.

no such single factor has been consistently identified in countries with high incidence.

Labouring work, particularly coal mining, is associated with a raised incidence of gastric cancer [12]. Not surprisingly, diet has received much attention. The many retrospective dietary surveys present many problems in interpretation and do no more than hint at a negative relationship between fresh vegetables, dairy milk and gastric cancer. This is given more weight by the only prospective dietary survey available—in a quarter of a million Japanese studied during 12 years Hirayama found a positive relationship between cigarette smoking and gastric cancer. Decreased gastric cancer risk followed regular consumption of fresh vegetables and dairy produce [26] (Fig. 28.3).

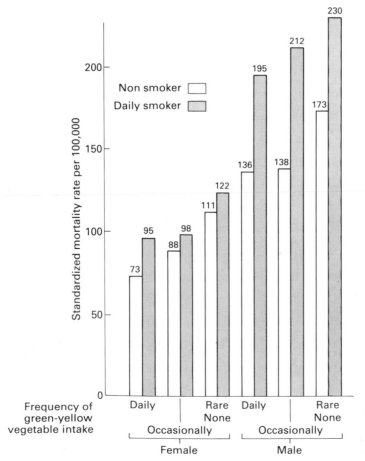

Fig. 28.3. Japanese prospective survey relating gastric cancer mortality to smoking and intake of vegetables [26].

A specific dietary factor has not yet been identified, but much attention is focused at present on N-nitrosamines [25], which are potent carcinogens in the experimental animal. N-nitrosamines arise from dietary nitrites, or from nitrates, which may be reduced by intragastric bacteria to nitrites. Nitrites then combine with secondary amines, amides or urea to form N-nitroso compounds. In the healthy stomach with a low pH and few bacteria high concentrations of nitrites do not occur. In the hypo- or anacidic stomach enough bacterial nitrate reductase exists to produce nitrites and thus allow N-nitrosamines to accumulate. This attractive, but unproven hypothesis suggests that stomach cancer may be related to nitrite/nitrate in the diet and to the gastric bacterial population.

Premalignant lesions

Chronic atrophic gastritis with intestinal metaplasia

Imai, Kubo and Watanabe in a world wide study have demonstrated a relationship between the national and regional incidences of chronic atrophic gastritis and of the intestinal types of gastric cancer [31]. A low incidence of gastric cancer is found in populations with a low (less than 20%) incidence of chronic atrophic gastritis, but populations with a high incidence of gastric cancer (Chile, Japan, Poland) have an incidence of chronic atrophic gastritis of more than 70%. The unknown, but presumably environmental determinants of chronic atrophic gastritis act in the earliest years of life; it can be found by the age of 15 in susceptible persons. Follow-up of patients with chronic atrophic gastritis reveals that approximately 10% will develop gastric cancer over 15 years [65].

There are several reports from Japan and the West of the strong topographic relationship between early gastric cancer and intestinal metaplasia [54]. However, the relationship is not yet too clear. Some histochemical studies show that several forms of intestinal metaplasia exist. The completely differentiated type is not as strongly related to gastric cancer as the incompletely differentiated type, which secretes sulphomucins and may be premalignant [33].

Dysplasia

Dysplasia is marked by atypical glandular formation, pleomorphic nuclei and increased mitotic figures (Fig. 28.4). It generally, but not invariably, arises from metaplastic gastric epithelium and can often be recognized at endoscopy as an elevated lesion—verrucous gastritis (Fig. 28.5). Even short follow-up for less than five years has shown progression from severe dysplasia to invasive gastric cancer in a number of patients [52].

Polyps

Malignancy rates of up to 60% have been reported in adenomatous gastric polyps [48], but far the commonest are hyperplastic polyps that have no malignant potential. As these two types cannot be distinguished at endoscopy from the much rarer adenomatous polyp, all must be excised for histological examination. (See Chapter 27.)

Ulcers

Malignant degeneration of a benign ulcer is very uncommon and difficult to show unequivocally, although coexistence of gastric cancer and benign ulcer is well recognized. The neoplastic component may remain small and confined to the mucosa for years, before becoming invasive.

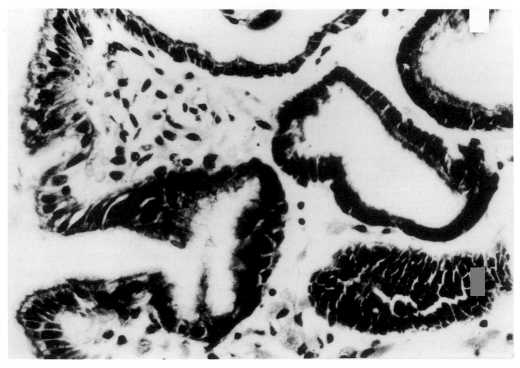

Fig. 28.4. Severe dysplasia of gastric mucosa.

Histogenesis

The statement that intramucosal cancers evolve from a premalignant state leaves unanswered the questions of how this change occurs. Study of microcarcinoma (less than 2 mm diameter) led Nagayo to suggest that in the immature dividing cells of the foveolar isthmus lay the origin of the malignancy [54]. Study of a large number of microcancers suggested that the neoplastic foci were always found in the transitional zone of the epithelium lying between the foveolar and gastric glands.

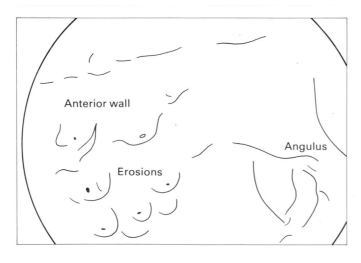

Fig. 28.5. Endoscopic appearance of verrucous gastritis—multiple small elevations of mucosa with central depressions.

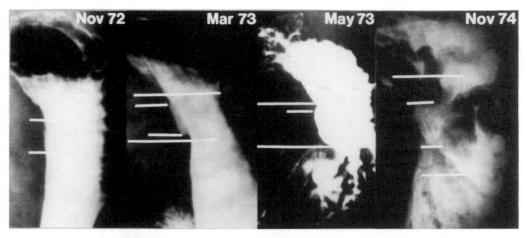

Fig. 28.6. After one and a half years dyspepsia a barium meal (Nov. 1972) was reported as normal. Antacids were prescribed with little improvement. A second barium meal (March, 1973) showed a probably benign gastric ulcer. Endoscopy confirmed this; four biopsies showed no malignant tissue. Carbenoxolone gave symptomatic relief—10 weeks later radiology and endoscopy confirmed healing of the ulcer. Symptoms recurred within one month and were palliated with antacids until November, 1974 when further radiology showed extensive ulceration and infiltration with carcinoma centred on the ulcer area. Total gastrectomy was performed—serosal and lymph node involvement was noted and the patient died with recurrent tumour two and a half years later. Note that none of the barium meals were double-contrast.

Autoradiographic and electron microscope studies of normal and metaplastic epithelium have given much insight into their cell kinetics and morphology [20] (Figs 28.7

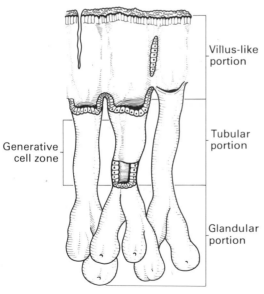

Fig. 28.7. Diagram of gastric gland—the generative zone lies in the middle level of the mucosa (the tubular portion).

and 28.8). At the generative region of the isthmus cells proliferate to move in two directions—upwards to form new epithelium, or downwards as newly formed glandular cells. Epithelial cells have a life span of some 14 days and glandular cells of 200 ± 100 days. In a normal mucosa a clone of cells cannot remain in one place, growing in numbers yet resisting the flow of normal cells. This poses problems in formulating hypotheses for the histogenesis of gastric cancer, because small collections of neoplastic cells would be pushed away by normal cells. In intestinal metaplasia, however, electron microscope studies show obliteration and embedding of glandular fragments in the lamina propria, while autoradiography shows a rapid turnover of the epithelium in these obliterated fragments. A captured clone of malignant cells may thus remain in the mucosa long enough to develop into an invasive intestinal-type of gastric cancer. Embedding of glandular fragments similarly occurs in gastric adenomas and may explain their

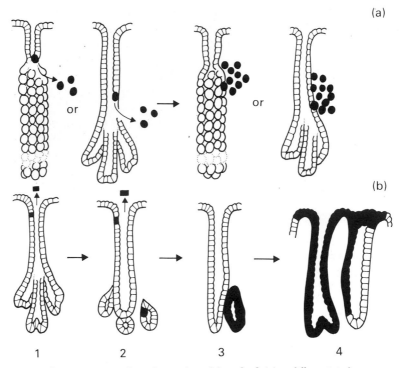

Fig. 28.8. Histogenesis of gastric cancer—hypothesis adapted from [20]. (a) undifferentiated cancers—neoplastic cells (darkened in diagram) arise in the generative cell zone and invade the lamina propria thus evading the stream of cell removal. (b) differentiated cancers—cancer cells arising in the fundic or pyloric glands are soon lost by the sloughing off mechanism ($b_1 b_2$) but if cancer cells arise in isolated cystic structures they may be captured to grow, spread and invade (b_2, b_3 and b_4).

malignant propensity. Undifferentiated cells of the generative zone are not so tightly bound to one another as those of the differentiated intestinal type and they may migrate into the lamina propria directly. Thus they will escape the stream of cell renewal and possibly develop into invasive undifferentiated gastric cancers.

Pathology

Invasiveness of gastric cancer is variable. The superficial spreading type may be confined to the mucosa, while the diffuse type spreads widely and horizontally within the submucosa. A small proportion, with a good prognosis, shows little tendency to invade and is surrounded by a pronounced plasma cell and lymphocytic reaction [67] but most invade through the stomach wall to adjacent organs. Prognosis may be better for tumours with a 'pushing' rather than with an infiltrating margin. Extension of the tumour is usually wider than its macroscopic margins and is not limited by the cardia or pylorus. Multiple tumours occur in about 10% of patients [63]. Lymphatic spread is common, increasing with the depth of invasion of the gastric wall, but may be present even in the most superficial tumours. The lymph nodes adjacent to the tumour are most likely to be involved, but it is not uncommon for only distant nodes to be infiltrated by the cancer [19].

The structural diversity of gastric cancers makes histological classification difficult and several classifications are in use, none of them ideal. The World Health Organization scheme describes papillary, tubular, mucinous and signet ring types based on the predominant cellular component [56]. Lauren's [38] classification is widely used by epidemiologists, but is less popular with pathologists and the two types—intestinal and diffuse, are not always easy to distinguish. The former tends to be related to intestinal metaplasia and to be localized, the

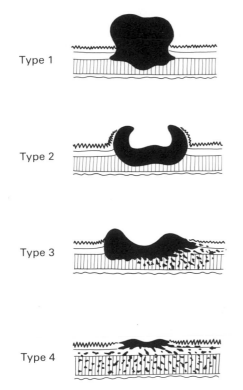

Type 1

Type 2

Type 3

Type 4

Fig. 28.9. Macroscopic classification of gastric cancer (adapted from [3]).

latter to be infiltrating. Another classification [49], is too new to have been well tested. It is based on biological behaviour and distinguishes two cancer types—expanding and infiltrative. Classification of cancer should be reproducible, it should be a prognostic aid and relate to aetiology and histogenesis of the cancer. None of the above satisfy these criteria. At present the best choices are the World Health Organization [66] and the Lauren [38] and Ming [49] classifications.

Another classification is based on gross morphology of gastric tumours (Fig. 28.9). In ascending order of malignancy:

    Type 1—solitary polypoid
    Type 2—sharply defined ulcers
    Type 3—less well defined ulcers with infiltrative margins
    Type 4—diffuse cancers (linitis plastica)

Diagnosis

The symptomatic patient

The earliest symptoms are slight, variable and uncharacteristic, but dyspepsia is present in most regardless of whether the disease is advanced or early [18]. The dyspepsia has no specific features—it may be mild upper abdominal discomfort, postprandial fullness or pain, or excessive belching. Unfortunately the diagnosis is seldom considered at this stage and delay is frequent, even when the symptoms are appreciable. The patient's optimistic or incurious attitude is often matched by the physician, who collaborates to achieve ready relief with antacids and anti-secretory drugs. Healing of an ulcerating gastric cancer occurs readily but temporarily when anti-ulcer treatment is given. Therefore misdiagnosis is common (5–14%) and to minimize this, careful endoscopic follow-up with multiple biopsies and cytological brushings is needed in all patients with gastric ulcers. Surgery is indicated for non-healing or recurring ulcers (see Fig. 28.6). It deserves emphasis that dyspepsia lasting longer than a few weeks in middle-aged or older patients demands a full investigation of the upper alimentary tract. Studies of dyspepsia in general practice assessed by endoscopy or radiology support this point [1].

When present, physical signs, such as an enlarged liver, or an epigastric mass, almost invariably indicate incurable disease, with the one exception of pyloric stenosis caused by a relatively early pyloric cancer.

Radiology

The conventional barium meal has little place in the diagnosis of gastric cancer—it has been replaced by the double-contrast barium meal, which allows study of fine mucosal detail. Neoplastic infiltration can be recognized by blunting, fusion, clubbing, or tapering of mucosal folds (Fig. 28.10). Particular diagnostic problems arise in distinguishing benign from malignant ulcers. The definite radiological diagnosis of gastric cancer can be an indication for surgical exploration without further investigation. Equivocal radiological diagnoses must be followed by endoscopic biopsy and cytology.

Endoscopy

Endoscopic inspection of the gastric mucosa is readily obtained in all patients with equivocal radiological diagnoses, but more importantly the fibreoptic endoscope allows target biopsy and direct brush cytology of all suspicious lesions. It needs to be emphasized that the small size of biopsy specimens and the frequently indeterminate or patchy nature of the lesion combine to produce a large sampling error. Six or more biopsies are needed for satisfactory diagnostic accuracy. The greatest yield of positive biopsies from a malignant ulcer are from its edge, but the malignant tissue is often confined to one part of the ulcer margin. Mucosal cancers of the diffuse type cause diagnostic difficulty—they are often flat or depressed and difficult to recognize macroscopically and the histological diagnosis is often difficult [47]. Biopsy evidence is often difficult to obtain in advanced cancers of the linitis plastica type, because the tumour may be confined to submucosal tissues.

The accuracy of endoscopic diagnosis can be increased by brush cytology. Diagnostic rates of more than 95% have been reported when this is combined with target biopsy [36]. It is helpful if the lesions are drawn by the endoscopist and the biopsy sites marked (Fig. 28.11). Repeat biopsies should be done when dysplasia is found and discrepancies between the endoscopic and

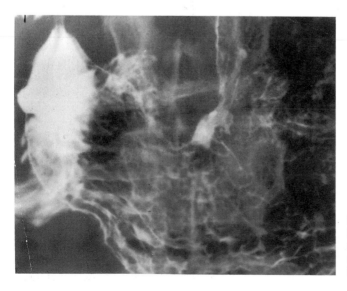

Fig. 28.10. Double-contrast barium meal demonstrating a neoplastic ulcer at the angulus surrounded by blunted mucosal folds.

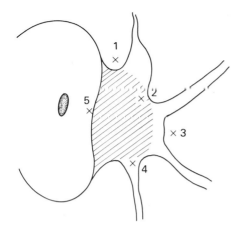

Fig. 28.11. Diagram of endoscopic appearances showing lesion and biopsy sites.

defined. Age is an obvious starting point because there is a rapid rise in incidence after 55 years. A family history of gastric cancer, pernicious anaemia, a gastrectomy more than 10 years before and chronic atrophic gastritis may all be high risk factors and pilot screening studies have been undertaken in some of these groups and asymptomatic cancers found in post-gastrectomy patients and in those with pernicious anaemia, or chronic atrophic gastritis (Table 28.1). However, it is possible to argue that deliberate endoscopic screening of the population with previous gastric surgery is poorly justified [42].

Early investigation

The Japanese programme of earlier diagnosis is nationwide and is often wrongly

pathological observations must be resolved by consultation and repeated examinations.

Early diagnosis

Early diagnosis can be approached either by population screening or through the early investigation of symptoms.

Population screening

Population screening can only be justified if the disease to be detected is common and shortens life, if a simple, safe, acceptable and cheap method indicates the presence of the disease and if early diagnosis and treatment can cure the disease. Simple, relatively inexpensive techniques such as urine dye test for anacidity, estimations of CEA antigens and gastric juice foetal sulphaglycoprotein antigen have been tried in the U.S., Hungary and Finland and have each been shown to have a low sensitivity and specificity. Rogers, *et al.* [59] have reported encouraging results using gastric juice lactic dehydrogenase and β-glucuronidase as screening markers for gastric cancer. If relatively expensive screening such as double-contrast radiology or endoscopy are to be used, then a high risk group has to be

Table 28.1. Screening of high risk groups.

High risk group	Reference	Diagnostic yield of cancers	Severe dysplasia
Pernicious anaemia	[2]	2/80	3/80
More than 15 years post gastrectomy	[30]	11/535	7/535
Chronic atrophic gastritis	[65]	10/116	?

referred to as a screening programme, as only a small fraction of the three million subjects seeking earlier diagnosis each year are asymptomatic.

The programme has evolved rapidly over 20 years and is now based on a limited double-contrast barium meal undertaken by a technician with follow-up, where indicated, by a radiologist's examination. Only in Japan, whose high incidence of gastric cancer ensures public acceptance for this uncomfortable and relatively expensive diagnosis, can such a complex method gain acceptance. The yield of cancers is not high—1,000 are found in every million examinees and of those only 40% are early cancers, but it has led to a startling increase in this more curable early stage of gastric cancer with a correspondingly decreased mortality in the population groups to whom earlier diagnosis was offered [27]. This emphasizes the difference between the Western and Japanese attitudes to the disease. In the West earliest symptoms are often ignored by the patient, misinterpreted by the doctor and inadequately investigated. In Japan there is a public awareness of the significance of gastric symptoms, advice is sought early, accurate investigation is common and improved treatment results follow. There is a need to establish whether early diagnosis could have such effects in the West. The dyspeptic patient aged 45 or above belongs to a well-defined and accessible risk group.

'Early' gastric cancer

'Early' gastric cancer is the term used to denote a stage of gastric cancer that is curable and can be recognized endoscopically. 'Early' does not imply a stage in the genesis of the cancer, but treatment results show that it is at a curable stage [50]. Five-year survival rates of more than 90% have frequently been reported and 10-year survival rates of more than 80% suggest that these are not the result of advancing the date of diagnosis to gain several years of 'lead time'.

The study of 'early' gastric cancers has shown the biological properties of these tumours. Their structure is more homogenous than that of the advanced cancer. Nagayo [54] showed that most differentiated cancers arise in areas of intestinal metaplasia and undifferentiated cancers in normal

Table 28.2. Clinicopathological differences in early gastric cancer.

	Undifferentiated	Differentiated
Histogenesis	From normal mucosa	From intestinal metaplasia
Growth	Infiltrative	Expansive
Age	Younger	Older
Sex M:F	1:1	2:1
Gross appearance	Excavated	Protuberant
Evolution into	[3] 4, 3*	[3] 1, 1, 3*

* See Fig. 28.9.

mucosa. These two types of cancer have different morphological, clinical and biological characteristics (Table 28.2). The commoner diffuse cancer produces a flat or ulcerated lesion when 'early'; it may contain 'sanctuary' areas of normal mucosa (Fig. 28.12) and often spreads horizontally to a wide extent. Its ulcerative characteristics produce dyspepsia, rendering earlier diagnosis more likely. The differentiated 'early' cancer tends to be asymptomatic, protruberant and associated with hypo- or anacidity. Strangely, venous metastases are noted in up to 10% of this type, even though they are confined to the mucosa or submucosa. Reports from the West have shown similar associations and suggest that Western gastric cancer is similar to Japanese [17].

Treatment

Surgery provides the only curative treatment and though attempted curative resection may be offered in the West to only 40–60% of patients, most of the remainder can, and should, be offered surgical

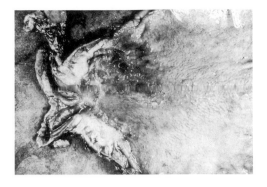

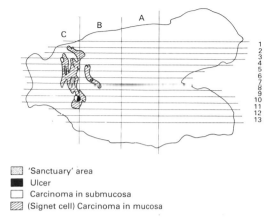

'Sanctuary' area
Ulcer
Carcinoma in submucosa
(Signet cell) Carcinoma in mucosa

Fig. 28.12. Resected specimen and reconstructed plan of early gastric cancer showing multiple lesions and 'sanctuary' areas. Note the lack of macroscopic change.

palliation. Only objective evidence of distant spread indicates incurability and clinical impressions are not an infallible guide; cervical ribs may simulate Virchow's node and a diverticular mass a rectal shelf. Decisions regarding inoperability must be based on histological evidence. Preoperative investigation such as angiography, CT, radionuclide or ultrasound scans are not reliable in determining either metastic spread or irresectability. Though grossly deranged liver function tests usually indicate metastic spread a laparotomy may be needed for palliation.

Preoperative preparation is important. Anaemia is common and demands blood transfusion. The equally common malnutrition demands preoperative hyperalimentation, preferably enteral, if the morbidity and mortality of gastric resection are to be diminished. Laparotomy should be seen as the essential guide to rational management. Though curative resection is impossible in the presence of peritoneal deposits, distant metastases, extension to irresectable adjacent structures and massive preaortic lymph node involvement, one should be aware that surgical evaluation of lymph nodes is frequently wrong.

The principles of surgical treatment

Attempted curative treatment should be guided by the following factors.

Routes of spread

Lymphatic and direct spread are common, followed by haematogenous spread and finally tumour cell implantation. Intramural lymphatics readily allow horizontal spread within the gastric wall. Neither the cardia, nor the pylorus is a barrier to this. The resection lines should be 5 cm clear of the tumour's macroscopic margin to ensure surgical clearance and some advocate intra-operative frozen section examination of the resection lines to ensure this. Extramural lymphatics carry tumour deposits to lymph nodes in more than 50% of operable cases. Those adjacent to the tumour are most often invaded, but several reports show that up to 25% of cancers have initial lymphatic spread to nodes distant from the tumour [19]. The Japanese Society of Gastric Cancer has defined first (N_1), second (N_2), third (N_3), and fourth (N_4) tier of nodes whose involvement, they claim, represents increasing advance of the disease (Fig. 28.13). Gastrectomies are defined as R_1, R_2 or R_3 resections according to the extent of the lymphadenectomy (a R_1 resec-

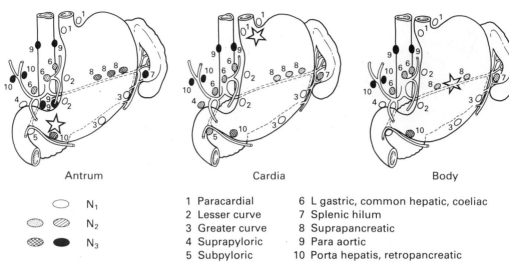

Antrum   Cardia   Body

	N₁

   N₁

   N₂

   N₃

1 Paracardial   6 L gastric, common hepatic, coeliac
2 Lesser curve   7 Splenic hilum
3 Greater curve   8 Suprapancreatic
4 Suprapyloric   9 Para aortic
5 Subpyloric   10 Porta hepatis, retropancreatic

Fig. 28.13. Lymph node 'tiers' surrounding cancer in various regions of the stomach.

tion includes excision of N₁ nodes, and so on). Miwa[50] reports on the treatment results in 6050 gastrectomied patients, defining curative resection as (a) no resection line involvement; (b) adequate lymphadenectomy (R number greater than N number); (c) no distant metastases; and (d) *en bloc* excision of involved adjacent structures. Though his view of gastric cancer spread is at variance with current knowledge of tumour growth and spread in other organs, a summary of results in Table 28.3

demonstrates an apparent soundness in his concepts.

Spread by continuity via the omenta to adjacent structures demands *en bloc* excision and five-year survivals will occur in this group. Implanted peritoneal deposits are not incompatible with curative gastrectomy if they are limited to the area to be resected[35]. Hepatic metastases will be obvious in 10–20% and indicate incurability, but the incidence of undetected liver metastases is, of course, unknown.

Table 28.3. Results of surgical treatment [50].

	No. patients	Five-year survival rate
¹Absolute curative resection	2010	77%
²Relative curative resection	1046	40%
³Relative noncurative resection	475	22%
⁴Absolute noncurative resection	1264	6%

1 *En bloc* resection with clear margins and including tiers of nodes beyond those involved.
2 As 1, but resection only to tier of involved nodes.
3 Residual tumour suspected.
4 Residual tumour proved.

Patterns of recurrence

Many authors[58] have shown that 10–20% of all resected gastric cancers will recur in the gastric stump—mainly because of inadequate excision or multicentric tumours. Since the 1950s surgeons have suggested that a policy of total gastrectomy would remove this cause of recurrence, but most found that the increased perioperative mortality which followed total gastrectomy adversely affected long-term survival figures. However, Pichlmayr and Meyer[58] report five-year survival rates of 42% after elective total gastrectomy, which is not worse than results after subtotal gastrectomy. On the other hand the University of Minnesota's unique reoperation data, which show recurrence in the gastric stump or gastric bed in 70% of 107 reoperated patients demonstrates that even the most radical resections are not immune from recurrence—extensive surgery frequently fails to control the local disease [23].

Postoperative mortality rates

Comparisons are hindered by varied definitions. The rates range up to 26% but some centres report a 3% mortality [11]. In all reports total gastrectomy had higher mortality rates than subtotal. The large variation in mortality rates suggest that standards of selection of patients, surgical technique and perioperative management are not uniform. There appears to be an inverse relationship between operability rates and operative mortality suggesting that the more aggressive surgeons are the best technicians.

Reconstructive techniques

After a subtotal gastrectomy either a gastroduodenal Billroth I or gastrojejunal Billroth II reconstruction may be undertaken. The latter is preferred by many surgeons in the unfounded belief that it minimizes the consequences of local recurrence. Billroth I reconstruction is more physiological—the advantages of the Billroth II reconstruction are more illusory than real.

It is generally accepted that after total gastrectomy oesophagoduodenostomy and end-to-side oesophagojejunostomy (even with an enteroanastomosis) should not be fashioned, because of the invariable consequences of severe reflux oesophagitis (Fig. 28.14(a)). This complication is overcome

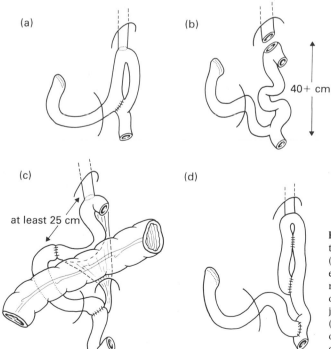

Fig. 28.14. Reconstruction after total gastrectomy:
(a) oesophagojejunostomy with entero anastomosis is not recommended. (b) Roux–en–Y oesophagojejunostomy with a jejunal loop of more than 40 cm. (c) interposition of a jejunal loop of at least 25 cm. (d) modification designed to produce a quasi gastric reservoir.

by a Roux-en-Y oesophagojejunostomy with a jejunal limb longer than 40 cm, or by the interposition of a jejunal loop of at least 25 cm (Fig. 28.14(b) and (c)). Several modifications, each designed to produce a quasi gastric reservoir have been proposed (Fig. 28.14(d)) but objective data on nutritional or other benefits are not available. After total gastrectomy all long-term survivors will need supplemental iron and vitamin B_{12}.

Attempted curative procedures

In the present state of knowledge the definitive radical surgical resection should be done for lesions confined to the stomach and neighbouring lymph glands. It should be the equivalent of the R_2 resection of Miwa with removal of the N_1 and N_2 tiers of nodes relevant to the primary (See Fig. 28.13). When the lesion is in the distal two-thirds of the stomach this involves a subtotal gastrectomy with omentum and the relevant nodes *en bloc*. Some evidence suggests that the spleen (and its nodes) should be included in the resection even when the lesion is in the distal one-third. A growth in the upper third needs a total gastrectomy with *en bloc* removal of the spleen and omentum. The pancreatic tail is not resected, unless extension to it or to the retropancreatic nodes is suggested. In all resections a 5 cm clearance of the tumour is required, unless frozen section confirms microscopic clearance. The procedures are described by Nakajima and Kajitani[55].

Palliation

Palliation is all that can be offered in 50–70% of patients. The median survival after diagnosis of incurability is measured only in months and palliative treatment should be offered in the knowledge of this. The symptoms usually requiring palliation are obstruction, haemorrhage and pain. Pallia-

tive resection, gastrenterostomy or intubation may each be successful.

In most incurable patients resection of the primary tumour, when possible, offers the best palliation in terms of length of survival and quality of life. The exceptions are proximal tumours for neither proximal, nor total gastrectomy offers much palliation and operative mortality rates are high. A palliative resection must be a subtotal or distal gastrectomy. Neither size, nor extension to neighbouring structures need preclude resection, but decisions about major and complicated resections must be taken in the clinical context. Palliative resections produce only limited benefits. The presence of extensive hepatic deposits usually precludes resection, but not if these are small and few in number. While the disability after total gastrectomy is a fair exchange for the hope of a cure, it is not advocated for incurable disease. Reconstruction after palliative surgery is probably best achieved by an antecolic Pólya gastrectomy, whose gastrojejunal anastomosis is sited away from the site of local residual tumour. When resection is neither possible nor advisable, a gastrenterostomy may relieve distal obstruction, while an indwelling Mousseau-Barbin, or Celestin tube may relieve a proximal obstruction, but neither produce as much symptomatic relief as resection.

All palliative surgery has high mortality rates of 11–18%[32]. Surprisingly, operative intubation appears at least as hazardous with mortality rates ranging from 11–45% and this has led to the suggestion that nonoperative endoscopic intubation, which was initially thought to have a lower mortality, is to be preferred, in the palliation of proximal gastric tumours[68]. While endoscopic intubation may represent an advance in the management of patients with objective evidence of widespread disease, it should be emphasized that clinical observations alone do not always provide reliable evidence of incurability; this must be decided on histological evidence.

In the absence of obstruction, antacids and the H_2-receptor antagonists are often successful in relieving the pain of an ulcerated cancer and may promote its temporary healing. Chronic blood loss can only be stopped by resection. Where this is not possible, temporary but worthwhile palliation may follow radiotherapy to the primary. Constant epigastric pain not responding to antisecretory drugs is likely to be due to extragastric extension or enlarging liver metastases. Where resection cannot be offered, analgesics and occasionally coeliac axis nerve block or radiotherapy should be used.

Results

One of the most remarkable facts about stomach cancer is the difference between the results of treatment reported from Japan and those from Europe, North America and Australia. While the former are tinged with optimism and report significant improvements in respectability rate, in resections for cure and in five- and 10-year survival rates, the latter remain pessimistic. Few of the Western studies report any improvement in results that could not be ascribed to advances in perioperative care[10]. In no other cancers do the results of treatment vary so much between one country and the rest of the world. Comparisons are hindered by the absence of standard definitions of operative mortality, surgical treatment, pathological staging, definitions of curative or palliative resection and the like. Nonetheless some attempt can be made to examine three prospective multicentre studies of gastric cancer treatment (Table 28.4).

Notwithstanding the difficulties, it is apparent that while the operability rates are comparable, resection was undertaken more frequently in Japan, with considerably less mortality and a higher 'curative' resection rate. A pathological comparison is difficult, but suggests that the percentage of early gastric cancer is higher in the Japan series (14%) than the United States (2·5%), or than the estimated rate in the European series (1–2%). The more favourable overall five-year survival rates in Japan therefore probably owe much to lower operative mor-

Table 28.4. Comparison of surgical treatment—results and pathological staging in three prospective studies of gastric cancer.

Country and years of study	No. patients	Operation rate	Resection rate (and operative mortality)	Curative resection rate (and five-year survival rate)	Overall five-year survival
Japan 1963–66 [58]	8401	94%	72% (4%)	37% (55%)	25%
USA 1951–56 [37]	1241	95%	66% (13%)	?% (?%)	10%
European 1966–68 [43]	903	91%	58% (21%)	28% (23%*)	9%

Pathological comparison					
	Japan	*USA*	*Europe*		
Mean tumour size (cm)	6 × 6†	?	8 × 6		
Node +ve	75%	76%	75%		
Hepatic 2°	7%	26%	25%		
Peritoneal 2°	25%		28%		
Early gastric cancer	14%	2.5%	?%		

* Forty year survival rate
† Calculated

tality and the higher number of early gastric cancers.

The causes of failure

Autopsy studies show that local and/or regional failure was present in more than three-quarters of the patients whose stomach cancer had not been cured by resection [45]. Distant metastases alone were uncommon. The University of Minnesota reoperation data revealed more importantly, that local and/or regional (gastric bed) failure was the _only_ site of recurrence in 53% of 86 patients [23]. None of the attempts made by Western surgeons to reduce local/regional failure by more extensive surgery has met with success [58]. Indeed there are many reports of extensive surgery yielding worse five-year survival figures, because of increased postoperative mortality rate [21].

Non-surgical treatment of gastric cancer

Chemotherapy—advanced disease

Trials of cytotoxic agents in gastric cancer are beset with difficulties. The mortality of advanced disease makes the therapeutic response difficult to define. When measurement of the tumour is possible, its burden is so large as to compromise the therapeutic potential of any agent. There are many reports of chemotherapy of gastric cancer, but most are uncontrolled series of no value and only 10 of the 30 or so established cytotoxic agents have been studied [9]. Single-agent therapy has no effect on survival. A combination of cytotoxic agents may be expected to increase response rates if all the drugs have some activity against the tumour and if their mode of action and toxicity are different. Trials containing 5 fluorouracil (5FU) with the nitrosoureas MeCCNU and BCNU were initially reported

to give higher response rates, but later reports did not confirm this. There are contradictory reports on the efficacy of 5FU, cyclophosphamide, vincristine and methotrexate. 5FU and adriamycin have been used together, or in combination with MeCCNU or Mitomycin C and in each a high response rate and significant improvement in survival of the responding patients is reported [40]. Further evaluations of these and other regimes in properly controlled trials are needed.

Surgical adjuvant studies

Cytotoxic agents should be most effective when the tumour burden is microscopic. The early trials of adjuvant chemotherapy were flawed in their design; there was no pretreatment randomization, single agents were used in low dosages and for too short a time. Those employing 5FU and thiotepa showed no benefit but two Japanese studies employing short course Mitomycin C reported significant improvement in survival at five and 10 years. These results must be treated with caution because there was no pretreatment stratification.

At present improvement in survival has not been demonstrated in any randomized controlled trial of surgical adjuvant therapy using various combinations of cytotoxic agents. Properly designed trials are only now emerging and much remains to be learnt of the effects of modifying combinations, their dosages and duration of treatment.

Radiotherapy

Radiation alone has rarely been used in gastric cancer, but has been shown to have a curative potential in a small proportion of patients with resected but residual, or irresectable but localized disease [69]. Results seem to be better when it is used with chemotherapy. Moertel, _et al._ showed a significant improvement in survival when irresectable stomach cancer was treated with radiotherapy and 5FU compared to those receiving radiation alone [51]; in a more recent randomized trial of the treatment of unresected stomach cancers XRT + 5FU followed by maintenance 5FU and MeCCNU was statistically superior to 5FU and MeCCNU alone for long-term survival.

II   GASTRIC LYMPHOMA

Although primary gastric lymphoma is rare, the stomach is the most frequent site for primary extranodal lymphoma, while gastric involvement in a more generalized lymphomatous process is not uncommon. Diagnosis is important, because treatment and prognosis are quite different from gastric adenocarcinoma, with an overall five-year survival greater than 50%.

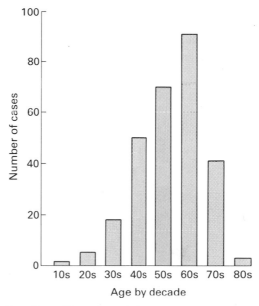

Fig. 28.15. Primary gastric lymphoma. Distribution by age in 280 patients.

Epidemiology

Primary gastric lymphoma accounts for less than 3% of all stomach neoplasms [13, 57] but during the past decade a rise to 5.5% has been recorded [57]. This may reflect a decline in the relative incidence of gastric carcinoma and improved diagnosis and classification. The overall incidence is therefore 1.0–1.5 per 100,000 of the population.

The incidence of secondary involvement of the stomach by lymphoma is 10–25%, depending on whether clinical or postmortem criteria are used [16, 60, 61]. There are no data on geographical variation of incidence and although the disease appears to affect predominantly Caucasians, this may reflect referral patterns and availability of medical care, rather than epidemiological significance.

Men seem to be affected more commonly than women in a ratio of 1.6:1 [15, 46] although this pattern is reversed for secondary gastric involvement. Primary gastric lymphoma most commonly affects patients in their fifth and sixth decades (Fig. 28.15),

although no age group is exempt including, rarely, children.

Aetiology

The aetiology of primary gastric lymphoma is unknown, although a recent case control study has suggested that a history of substantial exposure to asbestos is associated with an increased risk [62].

Pathology

Malignant lymphomas of the stomach originate in the lymphoid tissue of the lamina propria and submucosa. Macroscopically the lymphoma may produce diffuse infiltration of the stomach with mucosal and submucosal thickening resembling linitis plastica (Fig. 28.16). Deep ulcers with proliferative rolled edges (Fig. 28.17), polypoid or exophytic masses with or without surface ulceration and thickened, hypertrophied mucosal folds, which are often due to oedema and not to tumour, also occur.

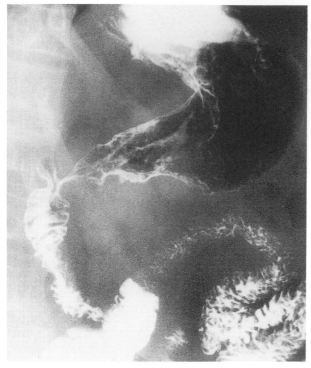

Fig. 28.16. Gastric lymphoma showing diffuse infiltration which extends across the pylorus into the duodenum.

Microscopically the tumours consist of cells derived from the follicle centre known as centrocytes and centroblasts. Classification is based on several features, including the predominant cell type present. A characteristic feature of these follicle centre cell

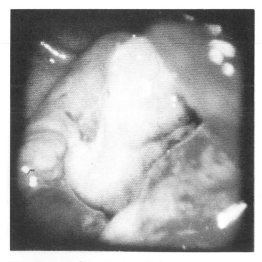

Fig. 28.17. Endoscopic view of a large lymphomatous gastric ulcer with florid rolled edges.

derived lymphomas is glandular invasion by malignant centrocytes (Fig. 28.18)[70]. Gastric lymphomas are usually of 'B' cell origin and 'T' cell tumours are uncommon.

Most lymphomas are ulcerated microscopically and 90% show tumour at the ulcer base. Fibrosis, necrosis and vascular invasion may all occur, while involvement of local or regional lymph nodes is present in over 60% of patients and may have prognostic implications[46]. As might be expected, smaller tumours (<7 cm diameter) often lack nodal involvement. It is important to exclude reactive lymphoid infiltration of the stomach, termed pseudolymphoma which is generally considered to be benign, although recent work suggests it may represent a precursor lesion with malignant potential[5].

Classification and staging

The original classification of lymphomas as lymphosarcoma, reticulum cell sarcoma,

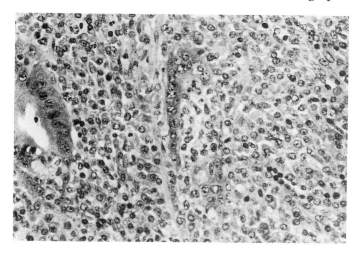

Fig. 28.18. Gastric gland showing invasion and partial effacement by malignant centrocytes (H&E × 165).

giant follicular lymphoma or Hodgkins disease was unsatisfactory and a number of newer classifications exist, many of which are based not only on morphology and histological cell type, but also on immunochemical and ultrastructural criteria [15]. The revised Rappaport classification and the working formulation of non-Hodgkins lymphomas are most commonly used, the former having the virtue of simplicity while the latter may be more helpful for determining prognosis [57]. Extent of disease is staged according to the modified Ann Arbor staging system [22] and is an important prognostic determinant.

Clinical features

The predominant symptoms of gastric lymphoma are abdominal pain and weight loss, although anorexia, nausea and vomiting, and gastrointestinal bleeding also occur (Table 28.5). Less common presentations include progressive dysphagia and free perforation. The mean duration of symptoms in older series is 30 months with an occasional history of similar symptoms for several years. However, less sophisticated investigative techniques may have led to inaccurate reporting. It appears that most patients have symptoms for less than two

Table 28.5. Symptoms in 557 patients with primary gastric lymphoma.

Abdominal pain	81%
Weight loss	57%
Nausea and vomiting	37%
Anorexia	25%
Haematemesis and/or melaena	24%
Weakness/fatigue	15%
Change in bowel habit	8%
Dysphagia	5%
Fever	4%

years and usually only for two to three months.

Abdominal pain is the most useful feature differentiating lymphoma from gastric carcinoma. Pain is similar to that of peptic ulcer with nocturnal waking, relief by antacids and a relationship to food in 50% of patients. Patients with a previous history of peptic ulcer are frequently unable to distinguish new symptoms related to a gastric lymphoma from their previous ulcer pain [34].

Weight loss is variable, but tends to correlate directly with the duration of symptoms. Patients with symptoms for less than six months averaged 7 kg, while those with a longer duration averaged 12 kg weight loss [64]. Overt gastrointestinal bleeding occurs in a quarter of patients, more often than with gastric adenocarcinoma. Patients

Table 28.6. Physical signs in 398 patients with primary gastric lymphoma.

Abdominal mass	30%
Epigastric tenderness	21%
Hepatomegaly	15%
Splenomegaly	6%
Peripheral lymphadenopathy	8%

with generalized lymphoma usually present with constitutional symptoms and lymphadenopathy. Gastrointestinal involvement is often late, although symptoms are similar. It is important to note however, that in most of these patients gastrointestinal bleeding arises from benign lesions [16].

Physical examination is often unrewarding, although weight loss may be apparent and an epigastric mass is palpable in one-third of patients. Only a small number of patients with primary gastric lymphomas have peripheral lymphadenopathy (Table 28.6).

Investigations

Routine investigations show microcytic, hypochromic anaemia in some 50% of patients (Table 28.7). A raised sedimentation rate is common, although liver function tests and protein electrophoresis are usually normal. Histamine fast anacidity is also common and reflects the presence of chronic gastritis in 60% of resected stomachs [4].

Barium studies are abnormal in 90–100% of patients with gastric lymphoma [15, 64] although the diagnosis is considered in less than 20%. There are no

Table 28.7. Laboratory investigations in patients with primary gastric lymphoma.

Anaemia	46%
Positive occult bloods	43%
Anacidity	46%
Positive cytology	45%
Positive biopsy	40%

radiographic features specific for gastric lymphoma, although a number of different lesions may suggest the diagnosis (Table 28.8). The diffuse type of lesion, particularly when umbilicated and nodular, while uncommon, is virtually diagnostic; so is the extension of the neoplasm across the pylorus (see Fig. 28.16).

Endoscopy combined with biopsy and brush cytology is the best investigation. The appearances may be indistinguishable from gastric carcinoma, although the possibility of a lymphoma is suggested by multiple

Table 28.8. Radiographic appearances suggesting gastric lymphoma (alone or in combination).

Posterior wall or greater curve ulcer with florid edges
Enlarged gastric rugae associated with polypoid mass or ulceration
Non-distensible thickened gastric wall
Multiple polypoid masses
Multiple malignant ulcerations
Extension of neoplastic appearance into duodenum

ulcerated nodules, large ulcers with florid edges (see Fig. 28.17) and giant infiltrated rugae. Lymphomas arise submucosally, so that superficial forceps biopsies are frequently negative. Ninety per cent of ulcerated lesions show tumour at the ulcer base, whereas the ulcer edge may not be infiltrated [4]—biopsies should therefore be directed accordingly. If lymphoma is strongly suspected, a biopsy of a florid lesion using snare diathermy harvests sufficient tissue for routine histology, electron microscopy and immunocytochemistry. Brush cytology by direct abrasion is also useful and in expert hands is positive in up to 75% of cases [8].

A bone marrow examination, lymphangiography and abdominal CT scan are important for accurate staging of the disease. The differential diagnosis of gastric lymphoma includes gastric adenocarcinoma, benign ulceration, Ménétrièr's disease,

Table 28.9. Treatment of gastric lymphomas.

Stage	Surgery	Radiotherapy	Chemotherapy
I_E	Limited resection	Postoperative to include liver	No
II or II_E	Nil or limited resection	Yes	Yes
III_E and IV	Only for life-threatening complications e.g. haemorrhage perforation and obstruction	Reserved for serious local problems only or equivocal residual disease following chemotherapy	Yes

leiomyosarcoma and benign nodular masses such as multiple polyps.

Treatment

The best treatment for primary gastric lymphoma is not established, although surgery, radiotherapy and chemotherapy either alone, or in combination, have all been shown to result in long term survival. Controlled trials are lacking in a disease which is uncommon and which has so many variables.

It has been suggested that for stage I and II disease elective resection is unnecessary before radiotherapy and that resection alone cannot be considered adequate treatment[24]. An alternative view is that resection should be the mainstay of therapy, with radiation given to patients with positive lymph nodes in resected specimens, or known residual intra-abdominal disease[57].

Chemotherapy is always used in patients with more widespread disease, although which is the best drug is undecided. The commonest regime consists of cyclophosphamide, adriamycin, vincristine and prednisone (CHOP).

In patients with diffuse lymphoma and secondary gastric involvement chemotherapy is the main treatment, with surgery reserved for life-threatening complications such as free perforation, massive haemorrhage, or obstruction. Radiotherapy for troublesome localized lesions may also be beneficial. The present concensus of opinion on treatment is outlined in Table 28.9 [22].

The **prognosis** of primary gastric lymphoma is dependent on the stage of the disease and to a lesser extent on its histological subtype, although long survival also correlates with young age at onset, small tumour size and degree of penetration through the gastric wall.

The probability of cure for patients with stage I_E disease is greater than 75%[7]. Long term control can be expected in 25–40% of patients with stage III_E or IV disease a proportion of whom will be 'cured' although recurrence may occur as late as 14 years after initial presentation.

Leiomyosarcoma

Gastric leiomyosarcomas are uncommon smooth muscle tumours accounting for less than 1% of all gastric malignancies. The sex incidence is approximately equal. The mean age at diagnosis is in the early 50s, although children may rarely be affected.

Aetiology

The aetiology of these tumours is unknown. The suggestion that they arise from pre-existing leiomyomas is unproven, but their relationship to these benign lesions is difficult to establish because sections from different parts of the same tumour often show considerable variation with benign and malignant elements present.

Pathology

Most leiomyosarcomas are submucosal and intramural, although they are occasionally attached to stomach but outside its lumen, or they may be dumb-bell shaped with an intraluminal and exogastric component. Distribution through the stomach is uniform. Although the tumours may be pedunculated, most lesions are sessile and may grow to a large size—35 cm in diameter and 5 kg in weight have been recorded [41]. The mucosa is often ulcerated, while the cut surface may show areas of central cavitation and necrosis. Histologically there are recognizable smooth muscle cells with elongated nuclei and abundant cytoplasm arranged in whorls and interlacing bundles. The gross size, number of mitotic figures and degree of infiltration of surrounding tissues are useful indicators of malignancy, although the presence of metastases is required for proof of malignant potential. The

liver is the commonest site of spread; lymph node metastases do not seem to occur [41].

Clinical features

There is wide variation in the length of history, from an acute onset to several years. The commonest symptoms are malaise, acute gastrointestinal bleeding, epigastric pain, discomfort or fullness and weight loss. Pain is less common and less severe than in gastric lymphoma and weight loss a less constant feature than in gastric carcinoma. Bleeding is common and may be severe and repeated. Prolapse of a pendunculated tumour through the pylorus can result in symptoms of pyloric stenosis (Fig. 28.19). Less commonly patients notice an epigastric mass or have no symptoms referrable to the gastrointestinal tract. Exogastric tumours present with a mass or bleeding into the peritoneal cavity.

Physical examination

Anaemia is common and an epigastric mass is palpable in 60% of patients [6]. There may be recent weight loss.

Investigations

A barium meal usually demonstrates the lesion, although surface ulceration may not always be seen. There are no radiological characteristics that enable a diagnosis of malignancy to be made. Endoscopically the tumours are readily apparent and surface ulceration may be visible. Endoscopic biopsy and cytology of the lesion are frequently negative due to its submucosal nature, although 'button hole' biopsies, through a previous biopsy site, may improve the pick up rate. Nevertheless the benign or malignant nature of the tumour is usually only established at surgery.

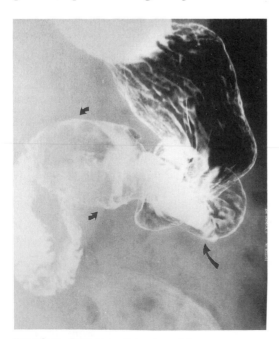

Fig. 28.19. Barium meal showing a leiomyosarcoma which has arisen on a stalk from the greater curve of the stomach (large arrow) and prolapsed through the pylorus to fill the duodenal bulb (small arrows).

Treatment

Resection is indicated for all smooth muscle tumours including tumours thought to be benign on endoscopy and biopsy. At surgery wide lymph node dissection is unnecessary, as lymph node spread is absent. Radiotherapy and chemotherapy have not been evaluated for this neoplasm, although it appears that radiotherapy is of little or no benefit, while chemotherapy is at best palliative.

Prognosis

The prognosis in leiomyosarcoma is variable, with a five-year survival rate of 30–50%. Some tumours are slow growing and long-term survivals, even in the presence of pulmonary and hepatic metastases, have been reported [41].

References

1 BARNES RJ, GEAR MWL, NOCOL A, DEW AB. Study of dyspepsia in a general practice as assessed by endoscopy and radiology. *Br Med J* 1974;4:214–218.

2 BORCH K, RENVALL H, LIEDBERG G. Gastric endocrine cell hyperplasia and carcinoid tumours in pernicious anaemia. *Gastroenterology* 1985;88:638–648.

3 BORRMAN R. Geschwulste des magens und duodenums. In: Henke F, ed. *Handbuch der speziellen pathologistchen anatomie, Vol. 4,* Berlin: Springer-Verlag, 1926.

4 BROOKS JJ, ENTERLINE HT. Primary gastric lymphomas: A clinicopathologic study of 58 cases with long term follow up and literature review. *Cancer* 1983;51:701–711.

5 BROOKS JJ, ENTERLINE HT. Gastric pseudolymphoma: Its three subtypes and relation to lymphoma. *Cancer* 1983;51:476–486.

6 BURGESS JN, DOCKERTY MB, REMINE WH. Sarcomatous lesions of the stomach, *Ann Surg* 1971;173:758–765.

7 BUSH RS, GASPODAROWICZ M, STURGEON J, ALISON R. Radiation therapy of localized non-Hodgkin's lymphoma. *Cancer Treat Rep* 1977;61:1129–1136.

8 CABRÉ-FIOL V, VILARDELL F. Progress in the cytological diagnosis of gastric lymphoma: A report of 32 cases. *Cancer* 1978;41:1456–1461.

9 CARTER SK, COMIS RL. Gastric cancer: current status of treatment. *J Natl Cancer Inst* 1977;58:567–578.

10 CRAVEN JL. International variation in the results of treatment of gastric cancer. In: Fielding JWL, *et al,* eds. *Gastric cancer.* Oxford: Pergamon Press, 1981;219–231.

11 CRAVEN JL, DAUM M, WEST RR. Variations in gastric cancer mortality in South Wales. *Clin Oncol* 1979;5:341–351.

12 CREGAN FT, HOOVER RN, FRAUMENI JF. Mortality from stomach cancer in coal mining regions. *Arch Environ Health* 1974;28:28–30.

13 CULVER GJ, BEAN BC, BERENS DL. Gastric lymphoma. *Radiology* 1955;65:518–529.

14 DOLL R, MUIR G, WALENHOUSE J. *Cancer Incidence in Five Continents.* Vol. 2 Berlin: Springer-Verlag, 1970.

15 DWORKIN B, LIGHTDALE CJ, WEINGRAD DN, *et al.* Primary gastric lymphoma: A review of 50 cases. *Dig Dis Sci* 1982;27:986–992.

16 EHRLICH AN, STALDER G, GELLER W, SHERLOCK P. Gastrointestinal manifestations of malignant lymphoma *Gastroenterology* 1968;54:1115–1121.

17 EVANS DMD, CRAVEN JL, MURPHY F, *et al.* Comparison of 'early gastric cancer' in Britain and Japan. *Gut* 1978;19:1–9.

18 FIELDING JWL, ELLIS DJ, JONES BG, *et al.* National history of 'early' gastric cancer—results of a 10 year regional survey. *Br. Med J* 1980;281:965–971.

19 FLY OA, WAUGH JH, DOCKERTY MB. Splenic hilar nodal involvement in carcinoma in the distal part of the stomach. *Cancer* 1956;9:459.

20 FUJITA S, HATTORI T. Cell proliferation, differentiation and migration in gastric mucosa: a study on the background of carcinogenesis. In: Farber E, *et al. Pathophysiology of carcinogenesis in digestive organs.* Tokyo: University of Tokyo Press, 1977:21–36.

21 GILBERTSON VA. Results of treatment of stomach cancer. *Cancer* 1969;23:1305–1308.

22 GRAY GM, ROSENBERG SA, COOPER AD, GREGORY PB, STEIN DT, HERZENBERG H. Lymphomas involving the gastrointestinal tract. *Gastroenterology* 1982;82:143–152.

23 GUNDERSON LL, SOSIN H. Adenocarcinoma of stomach: areas of failure in a reoperation series. Implications for adjuvant therapy. *Int J Radiat Oncol Biol Phys* 1982;8:1–11.

24 HERRMANN R, PANAHON AM, BARCOS MP, WALSH D, STUTZMAN L. Gastrointestinal involvement in non-Hodgkin's lymphoma. *Cancer* 1980;46:215–222.

25 HILL M. Nitrates and Bacteriology. Are these important aetiological factors in gastric carcinogenesis? In: Fielding JWL, *et al.* eds. *Gastric Cancer.* Oxford: Pergamon Press, 1981:35–44.

26 HIRAYAMA T. Methods and results of gastric cancer screening. In: Fielding JWL *et al.* eds. *Gastric Cancer.* Oxford: Pergamon Press, 1981: 77–84.

27 HIRAYAMA T. Changing patterns in the incidence of gastric cancer. In: Fielding JWL *et al.* eds. *Gastric Cancer* Oxford: Pergamon Press, 1981:1–16.

28 HOERR SO. Prognosis for carcinoma of the stomach. *Surg Gynecol Obstet* 1973;**137**:204–209.

29 HOWE GM. *Regional atlas of disease mortality in the United Kingdom.* London: Nelson, 1970.

30 HUIBREGTSE K. Endoscopic screening for malignancy in the gastric remnant. In: Cotton PB, ed. *Early gastric cancer, 2nd B.S.G.* International Workshop 1981; London, S.K.F., 58–59.

31 IAMI T, KUBO T, WATANABE H. Chronic gastritis in Japanese with reference to high incidence of gastric carcinoma. *J Nat Cancer Inst* 1971;**47**:179–195.

32 INBERG MV, HEINONON R, RANTAKOKKO V, *et al.* Surgical treatment of gastric carcinoma. *Arch Surg* 1975;**110**:703–707.

33 JASS JR, FILIPE MI. A variance of intestinal metaplasia associated with gastric carcinoma: a histochemical study. *Histopathology* 1979;**3**:191–199.

34 JOSEPH JI, LATTES R. Gastric lymphosarcoma: Clinicopathologic analysis of 71 cases and its relation to disseminated lymphosarcoma. *Amer J Clin Pathol* 1966;**45**:653–669.

35 KAJITANI T. Results of surgical treatment of gastric cancer. *Gann Mono Gast Res* 1968;**3**:245–251.

36 KEIGHLEY MRB, THOMPSON H, MOORE J, *et al.* Comparison of brush cytology before and after biopsy for the diagnosis of gastric carcinoma. *Br J Surg* 1979;**66**:246–247.

37 KENNEDY BJ. T.N.M. classification for stomach cancer. *Cancer* 1970;**26**:971–983.

38 LAUREN P. The two histological main types of gastric carcinoma: diffuse and so-called intestinal type carcinoma. *Acta Path et Microbiol Scand* 1965;**64**:31–49.

39 LEADING ARTICLE: Screening for gastric cancer in the West. *Lancet* 1978;**i**:1023–1024.

40 LEVI JA, DARLEY DN, ARONEY RS. Improved combination chemotherapy in advanced gastric cancer. *Br Med J* 1979;**2**:1471–3.

41 LINDSAY PC, ORDONEZ N, RAAF JH. Gastric leiomyosarcoma: Clinical and pathological review of 50 patients. *J Surg Oncol* 1981;**18**:399–421.

42 LOGAN RFA, LANGMAN MJS. Screening for gastric cancer after gastric surgery. *Lancet* 1983;**ii**:667–670.

43 LUNDH G, BURN JI, KALIG G. *et al.* A cooperative international study of gastric cancer. *Ann R Coll Surg Engl* 1974;**54**:219–228.

44 MACDONALD I, KALIN P. Biologic predeterminism in gastric carcinoma as the limiting factor of curability. *Surg Gynaecol Obstet* 1954;**98**:148–152.

45 MCNEER G, BOOHER RJ, BOWDEN L. The resectability of recurrent gastric carcinoma. *Cancer* 1950;**3**:43–55.

46 MCNEER G, PACK GT. Malignant gastric tumours of mesodermal origin. In: *Neoplasms of the stomach.* Philadelphia: Pitman Medical Publishing and J.B. Lippincott, 1967.

47 MARUYAMA M. Diagnostic limits for early gastric cancer by radiology. Murakami T. ed. *Gann Monograph on Cancer Research 11.* Tokyo: University of Tokyo Press, 1970: 119–130.

48 MING SC. Malignant potential of gastric polyps. *Gastrointest Radiol* 1976;**1**:121–125.

49 MING SC. Gastric carcinoma. A pathobiological classification. *Cancer* 1977;**39**:2475–2485.

50 MIWA K. Cancer of the stomach in Japan. *Gann Monogr Cancer Res* 1979;**22**:61–75.

51 MOERTEL CG, CHILDS DS, REITEMEIER RJ, *et al.* Combined 5FU and supervoltage radiation therapy of local unresectable gastrointestinal cancer. *Lancet* 1969;**ii**:865–867.

52 MORSON BC, SOBIN LH, GRUNDMANN E, *et al.* Precancerous conditions and epithelial dysplasia in the stomach. *J Clin Pathol* 1980;**33**:711–718.

53 MUNOZ N, CORREA P, CUELLO C, DUQUE E. Histologic types of gastric carcinoma in high and low risk areas. *Int J Cancer* 1968;**3**:809–818.

54 NAGAYO T. Microscopical cancer of the stomach—a study on histogenesis of gastric carcinoma. *Int J Cancer* 1975;**16**:52–60.

55 NAKAJIMA T, KAJITANI T. Surgical treatment of gastric cancer with special reference to lymph node dissecton. In: Friedman M, *et al.* eds. *Diagnosis and treatment of upper gastrointestinal tumours.* Amsterdam: Excerpta Medica 1981: 207–225.

56 OOTA K. *Histological typing of gastric and oesophageal tumours.* Geneva: World Health Organization, 1977.

57 ORLANDO R, PASTUSZAK W., PREISSLER PL, WELCH JP. Gastric lymphomas: A clinicopathologic reappraisal *Amer J Surg* 1982;**143**:450–455.

58 PICHLMAYR R, MEYER MJ. Patterns of recurrence in relation to therapeutic strategy. In: Fielding JWL *et al.*, eds. *Gastric cancer.* Oxford: Pergamon Press, 1981: 171–190.

59 ROGERS K, ROBERTS GM, WILLIAMS GT. Gastric juice enzymes—an aid in the diagnosis of gastric cancer. *Lancet* 1981;**i**:1124–1126.

60 ROSENBERG SA, DIAMOND HD, JASLOWITZ B, CRAVER LF. Lymphosarcoma: A review of 1269 cases. *Medicine* 1961;**40**:31–84.

61 ROSENFELT F, ROSENBERG SA. Diffuse histiocytic lymphoma presenting with gastrointestinal tract lesions: The Stamford experience. *Cancer* 1980; **45**:2188–2193.

62 ROSS R, DWORSKY R, NICHOLLS P *et al.* Asbestos exposure and lymphomas of the gastrointestinal tract and oral cavity. *Lancet* 1982;**ii**:1118–1120.

63 SANO R. Pathological analysis of 300 cases of early gastric cancer with special reference to cancer associated with ulcers. In: Murakami T., ed. Early Gastric Cancer. *Gann Monogr Cancer Res.* Tokyo: University of Tokyo Press, 1971: 81–89.

64 SHERRICK DW, HODGSON JR, DOCKERTY MB. The roentgenologic diagnosis of primary gastric lymphoma. *Radiology* 1965;**84**:925–932.

65 SIURALA M, VARIS K, WILJASSALO M. Studies of patients with atrophic gastritis: a 10–15 year follow-up. *Scand J Gastroenterol* 1966;**1**:40–51.

66 TSUKAMOTO K, GALLAN-VANGUAS M. A system for registration and classification of stomach cancer for WHO-IRC. *Jpn J Clin Oncol* 1973;**12**:117–128.

67 WATANABE HM, ENJOJ I, IMAI T. Gastric carcinoma with lymphoid stroma. Its morphological characteristics and prognostic correlations. *Cancer* 1976;**38**:232–243.

68 WATSON A. A study of the quality and duration of survival following resection, endoscopic intubation and surgical intubation in oesophageal carcinoma. *Br J Surg* 1982;**69**:585–588.

69 WIELAND C, HYMMEN U. Megavoltage therapy for malignant gastric tumours. *Strathlentherapic* 1970;**140**:20–26.

70 WRIGHT DH, ISAACSON PG. *Biopsy pathology of the lymphoreticular system.* London: Chapman and Hall, 1983.

Chapter 29
Diseases of the Duodenum

R. COCKEL

Although peptic ulceration in the duodenal cap is one of the commonest diseases of the alimentary tract, other disorders of the duodenum are rare. The reasons for this are obscure. Futhermore, few diseases are peculiar to the duodenum though it is involved by pathological processes occurring simultaneously elsewhere in the gut.

The dominant symptoms of duodenal disease are epigastric pain, perhaps related to ingestion of food, and vomiting, especially if there is narrowing of the lumen. Abnormal physical findings are rare except in duodenal obstruction, when there may be gastric distension with a succussion splash.

Barium meal radiography and the more specialized hypotonic duodenography allow good demonstration of duodenal anatomy and recognition of major structural abnormalities. Fibreoptic endoscopy enables the mucosa of the proximal duodenum to be examined directly and provides access to tissue for histological, cytological and biochemical investigation. The transverse duodenum is less frequently reached by endoscopy and the small bowel distal to the duodenojejunal flexure only rarely, except with a purpose designed enteroscope.

Structural abnormalities

Congenital

Duodenal atresia

Duodenal atresia, failure of the lumen to develop, (usually in the infrapapillary region) may be partial or complete. It generally presents with bile stained vomiting in the neonatal period. A plain X-ray of the abdomen is often diagnostic and shows

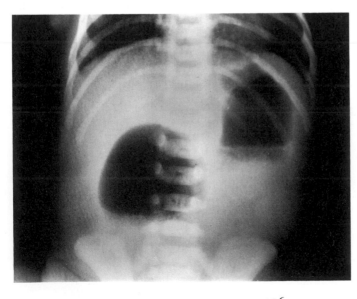

Fig. 29.1. Neonatal duodenal obstruction showing 'double-bubble' appearance and absent small bowel gas-duodenal atresia (courtesy Dr K.J. Shah).

406

absence of intestinal gas distal to the duodenum (Fig. 29.1). Antenatal diagnosis is sometimes possible in presence of polyhydramnios by ultrasonic scanning [11]. Partial atresia, although normally recognized early in life, can be asymptomatic until adulthood [4]. Incomplete upper small intestinal obstruction may cause recurrent vomiting and pain. Diagnosis is made by barium meal examination which shows a stricture, often of diaphragmatic type. Differential diagnosis includes malrotation with a duodenal band and annular pancreas in childhood, postbulbar duodenal ulceration, involvement by tumour and Crohn's disease in the adult. Treatment is surgical, usually by excision, gastroenterostomy or duodenojejunostomy.

Annular pancreas

Annular pancreas results when the ventral portion of the embryonic pancreas rotates incorrectly and encircles the duodenum in its second part. Clinical presentation is usually with obstruction of the descending duodenum at the level of the papilla. Rarely, acute pancreatitis affecting an annular pancreas may bring this congenital anomaly to clinical significance.

If required, treatment of the duodenal stenosis is surgical with a bypass, usually gastroenterostomy or duodenojejunostomy [14].

Congenital or acquired

Megaduodenum

Striking dilatation of the first part (megabulbus) or whole of the duodenum may be an incidental finding, but can on occasions be associated with abdominal pain or symptoms suggestive of obstruction. The cause is unknown although sometimes there are grounds for suspecting a congenital or hereditary origin. Abnormalities of duodenal

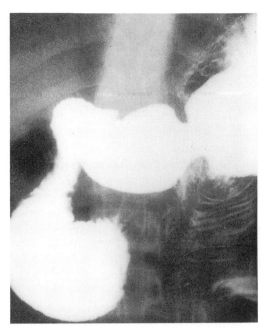

Fig. 29.2. Megaduodenum with dilatation of second and third parts of duodenum in idiopathic intestinal pseudo-obstruction.

musculature or of the myenteric plexus have been described, occasionally in association with disorders of other muscular organs (for example megacystis) or the central nervous system. Dilatation of the duodenum is often the first radiological indication of involvement of the small intestine by systemic sclerosis, with subsequent involvement of more distal parts of the gut. Amyloidosis of the small intestine can cause similar appearances.

Idiopathic intestinal pseudo-obstruction [5] (which may be familial), causes widespread dilatation of the bowel (Fig. 29.2). Episodes of obstruction, ileus and sometimes malabsorption occur [24].

Dilatation of the duodenum down to the region where it passes between the aorta and superior mesenteric vessels may be discovered accidentally, but occasionally produces symptoms of obstruction. Some authors have blamed an acute angle between those vessels for organic constriction of the duodenal lumen at this point (arteriomesenteric occlusion). Hold-up of barium is noted with the patient erect or supine, but prone position widens the angle and generally allows rapid emptying of the proximal duodenum [1].

Careful evaluation is of paramount importance in management of megaduodenum. Every effort must be made to ensure that the anomaly is the cause of symptoms and to arrive at an accurate diagnosis. Hasty bypass surgery for presumed organic obstruction may not only fail to improve symptoms, but may even worsen the situation by causing a poorly draining loop of duodenum with resultant bacterial overgrowth.

Diverticulosis

True **diverticula**, herniations of mucosa through the muscle coat of the bowel wall, are fairly common in the duodenum beyond the first part, being found in about 2% of barium meal examinations. The diverticula are most often single, although many may occur simultaneously. There is a predilection for the concavity of the duodenal loop, especially near the papilla of Vater (periampullary diverticula), which is commonly sited on the edge of, or even within a diverticulum.

As elsewhere in the gastrointestinal tract diverticula may be symptomless or liable to the complications of inflammation, perforation or haemorrhage [6]. Dyspepsia is rarely attributable to duodenal diverticula, although pain may result from common bile duct stones which are probably significantly associated. Fistulation through a diverticulum into another loop of bowel, especially the colon, may cause malabsorption.

Most duodenal diverticula are widemouthed and so fill and drain easily. Sometimes stagnation occurs with proliferation of bacteria, which can give rise to the contaminated bowel syndrome (see Chapter 44). A solitary diverticulum may be respon-

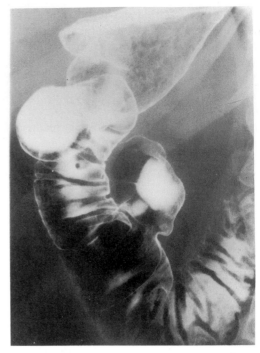

Fig. 29.3. Duodenal diverticulosis—two diverticula in second part of duodenum (courtesy Dr J.R. Lee).

sible for this [12]. Diagnosis of duodenal diverticulosis is usually made by barium radiography (Fig. 29.3) or duodenoscopy (Fig. 29.4), when typical outpouchings, sometimes multilocular, are demonstrated.

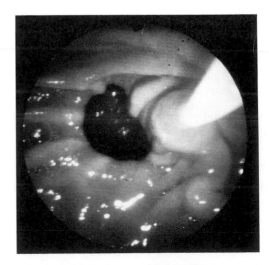

Fig. 29.4. Endoscopic view of periampullary diverticulum—papilla cannulated at ERCP.

Symptomless diverticula need no treatment, but complications may occasionally demand surgical excision, which can be technically difficult, especially when the diverticulum is within the substance of the pancreas, or adjacent to the common bile duct. Investigation and treatment of the contaminated bowel syndrome is considered in Chapter 44.

The cause of diverticula is obscure, though usually they occur in relation to vessels penetrating the muscular wall of the duodenum—especially along branches of the pancreaticoduodenal artery. Most are acquired, the condition being rare in childhood. Colonic diverticula often coexist, but as they are common the relationship may be coincidental. There is no evidence to implicate a fibre-depleted diet.

Intraluminal duodenal diverticulum is a rare condition where a wind-sock-like pouch is formed within the bowel from a mucosal fold or diaphragm. Food residues may collect within the diverticulum causing obstruction, sometimes bleeding, and rarely, acute pancreatitis. Treatment is generally surgical, although endoscopic excision with diathermy snare has been reported [13].

Pseudodiverticula including all layers of the duodenum occur in the bulb as a result of deformity caused by chronic peptic ulceration—this may give the typical 'trefoil' deformity shown by barium meal. Occasionally a surgically created choledocho-duodenostomy may be mistaken at endoscopy for a diverticulum.

Inflammatory diseases

Duodenitis

Duodenitis is usually recognized endoscopically but needs histological confirmation for certain diagnosis [27]. Inflammation of the mucosa and submucosa may result from known causes (for example infection, usually as part of a more generalized disease of the bowel) or more commonly is of unknown aetiology—non-specific duodenitis. Inflammatory changes may be restricted to the first part or may be more widespread. Distribution of changes as well as histological features aid diagnosis.

Bacterial

Acute duodenitis

Sometimes enteropathogenic bacteria cause inflammation of the duodenum as well as the more widely recognized jejunoileal or colonic lesions; there are no specific duodenal findings. Clinical features and microbiological examination usually make the diagnosis obvious, so investigation of the duodenum is rarely undertaken.

Tuberculosis

Tuberculosis of the duodenum is very rare—it causes ulceration and stricture. There is usually other evidence of abdominal tuberculosis and simultaneous pulmonary involvement is present in some patients. Clinical features may suggest Crohn's disease, but the presence of tuberculosis elsewhere should prompt the correct diagnosis. Treatment with antituberculous drugs is normally successful, unless a fibrous stricture demands surgery.

Viral disease

In immunodeficient or immunosuppressed patients viruses, notably cytomegalovirus, may cause inflammatory changes in the proximal duodenum (Fig. 29.5)—virus inclusions can be shown histologically [10]. Endoscopic appearances may be normal, although coarse nodulation can occur. It is uncertain whether this disease causes dyspepsia after renal transplantation, but it is frequently discovered. A relationship

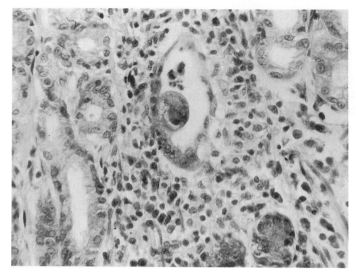

Fig. 29.5. Specific duodenitis in renal transplant patient— cytomegalic inclusion body in crypt at centre of field (courtesy Dr A.M. Hoare).

between duodenal ulceration and herpes simplex has been observed and a possible aetiological role postulated [17].

While not predominantly disorders of the duodenum, rotavirus infection in childhood, hepatitis A and probably other viruses may cause abnormalities of villous architecture with loss of the normal digitate form. Diarrhoea and malabsorption can result.

Parasitic disease (see Chapter 43)

Giardiasis

Infestation with *Giardia lamblia* [3] is rarely acquired by adults in the United Kingdom, but is commonly responsible for travellers' diarrhoea in those returning from high risk areas. It usually causes a self-limiting illness, although sometimes chronic diarrhoea, possibly with steatorrhoea, results. The organisms live predominantly in the lumen of the duodenum and jejunum and in some cases in the mucosa. Partial villous atrophy can occur and the lamina propria is infiltrated with acute and chronic inflammatory cells.

The diagnosis is made by demonstrating vegetative forms or cysts in the faeces, vegetative forms in aspirated duodenal juice

(the best method), or by small intestinal biopsy.

Treatment with metronidazole 400 mg three times a day for five days usually eradicates giardiasis. Villous structure rapidly returns to normal with clinical improvement.

Nematodes

Strongyloides stercoralis has been reported as causing severe duodenitis [2] spreading distally with narrowing of the lumen. Endoscopic biopsy can show the causative organism (Fig. 29.6). Hookworm and other parasites may cause similar changes [29].

A word of caution is appropriate, as strongyloidiasis has been transferred between patients by inadequate disinfection of endoscopes. It is probable that spread of parasites by this means is more common than published reports would suggest, as most studies of endoscopic cross-infection have come from temperate climates, where parasitic diseases are rare.

Non-specific duodenitis

Inflammatory changes are commonly found in the duodenal cap at endoscopy during

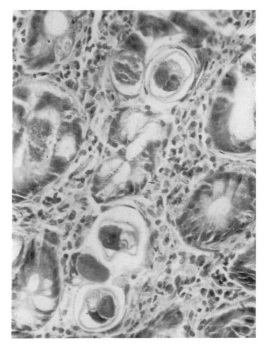

Fig. 29.6. Specific duodenitis—*Strongyloides stercoralis* in duodenal biopsy from second part (courtesy Dr P. Asquith and colleagues).

investigation of patients with dyspepsia. Symptoms are often similar to those of peptic ulceration, although sometimes duodenitis is discovered incidentally. The mucosa

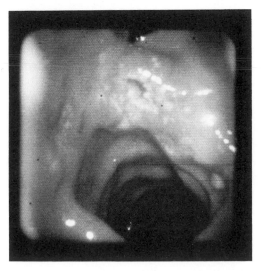

Fig. 29.7. Non-specific duodenitis—endoscopic view showing 'pepper and salt' erosions.

may be diffusely reddened or patchily inflamed, especially on the folds. In more severe cases erosions are present ('pepper and salt' duodenitis) (Fig. 29.7) and the mucosa can be coarsely nodular (Fig. 29.8). The second part is usually normal. Similar appearances are often found adjacent to duodenal ulceration.

Histological features include acute inflammation with capillary dilatation, resulting in migration of neutrophils into the lamina propria and the epithelium. Inflammatory erosion of the surface epithelium may be present. With more chronic disease villous abnormalities occur and the cellular infiltrate includes lymphocytes, plasma cells and eosinophils [27] (Figs 29.9, 29.10, 29.11 and 29.12).

Correlation between endoscopic and histological appearances is variable [26]. Undoubtedly disparity arises when tissue samples are taken carelessly, yet allowing for this, concordance is often imperfect. Histological findings are usually regarded as the final arbiter.

The cause of non-specific duodenitis is unknown, although there seems in many cases to be a relationship to duodenal ulcer disease [16]. When an ulcer heals, duodenitis may persist and sometimes frank peptic ulceration develops in patients with previous inflammatory changes. Gastric acid secretion and serum gastrin concentrations are normal [7]. Other intra-abdominal diseases, or exogenous irritants such as drugs and alcohol perhaps cause duodenitis in some patients, but most instances are unexplained.

Treatment is often unsatisfactory. Potential irritants should be withdrawn and associated diseases which may be the cause of symptoms should, where possible, be treated. Only when no other cause is found should treatment be directed at the duodenitis. Responses to alkalis, H_2-receptor antagonists and mucosal protectives are unpredictable. Ulcer-curing surgery is rarely

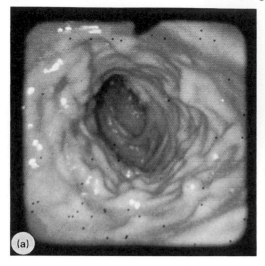 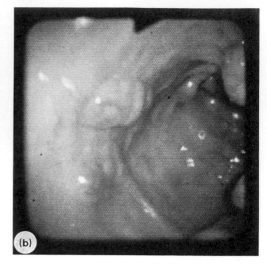

Fig. 29.8. (a) non-specific duodenitis—coarsely nodular appearance of cap with erythema on crests of mucosal folds. (b) non-specific duodenitis showing nodular appearance—erosions on crest of mucosal folds.

indicated, unless frank peptic ulcer disease is proved.

Coeliac disease

Although coeliac disease is usually diagnosed by jejunal biopsy, the typical changes are also found in the duodenum. Endoscopy may show a featureless atrophic-looking mucosa, which on close examination reveals loss of the normal velvety villous pattern; sometimes a 'mosaic' appearance can be discerned. Vital staining with, for example, methylene blue, enables easier distinction between normal and abnormal. Small endoscopic biopsies taken from the second part of the duodenum are adequate to confirm the diagnosis of coeliac disease by the appearance of subtotal villous atrophy [18, 23] and confusion with duodenitis should not occur if the pathologist is given full clinical details and endoscopic findings (see Chapter 42).

In ulcerative jejunoileitis, which is probably a variant of coeliac disease, strictures or even multiple mucosal diaphragms may develop in the duodenum or jejunum. Obstructive symptoms can result. Radiology

may demonstrate the strictures and ulceration is occasionally visible endoscopically. Despite a morphological response of the mucosa to gluten withdrawal, surgical resection may be required for symptoms of obstruction.

Crohn's disease (see Chapter 52)

The duodenum is affected in 2–4% of patients with ileal and/or colonic Crohn's disease [19]. Isolated involvement of the duodenum is exceedingly rare. Recognition is usually incidental during a barium meal examination performed to evaluate ileal disease. Coarse mucosal folds, deformity (Fig. 29.13), ulceration or stenosis (Fig. 29.14) of the duodenum may be present. Ulcer-type dyspepsia, or vomiting if the duodenum is narrowed, can occur. Some authors have suggested that there is an increased incidence of peptic ulceration in association with ileal Crohn's disease [9].

Endoscopy may be needed to differentiate peptic ulcer from duodenal Crohn's disease. Widespread patchy or confluent inflammatory changes, aphthoid (Fig. 29.15) or linear ulceration spreading beyond the cap

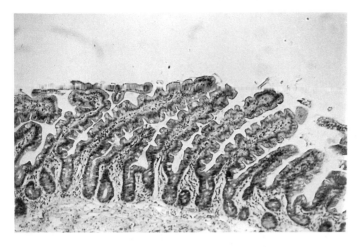

Fig. 29.9. Normal duodenal mucosal biopsy—digitate villi with no inflammatory cell infiltrate.

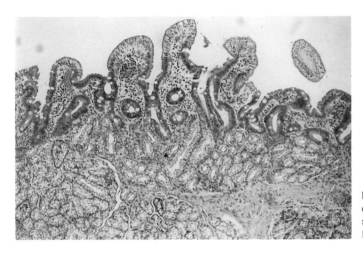

Fig. 29.10. Mild non-specific duodenitis with broadened and shortened villi containing inflammatory cells.

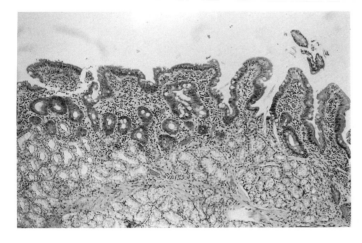

Fig. 29.11. Mild–moderate duodenitis with appearance similar to Fig. 29.10. On left—loss of villous structure; on right—marked cellularity.

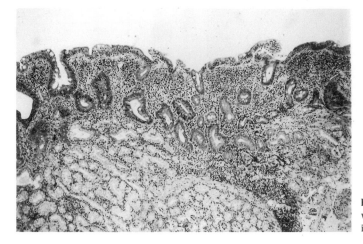

Fig. 29.12. Severe duodenitis—villous structure lost and intense inflammatory cell infiltrate.

suggest Crohn's disease. Mucosal biopsies sometimes show typical non-caseating granulomata, but usually non-specific changes are found. There may be similar appearances in the gastric antrum.

Precise diagnosis is essential to make decisions about treatment with ulcer-healing drugs, steroids or surgery. If duodenal obstruction results from Crohn's disease a gastroenterostomy provides good symptomatic relief and may allow regression of inflammatory changes.

Tumours of the duodenum

Most tumours of the duodenum are benign, carcinoma accounting for only 0.3% of all gastrointestinal malignancies [25].

Duodenal ulcers never undergo malignant change. Routine biopsy of duodenal ulcers is not necessary, although this should be done if appearances at endoscopy are unusual or healing is slow.

Benign tumours

Polypoid lesions in the duodenal cap are usually inflammatory, resulting from duodenitis, hypertrophy of Brunner's glands or

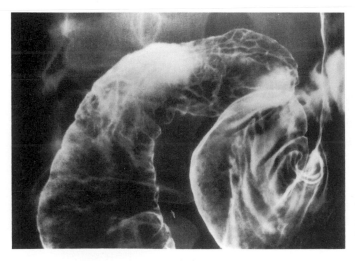

Fig. 29.13. Crohn's disease of proximal duodenum. Gross distortion of mucosal pattern (courtesy Dr J.R. Lee).

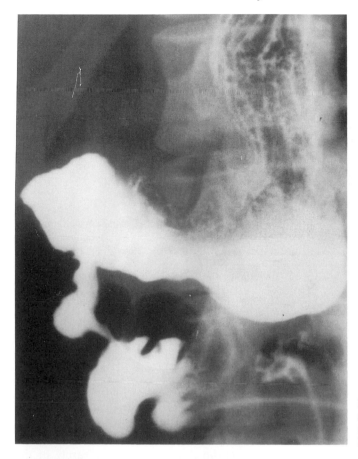

Fig. 29.14. Crohn's disease showing stricture of second and third parts of duodenum (courtesy Dr D.K.M. Toye).

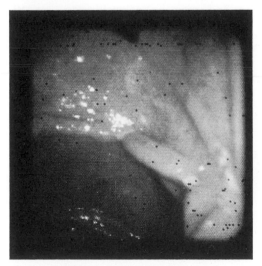

Fig. 29.15. Endoscopic view of Crohn's disease showing discrete ulceration on mucosal folds of the second part of the duodenum.

nodular lymphoid hyperplasia (Fig. 29.16). Neoplastic tumours in this region are very rare.

Adenoma, fibroma, leiomyoma, lipoma or lymphangioma may be found more distally, especially in the periampullary region. Usually discovery is incidental and rarely do such tumours cause pain, bleeding or obstruction. Exceptionally a polypoid tumour may form the apex of an intussusception. Precise diagnosis is not usually possible radiographically or by inspection at endoscopy. Mucosal, or snare loop biopsy can give the tissue diagnosis, but caution should be exercised lest over-enthusiastic diathermy excision of sessile polyps causes perforation or pancreatitis. Pedunculated adenomata (Fig. 29.17), if few in number, are removed by endoscopic polypectomy.

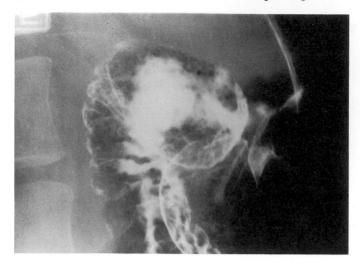

Fig. 29.16. Multiple 'polyps' in duodenal cap—nodular lymphoid hyperplasia (courtesy Dr J.R. Lee).

Surgical treatment is needed rarely, so provided malignancy is confidently excluded precise diagnosis of cell type of duodenal tumours may be regarded as unnecessary.

Duodenal polyps may be found as part of one of the rare diffuse intestinal polyposis syndromes. In the Peutz-Jeghers syndrome hamartomatous intestinal polyps are associated with circumoral pigmentation. Adenomatous polyps, sometimes only millimetres in diameter, occur in a large proportion of cases of familial polyposis coli [21]. Hypoplastic nails and malabsorption are found additionally in the Cronkhite-Canada syndrome.

Malignant tuomour

Carcinoma of the duodenum usually causes obstruction and more rarely, gastrointestinal haemorrhage, overt or occult. Carcinoma may occur anywhere in the duodenum, but exceptionally rarely in the cap and may be polypoid (Fig. 29.18),

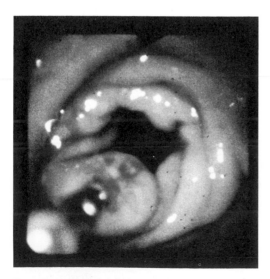

Fig. 29.17. Benign pedunculated adenoma just distal to superior duodenal angle—grasped in biopsy forceps.

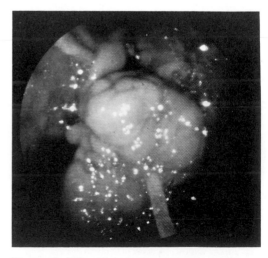

Fig. 29.18. Polypoid carcinoma adjacent to papilla—cannula passed between lobules.

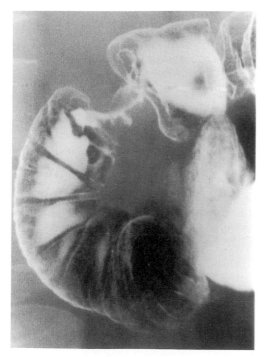

Fig. 29.19. Carcinoma in proximal duodenum causing 'apple core' appearance (courtesy Dr J.R. Lee).

ulcerated or stenosing (Fig. 29.19). Barium meal examination or hypotonic duodenography suggests the diagnosis, but endoscopy with biopsy and cytology is required for confirmation. Aetiology is obscure, although there is probably an increased incidence in patients with coeliac disease [15], Crohn's disease and certain types of intestinal polyposis, including familial polyposis coli [22].

Carcinoma of the duodenum occurring in the periampullary region may cause obstructive jaundice or pancreatic steatorrhoea. Bleeding from an ulcerated carcinoma here may darken otherwise pale faeces causing the so-called 'silver stool' with positive occult blood tests. Treatment is surgical by resection if technically feasible, or by palliative gastrojejunostomy.

More common than primary duodenal carcinoma is local invasion or discrete metastasis from pancreatic tumour. Differentiation is often impossible by histological means, so imaging of the pancreas by ultrasound, computerized tomography or ERCP is an essential part of evaluation.

Other malignant tumours occasionally found in the duodenum include carcinoid, lymphoma and various sarcomata.

Miscellaneous

Aortoduodenal fistula

If infection of an aortic prosthesis inserted for aneurysm occurs, an aortoduodenal fistula may develop where the transverse duodenum crosses the aorta. The fistula causes either massive or recurrent small gastrointestinal haemorrhages. Systemic symptoms due to the infection may be present. Anaemia and raised ESR are usual [20].

Diagnosis can be made by barium radiology if characteristic transverse banding of the prosthesis is seen. Distal duodenoscopy following haemorrhage locates the bleeding site and in a patient who has undergone aortic surgery a fistula should be suspected.

Treatment is surgical either by replacement of the prosthesis under antibiotic cover, or by excision of the graft and insertion of an axillofemoral by-pass. An aortic aneurysm can rupture spontaneously into the transverse duodenum.

Duodenal haematoma

Rarely an haematoma in the wall or behind the duodenum may cause pain and/or obstruction. This results from bleeding diatheses (excessive therapeutic anticoagulation, haemophilia), as part of the Henoch–Schöenlein syndrome or from trauma. The condition usually resolves spontaneously, if necessary after correction of the abnormality of coagulation; surgery is rarely required [28].

Vascular malformations

Obscure gastrointestinal bleeding may originate from vascular lesions of the duodenum, similar in appearance to angio dysplasia of the colòn. The aetiology of this disorder is unknown—it is not associated with any other pathology. Electrocoagulation with hot biopsy forceps usually controls bleeding [8].

References

1 BOCKUS HL. Chronic intermittent arteriomesenteric occlusion of the duodenum. In: Bockus HL, ed. *Gastroenterology Vol. II.* Philadelphia: W.B. Saunders, 1976:418–428.

2 BONE MF, CHESNER JM, OLIVER R, ASQUITH P. Endoscopic appearances of duodenitis due to strongyloidiasis. *Gastrointest Endosc* 1982; 28:190–191.

3 BRANDBORG IL. Giardiasis and traveler's diarrhoea. *Gastroenterology* 1980;78:1602–1614.

4 COOPERMAN AM, ADACHI M, RANKIN GB, SIVAK M. Congenital duodenal diaphragms in adults. *Ann Surg* 1975;182: 739–742.

5 CRANE SA, FAULK DL, HUBEL KA. Intestinal pseudo-obstruction. *Gastroenterology* 1978;74: 1318–1324.

6 DONALD JW. Major complications of small bowel diverticula. *Ann Surg* 1979;190:183–188.

7 DONOVAN IA, GREEN G, DYKES PW, OWENS C, CLENDINNEN BG, ALEXANDER-WILLIAMS J,The pathophysiology of duodenitis. *Gut* 1975;16:395.

8 FARUP PG, ROSSELAND AR, STRAY N, PYTTE R, VALNES K, RAND AA. Localised telangiopathy of the stomach and duodenum diagnosed and treated endoscopically. *Endoscopy* 1981;13:1–6.

9 FIELDING JF, COOKE WT. Peptic ulceration in Crohn's disease (Regional enteritis). *Gut* 1970;11: 998–1000.

10 FRANZIN G, NOVELLI P, FRATTON A. Histologic evidence of cytomegalovirus in the duodenal and gastric mucosa of patients with renal allograft. *Endoscopy* 1980;12(117):120.

11 GEE H, ABDULLA U. Antenatal diagnosis of fetal duodenal atresia by ultrasonic scan. *Br Med J* 1978;ii:1265.

12 GOLDSTEIN F, COZZOLINO HJ, WIRTS CW. Diarrhoea and steatorrhoea due to a large solitary duodenal diverticulum. *Am J Dig Dis* 1963;8:937.

13 HAJIRO K, YAMAMOTO H, MATSUI H, YAMAMOTO T. Endoscopic diagnosis and excision of intraluminal duodenal diverticulum. *Gastrointest Endosc* 1979; 25:151–154.

14 HARBERG FJ, POKORNY WJ, HAHN H. Congenital duodenal obstruction. *Am J Surg* 1982;11:593–608.

15 HOLMES GKT, DUNN GL, COCKEL R, BROOKES VS. Adenocarcinoma of the upper small bowel complicating coeliac disease. *Gut* 1980;21:1010–1016.

16 JOFFE SN, LEE FD, BLUMGART LH. Duodenitis. *Clin Gastroenterol* 1978;7:635–650.

17 LANCET EDITORIAL. Viruses and duodenal ulcer. *Lancet* 1981;i:705–706.

18 MEE AS, BURKE M, VALLON AG, NEWMAN J, COTTON PB. Small bowel biopsy for malabsorption: comparison of the diagnostic adequacy of endoscopic forceps and capsule biopsy specimens. *Br Med J* 1985;291:769–773.

19 NUGENT FW, RICHMOND M, PARK SK. Crohn's disease of the duodenum. *Gut* 1977;18:115–120.

20 PERDUE GD, SMITH RB, ANSLEY JD, CONSTANTINO MJ. Impending aortoenteric hemorrhage. *Ann Surg* 1980;192:237–243.

21 RANZI T, CASTAGNONE D, VELIO P, BIANCHI P, POLLI EE. Gastric and duodenal polyps in familial polyposis coli. *Gut* 1981;22:363–367.

22 SCHNUR PL, DAVID E, BROWN PW, BEAHRS OH, REMINE WH, HARRISON FG. Adenocarcinoma of the duodenum and the Gardner syndrome. *JAMA* 1973;223:1229–1232.

23 SCOTT BB, JENKINS D. Endoscopic small intestinal biopsy. *Gastrointest Endosc* 1981;27:162–167.

24 SNAPE WJ. Pseudo-obstruction. *Clin Gastroenterol* 1982;11:593–608.

25 SPIRA IA, GHAZI A, WOLFF WI. Primary adenocarcinoma of the duodenum. *Cancer* 1977;39:1721–1726.

26 STEPHEN JG, LESNA M, VENABLES CW. Endoscopic appearances and histological changes in ulcer-associated duodenitis. *Br J Surg* 1978;65:438–441.

27 THOMPSON H. Duodenitis. The pathologists contribution to endoscopic diagnosis. In: Schiller KFR, Salmon PR, eds. *Modern topics in gastrointestinal endoscopy.* London: Heinemann, 1976:188–190.

28 VELLACOTT KD. Intramural haematoma of the duodenum. *Br J Surg* 1980;67:36–38.

29 WITHAM RR, MOSSER RS. An unusual presentation of schistosomiasis duodenitis. *Gastroenterology* 1979;77:1316–1318.

SECTION V
GASTROINTESTINAL BLEEDING

Chapter 30
Upper Gastrointestinal Bleeding

M.W. DRONFIELD

Acute upper gastrointestinal haemorrhage is a common medical emergency. In the United Kingdom the annual incidence, as measured by hospital admission, is between 50 and 100 per 100,000, with around 3,500 deaths. The critical factors determining outcome are the patient's age, the site of bleeding, and the presence or absence of other diseases [25, 37, 38].

Epidemiology

Incidence

Acute upper gastrointestinal bleeding is a complication of a wide variety of disorders, and its incidence depends on the prevalence of the underlying causes. For example, in countries where alcoholic liver disease is common bleeding from oesophageal varices will also be common. In Britain chronic peptic ulceration is the commonest cause of acute upper gastrointestinal bleeding. A district general hospital will admit several patients with an upper gastrointestinal haemorrhage each week. Figures from Oxford [52], Birmingham [1] and Nottingham [16] indicate an annual admission rate of around 50 per 100,000 population—a figure that has not changed appreciably over the past 30 years. In Scotland, where duodenal ulcer is more prevalent, the annual admission rate for patients with acute upper gastrointestinal bleeding was 116 per 100,000 population during 1967–68 [31].

Sex ratio

No consistent difference in the incidence of acute upper gastrointestinal bleeding in men and women has been found, other than that which reflects differences in prevalence of the underlying pathology.

Age

The number of elderly patients admitted with acute upper gastrointestinal bleeding has increased steadily over the past 60 years. In series recorded in the 1920s, around 10% of patients were over 60, increasing to 20–30% in the 1940s, and 50–60% in the 1970s [1] (Fig. 30.1). As would be expected, mortality is highest in these elderly patients. For example in a recent study in which about 60% of patients were

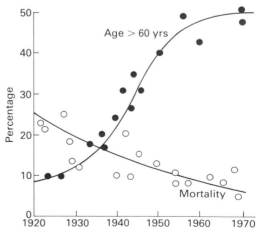

Fig. 30.1. Percentage of patients over 60 years and mortality rate from gastrointestinal bleeding in major European studies 1920–70 [1].

421

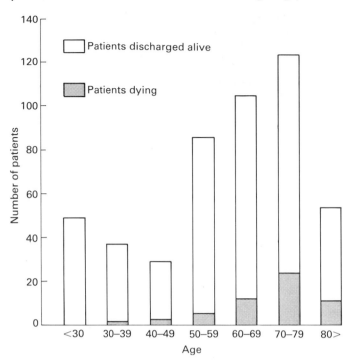

Fig. 30.2. Age distribution of patients admitted with, and dying from, acute upper gastrointestinal bleeding [15].

over 60 years old, mortality rates were only 4% in patients under 60, compared with 20% in patients over 70 (Fig. 30.2) [14]. Over the last 40 years overall mortality rates in most large series have been around 10% (Fig. 30.1). It is disappointing that figures have not improved despite changes in investigation and management. It seems likely, however, that the benefits of improved management have been masked by the gradually increasing proportion of elderly patients. Children may present with upper gastrointestinal haemorrhage [28, 49].

Pathophysiology

The effects of acute upper gastrointestinal bleeding are similar to those of acute blood loss from any cause. These effects will depend on the severity and speed of blood loss, and also on whether there are any pre-existing disorders such as anaemia, dehydration or atherosclerosis. The fall in blood vol-ume following a major bleed will lead to decreased venous return, cardiac output and blood pressure, which will result in peripheral vasoconstriction causing pallor, peripheral cyanosis and oliguria. If a severe reduction of blood volume is not corrected rapidly, lowered perfusion may cause acute tubular necrosis, mesenteric infarction, retinal artery occlusion or myocardial infarction.

In the absence of intravenous infusions, blood volume restoration after an acute bleed depends on the shift of extravascular fluid into the vascular compartment and a reduction of urine output. These fluid shifts cause a fall of haemoglobin concentration. The rate of these compensatory responses varies considerably from patient to patient, thus the lowest haemoglobin value may be found within a few hours, or as long as several days, after an acute bleed.

Table 30.1. Relative frequency of endoscopically-diagnosed causes of acute upper gastrointestinal bleeding.

Reference	UK [13]	USA [35]	USA [50]	UK [16]
Number of patients	208	149	100	526
% Bleeding from				
Oesophagus				
Oesophagitis/ulcer	8	3	0	6
Varices	3	13	20	2
Mallory–Weiss syndrome	1	3	16	6
Stomach				
Gastritis/erosions	9	45	6	5
Ulcer	30	3	18	25
Tumours	2	0	2	3
Duodenum				
Ulcer	21	8	22	23
Duodenitis	4	9	0	2
Others	2	2	0	1
No lesion found	20	14	16	27

Aetiology

The source of bleeding can be identified accurately at endoscopy in most patients; the relative frequency of the common causes varying between different studies (Table 30.1).

Peptic ulceration

Most recent British series, using either barium radiology or fibreoptic endoscopy, agree that around half of the patients admitted have chronic peptic ulcers, and duodenal ulcer is approximately twice as common as gastric ulcer (Table 30.2).

Oesophageal disease

Bleeding from oesophageal lesions is now recognized to be common. Oesophagitis accounts for up to 10% of all bleeding episodes, but the demonstration of a hiatus hernia alone cannot be taken as a potential source of bleeding unless oesophageal inflammation or ulceration is also found.

Table 30.2. Proportion of patients with acute upper gastrointestinal haemorrhage due to chronic peptic ulceration in British series.

Reference	Number	Chronic peptic ulcers (%)	Duodenal: gastric ulcers
[32]	673	47	1.94
[8]	238	49	1.88
[52]	2149	44	1.93
[31]	817	58	6.22
[13]	208	52	0.86
[22]	112	54	1.70
[1]	300	49	1.58
[59]	66	47	1.35
[16]	1037	48	1.30

Mallory–Weiss syndrome

The Mallory–Weiss syndrome is now recognized as a common cause of acute upper gastrointestinal bleeding. This syndrome was originally described in alcoholics who vomited severely after a bout of heavy drinking, with haematemesis developing due to a mucosal tear at the oesophagogastric junction [42]. It has since been realized that such mucosal tears often develop without the classical history of recurrent vomiting followed by haematemesis, occasionally it presents with melaena alone. Barium radiology rarely identifies these tears but fibreoptic endoscopy has shown that around 10% of patients with acute upper gastrointestinal bleeding have a Mallory–Weiss tear [20, 36].

Oesophageal varices (see Chapter 31)

In Britain bleeding from oesophageal varices is less common than in most other western countries, accounting for less than 5% of admissions. It is important to realize that patients with varices, and particularly those with alcoholic cirrhosis, may have other potential sites of bleeding in the upper gastrointestinal tract, particularly gastric erosions or chronic peptic ulcers [67]. In these patients endoscopy will usually identify which lesion has bled.

Gastric erosions

When radiology was the main diagnostic technique it was widely assumed that bleeding from gastric erosions accounted for many of the cases where the barium meal was negative. In most recent endoscopic studies erosive bleeding from the stomach is less common than was previously assumed—less than 10%. However, in some American series erosive bleeding is much commoner. The cause of these gastric erosions is unknown. In some cases drug therapy and/or alcohol ingestion have been incriminated.

Tumours

Malignant tumours of the oesophagus and stomach, usually a carcinoma but occasionally a lymphoma or sarcoma, may present with acute upper gastrointestinal bleeding. The commonest benign tumour of the upper gastrointestinal tract is the leiomyoma, usually found in the stomach although it can occur in the oesophagus or duodenum. This usually presents with acute upper gastrointestinal bleeding due to ulceration on its surface.

Rare causes of bleeding

The disorders discussed above and listed in Table 30.2 will account for at least 98% of identified causes of acute upper gastrointestinal bleeding, but some rare causes of the remaining 2% are listed in Table 30.3.

Table 30.3. Some rare causes of acute upper gastrointestinal bleeding.

Aneurysms.
Arterial malformations.
Pancreatic tumours, chronic pancreatitis and
    pseudocysts.
Various malignant tumours.
Haemobilia.
Hereditary haemorrhagic telangectasia.
Pseudoxanthoma elasticum.
Haemostatic disorders.
Association with aortic stenosis.

Bleeding from **aneurysms** is usually catastrophic and often rapidly fatal—they usually occur from thoracic or abdominal aortic aneurysms (often after a previous resection) which erode into the upper gastrointestinal tract, particularly into the duodenum. Bleeding may also occur from aneurysms at other sites, notably the splenic artery or pancreaticoduodenal artery in patients with **chronic pancreatitis.**

Vascular malformations may be found at any site in the gastrointestinal tract—in the upper gastrointestinal tract they are mainly found in the stomach where arterial malformations may cause severe bleeding and are often difficult to identify [24, 41].

Pancreatic malignant tumours may erode into the duodenum and bleed.

Haemobilia most commonly follows abdominal injuries, surgical treatment of biliary disease or liver biopsy [34]. It may also be due to bleeding aneurysms or vascular tumours in the liver, and in these circumstances diagnosis can be very difficult and depends on selective angiography.

Two very rare genetic conditions are important as they may be diagnosed on physical examination by an alert physician—telangiectasia around the lips and mouth suggests **hereditary haemorrhagic telangiectasia;** yellow, lax skin in the axillae, groins and neck suggests **pseudoxanthoma elasticum.**

Patients with **chronic renal failure** frequently bleed from angiodysplastic vessels in the stomach or duodenum [71].

Haemostatic disorders are rare causes of acute upper gastrointestinal bleeding which may be overlooked. Thrombocytopenia is the commonest such haematological condition, and bleeding is most likely when the platelet count has fallen rapidly, for example in acute leukaemia or after cytotoxic therapy. Patients with chronic thrombocytopenia usually tolerate a low platelet count. Defective platelet function may also cause bleeding, for example in patients with uraemia or myeloproliferative disorders such as primary polycythaemia or thrombocythaemia. This can also occur as an idiosyncratic reaction to aspirin. Congenital bleeding disorders rarely cause gastrointestinal bleeding except von Willebrand's disease, in which a reduction of factor VIII is combined with an endothelial cell defect [45]. In patients with liver disease there is a complex coagulopathy including depletion of clotting factors and thrombocytopenia; acute upper gastrointestinal bleeding is a common terminal event in patients with fulminant hepatic failure. Finally there is an unexplained association between aortic stenosis and acute upper gastrointestinal bleeding of undetermined cause [53].

Non-steroidal anti-inflammatory drugs and gastrointestinal haemorrhage [57]

Aspirin therapy has long been thought to cause acute upper gastrointestinal bleeding either by causing erosions or chronic ulcers, or by making established ulcers bleed. This supposition arises from the observation that in man aspirin ingestion will cause occult gastrointestinal bleeding of about 5 ml of blood daily. This bleeding seems to be due to depletion of prostaglandins in the gastric mucosa which have a 'cytoprotective' role; it is an effect that may be shared by many other anti-inflammatory drugs.

Whether aspirin causes acute major upper gastrointestinal bleeding remains controversial. Several studies have shown that there is a higher aspirin intake among patients admitted with acute upper gastrointestinal bleeding than in various control groups. There is also a higher incidence of paracetamol ingestion in patients admitted with bleeding, a drug that may even protect the gastric mucosa [59] and would not be expected to cause bleeding. In some patients it is likely that analgesic consumption just prior to admission is to relieve the 'flu-like' symptoms of early bleeding [10]. Corticosteroid drugs are also conventionally thought to induce acute upper gastrointestinal bleeding, but in an extensive review of 42 trials involving over 5,000 patients who had been allocated to corticosteroid or placebo therapy for a variety of disorders no more bleeding was found in treated patients than in controls [12]. A more recent review has calculated a 1.7-fold increase in peptic ulceration during steroid therapy [43]. There are many anecdotal reports of various non-steroidal anti-inflammatory drugs causing an acute upper gastrointestinal bleeding [47]. However, in Nottingham non-aspirin non-steroidal anti-inflammatory drugs were taken over twice as often by patients with bleeding peptic ulcers as by community or hospital controls [57].

Clinical features

Presentation

In most patients the presenting symptom will be haematemesis and/or melaena. Occasionally a patient may present with syncope or shock due to acute blood loss which has not immediately appeared from either end of the gastrointestinal tract. An assessment of the severity of blood loss is the first and most important priority. It depends almost entirely on the history and physical examination, which may also provide some clues as to the origin of the bleeding.

Assessment of blood loss

It is only possible to guess how much blood has been lost, nevertheless this estimate is a most important part of management because it dictates transfusion requirements and influences attitudes about possible surgery. A history of haematemesis with melaena implies considerably greater blood loss than haematemesis or melaena alone, and carries twice the mortality rate[52]. The volume of any haematemesis gives some guide to the amount of blood lost but the patient's account is often inaccurate. Similarly, the volume, frequency and appearance of melaena stools will help in assessing the severity of haemorrhage; major bleeding is likely if red blood appears *per rectum*. Patients may occasionally have a major bleed with little immediate visible evidence, but a history of faintness suggests rapid and significant bleeding.

Physical examination provides the most useful information about the severity of bleeding. The shocked patient with cold peripheries, thready pulse and low blood pressure has obviously lost a lot of blood. Where blood loss is less extreme, blood volume can be crudely assessed by examination of pulse, blood pressure and jugular venous pressure. After a large bleed, patients often have a fairly normal pulse and blood pressure when resting in bed, but the former rises and the latter falls abruptly on sitting or standing up. An invisible jugular venous pressure when the patient is lying flat also indicates a depleted blood volume. Thus if there is a normal jugular venous pressure and no significant postural change in pulse or blood pressure it is unlikely that there has been a major acute bleed. It should be remembered that a patient taking a beta adrenergic blocking drug will not always develop a tachycardia despite substantial blood loss. A careful drug history is therefore essential.

History

The history is unreliable for determining the exact source of bleeding. It may provide some help—for example dyspepsia suggests peptic ulcer, vomiting culminating in haematemesis suggests the Mallory–Weiss syndrome, and a history of liver disease suggests varices. However, in over 30% of patients with peptic ulcer (and in 50% of all patients) no symptoms relevant to the cause of bleeding are found[1]. Even in patients with the Mallory–Weiss syndrome less than half have the typical history of repeated vomiting followed by haematemesis[20]. Only investigation will determine the precise site of bleeding.

Physical examination

Physical examination is rarely useful in determining the site of bleeding, but there are occasional patients in whom examination provides very important information. In liver disease hepatosplenomegaly, ascites, liver flap or spider naevi will suggest the possibility of variceal bleeding. In carcinoma an epigastric mass, signs of metastatic disease may indicate the diagnosis. In patients with coagulopathy skin purpura and bleeding from other sites may occur. Lymphadenopathy or splenomegaly may be found in various haematological disorders. Two very rare causes of bleeding may be diagnosed on physical examination—hereditary haemorrhagic telangiectasia and pseudoxanthoma elasticum.

Course

Most patients admitted to hospital with acute upper gastrointestinal bleeding will have stopped bleeding by the time of admission and only a minority will bleed again. Certain causes of bleeding are rarely associated with severe or recurrent blood loss and their early identification may be of value in deciding which patients may be discharged early. Lesions that rarely cause severe bleeding are mainly superficial, such as oesophagitis, gastric erosions and the Mallory–Weiss syndrome. Patients with oesophageal varices often have severe recurrent bleeding.

Recent studies indicate that rebleeding after admission to hospital occurs in about 25% of patients with chronic peptic ulcers [5, 33]. Rebleeding is a serious matter in these patients and is associated with a mortality rate approaching 30%, compared with less than 10% in patients who do not rebleed [33].

Few studies have looked at the long-term risk of readmission with further bleeding following an episode of acute upper gastrointestinal bleeding. In patients with acute mucosal lesions the risk of further bleeding is low, while in patients with oesophageal varices further episodes of bleeding are almost invariable. In patients with bleeding duodenal ulcer treated non-surgically the risk of further bleeding is about 20% over the next 5–10 years which compares with 5% in those treated surgically [26]. This study was completed before potent ulcer

healing drugs were available and it could be that the incidence of rebleeding is now lower.

Investigations

Laboratory studies

These are directed mainly at assessing the severity of the bleed. Measurement of blood volume is of little value in such a patient as one does not normally know the patient's original blood volume. Therefore one has to rely on clinical assessment. The haemoglobin concentration is of little value in assessing acute blood loss, as it takes some hours for haemodilution to occur. It is of more value in patients who have chronic bleeding, and in the days after admission. Neutrophilia and thrombocytosis are often found soon after a major bleed; the blood urea also rises within a few hours due to renal hypoperfusion and the protein load from blood in the gastrointestinal tract. A high blood urea concentration on admission can be valuable evidence of severe bleeding, providing renal function was previously normal [55].

In all patients the possibility of an underlying haematological disorder should be considered; a platelet count, white cell count and blood film inspection should be routine. Routine tests of coagulation are not necessary, but should be done in patients with evidence of liver disease or where the cause of bleeding is obscure. A prothrombin time and kaolin partial thromboplastin time will identify most coagulopathies that may cause bleeding [45].

Identification of the site of blood loss

The two principal techniques are barium radiology and fibreoptic endoscopy. Many studies have now shown that endoscopy provides a substantially higher diagnostic yield than barium radiology, although double-contrast barium radiology compares well with endoscopy in the identification of chronic peptic ulcers [16, 59]. The higher diagnostic yield of endoscopy is largely due to the recognition of superficial lesions, such as gastric erosions and Mallory–Weiss tears, that are difficult to demonstrate radiologically—such lesions rarely bleed severely so this advantage is of questionable importance. Indeed, the increased accuracy of endoscopy does not seem to confer any advantage in terms of improved management or survival, when compared with investigation by barium radiology [16].

There are, however, a number of other advantages of fibreoptic endoscopy that makes it the investigation of choice. Firstly, endoscopy is performed with the patient supine, thus avoiding any problems due to postural hypotension. Secondly, endoscopy provides information that is of prognostic importance—if a chronic ulcer is seen with a visible vessel in its base (Table 30.4) there

Table 30.4. The stigmata of recent haemorrhage.

Fresh blood in stomach or duodenum.
A visible blood vessel in ulcer base.
Clot adhering to ulcer (black dots on ulcer base).

---

is a very high chance of rebleeding, whereas if the ulcer shows no sign of recent haemorrhage the chance of rebleeding is remote (Table 30.5) [6, 21, 29, 69]. Thirdly, endoscopy will also determine which of two potential bleeding sites has haemorrhaged—for example, in a patient with both varices and a peptic ulcer. The main disad-

vantage of endoscopy is that it carries a very small risk, although serious complications are exceedingly rare. Endoscopy does not seem to cause rebleeding; in a comparison of endoscopy and radiology the incidence of rebleeding was similar in the two groups of patients [16].

The ideal instrument for use in acute upper gastrointestinal bleeding is a forward viewing fibreoptic endoscope with a wide suction channel for aspiration of blood. Intravenous sedation should be given cautiously as aspiration of vomit is more likely to occur in a heavily sedated patient. Unlike the patient fasted for an elective endoscopy, the patient with a history of recent gastrointestinal haemorrhage often has a fluid-filled stomach. The optimal timing of endoscopy will vary from patient to patient and will depend on local circumstances. It is best done within 24 hours of admission when the diagnostic yield is highest, but should be left until the patient has been adequately resuscitated. Usually it is performed most conveniently on the morning after admission, although earlier endoscopy may be indicated if bleeding is rapid; this strategy provides as good results as when endoscopy is performed within a few hours of admission [70]. An adequate view can usually be obtained without prior gastric lavage. Occasionally, large volumes of blood may obscure the view but altering the patient's position may help—for example moving from the left to the right lateral position.

Table 30.5. Rebleeding rates of chronic peptic ulcers according to endoscopic appearances.

Reference	Total no. of patients	Patients with stigmata of bleeding		Patients without stigmata of bleeding	
		No.	No. rebleeding (%)	No.	No. rebleeding (%)
[21]	89	60	25 (42)	29	1 (3)
[60]	87	47	20 (43)	40	0 (0)

Unexplained upper gastrointestinal haemorrhage

No bleeding site will be found in about 20% of patients investigated by early endoscopy (40% by barium radiology). Many of these patients may have bled from superficial lesions which have healed and no further action is required unless bleeding recurs. If serious bleeding recurs after negative endoscopy then a number of possibilities arise. The most likely explanation is that a common cause of blood loss, for example a peptic ulcer, has been missed and a repeat endoscopy should be performed. If this is again negative then a rare cause of gastrointestinal bleeding must be considered, particularly a haemostatic disorder. The possibility that bleeding is coming from a site distal to the proximal duodenum should be considered—for example, the small intestine, biliary tree etc. (see Chapter 32).

Arteriography is indicated in patients with unexplained episodes of severe bleeding [2]. Considerable skill is required in both performing angiography and in interpreting the result, but in experienced hands the diagnostic yield can be high [25]. It is of most value when performed as the patient is actually bleeding; there is little point in doing it if the bleeding has stopped. The rate of bleeding must be at least 0.5 ml/min if injected contrast material is to enter the gastrointestinal tract. Arteriography is particularly useful in identifying small vascular malformations that are difficult to diagnose by other methods; it is the only technique that will reliably diagnose haemobilia. In certain circumstances (notably patients with vascular malformations) bleeding can be controlled by the injection of embolic materials at arteriography.

In a few patients with severe continuous bleeding emergency surgery will be necessary before the bleeding site has been identified. In these circumstances fibreoptic endoscopy should be done either before or just after the anaesthetic is given, providing haemorrhage is not torrential, to exclude an oesophageal source of bleeding. Large volumes of blood in the stomach may prevent identification of the bleeding site, but the surgeon will be reassured to know that the patient has not got oesophageal varices. The source of bleeding will often be readily apparent at laparotomy, but if the bleeding site is not identified, even after gastroduodenotomy, a blind gastric resection should not be performed.

Differential diagnosis

Patients with haematemesis usually give a clear history, although occasionally it is difficult to distinguish haematemesis from haemoptysis. Bleeding disorders of the mouth and nasopharynx may also be confused with haematemesis, particularly if blood is swallowed and then vomited. This possibility should always be considered, particularly when investigations are negative.

Haematemesis usually implies a bleeding site above the ligament of Treitz, but melaena alone can be due to lesions of the small intestine or the proximal colon. Fresh red blood may be passed rectally by patients with rapid upper gastrointestinal bleeding leading to confusion with a colonic site of bleeding. Melaena is usually unmistakable, but it should be remembered that various medications can blacken the stools, particularly iron and bismuth.

Occasional patients with severe gastrointestinal bleeding may present with shock alone, without immediate haematemesis or melaena, and this should be considered as a cause of shock among other common conditions such as myocardial infarction, pulmonary embolism and septicaemia. Overactive bowel sounds may provide a clue before the haemorrhage is apparent.

Prevention

It is not known why chronic lesions such as peptic ulcers and oesophageal varices bleed in some patients, and not in others. Peptic ulcer is a common condition and gastrointestinal bleeding is relatively rare. The role of anti-inflammatory drugs in the causation of gastrointestinal bleeding remains controversial [57]. If there is circumstantial evidence that non-steroidal anti-inflammatory drug consumption was associated with upper gastrointestinal bleeding, it is sensible to advise avoidance of these preparations.

One would hope that with improved management of the underlying disease that bleeding would occur less often. For example, the widespread use of ulcer healing drugs might reduce bleeding from chronic peptic ulcers although there is, as yet, no sign of this happening.

Prevention of acute upper gastrointestinal bleeding due to stress ulceration in seriously ill hospital inpatients may be possible. Patients most at risk are those with combinations of several serious complications, particularly respiratory failure, hypotension, sepsis and jaundice [54]. Bleeding in these patients is usually due to gastritis or gastric erosions; factors that may be important in the pathogenesis of these lesions include gastric acid, bile salts, the secretory state of the gastric mucosa, gastric blood flow, poor nutrition, drug treatment and coagulation defects. Even in the most seriously ill patient, severe upper gastrointestinal bleeding is not common and hence results of trials using prophylactic regimens have been inconclusive. Studies suggest that an H_2-blocker or large doses of antacids may reduce the risk of minor bleeding.

There are three situations where acute upper gastrointestinal bleeding is particularly common and can be prevented in most patients by intravenous cimetidine or ranitidine. In patients with fulminant hepatic failure, acute upper gastrointestinal bleeding occurs in 50% of patients and can be virtually abolished by intravenous cimetidine although overall survival is not affected [40]. In patients with severe head injury acute upper gastrointestinal bleeding is very common, occurring in up to 80% of patients (and may be due in part to gastric acid hypersecretion), intravenous cimetidine causes a substantial reduction in bleeding in these patients [27]. H_2-blockade has also reduced the incidence of post-transplant gastrointestinal haemorrhage in renal transplant recipients [68].

Medical treatment

Most patients with acute upper gastrointestinal haemorrhage will have stopped bleeding by the time of hospital admission and only a minority will bleed again. Thus simple supportive treatment is sufficient for the majority of patients. Medical treatment of these patients can be conveniently considered under three headings—resuscitation, patient monitoring, and measures to stop bleeding.

Resuscitation

This is the most important part of management and should take precedence over all investigations. Unless bleeding is trivial an intravenous infusion of dextrose or saline should be established. If there is significant hypovolaemia this should be corrected by blood transfusion as soon as crossmatched blood is available. Caution must be exercised that not too much saline is given before the blood is available as it may precipitate pulmonary oedema. It is not possible to give absolute rules that are valid for all patients to guide the necessity for blood transfusion (Table 30.6). If examination of pulse, blood pressure and jugular venous pressure suggests the blood volume to be

Table 30.6. A ready-reckoner for ordering blood at time of hospital admission [44].

Clinical condition	Admission haemoglobin	Blood requirements (500 ml packs)			
		For resuscitation	For anaemia	For rebleeding	Total
Not shocked	10.0 g/dl	0	0	+2	2
Shocked	10.0 g/dl	4	0	+2	6
Not shocked	*X g/dl	0	+10−X*	+2	10−X+2
Shocked	*Y g/dl	4	+10−Y*	+2	10−Y+6

*X and Y represent values of Hb < 10 g/dl

depleted, a transfusion of blood should be started. Similarly, patients with haemoglobin levels below 10 g/dl usually require transfusion. It is sensible to keep two units of blood cross-matched for 48 hours after the cessation of active bleeding in case of further haemorrhage.

Blood volume studies have shown that the loss in patients with acute upper gastrointestinal bleeding tends to be more severe than suspected clinically [63] and this should be remembered when planning blood transfusion requirements. For example, in one study it was found that 18 out of 30 patients with acute upper gastrointestinal bleeding had lost more than half their red cell volume [64]. The quantity of blood to be transfused depends partly on the estimate of loss and partly on frequent observation of the patient, paying particular attention to clinical measures of blood volume and evidence of recurrent or continued haemorrhage. Central venous presure measurement is of little value in assessing initial blood loss, but is very useful when monitoring transfusion in patients with severe bleeding, particularly the elderly or those with cardiac, renal or liver disease. If the patient has an elevated central venous pressure due to pre-existing water and salt overload, frusemide should be given to 'create a space' for packed red blood cells.

Patient monitoring

The aim is to identify as early as possible, patients with continuous or recurrent bleeding, since the mortality rate in patients who rebleed is greatly increased. Any material vomited or passed rectally should be examined carefully. Nasogastric tubes are widely used in the United States but not in Britain. They provide a potential means for early detection of rebleeding but can be misleading—large blood clots may not be aspirated up the tube, blockage of the tube or faulty placement may occur, and duodenal ulcers may bleed without blood refluxing into the stomach. Nasogastric tubes can also cause oesophageal or gastric trauma which makes endoscopic findings difficult to interpret. On balance, nasogastric tubes are best avoided—to the patients' great relief.

Careful clinical observation is the most reliable means for detecting rebleeding— frequent measurement of pulse and blood pressure by nursing staff, and regular examination of postural changes in pulse, blood pressure and jugular venous pressure by medical staff. Central venous pressure measurement will detect rebleeding earlier than clinical methods, but is not necessary in most patients and it should never be allowed to replace regular clinical observation by nursing and medical staff.

Most patients can be adequately monitored on acute general medical wards, and specialist units for these patients would be impractical in most hospitals. In most district general hospitals in the United Kingdom, expertise in nursing severely ill patients is concentrated in intensive care units, and the few patients with established severe bleeding are best cared for there, particularly if central venous pressure monitoring is required.

Measures to stop the bleeding

A variety of non-surgical techniques have been tried to stop bleeding or prevent further blood loss and, except in patients with oesophageal varices, none has yet proved to be effective. Histamine H_2-receptor antagonists, particularly cimetidine, have been tried in the hope that they might prevent further bleeding, perhaps by reducing the gastric acid and pepsin which may dissolve the clot overlying the ulcer [51, 72]. Several trials have been reported, but few have included adequate patient numbers and results have been inconclusive; combining the results of all trials suggests that H_2-blockade may decrease rebleeding from gastric ulcers [11]. Somatostatin is of no benefit [56]. Tranexamic acid, an oral antifibrinolytic agent, has also been tried and initial results are encouraging [5].

A variety of other methods to control bleeding have been tried—gastric cooling [23], tissue adhesives and injection of alcohol into the ulcer [3] have been advocated but not tested adequately. Arterial embolization during coeliac axis arteriography has been used to control bleeding from rare lesions, such as arterial malformations in the pancreas or liver [25]. Control of bleeding using angiographic techniques has not been shown to be of value in the common causes of bleeding, such as peptic ulcer.

There has been considerable recent interest in endoscopic techniques to control bleeding. These methods depend on using a probe passed down the biopsy channel of the endoscope which can transmit a source of energy onto the bleeding point and cause coagulation. Methods used have included electrocoagulation, thermal probes and lasers [30, 48, 62]. About 10% of patients presenting with a bleeding ulcer have a blood vessel that is clearly visible in the ulcer base; in this small minority laser photocoagulation may control bleeding and prevent the need for emergency surgery [7, 18, 19, 41, 61]. Further studies are required before such treatment can be recommended for general use.

Surgical treatment

There have been no controlled trials comparing different operation policies in acute upper gastrointestinal bleeding, indications for surgery having evolved mainly from personal experience and retrospective studies. Operation rates have tended to fall in recent years, probably due to the availability of effective ulcer healing drugs which provide an alternative to surgery for the long-term management of chronic peptic ulcers.

Factors influencing the decision to operate

Amount and duration of bleeding

The most important single factor when considering the use of surgical treatment is the severity of bleeding. It is not possible to define precisely how much bleeding should be allowed before operation is performed. In a minority of patients severe continuous bleeding from the moment of presentation will lead to early surgery. However, most patients have spasmodic bleeding and opinions on the optimal timing of surgery differ widely. Some consider a single large bleed is sufficient to justify surgery on the grounds that a further similar bleed may be fatal; others wait for two large bleeds to occur before recommending surgery; some use surgery only as a last resort for patients with many episodes of severe bleeding.

There is now a good deal of modern evidence to indicate that emergency surgery for acute upper gastrointestinal bleeding carries a high risk, suggesting that a more conservative surgical approach could lead to better overall mortality figures [1, 15, 39]. Studies comparing different surgical policies have shown, if anything, a trend towards improved overall survival with a conservative surgical approach. For example, in a study comparing patients randomly admitted to one of two hospitals with very different surgical policies, overall mortality was lower where surgery was performed less often (Fig. 30.3). In another study operation rates were found to fall substantially from 1975 to 1980, but during this time overall mortality rates were unchanged (Fig. 30.3). However, when 'aggressive' surgery was compared with 'conservative' surgery in Birmingham, death rates were 2% and 13%, respectively [46].

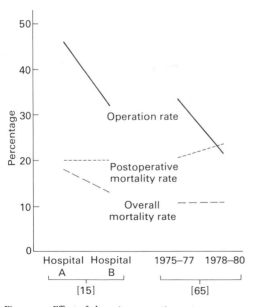

Fig. 30.3. Effect of changing operation rates on mortality in acute upper gastrointestinal bleeding.

If surgery is delayed until several severe bleeding episodes have occurred then some patients will inevitably die of uncontrolled haemorrhage. Such deaths are often regarded as therapeutic failures whereas post-operative deaths occurring several days after operation (for example, from heart failure, pneumonia or pulmonary emboli) may be thought of as unrelated to the bleeding, or just bad luck. When deciding on the optimum surgical policy, it is the overall mortality figures that are important and not the mode of death. Aggressive early surgery has not been shown consistently to improve overall mortality. As there are now alternatives to surgery for the long-term control of peptic ulcer disease, a conservative late surgical policy is recommended.

Diagnosis

Virtually any bleeding lesion in the upper gastrointestinal tract may require operative therapy to control blood loss, but the diagnosis is rarely important when deciding whether to operate. The major exception is bleeding from oesophageal varices which may be controlled by non-surgical means (see Chapter 31). An exact diagnosis may help to predict which patients could require operation because of further bleeding—superficial lesions, such as osophagitis, gastric erosions or Mallory–Weiss tears, rarely bleed sufficiently to justify surgery. Nearly all emergency operations are for recurrent bleeding from chronic peptic ulcer; duodenal and gastric ulcers are equally likely to require surgery [65]. Occasionally the identification of a bleeding lesion that is difficult to treat surgically, for example, diffuse haemorrhagic gastritis or an oesophageal ulcer, may lead to more prolonged medical therapy. Surgery will almost certainly be required in the rare cases where bleeding is from a gastric arterial malformation.

Endoscopic appearances

A chronic ulcer without any stigma of recent bleeding will rarely bleed again (Table 30.5). If stigmata are present (that is fresh arterial bleeding, as black dots on the ulcer base or a visible blood vessel), then a substantial proportion will rebleed and require surgery [6, 29, 69]. There is some uncertainty as to what a visible blood vessel looks like in an ulcer base, but in one recent report emergency surgery was required for all patients with visible arterial bleeding [41]. The predictive value of the endoscopic appearance of chronic ulcers has been under-used and further studies may lead to more accurate identification of those patients who will need surgery. At present, if stigmata of recent bleeding are seen in a chronic ulcer then close observation is essential as the patient has a 50/50 chance of a further major bleed. It is the duty of the endoscopist to emphasize to non-specialist colleagues the prognostic importance of this finding.

Age

There is a 20–30% post-operative mortality rate in patients over 70-years-old who have surgery for acute upper gastrointestinal bleeding [1, 15]. Mortality rates are likely to be high in this age group whatever is done, but in view of this high post-operative mortality rate it would seem wise to withhold surgical treatment in the elderly unless bleeding is very severe.

Previous history

In some patients with a bleeding chronic peptic ulcer, surgical therapy may be indicated because of previous uncontrollable symptoms. The risks of emergency surgery are far greater than those of elective surgery. The best approach is to allow the bleeding to settle and to arrange an elective operation at a later date, preferably after a few weeks of mobilization at home.

Coincident medical conditions

Patients with severe coincident cardio-respiratory or other serious disease will tend to do badly whatever course is adopted. In such circumstances, where bleeding is severe and continuous, operative treatment is potentially life-saving and surgery should not be postponed or delayed unnecessarily.

Likelihood of recurrence of bleeding

If most patients with bleeding peptic ulcers were likely to suffer recurrent bouts of bleeding, operation after the first bleed would be sensible. However, this does not appear to be the case—at least in patients with duodenal ulcer. In one study of 278 patients with bleeding duodenal ulcers, recurrent bleeding occurred in 20% of those treated medically over a 5–10 year follow-up period [26]. Although it was much lower (4.5%) in patients treated operatively, a 1-in-5 chance of recurrent bleeding over a 5 to 10-year period does not itself constitute an indication for operation.

Choice of operation

The principal aim of surgery is to stop the patient bleeding to death; the secondary aim is to prevent recurrence. Most patients coming to theatre will have had an accurate preoperative diagnosis made endoscopically or radiologically but sometimes this is not the case. The surgeon must first confirm or find the bleeding site. Most chronic peptic ulcers are palpable, but some are not and a gastrotomy or duodenotomy may be necessary—particularly to find acute ulcers [4]. Alternatively, a sigmoidoscope may be introduced through a small hole in the stomach for examination of the gastric mucosa [17] or fibreoptic endoscopy (through the mouth) may be performed during the laparotomy. Gastric ulcers high in the stomach and oesophageal tears in the Mallory–Weiss syndrome may be difficult to locate and, if the bleeding point has not been found, the region of the cardia should be examined carefully through an oblique gastrotomy. Once identified the bleeding point should be oversewn with a nonabsorbable suture, and a more definitive procedure can then be performed.

Duodenal ulcer

Oversewing the ulcer together with vagotomy and pyloroplasty is the best operation for most cases of duodenal ulcer. It has the advantage over gastrectomy of a lower postoperative mortality rate, especially in the elderly. Schiller, *et al.* [52] found that the postoperative mortality rate of vagotomy and pyloroplasty ulcer was 5.5% compared with 16.7% for Billroth I gastrectomy and 14.3% for Pólya's gastrectomy; the excess mortality after gastrectomy was confined to patients over 60-years-old. Clark reported similar findings, postoperative mortality falling from 16% to 5% on changing his operating policy from partial gastrectomy to vagotomy and pyloroplasty [9]. Furthermore the recurrent bleeding rate after vagotomy and pyloroplasty is no greater than after gastrectomy in duodenal ulcer patients [52].

Highly selective vagotomy is not appropriate for the treatment of ill patients, but may be the best procedure if the operation is semi-elective.

Gastric ulcer

Billroth I gastrectomy remains the most popular operation. Wedge resection of the ulcer along with vagotomy and pyloroplasty has been advocated as an alternative, but it may be technically difficult and may be associated with a greater recurrence rate. Ulcers high on the lesser curve are a difficult surgical problem which may be solved by performing a distal gastrectomy, with resection of a sleeve of lesser curve up to and including the ulcer [66].

Other lesions

Acute mucosal lesions such as those of the Mallory–Weiss syndrome or gastric erosions rarely require surgery. However if operation is necessary oversewing may be sufficient to control the bleeding although gastric erosions may require more radical surgery [66]. Gastric carcinomas seldom cause bleeding of sufficient severity to justify emergency surgery but when they do resection should be performed if feasible. Occasionally no bleeding lesion is found at laparotomy despite a gastroduodenotomy and careful examination of the gastric and duodenal mucosa. Blind gastrectomy is rarely indicated in these circumstances because of its high postoperative morbidity and mortality.

Prognosis

About 10% of patients with acute upper gastrointestinal bleeding die in hospital and this figure has not changed for over 30 years. Most deaths occur in elderly patients, and the failure to improve survival figures is almost certainly due to the increasing proportion of elderly patients admitted with bleeding [1]. Over half the deaths are unrelated to upper gastrointestinal bleeding, for example in patients with inoperable malignancies or severe cardiorespiratory disease where gastrointestinal bleeding has been trivial and irrelevant. Most of the remaining deaths occur postoperatively; death from uncontrolled bleeding in unoperated patients is uncommon. It is likely that many of the patients who die postoperatively will die whatever is done. While mortality rates overall are disappointingly high, patients under 65 with non-malignant disease do extremely well with a mortality rate substantially less than 5%.

References

1 ALLAN R, DYKES P. A study of the factors influencing mortality rates from gastrointestinal haemorrhage. *Q J Med* 1976;**45**:533–550.

2 ALLISON DJ, HEMINGWAY AP, CUNNINGHAM DA. Angiography in gastrointestinal bleeding. *Lancet* 1982;**ii**:30–33.

3 ASAKI S, NISHIMURZA T, SATOH A, *et al*. Endoscopic hemostasis of gastrointestinal haemorrhage by local application of absolute ethanol: a clinical study. *Tohoku J Exp Med* 1983;**141**:373–383.

4 BANNING A, BARON A, KOPELMAN H, LAM KL, WARREN P. Bleeding peptic ulcer. *Br Med J* 1965; **2**:781–784.

5 BARER D, OGILVIE AL, HENRY DA, *et al*. Cimetidine and tranexamic acid in the treatment of acute upper gastrointestinal bleeding. *New Engl J Med* 1983;**308**:1571–1575.

6 BORNMAN PC, THEODOROU NA, SHUTTLEWORTH RD, ESSEL HP, MARKS IN, Importance of hypovolaemic shock and endoscopic signs in predicting recurrent haemorrhage from peptic ulceration: a prospective evaluation. *Brit Med J* 1985;**291**:245–247.

7 BROWN SG, SWAIN CP, STOREY DW, *et al*. Endoscopic laser treatment of vascular anomalies of the upper gastrointestinal tract. *Gut* 1985;**26**:1338–1348.

8 CHANDLER GN, WATKINSON G. The early diagnosis of the causes of haematemesis. *Q J Med* 1959; **28**:371–395.

9 CLARK CG. Surgical aspects of gastrointestinal haemorrhage. *Postgrad Med J* 1968;**44**:590–598.

10 COGGON D, LANGMAN MJS, SPIEGELHALTER D. Aspirin, paracetamol and haematemesis and melaena. *Gut* 1982;**23**:340–344.

11 COLLINS R, LANGMAN M. Treatment with histamine H₂ anatagonists in acute upper gastrointestinal hemorrhage. *New Engl J Med* 1985;**313**:660–663.

12 CONN HO, BILTZER BL. Nonassociation of adrenocorticosteroid therapy and peptic ulcer. *New Engl J Med* 1976;**294**:473–479.

13 COTTON PB, ROSENBERG MT, WALDRAM RPL, AXON ATR. Early endoscopy of oesophagus, stomach and duodenal bulb in patients with haematemesis and melaena. *Br Med J* 1973;**2**:505–509.

14 DRONFIELD MW Medical or surgical treatment of haematemesis and melaena. *J R Coll Phys Lond* 1979;**13**:84–86.

15 DRONFIELD MW, ATKINSON M, LANGMAN MJS. Effect of different operation policies on mortality from bleeding peptic ulcer. *Lancet* 1979;**i**:1126–1128.

16 DRONFIELD MW, LANGMAN MJS, ATKINSON M, *et al*. Outcome for endoscopy and barium radiography for acute upper gastrointestinal bleeding: controlled trial in 1037 patients. *Br Med J* 1982;**284**:545–548.

17 DUTHIE HL. Surgical treatment of upper alimentary bleeding. *Br Med J* 1967;**4**:790–792.

18 FLEISCHER D. Endoscopic therapy of upper gastrointestinal bleeding in humans. *Gastroenterology* 1986;**90**:217–234.

19 FLEISCHER D. Endoscopic laser therapy for gastrointestinal disease. *Arch Intern Med* 1984;**144**:1225–1233.

20 FOSTER DN, MILOSZEWSKI K, LOSOWSKY MS. Diagnosis of Mallory-Weiss lesions. A common cause of upper gastrointestinal bleeding. *Lancet* 1976;**ii**:483–485.

21 FOSTER DN, MILOSZEWSKI KJA, LOSOWSKY MS. Stigmata of recent haemorrhage in diagnosis and prognosis of upper gastrointestinal bleeding. *Br Med J* 1978;**i**:1173–1177.

22 FRASER GM, RANKIN RN, CUMMACK DH. Radiology and endoscopy in acute upper gastrointestinal bleeding. *Br Med J* 1976;**i**:270–271.

23 GILBERT D, SAUNDERS D. Iced saline lavage does not slow bleeding from experimental canine gastric ulcers. *Dig Dis & Sci* 1981;**26**:1065–1069.

24 GOLDMAN RL Submucosal arterial malformation ('aneurysm') of the stomach with fatal haemorrhage. *Gastroenterology* 1964;**46**:589–593.

25 GOLDMAN R, HERLINGER H, BAUM S. In: Dykes PW, Keighley MRB, eds. *Gastrointestinal haemorrhage*. Littleton, MA: Wright–PSG, 1981:209–231.

26 HARVEY RF, LANGMAN MJS. The late results of medical and surgical treatment for bleeding duodenal ulcer. *Q Med J* 1970;**39**:539–547.

27 HALLORAN LG, ZFASS AM, GAYLE WE, WHEELER CB, MILLER JD. Prevention of acute gastrointestinal complications after severe head injury: a controlled trial of cimetidine prophylaxis. *Am J Surg* 1980;**139**:44–48.

28 HYAMS JS, LEICHTNER AM, SCHWARTZ AN. Recent advances in diagnosis and treatment of gastrointestinal hemorrhage in infants and children. *J Pediatr* 1985;**106**:1–9.

29 JOHNSTON JH. The sentinel clot and invisible vessel: pathologic anatomy of bleeding peptic ulcer. *Gastro Intest Endosc* 1984;**30**:313–314.

30 JOHNSTON JH, SONES JQ, LONG BW, POSEY EL. Comparison of the heater probe and YAG laser in endoscopic treatment of major bleeding from peptic ulcers. *Gastrointest Endosc* 1985;**31**:175–181.

31 JOHNSTON SJ, JONES PF, KYLE J, NEEDHAM CD. Epidemiology and course of gastrointestinal haemorrhage in north-east Scotland. *Br Med J* 1973;**3** 655–660.

32 JONES FA. Haematemesis and melaena with special reference to bleeding peptic ulcer. *Br Med J* 1947;**2**:441–446.

33 JONES PF, JOHNSTON SJ, McEWAN AB, KYLE J, NEEDHAM CD. Further haemorrhage after admission to hospital for gastrointestinal haemorrhage. *Br Med J* 1973;3:660–664.

34 KAPLAN RP, KAPLAN L, PARISH J, TREIMAN R. Hemobilia *Dig Dis Sci* 1980;25:140–144.

35 KATZ D, PITCHUMONI CS, THOMAS E, ANTONELLE M. The endoscopic diagnosis of upper gastrointestinal haemorrhage. Changing concepts of aetiology and management. *Dig Dis Sci* 1976;21:182–189.

36 KNAUER CM. Mallory-Weiss Syndrome. Characterisation of 75 Mallory-Weiss lacerations in 528 patients with upper gastrointestinal haemorrhage. *Gastroenterology* 1976;71:5–8.

37 LANGMAN MJS. Upper gastrointestinal bleeding. In: Pounder RE, ed. *Recent advances in gastroenterology-6.* Edinburgh: Churchill Livingstone, 1986:1–16.

38 LEADING ARTICLE. Bleeding Ulcers: scope for improvement? *Lancet* 1984;i:715–16.

39 LOGAN RFA, FINLAYSON NDC. Death in acute upper gastrointestinal bleeding. Can endoscopy reduce mortality. *Lancet* 1976;1:1173–1175.

40 MacDOUGALL BRD, BAILEY RJ, WILLIAMS R. H₂-receptor antagonists and antacids in the prevention of acute gastrointestinal haemorrhage in fulminant hepatic failure. *Lancet* 1977;i:617–619.

41 MacLEOD IA, MILLS PR, MacKENZIE JF, JOFFE SN, RUSSELL R, CARTER DC. Neodymium yttrium aluminium garnet laser photocoagulation for major haemorrhage from peptic ulcers and single vessels: a single blind controlled study. *Br Med J* 1983;286:345–348.

42 MALLORY GK, WEISS S. Haemorrhages from lacerations of the cardiac orifice of the stomach due to vomiting. *Am J Med Sci* 1929;178:506–515.

43 MESSER J, REITMAN D, SACKS HS, SMITH H, CHALMERS TC. Association of adrenocorticoid therapy and peptic-ulcer disease. *New Engl J Med* 1983;309:21–24.

44 MISIEWICZ JJ, POUNDER RE. Peptic Ulcer. In: Weatherall DJ, Ledingham JGG, Warrell DA, eds. *The Oxford textbook of medicine.* Oxford: Oxford University Press, 1983:1257–1270.

45 MITTAL R, SPERO JA, LEWIS JH, *et al.* Pattterns of gastrointestinal hemorrhage in hemophilia. *Gastroenterology* 1985;88:515–522.

46 MORRIS DL, HAWKER PC, BREARLEY S, SIMMS M, DYKES, P, Keighley MRB. Optimal timing of operation for bleeding peptic ulcer: prospective randomised trial *Br Med J* 1984;288:1277–1280.

47 O'BRIEN JD, BURNHAM WR. Bleeding from peptic ulcers and use of non-steroidal anti-inflammatory drugs in the Romford area. *Brit Med J* 1985;291:1609–1610.

48 O'BRIEN JD, DAY SJ, BURNHAM WR. Controlled trial of small biopolar probe in bleeding peptic ulcers. *Lancet* 1986;i:464–466.

49 OLDHAM KT, LOBE TE. Gastrointestinal hemorrhage in children. A pragmatic update. *Pediatr Clin North Am* 1985;32:1247–1263.

50 PETERSON WL, BARNETT CC, SMITH HJ, ALLEN MH, CORBETT DB. Routine early endoscopy in upper gastrointestinal tract bleeding. A randomised controlled trial. *New Engl J Med* 1981;304:925–929.

51 PEURA DA, JOHNSON LF. Cimetidine for prevention and treatment of gastroduodenal mucosal lesions in patients in an intensive care unit. *Ann Int Med* 1985;103:173–177.

52 SCHILLER KFR, TRUELOVE SC, WILLIAMS DG. Haematemesis and malaena, with special reference to factors influencing the outcome. *Br Med J* 1970;2:7–14.

53 SHOENFELD Y, ELDAR M, BEDAZOVSKY B, LEVY MJ, PINKAS J. Aortic stenosis associated with gastrointestinal bleeding. A survey of 612 patients. *Am Heart J* 1980;100:179–182.

54 SKILLMAN JJ, BUSHNELL LS, GOLDMAN H, SILEN W. Respiratory failure, hypotension, sepsis and jaundice. A clinical syndrome associated with lethal haemorrhage from acute stress ulceration of the stomach. *Am J Surg* 1969;117:523–529.

55 SNOOK JA, HOLDSTOCK GE, BAMFORTH J. Value of a simple biochemical ratio in distinguishing upper and lower sites of gastrointestinal haemorrhage. *Lancet* 1986;i:1064–1065.

56 SOMERVILLE K, DAVIES J, HAWKEY C, *et al.* Somatostatin in treatment of haemtemesis and melaena. *Lancet* 1985;i:130–132.

57 SOMERVILLE K, FAULKNER G, LANGMAN M. Non-steroidal anti-inflammatory drugs and bleeding peptic ulcer. *Lancet* 1986;i:462–466.

58 STERN AI, HOGAN DL, KAHN LH, ISENBERG JJ. Protective effect of acetaminophen against aspirin- and ethanol-induced damage to the human gastric mucosa. *Gastroenterology* 1984;86:728–733.

59 STEVENSON GW, COX RR, ROBERTS CJC. Prospective comparison of double contrast barium meal examination and fibreoptic endoscopy in acute upper gastrointestinal bleeding. *Br Med J* 1976;2:723–724.

60 STOREY DW, BROWN SG, SWAIN CP, *et al.* Endoscopic prediction of recurrent bleeding in peptic ulcers. *New Eng J Med* 1981;305:915–916.

61 SWAIN CP, KIRKHAM JS, SALMON PR, BOWN SG, NORTHFIELD TC. Controlled trial of Nd-YAG laser photocoagulation in bleeding peptic ulcers. *Lancet* 1986;ii:1113–1116.

62 SWAIN CP, MILLS TN, SHEMESH E, *et al.* Which electrode? A comparison of four endoscopic methods of electrocoagulation in experimental bleeding ulcers. *Gut* 1984;25:1424–1431.

63 TIBBS DJ, LESLIE WG. Blood volumes in gastroduodenal haemorrhage. *Lancet* 1956;ii:266–274.

64 TUDHOPE GR. The loss and replacement of red cells in patients with acute gastrointestinal haemorrhage. *Q J Med* 1958;27:543–560.

65 VELLACOTT KD DRONFIELD MW, ATKINSON M, LANG-

MAN MJS. Comparison of surgical and medical management of bleeding peptic ulcers. *Br Med J* 1982;**284**:548–550.

66 VENABLES CW. In: Dykes PW, Keighley MRB, eds. *Gastrointestinal Haemorrhage.* Littleton, MA: Wright PSG, 1981:337–356.

67 WALDRAM R, DAVIS M, NUNNERLEY H, WILLIAMS R. Emergency endoscopy after gastrointestinal haemorrhage in 50 patients with portal hypertension. *Br Med J* 1974;**4**:94–96.

68 WALTER S, ANDERSON JT, CHRISTENSEN U. Effect of cimetidine on upper gastro-intestinal bleeding after renal transplantation: a prospective study. *Br Med J* 1974;**4**:94–96.

69 WARA P. Endoscopic prediction of major rebleeding—a prospective study of stigmata of hemorrhage in bleeding ulcer. *Gastroenterology* 1985;**88**:1209–1214.

70 WHORWELL PJ, EADE OE, CHAPMAN R, SMITH CL, FISHER JA. Comparison between admission and next-day endoscopy in the management of acute upper gastrointestinal haemorrhage. *Digestion* 1981;**21**:18–20.

71 ZUCKERMAN GR, CORNETTE GL, CLOUSE RE, HARTER HR. Upper gastrointestinal bleeding in patients with chronic renal failure. *Ann Int Med* 1985;**102**:588–592.

72 ZUCKERMAN G, WELCH R, DOUGLAS A, *et al.* Controlled trial of medical therapy for active upper gastrointestinal bleeding and prevention of rebleeding. *An J Med* 1984;**76**:361–366.

Chapter 31
Variceal Haemorrhage

A. K. BURROUGHS

The treatment of variceal haemorrhage is directed not only at stopping bleeding but also at minimizing deterioration of liver function. The ideal management has yet to be established [14]. However the resurgence and development of emergency variceal sclerotherapy has meant that arrest of haemorrhage without surgery can be achieved in most patients. Even so, the severity of liver disease remains the prime factor determining survival; the method used to stop bleeding is less important [68].

Portal-systemic shunts prevent rebleeding but do not increase survival, and hepatic encephalopathy may be a serious complication. Repeated endoscopic sclerotherapy of varices and pharmacological control of portal hypertension are newer methods to prevent rebleeding. Their long-term efficacy and complications are still being assessed.

Introduction

Haemorrhage from varices is the most serious complication of portal hypertension. Variceal veins in the oesophageal and gastric submucosa are part of the portal-systemic channels which develop when pressure rises in the portal system (Fig. 31.1). In these positions the varices may rupture and bleed, irrespective of the type of liver disease or primary site of resistance in the portal system [23, 66].

There is little evidence to support mucosal erosion in the pathogenesis of variceal rupture [61]. An eruptive process is more likely, but portal vein pressure has not been shown to be directly related to risk of bleeding once varices are present [61]. Palmer and Brick [53] could not correlate intravariceal pressure with the likelihood of bleeding, but this has not been confirmed prospectively.

Patients with large varices are more likely to bleed than those with smaller ones [53]—abstinence by alcoholic cirrhotics leads to smaller varices, while continued drinking leads to larger ones [13]. In cirrhotics, the size of varices is partly related to the severity of liver disease [1] and deterioration of liver function often precedes bleeding [45]. The bleeding point is nearly always within 3 cm of the gastro-oesophageal junction [48, 52]. Bleeding from gastric varices is uncommon.

About 30–50% of cirrhotics with varices will eventually bleed from them [1, 20]. Immediate and long-term survival following variceal bleeding is directly related to the severity of liver disease [45]. Patients with non-cirrhotic intrahepatic or extrahepatic portal hypertension (the latter usually due to portal or splenic vein thrombosis) have normal or very well-compensated liver function, and therefore a much better prognosis [67].

Clinical features

Gastrointestinal bleeding from any source is an important cause of death in cirrhotic patients [20, 45]. Most bleed from gastro-oesophageal varices but up to 30% of haemorrhagic episodes are due to peptic ulcers or gastric erosions (Fig. 31.1(b)) [33].

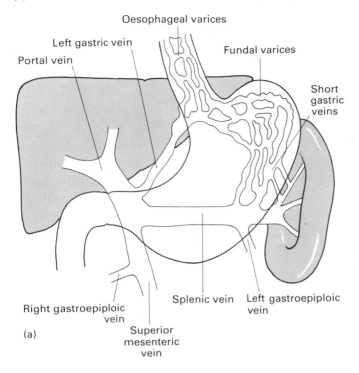

Oesophageal varices

Left gastric vein

Portal vein

Fundal varices

Short gastric veins

Right gastroepiploic vein

(a)

Superior mesenteric vein

Splenic vein

Left gastroepiploic vein

Fig. 31.1 (a). oesophageal and gastric varices, arising from left and short gastric veins. (b) post mortem specimen: the patient was thought to have died from bleeding varices, but in fact exsanguinated from a gastric ulcer. (c) endoscopic view of oesophageal varices.

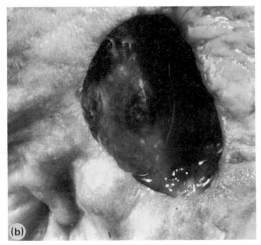

(b)

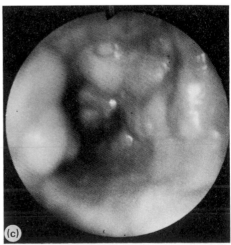

(c)

Variceal bleeding may be the first manifestation of chronic liver disease or may complicate previously diagnosed cirrhosis. Most patients have a haematemesis and melaena. In some bleeding may be 'silent', presenting with anaemia or portal-systemic encephalopathy.

In children, varices are commonly due to portal vein thrombosis. There is often a history of umbilical vein sepsis or catheterization. Examination is normal except for a large spleen.

In adults portal or splenic vein thrombosis without cirrhosis is a less common cause of variceal bleeding. It may be associated with abdominal sepsis, trauma, biliary surgery, splenectomy, haematological malignancies or pancreatic disease. In cirrhotics, direct invasion of the portal vein by primary liver cell carcinoma is not uncommon, and often first presents as variceal bleeding.

In a patient with gastrointestinal bleeding, clinical evidence of chronic liver disease should always suggest the presence of varices, but absence of a palpable liver or spleen does not exclude them. In these patients specific details should be asked regarding the likelihood of hepatitis B antigen related liver disease (parenteral drug abuse, homosexuality, transfusion of blood products and ethnic origin).

The patient's clinical condition prior to the haemorrhage, and details of any previous bleeding episodes including the degree of hepatic decompensation induced, must be recorded. These factors influence subsequent management. Recent, rapid clinical deterioration in a cirrhotic may be due to primary liver cell carcinoma.

Careful observation for impending alcohol withdrawal will be required in alcoholics, especially those with a history of withdrawal symptoms. Bleeding from drug- or alcohol-induced erosions is just as likely in the cirrhotic as non-cirrhotic. Symptoms or a history of ischaemic heart disease will limit the use of vasopressin.

The initial and subsequent physical examinations should include not only assessment of cardiovascular status but also the severity of liver impairment. This is best judged by depth of jaundice, amount of peripheral oedema and/or ascites, and the degree of hepatic encephalopathy. The latter signs, together with the level of serum albumin, bilirubin and prothrombin time can be used in a numerical scoring system classifying patients into three grades of severity (A, B, and C, Table 31.1) [59]. These correspond closely to Child's original grades, and correlate with short- and long-term survival. Mortality following variceal bleeding is about 5% in grade A, 20% in grade B, and greater than 40% in grade C patients. Rebleeding during hospitalization is seen more often in grade C, than grade A, patients.

Complications are far more frequent in patients with poor hepatic reserve. Hypovolaemia leads to deteriorating hepatocyte function so that ascites, jaundice and encephalopathy can develop rapidly. Fluid retention is made worse by the sodium load of transfused blood. Renal failure is a bad prognostic sign. Severe oliguria with a low urinary sodium concentration (<10 mmol/l) and a urine/plasma osmolarity ratio of 1.1 to 1.15 often persists, despite correction of hypovolaemia. Occasionally, a mixed picture with acute tubular necrosis is seen which may be precipitated by the X-ray contrast media used at portography. Encephalopathy is aggravated by the absorption of a substantial nitrogen load from the blood in the gut. Other complications such as ascitic infections, septicaemia, hypoglycaemia, stress erosions and severe

Table 31.1. Pugh's modification of Child's criteria [59].

	Score 1 point	Score 2 points	Score 3 points
Bilirubin (μmol/l)	17–34	34–51	>51
(if primary biliary cirrhosis)	(17–68)	(68–70)	(>170)
Prolongation prothrombin time (sec)	1–4	4–6	6
Albumin (g/l)	>35	28–35	<28
Ascites	None	Slight	Moderate +
Porto-systemic encephalography (grade)	None	1 and 2	3 and 4

Grade A = 5 or 6 points; Grade B = 7–9 points; Grade C = 10–15 points.

disseminated intravascular coagulation can occur, but are more often seen in the severely ill cirrhotic.

Management of acute variceal haemorrhage

Patients with known or suspected varices should receive intensive nursing care and be treated by a combined medical/surgical team experienced in dealing with these patients. When local expertise is not available, liaison with a referral centre should be established immediately and transfer arranged if necessary.

Treatment consists of general measures to prevent deterioration of liver function and specific measures to arrest haemorrhage. Diagnosis of the bleeding lesion is made by endoscopy after resuscitation. The patency of the portal vein should be established early on. Visualization of the complete portal anatomy, and investigation of the type of portal hypertension can usually be deferred.

If infection with the hepatitis B virus is known, or suspected, the patient should be nursed in a single room, and all attendants should wear gloves and protective gowns. In the event of accidental innoculation to a member of staff, hyperimmune globulin (500 mg in 5 ml) and hepatitis B vaccine (20 μg) should be administered immediately [8]. Before administration, 10 ml of blood should be taken to check baseline antibody to hepatitis B surface antigen. If this later proves to be positive the full course of vaccination need not be completed.

General measures

Investigations

An intravenous line is established with 5% dextrose pending plasma or blood replacement. Saline or dextran solutions must not be used. Blood should be withdrawn for cross matching six units of blood, a full blood count (including platelet count), prothrombin time, blood glucose, plasma creatinine, urea and electrolytes, hepatitis B antigen, biochemical liver function tests and baseline blood cultures. A coagulation screen is needed if the prothrombin time is prolonged. A chest X-ray and electrocardiogram are performed as soon as initial resuscitation is satisfactory. A diagnostic tap of ascitic fluid is made for total and differential white cell count, protein content, culture and haemoglobin level if blood-stained. Intraperitoneal bleeding in this context is usually secondary to primary liver cell carcinoma.

Baseline urinary sodium concentration is measured, and 24-hour sodium excretion monitored daily. Other daily tests should include a full blood count, prothrombin time, and plasma urea and electrolytes. Hypoglycaemia is detected by regular blood sampling using blood glucose capillary sticks.

Blood products

Whole blood transfusion requirements are dictated by the adequacy of circulating blood volume. Central venous lines may be necessary to monitor transfusion; they should be inserted only by experienced operators as iatrogenic complications, especially bleeding, are particularly dangerous in patients with chronic liver disease. Fresh frozen plasma (400 ml) and 10% calcium gluconate (10 ml) should be given for every 4 to 6 units of stored blood. Vitamin K_1 (10 mg) is given daily for 3 days by slow intravenous injection. Platelet transfusions may be required. Over-transfusion should be avoided as rapid expansion of plasma volume increases portal pressure which may worsen bleeding. As a guide, blood replacement should be aimed at maintaining the haemoglobin at 10 g/dl.

Prevention of encephalopathy

Twice daily sodium phosphate or lactulose enemata, plus oral lactulose (10 ml four times daily), should be used to evacuate the bowel and minimise hepatic encephalopathy. Oral neomycin (1g four times daily), for five days only, may be added in cases of profound coma. Patients should eat as soon as the initial haemorrhage has been controlled. Depending on the severity of liver disease and encephalopathy, dietary protein should be restricted (20 or 40 g/day) or withdrawn completely for a few days, maintaining caloric intake with glucose administered intravenously or by mouth.

Electrolytes

Dietary sodium should be restricted (22 mmol/day) in all patients with severe liver disease and fluid retention. Every litre of transfused blood has approximately 140 mmol of sodium, and many oral and parenteral drug formulations contain substantial amounts of sodium. Saline infusions should not be used. Accurate fluid balance, with daily combined bed and patient weighing, provide the best guide to fluid retention. Hypokalaemia should be corrected.

Control of gastric acid

Although antacids and H_2-receptor antagonists decrease gastric acidity they have not been shown to arrest upper gastrointestinal bleeding, or variceal bleeding [22]. However, stress erosions may be prevented by H_2-receptor antagonists in patients with fulminant liver failure [42], and in the severely ill cirrhotic. Ranitidine, which does not affect the hepatic microsomal enzyme system, is preferable to cimetidine. Ranitidine should be given as a continuous infusion: 50 mg eight hourly.

Sedative drugs

Sedative drugs worsen hepatic encephalopathy and should be avoided at all costs, even for endoscopic procedures. If a patient is suffering from alcohol withdrawal, a controlled intravenous infusion of 0.8% chlormethiazole (this has a shorter life than any parenteral benzodiazepine) should be used to achieve the minimum necessary sedation.

Diagnosis

Endoscopy

Endoscopic diagnosis of a bleeding lesion in patients with liver disease permits appropriate management and increases confidence and understanding of the clinical situation [33] (Fig. 31.1 (c)). Endoscopy is performed without sedation, as soon as initial resuscitation is complete. Even with prompt endoscopy, four to five hours after admission, active variceal bleeding is seen in less than 20% of patients. If a patient with varices rebleeds in hospital, then endoscopy within two hours identifies active variceal bleeding in 75% of patients [48]. Many centres perform endoscopy the morning after admission, unless the patient's clinical course requires balloon tamponade, sclerotherapy or surgery to arrest haemorrhage. Visualization is often improved by endoscoping after a short infusion of vasopressin.

If quiescent varices are seen, but no other bleeding site is detected, then it is accepted that bleeding has probably arisen from the varices. If other lesions coexist with the varices then re-endoscoping is mandatory if bleeding recurs. When erosions and varices coexist in alcoholic cirrhotic patients the course and prognosis is the same as that seen with varices alone [63]. Erosions are more common in the alcoholic cirrhotic and patients with severe liver failure.

Ultrasound

Ultrasonography is a non-invasive method of visualizing the portal vein. This enables one to distinguish between extrahepatic portal venous thrombosis and intrahepatic portal hypertension [78] and it may also detect a hepatocellular carcinoma.

Radiology

A patent portal vein is a prerequisite for percutaneous transhepatic obliteration of varices. Patency of the portal vein can be observed during the venous phase of a splanchnic arteriogram, or by transhepatic or splenoportography. The latter should not be attempted if there is severe coagulopathy but it provides the best images of the portal system, and allows measurement of the portal pressure. Portography is required as a preliminary to shunt surgery or transhepatic obliteration of varices. A liver tumour may be demonstrated by computed tomography (CT) or splanchnic arteriography.

Specific measures

Vasoconstrictive therapy

Vasopressin

In therapeutic doses vasopressin constricts splanchnic arterioles, thus decreasing splanchnic blood inflow, leading to a reduction in portal pressure and flow [64]. This should lead to adequate clot formation at the bleeding point, but further compromises hepatic function by reducing portal flow and hepatic arterial flow. A reduction in portal pressure is maintained for no more than 30 minutes after the infusion.

Vasopressin causes a systemic vasoconstriction, including the coronary circulation, with a reduction of cardiac output which may be complicated by arrhythmias, angina or myocardial infarction. Its antidiuretic action contributes to cardiac failure

and acute pulmonary oedema. Recent myocardial infarction or angina are absolute contraindications to the use of vasopressin. A baseline ECG and electrocardiographic monitoring are required in middle-aged and elderly patients.

Vasopressin is administered into a peripheral vein using either of two regimens.
1. Short infusion: 20 units in 100 ml of 5% dextrose given over 20 minutes. There is no benefit in repeating it more than three times within 24 hours.
2. Prolonged infusion: this starts at 0.4 units/min in 5% dextrose. The duration of infusion varies between four to 24 hours in different centres, unless bleeding has stopped earlier. The infusion is then reduced to 0.2 units/min for a further four to 24 hours.

No controlled study has compared these two regimens. Prolonged infusion might be more effective, lengthening the period of lowered portal pressure, but side-effects are more common. Infusion into the superior mesenteric artery does not improve efficacy and complications of arterial catheterization are a disadvantage [9].

The patient becomes pale, develops abdominal cramps and defaecates involuntarily. If this is not seen, the vasopressin has become pharmacologically inactive during storage.

The clinical efficacy of vasopressin leaves room for improvement [57]. A recent review [10] showed that vasopressin achieved control of bleeding in 57% of episodes, but caused death in 3% and major complications in 17%. Only two placebo-controlled trials are published [17, 45], and in one the placebo was as effective as vasopressin [17]. All studies agree that the use of vasopressin does not improve patient survival. Efficacy in controlling bleeding is partly related to severity of liver disease—grade C patients tend not to respond.

Intravenous vasopressin should be used as a temporizing emergency measure for no longer than 24 hours. Patients who show no response, or rebleed, should rapidly be treated by an alternative method to control haemorrhage.

Sublingual nitroglycerin minimizes the systemic effects of vasopressin and potentiates a reduction in portal pressure in stable cirrhotics [24]. It is presently being studied in patients with active haemorrhage, and should not be used until such studies confirm its safety.

Glypressin

Glypressin is a long acting analogue of vasopressin. An intravenous 1 mg bolus reduces portal pressure for over one hour. It has intrinsic vasoconstrictor activity, as well as being converted slowly to lysine vasopressin by vascular endothelial cells [58]. Unlike vasopressin it has no adverse effects on factor VIII complex and plasminogen activator [58].

Glypressin (2 mg every six hours as intravenous bolus) was more effective than synthetic vasopressin (0.4 units/min) in one small controlled trial [18].

Somatostatin

Somatostatin also lowers portal pressure, and it is as effective as vasopressin in controlling haemorrhage [31, 36]. It requires continuous infusion as the half-life is under three minutes [65].

Balloon tamponade

The tubes

The Sengstaken–Blakemore tube (three lumen) is a wide-bore nasogastric tube with two inflatable balloons. The gastric balloon compresses the cardia and fundal varices, preventing blood flow to the oesophageal varices. The oesophageal balloon compresses oesophageal varices. The Minnesota

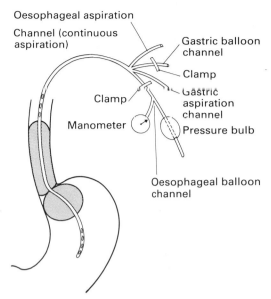

Fig. 31.2. A four lumen tube for oesophago-gastric balloon tamponade.

tube (four lumen) has an extra channel which allows aspiration above the oesophageal balloon and is marked at 5 cm intervals (Fig. 31.2). A three lumen tube should have an extra nasogastric tube taped alongside it, to act as the oesophageal aspiration channel. Paediatric tubes are available. The Linton–Nachlas tube has a single large gastric balloon. Compared with the Sengstaken tube, it is more effective for controlling haemorrhage from gastric than from oesophageal varices [77].

Indications

Tamponade should be used to reduce excessive blood loss, or if there is insufficient compatible blood, or for patient transfer if there is active bleeding. Some centres use it routinely before endoscopic sclerotherapy.

Inserting the tube

The tube is easier to pass if kept in an ice box, as the rubber is temporarily stiffened. All the equipment should be kept in a box ready for use in an emergency. Prior to its use the balloons must be tested, aspiration channels checked and the tube lubricated. Resuscitation equipment should be at hand. With the patient positioned head down on his left side, and with two assistants performing continuous pharyngeal aspiration, the tube is inserted through the mouth. A Maghill forceps is useful to feed the tube down. If the tube fails to pass, it should be inserted with the patient intubated and lightly anaesthetized. The airway must always be protected by insertion of a cuffed endotracheal tube in semi-comatose or comatose patients. Intravenous sedation alone should never be used.

Inflating the balloons

With the tube in the stomach, the gastric channel is aspirated and air blown through to check its position. The gastric balloon is then inflated with 250–400 ml of air and double clamped. Excessive resistance to inflation suggests that the gastric balloon is in the oesophagus. After inflation the tube is pulled back gently against the cardia. The oesophageal balloon is then inflated to between 30 and 40 mmHg on a manometer (that is, slightly greater than that known or expected in the portal vein) (Fig. 31.2), and is then clamped.

Balloon management

The gastric balloon's position is checked by X-ray and if satisfactory the tube is marked and taped firmly to the side of the mouth. No traction is necessary. Trained personnel must be at the bed-side at all times, with a pair of scissors to cut through the tube if respiratory distress occurs. The tube position (using the marking at the mouth), and oesophageal balloon pressure are checked hourly. The gastric balloon is checked if aspirations indicate fresh bleeding, or if its position is in doubt. The oesophageal lumen

is continuously aspirated. Gastric aspiration is done hourly or more frequently if continued bleeding is suspected. Medications can be given through the gastric aspiration channel.

Results

When used correctly, balloon tamponade provides effective control of haemorrhage [49]. If aspirations suggest persistent, fresh bleeding, the source of bleeding may be other than varices.

Potentially serious complications are usually associated with inexperienced attendants—pharyngeal obstruction and asphyxia (excessive traction of under-inflated or burst gastric balloon); oesophageal ulceration (prolonged compression); aspiration pneumonia (inhalation of blood and inadequate aspiration); oesophageal rupture (over-inflation of either balloon in the oesophagus).

Review of the literature shows that balloon tamponade controls haemorrhage in 77% of episodes, with fatal complications in 5% [10]. However, rebleeding occurs in 46% and death in 51%.

Because rebleeding occurs so frequently, particularly in the severely ill, balloon tamponade is not definitive treatment but a holding measure until a further procedure can be done, or a decision taken to treat with conservative measures alone. Ideally a management plan should be made before using tamponade [55].

Balloon deflation

Tamponade should last for no more than 24 hours, preferably for less. The oesophageal balloon is deflated first, then the gastric balloon one to two hours later. The deflated tube can be left *in situ* if there is delay before surgery or sclerotherapy.

Emergency sclerotherapy

Endoscopic injection sclerotherapy [16]

The optimal method for sclerosis of varices remains unclear. There are variations in anaesthetic technique, type of endoscope, use of local oesophageal compression, site of injection, and finally the sclerosant (Table 31.2) (Fig. 31.3).

sheath [80] gives better control than free-hand injection with fibreoptic endoscope. Firstly, the rigid endoscope or sheath compresses the varices, providing haemostasis and improving visualization. Secondly, by rotation of the slot or the window in the sheath, each varix is made to protrude in turn and can be injected with small volumes (2–8 ml) of sclerosant just above the gastro-oesophageal junction. Retrograde

Table 31.2. Different methods for endoscopic injection sclerotherapy of oesophageal varices.

Anaesthesia	Endoscope ($\pm$ local compression)	Injection site	Sclerosant
None	Fibreoptic $\pm$ flexible sheath	Intravariceal	5% ethanolamine
Local	Fibreoptic $\pm$ proximal balloon	Submucosal	5% sodium morrhuate
General	Fibreoptic $\pm$ distal balloon	Combined	1%/3% polidokanol
	rigid $\pm$ slot		0.5–1.5% sodium tetradecyl sulphate

During active bleeding visualization of the varices can be difficult. For this reason many centres inject varices immediately after deflation and removal of a Sengstaken tube—a combined approach to control haemorrhage [2, 15, 56, 76].

When there is active bleeding, the rigid Negus oesophagoscope modified with a distal slot or fibreoptic endoscope with flexible

propagation of sclerosant to gastric varices does occur and in some patients these veins will thrombose. Sclerotherapy can be repeated if there is rebleeding.

In most published series control of haemorrhage is achieved in around 70% by a single injection and in over 90% with repeated injection sessions [38].

Complications and mortality increase

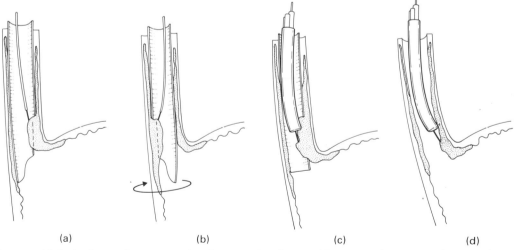

(a)   (b)   (c)   (d)

Fig. 31.3. Methods of variceal injection with endoscopic sclerotherapy. (a) injection of varix protruding into the slot of a rigid Negus oesophagoscope. (b) rotation of oesophagoscope compresses injected varix and another varix protrudes into slot. (c) flexible sheath with window allowing protrusion of varix. Injection with fibreoptic endoscope. (d) free-hand, direct injection with fibreoptic endoscope.

with repeated injections. Complications range from prolonged substernal pain, dysphagia, oesophageal bleeding, ulceration, perioesophageal leakage to perforation, thoracic empyema and pleural effusion. Delayed oesophageal necrosis is documented and oesophageal stenosis requiring bougienage is well-recognized. In the largest prospective emergency study complications occurred in 21% of patients, 5% being fatal [76].

Endoscopic sclerosis has several important advantages. It is a non-operative technique that can be performed without general anaesthesia, repeated to control any rebleeding, and is relatively easy to perform. However controlled studies are required to establish if it reduces rebleeding or improves survival more than other methods of acute treatment.

Percutaneous transhepatic obliteration of varices

Before attempting this technique, a patent portal vein must be demonstrated by contrast radiology. Using local anaesthesia, 50–100 mg of intravenous pethidine and 5–15 mg intravenous diazepam, a catheter is inserted percutaneously in the right mid-axillary line, under X-ray screening control, into the liver to enter the intrahepatic portion of the portal vein. The left gastric and short gastric veins feeding the varices are cannulated (Fig. 31.4). Thrombotic agents (such as 50% dextrose, gelatine foam, thrombin, isobutyl 2 cyanoacrylate or absolute alcohol) are injected to produce total occlusion of these feeding veins.

Although this procedure requires considerable technical skill and is used only in specialist centres, the development of a 'bridge-technique' modified from Okuda [50] together with preformed catheters, has

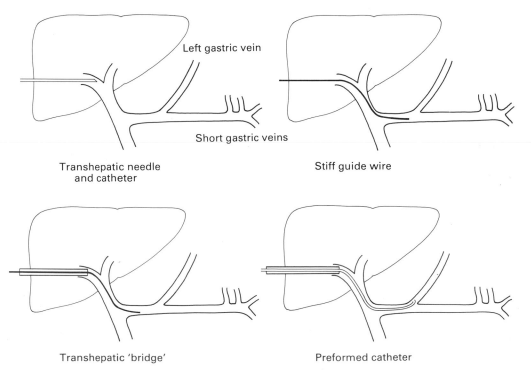

Fig. 31.4. Modified Okuda technique for transhepatic obliteration of varices.

made it a shorter procedure that is easier to teach and perform. The track in the liver is carefully sealed with gelatine foam on withdrawing the 'bridge' and catheter.

Thrombosis in the portal vein occurs in less than 5% of procedures [44, 69] and is often transient. Right pleural effusions are common in patients with ascites but rarely require drainage. Fatal or major complications occur in 4% or 17% of procedures, respectively.

Control of haemorrhage is achieved in only 75% of patients mainly due to a technical failure rate of 10–20%.

Recanalization of obliterated vessels is rare, but development of new smaller variceal vessels from the portal and splenic veins are common. Repeated obliteration is impractical. Rebleeding is as frequent as in patients treated with conservative measures alone [69], therefore this technique's role is only in the emergency treatment of variceal bleeding. Its advantages are that general anaesthesia is never required and bleeding gastric varices can be treated.

Emergency surgery

Oesophageal stapling transection

Transection of the oesophagus, using a staple gun, has replaced transthoracic transection of the oesophagus in most centres [21]. The operation time is an hour or less, and the EEA staple gun (Fig. 31.5) misfires very rarely. A 100% efficacy is reported in the literature with no patient rebleeding during the same hospital admission [4]. When the transection is accompanied by devascularization of the para-oesophageal collaterals and the left gastric vein rebleeding from varices is less than 5% in the long-term [32]. Technical failure can be anticipated in patients with previous high gastric surgery, where adhesions containing collateral veins make dissection difficult.

Selection of patients for surgery is crucial.

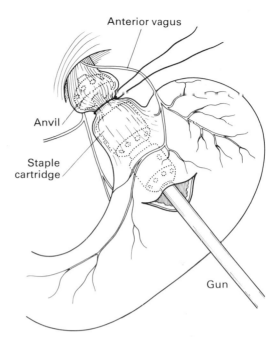

Fig. 31.5. Oesophageal transection with a staple gun.

For patients with less severe liver disease, emergency staple transection and percutaneous transhepatic obliteration are equally effective, and have a low mortality [4]. In severely ill cirrhotics, staple transection and endoscopic sclerotherapy have an equally high mortality [6]. In these small studies the severity of liver disease was the prime factor determining survival.

Portal-systemic shunts

Emergency shunts control variceal bleeding—96% of 582 episodes in one review [11] but mortality is 42% [19]. Severe portal-systemic encephalopathy, in around 20% of the patients, is such a serious problem that it outweighs the shunt's effectiveness in controlling bleeding. Emergency shunt operations are now rarely performed routinely, except in one major centre [51]. An end-to-side porta-caval shunt is the best emergency procedure.

Prevention of variceal rebleeding

Following recovery from variceal bleeding, the factors influencing survival are the same as those affecting survival during the acute bleed—the prognosis is far better for those patients with stable, well-compensated liver function or the potential for improvement (for example, abstinence from alcohol), than in those with deteriorating liver disease [68].

Three strategies have been assessed for the prevention of variceal bleeding—surgical shunting, injection sclerotherapy, and beta-adrenergic blockade with oral propranolol.

Portal-systemic shunts

Surgical decompression of varices can be achieved by a number of procedures (Fig. 31.6). The **end-to-side porta-caval shunt** is a total shunt, diverting all blood from the portal system and thus from the varices, into the systemic circulation. This diverted blood contains hepatotrophic and 'toxic' substances. The diversion may lead to deterioration of liver function and encephalopathy. To minimize these complications partially diverting shunts were devised. The **side-to-side porta-caval shunt**, and the **mesocaval shunt with interposition Dacron graft**, have lost popularity due to poor maintenance of portal flow and poor shunt patency, respectively. The proximal **splenorenal shunt** gave better results than the end-to-side porta-caval shunt in two studies [37, 41].

Selective shunts are designed to decompress varices without portal diversion. The **distal splenorenal shunt** [18, 62] is based on the premise that gastro-splenic (low

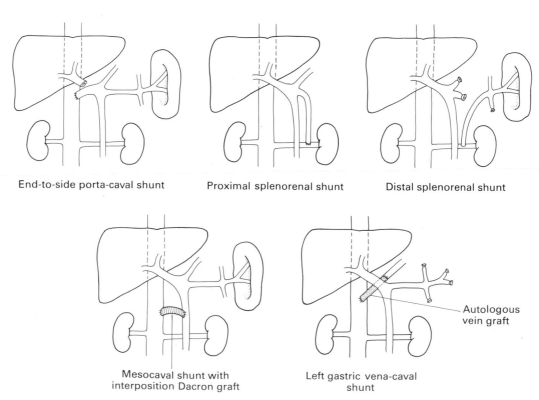

End-to-side porta-caval shunt   Proximal splenorenal shunt   Distal splenorenal shunt

Mesocaval shunt with interposition Dacron graft

Left gastric vena-caval shunt

Autologous vein graft

Fig. 31.6. Types of surgical portal-systemic shunts.

pressure) and mesenteric-portal (high pressure) circuits are functionally separate in normal man, but in portal hypertension collaterals develop between the two. This increased pressure in the gastro-splenic circuit is transmitted to the oesophageal varices. The key feature of the operation is meticulous ligation of all collaterals between these two circuits, including left gastric, umbilical and right gastroepiploic veins. The distal end of the splenic vein is anastomosed to the left renal vein and the spleen is left in place. The short gastric collaterals remain as venous conduits decompressing the oesophageal varices.

The **left gastric vena-caval shunt** is another selective shunt devised by Inokuchi [29, 30] but its use is reported solely from Japanese centres. Operative and long-term survival are very good with only 10% of patients rebleeding, but a 10% technical failure rate in constructing the shunt.

In patients who have bled from varices, all the four randomized controlled trials [10] comparing porta-caval anastomosis with conservative treatment show that in the shunted group, the risk of rebleeding is virtually eliminated. However, the incidence of severe encephalopathy is increased and there is no statistically increased survival.

The distal splenorenal shunt, although reducing the incidence of porta-systemic encephalopathy in most studies in the early years after shunting [27], does not increase patients' survival when compared to other shunts in controlled studies [10]. The shunt loses its selectivity with time [47] as it is very difficult to establish complete separation between the mesenteric-portal and gastro-splenic systems, and major collaterals slowly develop between the two.

About 25% of all shunted patients develop portal-systemic encephalopathy as a recurrent or incapacitating problem requiring hospital treatment. Only patients with non-cirrhotic portal hypertension, or stable well-compensated cirrhosis, remain good candidates for a shunt operation. The four controlled studies of prophylactic portacaval shunts (i.e. before patients have bled) have shown dramatic reduction in bleeding episodes but no increase in survival, and hepatic encephalopathy as a serious complication. There is no indication for a prophylactic shunt [60].

Endoscopic injection sclerotherapy [16, 72, 79, 81]

The disappointment with therapeutic shunts has led to the use of repeated endoscopic injection sclerotherapy as a preventive measure against variceal rebleeding [7, 34]. It does not alter portal flow so that hepatic function is preserved and no encephalopathy is precipitated by the technique. Endoscopic sclerotherapy is easier to perform electively than during an active bleeding episode. Most centres now perform repeated injections with fibreoptic endoscopy without general anaesthesia [12].

Repeated sessions of injection sclerotherapy completely obliterate oesophageal varices in most patients, preventing further haemorrhage [43, 75]. Rebleeding does occur, but this usually happens before all the varices have been obliterated. Follow-up endoscopy after obliteration should be performed every nine to 12 months, as some patients will re-develop varices that need further injections [43].

A minority of patients may rebleed from gastric varices after the oesophageal varices have been obliterated. However, retrograde flow of sclerosant has been observed during injection of oesophageal varices, with subsequent disappearance of gastric varices [73].

Short- and long-term complications are the same as those described for emergency injection sclerotherapy, with major complications being reported in 10–28% of patients [43, 54].

Despite control of haemorrhage, no improvement of survival with repeated injections has been demonstrated in one study at two [75] or five years [74]. Another centre has reported increased survival in a group treated with sclerotherapy, compared with a control group which was not treated with emergency sclerotherapy at the time of rebleeding [43, 79].

Should prophylactic endoscopic sclerotherapy be offered to a patient with varices that have never bled? Only one controlled trial is published in selected patients with moderate or large varices, considered at greater risk of bleeding from poor coagulation or 'erosions' overlying varices on endoscopy [54]. These erosions may not be true erosions but probably correspond to the red colour, red wheal or cherry red spot sign defined by the Japanese Research Society for Portal Hypertension [3]. These signs are considered risk factors for variceal haemorrhage. The prophylactic study reported a significant difference in bleeding and survival between patients who had their varices repeatedly sclerosed and those who did not. All deaths in the control group were due to haemorrhage. However, the difference in survival should be interpreted with the knowledge that patients in the control group were only treated with conservative measures when they bled—in clinical practice a further procedure would have been used when these measures had failed, which might have improved survival.

Beta-adrenergic blockade

Continuous oral propranolol reduces portal blood pressure [39] by reducing cardiac output and by a vasoconstrictive effect on the splanchnic circulation induced by blocking B_2-receptors [28].

The first randomized, controlled trial [40] showed that twice daily oral propranolol prevented recurrence of haemorrhage from both acute gastric erosions and varices in cirrhotic patients, when compared with placebo-treated patients. All the patients had good liver function and most had large varices and alcoholic cirrhosis. However, in unselected cirrhotics of various aetiologies with different degrees of hepatic impairment, who had survived variceal haemorrhage, no difference was shown between patients randomized to propranolol or placebo [5]. Serious resuscitation problems were encountered in some patients bleeding while on beta-blockers.

At present propranolol should not be used as a routine measure for prevention of variceal rebleeding [11].

Other surgical procedures

These are primarily devascularization procedures. The two stage Suguira operation is popular in Japan consisting of thoracic and abdominal stages. Rebleeding occurs in up to 7% of patients [35, 70, 71]. The Hassab procedure is similar [25] but does include oesophageal transection. It has been used predominantly in patients with schistosomal portal hypertension with a variceal rebleeding rate of 4%.

Despite the good results of these operations in terms of rebleeding, it is difficult to assess their potential for widespread use as the patient populations described in these papers were very selected.

References

1 BAKER LA, SMITH C, LIEBERMAN G. The natural history of oesophageal varices. A study of 115 cirrhotic patients in whom varices were diagnosed prior to bleeding. *Am J Med* 1959;**26**:228–237.
2 BARSOUM MS, BOLOUR FI, EL-ROOBY AA, RIZK ALLAH MA, IBUAHIM AS. Tamponade and injection sclerotherapy in the management of bleeding oesophageal varices. *Br J Surg* 1982;**69**:76–78.
3 BEPPU K, INOKUCHI K, KOYANAGI N, *et al*. Prediction of variceal haemorrhage by esophageal endoscopy. *Gastrointest Endosc* 1981;**27**:213–218.
4 BURROUGHS AK, BASS NM, OSBORNE D, DICK R, HOBBS KEF, SHERLOCK S. Randomised controlled

study of percutaneous transhepatic obliteration of varices and oesophageal stapling transection in uncontrolled variceal haemorrhage. *Liver* 1983;3:122–128.

5 BURROUGHS AK, JENKINS WJ, SHERLOCK S, *et al.* Controlled trial of propranolol for the prevention of recurrent variceal haemorrhage in patients with cirrhosis. *N Engl J Med* 1983;309:1539–1548.

6 CELLO JP, CRASS R, TRUNKEY DD. Endoscopic sclerotherapy versus oesophageal transection of Child's class C patients with variceal haemorrhage. Comparison with results of porta-caval shunt: a preliminary report. *Surgery* 1982;91:333–338.

7 CELLO JP, GRENDELL JH, CRASS RA, TRUNKEY DD, COBB EE, HEILBRON DC. Endoscopic sclerotherapy versus porta caval shunt in patients with severe cirrhosis and variceal haemorrhage. *N Engl J Med* 1984;311:1589–1594.

8 CENTERS FOR DISEASE CONTROL. Postexposure prophylaxis of hepatitis B. *Ann Intern Med* 1984;101:351–354.

9 CHOJKIER M, GROSZMANN RJ, ATTERBURY C, *et al.* A controlled comparison of continuous intra-arterial and intravenous infusions of vasopressin in haemorrhage from oesophageal varices. *Gastroenterology* 1979; 77:540–546.

10 CONN HO. A plethora of therapies. In: Westaby D, MacDougall BRD, Williams R, eds. *Variceal Haemorrhage*. London: Pitman Books Ltd, 1982: 225–226.

11 CONN HO. Propranolol in the treatment of portal hypertension: a caution. *Hepatology* 1982;2:641–644.

12 COPENHAGEN ESOPHAGEAL VARICES PROJECT. Sclerotherapy after first variceal haemorrhage in cirrhosis. *N Engl J Med* 1984;311:1594–1600.

13 DAGRADI AE. The natural history of esophageal varices in patients with alcoholic liver cirrhosis: An endoscopic and clinical study. *Am J Gastroenterol* 1972;57:520–540.

14 EDITORIAL. Bleeding oesophageal varices. *Lancet* 1984; i:131–141.

15 ESOPHAGEAL VARICES AND SCLEROTHERAPY PROGRAMME (EVASP) STUDY GROUP (DENMARK). Randomised trial of endoscopic sclerotherapy as a supplement to balloon tamponade for bleeding esophageal varices. *Scand J Gastroenterol [Suppl 78]* 1982;17:20.

16 FLEISCHER D. Endoscopic therapy of upper gastrointestinal bleeding in humans. *Gastroenterology* 1986; 90:217–234.

17 FOGEL MR, KNAUER M, ANDRES LL, *et al.* Continuous intravenous vasopressin in active upper GIT bleeding. *Ann Intern Med* 1982;96:565–569.

18 FREEMAN JG, COBDEN I, LISHMAN AH, RECORD CO. Controlled trial of terlipressin (glypressin) versus vasopressin in the early treatment of bleeding oesophageal varices. *Lancet* 1982;ii:66–68.

19 GALAMBOS JT. Esophageal variceal haemorrhage: diagnosis and an overview of treatment. *Semin Liver Dis* 1982;2:211–226.

20 GARCEAU AJ, CHALMERS TC. The natural history of cirrhosis. I. Survival and oesophageal varices. *N Engl J Med* 1963;268:469–473.

21 GEORGE P, BROWN L, RIDWAY G, CROFTS D, SHERLOCK S. Emergency oesophageal transection in uncontrolled variccal haemorrhage. *Br J Surg* 1973;60:635–640.

22 GRACE ND. The misuse of cimetidine in patients with cirrhosis. *Hepatology* 1983;3:124–125.

23 GROSZMANN RJ, ATTERBURY CE. The pathophysiology of portal hypertension. A basis for classification. *Semin Liver Dis* 1982;2:177–186.

24 GROSZMANN RJ, KRAVETZ D, BOSCH J, *et al.* Nitroglycerin improves the haemodynamic response to vasopressin in portal hypertension. *Hepatology* 1982;2:757–762.

25 HASSAB MA. Gastroesophageal decongestion and splenectomy in the treatment of oesophageal varices in bilharzial cirrhosis. *Surgery* 1967;61:169–176.

26 HENDERSON JM, MILLIKAN WJ, WARREN WD. The distal splenorenal shunt: an update. *World J Surg* 1984;8:722–732

27 HENDERSON JM, WARREN WD. The current status of the distal splenorenal shunt. *Semin Liver Dis* 1983;3:251–263.

28 HILLON P, LEBREC D, MUNOZ C, JUNGERS M, GOLDFARB G, BENHAMOU J-P. Comparison of the effects of cardio-selective and non-selective beta blocker on portal hypertension in patients with cirrhosis. *Hepatology* 1982;2:528–531.

29 INOKUCHI K, BEPPU K, KOYANAGI N, *et al.* Fifteen years' experience with left gastric venous caval shunt for esophageal varices. *World J Surg* 1984;8:716–721

30 INOKUCHI K, KOBAYASHI M, OGAWA Y, *et al.* Results of left gastric venacaval shunt for oesophageal varices. Analysis of one hundred cases. *Surgery* 1975;78:628–636.

31 JENKINS SA, BAXTER JN, CORBETT W, DEVITT P, WARE J, SHIELDS R. A prospective randomised controlled clinical trial comparing somatostatin and vasopressin in controlling acute variceal haemorrhage. *Br Med J* 1985;290:275–278.

32 JOHNSTON GW. Six years' experience of oesophageal transection for oesophageal varices using a circular stapling gun. *Gut* 1982;23:770–773.

33 KOFF RS. Benefit of endoscopy in upper gastrointestinal bleeding in patients with liver disease. *Dig Dis Sci* 1981;26:125–155.

34 KORULA J, BALART LA, RADVAN G. A prospective, randomized controlled trial of chronic esophageal variceal sclerotherapy. *Hepatology* 1985;5:584–589.

35 KOYAMA K, TAKAGI Y, OUCHI K, SATO T. Results of oesophageal transection for oesophageal varices:

experience in 100 cases. *Am J Surg* 1980;
139:204–209.

36 KRAVETZ D, BOSCH J, TERES J, BRUIX J, RIMOLA A,
RODES J. A controlled comparison of continuous
somatostatin and vasopressin infusion in the treatment of acute variceal haemorrhage. *Hepatology*
1984;**4**:99—104.

37 LANGER B, TAYLOR BR, MACKENZIE DR, GILAS T,
STONE RM, BLENDIS L. Further report of a prospective randomized trial comparing distal splenorenal
shunt with end-to-side portacaval shunt. An
analysis of encephalopathy, survival, and quality
of life. *Gastroenterology* 1985;**88**:424–429.

38 LARSON AW, COHEN H, ZWEIBAN B, *ET AL*. Acute
esophageal variceal sclerotherapy. Results of a
prospective randomized controlled trial. *JAMA*
1986;**255**:497–500.

39 LEBREC D, CORBIC M, NOVEL O, BENHAMOU J-P. Propranolol—a medical treatment for portal hypertension? *Lancet* 1980;ii:180–182.

40 LEBREC D, POYNARD T, HILLON P, BENHAMOU J-P.
Propranolol for prevention of recurrent gastro-
intestinal bleeding in patients with cirrhosis. *N
Engl J Med* 1981;**305**:1371–1374.

41 LINTON RR, ELLIS DS, GEARY JE. Critical comparative
analysis of early and late results of splenorenal
and directal portacaval shunts performed in 169
patients with portal cirrhosis. *Ann Surg* 1961;
154:446–549.

42 MACDOUGALL BRD, BAILEY JR, WILLIAMS R. H₂ receptor antagonists and antacids in the prevention
of acute gastrointestinal haemorrhage in fulminant hepatic failure. *Lancet* 1977;i:617–619.

43 MACDOUGALL BRD, WESTABY D, THEODOSSI A. Increased long-term survival in variceal haemorrhage using injection sclerotherapy. *Lancet* 1982;
i:124–127.

44 MENDEZ G, RUSSELL E. Gastrointestinal varices: percutaneous transhepatic therapeutic embolisation
in 54 patients. *Am J Roentgenol* 1980;**135**:1054–
1050.

45 MERIGAN TC, HOLLISTON RM, GRYSKA PF, STARKEY
GWB, DAVIDSON CS. Gastrointestinal bleeding with
cirrhosis. A study of 172 episodes in 158 patients.
N Engl J Med 1960;**263**:579–585.

46 MERIGAN TC, PLOTKIN GR, DAVIDSON CS. Effect of
intravenously administered post pituitary extract
on haemorrhage from bleeding oesophageal
varices. A controlled evaluation. *N Engl J Med*
1969;**266**:134–135.

47 MIALLARD JN, FALMANT YM, HAY JM, CHANDLER
JG. Selectivity of the distal splenorenal shunt. *Surgery* 1979;**86**:663–671.

48 MITCHELL KJ, MACDOUGALL BRD, SILK DBA,
WILLIAMS R. A prospective re-appraisal of emergency endoscopy in patients with portal hypertension. *Scand J Gastroenterol* 1982;**17**:965–968.

49 NOVIS BH, DUYS P, BARBEZAT GO, *et al*. Fibreoptic
endoscopy and the use of the Sengstaken tube in

acute gastrointestinal haemorrhage in patients
with portal hypertension. *Gut* 1976;**17**:258–263.

50 OKUDA K, KIMURA K, TAKAYASO K. Percutaneous
transhepatic portography and sclerotherapy. *Semin
Liver Dis* 1982;**2**:61–70.

51 ORLOFF MJ, BELL RH, HYDE PV, SKIVOLOCKI WP.
Long term results of emergency portacaval shunt
for bleeding oesophageal varices in unselected
patients with alcoholic cirrhosis. *Ann Surg* 1980;
192:325–340.

52 ORLOFF MJ, THOMAS HS. Pathogenesis of esophageal varix rupture. *Arch Surg* 1963;**87**:301–337.

53 PALMER ED, BRICK IB. Correlation between the
severity of oesophageal varices in portal cirrhosis
and their propensity towards haemorrhage. *Gastroenterology* 1956;**30**:85–90.

54 PAQUET K-J. Prophylactic endoscopic sclerosing
treatment of the oesophageal wall in varices—a
prospective controlled randomised trial. *Endoscopy*
1982;**14**:4–5.

55 PAQUET K-J, FEUSSNER H. Endoscopic sclerosis and
esophageal balloon tamponade in acute hemorrhage from esophagogastric varices: a prospective
controlled randomized trial. *Hepatology* 1985;
5;580–583.

56 PAQUET K-J, OBERHAMMER E. Sclerotherapy of
bleeding oesophageal varices by means of endoscopy. *Endoscopy* 1978;**10**:7–12.

57 PINTO-CORREIA J, MARTINS ALVES M, ALEXANDRINO
P, SILVEIRA J. Controlled trial of vasopressin and
balloon tamponade in bleeding esophageal varices.
Hepatology 1984;**4**885–888

58 PROWSE CV, DOUGLAS JG, FORREST JA, FORSLING ML.
Haemostatic effects of lysine vasopressin and tri-
glycyl lysine vasopressin infusion in patients with
cirrhosis. *Eur J Clin Invest* 1980;**10**:49–54.

59 PUGH RN, MURRAY-LYON IM, DAWSON JL, PIETRONI
MC, WILLIAMS R. Transection of the oesophagus
for bleeding oesophageal varices. *Br J Surg* 1973;
60:646–649.

60 RESNICK RH, CHALMERS TC, ISHIHARA AM. Controlled study of the prophylactic porta-caval shunt.
A final report. *Ann Intern Med* 1969;**70**:675–688.

61 REYNOLDS TB. Why do varices bleed? In: Westaby
D, MacDougall BRD, Williams R, eds. *Variceal
Haemorrhage*. London: Pitman Books Ltd, 1982:3–
12.

62 SALAM AA, WARREN WD. Anatomic basis of the
surgical treatment of portal hypertension. *Surg Clin
North Am* 1974;**54**:1247–1257.

63 SARFEH IJ, TABAK C, EUGENE J, JULER G. Clinical
significance of erosive gastritis in patients with
alcoholic liver disease and upper gastrointestinal
haemorrhage. *Ann Surg* 1981;**194**:149–151.

64 SHALDON S, DOLLE W, GUEVARA L, IBER F, SHERLOCK
S. Effect of pitressin on the splanchnic circulation
in man. *Circulation* 1961;**24**:797–807.

65 SHEPPARD M, SHAPIRO B, PIMSTONE B, *et al*. Metabolic clearance and plasma half disappearance

time of exogenous somatotropin in man. *J Clin Endocrinol Metab* 1979;**48**:50–53.

66 SHERLOCK S. The portal venous system and portal hypertension. In: *Diseases of the liver and biliary system*. 7th ed. Oxford: Blackwell Scientific Publications, 1985:135–181.

67 SHERLOCK S. Non-cirrhotic extrahepatic and intrahepatic portal hypertension. *Semin Liver Dis* 1982;**2**:202–210.

68 SMITH JL, GRAHAM DY. Variceal haemorrhage. A critical evaluation of survival analysis. *Gastroenterology* 1982;**82**:969–973.

69 SMITH-LAING G, SCOTT J, LOND RG, DICK R, SHERLOCK S. Role of percutaneous transhepatic obliteration of varices in the management of haemorrhage from gastro-esophageal varices. *Gastroenterology* 1981;**80**:1031–1036.

70 SUGIURA M, FUTAGAWA S. Further evaluation of the Sugiura procedure in the treatment of oesophageal varices. *Arch Surg* 1977;**112**:1317–1321.

71 SUGIURA M, FUTAGAWA S. Esophageal transection with paraesophagogastric devascularizations (the Sugiura Procedure) in the treatment of esophageal varices. *World J Surg* 1984;**8**:673–682.

72 TERBLANCHE J. Sclerotherapy for prophylaxis of variceal bleeding. *Lancet* 1986;**i**:961–963.

73 TERBLANCHE J, BORNMAN JC, JONKER MAT, KIRSCH RE, SAUNDERS SJ. Injection sclerotherapy of oesophageal varices. *Semin Liver Dis* 1982;**2**:233–241.

74 TERBLANCHE J, BORNMAN JC, KAHN D, *et al.* Failure of repeated injection sclerotherapy to improve long term survival after oesophageal variceal bleeding. *Lancet* 1983;**ii**:1328–1332.

75 TERBLANCHE J, NORTHOVER JMA, BORMAN P, *et al.* A prospective controlled trial of sclerotherapy in the long term management of patients after esophageal variceal bleeding. *Surg Gynecol Obstet* 1979; **148**:323–333.

76 TERBLANCHE J, YAKOOB HI, BORNMAN PC, *et al.* A five year prospective evaluation of tamponade and sclerotherapy. *Ann Surg* 1981;**194**:521–530.

77 TERES J, CECILIA A, BORDAS JM, *et al.* Esophageal tamponade for bleeding varices. Controlled trial between Sengstaken–Blakemore tube and the Lington–Nachlas tube. *Gastroenterology* 1978;**75**:566–569.

78 WEBB LJ, BERGER LA, SHERLOCK S. Grey-scale ultrasonography of portal vein. *Lancet* 1977;**ii**:275–277.

79 WESTABY D, MACDOUGALL BRD, WILLIAMS R. Improved survival following injection sclerotherapy for esophageal varices: final analysis of a controlled trial. *Hepatology* 1985;**5**:827–830.

80 WILLIAMS KGD, DAWSON JI. Fibreoptic injection of oesophageal varices. *Br Med J* 1979;**2**:766–767.

81 WITZEL L, WOLBERGS E, MERKI H. Prophylactic endoscopic sclerotherapy of esophageal varices. A prospective controlled study. *Lancet* 1985;**i**:733–736

Chapter 32

Bleeding from the Small or Large Intestine

J. D. HARDCASTLE

Bleeding from the small bowel or the large intestine can cause major diagnostic and management problems which can usually be overcome by orderly and well-conceived investigations.

Causes of bleeding in children

Approximately 2% of the population have a **Meckel's diverticulum**, but Soltero and Bill [95] have calculated that only one diverticulum in 25 causes symptoms during life. Symptoms usually occur during childhood or adolescence, the complication rate in the elderly being very low. Bleeding is due to acid secretion by heterotopic gastric epithelium in the diverticulum, which causes peptic ulceration of the mucosa of either the diverticulum or the adjacent ileum. It is usually episodic but can be severe. The rectal bleeding is usually dark-coloured but it may be bright red, depending upon the speed of transit through the bowel. Tarry stools are unusual [87]. A past history of previous episodes of bleeding is obtained frequently. Barium follow-through examination of the ileum seldom identifies a diverticulum. A ^{99m}Tc pertechnetate scan may allow visualization of the diverticulum, because of increased uptake of the isotope in the gastric ectopic mucosa when compared with the surrounding small bowel [11, 41, 90].

Juvenile polyps are a common cause of intermittent rectal bleeding in the first decade of life [54]. They may occasionally be associated with severe bleeding. The polyps are composed of a fibrous stroma, infiltrated with inflammatory cells and contain cystic spaces lined by mucus-secreting cells. They are mainly found in the rectum and left side of the colon [40]. Occasionally they outgrow their blood supply and slough into the lumen. Treatment is by removal, either through a sigmoidoscope or colonoscope; colotomy is rarely indicated. Multiple juvenile polyps may be present in the large bowel [66] and are rarely found throughout the whole gastrointestinal tract [88].

Hamartomas of the Peutz-Jeghers type may cause chronic blood loss and anaemia.

Intestinal haemangiomas are a rare but important cause of chronic bleeding in childhood and adolescence. In a review of 65 patients, Abrahamson and Shandling [1] found that many patients had associated cutaneous lesions and pleboliths visible on abdominal X-ray. Most haemangiomas are submucosal and cannot be diagnosed by conventional barium studies—superior or inferior mesenteric arteriograms are necessary for their identification. When haemangiomas are multiple, thrombocytopenia may be a complication due to sequestration of platelets in the lesions [73].

Intussusception is a common emergency in infants and young children, usually presenting as colic with the passage of blood and mucus *per rectum* [45, 62].

Causes of bleeding in adults [24]

Seventy per cent of **colorectal cancers** occur within the rectum, recto-sigmoid and sigmoid colon, and many of these tumours present with intermittent rectal bleeding

[97]. The amount of bleeding is usually small, but there are large day-to-day variations [29]. The mean blood loss from caecal and ascending colon tumours was found to be 9.3 ml/day compared with 1.5 ml/day to 1.9 ml/day for tumours in the transverse and sigmoid colon [69]. Using faecal occult blood tests, poorly differentiated or Dukes' stage B or C tumours are more likely to be positive than well-differentiated and Dukes' stage A tumours.

Blood loss from **colonic adenomas** is also small, with a mean of 1.3 ml/day in adenomas in the ascending and transverse colon, compared with 1.4 ml/day in the descending and recto-sigmoid region [53]. Large adenomas are more likely to bleed than small ones, particularly those over 2 cm in size [69].

Rectal bleeding is a common symptom of **ulcerative colitis,** but it is usually of a chronic nature. Severe bleeding is limited to those with extensive disease and is only seen in around 3–4% of patients [33].

Intermittent rectal bleeding is a less common symptom in **Crohn's disease,** occurring in 46% of colonic, 22% of ileocolonic and in only 10% of patients with ileal Crohn's disease [35]. Severe haemorrhage is rare [56] but in some patients it may be the only manifestation of the disease [25].

Jejunal diverticula may be complicated by severe haemorrhage [23], often mimicking a bleeding duodenal ulcer. Superior mesenteric angiography may occasionally show pooling of contrast in the diverticulum [96].

The major causes of bleeding from the small bowel in adults are tumours and lymphomas. **Lymphomas** can be associated with considerable damage to the bowel wall so that perforation and haemorrhage are not uncommon emergency presentations [65]. **Leiomyosarcomas,** which arise from the muscle of the small bowel, represent about 10% of malignant small bowel neoplasms. They may become polypoid and develop an area of central mucosal ulceration causing gastrointestinal bleeding [98]. Most **adenocarcinomas** grow in an annular constricting fashion causing obstruction; but chronic blood loss can occur although severe haemorrhage is unusual. **Carcinoid tumours** have been reported to bleed but this is unusual [82].

Gastrointestinal bleeding may occur from the **mucosal telangiectasia** of hereditary haemorrhagic telangiectasia or the Rendu-Osler-Weber syndrome [93]. The majority of patients have a family history with cutaneous or oral telangiectasia. Not all patients have the typical oral manifestations of the syndrome, making diagnosis more difficult. Telangiectasia of the small bowel cannot be diagnosed by barium studies, but gastroscopy may show typical lesions in the stomach. Identification of small bowel lesions is dependent upon angiography or endoscopy, possibly at the time of laparotomy [49]. Haemophiliacs bleed most frequently from the stomach and duodenum [79].

Cavernous haemangiomas of the small bowel or colon may present in adult life with chronic blood loss [101, 108, 112] or occasionally with more severe haemorrhage.

Aorto-enteric fistulae are usually associated with aortic aneurysms or previous aortic surgery. The site of rupture is usually into the duodenum, but fistulae from the aorto-iliac vessels into the ileum or colon have been reported [86]. A pulsatile mass is usually present in the abdomen, associated with a bruit. Definitive diagnosis can be made by aortography [59]. Rupture is not usually immediately fatal, so that a preoperative diagnosis can be made. In those patients in whom surgical treatment is possible, long-term survival has been reported [86].

Ischaemic colitis usually presents in the middle-aged or elderly, the patients often having other evidence of arterio-sclerosis, for example, ischaemic heart disease or peripheral arterial insufficiency. The clinical picture is usually one of lower abdominal pain and tenderness followed by the passage of one or two loose motions, characteristically containing dark blood and clots (see Chapter 69). Submucosal haemorrhage and oedema appear as thumb-printing on barium enema, and may appear within three days of the onset of symptoms [115]; stricture formation may occur later. Approximately one-third of patients will require urgent operation because of gangrene of the colon or continued bleeding. The remainder will improve spontaneously and either return to normal, needing no further treatment, or require elective therapy for a late stricture [70].

Bright red rectal bleeding is a very common symptom of **perianal conditions,** such as haemorrhoids, fissure, or rectal prolapse (see Chapter 66).

Angiodysplasia is a vascular malformation associated with ageing and should not be confused with congenital haemangiomas [13]. The disease has been recognized since the introduction of intestinal angiography and colonoscopy [57, 89]. Angiodysplasias particularly occur in the ascending colon and caecum of elderly patients over the age of 60 years; they are not associated with cutaneous lesions [109]. The venous malformations consist of dilated tortuous submucosal vessels and in severe cases the mucosa is replaced by a mass of dilated deformed vessels [15]. Histological examination shows the vascular ectasias to be made up of dilated distorted thin-walled vessels, with only scanty amounts of muscle in their walls [78]. In some cases the veins are so dilated that they resemble dilated lymphatic vessels. Inspection of the mucosa is often unremarkable. The lesions are only a few millimetres in size and appear as reddish raised areas in the mucosa. The morphology of the vascular malformation can best be identified by intra-

arterial injection of silicone rubber into the resected specimen followed by examination under the dissecting microscope [15]. The lesions appear elevated above the normal mucosa, the surface of the ectasia consisting of areas where the mucosa is lost and the dilated vessels are exposed. Bleeding is usually chronic and intermittent, but can be severe. There is no doubt that many patients, previously thought to have bled from diverticular disease, have probably been bleeding from angiodysplasia in the caecum. Asymptomatic submucosal ectasias have been found in 53% of colons excised for carcinoma [15]. An association of aortic stenosis with bleeding from angiodysplasia of the caecum is recognized [17, 43].

Angiodysplasias cannot be palpated at laparotomy, therefore preoperative diagnosis is essential. Fortunately, the bleeding stops spontaneously in most patients, allowing time for elective investigation. Barium enema examination is unhelpful and should be avoided. The important diagnostic investigations are colonoscopy and angiography. Colonoscopy may show 0.5–1 cm areas of haemorrhage in the mucosa of the caecum or ascending colon [116]. Selective angiography of the mesenteric arteries using subtraction techniques has proved to be useful. The angiographic signs include densely opacified, dilated tortuous, slowly-emptying intramural veins, usually seen in continuity with the ileocolic vein, and clusters of vessels best identified in the arterial phase which empty slowly and can be observed in association with the dilated intramural veins. Early filling of veins, visualized within six to eight seconds, is very suggestive of angiodysplasia and is probably due to the development of arterio-venous communications. Active bleeding may result in intraluminal extravasation of contrast [14].

In the past, severe bleeding from the colon was often attributed to **diverticulosis of the colon** (see Chapters 60 and 61). Use of selective angiography has enabled a more precise diagnosis to be made. For example, in 99 patients admitted with severe lower gastrointestinal haemorrhage, 43 were found to be bleeding from diverticulosis and 20 from angiodysplasia of the right colon [14]. It is unwise to attribute bleeding to either angiodysplasia or diverticulosis when a precise diagnosis has not been made by angiography or endoscopy. Diverticulosis is present in 48% of the population over the age of 50 years [58] and mucosal vascular ectasia is probably present in at least 25% of persons of the same age [15].

Bleeding from diverticular disease occurs mainly in elderly patients and, when diagnosed angiographically, has been shown to occur more commonly on the right side of the colon [5, 9, 74]. The only radiographic abnormality is pooling of contrast in the diverticulum during the arterial phase of the injection. No arterio-venous shunting or abnormal vascularity is seen. Bleeding in diverticular disease is usually from only one diverticulum and in most patients it stops spontaneously. Diverticula have a consistent relationship to the vasa recta vessels of the colon, which are stretched over the dome of the diverticulum and hence in very close contact with the mucosa. When the site of bleeding has been investigated it is more commonly found in the base of the diverticulum than at the neck [74]. The initial bleeding episode is usually more severe than in angiodysplasia [14].

Marathon runners may develop iron deficiency anaemia due to occult gastrointestinal blood loss, but the precise mechanism remains unclear [61, 99].

Severe lower intestinal bleeding in adults

Investigations

On admission the patient with lower intestinal bleeding is resuscitated and **blood tests** performed including coagulation studies, haemoglobin, and plasma urea and creatinine concentrations [94]. A history is taken, with particular reference to previous episodes of bleeding and drug therapy, the abdomen is examined for masses and bruits, and the skin for the presence of haemangiomas. After adequate resuscitation, **gastroduodenoscopy** should be performed to exclude a gastric or duodenal cause of the bleeding.

Rigid sigmoidoscopy should be performed to exclude an anal or rectal cause of bleeding such as a carcinoma or proctitis. Suction and washout facilities are essential. In patients who are bleeding severely, **fibreoptic sigmoidoscopy** or **colonoscopy** is not recommended as it is difficult to remove large quantities of blood and clots through the small suction channels. When the bleeding is not severe it may be possible for a skilled colonoscopist to obtain useful information, especially in the left side of the colon [21, 26, 117]. The blood may be dispersed with water using a double channel instrument [38]. Electro- or photo-coagulation down the colonoscope may occasionally be useful in controlling bleeding (for example the base of a polyp, a vascular malformation, or telangiectasia).

The next stage in the investigation is to attempt to identify the source of the bleeding by **selective arteriography** [5, 34]. Preliminary screening with [99m]**Technetium sulphur colloid** is recommended by some radiologists to identify those patients bleeding with sufficient severity to show angiographic abnormalities—a [99m]Technetium sulphur colloid scan is only positive if the patient is actively bleeding at the time of investigation. In 43 patients bleeding at the time of investigation a sulphur colloid scan was positive in 23, and angiography showed an abnormality in 10 [4]. Angiograms of the superior mesenteric system are performed first; if no site of bleeding is demonstrated the inferior mesenteric arterial circulation is then examined. Extravasation of contrast medium can identify the site of the bleeding; in addition angiographic signs of a tumour, vascular malformation, or angiodysplasia may also be demonstrated. This investigation is particularly useful in identifying bleeding from a colonic diverticulum, as pooling of contrast medium in the diverticulum may be seen [110]. Extravasation of contrast in angiodysplasia of the colon is less common [110].

If a bleeding site is not found on angiography, but slow or intermittent bleeding is continuing, a **Technetium labelled blood cell scan** may be of value. *In vitro* labelling should be used to reduce the artefact produced by gastric secretion of free ^{99m}Tc pertechnetate [19]. In one study using labelled red cells [68] 15% of the scans were positive in the first 15 minutes, 30% at one hour and 65% at 24 hours. Localization of the site of bleeding is only possible if extravasation is observed shortly after injection.

If no source of bleeding is identified by angiography or scintigraphy, **barium studies** of the small bowel and colon should be undertaken. A barium follow-through or enteroclysis should demonstrate lymphomas or tumours of the small bowel. When the bleeding is thought to be due to colitis, an 'instant' enema can provide useful information [105].

Using the above methods it should be possible to establish the cause of the haemorrhage in around 80% of patients [44]. If the bleeding stops spontaneously the patient should be investigated in the same way as those presenting with chronic intermittent haemorrhage.

Conservative management

Approximately 80% of episodes of severe bleeding from the bowel stop spontaneously. Adequate **blood replacement** is necessary to maintain a normal circulating blood volume and urine output.

If the site of the bleeding can be determined by selective angiography, particularly if the source is shown to be a bleeding colonic diverticulum, attempts may be made to control the bleeding by **intra-arterial infusions of vasopressin** [6, 44] or **selective embolism** of the blood supply with gel foam [16, 72, 80, 103].

Surgical management

Thorough investigation of the patient should identify the cause of the bleeding, allowing the surgeon to plan the operation. Emergency surgery is indicated for continuing haemorrhage, especially if the site has been identified.

Bleeding from the right colon can be treated by a right hemi-colectomy even in the presence of left-sided diverticular disease [14]. Segmental resection has a lower mortality rate than sub-total colectomy in such patients and the incidence of recurrent bleeding is low [110].

Occasionally it may be necessary to operate on a patient with exsanguinating haemorrhage when the bleeding site has not been identified. An adequate mid-line incision is essential to allow access to all regions of the large and small bowel. The distribution of blood in the large and small bowel should be noted, blood in the lumen of the small bowel appearing as dark-coloured fluid. If there is doubt, needle aspiration of the luminal contents can be undertaken. Most small bowel causes of bleeding are obvious at the time of surgery, for example a Meckel's diverticulum or a tumour of the small bowel. Care should be taken not to miss a jejunal diverticulum, as it may be hidden by peritoneal folds in the region of the ligament of Treitz or within the mesentery. Angiomatous malformations can sometimes be felt through the bowel wall. If no palpable lesion is found the mucosa can be inspected through an enterostomy using a rigid or flexible sigmoidoscope. A colonoscope can also be passed through the mouth and manipulated through the duodenum by the surgeon, to examine the small bowel [49].

In a patient bleeding from the colon, the use of multiple colotomies to try and localize the site of the bleeding is not recommended. It is seldom successful [31] and increases the risk of infection in an already ill patient. Although the cause of the bleeding may often be in the right side of the colon, segmental resection is not recommended as it can be followed by recurrent bleeding with serious consequences. Under these circumstances colectomy with ileorectal anastomosis is the most satisfactory procedure. It can be performed with a mortality rate of only 11% [30, 67].

Chronic or intermittent haemorrhage

Intermittent rectal bleeding is a very common symptom—in a group of 700 patients chosen randomly from general practitioners' lists, 6.4% had noticed rectal bleeding in the previous six months [22].

The majority of bright red bleeding originates from the anal canal but it may also be due to lesions on the left side of the colon; a careful history and examination is important. Haemorrhoidal bleeding is usually associated with blood splashing on the sides of the pan and, if this history is given, it is unlikely that the bleeding is coming from higher in the bowel. Careful examination of the anal margin is needed to diagnose an anal fissure or mucosal prolapse. At least 40% of rectal cancers can be felt digitally and abnormalities may also be felt in inflammatory bowel disease and solitary ulcer. After rectal examination the glove should be inspected for the presence of blood. A full blood count should be performed, particularly looking for iron deficiency anaemia or a microcytosis (MCV < 77 fl).

Investigation (see Chapter 58)

The patient should be examined initially using the **rigid sigmoidoscope** without bowel preparation to inspect the rectal mucosa and to assess whether blood can be seen in the lumen [28]. Proctitis, carcinoma of the rectum, solitary ulcer of the rectum, mucosal and rectal prolapse should all be excluded by sigmoidoscopy. Rigid sigmoidoscopy should be followed by **proctoscopy** to diagnose haemorrhoids and anal fissures, the main causes of intermittent rectal bleeding. Approximately 35% of colorectal cancers are within range of the rigid sigmoidoscope—the prevalence of rectal cancer in the population over the age of 45 is 1.2–1.3 per 1,000 [50]. Adenomatous polyps are found in 3.1–3.8% of the population over 45 [81, 84].

The introduction of **flexible sigmoidoscopy** has been one of the major advances in the investigation of patients with rectal bleeding. The standard instrument is 60 cm long, more robust than a colonoscope, with a wider suction channel making it easier to suck out mucus and faecal fluid. A preliminary phosphate enema is necessary but no sedation is required; an anti-spasmodic such as hyoscine butylbromide may be helpful if spasm of the sigmoid colon is encountered during the examination. The examination can usually be completed in six to eight minutes [12, 39]. In a comparison of rigid and fibreoptic sigmoidoscopy in 350 patients attending a gastrointestinal clinic, the yield from rigid sigmoidoscopy was 6.5% compared with 30% from fibreoptic sigmoidoscopy [107]. Bowel preparation with a single phosphate enema was adequate in over 90% of patients.

Sixty to seventy per cent of colorectal tumours occur within the range of the fibreoptic sigmoidoscope, as do the majority of large adenomas containing areas of invasive carcinoma [47].

Barium enema examination must be performed using an air contrast technique in a bowel empty of faecal residue [75]. Many carcinomas are missed because of poor bowel preparation [27]. Even with good technique, the interpretation of a double-contrast barium enema in patients with diverticular disease may be extremely difficult because of overlying loops of bowel. Diverticular disease is so common in middle age that it is unwise to attribute bleeding to it until all other lesions have been excluded by endoscopy. In a comparison of endoscopy with double-contrast barium enema in a group of 1245 patients, seven Stage A carcinomas, three of which were arising in adenomatous polyps, were missed by barium enema; six of the tumours were in the sigmoid colon [36]. Flat villous adenomas are especially difficult to detect by barium enema [18] partly because the mucus produced by the tumour causes poor coating of the bowel by the barium. A barium enema can provide diagnostic information about inflammatory bowel disease and the early and late stages of ischaemic colitis.

Colonoscopy is an essential investigation for the patient with unexplained rectal bleeding and a normal barium enema. Colonoscopy will find the cause of bleeding in 40% of such patients [102]. The most likely lesions missed by barium enema are adenomatous polyps, inflammatory bowel disease and polypoid carcinomas. In 40 patients with rectal bleeding and diverticular disease, four had a carcinoma and nine were found to have adenomatous polyps. It is dangerous to attribute rectal bleeding to diverticular disease. Lesions may, however, be missed on colonoscopy and a double-

contrast barium enema is a complimentary investigation [104]. Angiodysplasia of the caecum cannot be detected by barium enema examination but may be seen by the endoscopist as small 5–10 mm lesions in the right colon. Electrocoagulation of the lesion can be undertaken by the hot biopsy technique [111]. Haemangiomas of the colon may also be seen as tortuous vessels under the mucosa. Lesions demonstrated by contrast radiology can be confirmed colonoscopically and biopsies taken.

Occult blood tests

Small amounts of blood lost from the rectum and sigmoid colon may be noted by the patient, but larger amounts may be lost from the right side of the colon or the small bowel before it becomes clinically apparent [92]. Normal faecal blood loss is, using a radiochromium red cell labelling technique, in the range of 1.2 ml per day [20, 32]. The upper limit of normal blood loss is 2 mg haemoglobin/g of stool, assuming a 150 g stool per day in a patient with haemoglobin of 15 g/dl [83].

Most chemical tests for occult blood are dependent upon the oxidation of a phenolic chromagen such as a guaiac reagent to a quinone structure which has a blue colour, the haematin component of haemoglobin catalysing the oxidation. The oxidation is also facilitated by the presence of hydrogen peroxide and also by naturally-occurring vegetable and bacterial peroxidases. Animal haemoglobins occurring in food products will also produce a false positive result. Ascorbic acid in large quantities may also cause a false negative result because of its reducing action interfering with the quinone reaction [60].

The guaiac reagent is very sensitive; a large number of false positive reactions make it unsuitable for screening purposes [71]. To improve the accuracy of the test, a less sensitive guaiac-impregnated electrophoresis paper has been developed (Haemoccult). The sensitivity of guaiac reagent and Haemoccult have been compared using a radiochromium-labelled red cell assay. The guaiac reagent yielded 72% false positive results compared with only 12% false positive results with Haemoccult [83]. On Haemoccult testing, 7.4% of faecal samples containing 0–2 ml of blood were positive, 67% when blood loss was over 10 ml per day, and 93% with losses over 30 ml per day [100].

The amount of bleeding from the upper gastrointestinal tract required to give a positive Haemoccult result is much greater than that from the colon—subjects given labelled blood orally had only one positive reaction when 30 ml were ingested despite a stool concentration of 23 mg haemoglobin/g [85].

When gastrointestinal blood loss does not exceed 2 ml per day, approximately 10% of stool samples collected from patients not on dietary restriction will be Haemoccult positive [100], this being reduced to about 2% by dietary restrictions [8]. The effect of diet, however, varies from country to country and appears to be small in England. In a recent British screening study [52] only 2% of the population were positive, despite no dietary restriction. Because blood loss from the left side of the colon and rectum is not evenly distributed in the stool, small blood losses may be detected by the Haemoccult method. The total blood loss from carcinomas in the rectum and sigmoid colon was found to be 1.8–1.9 ml/day [69] but in spite of this small loss, 70% of the tumours were detected during three days of testing with Haemoccult. In another study after three days of Haemoccult testing 73% of colorectal tumours were positive, rising to 91% when tested for six days, indicating the intermittent nature of colonic tumour bleeding and the sampling error that is involved.

Using the more sensitive guaiac impregnated paper test, Fecatest, which will detect 2.5–3 mg haemoglobin/g of homogenized stool [2], 91% of colorectal tumours when tested over three days were positive but the false positive rate on an unrestricted diet is high [10].

The immunological testing of human haemoglobin eliminates most false positive reactions obtained with chemical tests [91]. Rabbit haemoglobin is the only common animal haemoglobin that cross-reacts with antibody to human haemoglobin. Tests involving radioimmunodiffusion plates [6, 105] have been developed but the methods are time-consuming and not suitable for population screening. Fecatest has been modified to include an immunological component (Feca EIA). A disc of filter paper is included in the slide to absorb moisture from the faecal specimen; if the guaiac test is positive the disc can then be tested for human haemoglobin, the immunological test having a sensitivity of 2 mg haemoglobin/g of stool [3].

Faecal occult blood tests in symptomatic patients

The diagnosis of colorectal cancer by the family doctor is not easy because bowel symptoms are so common. Indeed the average delay in treatment after the onset of symptoms has been shown by a prospective study to be 34 weeks, most of this delay being by the patient before presenting to his family doctor, and by the family doctor before referring to hospital [55].

Once the patient has been referred to hospital, it has been shown, in a controlled study of faecal occult blood testing in a gastrointestinal clinic, that the time taken to reach diagnosis was equal in both the test and control groups. This may of course be due to the greater awareness of symptoms in a gastrointestinal clinic, and the liberal use of endoscopy in all patients with symptoms. In a study of 802 symptomatic patients attending general medical and surgical outpatient clinics, faecal occult blood testing was undertaken using the Haemoccult faecal occult blood test—18.9% were positive, this high rate being partly due to the inclusion of patients with symptomatic bleeding in the study group. 140 patients were found to be positive, and all were investigated by colonoscopy and barium enema. No significant disease was found in twelve patients, a false positive rate of 8.6%. The test was positive in 22 of 26 colonic cancers, a false negative rate of 15%, but only 6 of 11 patients with rectal cancer had a positive test, a false negative rate of 45.4%. Thus a positive Haemoccult test indicates a group of patients worthy of further investigation but a negative test is unhelpful [64].

The real value of faecal occult blood testing in symptomatic patients lies in general practice where the patients are seen at a much earlier stage of their disease process. The general practitioner sees many patients with abdominal symptoms and may have difficulty in deciding which patients should be further investigated or referred to hospital for investigation. A controlled trial of faecal occult blood testing is at present being undertaken in patients over the age of 40, with abdominal and bowel symptoms. The test group is offered Haemoccult testing, and, if positive, fibreoptic sigmoidoscopy. The control group is treated by the general practitioner in the usual symptomatic fashion. Four carcinomas and two adenomas have been diagnosed in the test group, with a median time to diagnosis of 13 days; the median time to diagnosis of the three carcinomas in the control group was 53 days. It would thus appear from these preliminary data that faecal occult blood testing, and access to a rapid endoscopy service, would be of value to the family doctor [52]

Faecal occult blood tests in screening asymptomatic patients [63]

Faecal occult blood tests have been extensively used to screen persons over the age of 45 for colorectal cancers. Numerous screening studies have been published, with a detection rate for invasive cancer of 1.9–4.4, and for adenomas of 1.9–16.4, per 1,000 persons screened [42, 48, 113].

Pilot studies in the United Kingdom have shown that faecal occult blood testing using Haemoccult can be performed in general practice [37, 51, 52, 71]. To obtain a true assessment of faecal occult blood screening in detecting colorectal cancer, controlled studies must be performed with individuals randomly allocated to either test or control groups, the test group being invited to take part in the screening study. The two groups can be compared for a number of carcinomas detected, the pathological stage of the tumours, and ultimately the survival of the persons within both groups. In such a study being undertaken in the United States [46] study and control groups have been selected from health-conscious volunteers, many of whom may be undertaking regular health checks. Preliminary results show that 65% of tumours detected by screening are localized to the bowel wall (Dukes' Stage A) but no information relating to the control groups is yet available. A controlled study which has recently been completed in England, in which 20,000 individuals identified from general practitioners' lists were randomly allocated into test and control groups. The test group was invited to perform Haemoccult tests over three days— 37% of those invited completed the test, and in this group 12 invasive cancers were detected (3.6/1,000 persons screened) and 40 adenomas in 27 persons (7.9/1,000 persons screened). Nine of the 12 carcinomas were Dukes' Stage A lesions, and 12 of the adenomas were over 2 cm in size. In the year following the screening test, one carcinoma has presented in the group that performed the test; 10 carcinomas have presented in the control group (1.0/1,000 persons)—four Stage B, two Stage C, and two Stage D. Screening using occult blood testing would thus appear to detect tumours at a more favourable pathological stage and at 3.6 times the year's incidence rate.

The success of a screening test is also dependent upon the compliance of those to whom it is offered. Persons who volunteer for screening have an 80–91% compliance rate [48, 113] as do those from institutions and military establishments [76]. High compliance may also be obtained using education by the mass media, and publicity in the form of meetings or newspaper advertisements [114]. In the four studies that have been completed in England, Haemoccult tests were sent through the post and compliance ranged from 27% to 45% [37, 51, 52, 77]. Compliance is improved by direct invitation from the general practitioner or by prior health education, either by letter or interview.

References

1 ABRAHAMSON J, SHANDLING B. Intestinal haemangiomata in childhood and a syndrome for diagnosis: A Collective Review. *J Paediatr Surg* 1973;8:487–495.

2 ADLERCREUTZ H, LIEWENDAHL K, VIRKOLA P. Evaluation of Fecatest a new guaiac test for occult blood in feces. *Clin Chem* 1978;24:756–761.

3 ADLERCREUTZ H, TURUNEN MJ, LEIWENDHAL P, *et al*. Is specific detection of human haemoglobin (h.Hb) in faeces a solution to the problem of occult blood (OB) testing for detection of colorectal cancer? *World Congress of Gastroenterology*, Stockholm 1982; Abs. 1306.

4 ALAVI A, RING EJ. Localisation of gastrointestinal bleeding. Superiority of ^{99m}Tc sulphur. *Am J Radiol* 1981;137:741–748.

5 ALLISON DJ, HEMINGWAY AP, CUNNINGHAM DA. Angiography in gastrointestinal bleeding. *Lancet* 1982;ii:30–33.

6 ARMITAGE NC, HARDCASTLE JD, BALFOUR TW, *et al*. A comparison of an immunological faecal occult blood test Fecatwin sensitive/Feca EIA with

7 ATHANASOULIS CA, BAUM S, ROSCH J, *et al*. Mesenteric arterial infusions of Vasopressin for haemorrhage from colonic diverticulitis. *Am J Surg* 1975;129:212–216.

8 BASSETT ML, GOULSTON KJ. False positive and negative Haemoccult reactions on a normal diet and effect of diet restriction. *Aust NZ J Med* 1980;10:1–4.

9 BAUM S, ROSCH J, DOTTER C, *et al*. Selective mesenteric arterial infusions in the management of massive diverticular haemorrhage. *New Engl J Med* 1983;288:1269–1272.

10 BERETTA KR, GULLER R, SINGEISEN M, STALDER GA. Occult blood in feces—a prospective study for comparison of Haemoccult and Fecatest. *Schweiz Med Wochenschr* 1978;108:1905–1907.

11 BERQUIST TH, NOLAN NG, STEPHENS DH, CARLSON HC. Specificity of ^{99m}Tc Pertechnetate in scintigraphic diagnosis of Meckel's diverticulum: a review of 100 cases. *J Nucl Med* 1976;17:465–469.

12 BOHLMAN TW, KATON RM, LIPSHUTZ GR, McCOOL MF, SMITH FW, MELNYCK CS. Fiberoptic pansigmoidoscopy: an evaluation and comparison with rigid sigmoidoscopy. *Gastroenterology* 1977;72:644–649.

13 BOLEY SJ, BRANDT LJ, MITSUDO SM. Vascular lesions of the colon. *Ann Intern Med* 1984;29:301–326.

14 BOLEY SJ, SAMMARTANO R, ADAMS A, DIBBIASE A, KLEINHAUS S, SPRAYREGEN S. On the nature and etiology of vascular ectasias of the colon. *Gastroenterology* 1977;72:650–660.

15 BOLEY SJ, DIBIASE A, BRANDT JL, SAMMARTANO RJ. Lower intestinal bleeding in the elderly. *Am J Surg* 1979;137:57–64.

16 BOOKSTEIN JJ, NADERI MJ, WALTER JF. Transcatheter embolisation for lower gastrointestinal bleeding. *Radiology* 1978;127:345–349.

17 BOSS EG, ROSENBAUM JM. Bleeding from the right colon associated with aortic stenosis. *Am J Dig Dis* 1971;16:269–275.

18 BRESNIHAN ER, SIMPKINS KC. Villous adenoma of the large bowel: benign and malignant. *Br J Radiol* 1975;48:801–806.

19 BUNKER SR, BROWN JM, McAULEY RJ, *et al*. Detection of gastrointestinal bleeding sites. *JAMA* 1982;247:789–792.

20 CAMERON AD. Gastrointestinal blood loss measured by radioactive chromium. *Gut* 1960;1:177–182.

21 CAMPBELL WB, RHODES M, KETTLEWELL MGW. Colonoscopy following intraoperative lavage in the management of severe colonic bleeding. *Ann Roy Coll Surg Eng* 1985;67:290–292.

22 CHAPPUIS PH, GOULSTON KJ, TAIT AD, DENT OF. Predictive value of rectal bleeding in screening

moccult in population screening for colorectal cancer. *BR J Cancer* 1985;51:799–804.

for rectal and sigmoid polyps. *Br Med J* 1985;**290**:1546–1548.

23 CIVETTA JM, DAGGETT WM. Gastrointestinal bleeding from jejunal diverticula. *Ann Surg* 1967; **166**:976–979.

24 COOK IJ, PAVLI P, RILEY JW, GOULSTON KJ, DENT OF. Gastrointestinal investigation of iron deficiency anaemia. *Br Med J* 1986;**292**:1380–1382

25 CORONA FE, DYCK WP. Massive gastrointestinal haemorrhage as the sole clinical manifestation of regional enteritis. *Am J Dig Dis* 1973;**18**:1001–1004.

26 DEHYLE P, BLUM AL, NUESCH HJ, JENNY S. Emergency colonoscopy in the management of the acute perianal haemorrhage. *Endoscopy* 1974;**6**:229–232.

27 DELACEY G, WIGNALL B, AMROSE J, BAYLIS K, BRIDGES C. The double contrast barium enema: improvements to lateral decubitus views including the use of a wedge filter. *Clin Radiol* 1978;**29**:197–199.

28 DONALD IP, FRASER JSF, WILKINSON SP. Sigmoidoscopy/proctoscopy service with open access to general practitioners. *Br Med J* 1985;**290**:759–761.

29 DORAN J, HARDCASTLE JD. Bleeding patterns in colorectal cancer: the effect of aspirin and the implications for faecal occult blood testing. *Br J Surg* 1982;**69**:711–713.

30 DRAPANAS T, PENNINGTON G, KAPPELMAN M, LINDSEY E. Emergency sub-total colectomy: preferred approach to management of massively bleeding diverticular disease. *Ann Surg* 1973;**177**:519–526.

31 EATON AC. Emergency surgery for acute colonic haemorrhage—a retrospective study. *Br J Surg* 1981;**68**:109–112.

32 EBAUGH FG, CLEMENTS T, RODNAN G, PETERSEN RE. Quantitative measurement of gastrointestinal blood loss. *Am J Med* 1958;**25**:169–181.

33 EDWARDS FC, TRUELOVE SC. The course and prognosis of ulcerative colitis. *Gut* 1964;**5**:1–22.

34 EMANUEL RB, WEISER MM, SHENOY SS, SATCHIDANAND SK, ASIRWATHAM J. Arteriovenous malformations as a cause of gastrointestinal bleeding: the importance of triple-vessel angiographic studies in diagnosis and prevention of rebleeding. *J Clin Gastroenterol* 1985;**7**:237–246.

35 FARMER RG, HAWK WA, TURNBULL RB. Clinical patterns in Crohn's disease: a statistical study of 615 cases. *Gastroenterology* 1975;**68**:627–635.

36 FARRANDS PA, CHAMBERLAIN J, MOSS S, HARDCASTLE JD. Factors affecting compliance with screening for colorectal cancer. *J Exper Clin Cancer Res* [suppl], 1983;**2**:31.

37 FARRANDS PA, GRIFFITHS RL, BRITTON DC. A practical solution to the diagnosis and treatment of colorectal cancer? *Lancet* 1981;**i**:1231–1232.

38 FORDE KA. Colonoscopy in acute rectal bleeding. *Gastrointest Endosc* 1981;**27**:219–220.

39 FOSTER GE, VELLACOTT KD, BALFOUR TW, HARDCASTLE JD. Outpatient flexible fibreoptic sigmoidoscopy; diagnostic yield and the value of glucagon. *Br J Surg* 1981;**68**:463–465.

40 FRANKLIN R, McSWAIN B. Juvenile polyps of the colon and rectum. *Ann Surg* 1972;**175**:887–891.

41 FREIS M, MORTENSON W, ROBERTSON B. Technetium pertechnetate scintigraphy to detect ectopic gastric mucosa in Meckel's diverticulum. *Acta Radiol Diag* 1984;**25**:417–422.

42 FRUHMORGEN P, DEMLING L. Erste Ergebnisse einer prospektiven Feldstudie mit einem modifizierten Guajak-test zum Nachweiss von okkultem Blut im Stuhl. In: *Kolorektale Krebsvorsorge*. Nurnberg: Verlag, Wacholz, 1978:68–72.

43 GALLOWAY SJ, CASARELLA WJ, SHIMKIN PM. Vascular malformations of the right colon as a cause of bleeding in patients with aortic stenosis. *Radiology* 1974;**113**:11–15.

44 GIACCHINO JL, GEIS WP, PICKLEMAN JR, DADO DV, HADCOCK WE, FREEARK FJ. Changing perspectives in massive lower intestinal haemorrhage. *Surgery* 1979;**86**:368–376.

45 GIERUP J, JORULF H, LIVADITIS A. Management of intussusception in infants and children: a survey based on 288 consecutive cases. *Paediatrics* 1972;**50**:535–546.

46 GILBERTSEN VA, McHUGH RB, SCHUMAN LM, WILLIAMS SE. The earlier detection of colorectal cancer: A preliminary report on the results of the occult blood study. *Cancer* 1980;**45**:2899–2901.

47 GILLESPIE PE, CHAMBERS TJ, CHAN K, DORONOZO F, MORSON BC, WILLIAMS CB. Colonic adenomas—a colonoscopy survey. *Gut* 1979;**20**:240–245.

48 GLOBER GA, PESKOE SM. Outpatient screening for gastrointestinal lesions using guaiac impregnated slides. *Dig Dis Sci* 1974;**19**:399–403.

49 GREENBERG GR, PHILLIPS MJ, TOVEE EB, JEEJEEBHOY KN. Fibreoptic endoscopy during laparotomy in the diagnosis of small intestinal bleeding. *Gastroenterology* 1976;**71**:133–135.

50 HARDCASTLE JD. Screening for colorectal cancer. In: Wright R, ed. *Recent advances in gastrointestinal pathology*. Philadelphia: Saunders, 1980:311–329.

51 HARDCASTLE JD, BALFOUR TW, AMAR SS. Screening for symptomless colorectal cancer by testing for occult blood in general practice. *Lancet* 1980;**i**:791–793.

52 HARDCASTLE JD, FARRANDS PA, CHAMBERLAIN J, BALFOUR TW, AMAR SS, SHELDON MG. A controlled trial of faecal occult blood testing in the detection of colorectal cancer. *Lancet* 1983;**ii**:1–4.

53 HERZOG F, HOLTERMULLER KH, PREISS J, *et al.* Fecal blood loss in patients with colonic polyps: a comparison of measurements with 51 chromium

labelled erythrocytes and with the Haemoccult test. *Gastroenterology* 1982;**83**:957–962.

54 HOLGERSEN LO, MILLER RE, ZINTEL HA. Juvenile polyps of the colon. *Surgery* 1971;**69**:288–293.

55 HOLLIDAY H, HARDCASTLE JD. Delay in diagnosis and treatment of symptomatic colorectal cancer. *Lancet* 1978;i:309–311.

56 HOMAN WP, CHIK-KWUN TANG, THORBJARNARSON B. Acute massive haemorrhage from intestinal Crohn's disease and review of the literature. *Arch Surg* 1976;**111**:901–905.

57 HOWARD OM, BUCHANAN JD, HURT R. Angiodysplasia of the colon. Experience of 26 cases. *Lancet* 1982;ii:16–18.

58 HUGHES LE. Post mortem survey of diverticular disease of the colon. *Gut* 1969;**10**:336–351.

59 JACKSON RS, CREMIN BJ. Angiographic demonstration of gastrointestinal bleeding due to aorto-duodenal fistula. *Br J Radiol* 1976;**49**:966–967.

60 JAFFE RM, KASTEN B, YOUNG DS, MALLOWRY JD. False negative stool occult blood tests caused by ingestion of ascorbic acid (vitamin C). *Ann Intern Med* 1975;**83**:824–826.

61 LEADING ARTICLE. Gastrointestinal bleeding in long-distance runners. *Ann Intern Med* 1984; **101**:127–128.

62 LEADING ARTICLE. Acute intussusception in childhood. *Lancet* 1985;ii:250–251.

63 LEADING ARTICLE. Questions about occult-blood screening for cancer. *Lancet* 1986;i:22.

64 LEICESTER RJ, LIGHTFOOT A, MILLAR J, COLIN-JONES DG, HUNT RH. Accuracy and value of the Haemoccult test in symptomatic patients. *Br Med J* 1983;**286**:673–674.

65 LOEHR WJ, MUJAHED Z, ZAHN D, GRAY G, THORBJARNARSON B. Primary lymphoma of the gastrointestinal tract: a review of 100 cases. *Ann Surg* 1969;**170**:232–238.

66 McCOLL I, BUSSEY HJR, VEALE AMO, MORSEN BC. Juvenile Polyposis Coli. *Proc R Soc Med* 1964; **57**:34–35.

67 McGUIRE HH, HAYNES BW. Massive haemorrhage from diverticulosis of the colon: guidelines for therapy based on bleeding patterns observed in 50 cases. *Ann Surg* 1972;**175**(6):847–855.

68 McKUSICK KA, FROELICH J, CALLAHAN RJ, WINZELBERG GG, STRAUSS HW. ^{99m}Tc red blood cells for detection of gastrointestinal bleeding: experience with 80 patients. *Am J Radiol* 1981:**137**:1113–1118.

69 MACRAE FA, ST JOHN DJB. Relationship between patterns of bleeding and Haemoccult sensitivity in patients with colorectal cancer or adenomas. *Gastroenterology* 1982;**82**:891–898.

70 MARCUSON RW. Ischaemic colitis. *Clin Gastroenterol* 1972;1:745–765.

71 MASON EW, BELFUSS N. Detection of occult blood as a routine office procedure. *JAMA* 1952;**149**: 1526–1528.

72 MATOLO NM, LINK DP. Selective embolisation for control of gastrointestinal haemorrhage. *Am J Surg* 1979; **138**:840–844.

73 MELLISH RWP. Multiple haemangiomas of the gastrointestinal tract in children. *Am J Surg* 1971;**121**:412–417.

74 MEYERS MA, VOLBERG F, KATZEN B, ALONSO D, ABBOT G. The angioarchitecture of colonic diverticula. *Radiology* 1973;**108**:249–261.

75 MILLER RE. Detection of colon carcinoma and the barium enema. *JAMA* 1974;**230**:1195–1198.

76 MILLER SF, KNIGHT AR. The early detection of colorectal cancer. *Cancer* 1977;**40**:945–949.

77 MILLION R, HOWARTH J, TURNBER G, TURNER LA. Faecal occult blood screening in general practice. *Practitioner* 1982;**226**:659–663.

78 MITSUDO SM, BOLEY SJ, BRANDT L, MONTEFUSCO CM, SAMMARTANO RJ. Vascular ectasias of the right colon in the elderly: a distinct pathologic entity. *Human Pathol* 1979;**10**:585–600.

79 MITTALL R, SPERO JA, LEWIS JH, et al. Patterns of gastrointestinal hemorrhage in hemophilia. *Gastroenterology* 1985;**88**:515–522.

80 MITTY H, EFREMIDIS S, KELLER R. Colonic stricture after transcatheter embolization for diverticular disease. *Am J Radiol* 1979;**133**:519–521.

81 MOERTEL CG, HILL JR, DOCKERTY MB. The routine proctoscopic examination: a second look. *Mayo Clin Proc* 1966;**41**:368–374.

82 MOGADAM M, KATZEN BT, BROWN JG. Recurrent massive lower gastrointestinal bleeding from carcinoid tumour of the ileum. *Am J Gastroenterol* 1981;**76**:56–58.

83 MORRIS DW, HANSELL JR, OSTROW JD, LEE CS. Reliability of chemical tests for fecal occult blood in hospitalised patients. *Am J Dig Dis* 1976;**21**:845–852.

84 PAYNE RA. The incidence and clinical significance of rectal polyps. *Ann R Coll Surg Engl* 1976;**58**:241–242.

85 RANSON MB, SHOULDER PJ, TULEY NJ, HUNT RH. Does upper gastrointestinal bleeding affect the Haemoccult slide test for faecal occult blood? *Br J Surg* 1980;**67**:818.

86 RECKLESS JPD, McCOLL I, TAYLOR GW. Aortoenteric fistula: an uncommon complication of abdominal aortic aneurysms. *Br J Surg* 1972;**59**:458–460.

87 RUTHERFORD RB, AKERS DR. Meckel's diverticulum: a review of 148 paediatric patients with special reference to the pattern of bleeding and to mesodiverticular vascular bands. *Surgery* 1966;**59**:618–626.

88 SACHATELLO CR, PICKREN JW, GRACE J. Generalised juvenile gastrointestinal polyposis. *Gastroenterology* 1970;**58**:699–708.

89 SALAM RR, WOOD CB, REES HC, KHESHAVARZIAN A, HEMINGWAY AP, ALLISON DJ. A comparison of colonoscopy and selective visceral angiography

in the diagnosis of colonic angiodysplasia. *Ann Roy Coll Surg Eng* 1985;**67**:225–226

90 SCHUSSHEIM A, MOSKOWITZ GW, LEVY LM. Radionuclide diagnosis of bleeding Meckel's diverticulum in children. *Am J Gastroenterol* 1977;**68**:25–29.

91 SCHWARTZ S, ELLEFSON M. Quantitative fecal recovery of ingested hemoglobin-heme in blood: comparisons by HemoQuant assay with ingested meat and fish. *Gastroenterology* 1985;**89**:19–26

92 SIMON JB. Occult blood screening for colorectal carcinoma: a critical review. *Gastroenterology* 1985;**88**:820–827.

93 SMITH CR, BARTHOLOMEW LG, CAIN JC. Hereditary hemorrhagic telangiectasia and gastrointestinal hemorrhage. *Gastroenterology* 1963;**44**:1–6.

94 SNOOK JA, HOLDSTOCK GE, BAMFORTH J. Value of a simple biochemical ratio in distinguishing upper and lower sites of gastrointestinal haemorrhage. *Lancet* 1986;i:1064–1065.

95 SOLTERO MJ, BILL AH. The natural history of Meckel's diverticulum and its relation to incidental removal. *Am J Surg* 1976;**132**:168–173.

96 SPIEGEL RM, SCHULTZ RW, CASARELLA WJ, WOLFF M. Massive hemorrhage from jejunal diverticula. *Radiology* 1982;**143**:367–371.

97 STANILAND JR, DITCHBURN J, DEDOMBAL FT. Clinical presentation of diseases of the large bowel; a detailed study of 642 patients. *Gastroenterology* 1976;**70**:22–28.

98 STARR GF, DOCKERTY MB. Leiomyomas and leiomyosarcomas of the small intestine. *Cancer* 1955;**8**:101–111.

99 STEWART JG, AHLQUIST DA, McGILL DB, ILSTRUP DM, SCHWARTZ S, OWEN RA. Gastrointestinal blood loss and anaemia in runners. *Ann Intern Med* 1984;**100**:843–845.

100 STROEHLEIN JR, FAIRBANKS VF, McGILL BD, GO VLW. Hemoccult detection of fecal occult blood quantitated by radioassay. *Am J Dig Dis* 1976;**21**:841–844.

101 SUTTON D, MURFITT J, HOWARTH F. Gastrointestinal bleeding from large angiomas. *Clin Radiol* 1981;**32**:629–632.

102 SWARBRICK ET, FEVRE DI, HUNT RH, THOMAS BM, WILLIAMS CB. Colonoscopy for unexplained bleeding. *Br Med J* 1978;**2**:1685–1687.

103 TADAVARTHY SM, CASTANEDA A, ZUNIGA W, *et al.* Angiodysplasia of the right colon treated by embolization with ivalon (polyvinyl alcohol). *Cardiovasc Intervent Radiol* 1981;**4**:39–42.

104 THEONI RF, MENUCK L. Comparison of barium enema and colonoscopy in the detection of small colonic polyps. *Radiology* 1977;**124**:631–635.

105 THOMAS BM. The instant enema in inflammatory disease of the colon. *Clin Radiol* 1979;**30**:165–173.

106 TURUNEN MJ LIEWENDAHL K, PARTANEN P, ADLER-CREUTZ H. Immunological detection of faecal occult blood in colorectal cancer. *Br J Cancer* 1984;**49**:141–148.

107 VELLACOTT KD, HARDCASTLE JD. An evaluation of flexible fibreoptic sigmoidoscopy. *Br Med J* 1981;**283**:1583–1586.

108 VESCIA FG, BABB RR. Colonic varices: a rare, but important cause of gastrointestinal haemorrhage. *J Clin Gastroenterol* 1985;**7**:63–65.

109 WEAVER GA, BORDLEY J, OLSON JE. Management of bleeding angiodysplasia of the upper small intestine. *J Clin Gastroenterol* 1985;**7**:145–151

110 WELCH CE, ATHANASOULIS CA, GALDABINI JJ. Haemorrhage from the large bowel with special references to angiodysplasia and diverticular disease. *World J Surg* 1978;**2**:73–83.

111 WILLIAMS CB. Diathermy-biopsy: a technique for the endoscopic management of small polyps. *Endoscopy* 1973;**5**:215–218.

112 WILSON JM, MELVIN DB, GRAY G, THORBJARNARSON B. Benign small bowel tumours. *Ann Surg* 1975;**181**:247–250.

113 WINAWER SJ, ANDREWS M, FLEHINGER B, SHERLOCK P, SCHOTTENFELD D, MILLER DG. Progress report on controlled trial of fecal occult blood testing for the detection of colorectal neoplasia. *Cancer* 1980;**45**:2959–2964.

114 WINCHESTER DP, SHULL JH, SCANLON EF, *et al.* A mass screening program for colorectal cancer using chemical testing for occult blood in the stool. *Cancer* 1980;**45**:2955–2958.

115 WITTENBERG J, ATHANASOULIS CA, WILLIAMS L, PAREDES S, O'SULLIVAN P, BROWN B. Ischemic colitis: radiology and pathophysiology. *Am J Roentgenol* 1975;**123**(2):287–300.

116 WOLFF WI, GROSSMAN MB, SHINYA H. Angiodysplasia of the colon: diagnosis and treatment. *Gastroenterology* 1977;**72**:329–333.

117 WRIGHT HK, PELLICCIA O, HIGGINS EF, SREENIVAS V, GUPTA A. Controlled semi-elective segmental resection for massive colonic haemorrhage. *Am J Surg* 1980;**139**:535–538.

SECTION VI

DISEASES OF THE PANCREAS

Chapter 33
Imaging the Pancreas

A. T. R. AXON

The introduction of effective new imaging techniques for the pancreas has revolutionized the assessment of pancreatic disease. Earlier attempts to image the pancreas with radioisotopes or arteriography have now given way to ultrasonography and computerized axial tomography, which are less invasive and provide useful information about the parenchyma. In addition, endoscopic retrograde pancreatography (ERCP) can demonstrate the whole of the pancreatic duct system.

Although more than one imaging technique may be required for full anatomical assessment of the pancreas, this is not always necessary. Choice of the imaging technique depends upon the clinical presentation, local expertise and availability. Results of pancreatic function tests and imaging techniques vary from centre to centre leading to discrepancies in published results, which are further complicated by the lack of a generally accepted standard test; there are also variations in the standard of radiological reporting and clinical definitions.

This chapter discusses the different imaging techniques available and attempts to provide a logical approach to their use in pancreatic investigation.

Standard radiological techniques

Plain abdominal X-ray

Calcification in chronic pancreatitis may be visible on a plain abdominal film and may render further investigation unnecessary.

However, if pain is the problem or if surgery is contemplated, more sophisticated imaging techniques are needed to detect co-existent biliary disease, structural changes in the pancreatic duct system and the presence of pseudocysts.

Barium studies

Hypotonic duodenography, which was widely employed in pancreatic assessment, is no longer used. Pancreatic disease may be suspected for the first time by the discovery, on barium meal, of a lesion indenting the posterior wall of the stomach or deforming the second part of the duodenum.

Ultrasonography

The image produced by an ultrasound scan represents a section through the patient (Fig. 33.1). A transducer emits high frequency ultrasound in the 3.5–5.0 megahertz range which is reflected at tissue interfaces; the incoming echo is converted electronically into an image. Ultrasound techniques are advancing very rapidly and 'real time' equipment with high resolution is now available in most district general hospitals. Ultrasound scanning is quick, cheap, safe, and non-invasive. The whole abdomen can be examined in one study demonstrating the pancreas, liver, biliary tree, kidney, retroperitoneal space and other organs. Intestinal gas or obesity can interfere with the technique and may prevent successful imaging.

Although the pancreatic duct is often

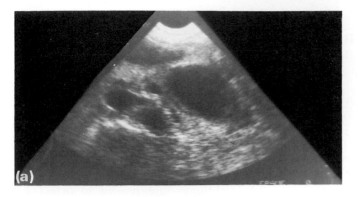

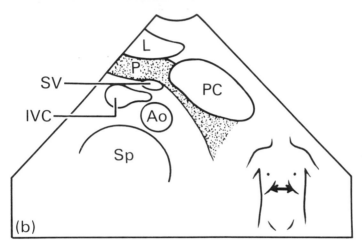

Fig. 33.1. (a) Ultrasound scan and (b) diagrammatic interpretation of pseudocyst following acute pancreatitis. Ao, Aorta; IVC, Inferior vena cava; SV, Splenic vein; PC, Pseudocyst; L, Liver; Sp, Spine (courtesy of Dr J. Watters).

seen at ultrasound examination [9, 12, 34], especially in a diseased gland, ultrasound is essentially a technique for demonstrating the parenchyma and identifying changes of shape, size or texture by alterations in echogenicity (Fig. 33.2) [9, 43].

In spite of improvements in hardware, the most important factors in ultrasound are the skill and experience of the ultrasonographer [28].

Applications

ACUTE PANCREATITIS

Ultrasound has made a valuable contribution to the management of acute pancreatitis [11, 44], often showing a reduction in echogenicity, poorly defined texture, and a generalized increase in size. Progress of the disease can be followed by serial examinations, which may help predict the formation of pseudocysts (Fig. 33.1) [18]. Such cysts can then be followed to determine whether they will resolve spontaneously or require percutaneous, ultrasound-guided, needle aspiration [30] or surgical drainage (see Chapter 35).

CHRONIC PANCREATITIS

In chronic pancreatitis the gland may show no change or be increased or decreased in size. The contour is irregular if an inflammatory mass is present [46]. The characteristic change is an alteration of echogenicity [43] due to fibrosis and calcification. Very high amplitude echoes may be seen when

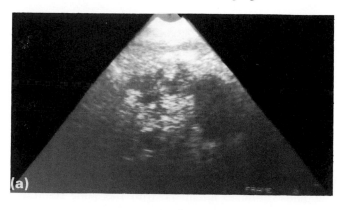

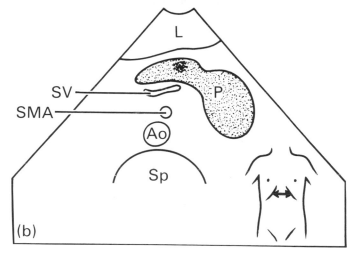

Fig. 33.2. (a) Transverse ultrasound scan and (b) diagrammatic interpretation of a case of chronic pancreatitis showing irregular outline and abnormal texture. Ao, Aorta; L, Liver; P, Pancreas; Sp, Spine; SV, Splenic vein; SMA, Superior mesenteric artery (Courtesy of Dr J. Watters).

extensive calcification is present. The normal pancreas has a 'cobblestone' appearance, but in chronic pancreatitis the pattern becomes coarse or patchy [25] and the echoes more heterogeneous. Although attempts are being made to quantify these differences in echo amplitude, interpretation is mainly subjective at present. Abnormal pancreatic ducts [27] are often seen and may help with diagnosis; changes may include dilatation, alteration in the walls and occasionally intra-duct calculi.

As it is relatively inexpensive, safe and quick ultrasound should be an ideal screening test for chronic pancreatitis and in expert hands it is as sensitive as computerized tomography and ERCP [9]. Most studies, however, have shown it to be relatively insensitive compared with other methods [16, 20, 23] and on its own it cannot be recommended for screening. Ultrasound is of particular value in assessing patients with relapsing pancreatitis prior to ERCP in order to detect pseudocysts and cholelithiasis.

CARCINOMA OF THE PANCREAS

The typical appearance of pancreatic cancer is a localized, well-defined mass with an echo pattern differing from that of the remaining gland [46]. There may, in addition, be secondary changes of chronic pancreatitis [47] and, if the tumour is in the head of the pancreas, upstream dilatation of the main pancreatic duct. The distinction between a benign and malignant mass can be difficult but fine needle aspiration, under ultrasound control, can provide cytological diagnostic information in around 80% of patients [21]. This technique is quick, simple and relatively safe; diagnostic rates improve with the number of passes—at least 4 passes are usually required [15].

Ultrasound tends to be the examination of first choice in non-specialized centres. It is particularly valuable in those presenting with an abdominal mass as it will readily show whether this arises from the pancreas, and whether it is cystic or solid.

Ultrasound is also useful in progressive jaundice where it will demonstrate a dilated biliary tree in patients with an obstructive lesion in the lower common bile duct. The presence of a mass in the pancreatic head area is very suggestive of a carcinoma but caution is required as ultrasound does not always detect stones in the bile duct; these require direct contrast cholangiography for diagnosis.

Computerized tomography (CT)

CT scanning of the abdomen is the most effective technique for demonstrating the pancreatic parenchyma. Its advantages are that it is less operator-dependent and produces an image with the same resolution throughout the gland (Fig. 33.3) providing a more objective assessment. Most recent studies [16, 23] have shown CT to be both more sensitive and specific in the detection of chronic pancreatic disease and cancer than is ultrasound.

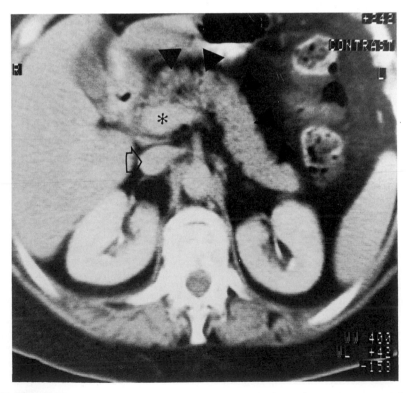

Fig. 33.3. CT scan showing a normal pancreas. Arrowheads, pancreas; *, portal vein; open arrow, inferior vena cava (With permission of Dr P.J. Robinson).

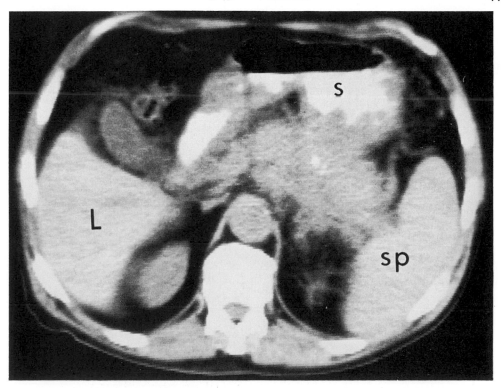

Fig. 33.4. CT scan showing changes of acute upon chronic pancreatitis. Note enlarged pancreas with irregular outline, flecks of calcification and inflammatory thickening of the posterior wall of the stomach. L, Liver; S, Stomach; Sp, Spleen (courtesy of Dr P. J. Robinson).

Applications

ACUTE PANCREATITIS

Whilst CT can provide similar, or even superior, information to ultrasound it is rarely used in acute pancreatitis because of logistic problems in the 'acute phase' of the illness. Pancreatic pseudocysts or abscesses (Fig. 33.5 and Fig. 33.6) can be demonstrated and percutaneous biopsy or aspiration carried out under CT control [32].

CHRONIC PANCREATITIS

The gland may be enlarged, normal or reduced in size but the shape is usually unaltered unless cysts, abscesses or inflammatory masses are present (Fig. 33.4) [13].

Parenchymal fibrosis and calcification show as alterations in attenuation giving rise to a heterogeneous or coarse appearance. Calcification may be seen as punctate areas of very high attenuation invisible on a plain X-ray of the abdomen [14]—intra-duct calculi or a dilated duct may be seen in advanced cases.

CARCINOMA OF THE PANCREAS

Neoplastic lesions (Fig. 33.7) usually show as a focal mass [28]. Occasionally tumours as small as 2 cm in size may be seen, particularly if there is surrounding oedema and intravenous contrast medium is used during the procedure [31]. A dilated main pancreatic duct upstream of the tumour may be seen. Evidence of spread may be

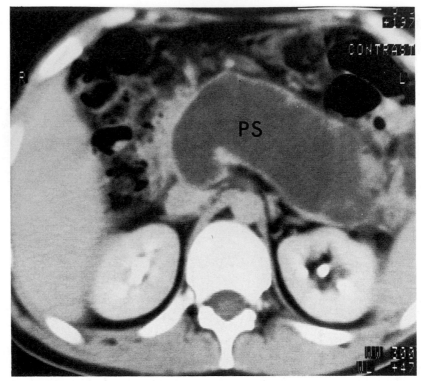

Fig. 33.5. CT scan of a patient with chronic pancreatitis showing replacement of the pancreas by a large pseudocyst, PS, (courtesy of Dr P. J. Robinson).

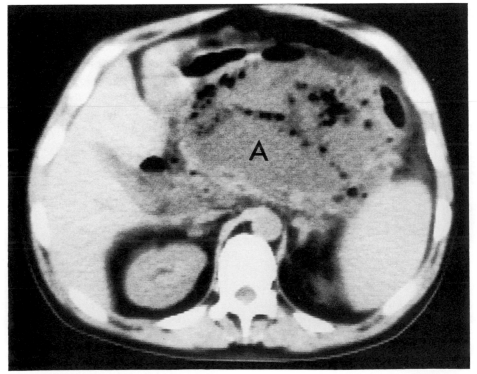

Fig. 33.6. CT scan showing a pancreatic abscess (A) with multiple pockets of gas and a small air-fluid level (courtesy of Dr P. J. Robinson).

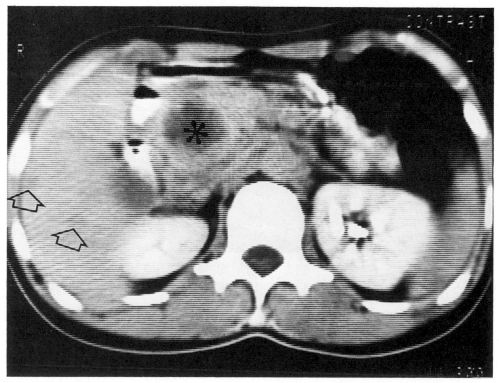

Fig. 33.7. CT scan showing a pancreatic carcinoma with a low density mass in the head of the pancreas (*) and small metastatic deposits within the liver (open arrows) (courtesy of Dr P. J. Robinson).

demonstrated by obliteration of the posterior fat plane, enlarged lymph nodes, or liver metastases.

Unfortunately pancreatic cancer is rarely resectable but CT may prove that a lesion is inoperable, where resection is being considered, avoiding an unnecessary laparotomy. This may be of particular value if endoscopic palliative procedures are being considered, or if radiotherapy or cytotoxic therapy is to be used. Most studies have shown that CT is more accurate than ultrasound [38] providing the correct diagnosis in over 90% of patients. However it is less sensitive than ERCP in chronic pancreatitis [9, 33].

Nuclear magnetic resonance (NMR)

This new imaging technique (Fig. 33.8) utilizes the energy emitted from the body as a result of re-alignment of protons after they have been subjected to changes in the magnetic field surrounding the body. A cross-section of the body similar to that of CT is shown. With current equipment the resolution is not as good as that with modern CT—but there is a greater contrast between different organs and between normal and abnormal tissues. There is little published work on its value in the pancreas. However some preliminary results [45, 48] suggest that it may become a valuable non-invasive imaging method demonstrating abnormalities that are not shown by current techniques.

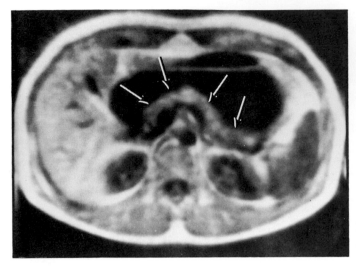

Fig. 33.8. NMR scan of a normal pancreas (arrowed) (courtesy of Dr G. Bydder).

Pancreatic angiography

The indications for pancreatic angiography have declined with the introduction of other imaging techniques. When required it should be carried out by an experienced radiologist using high quality equipment. Under these circumstances sensitivities and specificities of up to 90% can be achieved [22].

Pancreatic angiography is not an appropriate screening test for pancreatic disease, but it remains useful when other investigations have failed or have given equivocal results [17]. Angiography remains the best imaging test for diagnosing islet cell tumours of the pancreas, particularly insulinoma.

Transhepatic portal and pancreatic venous sampling may enable the site of origin of an insulinoma or gastrinoma to be identified by mapping the blood concentrations of the hormone [24] (Chapter 39).

Radioisotope scanning

Although radioisotope scanning is usually classified as an imaging test it is, in reality, a test of pancreatic function as it relies on the uptake of Se_{75}-selenomethionine by pancreatic acinar cells during protein synthesis. The radioactive emission produces an image of the metabolically active parts of the gland. As other intra-abdominal organs also incorporate this isotope a technetium scan is performed at the same time; this is subtracted to leave only the pancreatic image. A normal scan is a reliable indicator of a normal pancreas, with a false negative rate of only 5% [1]. Unfortunately there is a high false positive rate of up to 30%. In addition it cannot distinguish between chronic pancreatitis and carcinoma [2] and carries a small radiation hazard. For these reasons radioisotope scanning of the pancreas is no longer widely used.

Endoscopic retrograde cholangio-pancreatography (ERCP)

This procedure was first introduced in 1969 [35]. Although relatively invasive it enables the entire pancreatic duct system to be visualized in over 90% of patients. There are two indications for its use: firstly as a diagnostic procedure; secondly to provide additional information in patients with known pancreatic disease.

Technique

ERCP is a demanding procedure and satisfactory results are only obtained when it is carried out by a 'team' which includes both an endoscopist and a radiologist with a particular interest in the technique. It is certainly not a suitable procedure for the occasional endoscopist. High quality radiological equipment is also essential.

Patients are sedated and a side-viewing duodenoscope is passed into the second part of the duodenum and the ampulla of Vater is identified. The patient is then turned prone and a 'control' radiograph is taken. A cannula is then passed into the ampulla and contrast is injected under screening control. Films are taken during the filling phase, on completion, and where indicated at a later time. The radiologist is responsible for seeing that there is complete filling of the main duct and side branches but parenchymal opacification is to be avoided. Good quality radiographs are essential for reporting and should include a 'control' film, plus adequate demonstration of the main and branch ducts to the second generation (Fig. 33.9). There should be no blurring from movement and air bubbles should be avoided.

Applications

ACUTE PANCREATITIS

This procedure is best avoided in acute pancreatitis as there are less invasive methods for assessing the state of the pancreas in the acute phase [32]. Its only role has been as part of a therapeutic endoscopic sphincterotomy when the acute pancreatitis is due to stones (see Chapter 35).

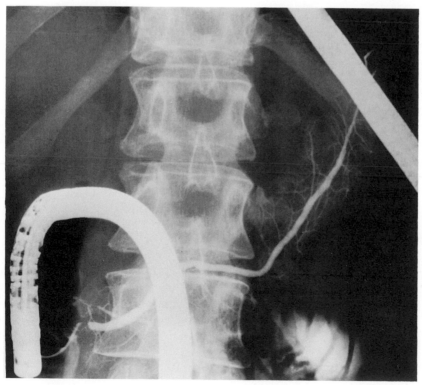

Fig. 33.9. A normal pancreatogram.

RECURRENT PANCREATITIS

In expert hands ERCP is probably the most sensitive method for diagnosing chronic pancreatitis [8], especially when pain is the presenting symptom, although CT will detect occasional cases missed by ERCP [16, 33]. Its major advantage over other methods is that it provides accurate information about the duct system which allows a rational surgical approach to be taken [73]. This is especially useful in recurrent pancreatitis or where biliary disease is thought to be the underlying cause [39]. Ultrasound and CT are of more value in the initial assessment of an abdominal mass; ERCP should not be performed in patients with pancreatic cysts unless expert surgical backup is available (see Chapter 37).

CHRONIC PANCREATITIS

Not all patients with chronic pancreatitis have an abnormal pancreatogram. A normal or equivocal appearance may be seen in up to 20% of cases [6]. The changes seen are classified as local or diffuse, and as mild, moderate or marked [4]. Abnormalities of the main duct [26, 42] include dilatation (Fig. 33.10), irregularity, stricturing and obstruction. Side branch changes include a reduced number, shortening, dilatation, narrowing or irregularity; all these changes may be localized or diffuse (Fig. 33.11).

Parenchymal opacification can occur if contrast is injected under too much pressure but when it occurs before full duct filling, it is a feature of acute inflammation [29]. It should be avoided, wherever

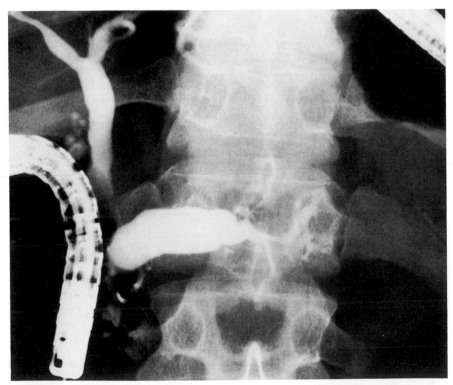

Fig. 33.10. A pancreatogram showing marked changes of severe chronic pancreatitis. Note the obstructed dilated duct in the body of the gland. This patient was suffering from chronic alcoholic pancreatitis.

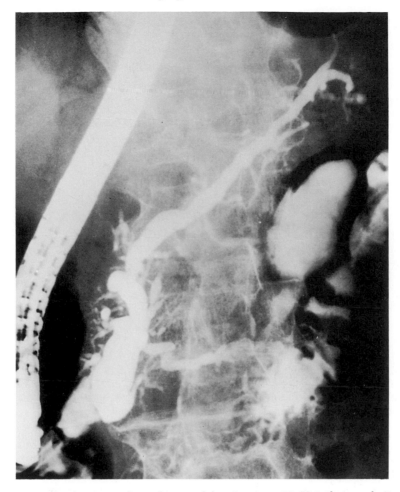

Fig. 33.11. A pancreatogram showing moderate changes of chronic pancreatitis. Note the irregularity of the main duct with shortening, dilatation and irregularity of the side branches. This patient had gallstone induced chronic pancreatitis.

possible, as it obscures duct detail and increases the risk of post-ERCP pancreatitis.

Cavities in the pancreas may fill with contrast or displace the main duct system, these may represent cysts, pseudocysts or abscesses (Fig. 33.12). There is a considerable risk of infection [10] if a cavity is filled with contrast, and urgent surgical treatment may be indicated.

The minimum criteria for diagnosing chronic pancreatitis on ERCP is the presence of at least three abnormal side branches. Mild changes of pancreatitis are present when only the side branches are affected, moderate changes when the main duct is affected and marked changes are implied by severe dilatation, irregularity, obstruction (Fig. 33.12) or intra-duct filling defects in the main duct, or the presence of a cavity. Such changes may be local (where less than one-third of the duct is involved) or diffuse. Another feature sometimes present in severe pancreatitis, which has surgical implications, is a delay in emptying of the duct system. Usually the duct empties within a few minutes but a delay in emp-

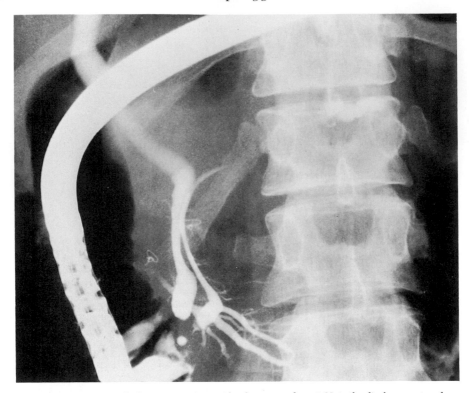

Fig. 33.12. The pancreatogram findings in a patient with a large pseudocyst. Note the displacement and obstruction of the main duct.

tying beyond 10 minutes suggests significant pancreatic disease.

Bile duct changes in chronic pancreatitis

The biliary system is often opacified at the same time as the pancreas during ERCP. Demonstration of the common bile duct, gall bladder and intra-hepatic ducts is particularly useful in chronic pancreatitis as other imaging techniques fail to detect calculi [19] in these areas (Fig. 33.13). An added advantage is that bile duct stones may be removed by endoscopic sphincterotomy at the same examination. [41].

Evidence of chronic pancreatitis at ERCP is common in patients with biliary disease, but is often asymptomatic [3]. Occasionally inflammation in the head of the pancreas affects the common bile duct leading to

rowing ('rat-tail' appearance) or even complete obstruction.

CARCINOMA OF THE PANCREAS

Ampullary area

Carcinoma of the ampulla of Vater (Fig. 33.14) is often first diagnosed at duodenoscopy for obstructive jaundice. It is usually easy for the experienced endoscopist to make the diagnosis on the macroscopic appearances. Biopsies should certainly be taken to confirm the diagnosis, where possible, but one needs to recognize that histological confirmation can be difficult as biopsies are small and representative samples may not be obtained. The major difficulty lies with the inflamed ulcerated papilla that is sometimes seen after the recent passage of a biliary calculus. Whenever

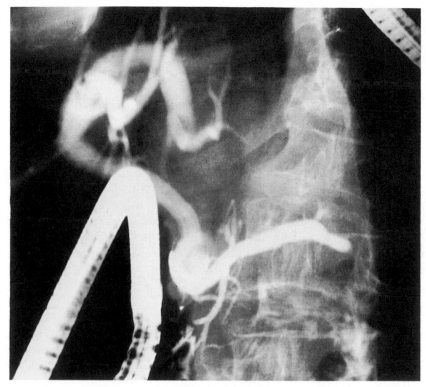

Fig. 33.13. A case of severe chronic pancreatitis with marked changes in the main pancreatic duct and side branches with a calculus at the lower end of the common bile duct.

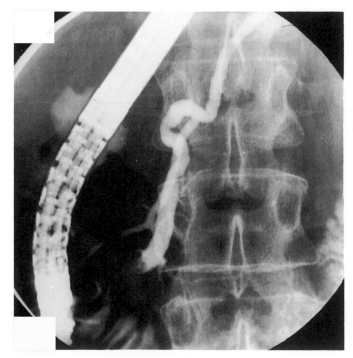

Fig. 33.14. A case of carcinoma of the ampulla. Note the frond-like filling defect at the ampullary end of the duct.

doubt remains it is wise to repeat the duo-denoscopy, after a few weeks, to re-assess the papilla.

Acinar and ductular cell tumours

Pancreatogram abnormalities are usually present by the time such patients present. The typical appearances [39] include ob-struction of the main duct (Fig. 33.15), or irregular narrowing of the duct with up-stream dilatation. Downstream from the block the duct system is relatively normal although, in the immediate vicinity of the tumour, contrast may be seen to seep out producing disorganized parenchymal opa-cification. Occasionally the main duct is dis-placed without being narrowed with a paucity of side branches in the area of the tumour.

Changes in the common bile duct are fre-quently seen when the tumour lies in the head; these include complete obstruction or irregular stricturing of the bile duct in its retro-pancreatic segment or as it passes under the first part of the duodenum.

Other tumours

Islet cell tumours are rarely diagnosed by ERCP because of their small size and lack of involvement of the duct system. Rarely they may be sufficiently large to distort the ducts around them.

Lower common bile duct tumours can mimic both acinar and ampullary tumours in their mode of presentation and their ERCP findings. About the only distinguish-ing feature is that the pancreatogram is often relatively normal in such patients.

Differential diagnosis

The distinction between chronic pancrea-titis and carcinoma of the pancreas can be very difficult. The pancreatogram findings can be similar and tumours can produce chronic pancreatitis downstream of them

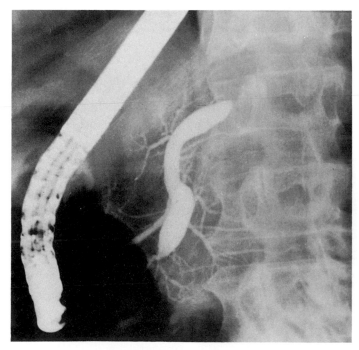

Fig. 33.15. The pancreatographic findings in a case of carcinoma of the pancreas. Note that the main duct is obstructed in the body but that the downstream duct and side branches are relatively normal.

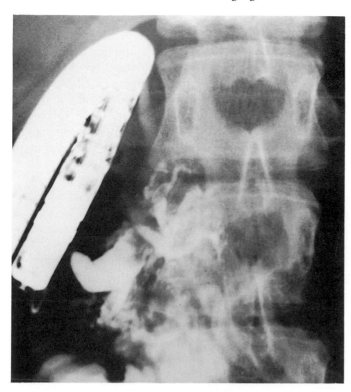

Fig. 33.16. The pancreatogram of a 16-year-old patient with familial chronic pancreatitis. Note that the main pancreatic duct and side branches are dilated and disorganized, appearances that can be difficult to distinguish from those of a carcinoma.

(Fig. 33.16). For these reasons it is important to interpret the pancreatogram findings in the light of the clinical history and to use alternative imaging tests where indicated. Further help may also be obtained by the collection of pure juice or the taking of brushings from the pancreatic duct for cytological examination [36].

Complications of ERCP

Endoscopic retrograde cholangio-pancreatography is a more invasive procedure than other imaging techniques. The major complications are sepsis and pancreatitis [5]. Sepsis arises from the introduction of infected material into partially obstructed bile and pancreatic ducts or into cysts. This danger can be minimized by careful disinfection of all endoscopic equipment and by the use of prophylactic antibiotics in patients at risk. Pancreatitis usually follows

repeated injections into the pancreatic duct or injection under excessive pressure causing parenchymal opacification. Complications are fewer when the examination is carried out by experienced operators.

Choice of imaging technique

The imaging method chosen by the physician depends upon the clinical presentation and local availability of techniques. Pancreatic disease may present as pancreatic insufficiency, acute or relapsing pancreatitis, chronic abdominal pain, an abdominal mass or as jaundice.

Pancreatic insufficiency

When steatorrhoea or other evidence of pancreatic insufficiency is present a pancreatic function test is often used to establish the diagnosis. However, in order to diagnose the pancreatic disease present an ERCP or CT, or a combination of both, may be required.

Acute or chronic pancreatitis

In acute pancreatitis there is little doubt that ultrasound is the safest and most appropriate technique.

In chronic pancreatitis the most useful method is ERCP. This not only establishes the diagnosis, but can also provide evidence for a rational surgical approach to the problem. It is particularly useful in patients who develop problems after previous cholecystectomy as, if these are due to a common bile duct stone, endoscopic sphincterotomy can be performed at the same time.

Chronic abdominal pain

One of the most difficult gastrointestinal problems is the patient with chronic abdominal pain in whom a pancreatic cause is suspected. The extent to which investigation is pursued will depend, to a large extent, on the clinical features. Young patients with a psychiatric history and symptoms stretching back over several years rarely have pancreatic pathology. However those with an alcoholic history, or elderly patients with a short history of pain and weight loss need more rigorous investigation [40]. A suitable screening combination is an oral pancreatic function test plus ultrasound. This will miss occasional patients with pancreatic disease, and if this is still suspected then a CT scan and ERCP may also be needed.

Abdominal mass

Patients presenting with an abdominal mass should first be examined by ultrasound. Additional CT scans and percutaneous aspirational biopsy may be needed to provide a final answer.

Jaundice

Ultrasound should be the first examination: if dilated intrahepatic ducts are present percutaneous cholangiography (PTC) should make the diagnosis. Occasionally it will be necessary to perform an ERCP to outline the pancreatic and bile ducts, to distinguish between an inflammatory or malignant cause or to insert a stent.

Conclusion

The plethora of available pancreatic investigations indicates that no single technique is ideal. A combination of tests will provide a precise diagnosis in the majority of patients with pancreatic disease. In chronic pancreatitis these investigations may suggest the need for a surgical approach, conversely they may show that surgery is not indicated for a patient with carcinoma of the pancreas. A preoperative diagnosis is becoming more important as radiological and endoscopic methods of palliation become established. They will become even more important in the future if radiotherapy or chemotherapy become an initial treatment for malignant disease.

References

1 Agnew JE, Youngs GR, Bouchier IAD. Conventional and subtraction scanning of the pancreas: an assessment based on blind reporting. *Br J Radiol* 1973;46:83–98.
2 Agnew JE, Maze M, Mitchell CU. Review article: pancreatic scanning. *Br J Radiol* 1976;49:979–995.
3 Axon ATR, Ashton MG, Lintott IJ. Pancreatogram changes in patients with calculous biliary disease. *Br J Surg* 1979;66:466–470.
4 Axon ATR, Classen M, Cotton PB, Cremer M, Freeny PC, Lees WR. Pancreatography in chronic pancreatitis: international definitions. *Gut* 1984;25:1107–1112.
5 Bilbao MK, Dotter CT, Lee TG, Katon RM. Complications of endoscopic retrograde cholangiopancreatography (ERCP): a study of 10,000 cases. *Gastroenterology* 1976;70:314–320.
6 Caletti G, Brocchi E, Agostinin D, Balduzzi A,

BOLONDI I, LABO G. Sensitivity of endoscopic retrograde pancreatography in chronic pancreatitis. *Br J Surg* 1982;**69**:507–509.

7 COTTON PB, BEALES JSI. Endoscopic pancreatography in the management of relapsing pancreatitis. *Br Med J* 1974;i:608–611.

8 COTTON PB, DENYER ME, KREEL L, HUSBAND J, MEIRE HB, LEES WR. Comparative clinical impact of endoscopic pancreatography, grey-scale ultrasonography, and computed tomography (EMI scanning) in pancreatic disease. *Gut* 1978;**19**:679–684.

9 COTTON PB, LEES WR, VALLON AG, COTTON M, CROKER JR, CHAPMAN M. Grey-scale ultrasonography and endoscopic pancreatography in pancreatic diagnosis. *Radiology* 1980;**134**:453–459.

10 DAVIS JL, MILLIGAN FD, CAMERON JL. Septic complications following endoscopic retrograde cholangiopancreatography. *Surg Gynecol Obstet* 1975; **140**:365–367.

11 DUNCAN JE, IMRIE CW, BLUMGART LH. Ultrasound in the management of acute pancreatitis. *Br J Radiol* 1976;**49**:858–862.

12 EISENSCHER A, WEILL F. Ultrasonic visualisation of Wirsung's duct: Dream or reality? *J Clin Ultrasound* 1979;**7**:41–44.

13 FAWCITT RA, FORBES WStC, ISHERWOOD I, BRAGANZA J, HOWAT HT. Computed tomography in pancreatic disease. *Br J Radiol* 1978;**51**:1–4.

14 FERRUCCI JT, WITTENBERG J, BLACK EB, KIRKPATRICK RH, HALL DA. Computed tomography in chronic pancreatitis. *Radiology* 1979;**130**:175–182.

15 FERRUCCI JT, WITTENBERG J, MUELLER PR, et al. Diagnosis of abdominal malignancy by radiologic fine needle aspiration biopsy. *Am J Roentgenol* 1980;**134**:323–330.

16 FOLEY WD, STEWART ET, LAWSON TL, et al. Computed tomography, ultrasonography and endoscopic retrograde cholangiopancreatography in diagnosis of pancreatic disease: A comparative study. *Gastrointest Radiol* 1980;**5**:29–35.

17 FREENEY PC, BULL JT, RYAN J. Impact of new diagnostic imaging methods on pancreatic angiography. *Am J Roentgenol* 1979;**133**:619–624.

18 GONZALES AC, BRADLEY EL, CLEMENTS JL. Pseudocyst formation: Acute pancreatitis: Ultrasonographic evaluation of 99 cases. *Am J Roentgenol* 1976;**127**:315–317.

19 GOODMAN MW, ANSEL HJ, VENNES JA, LASSEN B, SILVIS SE. Is intravenous cholangiography still useful? *Gastroenterology* 1980;**79**:642–645.

20 GOWLAND M, WARWICK F, KALANTZIS N, BRAGANZA J. Relative efficiency and predictive value of ultrasonography and endoscopic retrograde pancreatography in diagnosis of pancreatic disease. *Lancet* 1981;ii:190–193.

21 HANCKE S, HOLM HH, KOCH F. Ultrasonically guided percutaneous fine needle biopsy of the pancreas. *Surg Gynecol Obstet* 1975;**140**:361–364.

22 HERLINGER H, FINLAY DBL. Evaluation and follow-up of pancreatic arteriograms. A new role for angiography in the diagnosis of carcinoma of the pancreas. *Clin Radiol* 1978; **29**:277–284.

23 HESSEL SJ, SIEGELMAN SS, McNEIL BJ, et al. A prospective evaluation of computed tomography and ultrasound of pancreas. *Radiology* 1982;**143**:129–133.

24 INGERMASSON S, KULAL C, LARSSON LI, LUNDERQUIST A, NOBIN A. Islet cell hyperplasia localised by pancreatic vein catheterisation and insulin radioimmunoassay. *Am J Surg* 1977;**133**:643–645.

25 JOHNSON ML, MACK LA. Ultrasonic evaluation of the pancreas. *Gastrointest Radiol* 1978;**3**:257–266.

26 KASGAI T, KUNO N, KIZU M. Manometric endoscopic retrograde pancreatocholangiography. Techniques, significance and evaluation. *Am J Dig Dis*, 1974;**19**:485–502.

27 LEES WR, VALLON AG, DENYER ME, VAHL SP, COTTON PB. Prospective study of ultrasonography in chronic pancreatic disease. *Br Med J* 1979;i:162–164.

28 LEES WR. Ultrasonography of the pancreas. In: Mitchell CJ, Kelleher J, eds. *Pancreatic disease in clinical practice.* London: Pitman, 1981:18–35.

29 LINTOTT DJ. Endoscopic retrograde cholangiopancreatography. In: Mitchell CJ, Kelleher J, eds. *Pancreatic disease in clinical practice.* London: Pitman, 1981.

30 MACERLEAN DP, BRYAN PJ, MURPHY JJ. Pancreatic pseudocyst: management by ultrasonically guided aspiration. *Gastrointest Radiol* 1980;**5**:255–257.

31 MARCHAL G, BAERT AL, WILMS G. Carcinoma of the pancreas. *J Comp Assist Tomography* 1979;**3**:727–730.

32 MOOSA RA. Diagnostic tests and procedures in acute pancreatitis. *N Engl J Med* 1984;**311**:639–643.

33 MOSS AA, FEDERLE M, SHAPIRO HA, et al. The combined use of computed tomography and endoscopic retrograde cholangiopancreatography in the assessment of suspected pancreatic neoplasm: a blind clinical evaluation. *Radiology* 1980;**134**:159–163.

34 OHTO M, SAOTOME N, SAISHO H, et al. Real-time sonography of the pancreatic duct: Application to pancreatic ductography. *Am J Roentgenol* 1980; **134**:647–652.

35 OI I, TAKEMOTO T, KONDO T. Fibreduodenoscope. Direct observation of the papilla of Vater. *Endoscopy* 1969;**1**:101–103.

36 OSNES M, SERCK-HANSSEN A, KRISTENSEN A, SWENSEN T, AUNE S, MYREN J. Endoscopic retrograde brush cytology in patients with primary and secondary malignancies of the pancreas. *Gut* 1979;**20**:279–284.

37 REUBEN A, COTTON PG. Endoscopic retrograde cholangiopancreatography in cancer of the pancreas. *Surg Gynecol Obstet* 1979; **143**:179–184.

38 ROBINSON PJA. Computed tomography of the pancreas. In: Mitchell CJ, Kelleher J, eds. *Pancreatic disease in clinical practice.* London: Pitman, 1981:35–55.

39 RUDDELL WSJ, LINTOTT DJ, ASHTON MG, AXON ATR. Endoscopic retrograde cholangiography and pancreatography in the investigation of postcholecystectomy patients. *Lancet* 1980;i:444–447.

40 RUDDELL WSJ, LINTOTT DJ, AXON ATR. The diagnostic yield of ERCP in the investigation of unexplained abdominal pain. *Br J Surg* 1983;70:74–75.

41 SAFRANY L. Duodenoscopic sphincterotomy and gallstone removal. *Gastroenterology* 1977; 72:338–343.

42 SALMON PR. Endoscopic retrograde cholangiopancreatography in the diagnosis of pancreatic disease. *Gut* 1975;16:658–663.

43 SARTI DA, KING W. The ultrasonic findings in inflammatory pancreatic disease. *Seminars in ultrasound* 1980;1:178–191.

44 SILVERSTEIN W, ISIKOFF MB, HALL MC, BARKIN J. Diagnostic imaging of acute pancreatitis: Prospective study using CT and sonography. *Am J Roentgenol* 1981;137:497–502.

45 SMITH FW, HUTCHINSON JMS, MALLARD JR. Nuclear magnetic resonance imaging of the pancreas. *Radiology* 1982;146:577–580.

46 WEINSTEIN DP, WOLFMAN NT, WEINSTEIN BJ. Ultrasonic characteristics of pancreatic tumours. *Gastrointest Radiol* 1979;4:245–251.

47 WEINSTEIN DP, WEINSTEIN BJ. Ultrasonic demonstration of the pancreatic duct. An analysis of 41 cases. *Radiology* 1979;130:729–734.

48 YOUNG IR, BAILES DR, BURL M, *et al.* Initial clinical evaluation of a whole body tomograph. *J. Comp Assist Tomography* 1982;6:1–18.

Chapter 34
The Assessment of Pancreatic Exocrine Function

E. J. S. BOYD & K. G. WORMSLEY

The aim of pancreatic exocrine function tests is to detect diagnostically and therapeutically relevant changes of pancreatic secretion in relation to disease of the pancreas. It is assumed that pancreatic diseases cause a reduction in the number, or functional capacity, of the pancreatic acinar and ductular cells which results in a decrease in the secretion of electrolytes and enzymes. The role of compensatory mechanisms (such as an increase in synthetic capacity or a lowering of the threshold to stimuli) in determining when detectable changes in secretion occur is unknown.

In general, the reserve secretory capacity of the pancreas is such that diagnostic changes in exocrine function are not found until anatomical changes are advanced: particularly as sequential measurements from a healthy state are rarely available for the individual patient. Therefore the value of pancreatic function tests in predicting 'normality' is not as satisfactory as their positive predictive power for detecting disease.

Classification of pancreatic function tests

Tests of pancreatic secretory cell function

Direct tests depend on the collection of the pancreatic secretions produced in response to exogenous secretagogues, either by aspirating from the duodenum, or, more rarely, by collecting pure pancreatic juice at endoscopic retrograde pancreatography (ERCP).

Indirect tests depend on the measurement of pancreatic enzymes in the serum or stool.

Tests of pancreatic secretion provide an index of the functional secretory cell mass. These are best for the detection of pancreatic disease and for monitoring its progress.

Tests of pancreatic digestive capacity

Direct tests involve the collection of duodenal contents after the administration of a test meal.

Indirect tests depend on the digestion of a substrate considered to be specific for pancreatic enzymes and the detection of its metabolites in urine or blood.

Tests of pancreatic digestion are related not only to pancreatic secretory function, but also depend on gastric, intestinal and hepatobiliary functions. This type of test is therefore less specific for pancreatic disease, but provides a more 'physiological' assessment of functional pancreatic secretion. It is also useful for monitoring the effects of therapy and assessing the need for enzyme replacement.

In both categories of pancreatic function test the higher specificity of direct tests (which need duodenal intubation) is sacrificed for greater applicability, acceptability, and convenience of indirect tests.

489

Tests of pancreatic cell function

Direct tests

In these tests the pancreatic secretion is measured in response to secretin, secretin plus cholecystokinin (CCK), or caerulein.

Technique

Studies are done after an overnight fast. Drugs that can affect gastrointestinal secretions (for example anti-cholinergics) should be withheld for at least 48 hours before the test.

It is essential that gastric secretion is aspirated separately from duodenal contents, in order to prevent contamination. Separate vented gastric and duodenal tubes can be used, or one tube constructed by cementing a polyvinyl gastric aspiration channel (2 mm diameter) with an air vent, to a 12 F.G. Salem duodenal sump tube, so that the gastric aspiration holes are 20 cm proximal to the duodenal tube tip (Fig. 34.1).

The position of the tube must be checked by fluoroscopy before starting to aspirate. The duodenal aspiration holes should be in the descending duodenum and the gastric holes in the antrum. Secretions are collected by continuous mechanical aspiration. Marker techniques are unnecessary when vented tubes are used, as more than 80% recovery is achieved [30].

Common technical problems include contamination of the duodenal aspirate with gastric juice and, more importantly, duodenogastric reflux. Contamination by acid is immediately apparent from cloudiness of the normally clear duodenal aspirate. If this occurs, the position of the tube should be reconfirmed by screening and adjusted if necessary. The patency of air vents and aspiration channels should also be checked and the collection vessel changed when clear secretions are again aspirated. Only clear secretion should be used for assay of

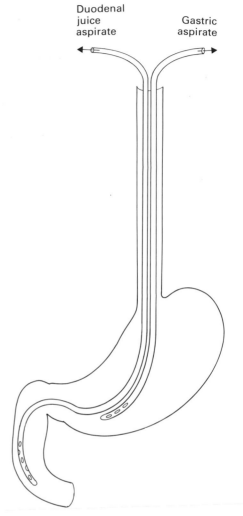

Duodenal juice aspirate

Gastric aspirate

Fig. 34.1. Position of double-lumen tube used for the secretin-pancreozymin test.

enzymes and electrolytes. If duodenogastric reflux occurs, tube patency and position should be checked and, if it persists, gastric contents should be collected separately and the volume, bicarbonate and enzyme concentrations measured. These results should be added to those of the duodenal aspirate analysis.

Choice of stimulant: dose and route of administration

Secretagogues are best given by a constant intravenous infusion, so that a steady rate of secretion is obtained. This permits calculation of output per unit time, as well as maximal secretory rate and concentration. A further advantage is that gastric secretion is inhibited more by a secretin infusion than by a bolus dose. Infusions should be given for at least 45 minutes, as maximal secretory rates are not achieved for at least 15 minutes. Highly purified secretin is available from Kabivitrum (AB Kabi Diagnostica, Nykoping, Sweden); synthetic secretin can be obtained from Roche (Roche Products Ltd., Welwyn Garden City, U.K.) and impure secretin from Boots (Boots PLC., Nottingham, U.K.). The dose of secretin that produces maximal bicarbonate secretion is 2–4 C.U./kg.h or 0.75–1.5 u/kg.h.

Cholecystokinin (CCK) is used by some investigators, either alone or with secretin [29]. When used alone secretory rates are low and the valuable index of bicarbonate secretory capacity is lost in favour of the less satisfactory index of enzyme secretion. When given in combination, bicarbonate and enzyme secretion are stimulated. However, measurement of enzyme secretion rarely provides additional useful information that is not obtained from bicarbonate measurement. Cholecystokinin can be obtained from Kabivitrum and from Boots. As an alternative, the octapeptide of CCK can be used in a dose of 30 ng/kg.h., or caerulein (Farmitalia Carlo Erba, Milan, Italy) in a dose of 75 ng/kg.h. Caerulein has the disadvantage that it also stimulates gastric secretion, which can contaminate duodenal secretion.

Whatever type of stimulant is used the dose should be 'maximal' in order to differentiate between impairment of function by disease and the low output produced by a sub-maximal stimulation.

Measurements on duodenal aspirate

Duodenal juice should be collected in 10 or 15 minute batches. The volume and bicarbonate concentration is measured in each sample. Hourly secretion rates are calculated from the sum of outputs during the two consecutive periods with the highest response. If enzyme activities are required, trypsin is the most satisfactory enzyme to measure because its output shows the greatest discrimination between patients with and without pancreatic disease [9]. Trypsin can be measured by the liberation of dye from benzoyl-arginine-p-nitranilide, liberation of hydrogen ions from benzoyl-arginine ethyl ester hydrochloride, or by radio-immunoassay. Unfortunately these methods give different results and no correlation, or definition of the limits of normality exists. For this reason each laboratory should establish its own reference range.

When appropriate, a fresh specimen of the initial sample of duodenal juice collected should be centrifuged so that the deposit can be examined for malignant cells [23]. Duodenal juice can also be assayed for lactoferrin [22], and carcino-embryonic antigen [20] using commercially available radio-immunoassay kits. These assays may assist in the diagnosis of malignancy.

Similar measurements have been made on pure pancreatic juice collected from a cannula inserted into the pancreatic duct at ERCP [5, 7, 12]. Unfortunately these studies have not provided any better discrimination between normality and disease. However, cytological examination of pure pancreatic juice for malignant cells can be valuable.

Interpretation of results

The ranges of maximal bicarbonate concentration and output regarded as normal and abnormal are given in Table 34.1. Enzyme secretion is much less reliable, as concentrations are very variable and outputs show

Table 34.1. Maximum bicarbonate and enzyme secretion.

		Normal	?Abnormal	Abnormal
Bicarbonate	Max. Conc.	> 100 mmol/l	50–100 mmol/l	< 50 mmol/l
	Max. Output	> 20 mmol/h	15–20 mmol/h	< 15 mmol/h
Enzymes	Max. Conc.	Too variable for discrimination.		
	Max. Output	Wide overlap with normality.		

a wide overlap between patients with and without pancreatic disease. At present, the maximal bicarbonate output is the best available functional discriminant between patients with and without pancreatic disease [29].

In a technically satisfactory secretin (or secretin-CCK) test an abnormal response has a predictive value of nearly 100%. False positive results are rare and only occur in coeliac disease or advanced malnutrition. They are probably due to pancreatic atrophy, which is sometimes reversible [24]. A 'normal' response has less predictive value, as 13–25% of patients with unequivocal pancreatic disease, determined by other diagnostic methods, have bicarbonate outputs within the normal range [28]. For example at least 5% of patients with pancreatic calcification have a normal response to secretin-CCK.

Carcinoma diagnosis

In over half of secretin-CCK tests no suitable material for cytological studies is obtained [6]. Malignant cells will be found in around 30% of those with suitable material and the chance is increased where the tumour is large, or in the head of the pancreas. The predictive value of positive cytology is high (78–86%). A small number of false positive results (about 5%) are found in patients with resolving acute and chronic pancreatitis. The absence of malignant cells is of no value in excluding malignancy [18].

Lactoferrin was first measured in pure pancreatic juice where concentrations > 900 ng/ml were claimed to provide complete discrimination between chronic pancreatitis and cancer [7]. It has also been measured in duodenal aspirate and similar claims have been made for discriminating between cancer and pancreatitis [22].

The levels of carcino-embryonic antigen (CEA) in pure pancreatic juice and duodenal aspirate show a wide overlap between patients with cancer and benign pancreatic disease. In addition very high levels can occur in benign disease. Such measurements are therefore of little diagnostic value.

Advantages and disadvantages

The secretin (or secretin-CCK) test is the most sensitive and specific method for detecting pancreatic disease. An abnormal result carries a positive predictive value of almost 100%. Unfortunately the test is relatively expensive (an ampoule of 75 C.U. costs £8.50) and technically demanding. It must be performed by a skilled operator if it is to be of any diagnostic value. Some patients find duodenal intubation very unpleasant and are unable to tolerate the procedure. In some patients, particularly those who have had a previous Pólya gastrectomy, it is impossible to position the tube within the duodenum.

A recent attack of acute pancreatitis is *not* a contra-indication for a secretin test. In such patients results are often normal, or demonstrate an increased electrolyte output. It is usual, however, to allow at least 6 weeks to elapse before attempting to ferentiate 'recurrent acute' from 'chronic' pancreatitis.

Indirect tests

Because of the unpleasant nature of direct tests of pancreatic secretion attempts have been made to assess pancreatic function indirectly.

Measurement of pancreatic enzymes in the blood

Trypsin, lipase, and amylase (either total or iso-enzymes) are all detectable in the serum of fasted subjects. In the absence of acute pancreatitis, or chronic renal failure (which reduces enzyme clearance), circulating levels of these enzymes are considered to reflect the functional pancreatic cell mass.

Trypsin is the most widely used enzyme for assessing pancreatic exocrine function and it can be measured by a commercially available immunoassay [16]. The normal range is 150–600 μg/l. and concentrations below 150 μg/l are indicative of pancreatic exocrine disease. However similar low concentrations can occur in non-pancreatic disease and the specificity of a low concentration is no better than 66% [25]. Many patients with proven chronic pancreatitis have serum trypsin concentrations within the normal range so a single fasting concentration is of little diagnostic value.

As fasting levels have failed to provide satisfactory discrimination between pancreatic exocrine diseases and other gastrointestinal diseases, attempts have been made to increase their diagnostic value by measuring the response to food [16], to CCK [14] and to physostigmine [17]. During these 'evocative' tests there is little or no rise in serum trypsin or isoamylase over fasting concentrations in 'normal' subjects. In some patients with chronic pancreatitis, or cancer, there may be a marked increase in circulating enzyme concentrations, often from abnormally low fasting ones. This is particularly the case where ductal obstruction, or stenosis, is demonstrated at ERCP.

Advantages and disadvantages

These tests are easy to do and can be repeated frequently. The predictive value of a marked rise in enzyme concentrations from a low fasting value seems to be high. Unfortunately this pattern is found in a relatively small group of patients who have marked ductal stenosis, or obstruction. The sensitivity of serum enzyme tests is low, because many patients with chronic pancreatitis have normal fasting and 'evoked' serum concentrations.

Measurement of pancreatic enzymes in the stool

Some pancreatic enzymes are detectable in the stool. Residual activities depend on diet, rate of intestinal transit, degradation and inactivation, and are only indirectly related to pancreatic output.

Oral pancreatic enzyme supplements must be stopped at least 4 days before stool collection. Chymotrypsin is the most frequently measured enzyme, as it is the least degraded during intestinal transit. Assay is usually performed on two stool specimens taken on separate days and the mean activity is expressed as units, or μg/g of stool [2]. Accuracy is improved by homogenizing a 24-hour stool collection and measuring enzyme concentration in an aliquot [21]. The lower limit of normal is 120 μg/g, with values between 70–120 μg/g being considered equivocal. When compared with secretin-CCK stimulation random stool samples have a sensitivity of 70–95% in the detection of 'severe' and 40–65% in 'slight' pancreatic insufficiency. The specificity of the test ranges from 70–100% with 30% false positives [1].

Advantages and disadvantages

Tests of pancreatic secretion based on stool enzyme concentrations are of limited diagnostic value. They are useful in detecting pancreatic insufficiency in young children with cystic fibrosis, where other tests are impractical. Faecal chymotrypsin may also be of limited value in assessing compliance with, and adequacy of, pancreatic replacement therapy in patients with steatorrhoea.

Tests of pancreatic digestion

Direct tests

The only direct test of pancreatic digestive function used routinely is the Lundh Test. This relies upon stimulation of pancreatic secretion by a mixed meal. It is therefore a physiological test dependent on the integrity of extra-pancreatic, as well as pancreatic functions.

Technique

The test is done after an overnight fast and avoidance of drugs that affect gastrointestinal secretion or motility for at least 48 hours. A vented 14 F.G. duodenal tube is positioned as for a secretin-CCK test. The patient then drinks a liquid test meal (18 g corn oil + 15 g Casilan and 40 g glucose in 300 ml water with a flavouring agent). Any drugs to be studied (for example pancreatic supplements) should be added to the meal before ingestion [26]. The duodenal contents are collected (usually in 4 × 30-minute samples) by mechanical suction into iced containers.

Measurements on duodenal contents and interpretation of results [11]

The mean activity of at least one enzyme is measured in pooled duodenal aspirate collected during the test. Usually trypsin is measured, as it has the best discriminatory value [9]. Most workers have used the liberation of hydrogen ions from benzoyl-arginine ethyl ester hydrochloride for trypsin estimation, expressing results as units (mmol of H^+/ml/min). Values above 8.8–10 units being interpreted as 'normal' pancreatic function. However, each laboratory needs to establish its own range.

The mean duodenal pH during a Lundh test should be 6.0–8.0. A lower pH implies gastric hypersecretion, increased gastric emptying, or diminished pancreatic bicarbonate secretion. Since pancreatic enzymes can be inactivated by a low pH and pepsin, this information may be helpful in planning therapy as well as in interpreting (sometimes spuriously) low enzyme concentrations.

Complete aspiration of the test meal is not possible, marker studies suggesting that only 10–15% of the meal is recovered. The Lundh test thus provides information on enzyme activity and not on enzyme, or bicarbonate output. Differentiation between patients with and without pancreatic disease is less satisfactory than with the secretin-CCK test. It cannot distinguish cancer from chronic pancreatitis.

As enzyme concentration is dependent on pancreatic function and the rate of gastric secretion and emptying, false positive results can occur in hypersecretion and/or increased gastric emptying (for example in duodenal ulcer and the Zollinger-Ellison syndrome).

Pancreatic secretion requires adequate stimulation by endogenous secretin and CCK, so the response may be impaired if there is disease, or anatomical by-pass, of the duodenum and upper jejunum. Up to 50% of patients after previous gastric surgery and 25% of patients with small intestinal disease will have abnormal Lundh test meal results.

False positive results may also occur in 25% of patients with obstructive jaundice of non-pancreatic aetiology and in 10–15% with chronic liver disease.

The Lundh test is reported to be abnormal in 75–90% of patients with chronic pancreatitis, or cancer, diagnosed by other means. This gives a sensitivity similar to that of secretin-CCK test, but with a lower predictive value because of the higher proportion of false positives.

Advantages and disadvantages

The Lundh test is cheap, easy to do and reasonably reproducible. It can be performed effectively by nursing staff without direct medical supervision. The test can be used to identify those patients requiring replacement therapy, thus permitting more rational treatment. It has also been used as a prognostic criterion, since enzyme activities can be shown to revert to normal after an attack of acute pancreatitis. Its major disadvantage is the number of false positives.

Indirect tests

Indirect tests have been devised to overcome the disadvantages of duodenal intubation. The two that have found a place in routine use are the N-benzoyl-tyrosyl-p-aminobenzoic acid test (PABA) and the fluorescein dilaurate test (FDL).

The PABA test (Fig. 34.2)

The rationale of the PABA test is that this peptide is hydrolysed in the upper small intestine by pancreatic chymotrypsin. Free PABA is liberated, absorbed, conjugated in the liver and excreted in the urine. The amount present in the urine is measured as

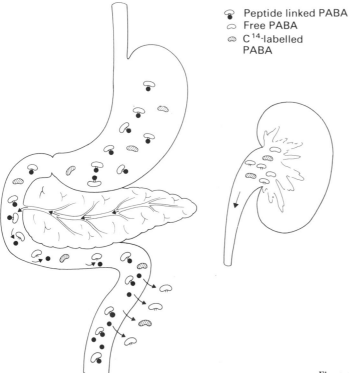

Peptide linked PABA
Free PABA
C^{14}-labelled PABA

Fig. 34.2. Principle of PABA single-day test.

total urinary aromatic amines. In order to allow for abnormalities of intestinal, liver, or renal function, either free PABA is given on a separate day [19], or C^{14}-PABA is given with unlabelled PABA-peptide in a single-day test. By calculating the ratio of free PABA (or C^{14}-PABA) to metabolized PABA as an excretion index, a correction for any functional problems can be made. The single-day test obviates problems caused by the different handling of PABA on separate days and also increases acceptability [27].

Technique

The PABA test is performed after an overnight fast. Pancreatic supplements should be withheld for at least four days (unless testing their effect), and drugs affecting motility, or secretion, for 48 hours beforehand. Certain drugs and foods result in a high urinary excretion of aromatic aminoacids (for example thiazides, paracetamol, sulphonamides, prunes and cranberries): these should be avoided for 48 hours before and during the test.

One gram of PABA-peptide (or 0.5 g PABA-peptide with 5 microcuries of C^{14}-PABA in a single-day test) is given with a standard meal (a Lundh meal or Carnation 'Instant Breakfast'); the bladder is emptied and the urine tested to exclude the presence of aromatic amines. Urine is then collected over the next 6 hours, encouraging urinary flow with a high fluid intake. The patient is allowed to eat a normal meal after 4 hours. A control test using PABA 1 g alone is performed the next day.

In the one-day test an aliquot of urine is counted in a scintillation counter to estimate the excretion of C^{14}-PABA. An excretion index is calculated as follows:

$$\text{Index} = \frac{\%\text{PABA excreted from PABA-peptide}}{\%\text{ Free PABA excreted on other day (or Free } C^{14}\text{-Labelled PABA)}} \times 100$$

Interpretation of results

A PABA excretion index of greater than 82% is considered normal. When compared with the secretin-CCK test the sensitivity varies from 52–74%, suggesting that many patients with mild pancreatic insufficiency are not detected [15]. The sensitivity or specificity of the test could be increased by choosing a higher (to increase sensitivity), or lower (to increase specificity) ratio for the excretion index.

As the PABA test is dependent upon the same extra-pancreatic factors as the Lundh test, false positive results can occur under the same circumstances.

Advantages and disadvantages

The PABA test is easy to do, acceptable to patients, shows a good correlation with the Lundh test and is very reproducible (coefficient of variation = 10%). It can be used to follow the progress of pancreatic disease and to monitor the effectiveness of replacement therapy [8].

The major disadvantage is drug or isotopic interference with the measurements, which can result in an unsatisfactory test in up to 12% of cases. The one-day test is unsuitable for children or pregnant women.

The fluorescein dilaurate test

Fluorescein dilaurate is a specific substrate for pancreatic aryl esterase. The principle of the test is similar to that of the PABA test, with fluorescein being excreted in the urine. Unesterified fluorescein is given on a separate day to correct for handling problems [3].

Technique

The test is performed after fasting and avoidance of pancreatic supplements and vitamin B preparations, which interfere with fluorescein measurements, for at least 4 days. A capsule containing 0.5 mmol fluorescein dilaurate (0.5 mmol fluorescein alone on control day) is given with a continental breakfast. The bladder is emptied and urine collected over the next 10 hours. Free fluids and a normal lunch (5 hours later) are given. Urinary fluorescein is measured by spectrophotometry at 492 nm and an excretion index calculated from:

$$\text{Index} = \frac{\text{Fluoroscein excretion on 'control' day}}{\text{Fluoroscein excretion on test day}} \times 100$$

Interpretation

An excretion index of 30% or more is regarded as 'normal'. Values below 20% are abnormal and those in between should have the test repeated—if still less than 30% the test can be assumed to be abnormal. Compared with secretin-CCK test the sensitivity is 100% with a high predictive value as false negative tests are extremely rare [4]. There is a high false positive rate with the same causes as for the Lundh test.

Advantages and disadvantages

The test is easy to do and measurements are simple with little interference. There are no contraindications. The high negative predictive value means that it is a good screening test—only abnormal results need further investigation. It can be used to follow progress of disease.

The test has been criticized for its low specificity [13]. It has been suggested that the test assesses the combined functional efficacy of secreted esterase and bile salts, rather than pancreatic function *per se*.

The place of pancreatic function tests in diagnosis and management of pancreatic disease

It is apparent that no one test is entirely satisfactory in differentiating patients with and without pancreatic disease. Pancreatic function tests may have a high predictive value when abnormal, but may fail to show any abnormality with small tumours or 'early' pancreatitis demonstrated at pancreatography.

References

1 AMMANN RW, AKOVBIANTZ A, HACKI W, LARGIADER F, SCHMIDT M. Diagnostic value of the faecal chymotrypsin test in pancreatic insufficiency, particularly chronic pancreatitis: correlation with the pancreozymin-secretin test. *Digestion* 1981;21:281–289.
2 AMMANN RW, TAGWERCHER E, KASHIWAGI H, ROSENMUND H. Diagnostic value of faecal chymotrypsin and trypsin assessment for detection of pancreatic disease. *Am J Dig Dis* 1968;13:123–146.
3 BARRY RE, BARRY R, ENE MD, PARKER G. Fluorescein dilaurate—tubeless test for pancreatic exocrine failure. *Lancet* 1982;ii:742–744.
4 BOYD EJS, CUMMING JGR, CUSCHIERI A, WOOD RAB, WORMSLEY KG. A prospective comparison of the fluorescein-dilaurate test with the secretin-CCK test for pancreatic exocrine function. *J Clin Path* 1982;35:1240–1243.
5 DENYER ME, COTTON PB. Pure pancreatic juice studies in normal subjects and patients with chronic pancreatitis. *Gut* 1979;20:97–98.
6 FARINI R, NITTI D, DEL FAVERO G, *et al.* CEA concentration and cytology in duodenal fluid collected during the secretin-pancreozymin test. *Hepato-Gastroenterol* 1980;27:213–216.
7 FEDAIL SS, HARVEY RF, SALMON PR, BROWN P, READ AE. Trypsin and lactoferrin levels in pure pancreatic juice in patients with pancreatic disease. *Gut* 1979;20:983–986.
8 FRIC P, MALIS F, KASAFIREK E, SLABY J. A new method of testing pancreatin therapy in vivo by the use of a peroral chymotrypsin substrate 4-N-acetyl-L-tyrosyl amino-benzoic acid. *Hepato-Gastroenterol* 1980;27:220–223.
9 GOLDBERG DM, SALE JK, FAWCETT N, WORMSLEY KG. Trypsin and chymotrypsin as aids in the diagnosis of pancreatic disease. *Am J Dig Dis* 1972;17:780–791.

10 GULLO L, COSTA PL, FONTANA G, LABO G. Investigation of exocrine pancreatic function by continuous infusion of cerulein and secretin in normal subjects and patients with chronic pancreatitis. *Digestion* 1976;**14:**97–107.

11 JAMES O. Progress report: The Lundh test. *Gut* 1973;**14:**582–591.

12 KAWANISHI H, SELL JE, POLLARD HM. Carcinoembryonic antigen and cytology of pancreatic fluid. *Gastroenterology* 1975;**68:**1033.

13 KAY G, HINE P, BRAGANZA J. The pancreolauryl test. A method of assessing the combined functional efficacy of pancreatic esterase and bile salts in vivo. *Digestion* 1982;**24:**241–245.

14 KIM, DK, SCHWARTZ MK, SHERLOCK P. The two-stage provocative test for pancreatic disease by serum enzyme measurements. *Surg Gynecol Obstet* 1980;**150** :49–53.

15 LANKISCH PG, ERHARDT-SCHMELZER S, KOOP H, CASPARY WF. Das NBT-PABA Test in der Diagnostik der exokrinen Pancreasinsuffizienz: ein Vergleich mit dem Sekretin-Pancreozymin Test, den Stuhlenzym-Bestimmungen und der quantitativen Stuhlfett-Analyse. *Dtsch Med Wschr* 1980;**105:**1418–1423.

16 LAKE-BAKAAR G, MCKAVANAGH S, REDSHAW M, WOOD T, SUMMERFIELD JA, ELIAS E. Serum immunoreactive trypsin concentration after a Lundh meal: Its value in the diagnosis of pancreatic disease. *J Clin Path* 1979;**32:**1003–1008.

17 LoGIUDICE JA, GEENEN JE, HOGAN WJ, DODDS WJ. Efficacy of the morphine-prostigmin test for evaluating patients with suspected papillary stenosis. *Dig Dis Sci* 1979;**24:**455–458.

18 MACKIE CR, COOPER MJ, LEWIS MH, MOOSA AR. Non-operative differentiation between pancreatic cancer and chronic pancreatitis. *Ann Surg* 1979;**189:**480–487.

19 MITCHELL CJ, HUMPHREY CS, BULLEN AW, KELLEHER J. Improved diagnostic accuracy of a modified oral pancreatic function test. *Scand J Gastroenterol* 1979;**14:**734–741.

20 MOLNAR, IG, VANDERVOORDE, JP, GITNICK, GJ, CEA levels in fluids bathing gastrointestinal tumours. *Gastroenterology.* 1976; **70:** 513–515.

21 MULLER L, WISNIEWSKI ZS, HANSKY J. The measurement of faecal chymotrypsin: a screening test for pancreatic exocrine insufficiency. *Aust Ann Med* 1970;**19:**47–49.

22 MULTIGNER L, FIGARELLA C, SARLES H. Diagnosis of chronic pancreatitis by measurement of lactoferrin in duodenal juice. *Gut* 1981;**22:**350–354.

23 NIEBURGS HE, DREILING DA, RUBIO C, REISMAN H. The morphology of cells in duodenal drainage smears: histologic origin and pathologic significance. *Am J Dig Dis* 1962;**7:**489–505.

24 REGAN PT, DiMAGNO EP. Exocrine pancreatic insufficiency in coeliac sprue: a cause of treatment failure. *Gastroenterology* 1980;**78:**484–487.

25 RUDELL WSJ, MITCHELL CJ, HAMINTON I, LEEK JP, KELLEHER J. Clinical value of serum immunoreactive trypsin concentration. *Br Med J* 1981;ii:1429–1431.

26 SAUNDERS JHB, DRUMMOND S, WORMSLEY KG. Inhibition of gastric secretion in treatment of pancreatic insufficiency. *Br Med J* 1977;i:478–479.

27 TETLOW VA, LOBLEY RW, HERMAN K, BRAGANZA J, A one-day pancreatic function test using a chymotrypsin-labile peptide and a radioactive marker. *Clin Trials J* 1980;**17:**121–130.

28 VALETINI M, CAVALLINI G, VANTINI I, *et al.* A comparative evaluation of endoscopic retrograde pancreatography and the secretin-cholecystokinin test in the diagnosis of chronic pancreatitis: a multicentre study in 124 patients. *Endoscopy* 1981;**13:**64–67.

29 WORMSLEY KG The response to infusion of a combination of secretin and pancreozymin in health and disease. *Scand J Gastroenterol* 1969;**4:**623–632.

30 WORMSLEY KG. Tests of pancreatic secretion. *Clin Gastroenterol* 1978;**7:**529–544.

Chapter 35
Acute Pancreatitis

M. J. McMAHON

Introduction

In 1925 Sir Berkeley Moynihan wrote 'acute pancreatitis is the most terrible of all calamities that occur in connection with the abdominal viscera. The suddenness of its onset, the illimitable agony which accompanies it and the mortality attendant upon it render it the most formidable of catastrophies' [12, 67].

This description remains true today, although we now recognize many more patients with less severe disease. There is still no specific treatment, but knowledge of aetiology and pathogenesis has advanced somewhat. In the last decade there have been advances in management of the early phases of an attack, but improved survival has not been achieved as many patients still die from the complications. In many patients with severe pancreatitis the pancreas is irreversibly damaged by the time treatment starts. Important aspects of management are control of the early shock-like illness, and anticipation, recognition and treatment of the serious local complications. There is no place for therapeutic nihilism in this disease, because patients who survive, even after prolonged hospitalization, usually return to a very acceptable quality of life.

Definition

Acute pancreatitis is an acute inflammation of the pancreas, characterized by upper abdominal pain with raised concentrations of pancreatic enzymes in blood and urine. It differs from chronic pancreatitis in that it is not associated with continuing pancreatic inflammation or irreversible morphological changes causing pain and/or loss of function.

Clearly some patients with chronic disease present with recurrent acute attacks. These are best regarded as 'acute' attacks, although further investigation is clearly required once the episode has subsided (see Chapters 36 and 37). These definitions differ from the traditional Marseilles classification [70] as the term 'relapsing pancreatitis' has been omitted.

Epidemiology

Prevalence (Table 35.1)

As there is no universally accepted definition of acute pancreatitis, collection of accurate prevalence data is difficult. In one study in England prevalence ranged from 32 to 389 cases per million in different districts [14]. The higher overall incidence in the United States and Scotland may reflect the greater incidence of alcohol-induced pancreatitis, in addition to other causes— for example, gallstones. One way to minimize the problem is to study only those with severe disease. Trapnel and Duncan [76] recorded in the Bristol area 6 to 12 deaths per million from acute pancreatitis, compared with 11.4 per million in England and Wales, during the same period. Statistics published by the Registrar General suggest that the disease is becoming commoner in the United Kingdom. (Fig. 35.1) [20].

499

Table 35.1. The prevalence of acute pancreatitis in different communities.

Location	Incidence per million of population (range gives data from different years)
Rochester, Minnesota, USA	100–115
Bristol Clinical Area, England [76]	32–79*
Nottingham, England [14]	21–83*
Glasgow, Scotland [30]	100

* Only first attacks of acute pancreatitis were included.

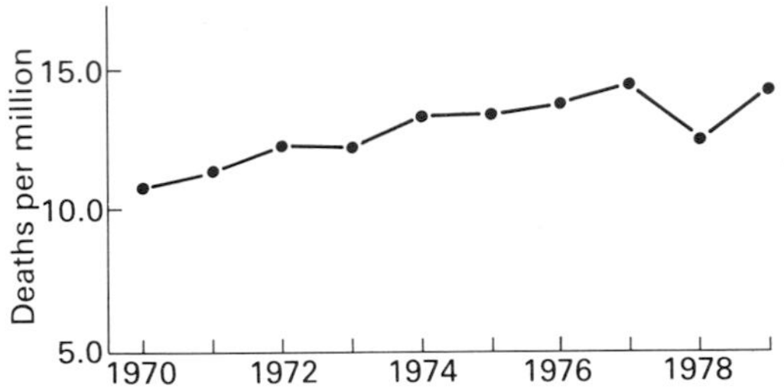

Fig 35.1. Annual death rate from acute pancreatitis in England and Wales.

Sex ratio

The sex ratio is affected by aetiology. In Bristol and Leeds where more than half of the attacks are associated with gallstones, the female-to-male ratios are 1.5:1 and 1.3:1 respectively. Although alcohol-induced pancreatitis is probably commoner in Glasgow than in England, 60% of attacks are associated with gallstone disease with a sex ratio of 1.3:1 [30]. By contrast, in one series from New York 74% of attacks were associated with ethanol and only 21% of the patients were women. The effect of alcohol on the sex ratio was shown in a longitudinal study from Gothenberg—between 1956–1960 68% of acute attacks were associated with gallstones and 47% of the patients were women; by 1974 66% of attacks of acute pancreatitis were associated with alcohol and only 23% occurred in women [74].

Age

Aetiology also influences the age distribution. The peak incidence of alcoholic pancreatitis is in the fifth decade, whereas pancreatitis associated with gallstones and other causes peaks in the seventh decade. Similar trends have been reported from North America where the peak age incidence of alcoholic pancreatitis was 44 years in New York [65] and 38 years in Atlanta [72]. In a multi-centre study of acute pancreatitis in the United Kingdom 57% of the patients were over 60 years [51]. It is important to consider the effect of age in reviews of mortality of acute pancreatitis of different types. Thus the death rate of gallstone-associated pancreatitis may be higher than that of alcoholic pancreatitis mainly because patients with gallstones are older.

Aetiology

Most cases of acute pancreatitis occur in association with gallstones or alcohol abuse. However an identifiable cause cannot be established in up to 30% of patients.

Alcohol

Abuse of alcohol is becoming increasingly important in the aetiology of acute pancreatitis in many countries [83]. In Sweden the association between ethanol and acute pancreatitis has risen from 14% to 66% during the last 20 years. In urban United States alcohol is the main aetiological factor in over 75% of patients.

All forms of intoxicating drinks appear capable of causing pancreatitis. It has been suggested that wine and spirits are more prone to do so than beer, but there is no evidence to confirm this. Most patients probably have chronic pancreatic damage underlying the acute episode. In most patients there is a history of alcohol consumption during the 48 hours before admission but the classical 'bender' probably precedes only a minority of acute attacks.

Alcoholic acute pancreatitis was believed to be the severest form of the disease with the highest mortality. In two large series [12, 31, 60] the mortality of alcoholic pancreatitis was less than that of pancreatitis caused by gallstones, operation, trauma or other unknown causes. This apparent change in the pattern of the disease may reflect different diagnostic criteria, different ages of the patients, a change in the disease itself, or greater success in managing the septic complications which appear more commonly in alcoholic pancreatitis.

How alcohol induces pancreatitis remains unclear. Possible mechanisms include a generalized action such as the solvent effect of ethanol upon cell components (causing interference with membrane potentials or active transport mechanisms), or a more specific effect upon pancreatic secretion (for example the deposition of protein as plugs within the minor ducts). Ethanol produces dose-related effects upon pancreatic secretion and can, under certain circumstances, result in an increase in enzyme secretion with a reduction in pancreatic protease inhibitor. This might result in premature enzyme activation within the pancreatic gland. Recent experimental work has suggested that zymogens may be activated by lysomal enzymes. A proportion of patients with alcoholic pancreatitis display hyperlipidaemia, this may result in the accumulation of free fatty acids which have a toxic effect upon the pancreas mediated by oxygen-derived free radicals.

Gallstones

The association between gallstones and acute haemorrhagic pancreatitis was beautifully illustrated by Opie [59] who described a case of fatal pancreatitis with a small stone impacted in the ampulla of Vater and intense bile staining of the pancreatic parenchyma. Over the intervening 85 years the association between gallstones and pancreatitis has been convincingly documented [6, 23]. Gallstones are six times more common in patients with pancreatitis than in the population at large [52]. In a later study gallstones were present in 56% of 179 autopsies for acute pancreatitis compared with only 22% out of 8,000 unselected post-mortems [9].

Further evidence is provided by the fate of patients who have undergone cholecystectomy. Of 160 patients undergoing cholecystectomy for gallstones 59 had one or more attacks of pancreatitis before operation but only seven (4%) had recurrent pancreatitis postoperatively over a seven-year follow-up period. Of these two had residual stones in the common bile duct, three had undergone a sphincterotomy and one was an alcoholic [29]. Similar reports have emerged from other centres.

The mechanism by which a gallstone causes acute pancreatitis remains unclear. Sieving the faeces of patients admitted with gallstone pancreatitis shows that gallstones are present in a high proportion of them, but not in patients with other clinical features of gallstone disease [1, 35]. It is now believed that acute pancreatitis arises when a gallstone becomes temporarily lodged in the ampulla of Vater. Supportive evidence for this has come from observations showing that such patients usually have rather wide patent cystic ducts and multiple small calculi in the gall bladder.

Most patients with gallstone-associated pancreatitis have a transient rise in plasma aspartate transaminase (AST) on presentation, this probably represents a temporary increase in common bile duct pressure [47].

Acute pancreatitis can be induced in animals by several agents injected into the pancreatic duct, which probably cause damage by a combination of chemical and physical effects. Toxic substances, such as infected bile, duodenal juice, or a combination of trypsin and enterokinase, induce severe pancreatitis when injected in small amounts at low pressure. However, even saline can cause pancreatitis if injected under sufficient pressure. The severity of the lesion is increased by ligation of the main duct or by stimulation of pancreatic secretion.

Conditions under which gallstones induce pancreatitis in man are difficult to simulate experimentally and it remains unclear how an impacted gallstone causes an attack. It is probable that a temporary obstruction of the pancreatic duct causes an increase in ductal pressure, oedema of the gland and leakage of enzymes into the circulation. Such changes, usually self-limiting, are found after ligation of the pancreatic duct in an animal. What determines the development of more severe pancreatitis remains unclear, but coexistent arterial disease, stimulation of secretion by food and drink, and retrograde flow of bile or bacteria along the pancreatic duct may all be involved. Some have argued in favour of duodenopancreatic reflux as an aetiological mechanism [42] but there is little evidence to support this theory in man.

Postoperative and traumatic pancreatitis

Postoperative pancreatitis accounts for about 6% of all episodes of acute pancreatitis [21], it most commonly follows gastric and biliary operations. Although the diagnosis often rests upon the finding of an inflamed or necrotic pancreas at re-laparotomy, or at post-mortem, it is diagnosed in some by the clinical features and a raised serum amylase [16]. Estimation of total serum amylase in the diagnosis of postoperative pancreatitis is unreliable as postoperatively hyperamylasaemia is often salivary in origin. The diagnosis of postoperative pancreatitis, in the absence of direct evidence, must rest on the demonstration of raised concentrations of pancreatic iso-amylase or lipase. The common cause is direct damage to the pancreas at operation, however, it can occur when the operation is remote from the pancreas [81]. One possible mechanism is pancreatic ischaemia due to hypotension during surgery.

Traumatic pancreatitis is associated with geographical variation. Blunt trauma from traffic accidents is the dominant cause in Europe while direct injury by a knife or bullet is more common in North America. The type and extent of the damage depends on the nature of the injury and the severity and mortality on the presence of other associated injuries [32, 84].

ERCP

ERCP can also cause acute pancreatitis. Hyperamylasaemia, with mild or relatively insignificant symptoms, is common after ERCP (in around 10% of patients) but severe pancreatitis only follows approximately 1% of examinations.

Other aetiological causes [21, 75]

There are many other causes of acute pancreatitis although all of these are relatively uncommon in clinical practice. It is important to exclude hyperparathyroidism and hyperlipidaemia and to recognize that pancreatic carcinoma can first present as acute pancreatitis, probably as a result of ductal obstruction. Many different drugs have also been implicated as causal agents [54] but evidence for many of these is circumstantial. There is mounting evidence to suggest that steroids, azothioprine and diuretics may cause acute pancreatitis.

Pathology

At laparotomy, in a mild case, a small amount of clear ascitic fluid with oedema of the fatty tissues around the pancreas and/or a swollen gland may be found. The characteristic white flecks of fat necrosis may also be seen (Fig. 35.2). In a severe attack there may be a large volume of dirty orange-brown peritoneal fluid ('prune juice' or 'motor oil'), marked oedema, haemorrhage and fat necrosis of the peripancreatic tissues with similar lesions at distant sites. Bruising may be apparent in the transverse mesocolon and the gland may be covered by haemorrhagic material, making the true extent of the necrosis difficult to determine.

If the patient survives the acute attack it is usual for the milder forms of pancreatitis to resolve completely. Areas of necrosis may form a sequestrum, with a relatively well-formed capsule consisting of the surrounding functioning pancreatic tissue, or form an abscess invading the peripancreatic tissues, particularly behind the duodenum, around the spleen, or within the mesentery.

Such abscesses are often sterile although they may later become secondarily infected. Necrosis involving the duct system can lead to a fluid collection, probably as a result of secretion leaking from a blocked main pancreatic duct. These are called pseudocysts as they have no epithelial lining. They can become very large and often extend outside the pancreas, commonly into the lesser sac, necrotic tissue is often present within the cyst.

Pathogenesis

Pathogenesis remains unclear [69]. It is generally assumed that autodigestion contributes to the lesions within the pancreas. The effect of the primary insult is to release activated pancreatic enzymes (trypsin, chymotrypsin, elastase, phospholipid A etc.) from the zymogen granules in the acinar cells. When locally released in amounts sufficient to overcome pancreatic protease inhibitors, which normally prevent activation until enzymes reach the duodenal lumen, the effect of these proteases is to accelerate and extend the damage within the pancreas in association with lipase and collagenase. Spasm and thrombosis of local blood vessels may be an important determinant of the extent and severity of the changes. Clinical

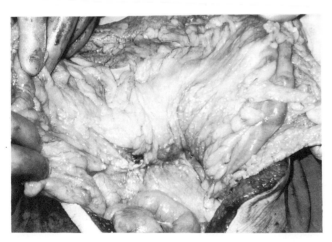

Fig 35.2. Specks of fat necrosis on the transverse mesocolon with oedema of the root of the mesentery.

evidence suggests that in most patients many of these changes are already established by the time treatment is started.

Raised concentrations of the proteolytic enzymes in the plasma occur in acute pancreatitis. This rise is usually confined to the zymogen form or a complex of the active enzyme with an inhibitor such as alpha$_1$-protease inhibitor. There is little direct evidence to suggest that free proteases circulate in active pancreatitis, although enhanced esterolytic activity has been demonstrated in the plasma of patients with pancreatitis and up to 30% of alpha$_2$-macroglobulin (the most potent and important circulating anti-protease) is complexed with trypsin in severe cases. Under normal circumstances activated proteases are rapidly complexed with alpha$_2$-macroglobulin, which is then cleared by the reticulo-endothelial system. The existence of such complexes is important because, although the enzyme can no longer hydrolyse its normal substrate, it may still retain the capacity to digest smaller peptide fragments. The possibility exists that in pancreatitis the reticulo-endothelial system is overwhelmed and clearance of complexes is delayed. Despite a recent vogue for antiproteinase therapy plasma reserves of alpha$_2$-macroglobulin are not exhausted in severe pancreatitis, even though they may fall to approximately half the normal concentrations [45].

What then causes the acute shock-like illness which can so rapidly lead to multi-organ failure in severe pancreatitis? There is increasing evidence to suggest that the agents causing these effects are produced within the peritoneal cavity, probably as a result of proteolytic activity within the enzyme-rich fluid that exudes from the pancreas. It takes time for alpha$_2$-macroglobulin to enter the peritoneal cavity in sufficient quantities to inhibit these enzymes, and even longer for the complexes formed to be cleared by intraperitoneal macrophages. There is, therefore, uninhibited proteolytic digestion within the peritoneal cavity, making peritoneal lavage and intraperitoneal antiprotease therapy logical treatments in acute pancreatitis.

Clinical features

Most patients have abdominal pain, usually continuous, although it can be colicky, centred in the epigastrium and right hypochondrium; in some 50% of patients the pain radiates into the back. Vomiting is frequent (75%) and diarrhoea, or haematemesis and melaena may occasionally occur. Prodromal symptoms of mild non-specific upper abdominal pain are not unusual.

Although the above symptoms are typical, an occasional patient, particularly in the older age group, may present with collapse and hyperglycaemia but without any pain.

Examination

Pain is usually obvious and severe and there may be a mild pyrexia—usually $< 38.5°C$. Clinically the patient may appear shocked. Tachycardia and peripheral vasodilation may be present but hypotension is infrequent. Epigastric and right hypochondrial areas may be tender to palpation and guarding is usual; occasionally generalized tenderness and rigidity are present. Some patients may be jaundiced and occasionally a mass may be palpable. Oliguria, though frequently regarded as an ominous sign, is usually pre-renal in origin. Tetany is rare, even though hypocalcaemia is common. Respiratory distress is common in severe pancreatitis, but may not be obvious until two or three days after admission. Other features that can appear at a later stage are mental confusion, particularly in the elderly patient, ascites, pleural effusions and intestinal ileus.

Diagnosis

It is important to bear in mind the protean manifestations of acute pancreatitis and to maintain a high index of suspicion. Plasma amylase concentration is a reliable diagnostic indicator and should be measured in anyone where the slightest suspicion exists, even when presentation is atypical.

The initial clinical features of pancreatitis are often a poor indicator of prognosis and half of severe attacks may appear relatively mild at the start [48]. The true severity of the attack may only become apparent a day or so later. Although local complications are more likely if the attack is severe on presentation they can complicate apparently mild attacks. Local complications (for example pseudocyst, abscess, necrosis) usually become apparent two or more weeks after the patient's admission [78]. The characteristic features are continuing or recurrent pyrexia, abdominal distension, an abdominal mass, hypotension, pneumonia, pleural effusion, or increasing multi-organ failure. With an abscess or pancreatic necrosis the toxic element predominates, but in patients with a pseudocyst an abdominal mass may be the only finding.

Investigations

Laboratory studies

Acute pancreatitis is associated with many laboratory abnormalities related to pancreatic [13], renal, hepatic or pulmonary function and coagulation disorders. Monitoring of these variables is necessary for correction of complications.

Since the original observations of Arnesen and Graham in 1929, the measurement of **serum amylase** has been the cornerstone of the diagnosis of acute pancreatitis. The pancreas produces a large number of enzymes but amylase and lipase [28, 39] have diagnostic advantages as they are not rapidly cleared by specific inhibitors. There is no specific discriminatory concentration of either enzyme which reliably provides an accurate diagnosis; if it is set high, specificity is good but sensitivity is poor and vice versa. A working definition of acute pancreatitis is a combination of suggestive clinical features with a **plasma amylase** or **lipase concentration** which is more than 10 standard deviations above the normal mean (five times upper limit of normal). Only a small proportion of patients with acute pancreatitis will be missed using these criteria [44]. Technical difficulties have limited lipase assays in the past, but reliable techniques are now available which may offer improved sensitivity and greater specificity than estimations of serum amylase.

Spurious elevations of amylase and lipase can result from a leak of upper gastrointestinal contents into the peritoneum (for example from a perforation or biliary peritonitis), and after intestinal infarction. Electrophoretic separation of the salivary and pancreatic amylase isoenzymes is too cumbersome for routine use but a simple assay based upon the selective inhibition of salivary isoenzyme by an inhibitor from wheat germ (Phadebas Isoamylase Test) has recently become available. Estimations of urinary amylase are not diagnostically superior to measurements of this enzyme in the serum. The amylase/creatinine clearance ratio is probably neither specific, nor sensitive enough for the diagnosis of acute pancreatitis [49]. There is no evidence to suggest that the measurement of immunoreactive trypsin in plasma provides any information additional to that obtained from the simpler assays of amylase or lipase.

Unfortunately serum enzyme levels may fall rapidly after the onset of acute pancreatitis, making the diagnosis difficult by biochemical techniques if more than 48 hours have elapsed. Blood for estimation of serum amylase should therefore be drawn as soon as possible after the patient's arrival in the hospital if the diagnosis of acute pancreatitis is suspected.

Detection of **hypocalcaemia** is the only other laboratory investigation which is in anyway specific for acute pancreatitis. Low serum calcium concentrations usually occur after severe attacks, the nadir being reached some five days after admission.

Other characteristic laboratory findings are an increased haematocrit, polymorph leucocytosis, raised urea and glucose and a fall in plasma phosphate and albumin. The magnitude of these changes is generally related to the severity of the attack. Gallstone induced pancreatitis is suggested by a plasma aspartate transaminase >60 i.u./l [11, 38, 47]. Jaundice occurs in 12–30% of patients with pancreatitis [15] from either a stone, ductal narrowing by pancreatic swelling, hepato-renal failure or from sepsis. In the majority it resolves spontaneously and only rarely is it an indication for operation.

A **pseudocyst** is associated with persistent hyperamylasaemia and necrosis-abscess is suggested by a pyrexia, leucocytosis or the presence of multi-organ failure. A persistent elevation of pancreatic iso-amylase [17], leucocytosis, or C-reactive protein [45] in someone who appears to be settling, suggests that a pseudocyst or even an abscess is developing.

In severe pancreatitis a **falling arterial oxygen tension** may indicate the onset of pulmonary insufficiency. This is thought to occur through an impairment of diffusion across the alveolar membrane as a result of oedema or toxic damage. It is important to check that oxygen therapy elevates the pO_2 to a satisfactory level as an occasional patient may need positive pressure ventilation.

Patients with severe pancreatitis may develop a **coagulopathy** manifested by a rise in fibrinogen, platelets, fibrinogen related antigen and an impairment of euglobulin lysis time [62].

A rise in plasma urea may indicate renal tubular necrosis, but is more commonly due to hypovolaemia.

Radiology and imaging

Plain X-rays of the abdomen and chest have little diagnostic value but may be useful in management. An erect chest film may show a large pleural effusion, which suggests a severe attack [50] although slight effusions are common with mild attacks.

Ultrasonography can be useful particularly when the plasma amylase level is not diagnostic. Gall bladder visualization can be difficult in the early stages of the disease but is nevertheless worthwhile in order to search for gallstones. The early appearance of a pancreatic mass suggests that a pseudocyst may follow [43]. Ultrasonography is particularly useful in diagnosing and monitoring pancreatic collections and should be repeated, at least weekly, in appropriate patients.

Despite the simplicity and reliability of ultrasound in the detection of fluid collections, it can be misleading in patients who have an abscess or necrosis. **Computerized tomography** (CT) provides more reliable information in such circumstances (Fig 35.3) [58, 62]. It is the author's preference to request a CT scan before surgery on all patients with pancreatic collections.

Radionuclide pancreatic scintiscanning has no role in the management of acute pancreatitis.

Endoscopic retrograde cholangio-pancreatography (ERCP) may be useful in acute pancreatitis. It must be used with circumspection, as ERCP can induce pancreatitis or introduce infection into a pancreatic cyst. This examination may demonstrate gallstones or a chronically diseased gallbladder previously missed [26]. When a pancreatic pseudocyst or pancreatic ascites is present ERCP can demonstrate the site of leakage from, or blockage of, the main

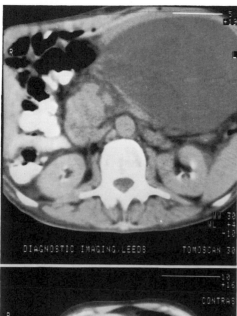

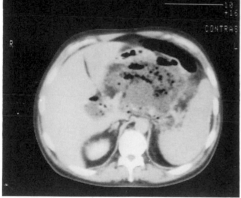

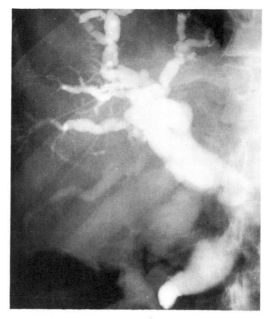

Fig 35.4. Percutaneous transhepatic cholangiography in a patient who developed obstructive jaundice after acute pancreatitis. The duct was obstructed by an ampullary neoplasm (courtesy of Dr J. Hogan).

Fig. 35.3. Computerized tomography scan of a large fluid filled pseudocyst (top) and pancreatic abscess in front of lumbar vertebra (bottom). Note the presence of numerous gas-filled spaces (courtesy of Dr P. J. Robinson).

pancreatic duct. This is useful in determining the need for pancreatic resection or distal duct drainage [26, 33, 57]. It is probably a reasonable policy to request ERCP in all patients with acute pancreatitis who do not have gallstones as the cause of the attack.

The development of jaundice during or after an attack of acute pancreatitis may indicate the need for **percutaneous cholangiography** (Fig. 35.4) or ERCP with endoscopic sphincterotomy if gallstones are present in the common bile duct.

Assessment of the severity of acute pancreatitis

Experimental studies suggest that the outcome of an attack of acute pancreatitis is improved by early treatment. Urgent treatment of severe pancreatitis might therefore improve the prognosis. Unfortunately severe pancreatitis can masquerade as a mild disease during the early phase [48]. Many attempts have thus been made to improve the recognition of a severe attack at the outset. There is some correlation between the severity of an attack and the abnormalities found in laboratory tests, for this reason such tests have been used to formulate prognostic systems [19].

Of particular importance is **methaemalbumin,** which is produced by a complex between haem and albumin. The detection of any methaemalbumin in plasma or peritoneal fluid suggests a severe attack of

Table 35.2. Multiple criteria for the prediction of severe acute pancreatitis. If three or more criteria are positive, the attack is predicted to be severe.

Reference [63]*	[30]*
On admission	*During the first 48 hours*
Age > 55 years	Age > 55 years
Blood glucose > 11.0 mmol	Serum albumin < 32 g/l
White cell count > 16 × 10⁹/l	Serum calcium < 2.0 mmol/l
S.G.O.T. (A.S.T.) > 120 i.u/l	White cell count > 15 × 19⁹/l
L.D.H. > 350 i.u./l	S.G.O.T. (A.S.T) > 100 i.u/l
	L.D.H. > 600 i.u./l
During the first 48 hours	Blood glucose > 10 mmol/l
Fall in haematocrit > 10%	Blood urea > 16 mmol/l
Serum calcium < 2.0 mmol/l	Arterial PO₂ < 7.5 kPa
Base deficit > 4.0 mmol/l	
Rise in blood urea > 1.0 mmol/l	
Fluid sequestration > 6l	
Arterial PO₂ < 7.5 kPa	

*Both systems have been modified to make them more suitable for patients with pancreatitis due to gallstones.

pancreatitis [15]. Unfortunately it may not appear until 24–48 hours after admission, by which stage the severity of the attack is already clinically apparent.

Prognostic systems using multiple laboratory criteria have been developed by several groups [3, 30, 63] (Table 35.2). The attack is likely to be severe if three or more of the variables reach a prescribed limit within 48 hours of admission. Although the correlation between such systems and severity is undisputed, it remains unclear whether they tell the doctor anything more than can be gathered by a careful clinical assessment of the patient [82].

Patients with severe pancreatitis frequently have 'prune juice' coloured peritoneal fluid, and it has been shown that the colour of the peritoneal fluid aspirated, before and after lavage with a litre of saline, can provide useful prognostic information. If more than 20 ml of free fluid is present, or if the colour of it or the lavage fluid reaches diagnostic limits (Fig. 35.5) then the attack is severe. This test appears to provide a more accurate prediction of the

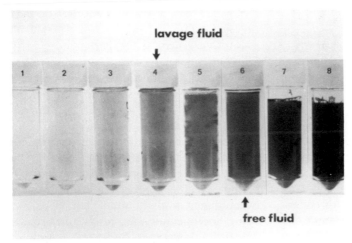

Fig. 35.5. Black and white photograph of a colour chart used to grade peritoneal fluid and lavage fluid for the prediction of severity. The arrows indicate the minimum colour for the prediction of severe pancreatitis (by permission of *British Journal of Surgery:* [47]).

shock-like illness than clinical examination within six hours of admission [46].

Differential diagnosis

This includes most other causes of the acute abdomen. Principal amongst these are **perforated peptic ulcer, biliary colic, acute cholecystitis and mesenteric infarction**. The diagnosis rests on the hyperamylasaemia. Unfortunately in some of these conditions the serum amylase may rise, although it is unusual for it to be over 1,000 i.u./l. In the author's experience only about 2% of patients with clinically apparent acute pancreatitis have an alternative intra-abdominal cause. Peritoneal lavage with saline may also reveal the diagnostic error by the appearance or odour of the fluid retrieved (in pancreatitis, the fluid is odourless and bacteria are barely seen on microscopy).

The diagnosis of acute pancreatitis should always be considered in patients admitted with **hypothermia or diabetic coma**. Pancreatitis can also occasionally mimic left ventricular failure due to myocardial infarction.

Prevention

This depends on prevention of diseases that cause acute pancreatitis. Abstinence from alcohol is important as is early surgery in those with gallstones.

Medical treatment

Management of the acute attack

Many treatments have been proposed for acute pancreatitis but few have been subjected to adequate clinical trials. Most studies have failed to differentiate between attacks of different severity. As most patients with mild pancreatitis will recover irrespective of treatment it is only in severe attacks that therapy is critical. An adequate trial needs to include at least 150 patients with severe pancreatitis to reach significant conclusions, and is therefore not easily achieved. Thus most of the measures used in acute pancreatitis are based on clinical common sense, or physiological principles, but have not been proved.

The mild attack

Treatment is aimed at the correction of abnormalities present on admission.

Pain is a dominant symptom, its severity is often remembered for many years, and a strong analgesic, such as pethidine (100–150 mg) should be given. Morphine causes spasm of the sphincter of Oddi and an elevation of plasma amylase—it is better avoided. Recently it has been shown that the additional use of indomethacin may reduce the amount of opiate analgesics required [22].

Vomiting is frequent in pancreatitis and the insertion of a nasogastric tube is an important aspect of management although there is no evidence that its presence affects the progress of the disease. Intravenous crystalloid solutions are adequate fluid replacement in mild cases, although the dangers of sodium overload in the elderly must be remembered.

These measures will suffice in most patients with a mild attack. As the patient's condition improves the nasogastric tube can be removed and oral fluid started. It is important to remember that an attack that seems mild on admission may worsen considerably during the first 48 hours.

Pharmacological treatment of acute pancreatitis

Enzyme inhibitors

If the manifestations of acute pancreatitis are due to circulating pancreatic enzymes it is logical to use intravenous inhibitors in treatment. The most widely used is an anti-kallikrein prepared from bovine lung (aprotinin–'Trasylol'). Aprotinin has been tested in a number of carefully conducted clinical trials with conflicting results. Trapnell, *et al.* [77] concluded that treatment with aprotinin significantly reduced mortality in acute pancreatitis, but two further studies failed to show this [30, 53]. As recent data suggests that in pancreatitis there is no overall deficiency of circulating anti-proteases it is not surprising that aprotinin did not have a dramatic effect. A more logical approach would be to put the anti-protease directly into the peritoneal cavity but trials to test this hypothesis are incomplete at the time of writing.

Anticholinergic drugs

Anticholinergics, such as atropine and propantheline, have been used in the treatment of acute pancreatitis for many years. They have not been shown to influence the outcome of acute pancreatitis and, because of unwanted side-effects, their continued use cannot be justified.

Inhibitors of pancreatic secretion

Glucagon, somatostatin, calcitonin, carbonic anhydrase inhibitors, vasopressin and isoprenaline all inhibit pancreatic secretion. All have been suggested as therapeutic agents. Calcitonin, glucagon and somatostatin have been tested in clinical trials but have not been shown to have any useful effect [53]. On present knowledge there would seem to be no rational basis for their use.

Oral enzyme supplementation

Evidence is emerging that pancreatic exocrine function is impaired for several weeks after an acute attack of pancreatitis [51].

Taken in conjunction with the observation that a small proportion of patients suffer recurrent attacks when they start to eat food it is possible that oral enzyme supplements may have a role during the convalescent phase. In animals the presence of intra-duodenal trypsin inhibits pancreatic enzyme secretion and the use of an effective pancreatic enzyme preparation in man might have a similar effect.

Antibiotics

There is no evidence that bacterial infection is important to the pathogenesis of acute pancreatitis. It is difficult, therefore, to justify the use of antibiotics unless septic complications have developed. Certainly there is no support for their use from therapeutic trials.

The management of the severe attack

Early treatment

Clearly such patients require the same initial treatment as those with a mild attack but additional measures are also required.

Oxygen

Oxygen will be required if the pO_2 level is low. The response to treatment should be monitored by repeated blood gas measurements—if there is no response positive pressure ventilation may be indicated. Pulmonary oedema can occur very readily in severe pancreatitis; fluid overload may exacerbate it and must be avoided.

Fluid replacement

In severe pancreatitis albumin is lost from the circulation into the peritoneal cavity through leaking capillary beds. This results in hypoalbuminaemia and a loss of fluid from the circulation. Restoration of blood volumes with large amounts of crystalloids will result in severe oedema. Adequate treatment requires regular monitoring of plasma volume by measurement of central venous pressure or, in extreme cases, by the use of a Swan-Ganz catheter in the pulmonary artery. The author prefers to replace the plasma volume with fresh frozen plasma or plasma protein fraction, and to provide sufficient intravenous fluid to cover other fluid losses from the body. It has recently been suggested [18] that fresh frozen plasma may confer certain specific advantages through its content of proteinase inhibitors, but large quantities of plasma or albumin should be avoided to minimize the danger of pulmonary oedema.

Diuretics

Catheterization of the bladder enables an accurate record of hourly urinary output to be determined providing useful information on the adequacy of peripheral perfusion. Diuretics should only be given to patients who were on them prior to admission. Most patients with oliguria produce a diuretic response once the hypovolaemia is corrected and adequate perfusion restored. Patients with pancreatitis can sustain proximal tubular damage and it is illogical to compound this by using a proximal tubular poison such as frusemide. An exception to this rule is the treatment of fluid overload with diuretics. Diuretic therapy of the pulmonary oedema associated with acute pancreatitis appears to be ineffective. It is more convenient to control fluid balance by peritoneal dialysis rather than with diuretics.

Peritoneal lavage

The accumulation of an enzyme-rich ascitic fluid in the peritoneal cavity probably plays an important part in the pathogenesis of the shock-like phase of acute pancreatitis.

For this reason peritoneal lavage has been advocated in the treatment of this condition [79]. Unfortunately most reports of the treatment, although favourable, have been anecdotal. A small controlled trial suggested that it might prevent death during the initial phase, but did not protect patients from the later septic complications of the disease [63]. Another trial, using 24–hour peritoneal lavage in alcoholic pancreatitis showed improved overall survival [72] but this has not been confirmed in a large multi-centre trial in 79 patients with severe acute pancreatitis, [41], although a minority of the patients had pancreatitis due to alcohol abuse. Nevertheless, some patients show marked improvement after lavage and further evaluation is needed.

TECHNIQUE

Peritoneal lavage should be used as therapy in patients with 'prune juice' peritoneal fluid. This can be done using standard dialysis fluid (for example 'Dialyflex', Boots plc) with 4 mmol of added potassium per litre. Two litres of this fluid are run into the peritoneal cavity through a dialysis cannula and allowed to remain for 20 minutes, before draining. Lavage is repeated at hourly intervals for 24 hours, or if the returned fluid remains prune coloured until this clears. Hyperosmolar peritoneal lavage may be used if fluid overload develops.

An added advantage is that peritoneal lavage can be used to treat associated renal failure. This is usually detected by a rising blood urea and creatinine in a patient whose hypovolaemia has been adequately corrected. The occasional patient may also need haemodialysis.

Diabetes

It is unusual for patients with severe pancreatitis to need insulin. If severe glucose intolerance develops insulin requirements are usually modest, unless septic complications occur.

Calcium

Although hypocalcaemia is common in severe pancreatitis, treatment is rarely necessary. Usually there is an intense renal conservation of calcium and only small doses (10 mmol calcium gluconate) are required to correct deficiency.

Later treatment

Nutritional support

Patients who are successfully resuscitated from a severe attack and then develop late complications rapidly become malnourished [10]. This may be an important determinant of outcome. Intravenous nutrition should be given if oral nutrition has not been restored by 6 to 10 days after admission, and continued until an adequate oral intake is possible. Despite the pancreatic lesion glucose intolerance is not usually a problem unless sepsis occurs. Feeding through a fine-bore nasogastric tube, or jejunostomy, is not usually appropriate. Some patients, whose initial attack is mild, may resist attempts to re-introduce feeding because of a recurrence of pain or nausea and hyperamylasaemia. This may be due to a return of pancreatic inflammation or to inflammation of the antrum or duodenum. It is clearly important to screen such patients with ultrasound and CT scanning, for a pancreatic collection. Intravenous feeding may be required for as long as 8 to 10 weeks in the occasional patient. With such a drawn out illness there is always the temptation to intervene surgically, particularly if gallstones are present. This must be resisted unless a specific complication such as abscess or pseudocyst is identified.

Management of the convalescent patient

There are few specific measures that are required at this stage. It is traditional to advise a low fat diet but there is no conclusive evidence of benefit from this regime. If gallstones are present these should be removed as soon as the patient is fit enough [40]. The problems of managing chronic alcoholism are beyond the scope of this text although it is clear that further alcohol should be avoided.

The most important aspect is to search for a cause for the attack and to treat it as appropriate (for example—removal of a parathyroid tumour). It is probably advisable to request ERCP for all patients in whom a definite cause for the attack has not been found. It is unnecessary to carry out a glucose tolerance test unless fasting hyperglycaemia is present. Even patients who recover from an extensive pancreatic necrosis seldom need long-term treatment for malabsorption or diabetes mellitus. Measurement of the percentage of glycosolated haemoglobin present in the blood can be a useful way of detecting the presence intermittent hyperglycaemia during follow-up. A level of over 7% may provide an early warning of diabetes.

Surgical treatment

Attitudes to early surgical intervention in acute pancreatitis vary but analysis of the results from different geographical areas suggest that early surgery does not increase survival [4, 8, 55].

If the diagnosis of acute pancreatitis is first made at laparotomy and the attack is mild no action is required [23]. If gallstones are present an opportunity exists to remove the gallbladder [37]. Whether this should be done is difficult to say, but the author prefers to leave the biliary tract alone unless the attack is very mild. If severe pancreatitis with necrosis and haemorrhage is present surgical treatment should be limited to the insertion of drains into the pelvis and paracolic gutters for subsequent peritoneal lavage. Lesser sac drainage has been advocated, but there is no objective evidence that it is necessary. It is possible to argue in favour of transduodenal sphincterotomy or exploration of the common bile duct if the biliary tract is engorged and tense, but it is probably better to leave well alone unless an experienced biliary surgeon is present.

There are two areas where surgery certainly plays an important role. The first is gallstones where, despite claims for endoscopic sphincterotomy, most patients will need a cholecystectomy. The second is in the management of local complications of pancreatitis which do not resolve spontaneously.

Management of gallstones after acute pancreatitis [23]

The traditional approach is to allow the attack of pancreatitis to resolve and to carry out cholecystectomy, with exploration of the common bile duct if indicated, at a later date. The disadvantage of this approach is that nearly half of these patients may have a further attack of acute pancreatitis before elective cholecystectomy [40]. It has become increasingly apparent that most patients with gallstones and pancreatitis can safely undergo cholecystectomy during the same admission. Exploration of the common bile duct is only indicated if preoperative cholangiography reveals stones in the duct. A recent study has confirmed that residual stones in the bile duct are a common cause of recurrent pancreatitis after cholecystectomy [36]. If the attack is severe, it is probably sensible to wait until serum biochemistry has returned to normal before undertaking cholecystectomy.

The concept that the surgical approach should be directed at the stone provoking the acute attack of pancreatitis has been widely advocated [2, 73]. It is argued that reducing the time a stone is impacted in the region of the papilla of Vater and the early establishment of free biliary drainage will arrest progress of the pancreatic lesion. In favour of this is the observation that the severity of the pancreatic lesion is correlated with the duration of ampullary obstruction [2]. There is one randomized study comparing the results of surgery within 72 hours of admission with those of operation three months later [73]. All patients underwent cholecystectomy, transduodenal sphinteroplasty and pancreatic duct septotomy and there was no overall difference in mortality or morbidity between the two groups. This would suggest that early surgery is safe.

If, however, there are patients who would benefit from early disimpaction of the ampulla then endoscopic sphincterotomy might be the logical approach. This has the advantage of avoiding major abdominal surgery in an ill patient. Reports of this technique are certainly encouraging [68].

There appear to be two main indications for urgent surgery or endoscopic sphincterotomy. The first is in patients with associated cholangitis, suggested by rapidly progressive jaundice, fever or rigors. The second is failure of pancreatitis to settle promptly in the presence of gallstones.

It is the author's practice to remove the gall bladder at emergency operations on the pancreas only if it is necessary to explore the common bile duct. It is reasonable to remove the gallbladder at an elective operation for a pseudocyst, if the patient is in good general health.

Surgical treatment of pancreatic complications

From the point of view of management it is probably irrelevant whether a pancreatic collection is an abscess, an area of necrosis or a pseudocyst [56, 78]. The aim is to allow all collections to mature for approximately six weeks before draining them by cystogastrotomy if possible.

Why wait six weeks? Experience has shown that it takes this long for a tough wall to form around the collection [80]. In addition, careful studies have shown that approximately one-third of cystic collections will resolve spontaneously during this period [5, 15]. Finally the incidence of serious complications appears to rise after six weeks.

There has been recent interest in percutaneous aspiration of pancreatic collections under ultrasound or CT scan control [27]. In the author's experience this is only successful in about 10% of cases and carries the risk of introducing infection or precipitating haemorrhage.

The technique of surgical cystogastrostomy is straightforward. Important points are to ascertain, by aspiration, that the posterior wall of the stomach is being opened in the correct place; that a disc of contiguous gastric and cyst wall is removed; and that a large number of interrupted sutures are placed around the opening to prevent secondary bleeding (Fig. 35.6). It is sensible to remove all necrotic tissue from the cyst and to treat the patient with cimetidine or ranitidine postoperatively to reduce the risk of ulceration at the stoma.

Nutritional support is often important in a patient with a relatively quiescent cyst but is vital in the presence of an abscess, or pancreatic necrosis. In these patients there is a considerable mortality if incorrectly treated [71] and it may be impossible to wait for the full six-week period before surgical intervention. Often surgery may be delayed for two to three weeks, by which stage an acceptable capsule may have formed. External drainage is usually necessary, the exploration being made easier by prior CT mapping of the collections.

TECHNIQUE

In the majority of patients with pancreatic necrosis or abscess, entry to the necrotic cavity is usually achieved by advancing the finger through the oedematous root of the transverse mesocolon. Once the cavity is located as much of the necrotic debris as possible is removed, sometimes a complete cast of the pancreas is removed. Cavities often extend into both the head and tail regions of the pancreas and drainage of these areas with wide sialastic drains through both flanks is advisable (Fig. 35.7). It is important to search carefully for any other abscesses within the abdomen at the same time. Drainage may be required for several weeks using tubograms to decide when the drains should be removed.

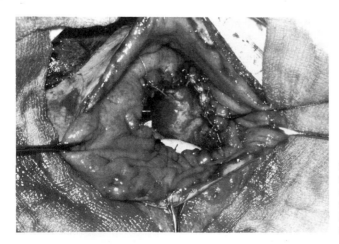

Fig. 35.6. Cystogastrotomy—through an anterior gastrostomy a disc of posterior wall is excised, the margins being sutured with a large number of polyglycolic acid sutures.

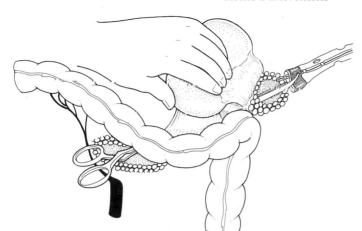

Fig. 35.7. Technique used to introduce a wide-bore sialastic drain into the necrotic cavity within the pancreas. A similar manoeuvre is used to drain the pancreatic head region, usually behind the duodenum.

Abscesses and necrosis of the pancreatic tail area may be susceptible to distal pancreatectomy. A cystojejunostomy, using a Roux-en-y loop, may occasionally be indicated in the management of a collection in the head of the pancreas. The more severe forms of pancreatic necrosis carry a mortality rate in excess of 50% and provide one of the greatest challenges to the pancreatic surgeon.

Complication of pancreatic collections

The most common complications are haemorrhage and rupture. Haemorrhage may be into the collection, or into the gastrointestinal tract through a fistulous connection. As such patients are also liable to bleed from erosive gastritis or ulceration, an accurate diagnosis is essential. Upper gastrointestinal endoscopy, with arteriography where this is not diagnostic, is usually adequate to locate the source of bleeding. The management of haemorrhage is complex and ranges from vagotomy, through local vascular control, to major pancreatic resection [15].

Rupture usually occurs in rapidly enlarging collections and is accompanied by an acute shock-like collapse often leading rapidly to multi-organ failure. Urgent operative intervention with peritoneal lavage and appropriate drainage procedures (for example cystogastrostomy) is the management of choice for this condition. The outcome is usually successful, but because of the risks of rupture all patients with pancreatic collections should be managed in hospital. Occasionally rupture may be relatively silent and may lead to pancreatic ascites or a pleural effusion. ERCP is useful to demonstrate the site of leakage and the type of surgical treatment required.

Sepsis, whether associated with bacterial infection of the collection or not, is the most common reason for urgent intervention.

Prognosis

One of the most gratifying aspects of managing acute pancreatitis is that many patients, even with the most severe disease, may ultimately have a good long-term prognosis. Clearly this will not be the case where the underlying aetiology is alcohol abuse, neoplasia or another chronic untreatable cause. It is obviously distressing if recurrent attacks occur, without any obvious cause, but usually these diminish in frequency and severity with time. The removal of gallstones guarantees freedom from further attacks in most patients where this has been the cause. Should recurrence happen in such a patient, a diligent search for further stones in the bile duct is clearly indicated. When an attack is precipitated by alcohol it is sound practice to advise the patient that further episodes are likely to occur if the patient continues to drink, even though in some it may only lead to chronic disease.

References

1 ACOSTA JM, LEDESMA CL. Gallstone migration as a cause of acute pancreatitis. *New Engl J Med* 1974; **290**: 484–487.

2 ACOSTA JM, PELLEGRINI CM, SKINNER DB Etiology and pathogenesis of acute biliary pancreatitis. *Surgery* 1980;**88**:118–125.

3 AGARWAL N, PITCHUMONI CS. Simplified prognostic criteria in acute pancreatitis. *Pancreas* 1986;**1**:69–73.

4 ALDRIDGE MC, ORNSTEIN M, GLAZER G, DUDLEY HAF. Pancreatic resection for severe acute pancreatitis. *Br J Surg* 1985;**72**:796–800.

5 ARANHA GV, PRINZ RA, ESGUERRA AC, GREENLESS HB. The nature and course of cystic pancreatic lesions diagnosed by ultrasound. *Arch Surg* 1983;**118**:486–488.

6 ARMSTRONG CP, TAYLOR TV, JEACOCK J, LUCAS S. The biliary tract in patients with acute gallstone pancreatitis. *Br J Surg* 1985;**72**:551–555.

7 ARNESEN H, FAGEROL MK. Alpha-macroglobulin, alpha₁-antitrypsin and antithrombin III in plasma and serum during fibrinolytic therapy with urokinase. *Scand J Clin Lab Invest* 1972;**29**:259–263.

8 BEGER HG, KRAUTZBERGER W, BITTNER R, BLOCK S, BUCHLER M. Results of surgical treatment of necrotizing pancreatitis. *World J Surg* 1985;**9**:972–979.

9 BELL ET. Pancreatitis. *Surgery* 1958;**43**:527–537.

10 BLACKBURN GL, WILLIAMA LF, BISTRIAN BR, et al. New approaches to the management of severe acute pancreatitis. *Am J Surg* 1976;**131**:114–124.

11 BLAMEY SL, OSBORNE DH, GILMOUR WH, CARTER DC, IMRIE CW. The early identification of patients with gallstone associated pancreatitis using clinical and biochemical factors only. *Ann Surg* 1983;**198**:574–578.

12 DE BOLLA AR, OBEID MI. Mortality in acute pancreatitis. *Ann R Coll Surg Engl* 1984;**66**:184–186.

13 BOUCHIER IAD. Biochemical tests for acute pancreatitis. *Brit Med J* 1985;**291**:1669–1670.

14 BOURKE JB. Variations in annual incidence of primary acute pancreatitis in Nottingham 1969–1974. *Lancet* 1975;**ii**:967–969.

15 BRADLEY EL. *Complications of pancreatitis. Medical and surgical management.* Philadelphia: W. B. Saunders 1982.

16 BRAGG LE, THOMPSON JS, BURNETT DA, HODGSON PE, RIKKERS LF. Increased incidence of pancreas-related complications in patients with postoperative pancreatitis. *Am J Surg* 1985;**150**:694–697.

17 COLLINS REC, FROST SJ, SPITTLEHOUSE KE. The P₃ iso-enzyme of serum amylase in the management of patients with acute pancreatitis. *Br J Surg* 1982;**69**:373–375.

18 CUSCHIERI A, WOOD RAB, CUMMING JRG, MEEHAN SE, MACKIE CR. Treatment of acute pancreatitis with fresh frozen plasma. *Br J Surg* 1983;**70**:710–712.

19 CORFIELD AP, COOPER MJ, WILLIAMSON RCN, et al. Prediction of severity in acute pancreatitis: prospective comparison of three prognostic indices. *Lancet* 1985;**ii**:403–407.

20 CORFIELD AP, COOPER MJ, WILLIAMSON RCN. Acute pancreatitis: a lethal disease of increasing incidence. *Gut* 1985;**26**:724–729

21 DURR GHK. In: Howat HT, SARLES H, eds. *The exocrine pancreas.* London: W. B. Saunders, 1979.

22 EBBEHOJ N, FRIIS J, SVENDSEN LB, BULOW S, MADSEN P. Indomethacin treatment of acute pancreatitis. *Scand J Gastroenterol* 1985;**20**:780–800.

23 FREI GJ, GREI VT, THIRLBY RC, McCLELLAND RN. Biliary pancreatitis: clinical presentations and surgical management. *Am J Surg* 1986;**151**:170–175.

24 GEOKAS MC, RINDEKNECHT H, WALBERG CB, WEISSMAN R. Methaemalbumin in the diagnosis of acute haemorrhagic pancreatitis. *Ann Intern Med* 1974;**81**:483–486.

25 HALL RI, LAVELLE MI, VENABLES CW. Use of ERCP to identify the site of traumatic injuries of the main pancreatic duct in children. *Br J Surg* 1986; **73**:411–412.

26 HAMILTON I, BRADLEY P, LINTOTT DJ, McMAHON MJ, AXON ATR. Endoscopic retrograde cholangiopancreatography in the management of patients with acute pancreatitis. *Br J Surg* 1982;**69**:504–506.

27 HANCKE S, HENRIKSEN FW. Percutaneous pancreatic cystogastrostomy guided by ultrasound scanning and gastroscopy. *Br J Surg* 1985;**72**:916–917.

28 HOLDSWORTH PJ, MAYER AD, WILSON DH, FLOWERS MW, McMAHON MJ. A simple screening test for acute pancreatitis. *Br J Surg* 1984;**71**:958–959.

29 HOWARD JM. In: Howard JM, Jordon GL, eds: *Surgical disease of the Pancreas.* London: Pitman Medical Books, 1960:169–189.

30 IMRIE CW, BENJAMIN IS, FERGUSON JC, et al. A single centre double-blind trial of trasylol therapy in primary acute pancreatitis. *Br J Surg* 1978;**65**:337–341.

31 JACOBS ML, DAGGETT WM, CIVETTA JM, et al. Acute pancreatitis: analysis of factors influencing survival. *Ann Surg* 1977;**185**:43–51.

32 JONES RC. Management of pancreatic trauma. *Am J Surg* 1985;**150**:698–704.

33 LAXSON LC, FROMKES JJ, COOPERMAN M. Endoscopic retrograde cholangiopancreatography in the management of pancreatic pseudocysts. *Am J Surg* 1985;150:683–686.

34 LEADER. Peritoneal lavage in severe acute pancreatitis. *Br J Surg* 1985;72:677.

35 KELLY TR. Gallstone pancreatitis: pathophysiology. *Surgery* 1976;80:488–492.

36 KELLY TR, SWANEY PE. Gallstone pancreatitis: the second time around. *Surgery* 1982;92:571–575.

37 MACKIE CR, WOOD RAB, PREECE PE, CUSCHIERI A. Surgical pathology at early elective operation for suspected acute gallstone pancreatitis: preliminary report of a prospective clinical trial. *Br J Surg* 1985;72:179–181.

38 MAYER AD, McMAHON MJ. Biochemical identification of patients with gallstones associated with acute pancreatitis on the day of admission to hospital. *Ann Surg* 1985;201:68–75.

39 MAYER AD, McMAHON MJ, HOLDSWORTH PJ, WILSON DH, FLOWERS MW, BROWN DA. Screening of acute pancreatitis: a rapid assay for plasma lipase. *Br J Surg* 1985;72:436–437.

40 MAYER AD, McMAHON MJ, BENSON EA, AXON ATR. Operations upon the biliary tract in patients with acute pancreatitis: aims, indications and timing. *Ann R Coll Surg Engl* 1984;66:179–183.

41 MAYER AD, McMAHON MJ, CORFIELD AP, et al. Controlled clinical trial of peritoneal lavage for the treatment of severe acute pancreatitis. *N Engl J Med* 1985;312:399–404.

42 McCUTCHEON AD. A fresh approach to the pathogenesis of pancreatitis. *Gut* 1968;9:296–310.

43 McKAY AJ, IMRIE CW, O'NEILL J, DUNCAN JG. Is an early ultrasound scan of value in acute pancreatitis? *Br J Surg* 1982;69:369–372.

44 McMAHON MJ. In: Mitchell CJ, Kelleher J, eds. *Pancreatic diseases in clinical practice.* London: Pitman Books Ltd, 1981:173–192.

45 McMAHON MJ, BOWEN M, MAYER AD, COOPER EH. Relationship of alpha$_1$-macroglobulin and other antiproteases to the clinical features of acute pancreatitis. *Am J Surg* 1983.

46 McMAHON MJ, MAYER AD. Determination of the prognosis of acute pancreatitis by peritoneal lavage. *Surgery* 1983.

47 McMAHON MJ, PICKFORD IR. Biochemical prediction of gallstones early in an attack of acute pancreatitis. *Lancet* 1978;ii:541–544.

48 McMAHON MJ, PLAYFORTH MJ, PICKFORD IR. A comparative study of methods for the prediction of severity of attacks of acute pancreatitis. *Br J Surg* 1980;67:22–25.

49 McMAHON MJ. PLAYFORTH MJ, RASHID SA, COOPER EH. The amylase to creatinine clearance ratio—a non-specific response to acute illness? *Br J Surg* 1982;69:29–32.

50 MILLWARD S, BREATNACH E, SIMKINS KC, McMAHON MJ. Do plain films of the chest and abdomen have a role in the diagnosis of acute pancreatitis. *Clin Radiol* 1983;34:133–137.

51 MITCHELL CJ, PLAYFORTH MJ. KELLEHER J, McMAHON MJ. Functional recovery of the exocrine pancreas after acute pancreatitis. *Scand J Gastroenterol.* 1983;18:5–8.

52 MOLANDER DW, BELL ET. Relation of cholelithiasis to acute haemorrhagic pancreatitis. *Arch Pathol* 1946;41:17–18.

53 M.R.C. MULTICENTRE TRIAL STUDY GROUP. Death from acute pancreatitis. M.R.C. multicentre trial of glucagon and aprotinin, *Lancet* 1977;ii:632–635.

54 NAKASHIMA Y, HOWARD JM. (1977) Drug-induced acute pancreatitis. *Surg Gynecol Obstet* 1977;145:105–109.

55 NORDBACK IH, AUVINEN OA. Long-term results after pancreas resection for acute necrotizing pancreatitis. *Br J Surg* 1985;72:687–689.

56 NORDBACK I, PESSI T, AUVINEN O, AUTIO V. Determination of necrosis in necrotizing pancreatitis. *Br J Surg* 1985;72:225–227.

57 O'MALLEY VP, CANNON JP, POSTIER RG. Pancreatic pseudocysts: cause, therapy and results. *Am J Surg* 1985;150: 680–682.

58 O'CONNOR M, KOLARS J, ANSEI H, SILVIS S, VENNES J. Preoperative endoscopic retrograde chlangiopancreatography in the surgical management of pancreatic pseudocysts. *Am J Surg* 1986;151:18–24.

59 OPIE EL. The aetiology of acute haemorrhagic pancreatitis. *Bull Hopkins Hosp* 1901;12:182–188.

60 RANSON JHC. The timing of biliary surgery in acute pancreatitis. *Ann Surg* 1979;189:654–663.

61 RANSON JHC. Acute pancreatitis. *Curr Probl Surg* 1979;16:1.

62 RANSON JHC, LACKNER H, BERMAN IB, SCHINELLA R. The relationship of coagulation factors to clinical complications of acute pancreatitis. *Surgery* 1977;81:502.

63 RANSON JHC, RIFKIND KM, TURNER JW. Prognostic signs and non-operative peritoneal lavage in acute pancreatitis. *Surg Gynecol Obstet* 1976;143:209–219.

64 RANSON JHC, RIFKIND KM, ROSES DF, FINK SD, ENG K, LOCALIO SA. Objective early identification of severe acute pancreatitis. *Am J Gastroenterol* 1974;61:443–451.

65 RANSON JHC, SPENCER FC. The role of peritoneal lavage in severe acute pancreatitis. *Ann Surg* 1978;187:565–575.

66 RANSON JHC, BALTHAZAR E, CACCAVALE R, COOPER M. Computed tomography and the prediction of pancreatic abscess in acute pancreatitis. *Ann Surg* 1985;201:656–665.

67 RENNER IG, SAVAGE WT, PANTOJA JL, RENNER VJ. Death due to acute pancreatitis. A retrospective analysis of 405 autopsy cases. *Dig Dis Sci* 1985;30:1005–18.

68 SAFRANY L, COTTON PB. A preliminary report: ur-

gent duodenoscopic sphincterotomy for acute gallstone pancreatitis. *Surgery* 1981;**189**:424–428.

69 SANFEY H,BULKLEY GB, CAMERON JL. The pathogenesis   of   acute   pancreatitis.   *Ann   Surg*
   1985;**201**:633–639.

70 SARLES H. *Pancreatitis. Symposium of Marseilles.*
   Basel: Karger, 1965.

71 SHI ECP, YEO BW, HAM JM. Pancreatic abscesses.
   Br J Surg 1984;**71**:689–691.

72 STONE HH, FABIAN TC. Peritoneal dialysis in the
   treatment of acute alcoholic pancreatitis. *Surg Gynecol Obstet* 1980;**150**:878–882.

73 STONE HH, FABIAN TC, DUNLOP WE. Gallstone pancreatitis. Biliary tract pathology in relation to time
   of operation. *Ann Surg* 1981;**194**:305–312.

74 SVENSSON J-O, NORBACK B, BOKEY EL, EDLUND Y.
   Changing pattern in aetiology of pancreatitis in an
   urban Swedish area. *Br J Surg* 1979;**66**:159–161.

75 TOOULI J, ROBERTS-THOMSON IC, DENT J, LEE J.
   Sphincter of Oddi motility disorders in patients
   with idiopathic recurrent pancreatitis. *Br J Surg*
   1985;**72**:859–863.

76 TRAPNELL JE, DUNCAN EHL. Patterns of incidence in
   acute pancreatitis. *Br Med J* 1975;**ii**:179–183.

77 TRAPNELL JF, RIGBY CC, TALBOT CH, DUNCAN EHL.
   A controlled trial of Trasylol in the treatment of
   acute pancreatitis. *Br J Surg* 1974;**61**:177–182.

78 WADE JW. Twenty-five year experience with pancreatic pseudocysts. Are we making progress? *Am
   J Surg* 1985;**147**:705–708.

79 WALL AJ. Peritoneal dialysis in the treatment of
   severe acute pancreatitis. *Med J Aust* 1967;**2**:281–
   283.

80 WARSAW AL, RATTNER DW. Timing of surgical
   drainage for pancreatic pseudocyst. *Ann Surg*
   1985;**202**:720–724.

81 WHITE TT, MORGAN A, HOPTON D. Postoperative
   pancreatitis. A study of seventy cases. *Surgery*
   1970;**120**:132–137.

82 WILLIAMSON RCN. Early assessment of severity in
   acute pancreatitis. *Gut* 1984;**25**:1331–1339.

83 WILSON JS, BERNSTEIN L, MCDONALD C, TAIT A,
   MCNEIL D, PIROLA RC. Diet and drinking habits in
   relation to the development of alcoholic pancreatitis. *Gut* 1985;**26**:882–887.

84 WYNN M, HILL DM, MILLER DR, WAXMAN K, ELS-
   NER ME, GAZZANIGA AB. Management of pancreatic and duodenal trauma. *Am J Surg*
   1985;**150**:327–332.

Chapter 36
Chronic Pancreatitis

R. LENDRUM

Chronic pancreatitis is an inflammatory process that results in permanent and irreversible damage to the pancreas. Its prevalence is increasing and diagnosis can be time consuming and expensive. The differential diagnosis includes all important causes of recurrent abdominal pain, malabsorption, weight loss and jaundice. Thus an uncommon condition assumes major importance in medicine. Several new classifications of pancreatis have been proposed recently [57,61]

Epidemiology

Prevalence

There is little reliable statistical information on prevalence. An autopsy series showed a five hundred-fold variation in prevalence in different parts of the world [58]. The highest prevalence is in the Kerala state of South India (5.4%) and the lowest in Japan (0.01%). Intermediate rates are encountered in France (0.4%), Brazil (0.4%), and South Africa (0.28%).

Incidence

Few surveys have been done. In Rochester, Minnesota, the incidence was estimated at 3.5 per 100,000 per year [49]. In Denmark the incidence of non-alcoholic pancreatitis has been estimated as 3.2 per 100,000 per year [4]. The proportion of alcohol-induced pancreatitis is increasing in England [36] suggesting that the overall incidence of the disease is increasing too. Between 1970 and 1979 there was a three-fold increase in alcoholic chronic pancreatitis in Copenhagen [4].

Sex ratio

Throughout the world chronic pancreatitis is commoner in men than women. This is particularly true of alcoholic pancreatitis. In Europe over 80% of cases occur in men; women account for nearly half the cases in Southern India [60].

Age of onset

The mean age at presentation in Europe is approximately 40 years in both sexes, but the range is wide. The first attack of pain, particularly in alcoholic disease, probably implies already well established disease. Hereditary pancreatitis and, rarely, that due to other causes may first occur in childhood, or adolescence.

Aetiology

Genetic factors

Hereditary pancreatitis

This condition was first recognized at the Mayo Clinic in 1952 [12]. Since then several affected families have been described throughout the world. Seventy-two patients from seven families in England and Wales were reported in 1978 [64]. Hereditary pancreatitis is an autosomal dominant condition with 80% penetrance. The pain begins in childhood, or the second decade of life. Lysine-cystine aminoaciduria was found in a few of these patients, but most do not have such abnormalities. The condition is usually a nuisance rather than life-threatening, attacks tending to become less severe, or disappear in middle life.

Human leucocyte antigens

No association with any particular HLA antigen is recognized. An increased frequency of HLA-B40 was found in patients with chronic alcoholic pancreatitis in France [21] and of HLA-B13 in Japan, where B5 was increased in non-alcoholic patients [34].

Congenital anatomical abnormalities

Annular pancreas

In this rare condition ectopic pancreatic tissue encircles the descending duodenum. This may result from persistence of the embryonic left ventral pancreatic bud. The anomaly predisposes to the development of acute and chronic pancreatitis which has been reported in 15–50% of such patients [17].

Pancreas divisum

This variant of pancreatic structure is much commoner than annular pancreas [16]. Its relevance to chronic pancreatitis is discussed later in this chapter.

Duodenal diverticula

These may be intra- or extra-luminal, the latter being commonest in the periampullary area. Diverticula near the ampulla seem to predispose to chronic disease of the biliary or pancreatic systems. Thus in one ERCP series they were found in 6% of patients with normal ducts, but occurred in 52% with abnormalities of both ducts [48].

Perhaps the diverticulum, or food debris within it, prevents adequate drainage of the duct.

Stenosis of the sphincter of Oddi

Chronic pancreatitis has been described in association with an apparent congenital hypertrophy of the sphincter [52, 69] and congenital obstruction of the main pancreatic duct [73].

Metabolic abnormalities

Gallstones

The importance of gallstones in chronic pancreatitis is difficult to define. While the association with acute pancreatitis is clearcut (Chapter 35), it is rare for such attacks to progress to a chronic condition unless severe pancreatic damage has occurred. On the other hand gallstones may be found in association with chronic pancreatitis in 2–93% of cases [36].

Hyperparathyroidism

Hyperplasia, adenoma, or malignancy of the parathyroid glands is found in association with 7% of all cases of pancreatitis, while chronic pancreatitis is found in 3% of patients with hyperparathyroidism [32].

Environmental factors

Alcohol

There is a strong correlation between the prevalence of chronic pancreatitis and the consumption of alcohol [18]. Apparently there is no safe, or 'threshold' level of alcohol ingestion below which pancreatitis does not occur. The incidence increases linearly with the amount drunk—even those consuming less than 20 g daily are at increased risk [60]. The type of alcohol consumed appears to be irrelevant. As alcoholism amongst the young is increasing in Western countries an increased incidence of chronic pancreatitis is to be expected.

Diet

Epidemiological studies show a correlation between chronic pancreatitis and a high protein and fat diet [1, 60]. In Japan, where chronic pancreatitis is rare, all these factors (including alcohol) are less common than in Europe. By contrast, evidence from Southern India where chronic calcific pancreatitis is common, suggests that protein and fat depletion in childhood may actually cause this. Prolonged protein depletion, as in kwashiorkor, can lead to pancreatic atrophy and exocrine insufficiency. This is entirely reversible if protein intake is increased and chronic calcific pancreatitis then does not result.

Pathogenesis

The mechanisms which initiate the sequence of events that lead to exocrine parenchymal destruction are far from clear. Several factors are thought to contribute, including the following.

Main duct obstruction

Obstruction of the main duct by stones, diverticula, anomalies of the papilla, tumours, or inflammatory stenosis can all lead to a sequence of changes in the gland of a chronic inflammatory nature. Relative obstruction at the minor papilla in pancreas divisum may also cause pancreatitis in the dorsal gland.

Intraduct obstruction

Alcohol in man and animals causes an increased concentration of pancreatic secre-

tion with the deposition of protein plugs [24, 46]. These plugs form a nidus for subsequent calcification. The duct adjacent to such plugs becomes fibrotic and so forms a stricture. The obstruction caused by these mechanisms results in dilatation of the distal duct and progressive acinar cell atrophy [57].

Reflux

Alcohol has been thought to cause spasm of the sphincter of Oddi either directly, or through duodenal inflammation. Recent evidence, however, suggests that intragastric alcohol relaxes the sphincter. This raises the possibility that reflux of bile, or duodenal juice into the pancreatic duct is important [70].

Immunology

There is no evidence for either anti-pancreatic or non-organ specific autoimmunity in this condition [39]. Knowledge of cell-mediated immunity in chronic pancreatitis is scanty. Islet-cell autoimmunity is not a feature of the diabetes that attends either chronic pancreatitis, or cystic fibrosis.

Pathology

The pancreas

Progressive exocrine atrophy and replacement by fibrous tissue leads to firm enlargement of the gland. The main duct becomes dilated, tortuous and strictured. Later on the fibrotic pancreas shrinks. Microscopically, islands of exocrine parenchyma become surrounded by expanding areas of fibrous tissue. The ducts dilate and fill with inspissated secretions which may later calcify. The islets are at first preserved, but later on their blood supply becomes compromised and they atrophy.

Organs adjacent to the pancreas

Sclerosis of tissues in the immediate vicinity of the pancreas can result in narrowing of the lower common bile duct, descending duodenum and colon. The portal vein, splenic vein and other blood vessels in the area may also become involved and thrombosis may occur. Nerves can also be damaged.

Pathophysiology

Destruction of the exocrine and ductular tissue leads to a progressive fall in bicarbonate and enzyme secretion (see Chapter 34). Malabsorption becomes important only when more than 90% of the normal output is lost [19].

Malabsorption of fat and protein

Malabsorption of protein is less of a problem than that of fat. Pancreatic lipase deficiency leads to severe steatorrhoea and calorie malnutrition, with unabsorbed triglyceride appearing as oil in the stool. Perhaps because free long-chain fatty acids are not released for conversion to hydroxy fatty acids by colonic bacteria, diarrhoea is not usually severe. Hydroxy fatty acids cause steatorrhoea of small intestinal origin by stimulating colonic secretion [8].

Malabsorption of vitamins A, D, E, K, calcium and magnesium

While low serum levels of these dietary components are often found, clinical evidence of metabolic bone disease and clotting disorders is unusual. Again the absence of free fatty acids, which can bind these components, may be a protective factor.

Absorption of vitamin B_{12}

Vitamin B_{12} is bound to the proteins in food and to the R-protein in intestinal secretions. Proteases are essential for its release [37]. In addition the pancreas may secrete cofactors essential for absorption of B_{12} [11]. In chronic pancreatitis low levels of serum B_{12} are often found, but severe deficiency is rare.

Absorption of iron

A proportion of patients with chronic pancreatitis have high iron absorption, which is corrected by giving pancreatic enzyme supplements. The mechanism is unknown and there are no known clinical consequences [37].

Endocrine secretion

Diabetes mellitus is a late complication of chronic pancreatitis as a result of islet destruction. Ketoacidosis is rare and insulin-treated patients are prone to hypoglycaemia, because the glucagon-secreting pancreatic cells are also destroyed. The physiological consequences of loss of somatostatin, pancreatic polypeptide and vasoactive intestinal peptide release, are uncertain.

Clinical features

Pain

This is the most troublesome aspect of chronic pancreatitis and the reason for consultation in most patients. Pain results from swelling of the gland, obstruction of the duct and involvement of nerves in the inflammatory reaction. The pain is usually felt anteriorly, over the most damaged part of the gland, but may also be felt in the back or left flank. This back pain may be worse on lying flat and relieved by leaning forward. Alcohol and food may aggravate the pain.

Painless chronic pancreatitis

Chronic pancreatitis can be found at post-mortem in patients who have never had symptoms during life—between 5% and 15% of patients with chronic pancreatitis may never experience pain [22]. Among patients with alcoholic cirrhosis the incidence of painless pancreatitis may be as high as 50% [43]. In one series three out of 30 patients with calcific pancreatitis and five out of 77 with non-calcifying pancreatitis (7% overall) did not have pain [36]. The severity of relapses and the amount of pain experienced in alcoholic pancreatitis may diminish, as exocrine function declines [25].

Malabsorption

Stools characteristic of severe fat malabsorption occur only in the later stages of the disease. Severe steatorrhoea, with oil on the water after a bowel action, is rarely caused by a non-pancreatic lesion. So in any patient with obvious steatorrhoea chronic pancreatic insufficiency should be suspected.

Weight loss

The combination of pain, anorexia and steatorrhoea leads to calorie malnutrition which results in severe weight loss. Overeating compensates for this in some patients.

Diabetes mellitus

Impaired insulin release leads to diabetes mellitus in 30% of patients with chronic pancreatitis. Oral hypoglycaemic agents are not very effective, but insulin requirements are usually modest, perhaps because there is no glucagon production either. Patients who develop diabetes are subject to all the vascular complications seen in other diabetics.

Jaundice

Constriction of the lower common bile duct may eventually result in permanent jaundice. Initially obstruction of the bile duct may be intermittent, occurring in association with acute exacerbations of pain. This obstruction is probably caused by oedema around the retro-pancreatic part of the common bile duct, which later may be replaced by fibrous tissue. Differentiation from carcinoma of the pancreatic head, or from obstruction of the lower bile duct by gallstones can cause problems [59].

Portal hypertension

The splenic, superior mesenteric and portal veins are all close to the pancreas and can thrombose if involved by peripancreatic inflammation. Obvious portal hypertension from this cause is uncommon, being found in only five out of 164 patients with chronic pancreatitis reported by Longstreth, Newcomer and Green [40]. Deformity of the splenic vein demonstrated by splenic venography is much commoner, but this investigation is seldom indicated.

Pancreatic cysts, ascites and pleural effusions

The pancreatic duct may be destroyed during an acute relapse, or in the course of the chronic disease. Pancreatic juice can then accumulate in a loculus adjacent to the pancreas or in the lesser sac (pseudocyst). It may leak freely into the peritoneal cavity causing painless ascites, or track upwards into the pleural cavities causing pleural effusion or a mediastinal cyst. The fluid in pancreatic ascites has a high protein and amylase content [10]. These patients can occasionally develop necrosis of the subcutaneous fat [20].

Cirrhosis of the liver

Only 2.3% of patients with alcoholic chronic pancreatitis have clinical evidence of cirrhosis, although histological features are found in 18.5% on liver biopsy [60]. The combination of alcoholism, splenomegaly, ascites and jaundice should not always lead to the automatic diagnosis of hepatic cirrhosis, as chronic pancreatitis can produce all of these.

Gastrointestinal haemorrhage

Haemorrhage can occur as a complication of chronic pancreatitis and may occasionally be the presenting feature. It can arise from oesophageal varices due to portal hypertension; from pseudo-aneurysms caused by vascular damage by pancreatitis and from increased vascularity of the stomach, colon, or duodenum secondary to peripancreatic inflammation [30]. Pseudo-aneurysms may bleed into the main pancreatic duct causing 'Wirsungorrhagia'. Finally bleeding can occur from duodenal ulceration which probably has an increased incidence in patients with chronic pancreatitis.

Cancer in chronic pancreatitis

Cancer developing on an established background of chronic pancreatitis is uncommon. However, carcinoma is frequently associated with segmental pancreatitis, presumably from obstruction of the main pancreatic duct.

Remote complications of chronic pancreatitis

Fat necrosis may occur during a relapse, or in association with pancreatic ascites. Lesions can occur in the subcutaneous fat layers, mainly in the lower limbs, and in bones, or adjacent to joints resulting in an inflammatory arthropathy.

Diagnosis

Clinical suspicion

Too often the diagnosis of chronic pancreatitis is made only after exclusion of many other conditions. This can produce considerable delays which should be avoidable by the judicious use of modern investigative techniques [47].

Investigation of pancreatic structure (see Chapter 33)

A **plain abdominal radiograph** is mandatory. Calcification occurs in less than one-third of patients seen in northern Europe, but is commoner in the south where it can be associated with normal function in 5% [60]. **Ultrasonography** should follow, to document abnormalities of shape, size, duct diameter and associated cysts.

ERCP will detect most patients with chronic pancreatitis (Figs 36.1 and 36.2) but the finding of 'minimal changes' should be followed by a pancreatic function test. Classifications of ERCP appearances in chronic pancreatitis are helpful in the interpretation and standardization of diagnosis [7].

^{75}**Se-selenomethionine scanning** has been abandoned in many centres because of its high false positive yield. However, pancreatic disease is unlikely if this is normal.

CT scanning and angiography may also be needed occasionally.

Investigation of pancreatic function (see Chapter 34)

The choice of test will be determined by local availability. Useful results will only be obtained by regular use and attention to detail. The **Lundh and PABA tests** are the easiest for routine use. Unfortunately differentiation between cancer and chronic

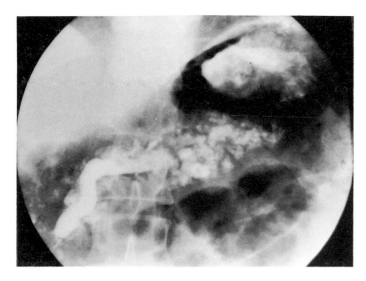

Fig. 36.1. ERCP picture showing chronic pancreatitis (with marked calcification) in the tail of the pancreas with a blocked main pancreatic duct in the body of the pancreas. Note the relative lack of calcification in the pancreatic head.

pancreatitis remains a problem with all of these tests.

Other tests

Measurement of **amylase** concentration in the serum is worth doing, as it may be raised during an acute relapse when the pancreatic duct is obstructed, or in the presence of extravasation of pancreatic juice. However, in the later stages of the disease the serum amylase may be normal, even when severe pain is present.

If an elevated serum amylase is found when the clinical features are inconsistent with the diagnosis of pancreatitis, macroamylasaemia should be suspected. This can be excluded by column chromatography and the presence of a normal 24-hour urine excretion of amylase in the urine.

Percutaneous aspiration cytology has been employed by some groups to assist in

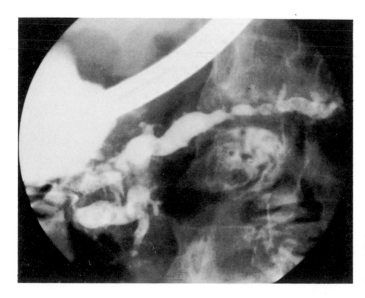

Fig. 36.2. Severe chronic pancreatitis affecting the whole pancreas with multiple filling defects within the ducts and 'chain-of-lakes' appearance of main pancreatic duct.

reaching a diagnosis. This is usually performed with CT or ultrasound scanning. Unfortunately there are very few centres with the necessary skilled cytologists available to make this a practicable proposition. In addition, since it is generally used to distinguish tumour from chronic pancreatitis, it suffers from the disadvantage that both can coexist in the same patient.

Liver function tests may show evidence of chronic liver disease or compression of the common bile duct.

Measurements of haemoglobin, mean corpuscular volume, leucocyte count, fasting blood glucose, serum calcium, proteins, prothrombin and serum B_{12} should also be done. **Random blood alcohol levels** may help to detect recidivist alcoholics. Steatorrhoea can be confirmed by measurement of the 72-hour faecal fat excretion with the patient on a 100 g fat diet. Ascitic fluid should be examined for protein and amylase content.

Differential diagnosis (Table 36.1)

The conditions that can be confused with chronic pancreatitis vary according to the coexisting complications present. It should be noted that pancreatic cancer may mimic each and every category shown in Table 36.1 and is the major differential

Table 36.1. A clinical classification and differential diagnosis of chronic pancreatitis and its complications.

Clinical features	Differential diagnosis
Painful chronic pancreatitis	
Uncomplicated	Gastric ulcer
	Gastric carcinoma
	Duodenal ulcer
	Mesenteric ischaemia
Complicated	
By steatorrhoea	Crohn's disease
By jaundice	Liver disease
	Biliary disease
By diabetes mellitus	Pancreatic carcinoma
By extrahepatic portal hypertension and/or ascites	Hepatic cirrhosis
	Malignant ascites
	Tuberculous peritonitis
By fat necrosis	
Subcutaneous	Erythema nodosum
	Weber-Christian disease
In bone	Other osteolytic lesions
	Other acute mono-arthropathies
Painful chronic pancreatitis	
(During a relapse)	
Uncomplicated	Acute peptic ulceration
	Cholecystitis
	Malingering, to obtain drugs
Complicated	As in complicated painful chronic
Painless chronic pancreatitis	*Other causes of painless malabsorption*
	Coeliac disease
	Post-gastrectomy
	Bacterial overgrowth
	Other causes of weight loss
	Malignancy
	Hyperthyroidism

diagnosis when diabetes is present. By definition 'uncomplicated' painless pancreatitis will not cause diagnostic problems.

Medical management

Recurrent attack

The management of an acute recurrent attack of pancreatitis is the same as that of the first attack (see Chapter 35). Avoidance of alcohol is the most important preventative measure.

Chronic pancreatitis

Pain

Chronic pain, which is sometimes very severe, is the predominant symptom in these patients. Avoidance of alcohol and rich meals may prevent exacerbations. Simple, non-opiate, analgesia is often inadequate and resorting to dihydrocodeine, pethidine, buprenorphine and even morphine may be needed. Drug addiction is a permanent risk in such patients.

Oral pancreatic enzyme supplements have been shown to reduce the pain of chronic pancreatitis significantly in double-blind randomized trials [35,65]. It is suggested that intra-duodenal proteases inhibit pancreatic secretion by a negative feedback mechanism. Antacids and anticholinergic agents may also sometimes decrease pain, perhaps by inhibiting pancreatic secretion. Treatment with inhibitory gastrointestinal hormones (somatostatin, glucagon, pancreatic polypeptide) is impractical at present.

Severe and persistent pain should be investigated by ultrasound and ERCP to detect the presence of cysts or ductal obstruction. Surgical treatment may be the most effective way of relieving the patient's pain in suitably selected cases and close collaboration between physician and surgeon is to be encouraged (see Chapter 37). There are still some physicians who believe that there is little role for surgery [71]. Coeliac axis block has been used for pain relief but is not recommended as it usually only lasts for a few months and can result in serious side effects, including impotence.

Irradiation of the pancreas has been used for pain relief, by accelerating pancreatic exocrine destruction [42], but has found little widespread acceptance. Ligation, or occlusion of the main pancreatic duct with glue has also been used to produce exocrine atrophy and pain relief, but has been associated with significant technical problems and surgical drainage is better.

Malabsorption

A low fat intake is the single most useful step in relieving troublesome steatorrhoea. Calorie supplementation by increased carbohydrate and medium chain triglyceride (MCT) preparations, which do not require lipase for digestion, may be required, although palatability is a problem. Medium chain triglyceride oil may also be used as a substitute for ordinary fat in the preparation of meals for such patients. Calcium and vitamin D supplements may also occasionally be required if there is evidence of calcium or vitamin D malabsorption. Protein malabsorption needs treatment by added dietary protein and oral enzyme preparations.

Three commonly used oral enzyme supplements are available in the U.K.— Cotazym (Organon), Pancrex (Paines and Byrne) and Nutrizym (Merck). In Nutrizym attempts have been made to overcome enzyme inactivation by a low duodenal pH by incorporating proteolytic enzymes of vegetable origin (bromelains from pineapple stems) which are active at a pH of 3 to 8 [38]. In practice there is little to choose between any of these preparations—all are helpful but none is able to correct malabsorption completely [27].

Pancreatic enzyme supplements should be taken together with and preferably dispersed through the food. They are rich in nucleic acids and, if taken in excess, can produce hyperuricosuria [66].

Enzyme activity in the duodenal lumen after taking pancreatic enzyme supplements correlates inversely with gastric acid secretion [56]. This has led to attempts to raise intraduodenal pH in order to prevent destruction of the enzymes by acid. Cimetidine has been shown to improve absorption in patients with severe exocrine pancreatic insufficiency [50, 74] and in cystic fibrosis [14]. However, other studies have shown cimetidine to be no better than placebo [28, 60]. Enhancement of the effect of pancreatic enzyme supplements occurred when sodium bicarbonate, or aluminium hydroxide was given with meals, although antacids containing calcium or magnesium salts caused increased steatorrhoea [28]. This latter finding is probably due to the formation of insoluble soaps and precipitation of glycine-conjugated bile acids by calcium and magnesium [29].

In practice if steatorrhoea fails to improve on supplements alone then cimetidine, ranitidine, or antacids (sodium bicarbonate or aluminium hydroxide) should be added to the meal. If this also fails, then an alternative cause for steatorrhoea such as small intestinal disease, or bacterial overgrowth, should be sought. Successful treatment will be reflected in weight gain. Repeated faecal fat estimations are not necessary.

Diabetes mellitus

The management of diabetes in patients with chronic pancreatitis is the same as in diabetes from other causes. It is, however, undesirable to restrict carbohydrate intake in the presence of malabsorption and weight loss. Insulin should be used with caution. Patients with chronic pancreatitis may be much more sensitive to it, with an increased risk of hypoglycaemia, because the release of glucagon may also be impaired by the damage to the islets of Langerhans.

Pancreatic calcification and stone dissolution

The calcium visible on plain abdominal radiographs is due to stones, or concretions within the ducts and ductular systems. As duct obstruction leads to pancreatic acinar damage it makes sense to attempt to dissolve these stones. Some success has been claimed following oral citrate therapy (citric acid 2.6 g; mono-potassium citrate 4 g; monosodium citrate 4 g) given three times daily with meals [55]. Our limited experience with this therapy has been disappointing and large randomized studies are needed before it can be recommended as a standard treatment for the dissolution of pancreatic stones and the control of pain.

Prevention

Alcohol is the predominant cause of chronic pancreatitis world-wide, but avoidance can only be achieved by better health education. While gallstones are an unusual cause of chronic pancreatitis, it would seem sensible to remove these if they appear to be of aetiological significance. The prevention of 'idiopathic' pancreatitis must await further work to determine the cause in such cases.

Prognosis

Male alcoholics seem to develop chronic pancreatitis after a mean interval of 18 years, females after 11 years of drinking. Occasionally pancreatitis occurs within one year of the onset of drinking [60]. Diabetes appears within 10 years of the start of pain in approximately one-third of patients [63].

Malabsorption may supervene in some 20% of patients.

The long-term prognosis of alcoholic pancreatitis is that of alcoholism. It is said that abstension will achieve pain relief in one-third of patients—the remainder showing no improvement, or continued deterioration in equal proportions. In the latter group drug addiction will affect the prognosis.

Longitudinal follow-up surveys are few. Of 56 patients first seen at the Mayo Clinic between 1939 and 1943 and reviewed in 1960, 20% were dead from complications of their pancreatitis [23]. In another series from Zurich 30% of 102 patients were dead in less than nine years [3].

Pancreas divisum

The normal pancreas is formed by fusion of dorsal and ventral pancreatic buds. Failed fusion results in pancreas divisum, found in 5–14% of individuals at post-mortem. At ERCP pancreas divisum is characterized by the 'ventral pancreas'—a small, but normal looking tree-like duct system filled from the main papilla. This configuration is found in some 5% of pancreatograms in Europe, but in less than 1% in Japan [13]. Whether it predisposes to pancreatic disease, remains uncertain.

Embryology

The pancreas arises during the fifth week of gestation from three outgrowths of the primitive duodenum (Fig 36.3). The dorsal pancreatic bud grows at first posteriorly in the midline and later comes to lie in the concavity of the duodenum. Two ventral buds develop slightly caudal to the dorsal bud and the left bud later atrophies. The right ventral bud develops in close association with the primitive bile-duct bud. Later on the ventral pancreas rotates posteriorly until it comes to lie on the left of the duodenum caudal to the dorsal pancreas. The duct systems then usually fuse together [41], the dorsal duct forming the major duct in the body and tail and the ventral duct that in the head of the pancreas. The major duct (Wirsung's duct) drains at the major papilla, while the dorsal duct forms the duct of Santorini, which drains through the minor papilla.

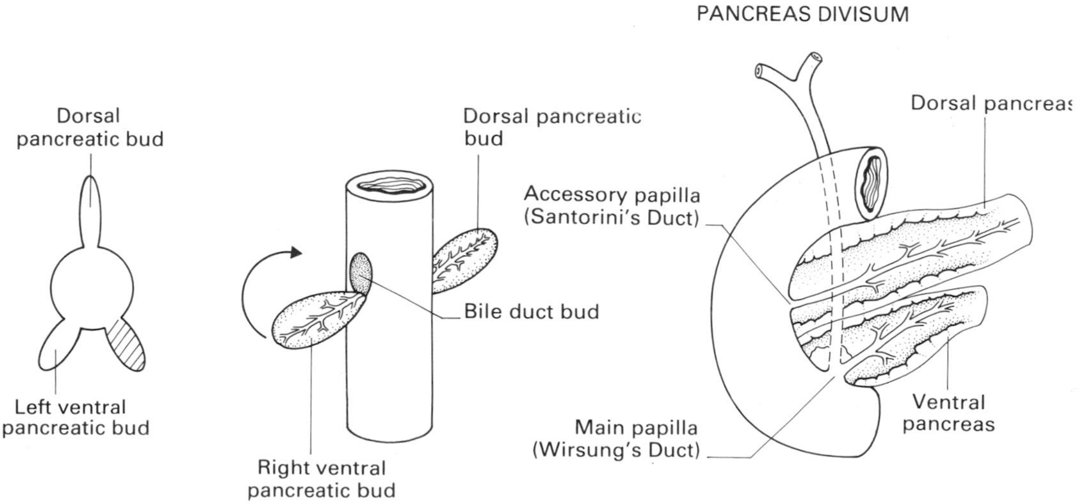

PANCREAS DIVISUM

Fig. 36.3. A diagrammatic illustration of the embryology of the pancreas at the 5th week of foetal development showing how pancreas divisum can occur.

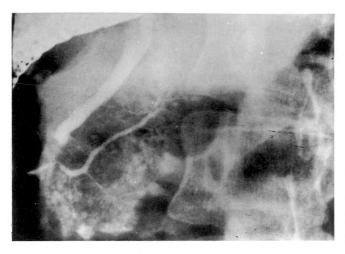

Fig. 36.4. Typical appearance of ventral pancreas at ERCP. Note the characteristic 'Christmas tree' appearance which distinguishes this from a block of the main pancreatic duct in the neck area.

The dorsal and ventral ducts may fail to fuse altogether (complete pancreas divisum), or be connected by a small communication (incomplete divisum). If this occurs then the main drainage of the body and tail of the pancreas is through the minor papilla (Figs 36.4 and 36.5).

Clinical importance of pancreas divisum

Pancreas divisum has been known for many years but the introduction of ERCP has greatly increased its importance. There are several reasons for this.

1. At ERCP a short ventral duct system may be mistaken for a main duct occluded by a carcinoma.

2. If the presence of a ventral duct system is not recognized rapidly at ERCP, inadvertent parenchymal filling can occur with subsequent pancreatitis.

3. Ultrasound or CT scanning may suggest pathology in the pancreatic head as it may appear 'bulky' or 'enlarged' when pancreas divisum is present [44].

4. At operation the surgeon may be unable to recognize the condition, because the gland looks outwardly normal. An operative pancreatogram through the tail, may also appear normal, unless concurrent biliary radiology is done demonstrating that the bile duct enters the duodenum separately and more distally [Fig. 36.5].

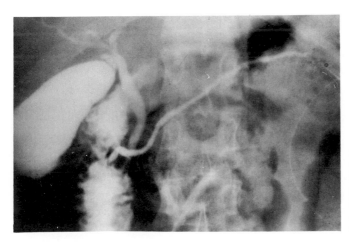

Fig. 36.5. An operative pancreatogram (through the tail) showing filling of the dorsal duct system which drains separately into the duodenum above the entry of the biliary system (filled via the gall bladder).

Does pancreas divisum cause pancreatitis?

Several authors have suggested that pancreas divisum may cause abdominal pain and pancreatitis but there is still disagreement over whether this is so.

In Leeds [45] pancreas divisum was found in 21 (4.7%) of 449 pancreatograms with pancreatitis in four (19%) of these. This compares with 116 cases (27%) of pancreatitis in 428 with normal anatomy. The authors conclude that pancreas divisum does not predispose to pancreatitis.

Contrary conclusions were reached in an analysis of 169 patients who had 'incidental' pancreatograms while undergoing billiary assessment. Six (3.6%) were found to have a pancreas divisum although this anomaly was found in 29 (16.4%) of 177 patients being assessed for recurrent pancreatitis and in 20 (25.6%) of 78 with 'idiopathic' pancreatitis [13]. This strong association, together with the known low incidence of pancreas divisum in Japan where pancreatitis is rare, seems strong evidence for a causal association.

Another study suggested that pancreas divisum was significantly more common in patients investigated for pancreatitis, than in those undergoing ERCP for biliary problems or unexplained abdominal pain. Among patients with pancreatitis those with the congenital abnormality were significantly younger than the others, as would be expected if it predisposes to this disease. The clinical pattern was that of relapsing acute pancreatitis [51]. Acute pancreatitis was also significantly associated with pancreas divisum in a series reported by Sahel, *et al.* [54] in 1982.

Does pancreas divisum cause abdominal pain?

Although most series suggest that there is an association, the question remains unresolved. Bias in referral to experienced ERCP centres may result in an excess of such patients. The difficulty in cannulating the minor papilla to exclude pancreatitis in the dorsal duct and the impossibility of performing 'split' pancreatic function tests means that the problem can only be resolved by direct surgical intervention.

If the pain is caused by impaired drainage of the dorsal duct (as has been suggested), it would seem logical to improve this drainage and see if the pain disappears. This can only be justified if symptoms are disabling. Endoscopic sphincterotomy of the minor papilla has been performed but the results are very disappointing and re-stenosis occurs. Operative sphincteroplasty of the minor papilla has produced good short-term results in a small number of patients with recurrent pancreatitis [9, 51] but long-term follow-up is not available. Another study has suggested that sphincteroplasty is only suitable for patients with recurrent attacks of acute pancreatitis and that once chronic pancreatitis occurs resection of the pancreas is required [72]. Distal drainage of the dorsal duct has also been tried but none of these surgical techniques has been shown to produce long-term improvement and, until this is so, management of these patients will continue to present a challenge to the physician [53].

Cystic fibrosis of the pancreas

Cystic fibrosis is the commonest inherited disorder in Caucasians. The condition is inherited as an autosomal recessive and affects 1 in 2,000 live births. Approximately 1 in 25 of the population are asymptomatic carriers of an abnormally viscous mucus secretion affecting various systems, leading to the alternative name of 'mucoviscidosis' [5]. This may result in neonatal intestinal obstruction (meconium ileus), progressive exocrine pancreatic insufficiency, cirrhosis and portal hypertension and chronic stasis and sepsis in the lungs

[62]. Occlusion of the vas deferens may cause aspermia in men. Cystic fibrosis is also characterized by a high electrolyte concentration in the sweat.

Pathology and pathophysiology

Blockage of the pancreatic duct by inspissated secretions leads to dilatation of the duct and destruction of exocrine function. Enzyme deficiency and ocasionally diabetes may follow. Pancreatic function tests show a low output of viscous duodenal fluid with a normal or low enzyme content. Marked fat and protein malabsorption follows.

Clinical features

Cystic fibrosis is usually diagnosed in infancy because of meconium ileus, failure to thrive, steatorrhoea and chronic respiratory problems. Milder cases may escape detection until later years when chronic pulmonary sepsis, portal hypertension, or delayed puberty with signs of malnutrition should suggest the diagnosis. Intestinal obstruction by solid bowel contents can also occur in adults [33].

Diagnosis

In infancy

The most important diagnostic procedure is the sweat chloride test [24]. Sweat is collected from a locally sealed area of skin into an absorbent pad after stimulation with pilocarpine by iontophoresis. A sweat chloride concentration of 60 mmol/l or more is diagnostic, except if there is adrenal insufficiency which may increase this level. Blood immunoreactive trypsin levels are high in the early stages and this has been used as a screening test [31]. Missed cases seem likely to continue to present diagnostic difficulties in later life. False positive diagnoses are common [15] and could be avoided by stricter adherence to established guidelines [6].

In adolescents and adults

The sweat chloride concentration tends to be higher in older individuals; even so, one of less than 60 mmol/l would exclude the diagnosis and one of greater than 110 mmol/l would confirm it. Between these levels there is no accurate diagnostic test. The clinical picture must, however, include chronic infective pulmonary disease and pancreatic exocrine deficiency. The lack of either of these features makes the diagnosis suspect.

Differential diagnosis

Conditions that may be confused with cystic fibrosis in patients with recurrent chest infections are coeliac disease and other pancreatic exocrine disorders presenting in childhood (for example isolated pancreatic enzyme deficiencies; enterokinase deficiency; the Shwachman-Diamond syndrome of pancreatic atrophy plus chronic neutropenia). In all these conditions the sweat chloride concentration is normal.

Treatment

The pancreatic exocrine deficiency is managed in the same way as in chronic pancreatitis. Oral enzyme supplements with or without antacids, fat restriction, medium-chain triglyceride and protein supplementation are important. Sodium supplements may be necessary to replace excess losses in sweat. Chest physiotherapy and antibiotics are often needed for respiratory complications. Rare cases of adult intestinal obstruction may respond to treatment with oral n-acetylcysteine (30 ml of a 20% solution three times daily) [33].

Prognosis

Before 1950, most of these patients died in childhood. Better initial management has led to almost 80% survival into early adult life [68]. Gastroenterologists must therefore be aware of this condition and be prepared to diagnose it in young adults presenting with appropriate symptoms.

References

1 ACHARYA SK, MISHRA PK. Chronic calcific pancreatitis of the tropics. *Trop Gastroenterol* 1984;5:124–134.

2 AMMANN RW, AKOVBIANTZ A, LARGIADER F, SCHUELER G. Course and outcome of chronic pancreatitis. Longditudinal study of a mixed medico-surgical series of 254 patients. *Gastroenterology* 1984;86:820–828.

3 AMMANN RW, HAMMER B, FUMAGALLI I. Chronic pancreatitis in Zurich 1963–1972. Clinical findings and follow-up studies of 102 cases. *Digestion* 1973;9:404–415.

4 ANDERSEN BN, PETERSEN NT, SCHEEL J, WORNING H. Incidence of alcoholic chronic pancreatitis in Copenhagen. *Scand J Gastroenterol,* 1982;17:247–252.

5 ANDERSON CM. Pancreatic disease in childhood. In: Howat HT, Sarles H, eds. *The exocrine pancreas.* London: W.B. Saunders, 1979:313–322.

6 ANDERSON CM, GOODCHILD MC. Clinical and diagnostic features of cystic fibrosis. In: *Cystic fibrosis. Clinical and diagnostic features.* Oxford: Blackwell Scientific Publications, 1976:24–44.

7 AXON ATR, CLASSEN A, COTTON PB, CREMER M, FREENY PC, LEES WR. Pancreatography in chronic pancreatitis: international definitions. *Gut* 1984;25:1107–1112.

8 BANKS PA. Clinical features of chronic pancreatitis. In: *Pancreatitis.* New York: Plenum Medical, 1979:189–194.

9 BRITT LG, SAMUELS AD, JOHNSON JW. Pancreas divisum: is it a surgical disease? *Ann Surg* 1983;197:654–662.

10 CAMERON JL. Chronic pancreatic ascites and pancreatic pleural effusions. *Gastroenterology* 1978;74:134–140.

11 CARMEL R, HOLLANDER D, GERGELY HM, RENNER JG, ABRAMSON SB. Pure human pancreatic juice directly enhances uptake of cobalamin by guinea pig ileum *in vivo. Proc Soc Exp Biol Med* 1985;178:143–150.

12 COMFORT MW, STEINBERG AG. Pedigree of a family with hereditary chronic relapsing pancreatitis. *Gastroenterology* 1952;21:54–63.

13 COTTON PB. Congenital anomaly of pancreas divisum as a cause of obstructive pain and pancreatitis. *Gut* 1980;21:105–114.

14 COX KL, ISENBERG JN, OSHER AB, DOOLEY RR. The effect of cimetidine on maldigestion in cystic fibrosis. *J Pediatr* 1979;94:488–492.

15 DAVID TJ, PHILLIPS BM. Overdiagnosis of cystic fibrosis. *Lancet* 1982;ii:1204–1205.

16 DELHAYE M, ENGELHOLM L, CREMER M. Pancreas divisum: congenital anatomic variant or anomaly? *Gastroenterology* 1985;89:951–958.

17 DHARMSATHAPHORN K, BURRELL M, DOBBINS J. Diagnosis of annular pancreas with ERCP. *Gastroenterology* 1979;77:1109–1114.

18 DI BISCEGLIC AM, SEGAL I. Cirrhosis and chronic pancreatitis in alcoholics. *J Clin Gastroenterol* 1984;6:199–200.

19 DIMAGNO EP, GO VLM, SUMMERSKILL WHJ. Relations between pancreatic enzyme outputs and malabsorption in severe pancreatic insufficiency. *N Engl J Med* 1973;288:813–815.

20 DONOWITZ M, KERSTEIN MD, SPIRO HM. Pancreatic ascites. *Medicine (Baltimore)* 1974;53:183–195.

21 FAUCHET R, GENETET B, GOSSELIN M, GASTARD J. HLA antigens in chronic alcoholic pancreatitis. *Tissue Antigens* 1979;13:163–166.

22 FITZGERALD O. Painless pancreatitis and other painless pancreatic disorders. *Clin Gastroenterol* 1972;1:195–218.

23 GAMBILL EE, BAGGENSTOSS AH, PRIESTLEY JT. Chronic relapsing pancreatitis. Fate of fifty-six patients first encountered in the years 1939 to 1943 inclusive. *Gastroenterology* 1960;39:404–413.

24 GIBSON LE, COOKE RE. A test for concentration of electrolytes in sweat in cystic fibrosis of the pancreas utilising pilocarpine by iontophoresis. *Pediatrics* 1959;23:545–549.

25 GIRDWOOD AH, MARKS IN, BORNMAN PC, KOTTLER RE, COHEN M. Does progressive pancreatic insufficiency limit pain in calcific pancreatitis with duct stricture, or continued alcohol insult? *J Clin Gastroenterol* 1981;3:241–245.

26 GIROGI D, BERNARD JP, DE CARO A, *et al.* Pancreatic stone protein. I. Evidence that it is encoded by a pancreatic messenger ribonucleic acid. *Gastroenterology* 1985;89:381–386.

27 GOODCHILD MC, SAGARO E, BROWN GA, CRUCHLEY PM, JUKES HR, ANDERSON CM. Comparative trial of Pancrex V Forte and Nutrizym in treatment of malabsorption in cystic fibrosis. *Br Med J* 1974;iii:712–714.

28 GRAHAM DY. Pancreatic enzyme replacement. The effect of antacids or cimetidine. *Dig Dis Sci* 1982;27:485–490.

29 GRAHAM DY, SACKMAN JW. Mechanism of increase in steatorrhoea with calcium and magnesium in exocrine pancreatic insufficiency: An animal model. *Gastroenterology* 1982;83:638–644.

534 Chapter 36

30 HALL RI, LAVELLE MI, VENABLES CW. Chronic pancreatitis as a cause of gastrointestinal bleeding. Gut 1982;23:250–255.

31 HEELEY AF, HEELEY ME, KING DN, KUZEMKO JA, WALSH MP. Screening for cystic fibrosis by dried blood spot trypsin assay. Arch Dis Child 1982;57:18–21.

32 HIRSKOVIC T, KEATING FR JR, GROSS JB. Coexistent pancreatitis and hyperparathyroidism. Observations in 15 cases. Gastroenterology 1967;52:1093.

33 HODSON ME, MEARNS MB, BATTEN JC. Meconium ileus equivalent in adults with cystic fibrosis of pancreas: a report of six cases. Br Med J 1976;ii:790–791.

34 HOMMA T, KUBO K, SATO T. HLA antigens and chronic pancreatitis in Japan. Digestion 1981;21:267–272.

35 ISAKSSON G, IHSE I. Pain reduction by an oral pancreatic enzyme preparation in chronic pancreatitis. Dig Dis Sci 1983;28:97–102.

36 JAMES O, AGNEW JE, BOUCHIER IAD. Chronic pancreatitis in England. A changing picture? Br Med J 1974;ii:34–38.

37 KELLEHER J. Nutritional status in chronic pancreatic steatorrhoea. In: Mitchell CJ, Kelleher J, eds. Pancreatic disease in clinical practice. London: Pitman, 1981:257–266.

38 KNILL-JONES RP, PEARCE H, BATTEN J, WILLIAMS R. Comparative trial of Nutrizym in chronic pancreatic insufficiency. Br Med J 1970;iv:21–24.

39 LENDRUM R. Immunology and the exocrine pancreas. In: Mitchell CJ, Kelleher J, eds. Pancreatic disease in clinical practice. London: Pitman, 1981: 240–256.

40 LONGSTRETH GF, NEWCOMER AD, GREEN PA. Extrahepatic portal hypertension caused by chronic pancreatitis. Ann Intern Med 1971;75:903–908.

41 MCLEAN JM. Embryology of the pancreas. In: Howat HT, Sarles H, eds. The exocrine pancreas London: W.B. Saunders, 1979:3–14.

42 MALLINSON CN. Medical treatment of chronic pancreatitis. In: Mitchell CJ, Kelleher J, eds. Pancreatic disease in clinical practice. London: Pitman, 1981: 337–345.

43 MARKS IN, BANK S, LOUW JH. The diagnosis and management of pancreatitis. In: Jerzy Glass G.B. Progress in gastroenterology. Vol 1. London: Grune and Stratton, 1968:412–472.

44 MITCHELL CJ. Pancreas divisum and pancreatitis. In: Mitchell CJ, Kelleher J, eds. Pancreatic disease in clinical practice. London: Pitman, 1981:404–414.

45 MITCHELL CJ, LINTOTT DJ, RUDDELL WSJ, LOSOWSKY MS, AXON ATR. Clinical relevance of an unfused pancreatic duct system. Gut 1979;20:1066–1071.

46 MULTINGNER L, SARLES H, LOMBARDO D, DE CARO A. Pancreatic stone protein. II. Implication in stone formation during the course of chronic calcifying pancreatitis. Gastroenterology 1985;89:387–391.

47 NIEDERAU C, GRENDELL JH. Diagnosis of chronic pancreatitis. Gastroenterology 1985;88:1973–1995.

48 OSNES M, MYREN J, LOTVEIT T, SWENSEN T. Juxtapapillary duodenal diverticula and abnormalities by endoscopic retrograde cholangio-pancreatography (ERCP). Scand J Gastroenterol 1977;12:347–351.

49 O'SULLIVAN JN, NOBREGA FT, MORLOCK CG, BROWN AL JR. Acute and chronic pancreatitis in Rochester, Minnesota 1940–1969. Gastroenterology 1972;62:373–379.

50 REGAN PT, MALAGELADA J-R, DIMAGNO EP, GLANZMAN SL, GO VLW. Comparative effects of antacids, cimetidine and enteric coating on the therapeutic response to oral enzymes in severe pancreatic insufficiency. New Engl J Med 1977;297:854–858.

51 RICHTER JM, SCHAPIRO RH, MULLEY AG, WARSHAW AL. Association of pancreas divisum and pancreatitis, and its treatment by sphincteroplasty of the accessory ampulla. Gastroenterology 1981;81:1104–1110.

52 ROBECHEK PJ. Hereditary chronic relapsing pancreatitis. A clue to pancreatitis in general? Am J Surg 1967;113:819–824.

53 RUSSELL RCG, WONG NW, COTTON PB. Accessory sphincterotomy (endoscopic and surgical) in patients with pancreas divisum. Br J Surg 1984;71:954–957.

54 SAHEL J, CROS R-C, BOURRY J, SARLES H. Clinicopathological conditions associated with pancreas divisum. Digestion 1982;23:1–8.

55 SAHEL J, SARLES H. Citrate therapy in chronic calcifying pancreatitis; preliminary results. In: Mitchell CJ, Kelleher J, eds. Pancreatic disease in clinical practice. London; Pitman, 1981:346–353.

56 SANDERS JHB, DRUMMOND S, WORMSLEY KG. Inhibition of gastric secretion in treatment of pancreatic insufficiency. Br Med J 1977;i:418–419.

57 SARLES H. Chronic calcifying pancreatitis. Scand J Gastroenterol 1985;20:651–659.

58 SARLES H, CROS RC, BIDART JM. A multicenter inquiry on the etiology of pancreatic diseases. Digestion 1979;19:110–125.

59 SARLES H, SAHEL J. Progress report. Cholestasis and lesions of the biliary tract in chronic pancreatitis. Gut 1978;19:851–857.

60 SARLES H, SAHEL J, STAUB JL, BOURRY J, LAUGIER R. Chronic pancreatitis. In: Howat HT, Sarles H, eds. The exocrine pancreas. London: W.B. Saunders, 1979;402–439.

61 SARNER M, COTTON PB. Classification of pancreatitis. Gut 1984;25:756–759.

62 SHWACHMAN H, HOLSCLAW DS. Complications of cystic fibrosis. New Engl J Med 1969;281:500–501.

63 SHEARMAN DJC, FINLAYSON NDC. Diseases of the pancreas. In: Diseases of the gastrointestinal tract and liver. Edinburgh: Churchill Livingstone, 1982: 790–791.

64 SIBERT JR. Hereditary pancreatitis in England and Wales. *J Med Genet* 1978;15:189–201.

65 SLAFF J, JACOBSON D, TILLMAN CR, CURINGTON C, TOSKES P. Protease-specific suppression of pancreatic enocrine secretion. *Gastroenterology* 1984;87:44–52.

66 STAPLETON EB, KENNEDY J, NOUSIA-ARVANITAKIS S, LINSHAW MA. Hyperuricosuria due to high-dose pancreatic extract therapy in cystic fibrosis. *New Engl J Med* 1976;295:246–248.

67 STAUB JL, SARLES H, SOULE JC, GALMICHE JP, CAPRON JP. No effect of cimetidine on the therapeutic response to oral enzymes in severe pancreatic insufficiency. *New Engl J Med* 1981;304:1364–1365.

68 STERN RC, BOAT TF, DOERSHUK CF, TUCKER AS, MILLER RB, MATTHEWS LW. Cystic fibrosis diagnosed after age 13. Twenty-five teenage and adult patients including three asymptomatic men. *Ann Intern Med* 1977;87:188–191.

69 TOOULI J, ROBERTS-THOMSON IC, DENT J, LEE J. Sphincter of Oddi motility disorders in patients with idiopathic recurrent pancreatitis. *Br J Surg* 1985;72:859–863.

70 VICONTE G. Effects of ethanol on the sphincter of Oddi: an endoscopic manometric study. *Gut* 1983;24:20–27.

71 WARSHAW AL. Pain in chronic pancreatitis. Patients, patience, and the impatient surgeon. *Gastroenterology* 1984;86:987–989.

72 WARSHAW AL, RICHTER JM, SCHAPIRO RH. The cause and treatment of pancreatitis associated with pancreas divisum. *Ann Surg* 1983;198:443–452.

73 WHITE TT, KAVLIE H. Congenital obstruction of the pancreatic duct at the duodenum. *Ann Surg* 1978;175:194–196.

74 ZENTLER-MUNRO PL, FINE DR, BATTEN JC, NORTHFIELD TC. Effect of cimetidine on enzyme inactivation, bile acid precipitation, and lipid solubilisation in pancreatic steatorrhoea due to cystic fibrosis. *Gut* 1985;26:892–901.

Chapter 37
Surgery for Chronic Pancreatitis

C. W. VENABLES

Introduction

The role of surgery in the management of patients with chronic pancreatitis remains controversial. There are some physicians who believe that surgery has no place in the treatment of this condition, claiming that avoidance of alcohol and adequate medical therapy will control most patients without the risks of operation [1]. In contrast, there are surgeons who believe that only radical surgery offers adequate control for the severe pain suffered by many of these patients.

Part of the reason for this controversy lies in the present disagreement as to what is 'chronic pancreatitis'. This makes comparison of results from different centres very difficult. Problems with the classification of pancreatitis have been referred to earlier (see Chapters 35 and 36), but they become particularly important in discussion of management and prognosis.

Classification of pancreatitis

If any classification of a disease is to be useful it should be easy to apply and should provide information that is useful in management and prognosis. At present the most commonly used classification of pancreatitis is that of the Marseille symposium [21] which divided pancreatitis into three groups.

Marseille classification

Acute pancreatitis

This is an acute inflammatory condition of the pancreas, which is followed by complete clinical and functional recovery after removal of the primary cause or factors.

Acute relapsing pancreatitis

Recurrent attacks of acute inflammation within the pancreas, with complete clinical and functional recovery between the attacks and no evidence of structural damage describe acute relapsing pancreatitis.

Chronic pancreatitis

This is a chronic inflammatory process within the pancreas associated with residual damage, either functional or anatomical, which persists even when the primary factors or causes are removed.

Revised classification

Although the Marseille classification was the best that could be achieved at that time, it is probably no longer ideal. It was devised before many of the modern, relatively non-invasive, imaging techniques for the pancreas became available (see Chapter 33). In 1963 the only way of assessing pancreatic damage was with a test of pancreatic exocrine function. It is now known that studies of exocrine function can be normal even with major structural damage, particularly

536

when the damage is in the distal duct system. The use of such tests for assessing the pancreas after an acute attack of pancreatitis must inevitably lead to an underestimate of structural damage.

With recognition of this problem there has been a recent attempt to reclassify pancreatitis [24]. Unfortunately it was decided to classify pancreatitis as either 'acute', or 'chronic' with no other sub-divisions. It was recognized that this classification was not ideal as it left a large group of patients in the grey-zone between the two extremes.

The author's centre has come to recognize an increasing number of patients whose *'chronic'* pancreatitis has followed an earlier episode of acute pancreatitis. Such patients were regarded as very uncommon [22]. The author believes that the original Marseille classification should be revised as follows (Table 37.1).

Table 37.1. Proposed classification of pancreatitis.

Major Type	Subtypes
Acute Pancreatitis	Initial attack
	Recurrent attack
	Complicated attack
Persistent Pancreatitis	
Chronic Pancreatitis	Painful
	Painless

Acute pancreatitis

This is an acute inflammatory condition of the pancreas which is followed by complete clinical and structural recovery.

The term 'relapsing acute pancreatitis' should be abandoned as confusing, because it contributes nothing to management, as each attack is handled in a similar manner. However, acute attacks may occur more than once and such patients can be labelled as having 'recurrent acute pancreatitis', the important point being that all such attacks should be followed by complete structural recovery.

Persistent pancreatitis

This is an inflammatory process within the pancreas, of sudden onset, associated with persistent or recurrent pain and clinical features of persistent pancreatic inflammation (for example, raised amylase, weight loss, malabsorption etc.).

Non-invasive imaging techniques (CT, ultrasound (US)) or ERCP will usually show evidence of structural damage in the pancreas. A combination of ERCP with CT, or US is best at demonstrating such damage. Studies of function may also be abnormal.

Painful chronic pancreatitis [30]

This is a chronic inflammatory process in the pancreas of insidious onset, associated with progressive functional and structural damage. Pain is a prominent feature in this condition—it is usually continuous and often punctuated by episodes of more severe pain. Pancreatic imaging studies will demonstrate structural damage and studies of function will usually be abnormal. Calcification may or may not be present.

Painless chronic pancreatitis

This is a chronic inflammatory process in the pancreas associated with marked functional and structural changes but without pain. It will often be diagnosed by the presence of calcification of the pancreas on a plain abdominal radiograph (although this is not a prerequisite). These patients frequently present with malabsorption and steatorrhoea—function studies are always abnormal.

Indications for surgery

This classification is useful in defining those who should be considered for surgery. There is clearly no place for pancreatic surgery in patients with uncomplicated 'acute pancreatitis', or 'recurrent acute pancreatitis', or in those with 'painless chronic pancreatitis' (Table 37.1).

In the other diagnostic groups the limitations of surgery have to be recognized before defining when it is indicated. The surgeon can only treat pancreatitis in three ways—he can resect diseased tissue, he can improve drainage of the main pancreatic duct system, or he can use a combination of these techniques. What he cannot

achieve is reversal of previous acinar, or islet cell damage. There is no place for surgery in the management of exocrine insufficiency or diabetes.

The major indication for surgery is the relief of **pain**—this is only likely to be successful if any aetiological cause, such as alcoholism, is removed, otherwise continued damage to the pancreas will cause a recurrence of symptoms. A lesser, but important indication for operation is the presence

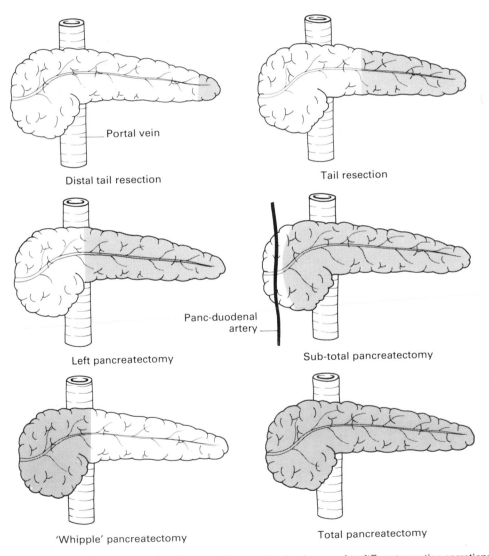

Fig. 37.1. Diagrammatic representation of amount of pancreatic gland removed in different resection operations

of a **cyst** or **pseudocyst**. The final indication is **recurrent gastrointestinal bleeding**—rare patients with chronic pancreatitis present with upper gastrointestinal bleeding associated with left loin or back pain [11].

Operative procedures

Pancreatic resections (Fig. 37.1)

These vary from a limited resection of the tail of the pancreas to complete removal of the gland.

Distal tail resection

This involves removal of the distal 2–3 cm of the pancreas in order to gain access to the main pancreatic duct. It is often undertaken for operative pancreatography, which is done more easily this way than through the papilla of Vater. Usually such a limited resection is appropriate for treatment only when combined with a distal drainage procedure.

Tail resection

This involves resection of the pancreatic tail up to the left border of the portal vein, the amount resected being determined by the extent of disease in the tail. It may, or may not be combined with duct drainage.

Left pancreatectomy

This involves resection of the tail and body of the pancreas up to the neck, with preservation of the head and uncinate process. This operation is often necessary in patients with acute onset persistent pancreatitis, because there has often been previous destruction of the neck of the pancreas, leading to severe inflammatory damage to the distal pancreas.

Sub-total Pancreatectomy

This procedure involves removal of most of the pancreatic head, body and tail. The only part of the pancreas left is the uncinate process and a narrow strip of pancreatic head along the inner loop of the duodenum, in order to preserve the pancreaticoduodenal arteries supplying the duodenum. This is a technically demanding procedure [27] and has the disadvantage of removing most of the islet cells, increasing the risk of diabetes.

Pancreaticoduodenectomy (Whipple's procedure)

This is performed exactly as for pancreatic carcinoma of the head (see Chapter 38) [16]. It has the disadvantage that the duodenum and the distal common bile duct have to be removed at the same time adding to the number of anastomoses. If the stomach is left intact postoperative stomal ulceration is very common, presumably because the residual pancreas produces insufficient bicarbonate for adequate neutralization of acid. The author prefers to add an antrectomy to the duodenal resection, but others claim that truncal vagotomy achieves the same objective. Recently it has been suggested that long-term results are improved by preserving the pylorus intact [4].

Total pancreatectomy

While there are advocates for this procedure, most surgeons would prefer to avoid it if at all possible. It has the distinct disadvantage of removing all the islet cell production of insulin and glucagon, so that diabetic control can prove extremely difficult. An alternative is to perform a pancreaticoduodenectomy in the standard way and then inject the pancreatic tail duct with a solution of prolamine [7, 9]. This leads to acinar atrophy in the pancreatic tail with preservation of the islets. This procedure re-

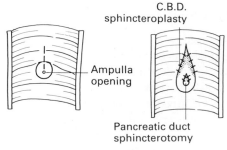

Sphincterotomy or sphincteroplasty

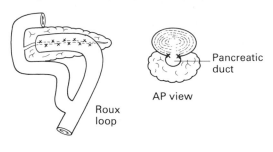

Lateral pancreaticojejunostomy

Fig. 37.2. Types of pancreatic duct drainage.

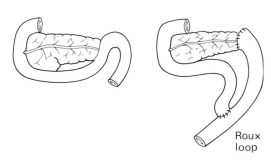

Caudal pancreaticojejunostomy

mains very experimental and cannot be recommended until greater experience has been obtained.

Pancreatic drainage procedures
(Fig. 37.2) [19, 20]

Sphincterotomy or sphincteroplasty of pancreatic duct

This used to be a popular method of treatment for chronic pancreatitis, avoiding the hazards associated with pancreatic resection, or duct drainage [2, 17]. It is now rarely done as the long-term results are poor and endoscopic retrograde pancreatography has shown that the strictures of the proximal part of the main duct are, in most patients, beyond the reach of this procedure.

Caudal pancreaticojejunostomy

This is an anastomosis between the distal pancreatic duct and a loop of jejunum [5]. The classical technique is to isolate a Roux-en-Y loop in the mid-jejunum and to anastomose the proximal end of this loop to the tail of the pancreas. In the author's experience an anastomosis to the duodeno-jejunal flexure is much easier and apparently as successful. The amount of pancreatic tail resected depends upon the severity of ductal damage.

Lateral pancreaticojejunostomy

In this procedure the aim is to marsupialize as much of the main pancreatic duct as is possible, while anastomosing the opened duct to a loop of jejunum (Fig. 37.2) [18].

Choosing the operation

There is no one operation that is appropriate for every patient with chronic pancreatitis. Any attempt to use a single procedure exclusively is bound to fail, as the nature of the structural damage in the gland varies considerably from one patient to the next.

Until the advent of endoscopic retrograde pancreatography (ERP) the only widely available imaging technique was operative pancreatography, either through the tail, or by cannulation of the ampulla of Vater through a duodenotomy. The disadvantages of this technique were that additional surgery was required, only static films were possible (which might be of poor quality) and a surgical decision had to be made immediately. Modern imaging techniques have enabled the selection of the most appropriate procedure for the individual patient to be planned preoperatively.

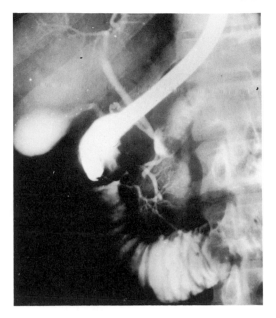

Fig. 37.3. Pancreatogram showing extravasation of the contrast medium from the main duct system in the neck area of the pancreas.

Acute onset persistent pancreatitis

The cause of the pancreatitis in such patients is frequently an area of localized necrosis within the pancreatic gland which leads to duct obstruction from fibrosis, extravasation of pancreatic secretion, or abscess formation (Fig. 37.3).

A persistent hyperamylasaemia ranging from slightly above normal to several thousand i.u./l is often, but not invariably, present in such patients. Other features include progressive weight loss, pain, malaise and, not infrequently, nausea with vomiting. While non-invasive imaging techniques (US and CT) may often help, endoscopic retrograde pancreatography is usually the best way to make the diagnosis. It may show oedematous changes in the second part of the duodenum, a stricture (with delayed disappearance of contrast from the distal pancreatic duct), obstruction of the pancreatic duct, extravasation of contrast from the duct system into the surrounding area, or an actual cyst cavity. If there is extra-ductal extravasation of the contrast medium, or the dye fills a cyst the surgical treatment should be performed within 24 hours as infection is inevitable, with a grave risk to the patient's life. Urgent operation is also recommended if there is a delay of over 30 min. in the disappearance of the contrast from the pancreatic duct, as infection is also a problem in such patients.

The operation performed depends partly upon the site of the lesion (for example distal resection when the tail is necrotic) and partly on the amount of normal duct system remaining (Fig. 37.4). The aim is to preserve as much functional pancreatic tissue as possible and to establish drainage of the distal duct, whenever there is doubt about the patency of the proximal duct beyond the point of resection. In addition, if a cyst is present then separate drainage of this into the stomach or intestine is necessary.

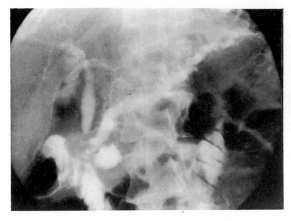

Fig. 37.4. Pancreatogram showing changes of chronic pancreatitis maximal in head of pancreas with intra-pancreatic cyst in the head.

Painful chronic pancreatitis

These patients present at any age and their treatment is difficult. Investigation usually shows diffuse changes throughout the gland, quite often associated with intra-ductular calculi which may or may not be calcified. The types of ductular changes found at endoscopic retrograde pancreatography vary considerably, ranging from diffuse dilatation of the whole of the major duct to areas of dilatation separated by multiple strictures ('chain-of-lakes'), often with calculi. The site and nature of the duct changes determine the type of operation (Table 37.2).

Perhaps the most difficult group of patients are those who have severe pain (and exocrine insufficiency), but without any obstruction or dilatation of the main duct. Such patients are rare in the author's experience. It has been suggested that they are most appropriately treated by sub-total pancreatectomy [10].

Table 37.2. Selection of operative procedure in relation to changes seen in pancreatogram.

Site/type of duct change	Operation(s)
Changes only in tail duct	Resection of tail
Changes maximal in tail (Fig. 37.1)	Resection tail + Pancreaticojejunostomy
Necrosis or stricture in body or neck of pancreas	Left pancreatectomy or distal tail resection + drainage
Changes maximal in head (Fig. 37.4)	Pancreaticoduodenectomy ('Whipple' procedure)
Diffuse dilated duct	Resection of distal tail + pancreaticojejunostomy
'Chain-of-lakes'	Lateral pancreaticojejunostomy
Narrow duct system	Sub-total pancreatectomy

Other surgery in chronic pancreatitis

Biliary tract

If the gall bladder contains stones it should be removed. Sometimes preoperative or intra-operative cholangiography will show a 'rat tail' stricture of the retropancreatic common bile duct with dilatation above it (Fig. 37.5). This may be due to oedema, but it is more often due to fibrosis. Under these circumstances separate biliary drainage is necessary, performing either a choledochoduodenostomy or choledochojejunostomy into a Roux-en-Y loop [14].

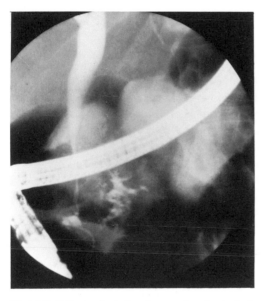

Fig. 37.5. Retrograde cholangiogram showing typical 'rat tail' stenosis of retropancratic duct system. Note blocked pancreatic duct in the head region.

Duodenal bypass

Occasionally there may be so much oedema or fibrosis around the duodenum that the lumen is obstructed, requiring a gastroenterostomy to be performed.

Cyst/abscess drainage

Small cysts or sterile abscesses are not infrequently found during mobilization of the pancreas, but they do not need specific treatment. If there is a large cyst or abscess, which is not drained adequately by the resection, separate drainage of the collection may also need to be done. The safest method is to drain it either into the nearby stomach (cystogastrostomy), or into a Roux-en-Y loop of jejunum (cystojejunostomy). Direct external drainage is not recommended, as a pancreatic fistula may follow.

Complications of pancreatic surgery

Perioperative complications

These include all those associated with any major abdominal surgery in addition to those specific to the operation itself. It is important to recognize that pancreatic surgery can be extremely difficult and should not be undertaken on an occasional basis, because the incidence of complications will directly reflect the experience of the operator. The common complications are the following.

Incidental splenectomy

As the splenic artery and vein are closely applied to the posterior surface of the pancreas, it is usually necessary to divide them in order to mobilize the tail of the gland. This can sometimes be done without damaging the short gastric branches of the splenic artery, thus preserving a blood supply to the spleen. Often the amount of peri-pancreatic and peri-splenic fibrosis makes this impossible, and the spleen has to be removed to mobilize the pancreatic tail.

Chapter 37

Haemorrhage

In chronic pancreatitis the amount of peri-pancreatic fibrosis and inflammation can be considerable and it may be difficult to find normal tissue planes. During dissection of the pancreas it is not unusual to find the portal vein, inferior mesenteric vein and middle colic artery all closely adherent to the pancreas so that damage to these vessels occurs readily. Experience is required to avoid or deal with these problems.

Ileus

Prolonged ileus often follows pancreatic surgery, perhaps due to the extensive intra-abdominal dissection. It may be made worse by the poor preoperative condition of the patient, who may already be severely malnourished. Most patients should therefore receive intravenous parenteral nutritional support starting within 24–48 hours of pancreatic surgery and continuing until an adequate intake by mouth is possible.

Sepsis

Septic complications, particularly a subphrenic abscess, are common after major pancreatic surgery. The risk of sepsis is probably increased by splenectomy and preoperative hypoalbuminaemia. Bacterial contamination is usually endogenous in type and is generally caused by the same bacterial species as are found in the biliary tree (for example, *E. coli*, *Pseudomonas*, or anaerobic bacteria). To decrease this risk all patients should receive perioperative prophylactic antibiotics—for example gentamicin 120 mg with the premedication and 80 mg eight-hourly for 2–5 days with metronidazole 400 mg six-hourly for 2–5 days.

Deep venous thrombosis and pulmonary embolus

This can be quite a problem as many of these patients have been in hospital for some time preoperatively. Prophylactic measures are appropriate, although the use of heparin may be restricted by the threat of intra- and postoperative bleeding.

Pancreatic fistula

If the operative procedure has been properly selected and the pancreatic duct (or cyst) has been drained into the gut if there is evidence of a proximal obstruction, a pancreatic fistula should be uncommon and self-limiting.

Mortality

Pancreatic surgery is associated with a higher operative mortality than most other abdominal operations. An overall mortality rate of around 5% can be expected even in experienced hands [15, 16, 23]. Resection appears to carry a greater risk than drainage—the larger the pancreatic resection the greater is the risk of death (up to 15% for total pancreatectomy).

Late complications

Diabetes mellitus

This is the commonest late complication of pancreatic surgery. Its development is related to some extent to the amount of pancreas removed, but this is not a universal finding. The risk of developing diabetes depends more on the amount of pre-existing islet cell damage from the inflammatory process and its effects upon the blood supply, than on the amount of gland removed surgically.

Malabsorption

Although this is a potential complication of pancreatic surgery it is relatively uncommon unless total pancreatectomy has been performed, or severe pancreatic insufficiency was present before operation. Usually surgical treatment results in a small improvement in absorption, with an associated increase of weight.

Recurrence of pancreatitis

If the correct operation has been done it is unusual for pancreatitis to recur unless the patient continues to drink alcohol. When a patient re-presents with recurrent symptoms one should always take care to exclude secret drinking. Rarely a pancreatic stone may form proximal to a pancreaticojejunostomy, or a bypass may have become blocked. An ERCP may assist in reaching a diagnosis if the pancreatic duct can be cannulated.

Late deaths

Most surgical series report a fairly high death rate during the follow-up period. Usually these deaths are from continued alcohol abuse, or from suicide in someone who is already psychologically disturbed. Total and sub-total pancreatectomy are, however, associated with a fairly high death rate from uncontrolled hypoglycaemia. For this reason there is considerable interest in trying to restore islet cell function by autotransplantation of islets in such patients [3, 12].

Results of surgical treatment (Table 37.3)

Review of the published results of surgery for chronic pancreatitis makes it immediately obvious that there is a desperate need for a better classification of the disease. No two series are exactly comparable with regard to the type of patients who are classified as having chronic pancreatitis and often acute pancreatic pseudocysts are included within this group. Furthermore few of the large series provide any clear reasons for selecting one operation over another. There are, however, a few general points that can be made.

Resection or drainage?

Bitter controversy rages as to which is better. Some believe that lateral pancreaticojejunostomy is the best procedure [13, 26, 29] while others argue in favour of resection [28]. However analysis of a number of published series shows that there is little difference between the two procedures as far as long-term results are concerned.

Table 37.3. Results of different surgical procedures (analysis of six reported series).

Procedure	None	Pain at follow-up Mild	Severe
Caudal pancreaticojejunostomy (n = 22)	59%	23%	18%
Lateral pancreaticojejunostomy (n = 209)	54%	30%	16%
Left pancreatectomy (n = 52)	48%	10%	42%
Sub-total pancreatectomy (n = 25)	56%	8%	36%
'Whipple' (n = 46)	63%	13%	24%

Table 37.4. Pain relief obtained more than one year after operation for persistent pancreatitis (n = 16; interval x̄ = 43.6; range 14–16 months).

Relief (analogue scale)	Number
100	10
76–99	0
50–75	4
1–49	0
0	2

Distal versus lateral pancreaticojejunostomy drainage

Again there are considerable arguments between those who favour the former and those who prefer the latter. Published comparisons are unsatisfactory [13, 25].

Partial (80%), versus sub-total, or total pancreatectomy

Direct comparisons are hindered by disparaties between different series. There is little doubt that mortality and the risks associated with diabetes are increased by sub-total or total pancreatectomy. Most surgeons would prefer to avoid these operations if possible [8].

Proximal (Whipple) versus distal pancreatic resection

Some claim that the best results are obtained by resection of the pancreatic head [28] and Gall, Gebhardt, and Zirngibl [7] have reported very good results for a combination of pancreaticoduodenectomy and occlusion of the distal pancreatic duct—which produces the equivalent of a total pancreatectomy.

Conclusion

Overall there seems to be general acceptance of the concept that the type of operation should be determined by the anatomy of the pancreatic duct system [6] and that, while a drainage procedure is acceptable for a dilated duct system, resection is best where the duct is small. Finally the long-term results obtained in our patients with 'acute onset persistent pancreatitis' are very good (Table 37.4). This group seems to be an ideal one for surgical management.

References

1 AMMANN RW, AKOVBIANTZ A, LARGIADER F, SCHUELER G. Course and outcome of chronic pancreatitis. Longitudinal study of a mixed medico-surgical series of 245 patients. *Gastroenterology* 1984;**86**:820–828.

2 ANDERSON TM, PITT HA, LONGMIRE WP. Experience with sphincteroplasty and sphincterotomy in pancreatobiliary surgery. *Ann Surg* 1985;**201**:399–406.

3 CAMERON JL, MEHIGAN DG, BROE PJ, ZUIDEMA GD. Distal pancreatectomy and islet autotransplantation for chronic pancreatitis. *Ann Surg* 1981;**193**:312–317.

4 COOPER MJ, WILLIAMSON RCN. Conservative pancreatectomy. *Br J Surg* 1985;**72**:801–803.

5 DUVAL MK. Caudal pancreatico-jejunostomy for chronic relapsing pancreatitis. *Ann Surg* 1954;**140**:775–785.

6 FREY CF. Role of subtotal pancreatectomy and pancreatico-jejunostomy in chronic pancreatitis. *J Surg Res* 1981;**31**:361–370.

7 GALL FP, GEBHARDT C, ZIRNGIBL H. Chronic pancreatitis—results in 116 consecutive partial pancreatico-duodenectomies combined with pancreatic duct occlusion. *Hepatogastroenterology* 1982;**29**:115–129.

8 GALL FP, MUHE E, GEBHARDT C. Results of partial and total pancreatico-duodenectomy in 117 patients with chronic pancreatitis. *World J Surg* 1981;**5**:269–275.

9 GEBHARDT C, GALL FP. Partielle duodenopankreatektomie mit intraoperativer pankreass-schwanzveröding bei chronischer pankreatitis. *Langebecks Arch Chir* 1980;**353**:57–62.

10 GRODSINSKY C, SCHUMAN BM, BLOCK MA. Absence of pancreatic duct dilatation in chronic pancreatitis: surgical significance. *Arch Surg* 1977; 112:444–449.

11 HALL RI, LAVELLE MJ, VENABLES CW. Chronic pancreatitis as a cause of gastrointestinal bleeding. *Gut* 1982;23:250–255.

12 HINSHAW DB, JOLLEY WB, HINSHAW DB, KAISER JE, HINSHAW K. Islet autotransplantation after pancreatectomy for chronic pancreatitis with a new method of islet preparation. *Am J Surg* 1981; 142:118–122.

13 JORDAN GJ, STRUG BS, CROWDER WE. Current status of pancreatojejunostomy in the management of chronic pancreatitis. *Am J Surg* 1977;133:46–51.

14 KIM U, SHEN H, ROMEU J. Biliary obstruction associated with chronic pancreatitis: surgical approaches. *Mt Sinai J Med (NY)* 1979;46:489–493.

15 KINAMI Y, KONISHI K, TAKESHITA Y. Effectiveness and limitation of surgical treatment for chronic pancreatitis. *Gastroenterol Jpn* 1982;17:334–340.

16 LONGMIRE WP JR. The vicissitudes of pancreatic surgery. *Am J Surg* 1984;147:17–24.

17 NARDI GL Transduodenal sphincteroplasty. 5–25 year follow-up of 89 patients. *Ann Surg* 1983;198:453–461.

18 PEUSTOW CB, GILLESBY WJ. Retrograde surgical drainage of pancreas for chronic relapsing pancreatitis. *Arch Surg* 1958;76:898–907.

19 PRINZ RA, GREENLEE HB. Pancreatic duct drainage in 100 patients with chronic pancreatitis. *Ann Surg* 1981;194:313–320.

20 PROCTOR HJ, MENDES OC, THOMAS CG, HERBST CA. Surgery for chronic pancreatitis: drainage versus resection. *Ann Surg* 1979;189:664–671.

21 SARLES H. *Pancreatitis: symposium in Marseille 1963.* Basel: S. Karger, 1965.

22 SARLES H, GEROI AMI-SANTANDREA A. Chronic pancreatitis. *Clin Gastroenterol* 1972;1:167.

23 SARLES J-C, NACCHIERO M, GARANI F, SALASC B Surgical treatment for chronic pancreatitis. *Am J Surg* 1982;144:317–321.

24 SARNER M, COTTON PB Classification of pancreatitis. *Gut* 1984;25:756–759.

25 SATO T, NOTO N, MATSUNO S, MIYAKAWA K. Follow-up results of surgical treatment for chronic pancreatitis: present status in Japan. *Am J Surg* 1981;142:317–323.

26 TAYLOR RH, BAGLEY FH, BRAASCH JW, WARREN KW. Ductal drainage or resection for chronic pancreatitis. *Am J Surg* 1981;141:28–33.

27 TRAPNELL JE. Subtotal pancreatectomy. *Br J Hosp Med* 1978;19:482–491.

28 TRAVERSO LW, TOMPKINS RK, URREA PT, LONGMIRE WJ. Surgical treatment of chronic pancreatitis. *Ann Surg* 1979;190:312–319.

29 WHITE TT, HART MJ Pancreaticojejunostomy versus resection in the treatment of chronic pancreatitis. *Am J Surg* 1979;138:129–132.

30 WONG DH, SCHUMAN BD, GRODSINSKY C. The value of endoscopic retrograde cholangiopancreatography in the surgical management of chronic pancreatitis. *Am J Gastroenterol* 1980;73:353–356.

Chapter 38
Carcinoma of the Pancreas and Ampulla of Vater

R. C. G. RUSSELL

Introduction

Carcinoma of the pancreas is now the fifth commonest cause of death from cancer in the United States, behind lung, bowel, breast and prostatic carcinomas—its incidence having increased threefold since 1930. In England and Wales the incidence of pancreatic cancer has doubled during the same time period. Although interest in this disease has increased since the early 1970s there have been few therapeutic advances.

Most patients still die within six months of diagnosis. Operative treatment appears ineffective despite a third of the tumours remaining localized up to the time of death. Ampullary tumours appear to have a more favourable outcome and therefore it is essential to determine the exact site of origin of a pancreatic carcinoma—the term 'periampullary' is unhelpful and should be abandoned. Tumours originating in the bile duct also appear to have a better prognosis and should therefore be demarcated from true pancreatic duct cancer.

Incidence

The incidence of carcinoma of the pancreas is around 9.5 per 100,000 *per annum* in the U.S.A. and Western Europe [33]. Its incidence is highest in males, with a ratio of about 1.5 to 1, and increases with age. Analysis of the effect of race is complicated by relative underdiagnosis of the condition in underdeveloped nations. Nevertheless the average annual age-adjusted incidence rate for the black community in the U.S.A. is 14.4 compared with 9.5 cases per 100,000 in the white community [34]. High incidence rates have been reported in Maoris in New Zealand, especially among males, and in females in Hawaii. International mortality rates [3] show a band of higher incidence rates (7.5 for males and 4.5 per 100,000 for females) in the northern latitudes, another band of intermediate rates and a band of low rates closer to the equator. In contrast to some other tumours (for example oesophagus) there are no areas with inordinately high prevalence of pancreatic cancer and the ratio of high to low incidence rates is small.

Pancreatic cancer appears to be commoner in urban than in rural areas but has no relation to social class. Neither genetic, nor familial factors are important [33].

Risk factors

Tobacco

The data pertaining to cigarette smoking are consistent and repeatable, demonstrating an increase in pancreatic cancer of 60–200% in cigarette smokers [43]. Smokers also die earlier from this disease than do non-smokers. The relationship of pancreatic cancer to smoking probably accounts for the rising incidence of the disease.

Alcoholism

The association between alcoholism and acute and chronic pancreatitis is well recognized. However, the relationship between alcohol and cancer is open to debate. No report has established alcohol as a risk factor, once smoking has been taken into account.

Diabetes

Mortality rates from pancreatic cancer correlate with diabetic mortality in women, but not men. Direct evidence that diabetes predisposes to pancreatic cancer comes from follow-up studies of deaths in diabetic patients [4]. No satisfactory mechanism to explain this association has been proposed.

Pancreatitis

There is no evidence that pancreatitis predisposes to carcinoma of the pancreas, although chronic inflammation in some part of the gland is commonly associated with such cancers. It is thought that this results from a downstream block of the main pancreatic duct (see Chapter 36). Carcinoma may rarely develop in patients with longstanding chronic pancreatitis, but this may be fortuitous.

Carcinogens

Carcinoma of the pancreas can be readily induced in experimental animals by implantation of carcinogens directly into the pancreas. Methylnitrosourea and some metabolites of di-n-propylnitrosamine, given systemically, will produce carcinoma in some animals but the mechanism by which this occurs is unknown.

Diet

Evidence suggesting the importance of diet in this condition comes from studies indicating a significant correlation between fat intake and the national incidence of pancreatic carcinomas. Studies in Japan have shown increased protein intake in patients

with this tumour. A significant correlation between the national consumption of coffee and the incidence of this cancer in men has been claimed but this is disputed. Nitrosamines have been implicated in the causation of pancreatic cancer, but the evidence for this is tenuous.

Pathology

Primary, non-endocrine tumours of the pancreas can be classified by their cell of origin into those of duct cell, acinar cell, connective tissue and uncertain histogenesis origins.

Duct cell adenocarcinoma

This is the commonest type of pancreatic cancer constituting 75% of all malignant epithelial tumours of the gland. It probably arises from the duct epithelium, an idea supported by the finding of *in situ* carcinoma in the duct epithelium adjacent to resected cancer in 24% of specimens.

The cancer originates in the head of the pancreas in 60%, the body in 13%, the tail in 5% and at multiple sites in 21% of patients [14] (Fig. 38.1). Few tumours are under 2 cm in diameter at presentation, the median being 5 cm. In a retrospective study

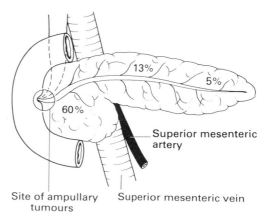

Fig. 38.1. Frequency distribution of adenocarcinoma in various areas of the pancreas.

14% of tumours were confined to the pancreas (Stage I), 21% showed invasion of local lymph nodes (Stage II) and around two-thirds had already developed metastases (Stage IV) at the time of diagnosis. A higher percentage of patients with tumours of the body and tail of the pancreas were Stage III on presentation. Only about 5% of patients with carcinomas of the head are Stage I at the time of diagnosis, lymph node involvement occurring in the superior and posterior pancreaticoduodenal nodes most commonly. Metastases occur in the liver, regional nodes, peritoneum, lungs and pleura in descending order of frequency. Invasion of nerve sheaths is found in 90% of patients and venous invasion in 50% [15].

In addition to the tumour, foci of haemorrhage with pancreatic cell and fat necrosis are frequently present. In association with, or probably as a result of, ductal obstruction atrophy of acinar cells is marked with duct and ductular dilatation.

Tumours of the **papilla of Vater** arise from the ampulla and usually project into the duodenum. Periampullary tumours probably arise from the pancreatic duct and should be considered as cancers of the pancreatic head. True ampullary tumours can be benign and when malignant are slow growing with a good prognosis, even if not resected.

Giant cell carcinoma (pleomorphic carcinoma, sarcomatoid cancer, carcinosarcoma)

This is distinguished by the presence of bizarre giant tumour cells and sarcomatous cells. Epithelial glands and mucin are present. Patients present with advanced disease and median survival is around two months.

Adenosquamous cancer

This rare tumour is recognized by the presence of glandular and squamous cells in equal distribution. Survival is average for pancreatic cancers.

Microadenocarcinoma

This consists of sheets of cells with uniform oval nuclei and pale staining cytoplasm. It resembles carcinoid in appearance, but has none of the characteristic staining properties. Survival is poor.

Mucinous adenocarcinoma

This consists of well differentiated adenocarcinomatous cells containing excessive amounts of mucin. It is often large and has a better prognosis than other pancreatic tumours.

Cystadenocarcinoma

This well known form of pancreatic cancer is distinct from a benign serous cystadenoma. It can grow to a large size and is commoner in women. Characteristically, there are multilocular cysts lined by tall columnar cells with prominent intracystic papillary projections. Prolonged survival is usual with or without resection.

Acinar cell origin

This has been recognized as a distinctive type of pancreatic tumour. These tumours are grey/tan in colour and firm in consistency with areas of necrosis. Characteristic acinar formation is present with a small central lumen. Median survival is similar to that of tumours of ductular origin.

Pancreatoblastoma

This group represents tumours of uncertain origin. They are extremely uncommon. Similarly, papillary cystic carcinoma, a tumour with a distinctive papillary appearance, is of unknown aetiology, rare, and with a low malignant potential.

Anaplastic carcinoma, mixed cell type, and connective tissue cancers are all very rare and experience with such tumours is limited.

Separation of these histological types has so far proved of little value either as an epidemiological tool, or as a guide to therapy or prognosis except for cystadenocarcinoma and ampullary tumours. A detailed pathological classification, based on that proposed by the American Joint Committee for Cancer Staging, has been suggested by Fitzgerald [17] (Table 38.1). This emphasizes the difference in prognosis among cancers 2–3 cm, 3–5 cm and of over 5 cm in diameter. As it is rare for involvement of adjacent organs to occur without local lymph node metastases no separation between local invasion and node involvement is proposed.

Clinical features

Carcinoma of the pancreas can develop in the head, body, or tail. To some extent the site of origin alters the mode of presentation, although the cardinal features of pain, weight loss and jaundice are similar.

Pain

Pain is a presenting symptom in 50–80% of patients and occurs at some stage in 75–90% [48]. It is variable in site and severity, but most frequently it is a dull aching, or boring pain in the epigastric region. Gambill [19] reported the site of pain in 239 patients with pancreatic cancer as mid-epigastric in 46%, upper abdominal in 23%, lower abdominal in 20%, right upper quadrant in 18% and left upper quadrant in 13%. Although 80% of the patients had abdominal pain at some time during their illness it was not a constant feature. The pain is often aggravated by ingestion of food and may be indistinguishable from that of a peptic ulcer; it is often mild for months and only elicited upon direct questioning. In tumours of the body and tail the pain may be altered by position, being worst when recumbent and eased by sitting forward. The classical severe penetrating pain is a late and uncommon symptom.

Table 38.1. Suggested TNM classification of pancreatic cancer [15].

Tumour	TX	= Not assessable
(Add 'i' if local organs infiltrated)	T1	= < 2 cm maximum diameter
	T2	= 2–3 cm maximum diameter
	T3	= 3–5 cm maximum diameter
	T4	= > 5 cm maximum diameter
Nodes	NX	= not assessable
	N0	= no nodal involvement
	N1	= anterior and/or posterior pancreaticoduodenal groups
	N2	= above + superior and/or inferior head nodes
	N3	= above + superior and/or inferior body lymph nodes
	N4	= above + other node groups
Metastases	MX	= not assessed
	M0	= no distant metastases
	M1	= distant metastases

Jaundice

This is the first symptom in 10–30% of all patients with carcinoma of the pancreas and the presenting symptom in 30–65%. It occurs at some time in up to 90% of cases. The jaundice is often accompanied by pain, which may be mild, and often preceeds the jaundice by many months. The classical painless jaundice of pancreatic carcinoma, so often described in textbooks, is fairly uncommon.

The jaundice is usually progressive, until relieved by surgery, but spontaneous fluctuations in severity, early in the course of the disease, are found in about 10% of patients. Pruritus commonly accompanies the jaundice. Jaundice occurs most often with tumours of the head, but is also found in 20–50% of patients with tumours of the body and tail, usually due to hepatic metastases, or obstruction of the bile duct by enlarged lymph nodes in the porta hepatis.

Weight loss

This is prominent, occurring as a presenting feature in over 90% of the patients [48]. It is generally rapid and progressive with an average weight loss of 11.9 kg. The cause is unclear. It cannot be due entirely to malabsorption from blockage of the pancreatic duct as it occurs with small tumours in the tail. Nor can it be entirely explained by anorexia, which is present in about 50% of patients on presentation, as some have an excessive appetite when first seen.

Other symptoms

Gambill [19] noted that weakness, fatigue or epigastric bloating was found in a third of patients. Diarrhoea and rarely, frank steatorrhoea occurs in about 25% and constipation in 10% of patients. Nausea, regurgitation and retching are common symptoms and vomiting, caused by duodenal obstruction, is present in approximately one-quarter of the patients.

It is important to recognize that the symptoms of pancreatic cancer are often mild and vague, so that early diagnosis rests on an awareness that this tumour is one of the causes of unexplained dyspepsia.

Physical signs

Most often there are no abnormal signs. When present, the commonest are jaundice, hepatomegaly, a palpable gall bladder and epigastric tenderness. Recurrent thrombophlebitis occurs in less than 10% of cases. Tumours of the body and tail often present with signs of distant spread—these include hepatomegaly, enlarged supraclavicular lymph nodes, pelvic metastases and ascites. The presence of diabetes is comparatively rare, although the observation that diabetes becomes unstable when cancer develops is well described. The sudden appearance of diabetes, in middle or late life, without a family history is rarely an indication of pancreatic cancer, unless accompanied by weight loss, or vague abdominal pain.

Investigations

The diagnosis of pancreatic disease, until recently, rested on the exclusion of other causes, but now there are a number of imaging techniques available [38] (see Chapter 33). The simplest is that of ultrasound, which achieves a 95% accuracy in diagnosing the presence of pancreatic disease in experienced hands, although distinguishing tumour from pancreatitis can be more difficult. Pathological confirmation of tumour may be obtained, in 80% of patients, by fine needle percutaneous aspiration cytology under ultrasound control, thus avoiding the need for more complex techniques [24].

Unfortunately such expertise is not yet universally available so that each clinician must decide what techniques available to him provide the best sensitivity, specificity and predictive value. Moossa and Levin [37] found that a combination of ultrasound and ERCP with cytology were the best way of diagnosing pancreatic cancer and provided the best discrimination between chronic pancreatitis and carcinoma. A similar study from the Mayo clinic showed that pancreatic function tests and ultrasonography had the highest sensitivities (72% and 84%) for detecting pancreatic disease with a specificity of 80%, while pancreatic scintiscanning had a high sensitivity (90%) with a low specificity (30%). ERCP had a sensitivity and specificity of 90% when successful, but arteriography had a lower sensitivity [16]. Their conclusion was that ultrasound and pancreatic function tests were the best way of diagnosing pancreatic disease without invasive techniques. A combination of these tests with ERCP identified 90% of all patients with significant pancreatic disease and 80% of those with cancer.

A possible sequence for the investigation of suspected carcinoma follows (see also Fig. 38.2).
1. Ultrasound with fine needle aspiration if a mass is detected [5].
2. ERCP to detect the presence of an ampullary tumour, assess the biliary and pancreatic duct systems, and to obtain samples for histological and cytological examination [40].
3. Computerized tomography for the occasional case where adequate delineation has not been obtained by other means. In some countries this may be used as an initial screening examination but in some parts of Britain this is impracticable because of poor access to such machinery.
4. Arteriography for cases where the other techniques have failed.

Pancreatic function tests are now rarely used for the diagnosis of pancreatic cancer because of the technical difficulties involved (see Chapter 34).

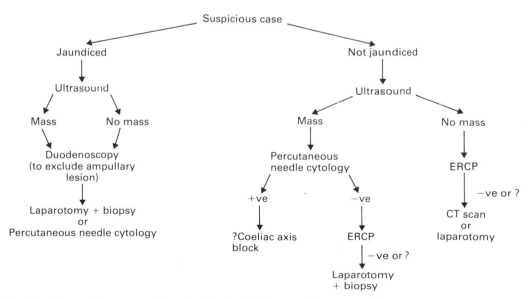

Fig. 38.2. A suggested sequence of investigations for the diagnosis of carcinoma of the pancreas. *Note:* CT scan can assist in diagnosing extent and spread of tumour *or* when ultrasound is difficult or impossible.

Tumour marker studies

Because of the vague symptoms and difficulty in early diagnosis of pancreatic cancer a specific tumour marker would be of considerable value [41].

Carcinoembryonic antigen (CEA)

Elevated plasma CEA concentrations are found in most patients with pancreatic cancer at some time during their disease [50]. Absolute values of CEA are variable and depend upon the rate of production, clearance and excretion. As clearance and excretion depend on hepatobiliary function, any impairment by metastases or bile duct obstruction will have an impact on CEA concentrations. Initial CEA concentrations are usually elevated, rising further with the development of metastases, yet in 20% of cases CEA is within the normal range, even when metastases are present [23]. As CEA is cleared by the liver, it is raised in the presence of jaundice and may be found in increased amounts in duodenal juice in non-jaundiced patients, even when plasma levels are normal. Surgical resection, even if not curative, reduces CEA which rises again as metastases develop. Unfortunately the measurement of CEA in plasma, or duodenal juice is not sufficiently sensitive for use as a screening test.

Pancreatic oncofoetal antigen (POA)

This is a glycoprotein found in foetal and cancerous pancreatic tissue, but not in the normal pancreas. Immunofluorescent studies have shown this antigen to be present in larger amounts in well differentiated cancer cells than in undifferentiated cells; it is mainly located in the cytoplasm. Elevated plasma concentrations are found in some 50% of pancreatic cancer patients, but it is also raised in biliary tract, lung and gastric cancers [30]. POA appears to be superior to CEA in the diagnosis of pancreatic cancer and used in conjunction with CEA may be a useful marker substance.

Serum carbohydrate antigenic determinant (CA19–9)

It has very recently been shown that this marker is raised in pancreatic cancer [50]. The authors have suggested that greater discrimination is achieved if this is measured simultaneously with alpha-foetal-protein (AFP) and CEA [9].

Other markers.

Other markers such as protein degradation products, leukocyte adherence inhibition and galactosyl transferase isoenzyme have been studied in pancreatic cancer, but none have proved useful.

Differential diagnosis

The symptoms of pancreatic cancer are vague and it can be confused with many upper abdominal diseases. However, with the use of modern diagnostic techniques the main difficulty is distinguishing cancer from chronic pancreatitis (see Chapters 33 and 36).

These conditions can resemble each other clinically and may produce similar appearances on imaging techniques. Even at laparotomy both may and frequently do coexist. The only certain way of separating the two is by biopsy and even then false negative results are not uncommon. Pancreatic biopsy has always had a bad reputation, but fine needle aspiration cytology [49] either percutaneously using ultrasound or CT control [5], or at laparotomy is without complication and provides a satisfactory diagnostic yield [42].

Finally if doubt remains the patient should be carefully watched and re-investigated at intervals, for many turn out to have a pancreatic cancer.

Treatment

Using modern techniques the diagnosis of pancreatic cancer should be made before a decision on treatment is reached. Treatment poses a dilemma between a nihilistic approach or unbounded optimism in the face of adverse statistical findings. Even the best surgical series show only a 5% five-year survival for true pancreatic cancer with an operative mortality of some 20%. Only ampullary tumours and tumours of the intra-pancreatic bile duct (often mistaken for pancreatic tumour) have an acceptable five-year survival rate following resection of between 30% and 50%; the operative mortality rate (5–10%) is also lower. While no other treatment has produced a cure for this disease, surgery is done at the expense of considerable morbidity from malabsorption and unstable diabetes in some patients. It is essential to achieve a balance between aggression and conservatism—careful preoperative assessment is therefore required.

Pretreatment assessment

Widespread metastases should be excluded by imaging techniques and a full medical assessment of lung, cardiac and renal function is needed. Hepatic function, including coagulation studies, requires evaluation and correction of any abnormalities. An assessment of the patient's fitness to undergo major surgery should then be made.

Radical surgery (Fig. 38.3)

This should only be considered in patients who are fit enough to tolerate the procedure, who are in the younger age group (under 60 years) and whose tumour appears small (< 3 cm) on imaging studies without any obvious metastases [35].

The traditional procedure for carcinoma of the head of the pancreas has been pan-creatoduodenectomy. However, resection can be incomplete in around one-third of cases, with histopathological studies showing carcinoma *in situ* in the remaining duct system, suggesting a multifocal origin of the tumour. Total pancreatectomy removes the risk of leaving disease behind in the remnant, enables better lymph node clearance and avoids the problems associated with the pancreatic anastomosis [36, 51]. In 1973 Fortner [18] proposed the super-radical or regional approach, in which the tumour was resected *en bloc* with the portal vein, superior mesenteric artery and coeliac artery with subsequent vascular reconstruction [16]. Follow-up studies have failed to confirm any long-term benefit of such radical dissections, in terms of survival, over that achieved by simpler techniques [11, 26]. In addition, total pancreatectomy is inevitably followed by diabetes which can prove difficult to control in many patients. It seems probable, therefore, that if surgery is going to cure the disease, pancreatoduodenectomy alone will achieve this [10].

Palliative surgery (Fig. 38.4)

The presence of carcinoma of the pancreas is not in itself an indication for surgery. The objective of palliative surgery is to relieve symptoms, of which jaundice and duodenal obstruction are those most readily relieved [35].

The ideal surgical biliary bypass is the simplest procedure which will adequately relieve the blockage with the lowest risk of re-obstruction. Late obstruction usually occurs as a result of metastatic glands around the porta hepatis, or from intra-hepatic metastases. The purists advise a Roux-en-Y choledochojejunostomy, but this seems an unnecessarily complicated operation for a patient with a median survival of less than six months. On the other hand the commonly performed cholecystenterostomy can easily re-obstruct from tumour exten-

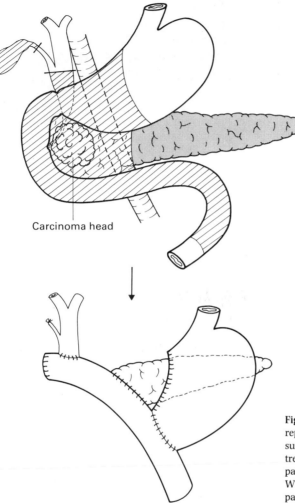

⬚⬚ Area resected in
pancreaticoduodenectomy

▨ Additional area
removed with
total pancreatectomy

Carcinoma head

Whipple reconstruction

Fig. 38.3. Diagrammatic
representation of the radical
surgical procedures used in the
treatment of carcinoma of the
pancreas. Top = areas resected in
Whipple operation and total
pancreatectomy;
bottom = reconstruction technique
after Whipple procedure.

sion up to the cystic duct, or by inspissated
mucus within the cystic duct. Probably the
best palliative procedure is an end-side or
side-side choledochoduodenostomy. The
former has the theoretical advantage of reducing the risk of tumour extension across
the anastomosis, but is technically more difficult.

In the presence of duodenal obstruction
there is no alternative to a gastric bypass,
which should be done at the same time as
the biliary bypass [6]. A long antecolic gastroenterostomy to the antrum of the stomach is the best operation [8]. This should
also be done at the time of biliary bypass if
duodenal infiltration has already occurred,
or if the tumour is close to the duodenal
wall.

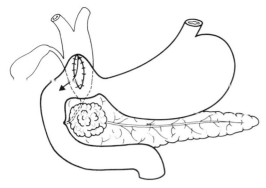

Fig. 38.4. Diagrammatic representation of choledochoduodenostomy.

Relief of jaundice with an endoprosthesis

An endoprosthesis can be inserted either via a percutaneous trans-hepatic route under radiological control [27] or endoscopically after duodenoscopic sphincterotomy [12, 13]. Either of these procedures should be considered in a patient with pancreatic cancer and obstructive jaundice [7].

Technique for percutaneous endoprosthesis insertion

An initial percutaneous trans-hepatic cholangiogram (PTC) is performed to ascertain the site of the obstruction and a 7 French gauge (FG) catheter is left above the obstruction to drain the biliary system for 24–48 hours. Then a 12 FG Lunderquist prosthesis is passed through the obstruction under biplane X-ray screening leaving a drainage catheter above the prosthesis until check X-rays have confirmed that the position is satisfactory.

Technique of endoscopic prosthesis insertion

Endoscopic prostheses are inserted under sedation after a preliminary duodenoscopic sphincterotomy has been performed. Either two double pigtail prostheses of 8 FG tubing

or, if a wide channel duodenoscope is available, two 10 FG prosthesis are inserted [25].

Choosing techniques

Either technique can be complicated by infective cholangitis; it is not certain which technique carries the greatest risk of this complication. The main disadvantage of both methods is blockage of the prosthesis by biliary sludge, this leads to recurrence of jaundice. With the endoprosthetic technique it is possible to overcome this problem by replacing the tube but this is very difficult to do if the tube has been inserted percutaneously.

Preoperative external biliary drainage in jaundiced patients [22] should be used with caution as the dangers of introducing infection into the liver and causing major electrolyte imbalance probably outweigh any advantage of operating upon a less jaundiced patient.

The main advantage of endoprostheses is lower morbidity and a shorter stay in hospital allowing the patient a longer period of normal life at home. There is no upper age limit for these procedures [32].

Control of pancreatic pain

Pancreatic pain is not so amenable to surgical treatment. When it results from obstructive pancreatitis, through obstruction of the main pancreatic duct, a pancreatic duct bypass may produce pain relief (see Chapter 37) although there is doubt as to whether this will remain open. Where the tumour is in the body of the pancreas and there is local invasion of surrounding tissues, infiltration of the coeliac axis with 70% alcohol at the time of surgery, may provide good palliation for a time. This is safer than percutaneous coeliac axis infiltration although the latter may have to be used if operation is not required [31].

Ampullary tumours

Ampullary tumours include all malignant lesions that appear endoscopically to be arising from the ampulla of Vater [46]. Usually there is little periampullary involvement and metastases occur relatively late. Provided that the patient is fit, resection of the head of the pancreas by pancreaticoduodenectomy is the preferred treatment, although local excision has been proposed by some as an acceptable alternative [28, 29]. Endoscopic sphincterotomy has been used to relieve the jaundice prior to pancreaticoduodenectomy, with apparent benefit [2]. In the old or infirm endoscopic sphincterotomy alone has been used to relieve the jaundice and to produce palliation. It can be repeated if necessary.

Complications of surgical treatment

As many patients with pancreatic cancer are elderly and in poor health at the time of operation, they are liable to a number of complications. Most are those one would expect at this age group, such as cardio-respiratory, septic and embolic complications. Renal failure may occur after surgery the presence of jaundice but it is preventaby careful management. The renal tubules are sensitive to low flow rates in the presence of hyperbilirubinaemia. Prophylaxis is therefore directed at maintaining a high urinary flow (>30 ml/h) by starting a 5% dextrose infusion 12 hours preoperatively and adjusting the infusion rate during the next 48 hours to maintain this flow rate. The use of mannitol or a diuretic, have the disadvantage that the diuresis may be followed by a period of oliguria, which can lead to renal failure if adequate fluid replacement is not given.

The incidence of septic complications can be decreased if prophylactic antibiotics, appropriate to the common bacteria found in bile (for example aminoglycosides), are used perioperatively in such patients.

Non-surgical management

Many patients will be diagnosed by imaging techniques before severe symptoms develop. This is particularly true with tumours of the body and tail of the pancreas. At that stage symptoms can be readily controlled by antacids, histamine H_2-receptor antagonists, pancreatic enzyme supplements, simple analgesics and, occasionally, small doses of corticosteroids. Such patients are often over 60 years of age and unsuitable for radical surgery, particularly as their medial survival is under six months. To spend over half of their remaining life recovering from major surgery which offers little chance of cure seems cruel, while other treatments may add to rather than decrease their symptoms. For these reasons conservative medical therapy is often the best way to manage such patients.

Pain may become severe as the tumour progresses. A coeliac axis block is one of the most effective ways of providing relief of pain over the long term. When 70% alcohol is used for the block pain relief may last for 4–6 months; it can be repeated if required although subsequent injections are less effective [31]. The procedure is difficult to do and not without serious complications (for example retroperitoneal haemorrhage, spinal root injuries, etc). It should be done under radiological control by an interested anaesthetist.

Radiotherapy and cytotoxic therapy

As adequate clinical trials of radio- and cytotoxic therapy have not been done in patients with pancreatic cancer suitable for assessment, their effectiveness in this disease remains unclear. Mitomycin C, 5 fluorouracil BCNU, methyl CCNU, streptozotocin, adriamycin and methotrexate have all been tested as single agents and have low response rates. A combination of 5 fluorouracil and BCNU has produced response rates of nearly 30% with those responding living twice as long as those who did not although without any overall increase in survival. Considerable interest has centred upon three-drug combinations, particularly the SMF regime of streptozotocin $1\,g/m^2$; mitomycin C $10\,mg/m^2$ and 5 fluorouracil $500\,mg/m^2$ given on weeks one, two, five and six and repeated in eight week cycles. Of 23 patients with measurable metastatic lesions four lived for one year or longer and one patient survived for five years despite hepatic metastases diagnosed at biopsy [52].

Chemotherapy may have a role in locally advanced disease [39]. The combination of 5 fluorouracil with radiotherapy appears to be better than radiotherapy alone, increasing survival from 6 to 10.4 months. Similar results have been reported by the Gastrointestinal Tumour Group [20]. Radiotherapy has been used preoperatively in a single large tumour dose, but this approach has yet to be fully evaluated [47]. Pancreatic carcinoma is not curable by radiotherapy but it does have a short-term response which can be used to relieve symptoms, such as intractable pain.

Prognosis (Fig. 38.5)

Most studies show that after diagnosis the mean survival is less than six months, with only a 10% one-year survival. The prognosis is worse in those patients with widespread dissemination at diagnosis, but in the 10% with Stage I disease (Table 38.1) at the time of diagnosis, only 40% live for six months, 20% for one year and 2% survive for five years.

Review of 61 reported series indicated that 78% of patients with pancreatic cancer underwent laparotomy, but resection was done in only 11%. The estimated overall

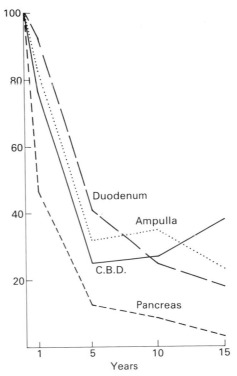

Fig. 38.5. Survival following radical resection depending upon site of primary 'pancreatic' tumour [45].

survival was 0.4% [21]. Bypass surgery appears to offer a modest increase in survival. Analysis of 17 series, summarizing experience of Whipple resections in 496 patients, showed that only 4% of the patients survived for five years and there was no significant improvement in length or quality of survival in comparison with simple bypass [45]. Comparison of pancreatoduodenectomy (92 patients) with total pancreatectomy (58 patients) showed no significant advantage for the latter in terms of survival (overall 5.7% at five years). The operative mortality was higher (26%), compared with 14% for Whipple's procedure [11]. Survival after radical pancreatoduodenectomy for true ampullary tumours is much better—56% at two and 34% at five years [1]. Inclusion of such tumours in studies of so called adenocarcinoma of the head of the pancreas may well lead to false conclusions.

Conclusion

Carcinoma of the pancreas has one of the poorest outlooks of any cancer. It is important to diagnose early in the young patient for whom surgical excision may offer the only hope of a cure. With others emphasis on a policy of minimal intervention with the selected use of palliative surgery, endoprostheses, coeliac axis block and symptomatic medical therapy will ensure the maximum of relief.

References

1 AKWARI OE, VanHEERDEN JA, ADSON MA, BAGGENSTOSS AH. Radical pancreatoduodenectomy for cancer of the papilla of Vater. *Arch Surg* 1977;112:451–456.
2 ANDERSON D, LAVELLE MI, VENABLES CW. Endoscopic sphincterotomy before pancreatoduodenectomy for ampullary carcinoma. *Br Med J* 1981; i:1109–1111.
3 AOKI K, OGAWA H. Cancer of the pancreas, international mortality trends. *World Health Stat Q* 1978 31:2.
4 ARMSTRONG B, LEA AJ, ADELSTEIN AM, DONOVAN JW, WHITE GC, RUTTLE S Cancer mortality and saccharin consumption in diabetics. *Br J Prevent Med* 1976;30:151–156.
5 BEAZLEY RM. Needle biopsy diagnosis of pancreatic cancer. *Cancer* 1981; 47:1685–1687.
6 BLIEVERNICHT SW, NIEFELD JP, TERZ JJ, LAWRENCE WJL The role of prophylactic gastrojejunostomy for unresectable periampullary carcinoma. *Surg Gynecol Obstet* 1980;151:794–796.
7 BORNMAN PC, HARRIES-JONES EP, TOBIAS R, van STIEGMANN G, TERBLANCHE J. Prospective controlled trial of transhepatic biliary endoprosthesis versus bypass surgery for incurable carcinoma of head of pancreas. *Lancet* 1986;i:69–71.
8 BROOKS DC, OSTEEN RT, GRAY EB, STEELE GD, WILSON RE Evaluation of palliative procedures for pancreatic cancer. *Am J Surg* 1981;141:430–433.
9 BUAMAH PK, CORNELL C, VENABLES CW, SKILLEN AW An initial assessment of the value of serum carbohydrate antigenic determinant (CA19-9) concentrations in patients with pancreatic cancer. *Gut* 1985:26:A577.
10 COOPER MJ, WILLIAMSON RCN. Conservative pancreatectomy. *Br J Surg* 1985;72:801–803.
11 COOPERMAN AM, HERTER FP, MARBOE CA. Pancreatoduodenal resection and total pancreatectomy—an institutional review. *Surgery* 1981;90:707–712.
12 COTTON PB. Duodenoscopic placement of biliary prostheses to relieve malignant obstructive jaundice. *Br J Surg* 1982;69:501–503.
13 COTTON PB. Endoscopic methods for relief of malignant obstructive jaundice. *World J Surg* 1984;8:854–861.
14 CUBILLA AL, FITZGERALD PJ. Pancreas cancer I. Duct adenocarcinoma. A clinical pathological study of 380 patients. In: *Pathology Annual part I.* New York: Appleton-Century-Crofts, 1978:241.
15 CUBILLA AL, FITZGERALD PJ. Surgical pathology of tumours of the exocrine pancreas. In: Moosa AR, ed. *Tumours of the pancreas.* Baltimore: Williams & Wilkins, 1980:159–193.
16 DiMAGNO EP, MALAGELADA J, TAYLOR WF, GO VLW. A prospective comparison of current diagnostic tests for pancreatic cancer. *New Engl J Med* 1977;297:737–742.
17 FITZGERALD PS. Pathology in pancreatic cancer—a series of workshops on the biology of human cancer. In: Cohen I, Hastings PR, eds. *Report No. 12.* Geneva: UICC, 1981:13–29.
18 FORTNER JG. Regional resection of cancer of the pancreas. A new surgical approach *Surgery* 1973;73:307–320.
19 GAMBILL EE. Pancreatic and ampullary carcinoma: diagnosis and prognosis in relation to symptoms, physical findings and elapsed time as observed in 255 patients. *South Med J* 1970;63:1119–1122.
20 GASTROINTESTINAL TUMOUR STUDY GROUP. A multi-institutional cooperative trial of radiation therapy alone and in combination with 5-fluorouracil for locally unresectable pancreatic carcinoma. *Ann Surg* 1979;189:205–208.
21 GUDJONSSON B, LIVSTONE EM, SPIRO HM. Cancer of the pancreas. Diagnostic accuracy and survival statistics. *Cancer* 1978;42:2492–2506.
22 HADFIELD ARW, TOBIAS R, TERBLANCH J, *et al.* Pre-operative external biliary drainage in obstructive jaundice. *Lancet* 1982;ii:896–899.
23 HOLYOKE ED, DOUGLAS HP, GOLDROSEN MH, *et al.* Tumour markers in pancreatic cancer. *Semin Oncol* 1979;6:347.
24 HOVDENAK N, LEES WR, PEREIRA J, BEILBY IOW, COTTON PB Ultrasound guided percutaneous fine needle aspiration cytology of pancreatic mass lesions. *Br Med J* 1982;2:1183–1184.
25 HUIBREGTSE K, TYTGAT GN. Palliative treatment of obstructive jaundice by transpapillary introduction of large bore bile duct endoprosthesis. *Gut* 1982;23:371–375.
26 IHSE I, LILJA P, ARNESJO B, BENGMARK S. Total pancreatectomy for cancer. An appraisal of 65 cases. *Ann Surg* 1977;186:675–680.

27 IRVING JD. Intervention radiology: relief of biliary obstruction. *Br J Hosp Med* 1981;**27**:329–333.

28 ISAKSSON G, IHSE I, ADREN-SANDBERG A, *et al.* Local excision for ampullary carcinoma. *Acta Chir Scand* 1982;**149**:163–165.

29 JONES BA, LANGER B, TAYLOR BR, GIROTTI M. Periampullary tumors: which ones should be resected? *Am J Surg* 1985;**149**: 46–52.

30 KLAVINS JV. Tumour markers of pancreatic carcinoma. *Cancer* 1981;**47**:1597–1601.

31 LEUNG JWC, BOWEN-WRIGHT M, AVELING W, SHORVON PJ, COTTON PB. Coeliac plexus block for pain in pancreatic cancer and chronic pancreatitis. *Br J Surg* 1983;**70**:730–732.

32 LEUNG JWC, EMERY R, COTTON PB, RUSSELL RCG, VALLON AG, MASON RR. Management of malignant obstructive jaundice at the Middlesex Hospital. *Br J Surg* 1983;**70**:584–586.

33 LEVIN DL, CONNELLY RR. Epidemiology in pancreatic cancer—a series of workshops on the biology of human cancer. In: Cohen I, Hastings PR, eds. *Report No. 12*. Geneva: UICC, 1981:5–12.

34 LEVIN DL, CONNELLY RR, DEVESA SS. Demographic characteristics of cancer of the pancreas. *Cancer* 1981;**47**:1456–1468.

35 LONGMIRE WP JR. Cancer of the pancreas: palliative operation, Whipple procedure or total pancreatectomy. *World J Surg* 1984;**8**:872–879.

36 MOOSSA AR. *Tumours of the pancreas.* In: Moossa AR, ed. Baltimore: Williams & Wilkins, 1980:443–467.

37 MOOSSA AR, LEVIN B. Collaborative studies in the diagnosis of pancreatic cancer. *Semin Oncol* 1979;**6**:298–308.

38 MORGAN RGH, WORMSLEY KG. Progress report—cancer of the pancreas. *Gut* 1977;**18**:580–596.

39 O'CONNELL MJ. Current status of chemotherapy for advanced pancreatic and gastric cancer. *J. Clin Oncol* 1985;**3**:1032–9

40 OSNES M, SERCK-HANSSEN A, MYREN J. Endoscopic brush cytology (ERBC) of the biliary tract and pancreatic duct. *Scand J Gastroenterol* 1975;**10**:829–831.

41 PODOLSKY DK. Serological markers in the diagnosis and management of pancreatic carcinoma. *World J Surg* 1984;**8**:822–830.

42 REUBEN A, COTTON PB. Operative pancreatic biopsy: a survey of current practice. *Ann R Coll Surg Engl* 1978;**60**:53–57.

43 ROGOT E, MURRAY JL. Smoking and causes of death among US veterans: 16 years of observation. *Pub Health Rep* 1980;**95**:213.

44 SARR MG, CAMERON JL. Surgical palliation of unresectable carcinoma of the pancreas. *World J Surg* 1984;**8**:906–918.

45 SHAPIRO TM. Adenocarcinoma of the pancreas. A statistical analysis of biliary bypass versus Whipple resection in good risk patients. *Ann Surg* 1975;**182**:715–721.

46 SHERLOCK S. Carcinoma in the region of the ampulla of Vater. In: Sherlock S, ed. *Diseases of the liver and biliary system.* Oxford: Blackwell Scientific Publications, 1985: pp 537–540.

47 SHIPLEY WV, NARDI GL, COHEN AM, *et al.* Iodine 125 implant and external beam irradiation in patients with localised pancreatic carcinoma: a comparative study to surgical resection. *Cancer* 1980;**45**:709–714.

48 SILVERSTEIN MD, RICHTER JM, PODOLSKY DK, WARSHAW AL. Suspected pancreatic cancer presenting as pain or weight loss: analysis of diagnostic strategies. *World J Surg* 1984;**8**:839–945.

49 SOREIDE O, SKAARLAND E, PEDESEN OM, LARSSEN TB, ARNESJO B. Fine-needle biopsy of the pancreas: results of 204 routinely performed biopsies in 190 patients. *World J Surg* 1985;**9**:960–965.

50 STEINBERG WM, GELFAND R, ANDERSON KK *et al.* Comparison of the sensitivity and specificity of the CA19-9 and carcinoembryonic antigen assays in detecting cancer of the pancreas. *Gastroenterology* 1986;**90**:343–9.

51 TREDE M. The surgical treatment of pancreatic carcinoma. *Surgery* 1985;**97**:28–35.

52 WIGGANS GR, WOOLLEY PV, MACDONALD JS, *et al.* Phase II trial of streptozolvein, mitomycin C and 5-fluorouracil (SMF) in the treatment of advanced pancreatic cancer. *Cancer* 1978;**41**:387–391.

SECTION VII

HORMONE SECRETING TUMOURS OF THE GUT AND PANCREAS

Chapter 39
Tumours of the Apud Cells

F. STADIL

Apud is an acronym introduced by Pearse [40] to describe a presumed system of endocrine cells with common cytochemical and ultrastructural properties. The name refers to the amine-handling characteristics of the cells (amine, precursor, uptake and decarboxylation). Pearse suggested that these cells had a common embryological origin from the neuroectoderm, but both of these assumptions have been challenged. According to some experiments the mucous and enterochromaffin cells of the mouse gut originate from the same stem cell [6, 37] and in embryos whose neural crest has been removed a normal proportion of endocrine cells still develops in their pancreas [41]. Although the common neural crest origin for apud cells remains controversial, the anatomical, functional and neurohormonal relationships still support an integrated apud cell concept.

Identification of apud cells

The term apudoma was first used by Cszij and associates to describe neoplastic lesions arising in the apud cell systems of the body [8, 11]. These tumours all have similar appearances and share a number of cytochemical and morphological characteristics which can assist the pathologist, who might otherwise miss the diagnosis (Table 39.1). At light microscopy level the cells are **argyrophilic**—the peptide-containing cell granules stain with silver when a reducing agent is used simultaneously [19]. Alternatively they stain with lead haematoxylin [50]. Some argyrophilic cells are also

Table 39.1. Main methods used for the pathological diagnosis of an apudoma.

Technique	Characteristics
Histology	Argyrophilia
	Lead haemotoxylin
Histochemistry	Formaldehyde-ozone induced fluorescence
Immunocytochemistry	Neuron specific enolase
	Specific gastrointestinal peptides
Electron microscopy	Neurosecretory granules

argentaffin (they stain with silver without a reducing agent), as in the enterochromaffin cells of a carcinoid tumour (see Chapter 40).

The apud cell can be shown histochemically, but it is normally easier to demonstrate **formaldehyde-ozone fluorescence**, which probably reflects the presence of peptides with end-terminal tryptophan [20]. When specific peptides are suspected these may be demonstrated by immunochemistry, but with improper fixation or in the absence of storage granules these methods may fail. **Neuron-specific enolase**, an isomer of the glycolytic enzyme, is found in the brain apud cells, and in various neurons [49]. This enzyme can be detected in apudomas and in the circulation by immunochemical techniques. In the future radioimmunoassays for this enzyme may be used as a marker for functioning and non-functioning tumours. Finally **neurosecretory granules**, seen at electronmicroscopy, may be diagnostic and allow differentiation into sub-types.

The secretory products of the cell can usually be identified by **immunochemistry**. However the tumours often contain different cell types and occasionally more than one type of peptide granule in the same cell. From this point of view most tumours are of mixed type even if, from a clinical and biological point of view, the disease appears to be due to hypersecretion of a single substance. It must be remembered that this mixed cell origin makes it theoretically possible for the apud tumour, or its secondaries to change their secretory pattern.

Classification

In view of the mixed cell populations of apudomas it is better to classify them according to biochemical and clinical features, than by morphology [11,28]. If a specific circulating peptide is present then the tumour is named after this peptide by adding 'oma' to it (for example gastrinoma). If more than one hormone is produced, the tumour is named after the hormone responsible for the clinical symptoms. Finally, when neither of the above applies, it is called a 'multiple hormone producing tumour'.

Non-functioning endocrine tumours of the pancreas have often been diagnosed in the past, but this label should become less frequent as diagnostic methods improve. In the gastrointestinal tract such tumours are often categorized as 'carcinoids'. Some pathologists use this term for all argyrophilic tumours of the gastrointestinal tract while others only use it for those of enterochromaffin origin. Enterochromaffinomas are usually derived from the mid-gut and are argentaffin because of their serotonin content. Amines are lacking in argyrophilic tumours of the fore- and hind-gut, or present in amounts too small for detection by staining. In this text these tumours are

still called 'carcinoids' because of their morphological similarity to those of mid-gut origin and because of the absence of a specific mode of presentation. As our knowledge of the composition and production of these tumours improves this classification may be changed.

Apudomas may be benign or malignant [58]. They are often small but may grow to huge dimensions and can give rise to many clinical syndromes. This chapter describes the main pathological and clinical characteristics of some established endocrine tumours. The syndromes associated with them are relatively rare but are being diagnosed more frequently, suggesting that their true incidence is higher than thought in the past.

Insulinoma

The insulinoma, first recognized in 1927, is the best known of the endocrine pancreatic tumours. The estimated incidence is about one or two per 1,000,000 inhabitants per year in Western countries.

Pathology

An insulinoma arises from the beta cells of the pancreatic islets; 90% are solitary measuring 2–50 mm in diameter. They can occur in all areas of the pancreas and, in a survey of 951 patients with insulinoma, metastases were found in only 5% [57].

Clinical features

The tumour is found equally in both sexes and no age is exempt, although most are first diagnosed in middle age. Symptoms are intermittent and are caused by hypoglycaemia which develops during fasting, or after severe exercise. Patients frequently fail to notice this relationship, although they are often aware of the relief obtained by eating. The hypoglycaemia can develop rapidly, but is more often gradual with neuroglycopenia presenting oddly with strange behaviour, automatism, confusion, epileptic fits, transient paralysis, or tremor. A diagnostic delay due to mistaken psychiatric, or neurological referral is quite common. Repeated attacks can lead to dementia.

Investigations

Whipple's triad

The diagnosis is made when symptoms are provoked by hypoglycaemia and relieved by intravenous glucose. This is the basis for the classical 'Whipple's triad' test. In this the patient fasts for up to 72 hours under careful observation in hospital. Patients with insulinomas, in contrast to normals, will develop hypoglycaemic symptoms during the first 24–48 hours [50, 51].

Plasma insulin

Constant hyperinsulinaemia is rare although relative hyperinsulinaemia is frequent. When the blood glucose falls insulin secretion normally decreases until it virtually stops when the glucose concentration falls below 1.7 mmol/l. This does not occur in patients with an insulinoma—the morning fasting plasma insulin concentration is often inappropriately high for the blood glucose concentration. The 'amended insulin/glucose ratio'

$$\frac{\text{Plasma insulin (mU/l)}}{\text{Plasma glucose (mmol/l)}} \div 1.7$$

is usually > 50 in patients with insulinoma and < 10 in normal subjects [59].

Measurements of plasma pro-insulin may also be diagnostic, as patients with insulinoma have relatively higher concentrations of the pro-hormone [7]. Insulin and C-peptide are stored in islet cell granules and released into the circulation on an equimolar basis. The concentration of C-peptide in the plasma is therefore an index of endogenous insulin secretion and measurements of this can be used to rule out factitious hypoglycaemia produced by exogenous administration of insulin. When this is suspected, analysis of the urine for sulphonylurea compounds may also be needed.

Localization of the tumour

The most valuable methods are **arteriography**, which can detect up to 90% of tumours [34, 45] and **percutaneous transhepatic portal vein catheterization**, to measure insulin concentrations in blood obtained from the portal vein and its tributaries. The latter technique identifies the part of the pancreas from which excess insulin is released.

Ultrasound and CT-scanning rarely identify a tumour that is less than 1 cm in diameter.

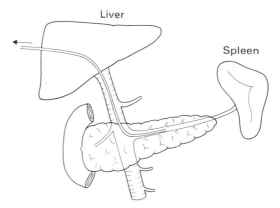

Fig. 39.1. Diagrammatic representation of method of percutaneous transhepatic portal venous sampling.

Differential diagnosis

The few other causes of fasting hypoglycaemia in adults are listed in Table 39.2. Extra-pancreatic tumours that may cause hypoglycaemia, for unknown reasons, include retroperitoneal sarcoma and primary liver cell tumours—the latter usually weighs at least 1 kg and is easily detected.

Chapter 39

Table 39.2. Classification of hypoglycaemia in fasting adults.

Pancreatic insulinomas (benign or malignant)
Mesenchymal or hepatic neoplasms
Endocrine deficiences (pituitary or adrenals)
Liver diseases (advanced)
Starvation
Factitious (exogenous hypoglycaemic agents)

Hypopituitarism and Addison's disease are easily diagnosed, as is alcohol induced hypoglycaemia or liver failure. Self-administration of insulin can cause problems.

In a hypoglycaemic child the differential diagnosis is more complicated due to various inborn errors of metabolism. Fortunately insulinomas are rare in the very young.

Treatment

Medical therapy

Hypoglycaemia can be controlled acutely by administration of glucose. **Diazoxide** inhibits the release of insulin from the granules in the tumour cells, but is only effective if normal storage mechanisms are maintained. The starting dose is usually 50 mg three times daily rising up to 1,000 mg daily in some patients. Unwanted effects are frequent and include water retention, oedema, dyspepsia, diarrhoea, skin reactions and depression of the bone marrow. **Streptozocin** alone, or in combination with 5-fluorouracil, may result in a remission in around 60% of patients [3]—it is usually given intravenously in doses of 1–4 g every six weeks. Adverse reactions include serious renal damage, which can occur even after the first dose.

Surgical therapy

Surgical removal of the tumour should be undertaken whenever possible. The tumour can be removed by enucleation, or by pan-creatic resection. When the tumour has not been localized preoperatively, mobilization of the whole pancreas may be necessary. If the tumour is not palpable, blind resection is not advised and a further attempt at localization 6 to 12 months later is recommended. Should this also fail, a 'second-look' operation after one or two years is indicated [38].

Operative mortality in insulinomas is low and cure is usually achieved. Mortality and morbidity are usually associated with re-operation, or surgery for malignant tumours, where pancreatoduodenectomy may be required.

Without surgery insulinomas can prove fatal, with death due to untreated hypoglycaemia. However the course may be protracted, the patient having attacks for many years. Delayed diagnosis frequently causes dementia.

Glucagonoma

Symptoms from a glucagonoma were first reported by McGavran in 1966 [32], but full recognition of the clinical presentation came with the publication of nine cases by Mallinson *et al.* in 1974 [36].

Pathology

This tumour arises from the A-cell of the pancreatic islets and is the rarest of the islet-cell tumours. Most, maybe all, are malignant, with metastases at the time of presentation [36]. Immunologically the cells react with most types of glucagon antisera but they appear to secrete mainly pancreatic glucagon.

Clinical features

The main symptoms are wasting, mild diabetes and a characteristic skin eruption (Fig. 39.2), which has been called necrotizing migratory erythema and consists of a

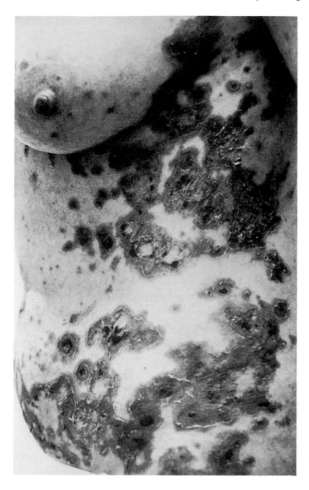

Fig. 39.2. Photograph of skin lesions in a patient with a glucagonoma (courtesy of Svein Helland).

superficial epidermal bullous lesion, with healing in its centre and a peripheral, spreading, well-defined edge. The eruption moves from one area to another, healing at the original location. It can occur any-where, but has a predilection for the lower abdomen, arms, legs and feet. Its patho-genesis is unknown. Additional features in-clude glossitis, cheilitis, anaemia, mild diar-rhoea and fatigue.

Investigations

The diagnostic feature is a marked elevation in plasma glucagon. Plasma insulin is also increased, which probably explains the mild nature of the diabetes. Slight hyperglycae-mia and hypoaminoacidaemia is usually found as well. The value of provocative tests, using tolbutamide or arginine, is based on anecdotal reports—they are rarely necessary as the plasma glucagon concen-tration is usually 5–10 times above normal.

Glucagonomas can be localized by trans-hepatic portal or pancreatic vein catheter-ization, with measurement of glucagon concentrations in blood samples [24]. In many patients the size of the tumours per-mits detection by ultrasonography or CT-scanning.

Treatment

Medical therapy

The skin condition may respond to intravenous aminoacids, but zinc supplements are of no value. Long-acting somatostatin analogues may depress the tumour secretion, but have little practical therapeutic value. Unresectable tumours can be treated with streptozocin alone, or in combination with 5-fluorouracil [5]. Favourable responses to dacarbazine (DTIC) have also been reported [60].

Surgical therapy

Removal of the tumour, with as much of the local and metastatic spread as is feasible, is the best treatment and will control the skin condition and normalize the blood sugar. In non-resectable, or metastatic tumours transcutaneous (or operative) implantation of radioactive seeds can be used [22].

Most tumours are slow growing and patients with unresectable lesions can survive for several years.

Vipoma

A syndrome that includes severe diarrhoea, hypokalaemia, and an islet cell tumour was described by Verner & Morrison in 1958 [61]. It is caused by hyperproduction of vasoactive intestinal polypeptide (VIP), although it has been suggested that more than one peptide may cause this syndrome.

Pathology

Most vipomas are found in the pancreas, although some neurogenic tumours can produce VIP (for example phaeochromocytoma, neurofibroma, neuroblastoma, ganglioneuronoma or ganglioneuroblastomas). VIP-secreting neuronomas are most frequently found in the retroperitoneum and thorax. No age is exempt, although neuronomas are found more often in children and pancreatic tumours in the middle-aged or elderly. Vipomas are usually malignant, and over half the patients have metastases at the time of diagnosis [62].

Clinical features

The syndrome has also been called the WDHA-syndrome (an acronym for watery diarrhoea, hypokalaemia and achlorhydria), or pancreatic cholera. Both these names are unfortunate as only half the patients are achlorhydric and the tumour is not always in the pancreas. About one patient per year per million population is diagnosed in Western countries.

The main symptom is **watery diarrhoea**, which is often intermittent and present for one or two years before diagnosis. In the active phase as much as 10 litres of fluid stool, with an appearance of weak tea or urine, may be passed per day. The potassium and bicarbonate content is high and potassium loss may exceed 200 mmol per day (> 10 times normal). The result is **severe hypokalaemia** with plasma concentrations below 3.0, or sometimes 2.0 mmol/l. The hypokalaemia is associated with **metabolic acidosis** due to loss of bicarbonate ions. Many patients have low gastric acid secretion; other features include decreased glucose tolerance, mild hypocalcaemia and occasional flushing.

The clinical presentation in patients with a neurogenic tumour can be more complicated as they may also produce excess amounts of catecholamines and other substances.

Investigations

In spite of reports that other peptides may cause the syndrome, the constant feature seems to be hypersecretion of VIP with elevated plasma concentrations of the hormone (>60 pmol/l). Concentrations 2–3 times above normal produce diarrhoea and are characteristic of the active phase of the disease [14]. Tumours may be localized by transhepatic catheterization of the portal vein, with blood sampling—larger tumours may be localized by ultrasound or CT-scanning, with percutaneous biopsy of the tumour mass. An X-ray of the chest, or even bronchoscopy, should be undertaken if the abdominal examinations are negative.

Differential diagnosis

The investigation of diarrhoea can be very demanding (see Chapter 4). Bacterial and parasitic causes can be excluded by microscopy and culture of the stool. Crohn's disease and ulcerative colitis can be eliminated by endoscopy and radiological studies. The osmotic diarrhoea in carbohydrate malabsorption will stop on fasting. Biliary, gastro-, and uro-colic fistulae, malabsorption of bile salts, intestinal polyps, drugs and laxative abuse must also be considered. A few endocrine diseases (such as Addison's disease, hyperthyroidism, and hypoparathyroidism) can also be associated with diarrhoea, as can other endocrine tumours (Table 39.3). Generally the volume of stool is highest in a patient with a vipoma.

Treatment

Medical therapy

Adequate fluid and electrolyte replacement can be difficult if the diarrhoea is severe, but usually the losses can be monitored continuously after a large cuffed endotracheal tube has been placed in the rectum. Emergency control of the diarrhoea can be achieved by the use of high dose steroids while confirmation of the diagnosis is obtained. Suppression of the diarrhoea has been observed after lithium, trifluoperazine, or somatostatin, but most patients respond within a few days, to intravenous infusions of streptozocin 1–2 g daily for some days. Renal function should be followed carefully during such treatment. Prolonged remissions after streptozocin, with or without 5-fluorouracil, may be attained but the diarrhoea usually recurs within three to six months [16].

Surgical therapy

Cure is possible by surgical excision, but this is feasible in only 30% of patients because of metastatic disease [62]. Symptoms can be controlled by palliative surgery, removing as much tumour as possible. Alternatively embolization of hepatic metastases, or interstitial irradiation (with radioactive seeds) can be tried [22].

Table 39.3. Endocrine tumours causing diarrhoea.

Diagnosis	Site of tumour	Specific parameter
Zollinger-Ellison syndrome	Usually in the pancreas	Gastrin
Medullary thyroid carcinoma	Thyroid gland	Calcitonin
Carcinoid syndrome	Liver	Urine 5-hydroxy-indolic acid (5-HIAA)
Verner-Morrison syndrome	Pancreas or neurogenic tumours	Vasoactive intestinal peptide (VIP)

Early diagnosis is essential for cure, but aggressive treatment of an unresectable tumour usually controls the diarrhoea.

Gastrinoma

Zollinger and Ellison [65] first suggested the concept of an ulcerogenic tumour when they speculated that the intractable ulcer disease and hypersecretion in two of their patients was due to the release of an ulcerogenic agent from their pancreatic tumours. Later developments proved this agent to be 'gastrin'. Gastrinomas are the commonest type of islet cell tumour and occur with an incidence of 2–3 cases per 1,000,000, per year in Western countries. Diagnosis of the condition is probably still low.

Pathology

When these tumours are found in the pancreas they arise from the D_1-cells of the islets of Langerhan's [28]. Occasionally gastrinomas are found in the duodenum and, more rarely, the antrum of the stomach. The tumour is often small—solitary gastrinomas are found in less than 30% of patients [13]. In one collected series 61% of the patients had malignant tumours [13]. This is probably an underestimate of malignancy, as metastases can be very small and are easily overlooked for many years [66, 67], in all probability most gastrinomas are malignant [54]. Even small tumours, of less than 2–3 mm diameter, can be associated with the full clinical syndrome.

Gastrin cells are not normally present in the adult pancreas, but can be demonstrated during a short period of foetal development.

Clinical features

Gastrinomas occur at any age and with equal frequency in both sexes. In one U.S. survey 8% of the patients were children [13]. According to the original description of the syndrome, all patients were suffering from a fulminant and intractable ulcer diathesis [65], but it is now known that the clinical picture varies and mild forms of the disease are often encountered [10, 56].

The most frequent symptom is ulcer type abdominal pain which occurs in approximately 75% of patients. The dyspepsia may be continuous or intermittent. Diarrhoea is present in some 60% of patients, and in 10% it is the only symptom [56]. The diarrhoea is caused by acid in the proximal jejunum which inactivates pancreatic lipase and deconjugates bile salts. A few patients present with peptic oesophagitis. Associated endocrinopathies and familial disease occur in 20–30% of the patients [18, 26, 66].

The diagnosis is missed in some 30% of patients with the result that they are subjected to one or more operations for peptic ulcer. Most of these patients do quite well for several years after each operation but eventually the ulcers recur.

In a minority the disease presents dramatically with perforation, haemorrhage, oesophageal stricture, jejunal ulceration or anastomotic breakdown as a result of hypersecretion of acid.

Investigations

The main diagnostic features are hypergastrinaemia and acid hypersecretion.

Acid secretion

In the author's experience of 44 patients, the median value for spontaneous overnight acid secretion was 41 mmol H^+/h and the peak for pentagastrin stimulation was 81 mmol H^+/h (the normal values being 3 and 25 mmol/h respectively). Unfortunately, because of marked variations in these measurements it is not possible to use them as absolute criteria for diagnosis

[1, 56]. A basal acid output of over 20 mmol/h is highly suggestive of a gastrinoma, but it is recommended that fasting serum gastrin be measured whenever basal secretion is > 10 mmol/h.

Serum gastrin

Fasting hypergastrinaemia is almost always present in this condition [63]. In our experience the median plasma gastrin concentration is 290 pmol/l, but the range is wide from 50–96,000 pmol/l. In our laboratory the upper limit of normal for plasma gastrin concentration is 46 pmol/l (1 pg = 0.5 pmol). Values around the upper limit of normal may be found in a few patients with the Zollinger-Ellison syndrome.

The molecular forms of circulating gastrin in gastrinoma patients are the same as those in normal subjects, but in some patients a single component may predominate. This stresses the importance of the antisera used for the gastrin immunoassay. An antisera which reacts with all forms of gastrin (G-14; G-17; G-34; and gastrin-component-I) is preferable [42, 43].

Serum gastrin provocation tests

When the fasting serum gastrin level is borderline, various provocative tests (using secretin, calcium, glucagon or a combination of these) may be required.

The **secretin provocation test** [33] relies on the fact that secretin stimulation causes the release of gastrin into the circulation from a gastrinoma. It is performed as follows:

Fasting blood is taken at −15 and 0 min. Secretin (Gastrointestinal Hormone Laboratory) 2u/kg is given intravenously as a bolus injection over 30 seconds.

Further blood samples are taken at 2, 5, 10, 15, 20, 25, 30, 45 and 60 minutes after the stimulus.

Note: G-I-H secretin is used as Boots' contains gastrin-like immunoreactive contaminants. The early blood samples are particularly important as most patients show a rapid response to the secretin (Fig. 39.3).

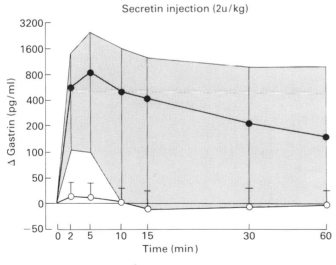

Secretin injection (2u/kg)

mean + range for 21 ZE patients

mean + 2SD for 16 DU patients

Fig. 39.3. Gastrin response to IV secretin (2 u/kg) in ZE patients compared with DU controls (after [10]).

The **calcium provocation test** relies on the fact that calcium stimulates the release of gastrin from all G cells and more is produced by a tumour. There are two methods: one is a slow calcium infusion given over three hours (at 5 mg/kg/h) with blood samples taken every 15 minutes [9] and the other is the recently described use of a rapid calcium infusion (2 mg Ca^{++} over one minute) with blood samples taken as for the secretin test [47].

Response to a standard meal relies on the fact that whereas the stomach shows a gastrin response to a meal, a gastrinoma rarely does. The recommended meal is one containing 20 g fat, 30 g protein and 25 g carbohydrate. Blood samples are taken before and after the meal for three hours [10].

Interpretation of these tests

A positive provocation test is one in which the serum gastrin rises over 200 pg/ml, or more than 100% over fasting gastrin concentration (Fig. 39.4). Unfortunately false positive and negative tests do occur although these are reduced when G-I-H secretin is used with careful attention to blood sampling times. The secretin test is generally preferred to the calcium test as it has less side-effects.

The major use of the meal test is in attempting to distinguish between a gastrinoma and antral G cell hyperplasia.

Endoscopic findings

Ulcers are found in the duodenum, jejunum and stomach in about half of the patients, but most have a single duodenal bulb ulcer. Multiple, or ectopic ulcers in the duodenum, or jejunum, are very suggestive of the diagnosis, as is marked irritation and small superficial erosions throughout the duodenum at endoscopy. A barium meal often demonstrates rapid intestinal transit with paradoxical fluid levels (duodenal ileus).

Localization of tumour

Selective angiography and CT scanning have proved to be of limited value in localizing the primary gastrinoma [21]. Percutaneous transhepatic portography, with venous blood sampling, is the most useful

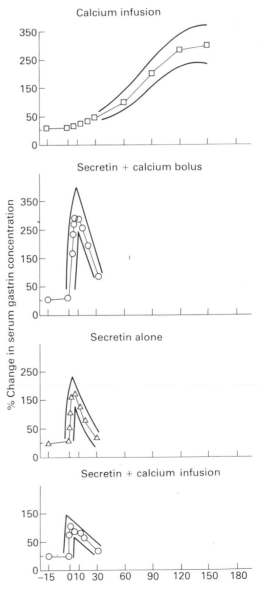

Fig. 39.4. Average percentage increase in serum gastrin in 13 patients with gastrinoma during four provocation tests (after [47]).

Table 39.4. Classification of hypergastrinaemia in fasting adults.

Disease or treatment	Degree of hypergastrinaemia
Pernicious anaemia	Moderate* to extreme
Atrophic gastritis	Moderate to extreme
Gastric ulcer	Moderate
Vagotomy	Moderate
Antacids and anticholinergics	Slight
Histamine H_2-receptor antagonists	Slight
Excluded antrum	Moderate
Severe gastric retention	Moderate to extreme
G-cell hyperplasia	Moderate to extreme
Gastrinomas	Moderate to extreme

*Moderate hypergastrinaemia is 1.5–3 times upper normal limit

localization technique. If the pancreatic veins can be selectively catheterized, it may be possible to determine if the tumour is of pancreatic origin and whether it is in an area that can be resected [46]. Selective catheterization of a number of vessels is essential. Ultrasonography or CT scanning may identify large tumours or metastases.

Differential diagnosis

Fasting hypergastrinaemia can occur in a number of clinical situations (Table 39.4). It is important to be able to distinguish the increased plasma gastrin found in these conditions from that produced by a gastrinoma.

Pernicious anaemia and **atrophic gastritis** cause hypergastrinaemia through the loss of the acid 'feedback' mechanism controlling the release of gastrin. These conditions are diagnosed by the presence of severe hypo- or achlorhydria on acid secretory studies.

The greatest diagnostic problem occurs when the fasting serum gastrin concentration is only marginally elevated and the patient is secreting acid at a normal rate. Under these circumstances provocation tests are used to ascertain the relevance of this finding. Unfortunately it is our experience that such tests are of limited value in the individual patient because of poor discrimination [56]. Recently it has been suggested that combining the rapid calcium infusion test with bolus secretin gives rise to fewer false positive or negative tests [47].

When doubt remains the patient should be carefully observed, with serial measurements of basal acid secretion and fasting serum gastrin concentration, for several weeks or months.

An important, although rare, cause of fasting hypergastrinaemia and peptic ulceration is **antral G-cell hyperplasia**. In this condition there is an abnormal release of gastrin by the G cells of the gastric antrum which is not inhibited by acid on the antral mucosa. The most useful test for this condition appears to be the response to a 'protein rich meal'. In G-cell hyperplasia there is a rapid and excessive serum gastrin response to the meal, which is absent in gastrinoma patients. Secretin usually results in inhibition of the serum gastrin concentration in this condition. **Bombesin stimulation** has also been reported to be useful in this condition as this agent results in a rapid rise in serum gastrin concentration in G-cell hyperplasia, which does not occur with a gastrinoma.

Treatment

Medical therapy

Complete control of symptoms follows inhibition of acid secretion. Until recently
only continuous treatment with **histamine
H₂-receptor antagonists** was sufficiently efficacious and safe for use in this condition.
The dose has to be tailored to the patient's
requirements, but usually a starting dose of
approximately twice that used for peptic
ulcer is required, taken in divided doses
throughout the 24 hours. Therapy must be
given permanently and the dose must be
adjusted in relation to clinical assessment,
serial acid secretion studies and endoscopic
findings at regular intervals. There is a tendency for the dose to increase with time. A
small number of patients cannot be controlled with these agents [23, 35, 39].

Recently a new group of drugs have been
developed. These directly inhibit the proton
pump (H^+, K^+ ATPase) within the parietal
cell for a prolonged period.

Omeprazole has been shown to virtually
abolish acid secretion in man with a single
daily dose of 30–60 mg. Initial studies with
omeprazole suggest it is effective, even
when histamine H₂-receptor antagonists
have failed [27, 30]. The long-term actions
and unwanted effects of omeprazole are still
being assessed, although initial results are
encouraging.

Treatment with antacids and anticholinergic agents alone produce only marginal
benefit. However, it may be useful to combine a histamine H₂-receptor antagonist
with an anticholinergic agent (for example
pirenzepine).

Cytostatic treatment with **streptozocin
alone, or in combination with 5-fluorour-
acil** may also produce symptomatic control.
Occasionally year-long remissions may be
induced by such therapy. Due to the
nephrotoxicity of the drug and the slow
growing nature of gastrinomas, such treatment should be restricted to patients with
advanced and uncontrolled metastatic disease.

Surgical therapy

The best treatment is excision of the gastrinoma before metastatic spread has occurred. Unfortunately gastrinomas are
usually difficult to find. Percutaneous transhepatic portal catheterization, with multiple blood sampling, may show that the
tumour is located in an area of the pancreas
which can be resected [46]. Only patients
with clear-cut gradients in the blood samples should be selected for operation. Based
on this method around 20% of patients can
probably have a curative operation [4].
Tumours located in the pancreatic tail
should always be resected as the risks of
surgery are small. Blind pancreatic resection should be avoided although careful exploration of the pancreas, in the area where
most such tumours occur, may be rewarding [21, 53].

In the past, surgery was directed at the
target organ—total gastrectomy improving
survival considerably over less extensive
operations, or attempts at removal of the
tumour [15]. This improved survival was
mainly because death from the complications of recurrent ulceration was avoided
rather than through tumour control [15].
The development of efficient medical inhibitors of acid secretion appears to have rendered total gastrectomy rarely necessary
[31, 55], although the occasional case may
still need it [2, 25, 53, 66].

The advent of better medical treatment
has reopened the question of lesser surgical
procedures. It has been suggested that proximal gastric vagotomy should be performed
at the time of a negative laparotomy to remove a tumour [12, 45]. This approach

may be followed by a period when continued use of acid inhibitors is unnecessary or the dose required to control ulceration is substantially reduced. Unfortunately it does result in considerable perigastric adhesions which may make a subsequent search for the primary tumour impossible [21] and the author cannot recommend this approach.

Somatostatinoma

Somatostatin was originally isolated from the hypothalamus and later from other parts of the central nervous system. It also occurs in the D-cells of the pancreatic islets and in the upper gastrointestinal tract. Somatostatin inhibits the secretion of many hormones including growth hormone, thyrotropin, insulin, glucagon, gastrin and renin. It also inhibits exocrine pancreatic and gastric secretion. About 10 patients with somatostatin-producing tumours in the pancreas have been reported since the initial reports [17, 29].

Pathology

These malignant tumours develop from the D-cells of the pancreatic islets; most have hepatic metastases at the time of diagnosis.

Clinical features

The clinical presentations have been characterized by mild diarrhoea, wasting, fatigue, anaemia, diabetes, and maldigestion with steatorrhoea. Most patients have gallstones and hypochlorhydria.

Investigations

Plasma concentrations of somatostatin are markedly raised in these patients. As the clinical presentation is so vague, it is unlikely that less advanced disease will be detected unless all diabetics are screened by somatostatin assay. Some patients have had evidence of multiple endocrine neoplasia with increased plasma concentrations of calcitonin or ACTH.

Treatment

Surgical removal of the tumour has relieved symptoms in a few patients. Streptozocin treatment can probably be used in metastatic disease.

Multiple endocrine adenomatosis

Multiple endocrine adenomatosis or neoplasia (MEA, MEN) is a familial condition with a dominant inheritance characterized by concurrent hyperplasia, adenoma, or carcinoma of several endocrine organs. Two

Table 39.5. Multiple endocrine adenomatosis syndromes (MEA).

	I (Wermer's syndrome)		IIa (Sipple's syndrome)		IIb (Schimke's syndrome)	
Inheritance	Dominant autosomal		Dominant autosomal		Dominant autosomal	
Organs involved	Parathyroid	90%	Medullary thyroid		Medullary	
	Pancreas	80%	carcinoma	100%	thyroid carcinoma	90%
	Pituitary	60%	Phaeochromocytoma	60%	Phaeochromocytoma	30%
	Adrenal cortex	30%	Parathyroid	50%	Ganglioneuromas of	
	Thyroid (non-				tongue, lips, etc.	100%
	functional)	20%			Skeletal	
	Carcinoid	5%			abnormalities	80%

main sub-groups are recognized.

MEA type I (Wermer's syndrome) consists of at least two of the following: primary hyperparathyroidism, pituitary hyperplasia or tumour and an endocrine pancreatic tumour.

MEA type II (Sipple's syndrome) is characterized by concurrent medullary carcinoma of the thyroid and phaeochromocytoma. There are two varieties of MEA type II—in some patients (MEA IIa) primary hyperparathyroidism is also present; other patients with Schimke's syndrome (MEA IIb) have mucosal neuromas around the mouth and eyes and a Marfan-like appearance [48].

The tumours in the MEA syndromes are often bilateral. The true incidence is uncertain but it is likely that more than 20% of patients with endocrine gastrointestinal tumours belong to a MEA family. For this reason associated endocrinopathies should always be looked for in such patients and a full family history should always be obtained. The features of the various syndromes are summarized in Table 39.5. For more details of these conditions the reader is referred to the review published by Greene, Golladay and Mollit [18].

References

1 AOYAGI T, SUMMERSKILL WHJ. Gastric secretion with ulcerogenic islet cell tumour. *Arch Intern Med* 1966;117:667–672.
2 BONFILS S, MIGNON M, GRATTON J. Cimetidine treatment of acute and chronic Zollinger-Ellison syndrome. *World J Surg* 1979;3:597–604.
3 BRODER LE, CARTER SK. Pancreatic islet cell carcinoma. Results of therapy with streptozotocine in 52 patients. *Ann Intern Med* 1973;79:108–118.
4 BURCHARTH F, STAGE JG, STADIL F, JENSEN LI, FISCHERMAN K. Localisation of gastrinomas by transhepatic portal catheterisation and gastrin assay. *Gastroenterology* 1979;77:444–450.
5 CHANDEKER JD, OYER D, MILLER HJ, VICK NA. Neurologic involvement in glucagonoma syndrome. Response to combination chemotherapy with 5-fluorouracil and streptozocin. *Cancer* 1979;44:2014–2016.

6 CHANG H, LEBLOND CP. Origin differentiation and renewal of the four main epithelial cell types in the mouse's small intestine—unitarian theory of the origin of the four epithelial cell types. *Am J Anat* 1974;141:537–562.
7 CREUTZFELDT W, ARNOLD R, FRERIHS H. Insulinomas and gastrinomas. In: Bloom SR, ed. *Gut Hormones*. New York: Churchill Livingstone, 1978:589–599.
8 CSZIJ I, CSAPO FA, LASZLO F, KOWACS K. Medullary cancer of the thyroid gland associated with hypercorticism. *Cancer* 1969;24:167–173.
9 DEVENEY CW, DEVENEY KS, JAFFE BM, et al. Use of calcium and secretin in the diagnosis of gastrinoma (Zollinger-Ellison syndrome). *Ann Intern Med* 1977;87:680–686.
10 DEVENEY CW, DEVENEY KS, WAY LV. The Zollinger-Ellison syndrome—23 years later. *Ann Surg* 1978;188:384–393.
11 DURNING P, GALLAND RB, NAGORNEY DM, WELBOURN RB. Neuroendocrine tumors of the gut. *World J Surg* 1985;9:348–360.
12 EDITORIAL. Vagotomy in the management of patients with Zollinger-Ellison syndrome: pros and cons. *Gastroenterology* 1985;89:435–437.
13 ELLISON EH, WILSON SD. The Zollinger-Ellison syndrome: Reappraisal and evaluation of 260 registered cases. *Ann Surg* 1964;160:512–520.
14 FAHRENKRUG J. Vasoactive intestinal polypeptide. *Clin Gastroenterol* 1980;9:633–643.
15 FOX PS, HOFFMAN JW, DECOSSE JJ, WILSON SD. The influence of the total gastrectomy on survival in malignant Zollinger-Ellison tumors. *Ann Surg* 1974;180:558–566.
16 GAGEL RF, CONSTANZA ME, DELDLIS RA, et al. Streptozocin-treated Verner-Morrison syndrome: Plasma vasoactive intestinal peptide and tumor responses. *Arch Intern Med* 1975;136:1429–1435.
17 GANDA OP, WEISS GC, STEWART-SOELDNER J, et al. Somatostatinoma: A somatostatin containing tumour of the endocrine pancreas. *N Engl J Med* 1977;286:963–967.
18 GREENE BM, GOLLADAY ES, MOLLITT DL. Multiple endocrine adenopathy (Review). *Surg Gynecol Obstet* 1983;156:665–678.
19 GRIMELIUS L. The argyrophil reaction in islet cells of adult human pancreas studied with a new silver nitrate procedure. *Acta Soc Med Upsal* 1968;73:271–294.
20 HAKANSON R, SUNDLER F. Formaldehyde condensation. A method for the fluorescence microscopic demonstration of peptides with NH_2-terminal tryptophan residues. *J Histochem* 1971;19:477–482.
21 HARMON JW, NORTON JA, COLLIN MJ, et al. Removal of gastrinomas for control of Zollinger-Ellison syndrome. *Ann Surg* 1984;200:396–404.
22 HOLM HH, STRYER I, HANSEN H, STADIL F. Ultrasonically guided percutaneous interstitial implantation

of iodine[125] seeds in cancer therapy. *Br J Radiol* 1981;**54**:665–670.

23 HOWARD JM, CHREMOS AN, COLLEN MJ, et al. Famotidine, a new, potent, long-acting histamine H₂-receptor antagonist: comparison with cimetidine and ranitidine in the treatment of Zollinger-Ellison syndrome. *Gastroenterology* 1985;**88**:1026–1033.

24 INGEMANSSON S, LUNDERQUIST A, LUNDERQUIST J, LOVDAHL R, TIBBLINS S. Portal and pancreatic vein catheterisation with radioimmunologic determination of insulin. *Surg Gynecol Obstet* 1975;**141**:705–711.

25 JENSEN RT. Zollinger-Ellison syndrome: current concepts and management (NIH Conference). *Ann Intern Med* 1983;**98**:59–75.

26 LAMERS CBH, STADIL F, VAN TONGEREN JHM. Prevalence of endocrine abnormalities in patients with the Zollinger-Ellison syndrome and their families. *Am J Med* 1978; **64**:607–612.

27 LAMERS CBH, LIND T, MOBERG S, JANSEN JBMJ, OLBE L. Omeprazole in Zollinger-Ellison syndrome. Effects of a single dose and of long-term treatment in patients resistant to histamine H₂-receptor antagonists. *N Engl J Med* 1984;**310**:758–761.

28 LARSSON L-I. Classification of pancreatic endocrine tumours. *Scand J Gastroenterol* [Suppl 53] 1979;**14**:15–18.

29 LARSSON L-I, HIRSCH MA, HOLST JJ, et al. Pancreatic somatostatinoma. Clinical features and physiological implications. *Lancet* 1977;**i**:666–668.

30 MCARTHUR KE, COLLEN MJ, MATON PN. et al. Omeprazole: effective, convenient therapy for Zollinger-Ellison syndrome. *Gastroenterology* 1985;**88**:939–944.

31 MCCARTY DM. Report on the United States' experience with cimetidine in Zollinger-Ellison syndrome and other hypersecretory states. *Gastroenterology* 1978;**74**:453–458.

32 MCGAVRAN MH, UNGER RH, RECANT L, POLCK HC, KILO C, LEVIN ME. A glucagon secreting alpha-cell carcinoma of the pancreas. *N Engl J Med* 1966; **274**:1408–1413.

33 MCGUIGAN JE, WOLFE MM. Secretin injection test in the diagnosis of gastrinoma. *Gastroenterology* 1980;**14**:1324–1331.

34 MADSEN B. Angiographic localisation of B-cell tumours. *Scand J Gastroenterol* [Suppl 53] 1979;**14**:101–109.

35 MALAGELADA J-R, EDIA AJ, ADSON MA, VAN HEERDEN JA, GO VLW. Medical and surgical options in the management of patients with gastrinomas. *Gastroenterology* 1983;**84**:1524–1532.

36 MALLINSON CN, BLOOM SR, WAREN AP, SALMON PR, COX B. A glucagonoma syndrome. *Lancet* 1974;**ii**:1–15.

37 MATSUYAMA MG, SUZUKI H. Differentiation of immature mucous cells into parietal, argyrophil, and chief cells in stomach grafts. *Science* 1970; **169**:385–387.

38 MENGOLI L, LEQUESNE P. Blind pancreatic resection for suspected insulinoma; a review of the problem. *Br J Surg* 1967;**54**:749–756.

39 PASSARO E JR, STABILE BE. Of gastrinomas and their management. *Gastroenterology* 1983;**84**:1621–1623.

40 PEARSE AGE. Common cytochemical properties of cells producing polypeptide hormones (the APUD series) and their relevance to thyroid and ultrimobranchial C-cells and calcitonin. *Proc R Soc Med (Biol)* 1968;**170**:71–80.

41 PITCHET R, RALL L, PHELPS P, RUTTER BJ. The neural crest and the origin of the insulin-producing and other gastrointestinal hormone-producing cells. *Science* 1976;**191**:191–192.

42 REHFELD JF, STADIL F. Gel filtration studies on immunoreactive gastrin in serum from Zollinger-Ellison patients. *Gut* 1973;**14**:369–373.

43 REHFELD JF, STADIL F, VIKKELSOE J. Immunoreactive gastrin components in human serum. *Gut* 1974;**15**:102–111.

44 RHYS-DAVIES E. The radiological and scintigraphic investigation of spontaneous hypoglycaemia. *Clin Radiol* 1973;**24**:177–185.

45 RICHARDSON CT, PETERS MN, FELDMAN M, et al. Treatment of Zollinger-Ellison syndrome with exploratory laparotomy, proximal gastric vagotomy, and H₂-receptor antagonists. A prospective study. *Gastroenterology* 1985;**89**:357–367.

46 ROCHE A, RAISONNIER A, GILLON-SAVOURET M-C. Pancreatic venous sampling and arteriography in localising insulinomas and gastrinomas: procedure and results in 55 cases. *Radiology* 1982;**15**:621–627.

47 ROMANUS ME, NEAL JA, DILLEY WG, et al. Comparison of four provocative tests for the diagnosis of gastrinoma. *Ann Surg* 1983;**197**:608–617.

48 SCHIMKE RN, HARTMANN WH, PROUT TE, RIMOIN DL. Syndrome of bilateral pheochromacytoma, medullary thyroid carcinoma and multiple neuromas. A possible regulatory defect in the differentiation of chromaffin tissues. *N Engl J Med* 1968;**279**:1–6.

49 SCHMECHEL D, MARRANGOS PJ, BRIGHTMAN M. Neuron-specific enolase is a molecular marker for peripheral and central neuroendocrine cells. *Nature* 1978;**276**:834–836.

50 SERVICE FJ, DALE JD, ELVEBACK LR, JIANG NS. Insulinoma: Clinical and diagnostic features of 60 consecutive cases. *Mayo Clin Proc* 1976;**51**:417–429.

51 SEYER-HANSEN K, LUNDBAEK K. The clinical diagnosis of insulinomas. *Scand J Gastroenterol* (Suppl, 53) 1979;**14**:39–42.

52 SOLCIA E, WASSALLO G, CAPELLA C. Selective staining of endocrine cells by basic dyes after acid hydrolysis. *Stain Technol* 1968;**43**:257–263.

53 STABILE BE, MORROW DJ, PASSARO E JR. The gastrinoma triangle: operative implications. *Am J Surg* 1984;**147**:25–31.

54 STABLE BE, PASSARO E. Benign and malignant gastrinoma. *Am J Surg* 1985;**149**:144–150.

55 STADIL F, STAGE JG. Cimetidine and the Zollinger-Ellison syndrome. In: Wastell C, Lance P. eds. *Cimetidine.* Edinburgh: Churchill Livingstone, 1978:91–100.

56 STAGE JG, STADIL F. The clinical diagnosis of the Zollinger-Ellison syndrome. *Scand J Gastroenterol* (Suppl 53) 1979;**14**:79–91.

57 STEFANINI P, CARBONI C, PATRASSI N, BASOLI A. Beta-islet cell tumours of the pancreas. *Surgery* 1974;**75**:597–609.

58 TOWNSEND CM JR, THOMPSON JC. Surgical management of tumors that produce gastrointestinal hormones. *Ann Rev Med* 1985;**36**:111–124.

59 TURNER RC, OAKLEY NW, NABARRO JDN. Control of the insulin secretion with special reference to the diagnosis of insulinomas. *Br Med J* 1971;ii:132–135.

60 VALVERDE J, LEMON HM, KINSINGER A, UNGER RH. Distribution of plasma glucagon immunoreactivity in a patient with suspected glucagonoma. *J Clin Endocrinol Metab* 1976;**42**:804–808.

61 VERNER JV, MORRISON AB. Islet-cell tumor and a syndrome of refractory watery diarrhea and hypokalemia. *Am J Med* 1958;**25**:374–380.

62 VERNER JV, MORRISON AB. Endocrine pancreatic islet disease with diarrhoea. *Arch Intern Med* 1974;**75**:492–499.

63 WOLFE MM, JAIN DK, EDGERTON JR. Zollinger-Ellison syndrome associated with persistently normal fasting serum gastrin concentrations. *Ann Intern Med* 1985;**103**:215–217.

64 ZOLLINGER RM, COLEMAN DV (1974). *Influence of pancreatic tumors in the stomach.* Springfield, Illinois: Charles C. Thomas, 1974.

65 ZOLLINGER RM, ELLISON EH. Primary peptic ulcerations of the jejunum associated with islet cell tumours of the pancreas. *Ann Surg* 1955;**142**:709–723.

66 ZOLLINGER RM, ELLISON EC, O'DORISIO TM, SPARKS J. Thirty years' experience with gastrinoma. *World J Surg* 1984;**8**:427–435.

67 ZOLLINGER RM, MARTIN EWJR, CAREY LC, SPARKES J, MENTON JP. Observations of the postoperative tumour growth behaviour of certain islet cell tumours. *Ann Surg* 1976;**184**:525–530.

Chapter 40
Carcinoid Syndrome

D. G. GRAHAME-SMITH & M. SCHACHTER

The carcinoid syndrome is a rarity. Odendorfer first coined the term 'carcinoid' in 1907 to describe a small intestinal tumour of relatively good prognosis despite its capacity for metastatic spread. In 1954 Thorson defined the relationship between the metastases and the symptoms produced by circulating products released from them [45]. It is now clear that the range of these pharmacologically active agents is very wide and that the clinical features are correspondingly complex, differing from one patient to the next.

Epidemiology and aetiology

Carcinoid tumours are rare and the syndrome even more so. Godwin [14] estimated that the prevalence of the tumour was 1.5 per 100,000 in Caucasians. Only a minority of these are functional although the proportion that are varies from one series to another. Functional carcinoid tumours account for 0.05–0.2% of all malignant tumours [30]. They are a common incidental finding at post-mortem with an incidence of 1 in 300 or higher [32]. In most of these cases there are no metastases.

In most series the sex incidence is equal, but in some women predominate. The age of onset is variable, but tends to be younger than in other gastrointestinal tumours. There is little information on the geographical distribution of the tumour, or on genetic or environmental factors in its aetiology.

Pathology

The sites of carcinoid tumours may conveniently be described according to their embryological origins as fore-, mid-, or hind-gut. Table 40.1 shows that mid-gut tumours are most common, whilst rectal tumours are the least likely to metastasize [10, 50]. Most studies agree that the occurrence of metastases depends to some extent upon the site of the primary tumour,

Table 40.1. Sites of carcinoid primary tumours, and incidence of the carcinoid syndrome for each site (after [34]).

Site of tumour	No. of patients	No. with carcinoid syndrome
Oesophagus	1	0
Stomach	98	7
Duodenum	80	1
Illeum, jejunum	992	39
Meckel's diverticulum	46	6
Appendix	1609	2
Caecum, ascending colon	59	3
Descending colon	35	0
Rectum	706	0

Table 40.2. Pathological characteristics of carcinoid tumours according to site of origin.

	Fore-gut	Mid-gut	Hind-gut
Histological structure	Similar to mid-gut but more trabecular. Can be pleomorphic.	Small round cells; clusters, acini	Often trabecular
Argentaffin reaction	Often negative	Positive	Often negative
Association with syndrome	Frequent	Frequent	None
Tumour 5-HT content	Low	High	None
Urinary 5-HIAA	High	High	Normal
5-HTP secretion	Frequent	Rare	None
Bone metastases	Common	Rare	Common
Polypeptide hormone secretion	Frequent	Very rare	None

although this relationship is not direct [7]. In general most tumours that metastasize are over 2 cm in diameter.

The cell from which the tumour derives its name is generally termed an 'enterochromaffin' or 'argentaffin' cell because of its histochemical properties. These cells form part of the neuroectodermal apud (amine, precursor, content and/or uptake, and decarboxylation) system described by Pearse & Takor [36]. Within this broad scheme there is considerable ultrastructural and histochemical variation in tumours from different sites (Table 40.2). This is paralleled by clinically important differences: for example fore-gut tumours frequently metastasize to bone with osteoblastic secondaries.

There has been controversy concerning the prognostic significance of histological classification [28]. However, a recent series of 138 patients showed that the relatively rare undifferentiated tumours have a much worse prognosis than those with a trabecular or acinar pattern of growth [22].

Gastrointestinal carcinoids metastasize most frequently to regional lymph nodes and almost as often to the liver. In general, the carcinoid syndrome occurs only in those patients with hepatic metastases. This is probably because the biologically active products of the tumour are normally detoxified by the liver as they circulate through the portal system. Nevertheless, there are well documented cases of the syndrome in patients with bronchial, testicular or ovarian tumours, some without metastases, where the venous drainage is direct into the systemic circulation [9].

A remarkable feature of such tumours is their association with widespread fibrosis. This is mainly confined to the area of the primary tumour, but may be much more generalized and extend into the peritoneum or pleura. Fibrotic changes in the endocardium of the right side of the heart produce some of the most characteristic clinical features of the syndrome. In the tumour itself there may be a fibrous pseudocapsule, or strands of collagen within the substance of the primary.

Clinical features

The clinical features of the carcinoid syndrome are summarized in Table 40.3. The 'classical carcinoid syndrome' is seen with a primary ileal tumour and hepatic secondaries [47]. However there are also variants of the classical picture, and other

Table 40.3. Clinical features of the carcinoid syndrome.

(a) Vasomotor—flushing, telangiectasiae, 'cyanosis'.

(b) Intestinal hypermotility—diarrhoea, pain, borborygmi, malabsorption[1].

(c) Cardiac involvement—endocardial fibrosis, stenosis/incompetence of pulmonary and tricuspid valves.

(d) Hepatomegaly.

(e) Bronchoconstriction.

(f) Skin changes in legs.

(g) Arthropathy.

(h) Psychiatric disturbance.

(i) Peyronie's disease.

---

[1] May involve factors other than hypermotility

clinical and pathophysiological issues need to be taken into account.

Classical carcinoid syndrome

Vasomotor changes

Flushing is the most consistent feature of the syndrome. Grahame-Smith [15] described 4 types of flush seen in such patients (Table 40.4). Many patients notice that

Table 40.4. Types of flushing in carcinoid syndrome (after [11]).

---

(1) Diffuse erythematous; mostly normal flushing area but may be more widespread. Paroxysmal, transient—up to 5 minutes.

(2) Violaceous colour. Similar distribution to type 1 but may last longer. May be permanent cyanotic skin colour of face, with telangiectasiae. May have associated conjunctival swelling and lacrimation.

(3) Flush may last hours or days. Erythematous, widespread, conjunctival injection, lacrimation. Facial swelling, sometimes swelling of salivary glands. May have associated palpitations, hypotension. Usually associated with bronchial carcinoids.

(4) Bright red, patchy flush, with interspersed white areas. Most obviously associated with histamine-secreting gastric carcinoids.

---

flushing is induced by certain foods, particularly highly spiced. Alcohol in small amounts (for example 5 ml of brandy or 10 ml of sherry) is a very common precipitant. The frequency and severity of the flush varies enormously. Some patients feel unwell during an attack while others are hardly aware of it.

Intestinal hypermotility

Diarrhoea is almost as common as the flush. The two often occur together, but may be dissociated. As with the skin changes, the severity of the diarrhoea is variable, ranging from 1–30 loose stools each day. In some patients it is episodic with several consecutive days of diarrhoea followed by days, or weeks of normal bowel function.

Borborygmi and colicky abdominal pain may occur because of the hypermotility. However the pain may also be due to sub-acute obstruction from the primary tumour or, more commonly, because of fibrosis causing intestinal kinking or narrowing. An uncommon cause of acute pain is segmental intestinal infarction.

Malabsorption is uncommon in patients with a carcinoid tumour although severe weight loss can be seen in advanced disease due to 'malignant cachexia'.

Cardiac involvement

A fibrotic reaction occurs in the internal elastic lamina, predominantly in the valves of the right side of the heart. It can also involve the walls of the right atrium and ventricle. These changes can lead to stenosis of the pulmonary valve with haemodynamically predominant tricuspid incompetence and occasional stenosis. Lesions may also involve the left side of the heart but are rare in the absence of right-sided abnormalities.

The symptoms of carcinoid heart disease

can be surprisingly mild even with severe valvular involvement. However, it often causes congestive cardiac failure with oedema, ascites, right ventricular hypertrophy and abnormal venous pulsations, particularly the characteristic 'V' waves of tricuspid incompetence. Some patients may have florid signs for years before symptoms develop, then they deteriorate rapidly.

Hepatomegaly

This almost always accompanies the carcinoid syndrome. The mass of the hepatic secondaries greatly exceeds that of the primary tumour. Liver secondaries can cause abdominal pain particularly if they undergo necrosis. This can lead to the release of enormous amounts of biologically active products which can result in a dramatic, although usually temporary, deterioration in the patient's general condition (a carcinoid crisis).

Bronchoconstriction

Bronchoconstriction has been reported in around 20% of patients with the carcinoid syndrome but may be much less common as in the authors' experience. In some patients it occurs in association with pre-existing asthma or bronchitis, but it can occur as an independent entity. Acute bronchoconstriction can also occur in association with anaesthesia.

Skin changes

Pellagra may be present in the carcinoid syndrome, presumably because disturbed tryptophan metabolism decreases nicotinamide synthesis. Very rarely a scleroderma-like change is seen in the skin of the lower leg, which becomes erythematous with brawny oedema, the dermis being replaced by dense collagen.

Arthropathy

An unusual erosive arthropathy is a very rare complication of the syndrome. In 5 patients X-rays of the hands showed erosion of the interphalangeal joint surfaces, multiple cystic areas in the phalanges and generalized loss of bone density in the juxta-articular areas [37].

Psychiatric disturbances

Dementia and confusion may be due to pellagra in these patients. However, disturbances of consciousness and hallucinations can occur without frank pellagra, due to tryptophan deficiency from diversion of dietary tryptophan to 5-hydroxytryptamine (5-HT) synthesis by the tumour, with decreased formation of 5-HT in the brain [23].

Peyronie's disease

Peyronie's disease of the penis has been described in carcinoid patients with induration and fibrosis of the corpora cavernosa. It has an interesting similarity with the fibrotic proliferation in the tumour, skin, peritoneum, retroperitoneum or pleura.

Variant syndromes

Bronchial carcinoid

Most bronchial carcinoids are non-functional. Those that are secretory have distinctive features. Symptoms occur more frequently in the absence of distant metastases. They may be very dramatic with extremely severe and prolonged flushing, facial and conjunctival oedema, sweating, lacrimation and salivation. There may also be associated anxiety and severe hypotension, occasionally leading to circulatory collapse. Left-sided cardiac lesions predominate, as would be expected from the venous drainage of such tumours. The tumour can also secrete other polypeptide hormones including parathyroid, growth and adrenocorticotrophic hormones. There is an obvious comparison with oat cell bronchial carcinomas, which are also thought to arise from neuroectodermal tissue [46]. Patients who survive for several years may develop marked facial skin thickening, and lacrimal and salivary gland enlargement. Headaches are also a prominent symptom. Osteoblastic bone secondaries are relatively common.

Gastric carcinoid [2]

The characteristic flush seen with gastric carcinoids (Table 40.4) is probably due to the release of histamine from the tumour. Flushing in association with certain foods is often very obvious, but diarrhoea and cardiac lesions are less common than with ileal tumours [34, 50].

There has been a renewed interest in gastric carcinoids after the finding that omeprazole (a potent long-acting gastric acid inhibitor) produces carcinoid-like lesions in the rat stomach after long-term administration [11]. It has been shown that this is due to a hyperplasia of ECL cells in the gastric mucosa. This hyperplasia has been shown to correlate with the level of the serum gastrin [19] and it has been concluded that this hyperplasia is a response to prolonged acid inhibition rather than a direct carcinogenic effect. Very recently similar lesions have been reported in patients with pernicious anaemia, in whom very high serum levels of gastrin are found [5, 6, 24]. From this evidence it seems likely that gastric carcinoid tumours are due to a hyperplasia of histamine secreting ECL cells in the gastric mucosa in response to a prolonged stimulus, such as hypergastrinaemia [11].

Pathophysiology and biochemistry

The best-known biochemical property of carcinoid tumours is their capacity for secreting 5-hydroxyindoles, sometimes in vast amounts. The most important of these is serotonin—5-hydroxytryptamine (5-HT) [45].

Serotonin is synthesized from the essential amino-acid tryptophan (Fig. 40.1). Normally only 1% of dietary tryptophan is converted into 5-hydroxytryptophan and then to 5-HT, but in carcinoid patients over 60% may be diverted along this pathway rather than into synthesis of protein and nicotinamide. This may be a factor in the nutritional disturbances seen in advanced carcinoid disease.

Excessive 5-HT secretion cannot account for all the clinical features of the syndrome. In particular there is little correlation between blood 5-HT levels and flushing. Infusions of 5-HT usually do not produce a flush, and when they do it is not characteristic [39]. Furthermore, drugs that reduce the synthesis or block the peripheral effects of 5-HT, have an inconsistent and generally disappointing therapeutic effect in patients with the syndrome. These agents, however, can greatly lower the frequency and severity of the diarrhoea, which would be expected as 5-HT is known to increase intestinal motility and secretion.

Other mediators must therefore be involved in the syndrome. Bradykinins (bradykinin, lysine-bradykinin) are important in inducing flushing. These peptides are formed from circulating alpha$_2$ globulin by the enzyme kallikrein, which has been detected in some carcinoid tumours. Catecholamines and alcohol can cause the release of kallikrein from tumour cells. The kinins are potent vasodilators causing hypotension and increased capillary permeability, which may account for some of the oedema in carcinoid patients who are not in cardiac failure. Some carcinoid tumours also secrete

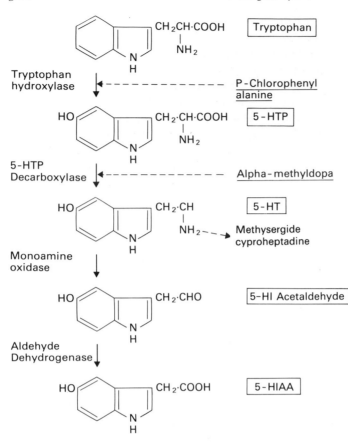

Fig. 40.1. Synthesis and metabolism of 5-hydroxytryptamine (serotonin). Enzyme inhibitors are underlined. 5-HTP = 5-hydroxytryptophan. 5-HT = 5-hydroxytryptamine. 5-HI acetaldehyde = 5-hydroxyindole acetaldehyde. 5-HIAA = 5-hydroxyindole acetic acid. Methysergide and cyproheptadine are serotonin receptor antagonists.

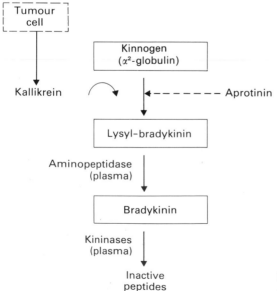

Fig. 40.2. Synthesis and metabolism of kinins. Aprotinin is an inhibitor of kallikrein.

prostaglandins E and F_2 alpha but the pathogenic role of these agents remains uncertain [21]. Gastrin may also be involved in certain patient's flush [13] and other peptides may be secreted causing ectopic humoral syndromes [8, 38].

Investigations

Special investigations

Urinary 5-hydroxyindoleacetic acid (5-HIAA)

A qualitative screening test for 5-HIAA is widely available, but a quantitative test is always better. Most patients with metastatic carcinoid disease excrete large amounts of 5-HIAA, usually in the range of 50–600 mg/24 h (0.3–3 mmol/24 h). The threshold for the qualitative test is about 30 mg/24 h but some patients, notably those with non-ileal tumours, may only secrete 10–30 mg/24h. Foods rich in 5-HT (walnuts, bananas, pineapples, avocados) should be avoided before a test, especially in borderline cases. Mephenesin and glycerol guaiacolate may also give falsely high values of 5-HIAA, while phenothiazines can cause false negative results.

Whole blood 5-HT

Whole blood 5-HT estimations are only available in a few centres, but can be useful when 5-HIAA concentrations in urine are equivocal. This test is effectively a measure of platelet 5-HT, as there is little or no free 5-HT in plasma. As with 5-HIAA the diet can cause large variations in concentration of 5-HT. The upper limit of normal is 300 ng/ml (1.7 μM/ml). The increasing use of high performance liquid chromatography (HPLC) in clinical laboratories will make this estimation easier to obtain in the future.

Flush provocation

Intravenous catecholamines usually provoke a flush, even when none occurs spontaneously. The usual doses are 1–5 μg of adrenaline or 5–10 μg of nor-adrenaline. This test is rarely used when quantitative 5-HIAA or 5-HT determination is feasible and has obvious risks in patients with heart disease. Another safer stimulant of the flush is pentagastrin (0.6 μg/kg i.v.); this will induce a flush in most patients with the syndrome [1]. In about one-third of cases alcohol (10 ml ethanol or equivalent) induces flushing and can be a useful confirmatory out-patient test.

Other investigations

Liver scan

In all patients with biochemical and clinical evidence of the carcinoid syndrome some form of liver scan is mandatory. With advances in imaging techniques progressively better demonstrations of the liver are obtainable using **isotope, ultrasound and computerized tomography (CT) scans**. While none of these techniques is entirely reliable they can usually detect the presence of significant metastases.

Barium radiology

An **endoscopic examination** is superior to a barium meal if a gastric carcinoid tumour is suspected. A **small bowel barium study** may identify an ileal tumour [50]; a **barium enema** may also be required when adequate visualization of the terminal ileum is not obtained.

Routine radiology and bone scanning

A **chest X-ray** should exclude a bronchial primary tumour, or lung secondaries. A **bone scan and skeletal X-ray survey** are indicated when bone secondaries are suspected, or probable.

Cardiac assessment

A full cardiac assessment is indicated in any patient with the carcinoid syndrome. An **electrocardiograph (ECG)** may show evidence of right ventricular hypertrophy, often with right bundle branch block. **Echocardiography** may be helpful in identifying and assessing the severity of any valvular lesions, although interpretation can be difficult with right-sided cardiac disease. Cardiac catheterization is seldom indicated.

Haematology and biochemistry

A **blood count** rarely contributes any useful information, other than the presence of anaemia from chronic blood loss, or malnutrition. In the presence of liver or bone secondaries the **alkaline phosphatase** will be raised, sometimes markedly, while the **transaminases** are usually less elevated. Hyperbilirubinaemia is rare. Plasma proteins are usually normal until late in the disease. Renal function is not generally affected unless there is retroperitoneal fibrosis, or severe dehydration as a result of the diarrhoea. Similarly plasma electrolytes are usually normal; if there is hypokalaemia and alkalosis an ectopic secretion of ACTH should be suspected.

Differential diagnosis

The diagnosis of the carcinoid syndrome is often delayed, sometimes for many years. Yet the characteristic syndrome of flushing, diarrhoea, hepatomegaly and sometimes secondaries in bone is mimicked by only two much rarer conditions—**medullary carcinoma of the thyroid** and **systemic mastocytosis**. Rarely 5-HT secretion may be increased in both of these conditions.

Flushing

This is usually very characteristic and can be distinguished from menopausal, or cirrhotic flushing by the elevated 5-HIAA urinary excretion or 5-HT blood levels and by the provocative tests described previously.

Diarrhoea

An isolated attack of diarrhoea does not suggest that the patient has the carcinoid syndrome. In the absence of infection, or infestation most patients would be first investigated for large bowel cancer or inflammatory bowel disease. Recurrent or chronic watery diarrhoea without blood, or mucus in the stool should certainly lead to a suspicion of carcinoid syndrome. Nevertheless many such patients are only diagnosed at the time of laparotomy. The same applies to those who present with acute, or sub-acute intestinal obstruction.

Hepatomegaly

This is unlikely to be present in isolation and one would expect the associated symptoms of flushing and/or diarrhoea. Clinically and on scanning secondaries of carcinoid cannot be distinguished from those of other tumours.

Pulmonary shadow

A non-functioning bronchial carcinoid tumour can usually be distinguished from other causes (e.g. carcinoma) by bronchoscopy and biopsy. Functioning tumours would usually produce raised urinary 5-HIAA and blood 5-HT concentrations.

Treatment

Considering its relative rarity a remarkable number of treatments have been tried in

Table 40.5. Modalities of treatment in carcinoid syndrome.

Pharmacological
Serotonin receptor antagonists (mainly anti-diarrhoeal)
Methysergide
Cyproheptadine[1]
Pizotifen
Chlorpromazine[2]

Serotonin synthesis inhibitors (mainly anti-diarrhoeal)
Parachlorophenylalanine
Alpha-methyldopa

Adrenergic receptor antagonists (mainly anti-flushing)
Phenoxybenzamine
Propranolol

Inhibitors of kinin synthesis
?Corticosteroids[3]

Cytotoxic drugs
5-Fluorouracil
Streptozotocin
Adriamycin

Miscellaneous
Cimetidine
Clonidine
Tamoxifen
Somatostatin

Surgical
Partial hepatectomy or enucleation of liver secondaries
± resection of primary

Devascularization
Ligation of branches of hepatic artery
Selective percutaneous angiographic
    embolization of branches of hepatic artery

[1] also antihistamine (H_1), anticholinergic.
[2] also alpha-adrenergic, dopaminergic antagonist.
[3] other possible mechanisms.

this condition (Table 40.5). This indicates that none is particularly satisfactory.

Medical therapy

Drugs that prevent the synthesis, or peripheral effects of 5-HT have long been standard treatment in this condition. Their effect on the flush is usually slight or non-existent, but diarrhoea generally responds well.

Methysergide is the traditional serotonin antagonist, although it may itself induce fibrotic changes, retroperitoneal fibrosis being particularly notorious. Other side-effects include sedation, nausea and confusion. It is usually given in a daily dose of 3–12 mg, in 3 divided doses.

Cyproheptadine is an alternative 5-HT antagonist, which also has marked histamine H_1 receptor blocking and anticholinergic activity. The latter may be a disadvantage, particularly in elderly men in whom urinary retention can occur. However, its antihistamine activity is an advantage, especially in histamine-secreting gastric carcinoids. A recent case report [18] suggests that cyproheptadine can induce tumour regression—the mechanism for this action is obscure. The usual daily dose is 12–32 mg, in divided doses 3–4 times daily.

Chlorpromazine, amongst its large range of pharmacological actions, is a 5-HT antagonist and alpha-adrenoreceptor blocker. Both effects can be useful in the management of the carcinoid syndrome.

Parachlorophenylalanine is not widely available, but can be useful where other peripheral antagonists are ineffective or have to be given in prohibitively high doses. Daily doses range from 750 mg to 4 g in 3–4 divided doses. Unwanted effects include depression, eosinophilia and sometimes pulmonary infiltration. Hypothermia is a rare complication.

Alpha-methyldopa is thought to inhibit the decarboxylation of hydroxytryptophan to 5-HT, but it may also act through an alpha-adrenergic mechanism. Like other drugs in the broadly 'anti-5-HT' category it may decrease the severity of the diarrhoea and occasionally of the flush. It is given in a daily dose of 750 mg to 2 g in 3–4 divided doses. The main unwanted effects are hypotension and sedation.

Corticosteroids appear to be useful in patients with severe or long-lasting flushing, particularly those due to bronchial tumours. How they work is unclear; they may prevent the release of lysosomal contents from the tumour cells, but the doses required for this effect are unlikely to be attained in clinical practice. More likely they interfere with the formation and, possibly, the release of kinins by kallikrein secreted by the tumour. Methylprednisolone has been used parenterally during surgery to overcome the effects of the massive release of 5-HT and other kinins that can occur.

Adrenergic blockade may alleviate flushing by preventing the release of kinins from the tumour cells. **Phenoxybenzamine** (10–60 mg daily) has been widely used, but has significant unwanted effects, including dizziness and nasal congestion; tolerance may develop. **Propranolol** is of limited value in the syndrome despite initial encouraging reports.

Cytotoxic therapy has proved very disappointing, presumably because of the slow growth of the tumour [17]. At least 24 drugs have been tried alone, or in combination, but only 10 have been tested on more than 5 patients; combination therapy has not proved better than single agents. **5-fluorouracil** appears to be the most effective, producing relief of symptoms and partial regression in some patients. **Streptozotocin** has similar efficacy, but is more toxic, especially on the kidney and causes nausea. In addition to the usual unwanted effects of cytotoxic therapy (suppression of the bone marrow and intestinal and skin damage, etc.) these agents can cause necrosis of the tumour with the release of large quantities of biologically active agents (carcinoid crisis) into the circulation, which can prove fatal.

Symptomatic therapy

Diarrhoea may be treated symptomatically with **codeine phosphate, diphenoxylate**, or **loperamide**. These may be as effective as specific blocking agents, although very large doses may be needed.

Tamoxifen, the anti-oestrogen agent, was reported to relieve the flush in one female patient. A combination of **cimetidine and clonidine** can prevent the flush induced by alcohol [49].

Other agents

Aprotinin can be shown to inhibit kinin synthesis *in vitro* but its clinical efficacy is doubtful. **Somatostatin**, a potent inhibitor of hormone release, alleviates the diarrhoea and flushing [25]. But unfortunately is limited by the fact that it has to be given intravenously, or subcutaneously and causes widespread other effects. An orally active analogue might prove valuable in this syndrome.

Surgical treatment

Resection

Surgical resection can be useful in the carcinoid syndrome, even when the tumour is very advanced. If the tumour is diagnosed before metastasizing (most often with bronchial lesions), resection may be curative. An intestinal primary tumour may be removed, or left *in situ* if surrounded by dense fibrosis, when an intestinal by-pass procedure is done to prevent later obstruction.

Even when there are large and numerous hepatic secondaries symptoms may be relieved by removal of some, or all of them. Relief may last for remarkably long periods even after palliative surgery. If metastases are localized to one lobe, hepatic lobectomy will be the preferred operation. When metastases are widespread it may be possible to remove them by enucleation [4, 44, 48].

The removal of carcinoid secondaries is associated with many complications [26]. Manipulation of large tumour masses can cause the release of tumour cell products which result in abrupt and unpredictable changes of blood pressure and bronchial tone. Blood loss from the liver can be substantial and fibrous adhesions are more likely to occur than after other abdominal surgery.

Tumour devascularization

Tumour devascularization may be achieved by selective arterial ligation [12], or selective arterial embolization of branches of the hepatic artery [3, 27]. The former carries a high risk of operative morbidity and mortality. Embolisation is safer and can produce very worthwhile responses. In a recent series [29], flushing and diarrhoea were controlled in four out of five patients, who had been resistant to pharmacological control. Complications of embolization are related to the sudden release of 5-HT and other kinins, as the tumour undergoes ischaemic necrosis. For this reason the procedure should be undertaken under close anaesthetic supervision.

Prognosis

The clinical course of carcinoid disease is very variable and unpredictable. Individual patients have survived for years, or even decades, with an enormous tumour load. The largest reported series of functioning tumours revealed a 50% survival at 3 years, 25% at 6 years and 15% at 10 years [9]. A more recent series of 30 patients gave very similar results with 40% survival at 5 years and 15% at 10 years [29]. It was also noted that half of the deaths occurred within the first year after diagnosis.

Medullary carcinoma of the thyroid

Medullary carcinoma of the thyroid is a rare tumour, accounting for less than 7% of all thyroid malignancies [51]. It is thought to arise from para-follicular C cells which, like enterochromaffin cells of the gut, are regarded as part of the apud system.

In some patients they occur as part of the multiple endocrine adenoma syndrome (MEA), most commonly being associated with either a parathyroid adenoma/hyperplasia, or a phaeochromocytoma [33]. The disease may be inherited as an autosomal dominant, or may occur spontaneously. The familial form is almost always bilateral and often multifocal. Characteristically the tumour secretes calcitonin, but it can also produce prostaglandins, histamine, ACTH, and occasionally other polypeptide hormones.

Gastrointestinal presentation

Medullary carcinoma may present to the gastroenterologist with diarrhoea. About 30% of such patients develop diarrhoea at some stage of their illness [43]. Most pass less than 5 loose stools per day, but occasionally the frequency may be up to twice this figure. Other features of the syndrome relate mainly to local invasion and the effects of the endocrine secretions. Interestingly, hypocalcaemia, as a result of calcitonin hypersecretion, is very rare.

Diagnosis

Sensitive and specific radio-immunoassays for calcitonin now exist and allow early diagnosis. Most such patients have fasting calcitonin concentrations above 0.38 ng/ml. In all patients the calcitonin concentration rises over 1 ng/ml in response to a calcium infusion (see Chapter 39). A more convenient provocation test is the response to pentagastrin (0.5 μg/kg i.v.), when peak calcitonin values are reached within 5 minutes of the injection [42]. In view of the strong genetic component of the disease, all relatives of the affected patient should be screened for elevated plasma calcitonin concentrations.

Treatment

Irradiation, either external or with radio-iodine, is totally ineffective in this disease.

Chemotherapy has not been extensively tested but appears ineffective. In some patients a prostaglandin inhibitor, such as indomethacin, may alleviate diarrhoea. The best treatment is surgery [31]. Total thyroidectomy with lymph node clearance of the central cervical and upper mediastinal nodes is recommended. Mediastinal clearance is probably not justified if scintiscanning, or a CT scan shows hepatic metastases, although solitary metastases may be amenable to local removal.

Prognosis

Prognosis is very variable, as with the carcinoid syndrome; it appears to be worse if the patient has a multiple endocrine adenoma syndrome. A few patients have survived for over a decade, while in others the tumour has proved to be rapidly fatal.

Systemic mastocytosis

Systemic mastocytosis is a malignant proliferation of mast cells in the skin, lymph nodes, bones, liver and intestine. The mast cells release histamine, causing headaches, flushing and diarrhoea. Malabsorption may be due to gastric hypersecretion, small intestinal infiltration, or villous atrophy [41].

The diagnosis should be considered in a patient with urticaria, hepatomegaly and diarrhoea. Although many of the symptoms are controlled by high dose histamine H_2 receptor blockade, most patients will die from the effects of tumour infiltration [20].

References

1 AHLMAN H, DAHLSTROM A, GRONSTAD K, *et al.* The pentagastrin test in the diagnosis of the carcinoid syndrome. *Ann Surg* 1985;**201**:81–86.
2 ALI MH, DAVIDSON A, AZZOPARDI JG. Composite gastric carcinoid and adenocarcinoma. *Histopathology* 1984;**8**:529–536.
3 ALLISON DJ, MODLIN IM, JENKINS WJ. Treatment of carcinoid liver metastases by hepatic artery embolisation. *Lancet* 1977;**ii**:1323–1325.

4 BERSOHN I, BLELOCK J. Right hemihepatectomy in secondary carcinoid of the liver: clinical course and liver function tests. *S Afr Med J* 1966;1:271–274.

5 BORCH K, RENVAL H, LIEDBERG G. Gastric endocrine cell hyperplasia and carcinoid tumours in pernicious anaemia. *Gastroenterology* 1985;88·638–648.

6 CARNEY JA, GO VLW, FAIRBANKS VF, MOORE SB, ALPORT EC, NORA FE. The syndrome of gastric argyrophil carcinoid tumours and nonantral gastric atrophy. *Ann Intern Med* 1983;99:761–766.

7 CONTI AR, CUSUMANO F, SALVADORI B. Clinical considerations on 8 cases of abdominal carcinoids. *Tumori* 1981;67:145–149.

8 DABEK FT. Bronchial carcinoid tumor with acromegaly in two patients. *J Clin Endocrinol Metab* 1974;38:329–334.

9 DAVIS Z, MOERTEL CG, ILLRATH DC. The malignant carcinoid syndrome. *Surg Gynecol Obstet* 1973;137:637–644.

10 DURNING P, GALLAND RB, NAGORNEY DM, WELBOURN RB. Neuroendocrine tumours of the gut. *World J Surg* 1985;9:348–360.

11 ELDER JB. Inhibition of acid and gastric carcinoids. *Gut* 1985;26:1279–1283.

12 FARNDON JR. The carcinoid syndrome: methods of treatment and recent experience with hepatic artery ligation and infusion. *Clin Oncol* 1977;3:265–272.

13 FROLICH JC, BLOOMGARTEN ZT, OATES JA, *et al.* The carcinoid flush. Provocation by pentagastrin and inhibition by somatostatin. *N Engl J Med* 1979;299:1055–1058.

14 GODWIN JD. Carcinoid tumours—an analysis of 2,837 cases. *Cancer* 1975;36:560–569.

15 GRAHAME-SMITH DG. The carcinoid syndrome. *Am J Cardiol* 1968;21:376–388.

16 GRAHAME-SMITH DG. *The carcinoid syndrome.* London: Heinemann Medical Books, 1972.

17 HARRIS AL. Chemotherapy for the carcinoid syndrome. *Cancer Chemother Pharmacol* 1981;5:133–138.

18 HARRIS AL, SMITH IE. Regression of carcinoid tumour with cyproheptadine. *Br Med J* 1982;285:475.

19 HARVEY RF, BRADSHAW MJ, DAVIDSON CM, WILKINSON SP, DAVIES PS. Multifocal gastric carcinoid t7umours, achlorhydria, and hypergastrinaemia. *Lancet* 1985; i: 951–952.

20 HIRSCHOWITZ BI, GROARKE JF. Effect of cimetidine in gastric hypersecretion and diarrhoea in systemic mastocytosis. *Ann Intern Med* 1979;90:769–770.

21 JAFFE BM. Prostaglandins and serotonin in diarrhoeogenic syndromes. Speranza V & Bono N, eds. *Gastrointestinal hormones and pathology of the digestive system.* New York: Plenum Press, 1978.

22 JOHNSON LA, LAVIN P, MOERTEL CG, WEILAND L, *et al.* Carcinoids: the association of histologic growth pattern and survival. *Cancer* 1983;51:882–889.

23 LEHMANN J. Mental disturbances followed by stupor in a patient with carcinoidosis. *Acta Psychiatr Scand* 1966;42:153–161.

24 LEHTOLA J, KARTTUNEN T, KREKELA I, NIEMELA S, RAGANEN O. Gastric carcinoids with minimal or no macroscopic lesion in patients with pernicious anaemia. *Hepatogastroenterology* 1985;32:72–76.

25 LONG RG, PETERS JR, BLOOM SR, *et al.* Somatostatin, gastrointestinal peptides and the carcinoid syndrome. *Gut* 1981;22:549–553.

26 MASON RA, STEANE PA. Carcinoid syndrome: its relevance to the anaesthetist. *Anaesthesia* 1976;31:228–242.

27 MATON PN, CAMILLERI M, GRIFFIN G, ALLISON DJ, HODGSON HJF, CHADWICK VS. Role of hepatic arterial embolisation in the carcinoid syndrome. *Br Med J* 1983;287:932–933.

28 MCDONALD RA. A study of 356 carcinoids of the gastrointestinal tract—report of four new cases of the carcinoid syndrome. *Am J Med* 1956;21:867–872.

29 MELIA WM, NUNNERLEY HB, JOHNSON PJ, WILLIAMS RJ. Use of arterial devascularisation and cytotoxic drugs in 30 patients with the carcinoid syndrome. *Br J Cancer* 1982;46:331–339.

30 MENGEL CE, SHAFFER RD. The carcinoid syndrome. In: Holbard JF & Frie E, eds. *Cancer medicine.* Philadelphia: Lea & Febiger, 1982:1584–1594.

31 MILLER HH, MELVIN KEW, GIBSON JM, TASHJIAN AH. Surgical approach to early medullary carcinoma of the thyroid. *Am J Surg* 1972;123:438–443.

32 MOERTEL GC, DOCKERTY MB, JUDD ES. Carcinoid tumors of the vermiform appendix. *Cancer* 1968;14:901–908.

33 NEWSOME HH. Multiple endocrine adenomatosis. *Surg Clin North Am* 1974;54:387–393.

34 OATES JA, BUTLER C. Pharmacological and endocrine aspects of the carcinoid syndrome. *Adv Pharmacol* 1967;5:109–132.

35 OLNEY JR, URDANETA LF, ALJURF AS, JOCHIMSE PR, SHIRAZI SS. Carcinoid tumours of the gastrointestinal tract. *Am Surg* 1985;51:37–41.

36 PEARSE AGE, TAKOR TT. Neuroendocrine embryology and the APUD concept. *Clin Endocrinol* 1976;5:229S–244S.

37 PLONK JW, FELDMAN JM. Carcinoid arthropathy. *Arch Intern Med* 1976;134:651–654.

38 POWELL D, CANUCK D, SKRABICH P. The pathophysiology of substance P in man. In: Bloom SR, ed. *Gut hormones.* London: Churchill Livingstone, 1978:521–529.

39 ROBERTSON JIS, PEART WS, ANDREWS TM. The mechanism of facial flushes in the carcinoid syndrome. *Q J Med* 1962;21:103–112.

40 SANDERS RJ. *Carcinoids of the gastrointestinal tract.* Springfield, Illinois: Charles C. Thomas, 1973.

41 Scott BB, Hardy GJ, Losowsky MS. Involvement of the small intestine in systemic mast cell disease. *Gut* 1979;16:918–924.

42 Sizemore GW. Stimulation tests for diagnosis of medullary thyroid carcinoma. *Mayo Clin Proc* 1975;50:53–56.

43 Steinfeld CM, Moertel CG, Woolner LB. Diarrhoea and medullary carcinoma of the thyroid. *Cancer* 1973;31:1237–1239.

44 Stephens J, Grahame-Smith DG. Treatment of carcinoid syndrome by local removal of hepatic metastases. *Proc R Soc Med* 1972;15:444–449.

45 Thorson A, Bjorck G, Bjorkmann G, Waldenstrom J. Malignant carcinoid of the small intestine with metastases to the liver, valvular disease of the right side of the heart, peripheral vasomotor symptoms, bronchoconstriction and an unusual type of cyanosis: Clinical and pathological syndrome. *Am Heart J* 1954;47:795–804.

46 Tischler AS, Dichter MA, Biales B, Greene LA. Neuroendocrine neoplasias and their cells of origin. *N Eng J Med* 1977;296:919–925.

47 Wareing TH, Sawyers JL. Carcinoids and the carcinoid syndrome *Am, J.Surg* 1983:145:769–772.

48 Welch JP, Malt RA. Management of carcinoid tumours of the gastrointestinal tract. *Surg Gynecol Obstet* 1977;145:223–227.

49 Wilkin JK, Rountree CB. Blockade of carcinoid flush with cimetidine and clonidine. *Arch Dermatol* 1982;118:109–111.

50 Woods HF, Bax NDS, Smith JAR. Small bowel carcinoid tumours. *World J Surg* 1985;9:921–929.

51 Woolner LB, Beanns CN, Black BM, McConahey WM, Keating FR. Classification and prognosis of thyroid carcinoma: A study of 885 cases observed in a thirty year period. *Am J Surg* 1961;102:354–388.

SECTION VIII

DISEASES OF THE SMALL INTESTINE

Chapter 41
Investigation of the Small Intestine

J. G. C. KINGHAM & P.D. FAIRCLOUGH

The major functions of the small intestine are digestive, absorptive and motor. In addition the small intestine has endocrine and immunological functions and it acts as a semi-permeable barrier between the environment and the internal milieu. Tests of the small intestine can reveal its anatomy, both gross and microscopical, and some of its functions. More than one test is usually required to make a satisfactory diagnosis, but sometimes a single test is crucial.

In the investigation of suspected disorders of the small intestine a series of screening tests are usually performed to determine whether significant nutritional deficiency has arisen. It is not easy to put forward a simple and logical plan for the subsequent investigation of all small intestinal disorders. The tests required will depend on the clinician's assessment of the problem, the results of initial screening tests, and a knowledge of the characteristics of the known disorders of the small intestine and associated organs (Table 41.1). In general, tests of structure—biopsy and barium studies, for example—are of more diagnostic help than tests of function.

Gross anatomy is best investigated radiologically, although endoscopy has a limited role.

Radiology

Plain abdominal X-rays

The main function of the plain film in investigating the small bowel is to diagnose obstruction or ileus, recognized by dilated bowel loops with fluid levels (Fig. 41.1).

Table 41.1. Principal causes of malabsorption.

Pancreatic exocrine insufficiency
Chronic pancreatitis
Carcinoma of pancreas
Cystic fibrosis
Pancreatectomy

Intraluminal bile salt deficiency
Biliary obstruction
Bacterial overgrowth in small bowel
Ileal resection
Ileal Crohn's disease

Brush border membrane diseases
Disaccharidase deficiency
Glucose-galactose malabsorption
Cystinuria
Hartnup disease

Small intestinal disorders
Massive resection
Coeliac disease/Dermatitis herpetiformis
Tropical sprue
Whipple's disease
Lymphangiectasia
Radiation enteritis
Intestinal ischaemia
Primary intestinal lymphoma
Hypogammaglobulinaemia
Eosinophilic gastroenteritis
Amyloidosis
Parasite infestation

Complex disorders
Post gastrectomy
Diabetes mellitus
Endocrinopathies
Scleroderma

Drugs
Cholestyramine
Neomycin
Mefenamic acid
Colchicine
Cathartics

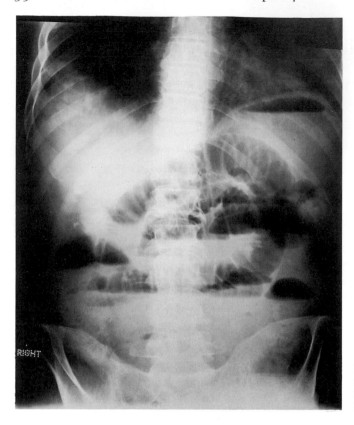

Fig. 41.1. Plain abdominal X-ray, showing features of small intestinal obstruction (courtesy of Dr J. Laidlow).

Barium studies [4, 31, 43, 49, 76]

Small bowel meal

This is a single-contrast procedure requiring a large volume (300–600 ml) of a dilute barium suspension. The patient should be fasted. Oral metoclopramide 10 mg may be given immediately beforehand to hasten the procedure. The whole volume of barium is swallowed rapidly so that it can pass along the bowel as a relatively unbroken column. Films are taken every 10–30 minutes until the barium reaches the caecum. Transit time is extremely variable (10 min–6 h) and of doubtful significance. It is important to see the terminal ileum which usually requires manipulation of the patient's abdomen by the radiologist. More detailed double-contrast views of the terminal ileal mucosa can be obtained by insufflation of air through a rectal catheter. The standard small bowel meal is a sensitive detector of the lesions shown in Table 41.2. A normal small bowel meal is shown in Fig. 41.2.

Table 41.2. Lesions readily detected by small bowel meal examination.

Areas of stricturing and dilatation (e.g. Crohn's disease)	Fig. 41.3
Deep ulceration (e.g. Crohn's disease)	Fig. 41.4
Discrete mass lesions greater than 2 cm diameter (e.g. tumour)	Fig. 41.5 Fig. 41.11
Proximal outpouchings (e.g. duodenal diverticulum)	Fig. 41.6
Fistulae (e.g. Crohn's disease)	Fig. 41.7
Generalized dilatation and disturbance of mucosal fold pattern (e.g. coeliac disease)	Fig. 41.8
Bowel wall thickening (e.g. radiation enteritis)	Fig. 41.9
Motility disturbance (e.g. scleroderma)	Fig. 41.10

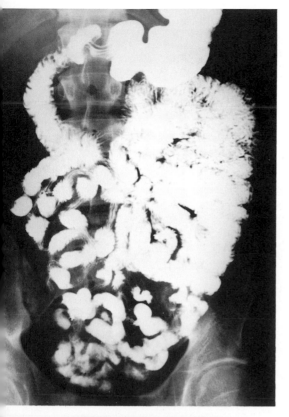

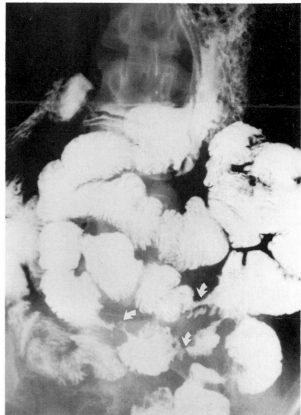

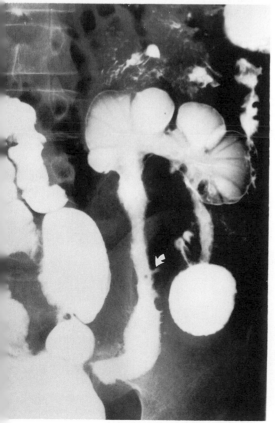

Fig. 41.2. (above left) Normal small bowel meal (courtesy of Dr C. Bartram).

Fig. 41.3. (above) Small bowel meal, showing Crohn's disease of the small intestine with areas of stricturing (arrowed) and dilatation (courtesy of Dr C. Bartram).

Fig. 41.4. (left) Small bowel meal showing deep ulceration (arrowed) due to Crohn's disease (courtesy of Dr C. Bartram).

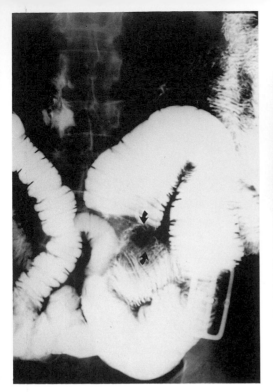

Fig. 41.5. Small bowel meal showing a tumour (2°
deposit, arrowed) obstructing the small intestine
(courtesy of Dr C. Bartram).

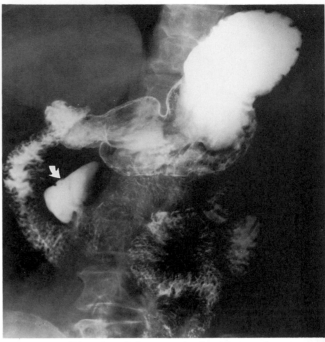

Fig. 41.6. Small bowel meal showing a duodenal diverticulum
(arrowed) (courtesy of Dr C. Bartram).

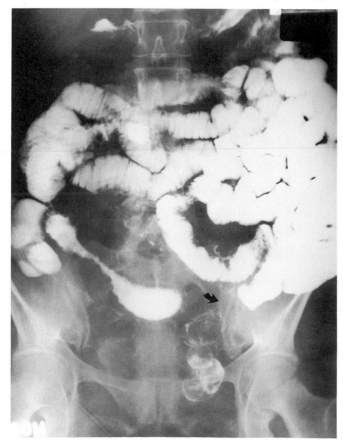

Fig. 41.7. Small bowel meal showing enterosigmoid fistula
(arrowed) due to Crohn's disease (courtesy of Dr C. Bartram).

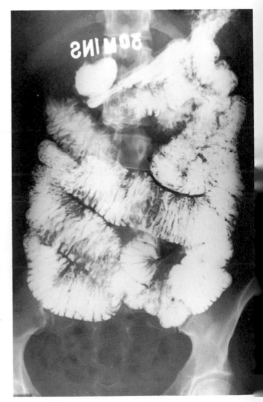

Fig. 41.8. Small bowel meal showing dilatation of
the intestine and loss of normal jejunal fold pattern
in coeliac disease (courtesy of Dr C. Bartram and Dr
P. J. Kumar, [4]).

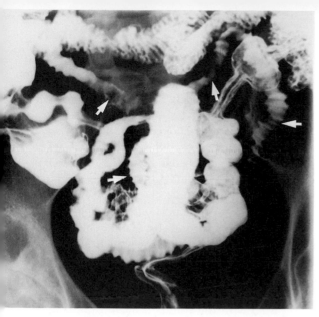

41.9. Small bowel meal showing thickening of the bowel and stricturing due to radiation enteritis (courtesy of Dr Bartram).

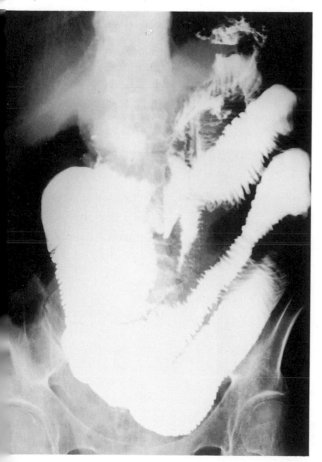

.10. Small bowel meal in a patient with intestinal scleroderma.

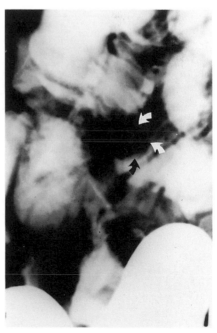

Fig. 41.11. Small bowel meal showing small (hamartomatous) polyp (arrowed) (courtesy of Dr C. Bartram).

Small bowel enema (enteroclysis)

This technique allows a greater volume of barium suspension to be administered at a rate faster than it could be swallowed. It requires prior emplacement of a tube in the fourth part of the duodenum. The suspension is more dilute (specific gravity 1.25) than that used in the standard small bowel meal and is infused at 80–100 ml/minute to a maximum of 1800 ml. This technique is particularly useful to identify lesions listed in Table 41.3. A normal small bowel enema is shown in Fig. 41.12.

Table 41.3. Lesions for which small bowel enema is particularly useful.

Strictures, especially short or solitary (e.g. adhesions)	Fig. 41.13
Small mass lesions (e.g. polyps less than 2 cm in diameter)	Fig. 41.11
Distal outpouchings (e.g. Meckel's diverticulum)	Fig. 41.14
Fine mucosal lesions (e.g. Crohn's aphthae)	Fig. 41.15

The disadvantages of the intubation over the standard study are that it is more uncomfortable for the patient and that it requires extra radiological skill. The small bowel enema should only be used when specifically indicated as it is not superior to the standard examination in most circumstances.

The range of normal values for transverse diameter and size of mucosal folds depends to some extent on which of the two techniques is used. In general, with the intubation technique transverse diameter is greater and mucosal folds less prominent than with the standard meal. Approximate ranges for normal values are given in Table 41.4.

Barium enema

Sometimes the terminal ileum may be seen better on barium enema than small bowel meal, particularly when looking for recurrent Crohn's disease immediately proximal to an ileocolic anastomosis.

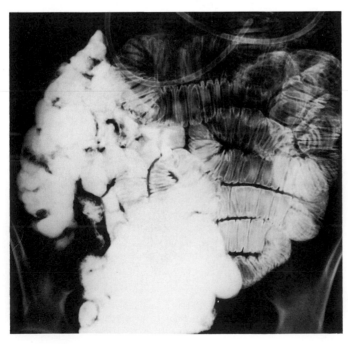

Fig. 41.12. Normal small bowel enema (courtesy of Dr C. Bartram).

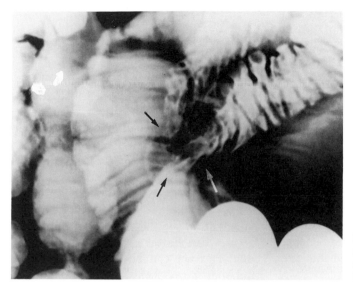

Fig. 41.13. Small bowel enema showing short stricture due to an adhesion (arrowed) (courtesy of Dr C. Bartram).

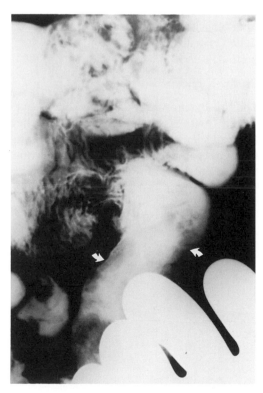

Fig. 41.14. Small bowel enema showing a Meckel's diverticulum (arrowed) (courtesy of Dr C. Bartram).

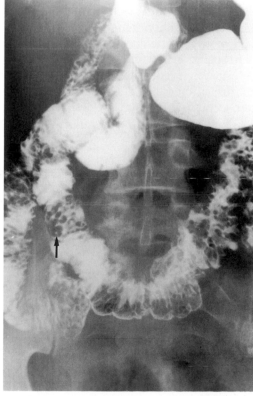

Fig. 41.15. Small bowel enema showing aphthous ulcers (arrowed) due to Crohn's disease (courtesy of Dr C. Bartram & Dr P. J. Kumar [4]).

Table 41.4. Morphometry of normal small bowel meal examination [4].

Jejunal diameter <40 mm
Ileal diameter <35 mm
Valvulae conniventes
Height (jejunum > ileum) 2–6 mm
Thickness (jejunum > ileum) 1–2 mm
Interval (ileum > jejunum) 1–10 mm
Bowel wall thickness (separation of adjacent
loops) < 2 mm

Ileostomy enema

Ileostomy dysfunction is often associated with a distal small bowel stricture and is investigated best by retrograde enema through a Foley catheter inserted into the stoma.

Endoscopy [20]

Endoscopy has little to offer in small intestinal investigation other than inspection and biopsy of the duodenum at gastroduodenoscopy or of the terminal ileum at colonoscopy. The latter may be useful to confirm a diagnosis of Crohn's disease. Enteroscopy with specially-designed fibrescopes is rarely performed.

Anatomy—microscopic

Small intestinal biopsy

Microscopic anatomy of the small intestinal mucosa can be assessed with relative ease by biopsy. Such biopsies can also be analysed biochemically, or put into cell culture. The most proximal and distal parts of the small intestine can be biopsied by forceps under direct endoscopic vision using standard fibrescopes. The advantages of endoscopy are speed, that the biopsy can be aimed at a specific lesion, that multiple biopsies can be taken, that the upper alimentary tract can be inspected en route, and that X-ray facilities are unnecessary. The disadvantages are the limited access, that the biopsies are small and poorly orientated and that endoscopy is a skilled, expensive and relatively invasive technique. The more conventional approach to small intestinal biopsy is by the use of specifically designed instruments.

Crosby-Kugler capsule [21]

The Crosby capsule is a metal cylinder (9 × 18 mm) with a single 3 mm port attached to a sufficient length of fine plastic tubing to allow passage into the small intestine. Suction on the tubing with a syringe draws

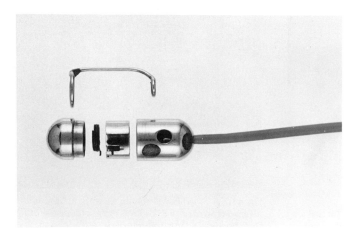

Fig. 41.16. Exploded view of Crosby-Kugler capsule used for small intestinal mucosal biopsy.

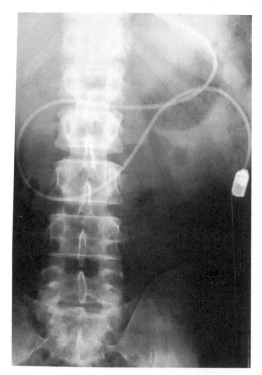

Fig. 41.17. Plain abdominal X-ray showing Crosby-Kugler capsule in position for a jejunal biopsy.

a bleb of mucosa through the port and activates a spring-loaded, rotating knife within the cylinder to slice off the biopsy (Fig. 41.16). A small capsule with a 2 mm port can be used in children. Most biopsies are taken in the jejunum just beyond the ligament of Treitz. This position is chosen as it is identified readily on X-ray screening (Fig. 41.17) and allows repeat biopsies to be taken from the same site. This is important when the lesion under study is unevenly distributed. Occasionally biopsies are required from the ileum; for this a greater length of tubing is needed.

Jejunal biopsy techniques

Traditional method

The fasted patient swallows the capsule and about 100 cm of tubing at bedtime and lies on his right side. The proximal end of the tube is securely fixed to the cheek. The following morning a plain X-ray of the abdomen should confirm that the capsule has passed into the jejunum. If it is too far advanced, it may be retracted to the desired position. The tubing and capsule port are cleared of any food debris by flushing through with a little water. The capsule is then fired by applying suction with a 20 ml syringe. The capsule is withdrawn by gentle traction and disassembled. The biopsy is removed with a needle and carefully spread out flat on a piece of ground glass. The villous morphology is examined under a dissecting microscope before the biopsy is put into fixative for histological processing. Well-orientated sections can only be obtained if the biopsy is correctly orientated before fixation. If enzyme analysis or tissue culture is to be performed, half the biopsy should be set aside for this purpose immediately after removal from the capsule.

Screening method [62, 75]

The capsule and 60–80 cm of tubing are swallowed. The abdomen is screened with the patient lying supine on the fluoroscopy couch. The tubing is manipulated so that there are no loops in the stomach and the capsule lies at the pylorus. The patient lies on his right side and periodic screening will show when the capsule enters the duodenum. Entry can be speeded by oral or intramuscular metoclopramide 10 mg. Once the capsule is in the duodenum a further 20–40 cm of tubing is fed in at the mouth and in most patients the ligament of Treitz is reached within half an hour. For greater speed a stiffening wire can be introduced down the tube and the capsule pushed round the duodenum [39].

Endoscopic method [58]

The patient is prepared as for a normal gastroscopy. The capsule is assembled and attached to a length of arteriography catheter 50 cm longer than the endoscope. The end of the tubing is fed retrogradely up the endoscopic biopsy channel until the capsule is hard up against the tip of the scope which is then passed in the conventional manner. With the endoscope positioned just proximal to the pylorus the capsule is threaded through into the duodenum and advanced a further 30 cm. The capsule is then fired and withdrawn with the endoscope [45]. Biopsies of the second part of the duodenum can also be conveniently obtained using routine endoscopic biopsy forceps [20].

Steerable biopsy instrument [72]

Various purpose-built steerable biopsy catheters have been designed but have not achieved general popularity. The technique to intubate the jejunum is similar to that used for the screening method.

Multiple biopsy instrument [11, 26]

The original apparatus was later modified to operate hydraulically and enables any number of rather small biopsies to be taken and delivered to the operator immediately. The instrument consists of a biopsy capsule, whose mechanics are similar to a Crosby capsule, affixed to a thick, semi-rigid tube. The capsule is positioned in the jejunum by X-ray screening [57].

Critique of methods

Of the methods described the traditional is the simplest, but time-consuming and not appropriate for out-patient investigation. It does not however require a skilled operator to pass the tube. The screening method is reasonably quick, but requires a skilled operator and X-ray screening. The endoscopic method is rapid, but has all the drawbacks of endoscopy. Both the steerable forceps and the multiple biopsy apparatus are expensive and unnecessary in general use. Personal preference will decide which method is used but, if X-ray screening is

Table 41.5. Diseases in which jejunal biopsy is helpful or essential in diagnosis.

Disease	Features
Coeliac disease/Dermatitis herpetiformis	'Flat' mucosa. Inflammatory cells. Jejunum more affected than ileum.
Tropical sprue	Like coeliac disease but less severe. Jejunum and ileum both affected.
Dietary protein intolerance (milk, soy)	Children only
Whipple's disease	Infiltration with foamy macrophages and bacillary structures.
Parasitic enteritis (e.g. giardiasis)	Mucosa normal or like mild coeliac disease. Parasites visible.
Intestinal lymphangiectasia	Mucosal normal. Dilated lymphatics.
Diffuse primary intestinal lymphoma	Infiltration with malignant histiocyte/plasma cells.
Primary disaccharidase deficiency	Children. Normal morphology. Diagnosis by enzyme analysis.
Allergic gastroenteropathy	Infiltration with eosinophils.
Abetalipoproteinaemia	Lipid vacuoles in enterocytes.
Hypogammoglobulinaemia	Mucosa normal or like coeliac disease. Lymphoid aggregates.
Amyloidosis	Normal mucosa. Infiltration of vessels with amyloid protein.

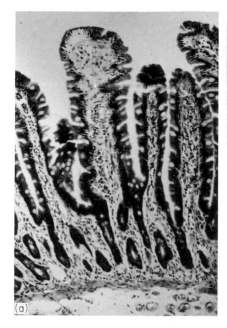

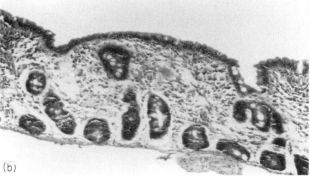

Fig. 41.18. Histological section of normal (a) and coeliac jejunal mucosa (b) (courtesy of Dr P. J. Kumar).

available, it has the most advantages. For the gastroenterologist working alone, endoscopy is perhaps the most convenient.

Precautions and complications

Although complications of small bowel biopsy are rare, haemorrhage [73], perforation [16], and bacteraemia [56] have been reported. Complications are probably more frequent using the multiple biopsy apparatus [61], although some have disputed this [64]. The procedure should not be undertaken if the prothrombin time and platelet count indicate a bleeding tendency.

Interpretation of the biopsy

Table 41.5 shows the principal conditions in which the jejunal biopsy is essential or helpful in making a diagnosis. In the United Kingdom the commonest of these is coeliac disease in which there is partial or complete villous atrophy associated with an inflammatory infiltrate (see Chapter 42). Biopsies of normal and coeliac jejunal mucosa are illustrated (Fig. 41.18). A number of conditions other than those shown in Table 41.5 are associated with varying degrees of villous atrophy (for example infective enteritis in young children [3], and Zollinger-Ellison syndrome [37]), but only rarely is the lesion as severe as in coeliac disease.

Tests of small intestinal function

Screening tests for nutritional deficiencies

A range of tests is available to measure various aspects of small intestinal function [60]. Nutritional deficiencies are sought by the simple laboratory tests indicated in Table 41.6. Useful normal values are given in Table 41.7.

Anaemia is common in small intestinal disorders, and may be due to deficiency of one or more haematinics, or to the 'anaemia of chronic disorder' (see Chapter 6). Serum B_{12}, and serum and red cell folate concentrations are best assayed microbiologically [19] but the assay takes two days.

Table 41.6. Screening tests for small intestinal disorders.

Parameter	Normal range	Interpretation
Haemoglobin	13.5–17.5 g/dl males 12.0–16.0 g/dl females	<13.5 g/dl ⎱ <12.0 g/dl ⎰ Anaemia
Mean corpuscular volume (MCV)	80–100 fl	<80—iron deficiency, chronic disorder? >100—B_{12} or folate deficiency, or alcoholism
Albumin	35–50 g/l (decreases with age)	<35 g/l—malnutrition, protein losing state
Globulin	29–33 g/l	<29 g/l—malnutrition, protein loss or hypoglobulinaemia
Ca^{2+}	2.1–2.55*mmol/l	$Ca^{2+} < 2.1$ mmol—malabsorption Ca^{2+} or vitamin D
Alkaline phosphatase	25–100 i.u./l	>100 i.u./l—Bone or liver disease?

Corrected to a serum albumin of 46 g/l, by addition (or subtraction) of 0.023 mmol/l of Ca^{2+} for every 1 g/l of serum albumin above (or below) 46 g/l.

A deoxyuridine suppression (D.U.) test on the marrow [48] will differentiate B_{12} and folate deficiency more rapidly, and is also of value when blood concentrations of B_{12} and folate are both low. The red cell folate concentration reflects body stores more accurately than the serum concentrations, which reflect recent dietary intake [32]. If the diagnosis of iron deficiency is still in doubt after blood tests, the state of iron stores in the bone marrow is the best arbiter.

A low serum albumin concentration may be due to advanced malnutrition, but more commonly is due to excessive loss of protein into the gut (see enteric protein loss). Serum IgG concentrations also fall in protein-losing states because IgG is a small molecule with a short half-life. Calcium, phosphate and alkaline phosphatase levels are useful for detecting vitamin D deficiency and osteomalacia, but trephine bone biopsy is the ultimate diagnostic tool in suspected osteomalacia.

Tests of specific functions

Fat absorption tests

Naked-eye and microscopic examination of stools for fat are unreliable except in gross steatorrhoea, and are not quantitative.

Faecal fat

A fat balance study is the standard measure of fat absorption (Fig. 41.19) [7, 70]. The patient is given a 100 g fat diet for seven days and the faeces collected over the last three days are taken for analysis [71]. This method is reliable and well-accepted, but is disliked in the laboratory because the workers have to handle the malodorous stools. Normal subjects excrete less than 7 g of faecal fat per day (<17 mmol, assuming

Table 41.7. Useful normal values.

Serum iron	8–28 μmol/l
Serum iron binding capacity	45–72 μmol/l
Serum ferritin	15–200 μg/l
Serum B_{12}	160–700 pg/ml
Serum folate	1.8–9 ng/ml
Red cell folate	150–450 ng/ml cells
Serum Total Globulins	
Serum IgG	600–1600 mg/dl
Serum IgA	60–380 mg/dl
Serum IgM	40–345 mg/dl
Plasma 1:25 dihydroxy cholecalciferol	60–110 nmol/l
25 hydroxy cholecalciferol	35–200 nmol/l

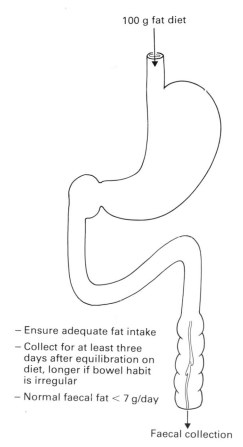

100 g fat diet

- Ensure adequate fat intake
- Collect for at least three days after equilibration on diet, longer if bowel habit is irregular
- Normal faecal fat < 7 g/day

Faecal collection

Fig. 41.19. Fat balance study.

an average molecular weight of stool fatty acids of 284). Moderate steatorrhoea (10–20 g per day) occurs in a wide variety of malabsorptive conditions; gross steatorrhoea (30–50 g per day) is suggestive of

pancreatic exocrine insufficiency. The method suffers from all the disadvantages of faecal collections. These can be overcome, but with some loss of accuracy, by the use of unabsorbed stool markers [41] which enable faecal fat to be estimated from a single stool. Faecal fat output is generally higher in patients with pancreatic steatorrhoea [9].

Breath tests

These tests depend on the measurement of $^{14}CO_2$ in the breath after giving oral ^{14}C-labelled substrates. In the tests of fat absorption, 2–5 μCi of ^{14}C-labelled substrate are given by mouth in an unlabelled carrier meal containing usually about 30 g of fat. Interval breath sampling is performed before and at intervals after the meal. Absorbed isotope is metabolized to $^{14}CO_2$ and expired with endogenous unlabelled CO_2. Suitable apparatus for collecting breath CO_2 is shown in Fig. 41.20. Using alcoholic thymolphthalein as indicator, 2 ml of 1 M hyamine will have trapped 2 mmol of CO_2 when the blue indicator turns colourless. This usually takes about a minute's normal expiration. Scintillation fluid is added to the hyamine and the $^{14}CO_2$ estimated by liquid scintillation counting. The same collection system is used for other breath tests using ^{14}C-labelled isotopes.

In initial studies the overlap with nor-

Expiratory valve   Calcium chloride drying chamber

Hyamine
+
thymolphthalein

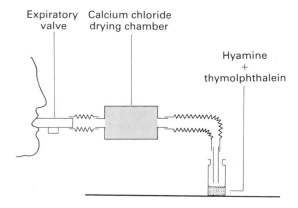

Fig. 41.20. Apparatus for collecting expired CO_2 for $^{14}CO_2$ breath tests.

mals was wide, but recently the ^{14}C-triolein breath test has been shown to compare well with faecal fat measurement in a variety of malabsorptive conditions [1, 5, 12]. Its great advantage is that it is simple, elegant and clean. A second test in which pancreatin is given with the isotope may differentiate pancreatic steatorrhoea from other causes [28]. Other triglycerides (tripalmitin, trioctanoin) seem to give less satisfactory results than triolein [51]. It seems likely that the ^{14}C triolein test will become more widely used.

Carbohydrate absorption tests

Xylose absorption

Oral xylose is given and the amount excreted in urine in the next five hours is measured. Excretion of more than 22% of a 5 g oral dose or 17% of a 25 g dose is normal. Normal results are rare in untreated coeliac disease or tropical sprue, but are the rule in pancreatic exocrine insufficiency. Capsule biopsy of the small bowel, which gives direct and structural information, has largely replaced the xylose test.

Glucose absorption

A standard glucose tolerance test is not of much value. A diabetic curve in a patient with gross steatorrhoea suggests pancreatic disease.

Lactose absorption

Constitutional hypolactasia is common, particularly in non-Caucasians, but rarely produces symptoms in adults [23, 65]. Secondary hypolactasia also occurs in many small intestinal disorders. Oral lactose 50 g is given and capillary blood is taken each half hour for two hours. A rise of blood glucose of less than 20 mg/dl sug-

gests hypolactasia. Many hypolactasic subjects develop abdominal rumbling, bloating and diarrhoea during the test. Many modifications of the basic test are described, but are rarely used.

Breath tests for carbohydrate malabsorption

There are two sorts of test which are quite different in principle. In the first, ^{14}CO$_2$ in breath is measured after oral ^{14}C-labelled sugar. The test depends upon *absorption* of the ^{14}C-labelled substrate which is then metabolized to ^{14}CO$_2$ and expired. Normals therefore excrete *more* ^{14}CO$_2$ than abnormals. By contrast, in the second type of test, breath hydrogen is measured (by gas chromatography or electrochemically) after giving the unlabelled sugar by mouth. The hydrogen is generated from the *unabsorbed* sugar which enters the colon and is fermented by bacteria. Normals therefore excrete *less* H$_2$ than abnormals. Both tests give false results in the blind-loop syndrome because of generation of the measured gas by bacteria in the proximal bowel, rather than by the expected mechanism.

In the ^{14}C **lactose test** 2–5 μCi of ^{14}C lactose are given by mouth with 50 g of unlabelled lactose. Breath ^{14}CO$_2$ is measured as described. The test performs well when compared to lactase assays in small bowel biopsies; a one hour sample detected 23 of 25 hypolactasic subjects [52].

To perform the **breath hydrogen test** hydrogen concentrations in alveolar air, collected using a modified Haldane-Priestley tube, are measured at intervals after an oral dose of sugar (for example, 50 g of lactose). This is probably the simplest and most accurate indirect method of detecting lactase deficiency; at two hours after oral lactose, hypolactasic subjects all excrete more H$_2$ than normals [52]. Extra-intestinal influences may affect the results [69].

Breath hydrogen measurements after ingestion of other sugars may be used, particularly in paediatric practice, to detect other disaccharidase deficiencies [50].

Vitamin B_{12} absorption tests

A low serum B_{12} concentration is good evidence of deficiency but speaks nothing of the cause. 'Schilling' tests [63] and whole body counting methods are used to define the absorptive defect.

Schilling tests (Fig. 41.21)

Part I—after an overnight fast the patient voids and discards bladder urine. $1 \mu Ci$ of ^{58}Co-B_{12} is given orally in 50 ml of water, followed by a 'flushing' dose of $100 \mu g$ of unlabelled B_{12} (cyanocobalamin) given intramuscularly. Urine is collected for 24 hours and the percentage of the oral dose excreted in the urine is estimated by gamma-counting.

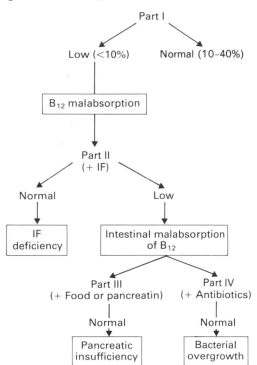

Part II—this is usually performed a week later. 50 mg of hog or human intrinsic factor are given mixed in water with the oral ^{58}Co-B_{12}. In all other respects the test is identical.

Normal subjects excrete 10–40% of the label within 24 hours. A low value in part I demonstrates B_{12} malabsorption, but not the cause. Correction by intrinsic factor implies intrinsic factor deficiency, usually due to chronic gastritis or pernicious anaemia. Persistently low excretion in Part II indicates intestinal malabsorption, usually due to ileal resection or disease and occasionally due to pancreatic insufficiency or bacterial overgrowth. Variable B_{12} malabsorption corrected by food or pancreatin (Part III Schilling Test) is characteristic of pancreatic insufficiency, and correction of B_{12} malabsorption after a course of an oral broad-spectrum antibiotic (Part IV Schilling Test—Fig. 41.21) suggests bacterial overgrowth in the small gut [2, 14].

Incomplete urine collection is the common source of error in Schilling tests. Falsely low values are found if renal function is poor. The use of the large flushing dose of B_{12} also treats the patient and prevents further studies using physiological doses of vitamin B_{12}.

Whole body B_{12} absorption [25]

The patient takes a dose of $1.0 \mu Ci$ of ^{58}Co-B_{12} in $1 \mu g$ of unlabelled B_{12} and is counted immediately, and again a week later. Normally 50% or more of the label is retained. Adaptations of the tests similar to those described for Schilling tests have been devised.

This method is simple and relatively fool-proof since it does not depend on urine collections, but it does depend on the availability of a whole-body counter.

Bile acids

^{75}Se-labelled bile acid (SeHCAT) given orally and measured by a simple gamma

Fig. 41.21. Principal features and interpretation of Schilling tests; IF = Intrinsic factor.

counter, can be used as a clinical test of terminal ileal function [24, 30, 46, 54].

Microbiological investigation of the small intestine

The small intestine is normally relatively sterile. Microbiological investigation is required in the diagnosis of primary infective enteritis (Table 41.8) and with secondary bacterial overgrowth (see Chapter 44).

Bacterial overgrowth [10, 34]

The normal upper small intestine is relatively sterile with low counts of predominantly salivary organisms, but higher counts of more colonic organisms in the ileum. Many intestinal organisms are anaerobic, which presents major difficulties with collection and culture. This in part explains the wide variation in normal values reported for bacterial flora.

Direct sampling

Direct sampling of small bowel contents by intubation is tedious, but is the best method if good anaerobic culture facilities are available and care is taken with the collection. No antibiotics should be given for a week prior to the test. Under fluoroscopy, the small bowel of the fasting patient is intubated with a sterile 3 m double-lumen mercury-weighted sump tube. The proximal end is clamped. Samples (1–2 ml) are aspirated at intervals into an infant sputum trap, allowing access of unpressurized nitrogen via the second lumen. Samples should be taken at different sites in the fasting and fed states and transported rapidly to the bacteriology laboratory. The range of values reported for bacterial counts in jejunal contamination [10] is shown in Table 41.9. More distally, the bacterial flora progressively approaches that of the colon. Overgrowth of *Escherichia coli* is often associated with vitamin B_{12} malabsorption, and anaerobes often show bile salt deconjugating activity.

Because of the complicated nature of anaerobic culture indirect tests on jejunal fluid have been used to indicate bacterial overgrowth, mainly through the presence of volatile fatty acids [15] or deconjugated bile salts [53].

Table 41.8. Diagnosis of the common enteric infections.

Pathogens		Clinical	Stool
Virus	Reo	Acute	Immunoelectron microscopy, culture
	Parvo		
Bacteria	*Salmonella*	Acute/	Microscopy, culture
	Campylobacter	sub-acute	
	E. coli		
Bacterial toxins	*V. cholerae*	Acute	Microscopy
	Staphylococcus aureus ⎫	Very acute	—
	C. Welchii ⎬		
	E. coli ⎭		
Protozoa	*Giardia lamblia*	Sub-acute/ chronic	Microscopy
Worms	Hook		
	Round	Chronic	Microscopy
	Strongyloides		

Table 41.9. Small intestinal bacterial flora in normal subjects and in bacterial overgrowth.

	Anaerobes		Aerobes	
	Gram +	Gram −	Gram +	Gram −
Normal				
Jejunum	0–3*	0–3	0–6	0–3
Proximal ileum	0–3	0–3	0–6	0–3
Distal ileum	2–8	3–8	2–8	2–8
Contaminated				
Jejunum	1–7	1–8	1–8	1–8

* Counts Log_{10}/ml

Indirect methods

Cholyl-^{14}C glycine breath test [27]

One to 2 μCi of cholyl-^{14}C glycine are given by mouth to the fasting patient in a standard Lundh meal. $^{14}CO_2$ in breath is measured before the dose and hourly for six hours. Bacterial deconjugation of the isotope releases ^{14}C-glycine which is metabolized to $^{14}CO_2$ and excreted in the breath (Fig. 41.22). Normal subjects excrete less than 0.1% of the dose/mmol CO_2 × the body weight (in kilograms) in any of the first three hours, and no more than 0.3% at any time up to six hours. Positive results indicate bacterial overgrowth or cholangitis, but also are seen in bile salt malabsorption due to ileal disease, or in resection when unabsorbed isotope is deconjugated by bacteria in the colon (Fig. 41.22). The onset of $^{14}CO_2$ excretion tends to be earlier in overgrowth than in bile salt malabsorption, but there is considerable overlap. Measurement of faecal ^{14}C by oxidation to $^{14}CO_2$ can aid interpretation (faecal ^{14}C high in malabsorption, low in overgrowth), but is messy and requires special apparatus. Because of these difficulties and the fact that not all bacteria can deconjugate bile salts, this test does not replace direct sampling. A low-dose (1 g) ^{14}C-D-xylose breath test, based on the fermentation of xylose by bacteria, may correlate better with jejunal bacteriology [35].

Breath hydrogen tests

Increased excretion of hydrogen in breath soon after small doses of oral glucose can be taken as evidence of bacterial over-

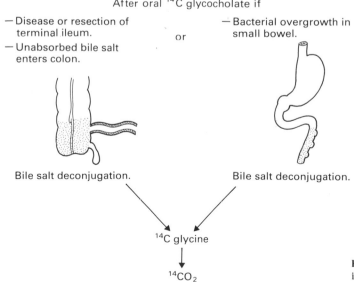

After oral ^{14}C glycocholate if

— Disease or resection of terminal ileum.
— Unabsorbed bile salt enters colon.

or

— Bacterial overgrowth in small bowel.

Bile salt deconjugation.

Bile salt deconjugation.

^{14}C glycine

$^{14}CO_2$ in breath

Fig. 41.22. Mechanism of increased breath $^{14}CO_2$ in the cholyl-^{14}C-glycine breath test.

growth in the proximal small gut, or mouth [47].

Urinary indican

Indoles produced by bacterial action on dietary tryptophan in the small bowel are excreted in excess in the urine of some patients with bacterial overgrowth. This test is too erratic to be useful [44].

Enteric protein loss

Excessive loss of plasma proteins into the small bowel occurs in many conditions (Table 41.10). The amount of loss can be determined by measurement of faecal radioactivity for four days after an intravenous injection of $^{51}CrCl_3$, which binds to serum proteins *in vivo* and is excreted into the gut with the proteins. Normals excrete 0.1–0.7% of the radioactivity in the four days after labelling, whereas patients with excessive protein loss excrete 2–40%. This

Table 41.10. Principal disorders associated with excessive enteric loss of plasma protein.

Mucosal ulcerative diseases
Gastric carcinoma
Gastric lymphoma
Multiple gastric ulcers
Colonic carcinoma
Crohn's disease
Diffuse non-granulomatous ileojejunitis

Mucosal disease without ulceration
Ménétrièr's disease
Coeliac disease
Tropical sprue
Whipple's disease
Eosinophilic gastroenteritis
Bacterial or parasitic enteritis
Gastrocolic fistula
Villous adenoma of colon

Lymphatic abnormalities
Primary lymphangiectasia
Lymphenteric fistula
Lymphoma
Constrictive pericarditis
Severe chronic heart failure

test is reliable [74], but not used often because quantification of the protein loss is usually not helpful to the clinician.

Endocrinology

A plethora of hormones has been described in the gut [67]. Alterations in the pattern of hormone release have been shown in various intestinal disorders [6] but these are as yet of little practical value [42]. In the investigation of patients with obscure diarrhoea, elevated plasma gastrin (normal < 50 pg/ml) or VIP (vasoactive intestinal polypeptide) concentrations may indicate a hormone producing tumour. Several samples should be sent for each hormone as secretion may be intermittent (see Chapter 39).

The small bowel, particularly the ileum, is the commonest primary site of carcinoids which later produce the carcinoid syndrome (see Chapter 40). Chemical diagnosis is by measurement of urinary 5-HIAA (normal < 25 mg/24 hours). Foods containing serotonin (bananas and tomatoes) and some drugs (phenothiazines and reserpine) should be avoided as these affect the results.

Immunological investigations [68]

The only immunological tests available in most hospital laboratories are the differential white cell count, serum immunoglobulin and complement concentrations and the detection of autoantibodies. Most of the other tests of immunological function described are research tools without agreed standardization.

Abnormalities of immunological tests in primary small bowel diseases

Abnormal serum immunoglobulin and complement concentrations may occur in coeliac disease (IgA↑; IgM, C_3, C_4, ↓) and

Crohn's disease (IgA,C_3,C_4↑) but these tend to revert to normal as the disease goes into remission. About one in 50 patients with coeliac disease has persistent selective IgA deficiency.

Most patients with untreated coeliac disease (75%) and some patients with Crohn's disease (25%) have anti-reticulin antibodies. IgA antibodies are more specific to coeliac disease.

The presence in the serum of the heavy chains of IgA is indicative of alpha chain disease.

Protein-losing enteropathy from any cause may lead to low concentrations of serum globulins, particularly IgG.

Primary immunological disorders with small intestinal involvement

Partial villous atrophy may be seen with acquired hypogammaglobulinaemia and nodular lymphoid hyperplasia. These two conditions often coexist and both predispose to infection with *Giardia lamblia*. It is unclear whether the immunological defect or the giardiasis is responsible for the mucosal abnormality.

Ultrasound and isotopic scanning of the small intestine

Neither of these techniques has much to offer in investigation of the small bowel. Ultrasound [8, 33] may sometimes demonstrate thickened bowel wall in Crohn's disease and abdominal gamma scanning after injection of indium-labelled white cells has been used to delineate its extent [66]. However, barium radiology remains the cornerstone of anatomical investigation.

The pertechnetate scan [18] is useful in the diagnosis of Meckel's diverticulum in childhood (Fig. 41.23). Gastric type mucosa, which is found in 50% of diverticula, will take up and excrete pertechnetate. The test is rarely positive in adults.

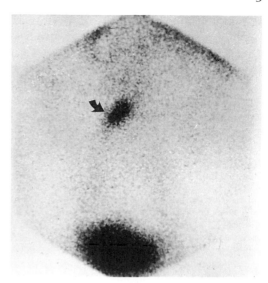

Fig. 41.23. Positive Tc^{99m} scan in a patient with a Meckel's diverticulum (arrowed). The isotope in the lower part of the scan is in the bladder.

Tests of small intestinal permeability [40]

An increase in permeability to certain polar solutes, particularly sugars, has been shown in coeliac disease although the finding is non-specific and of little clinical value. Such tests have been used in screening for coeliac disease [22, 29, 55], but should not be regarded as a substitute for biopsy.

Tests of small intestinal motility [17]

Investigation of small bowel motility is unsatisfactory. The radiologist may gain an impression of disordered peristalsis during a small bowel meal and can measure the transit time of the barium. The former is too subjective, and the latter is unphysiological and too variable to be of much value. Small bowel transit time can be measured more physiologically using radio-opaque or isotopic markers mixed with food [13].

Hydrogen breath tests using a non-absorbed sugar such as lactulose can assess mouth to caecum transit time. In all transit studies the overlap between normal and abnormal is wide. Measurement of small bowel pressure and electrical activity is still a research tool of no proven diagnostic value [36, 59].

References

1 AKESSON B, FLOREN CH. Use of the triolein breath test for the demonstration of fat malabsorption in coeliac disease. *Scand J Gastroenterol* 1984;**19**:307–314.

2 BADENOCH J, BEDFORD PD, EVANS JR. Massive diverticulosis of the small intestine with steatorrhoea and megaloblastic anaemia. *Q J Med* 1955;**24**:321–330.

3 BARNES GL, TOWNLEY RRW. Duodenal mucosal damage in 31 infants with gastroenteritis. *Arch Dis Child* 1973;**48**:343–349.

4 BARTRAM CI, KUMAR PJ. *Clinical radiology in gastroenterology*. Oxford: Blackwell Scientific Publications, 1981.

5 BENINI L, SCURO LA, MENINI E, *et al.* Is the ^{14}C-triolein breath test useful in the assessment of malabsorption in clinical practice? *Digestion* 1984; **29**: 91–97.

6 BESTERMAN HS, SARSON DL, JOHNSTON DI, *et al.* Gut-hormone profile in coeliac disease. *Lancet* 1978;i:785–788.

7 BIN TL, STOPARD M, ANDERSON S, *et al.* Assessment of fat malabsorption. *J Clin Pathol* 1983;**36**:1362–1366.

8 BLUTH EI. Ultrasound evaluation of small bowel abnormalities. *Am J Gastroenterol* 1983;**78**:788–793.

9 BO-LINN GW, FORDTRAN JS. Faecal fat concentration in patients with steatorrhea. *Gastroenterology* 1984; **87**:319–322.

10 BORRIELLO P, HUDSON M, HILL M. Investigation of the gastrointestinal bacterial flora. *Clin Gastroenterol* 1978;**7(2)**:329–350.

11 BRANDBORG LL, RUBIN CE, QUINTON WE. A multipurpose instrument for suction biopsy of the oesophagus, stomach, small bowel and colon. *Gastroenterology* 1959;**37**:1–16.

12 BUTLER RN, GEHLING NJ, LAWSON MJ, GRANT AK. Clinical evaluation of the ^{14}C triolein breath test: a critical analysis. *Aust NZ J Med* 1984;**14**:111–114.

13 CARIDE VJ, PROKOP EK, TRONCALE FJ, BUDDOURA W, WINCHENBACH K, McCALLUM RW. Scintigraphic determination of small intestinal transit time: comparison with the hydrogen breath technique. *Gastroenterology* 1984;**86**:714–720.

14 CHANARIN I. *The megaloblastic anaemias*. Oxford: Blackwell Scientific Publications, 1979.

15 CHERNOV AJ, DOE WF, GOMPERTZ D. Intrajejunal volatile fatty acids in the stagnant loop syndrome. *Gut* 1972;**13**:103–106.

16 CLARKE SW. Jejunal perforation with the Crosby capsule. *Lancet* 1964;ii:727–728.

17 CONNELL AM. Motility and its disturbances. *Clin Gastroenterol* 1982;**11(3)**:665–672.

18 CONWAY JJ. Radionuclide diagnosis of Meckel's diverticulum. *Gastrointest Radiol* 1980;**5**:209–216.

19 COOPER BA, WHITEHEAD VM. Evidence that some patients with pernicious anaemia are not recognised by radiodilution assay for cobalamin in serum. *New Engl J Med* 1978;**299**:815–818.

20 COTTON PB, WILLIAMS CB. *Practical gastrointestinal endoscopy*. Oxford: Blackwell Scientific Publications, 1982.

21 CROSBY WH, KUGLER HW. Intraluminal biopsy of the small intestine; the intestinal biopsy capsule. *Am J Dig Dis* 1957;**2**:236–242.

22 EDITORIAL. Sugaring the Crosby capsule. *Lancet* 1981;i:593–594.

23 FERGUSON A, MacDONALD DM, BRYDON WG. Prevalence of lactase deficiency in British adults. *Gut* 1984;**25**:163–167.

24 FERRARIS R, JAZRAWI R, BRIDGES C, NORTHFIELD TC. Use of a γ-labelled bile acid (^{75}Se HCAT) as a test of ileal function. Methods of improving accuracy. *Gastroenterology* 1986;**90**:1129–1136.

25 FINLAYSON NDC, SHEARMAN DJC, SIMPSON JD, GIRDWOOD RH. Determination of vitamin B_{12} absorption by a simple whole-body counter. *J Clin Pathol* 1968;**21**:595–598.

26 FLICK AL, QUINTON WE, RUBIN CE. A peroral hydraulic biopsy tube for multiple sampling at any level of the gastrointestinal tract. *Gastroenterology* 1961;**40**:120–126.

27 FROMM H, HOFMANN AF. Breath test for altered bile acid metabolism. *Lancet* 1971;ii:605–607.

28 GOFF JS. Two-stage triolein breath test differentiates pancreatic insufficiency from other causes of malabsorption. *Gastroenterology* 1982;**83**:44–46.

29 HAMILTON I. Small intestinal permeability. In: Pounder RE, ed. *Recent advances in gastroenterology*. Edinburgh: Churchill Livingstone, 1986:73–91.

30 HEATON KW. Functional diarrhoea: the acid test. *Br Med J* 1985;**290**:1298–1299.

31 HERLINGER H. Small bowel. In: Laufer I, ed. *Double contrast gastrointestinal radiology*. Philadelphia: W.B. Saunders Co, 1979.

32 HOFFBRAND AV, NEWCOMBE BFA, MOLLIN DL. Method of assay of red cell folate activity and the value of the assay as a test for folate deficiency. *J Clin Pathol* 1966;**19**:17–28.

33 HOLT S, SAMUEL E. Grey-scale ultrasound in Crohn's disease. *Gut* 1979;**20**:590–595.

34 KING CE, TOSKES PP. Small intestine bacterial

overgrowth. *Gastroenterology* 1979;**76**:1035–1055.

35 KING CE, TOSKES PP, SPIVEY JC, LORENZ E, WELKOS SS. Detection of small intestine bacterial overgrowth by means of a [14]C D-xylose breath test. *Gastroenterology* 1979;**77**:75–82.

36 KINGHAM JGC, BOWN R, COLSON R, CLARK ML. Jejunal motility in patients with functional abdominal pain. *Gut* 1984;**25**:375–380.

37 KINGHAM JGC, LEVISON DA, FAIRCLOUGH PD. Diarrhoea and reversible enteropathy in Zollinger-Ellison syndrome. *Lancet* 1981;**ii**:610–611.

38 LAMBERT HP. Infections of the gastrointestinal tract. *Clin Gastroenterol* 1979;**8**:3.

39 LAW RL. Guide wire manipulation of Crosby jejunal biopsy capsule under fluoroscopic control. *Br Med J* 1984;**288**:286–287.

40 LEADER. Intestinal permeability. *Lancet* 1985;**i**:256–257.

41 LEE MF, TEMPERLEY JM, DICK M. Estimation of faecal fat excretion using cuprous thiocyanate as a continuous marker. *Gut* 1969;**10**:754–759.

42 McFARLAND RF. Gastrointestinal hormones and diseases of the gastrointestinal tract. *Clin Endocrinol Metab* 1979;**8**:331–347.

43 MARSHAK RH, LINDNER AE. *Radiology of the small intestine*. Philadelphia: W.B. Saunders Co, 1979.

44 MAYER PJ, BEEKEN WZ. The role of urinary indican as a predictor of bacterial colonisation in the human jejunum. *Am J Dig Dis* 1975;**11**:1003–1009.

45 MEE AS, BURKE M, VALLON AG, NEWMAN J, COTTON PB. Small bowel biopsy for malabsorption: comparison of the diagnostic accuracy of endoscopic forceps and capsule biopsy specimens. *Br Med J* 1985;**291**:769–772.

46 MERRICK MV, EASTWOOD MA, FORD MJ. Is bile acid malabsorption underdiagnosed? *Br Med J* 1985;**290**:665–668.

47 METZ G, GASSULL MA, DRASAR BS, JENKINS DJA, BLENDIS LM. Breath hydrogen test for small-intestinal bacterial colonisation. *Lancet* 1976;**i**:668–669.

48 METZ J, KELLY A, SWETT VC, WAXMAN S, HERBERT V. Deranged DNA synthesis by bone marrow from vitamin B[12] deficient humans. *Br J Haematol* 1968;**14**:579–592.

49 MILLER RE, SELLINK JL. The small bowel enema—how to succeed and how to fail. *Gastrointest Radiol* 1979;**4**:269.

50 NEWCOMER AD. Screening tests for carbohydrate malabsorption. *J Pediatr Gastroenterol Nutr* 1984;**3**:6–8.

51 NEWCOMER AD, HOFMANN AF, DI MAGNO EP, THOMAS PJ, CARLSON GL. Triolein breath test; a sensitive and specific test for fat malabsorption. *Gastroenterology* 1979;**76**:6–13.

52 NEWCOMER AD, McGILL DB, THOMAS PF, HOFFMANN AF. Prospective comparison of indirect methods for detecting lactase deficiency. *N Engl J Med* 1975;**293**:1232–1236.

53 NORTHFIELD TC, DRASAR BS, WRIGHT JT. Value of small intestinal bile acid analysis in the diagnosis of stagnant loop syndrome. *Gut* 1973;**14**:341–347.

54 NYHLIN H, BRYDON G, DANIELSSON A, WESTMAN S. Clinical application of a selenium (^{75}Se)-labelled bile acid for the investigation of terminal ileal function. *Hepatogastroenterology* 1984;**31**:187–191.

55 PEARSON ADJ, EASTHAM EJ, LAKER MF, CRAFT AW, NELSON R. Intestinal permeability in children with Crohn's disease and coeliac disease. *Br Med J* 1982;**ii**:20–21.

56 PETTY AN, WENGER J. Bacteraemia following peroral biopsy of the small intestine. *Gastroenterology* 1970;**59**:140–143.

57 PRICE AB. Small intestinal biopsy. In: Booth CC, Neale G, eds. *Disorders of the small intestine*. Oxford: Blackwell Scientific Publications, 1986: 19–20.

58 PROUT BF. A rapid method of obtaining a jejunal biopsy using a Crosby capsule and a gastrointestinal fibrescope. *Gut* 1974;**15**:571–572.

59 READ NW, AL-JANABI MN, EDWARDS CA, BARBER DC. Relationship between postprandial motor activity in the human small intestine and gastrointestinal transit of food. *Gastroenterology* 1984;**86**:721–727.

60 RINSLER MG, BOOTH CC. Intestinal function tests. In: Booth CC, Neale G. *Disorders of the small intestine*. Oxford: Blackwell Scientific Publications, 1986:21–28.

61 RUBIN CE, DOBBINS WO. Peroral biopsy of the small intestine; a review of its usefulness. *Gastroenterology* 1965;**49**:676–697.

62 SALTER RH, GIRDWOOD TG. Peroral jejunal biopsy with Watson capsule and Scott-Harden duodenal intubation tube. *Lancet* 1983;**ii**:1460–1469.

63 SCHILLING RF. Intrinsic factor studies II. The effect of gastric juice on the urinary excretion of radioactivity after the oral administration of radioactive vitamin B[12]. *J Lab Clin Med* 1953;**42**:860–866.

64 SCOTT BB, LOSOWSKY MS. Peroral small intestinal biopsy: experiences with the hydraulic multiple biopsy instrument in routine clinical practice. *Gut* 1976;**17**:740–743.

65 SEDAL I, GAGJEE PP, ESSOP AR, NOORMOHAMED AM. Lactase deficiency in the South African black population. *Am J Clin Nutr* 1983;**38**:901–905.

66 SEGAL AW, ENSELL J, MUNRO JA, SARNER M. [111]Indium-tagged leukocytes in the diagnosis of inflammatory bowel disease. *Lancet* 1981;**ii**:230–232.

67 SJÖLUND K, SANDEN G, HÅKANSON R, SUNDLER F. Endocrine cells in human intestine: an immunocytochemical study. *Gastroenterology* 1983;**85**:1120–1130.

68 THOMAS HC, JEWELL DP *Clinical gastrointestinal im-*

munology. Oxford: Blackwell Scientific Publications, 1979.

69 THOMPSON DG, BINFIELD P, DE BELDER A, O'BRIEN J, WARREN S, WILSON M. Extra intestinal influences on exhaled breath hydrogen measurements during the investigation of gastrointestinal disease. *Gut* 1985;**26**:1349–1352.

70 THORSGAARD PEDERSEN N, HALGREEN H. Faecal fat and faecal weight-reproducibility and diagnostic efficiency of various regimens. *Scand J Gastroenterol* 1984;**19**:350–354.

71 VAN DE KAMER JH, TEN BOKKEL HUININK H, WEYERS HA. Rapid method for determination of fat in faeces. *J Biol Chem* 1979;**177**:347–355.

72 VANDERHOOF JA, HUNT LI, ANTONSON DL. A rapid procedure for small intestinal biopsy in infants and children. *Gastroenterology* 1981;**80**:938–941.

73 VIDINLI N, FINLAY JM. Masssive haemorrhage following small bowel biopsy. *J Can Med Assoc* 1964;**91**:1223–1225.

74 WALDMANN TA, WOCHNER RD, STROBER W. The role of the gastrointestinal tract in plasma protein metabolism. *Am J Med* 1969;**46**:275.

75 WICKS T, CLAIN D. A guide wire for rapid jejunal biopsies with the Crosby capsule. *Gut* 1972;**13**:571.

76 WILKINS R, GARVEY C, DE LACEY G. Radiological examination. In: Booth CC, Neale G, eds. *Disorders of the small intestine.* Oxford: Blackwell Scientific Publications, 1986:5–11.

Chapter 42
Coeliac Disease

M. D. HELLIER

Coeliac disease is the commonest and most important cause of malabsorption in the West[10, 19]. Although first described a century ago the precise cause of the mucosal damage remains uncertain. However, astute clinical observations coupled with the development of intestinal biopsy techniques have lead to great advances in our understanding of the environmental and genetic factors which are the essential ingredients for the development of the disease.

Probably the most important of these observations was made by the Dutch paediatrician, Dicke, who noticed in 1950 that the incidence of coeliac disease in children in Holland decreased and that patients with coeliac disease improved during the second World War, a period when cereal grain products were in short supply[21]. He suggested a link between certain cereals and coeliac disease and proceeded to show that a water-insoluble protein of gluten was responsible. These observations were closely followed by the development of jejunal biopsy techniques (see Chapter 41) which led to an explosion of information about the lesion. What was thought to be a condition confined to children was recognized to be the condition previously called idiopathic steatorrhoea of adults.

Synonyms for coeliac disease include Gee-Thayson disease, idiopathic steatorrhoea, gluten-induced enteropathy, coeliac syndrome, non-tropical sprue and coeliac sprue. Coeliac disease is now the most widely-accepted name, although it implies that the disease is a single entity. This is as yet to be proven.

Coeliac disease is defined as a condition in which there is an abnormal jejunal mucosa which improves morphologically when treated with a gluten-free diet and which deteriorates again on the reintroduction of gluten[67]. Re-challenge with gluten is considered necessary for the diagnosis in children to differentiate from soya protein or milk intolerance, but there is dispute as to its necessity in adults[41].

Epidemiology

Prevalence

This varies considerably in different parts of the world, being highest in Galway, Ireland (1:300) and as low as 1:6500 in Sweden[54]. On the basis of symptomatic patients presenting to hospital in the United Kingdom an overall prevalence of 1:1800 is estimated[50]. In the last three decades there appears to have been a substantial increase in prevalence but this is probably more apparent than real, reflecting changes in diagnostic techniques and a greater awareness of the disease[47].

The need for a biopsy to confirm the diagnosis and the frequent presentation in later life[24] suggest these figures substantially underestimate true prevalence.

Sex ratio

Coeliac disease in adults appears to be more common in women than men and amongst 1075 new adult members of the Coeliac Society the ratio of women to men was 2:1.

However, the ratio of 1:1 for childhood coeliac disease found in most studies suggests that the adult ratio reflects a difference in diagnostic rate between women and men rather than in true incidence [49].

Geographical distribution

Originally thought to be a European disorder, coeliac disease is now known to occur everywhere. Though rare in indigenous Indians, the incidence amongst Indians in the United Kingdom approaches that of the local population, suggesting that Indians have the genetic predisposition for coeliac disease, but are protected from it by the preponderance of rice in their natural diet. Though a few cases have been described in the Sudan, coeliac disease is extremely rare in the rest of the indigenous African population; it has not been described in China or the Caribbean.

Aetiology

The clinical expression of coeliac disease requires the interaction of an environmental factor with a genetic factor. Without both factors the clinical condition does not occur.

Environmental factors

Gluten, the toxic factor, is the water-insoluble protein fraction of cereal grain. The toxicity of cereals is shown in Table 42.1. Although indirect evidence has sug-

Table 42.1. Toxicity of different cereals in coeliac disease.

Cereal	Toxicity
Wheat	+
Barley	+
Rye	+
Oats	±?
Rice	−
Maize	−

gested oats may be harmful, studies based on the direct effect of oats on the mucosa of treated coeliac patients have failed to show any damage. Gluten consists mainly of glutenins and several ethanol-soluble gliadins (alpha, beta, gamma and omega) [9, 35]. Gliadin (mol. wt 50,000) is toxic, but hydrolysis to free amino acids and small peptides renders it non-toxic. Recent *in vivo* studies using an improved separation technique suggest toxicity is confined to a mixture of alpha and beta 1-3 gliadins [62]. Fractionation of gliadin has revealed that a subfraction rich in glutamine, glutamic acid and proline is toxic. This has an apparent molecular mass of less than 1500 daltons [14]. Factors other than gluten may also be important [46].

Genetic factor

Though mystery still surrounds the genetic component, there is strong evidence for its existence. Family studies show that siblings and progeny have a 2–5% risk of developing overt coeliac disease. Ten per cent of asymptomatic first degree relatives have sub-total villous atrophy. This data suggests that recessive genes are not the determinants of susceptibility because if they were, a higher prevalence would be expected in siblings than offspring. The data are compatible with modified dominant or polygenic inheritance [2].

More identical twin studies have shown concordance [38]. The demonstration in 1972 of the association with the histocompatibility antigen HLA B8 established coeliac disease as a genetic disease. HLA B8 is found in 80–90% of patients compared with 20% in the general population [25].

More recently new antigens, B cell, HLA DW3 and HLA DR3 have been demonstrated in higher frequencies in association with coeliac disease suggesting that these, rather than HLA B8 might be the primary determinants. A recent study suggested the disease would occur within families when two conditions were fulfilled. Firstly the family member was homozygous for the coeliac-associated B cell antigen. Secondly the family member also carried the HLA DW3 antigen. Results suggested that the gene(s) controlling the DW3 antigen and the coeliac-associated B cell antigen were separate non-linked genetic foci supporting a genetic basis for coeliac disease on at least two genes [57].

Pathogenesis

How does gluten damage the mucosa?

Two main theories have been suggested— either a defect of gluten digestion due to an enzyme deficiency leads to accumulation of a toxic factor which damages the mucosa [31], or an immunological reaction with gluten at the level of the mucosa causes mucosal damage.

Enzyme defect

There is continued, though dwindling, support for this theory. Peptidase assays have demonstrated low mucosal enzyme concentrations and a toxic gliadin fraction has been shown to be incompletely digested by untreated coeliac mucosa, but digested to free amino acids by normal mucosa [15]. However, no specific peptidase deficiency has so far been demonstrated and the peptidase concentrations return to normal after treatment. Recent studies have revived interest in this theory. A toxic fraction of gliadin was shown to be incompletely digested *in vitro* by coeliac mucosa even during remission when the mucosa was histologically normal. Defective digestion was also seen in first degree relatives without clinical disease or mucosal abnormality [14].

Immunological response to gluten

By contrast with the enzyme theory, there is a wealth of data showing abnormalities of humoral and cellular immunity, suggesting that an immune mechanism is responsible for mucosal damage (Table 42.2).

Table 42.2. Evidence for an immunological response in coeliac disease.

Indirect
Immunocompetent cells increased in mucosa.
Splenic atrophy.
Mesenteric node hypertrophy.
Peripheral node hypoplasia.
Increased incidence of lymphoma.
Improvement on steroids.
Associated IgA deficiency.

Direct
Humoral—Arthus type III skin reaction to gluten.
  Increased mucosal production of immunoglobulins.
  Presence of specific antibodies in the blood.
  Changes in complement levels.
  Association with other autoimmune disorders.
  Circulating antigen-antibody complexes.
  Lymphocyte surface receptors for gliadin.
Cellular
Delayed hypersensitivity to recall antigens.
Impaired lymphocyte transformation.
Epithelial lymphocyte infiltration.
Leucocyte migration inhibition by lymphokines.

Immunoglobulins

Exposure to gliadin results in increased production of local and circulatory antibodies. Serum concentrations of IgA are increased and IgM reduced, while IgA and IgM concentrations are increased in intestinal secretions. The specificity of these changes for gliadin is less clear. Early studies suggested 50% of the rise was due to anti-gliadin antibodies [45]. However, subsequent studies have indicated a much lower proportion (7%) with a pattern not specific for coeliac patients ingesting gluten [4]. Furthermore, anti-gliadin antibodies do not occur in all coeliacs or correlate with disease activity and can be directed against one or many gliadin fractions [44].

Antigen-antibody complexes

Importance has been attached to antigen-antibody complexes in coeliac patients, but they have been detected in less than 50% of patients and their nature is not clear. The fact that complexes to bovine antigens occur in control subjects throws doubt on their significance and they may well be quite non-specific.

Complement

C_3 and C_4 components of complement may be low in untreated coeliac disease and complement breakdown products increase after gluten challenge. Ultrastructural and immunofluorescent studies in coeliac children have shown complement fixing IgA complexes in the basement membrane following gluten challenge [59].

Other factors

1. Isolated IgA deficiency occurs in 1:50 coeliacs compared with 1:700 normals.
2. Cryoglobulinaemia occasionally occurs, possibly due to circulating gluten immune complexes.
3. There is an association between coeliac disease and autoimmune disease (thyroiditis, diabetes mellitus, alveolitis, chronic liver disease) [3].
4. B lymphocytes have a surface receptor for gliadin [66].
5. Reticulin antibodies occur in between 36–75% of patients [42].
6. Coeliac disease responds to corticosteroids which are known to inhibit development of an Arthus type III reaction.

Type of immunological response

Evidence from skin tests, and immunofluorescent studies examining the type and timing of the reaction following gluten challenge suggests an Arthus type III reaction [1].

Evidence for cell-mediated immunity

1. Delayed hypersensitivity to recall antigens and lymphocyte transformation responses to plant mitogens have been shown to be impaired in untreated coeliac disease. However, these are non-specific changes which improve with treatment and may simply reflect malnutrition or enteric loss of lymphocytes. Skin tests with gluten subfractions have shown no evidence of delayed hypersensitivity to gluten in coeliac disease [60].
2. Mucosal biopsies of untreated coeliacs show abnormal infiltration of the epithelium by lymphocytes.
3. Culture of small intestinal mucosa of untreated coeliac disease in the presence of gliadin produces a factor which inhibits migration of normal leucocytes (lymphokine) [29]. This is assumed to be produced by T lymphocytes and indicative of a local cell mediated immune reaction. However, recent studies cast doubt on this interpretation, suggesting that inhibition of leucocyte migration might be due to a serum factor, possibly cytophilic antibody rather than a T lymphocyte lymphokine. At present cell-mediated immunity to gluten in coeliac disease cannot be regarded as established. Although a unifying concept of pathogenesis remains to be found, an immunological cause for the mucosal damage in coeliac disease remains most likely.

The main unanswered question is whether a primary immunological difference exists between coeliac patients and normal subjects, or whether the above changes are a secondary phenomenon. It remains possible that the primary difference between these two groups is after all an enzyme defect, and the mucosal damage is the result of a secondary immunological response.

Pathology

Damage to the mucosa of the upper small intestine is the cardinal anatomical feature of coeliac disease. As the severity of the disease increases the lesion extends distally, but rarely is the whole of the ileum involved. There is a long transitional zone between abnormal and normal mucosa. Mucosal changes are patchy, especially in mild disease and biopsy findings vary depending on the site in relation to the mucosal folds. Most marked changes occur at the crest of the folds, presumably a site more exposed to luminal trauma. Although originally described in dermatitis herpetiformis, this patchiness also occurs in coeliac disease.

Macroscopical changes

Macroscopic assessment of the jejunal mucosal biopsy by dissecting microscope is important. Characteristically the mucosa appears smooth or flat with complete loss of villi and visible crypt orifices on the surface (total villous atrophy), or as a convoluted pattern of ridges, which are the broadened and joined bases of villi (sub-total villous atrophy) (Figs 42.1 and 42.2).

For practical purposes a 'flat' biopsy in an adult in the United Kingdom means coeliac disease. This is not true in infants where cows' milk and soya protein allergy can also result in a flat biopsy.

Milder changes in villous structure, with shortening and broadening of the villi forming leaves and ridges (partial villous atrophy), are less specific and seen in a wide range of conditions (Table 42.3).

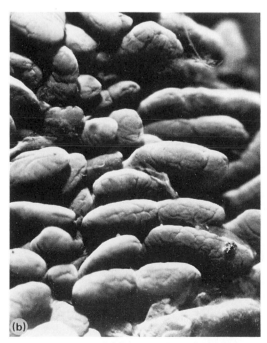

Fig. 42.1. Dissecting microscope appearance of normal jejunal mucosa. (a) finger shaped villi. (b) leaf shaped villi (with kind permission of Dr B. Creamer).

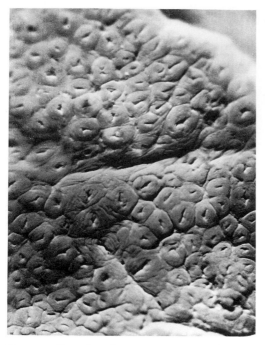

Fig. 42.2. Dissecting microscope appearance of jejunal mucosa from untreated coeliac disease showing sub-total villous atrophy (with kind permission of Dr B. Creamer).

Table 42.3. Other causes of an abnormal small intestinal mucosa.

Acute infectious enteritis
Bacterial overgrowth
Giardiasis
Immunodeficiency syndromes
Cows milk protein sensitivity
Soya protein enteropathy
Tropical sprue
Tropical enteropathy
Kwashiorkor
Eosinophilic gastroenteritis
Radiation

Histological changes

Light microscopy reveals a hypertrophied mucosa with shortened villi and lengthened crypts (Figs 42.3 and 42.4). There is an increase in crypt cell mitotic index and crypt cell production is greatly increased. The absorptive columnar cells become shor-

tened and cuboidal and the cytoplasm more basophilic with loss of the basal polarity of the nucleus. The lamina propria is markedly infiltrated by plasma cells, mainly IgA and IgM in type, and numbers of eosinophils and mast cells are increased. Migration of lymphocytes through the intercellular spaces of the surface epithelial cells (lymphocyte traffic) is an important diagnostic feature, the ratio of lymphocytes to surface epithelial cells showing a clear separation between coeliac disease and other gastrointestinal disorders (Figs 42.5 and 42.6). After recovery on a gluten-free diet, mucosal damage occurs within three to four hours after a gluten challenge.

Electron microscopy changes

The brush border shows striking attenuation with shortening and fusion of microvilli. Free ribosomes are increased and degenerative changes, such as cytoplasmic and mitochondrial vacuolation, are seen. Many cells contain large lysosomes.

The damaged surface cells are desquamated at 5–6 times the normal rate resulting in compensatory crypt cell proliferation. This alteration in cell dynamics appears to lead to the macroscopic mucosal appearance.

By contrast in the small group of unresponsive coeliacs, cell turnover is decreased, possibly indicating a phase of turnover exhaustion. With increasing severity of the disease collagen deposition occurs in the basement membrane. The term 'collagenous sprue' was coined to describe a particularly severe malabsorption associated with a flat mucosa, failure to respond to diet, a very poor prognosis and characterized by massive collagen deposition. It now seems unlikely that this is a separate entity and subsequent studies have shown collagen deposition in most coeliac patients.

Recent studies following gluten exposure indicate that damage occurs first on the

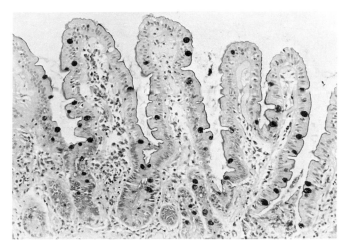

Fig. 42.3. Normal jejunal mucosa (PAS stain × 50) (with kind permission of Dr R.I. Vanhegan).

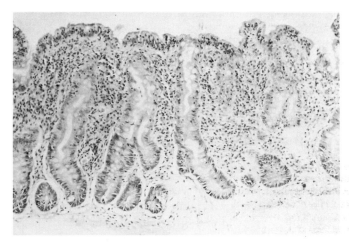

Fig. 42.4. The mucosa in untreated coeliac disease showing absence of villi and elongated crypts and cellular infiltration (H and E stain × 50) (with kind permission of Dr R.I. Vanhegan).

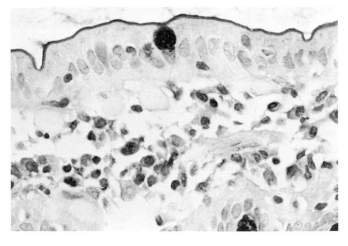

Fig. 42.5. Normal villous epithelium showing the regular arrangement of the cells and their nuclei (PAS stain × 200) (with kind permission of Dr R.I. Vanhegan).

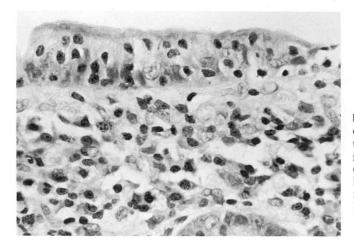

Fig. 42.6. Histological appearance of the surface epithelium in untreated coeliac disease showing gross disorganization with intra-epithelial migration of lymphocytes and increased numbers of plasma cells in the lamina propria (H and E stain × 200) (with kind permission of Dr R.I. Vanhegan).

minal aspect of the cell followed by intra-cellular organelle changes, cellular infiltration into the epithelium and later basement membrane changes. On gluten withdrawal, surface cells are the first to recover over a few days. The distal bowel recovers before the proximal bowel and full recovery to macroscopic normality may take months or years and occasionally is never complete.

Other changes

Mild rectal changes have been described in some patients with coeliac disease resembling a mild proctitis, and histological gastritis is commoner in coeliac patients than normal people.

Pathophysiology

The malabsorption of coeliac disease is complex and not solely the result of mucosal damage. Secretion of bile and pancreatic juice is under the control of hormones produced by endocrine cells of the upper small bowel. Their production is impaired in coeliac disease [6]. There is gall bladder inertia, and a sluggish extrahepatic circulation of bile salts probably due to impaired cholecystokinin secretion [20, 22]. This may account for the defective lipolysis and mi-

celle formation demonstrated in coeliac disease. Levels of pancreozymin and secretin are lowered and may contribute to the exocrine pancreatic insufficiency seen in some patients.

Undoubtedly mucosal damage with the consequent loss of surface area and reduction in brush border enzymes results in true malabsorption, but loss from the mucosa to the lumen compounds the problem. Cell loss may increase sixfold leading to protein and fat loss. Exudation across the damaged mucosa results in the loss of protein and other plasma constituents [17]. Finally, appetite plays a crucial role in the clinical results of the disease. Some patients eat sufficiently to compensate for the malabsorption, others do not. Surprisingly, weight loss in coeliac patients correlates more closely with appetite than with steatorrhoea [33].

Clinical features

Presentation

Coeliac disease may present at any time from the first months of life to the eighth decade.

In childhood clinical features are more uniform and the course more predictable

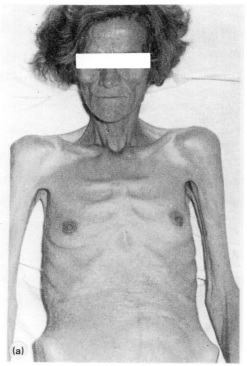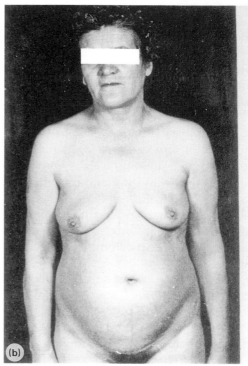

Fig. 42.7. (a) Severe emaciation in a patient with untreated coeliac disease. (b) The same patient following response to gluten withdrawal (with kind permission of Dr M.L. Clark).

than in adults. The cardinal features are poor growth, abdominal distension, pale, bulky stools, wasting and loss of appetite [8]. The trend for the disease to present earlier in life may reflect the practice of earlier introduction of cereals into the diet on weaning.

By contrast, adult coeliac disease may present in an extraordinary variety of ways. Diagnosis may be extremely difficult and is frequently overlooked for many years after the onset of symptoms. The peak period of presentation is between 20 and 40 years. The most characteristic features are diarrhoea, weight loss and anaemia (Fig. 42.7). However, this classical presentation is now less common, anaemia being the most frequent presentation. This probably reflects a greater awareness of the diagnosis and the increasing use of routine screening tests.

The clinical diversity of coeliac disease can be illustrated by considering recognized modes of presentation. These can occur singly or in combination.

Common modes of presentation

1. Anaemia. This is often a chance finding, due to either folate deficiency, iron deficiency or a combination of the two. Unlike tropical sprue, B_{12} deficiency is uncommon and anaemia due to B_{12} deficiency rare. Glossitis and angular stomatitis occur commonly.
2. Weight loss. Though not invariable, this is a common feature and may dominate the picture in severely ill and unresponsive patients.
3. Diarrhoea. Pale, bulky, frequent stools are the rule, profuse watery diarrhoea being

a feature of more advanced disease. Occasionally there is no history of bowel disturbance.

4. Oedema. Mild ankle oedema is common and a result of hypoproteinaemia. Generalized oedema and ascites signify advanced disease.

5. Weakness and lassitude. These common but vague symptoms may be the consequence of any one or a combination of the following: anaemia, weight loss, hypotension, muscle wasting and osteomalacia.

6. Skin lesions. A variety of skin lesions, including eczema and pigmentation, are common in coeliac disease. The association with dermatitis herpetiformis is considered later.

7. Psychiatric disturbance. Psychiatric features are frequent, depression predominating.

8. Mouth ulcers. Aphthous ulcers occur in 25% of patients, disappearing on gluten withdrawal. Their cause is unknown.

9. Abdominal pain. Abdominal discomfort, distension, rumbles (borborygmi) and mild colic are common. On the other hand severe pain is rare and may signify serious complications.

10. Amenorrhoea. Whether primary or secondary this usually responds quickly to gluten withdrawal.

Nutritional deficiencies

Tetany, due to low calcium or magnesium, is a feature of severely ill patients. Bruising, due to hypoprothrombinaemia, is extremely rare. Osteomalacia, due to vitamin D and calcium malabsorption occurs, particularly in the elderly. Weakness, especially limb girdle, may cause difficulty in standing up and climbing steps. Bizarre muscle and bone pain and overt fractures occur. Night blindness due to vitamin A deficiency is rare.

Table 42.4. Clinical features of coeliac disease.

Common
    Weight loss
    Pallor
    Oedema
    Angular stomatitis
    Glossitis
    Abdominal distension
    Pigmentation
    Aphthous ulceration
    Muscle wasting

Uncommon
    Clubbing
    Hypotension
    Bruising
    Ascites
    Neuropathy
    Ataxia
    Tetany

Physical findings (Table 42.4)

Clinical findings in coeliac disease are entirely non-specific. Examination is often normal. When abnormal, features include weight loss, pallor, angular stomatitis, glossitis, oedema, skin pigmentation and abdominal distension with accentuated bowel sounds.

Associated features and diseases

Hyposplenism

This is a now well-recognized and common association of coeliac disease occurring in 30–50% of patients. It is detected by the presence of target cells and Howell Jolly bodies recognized in the blood film and can be quantified by measuring the half-life of chromium-labelled heat-damaged red blood cells. The spleen becomes increasingly atrophic with the duraton of disease. Whether the hyposplenism is reversed by diet is uncertain, but a recent study showed improvement after gluten withdrawal suggesting environmental factors may be important in determining and maintaining hyposplenism [12]. The absence of hyposplenism in childhood suggests that it results from prolonged exposure to gluten[13]. It does not appear to predispose to malignancy.

Endocrine abnormalities

Hypogonadism

Sexual dysfunction is recognized in men and women with coeliac disease. Infertility in women has been reversed after gluten withdrawal[53]. Impotence and infertile marriages appear commoner in coeliac patients than in the normal population or a matched group of patients with Crohn's disease. The impotence improves on gluten withdrawal[26].

Altered plasma testosterone and luteinizing hormone concentrations indicate androgen resistance, and they return to normal on gluten withdrawal. These changes appear to be relatively specific to coeliac disease and unrelated to chronic ill-health[28].

Hypothalamic-pituitary dysfunction

Disturbance of growth hormone secretion and the regulation of thyroid function have been described in coeliac disease[27, 65].

Diabetes mellitus

There have been many reports of the co-existence of diabetes and coeliac disease in children and adults and the antigen HLA B8 is commoner in juvenile diabetes and coeliac disease than in the general population. Although there is no clear evidence that this is more than a chance association, it has important clinical implications. Diarrhoea due to coeliac disease in a patient with coexisting diabetes may be mistakenly diagnosed as diabetic diarrhoea. Control of diabetes in the presence of undiagnosed coeliac disease may be difficult and compli-

cated by episodes of profound hypo-glycaemia. Treatment of coexisting coeliac disease increases insulin requirements[68].

Adrenal insufficiency

Addison's disease has been described in association with coeliac disease on several occasions. Certain features, i.e. weakness, lassitude, dizziness, hypotension and pigmentation are common to both conditions. Though rare, clinical awareness of this possible association is important.

Involvement of the nervous system

Various abnormalities of the nervous system have been described in coeliac disease: encephalopathy[11], cerebellar abnormalities[30], psychiatric disorders, myelopathy, myopathy and peripheral neuropathy[56].

A review of 10 coeliac patients who developed progressive central nervous system disorders reported that every patient had ataxia. Other features included dementia, involuntary movements, myoclonus, seizures, hyper-reflexia and cranial nerve abnormalities. Clinical and pathological features were those of a degenerative state developing at any time during the course of coeliac disease. The illness pursued a relentless and ultimately fatal course, regardless of dietary and nutritional measures. The cause is unknown but the relationship with coeliac disease seems unlikely to be coincidental[39]. Psychiatric upsets are common, especially depression. There now seems little sound evidence to support the view that schizophrenia is commoner in coeliac disease or improved by gluten withdrawal.

Lung disease

An association has been described between coeliac disease and the following disorders—diffuse interstitial pulmonary fibrosis, bird fancier's lung, sarcoidosis [23] and cryptogenic fibrosing alveolitis. The significance of these associations is not clear.

Inflammatory bowel disease

Inflammatory bowel disease and coeliac disease have been described in four patients, an association thought not to be due to chance. Similarity between the symptoms could result in one or other disease being overlooked [40].

Dermatitis herpetiformis

The presence of jejunal mucosal abnormalities in dermatitis herpetiformis (DH) was first recognized in 1966 [52]. Great variability is quoted in the incidence of these abnormalities, but it now appears that almost all patients have some degree of mucosal lesion. The florid lesion is indistinguishable from that of coeliac disease and its response to gluten withdrawal now leaves few in doubt that it is indeed coeliac disease associated in some way with DH.

In a recent study of DH patients only 19% showed no evidence of coeliac disease. HLA 8 antigen was positive in 78%, a figure comparable to coeliac disease.

It is puzzling that the clinical features of malabsorption in dermatitis herpetiformis patients with coeliac disease are mild or absent, a fact which may explain why DH is rare amongst coeliac patients presenting to gastrointestinal clinics.

It has been suggested that these are two quite separate conditions, genetically linked, and this is supported by family studies. However, prolonged gluten withdrawal has been shown to correct the mucosal lesion and to clear the skin lesion [32], while sulphone treatment for the skin has no effect on the mucosa. Furthermore, the IgA deposits in the upper dermis of involved skin, a diagnostic feature of DH, have been shown to be dimeric, suggesting small intestinal origin [64]. These observations raise the possibility that DH might be a rare skin manifestation of coeliac disease.

The association between DH and malignancy is now well-established. In a recent study seven of 109 DH patients had developed malignant tumours, three of which were lymphomas, giving a relative risk a little over half that seen in coeliac disease [43].

The practical dilemma is whether all patients with DH should be investigated and treated for a mucosal lesion as symptoms are usually mild or absent. The above observations regarding lymphomas, and the suggestion that treatment by gluten withdrawal reduces this risk coupled with the fact that gluten withdrawal is also beneficial for the skin lesion, suggests that a gluten-free diet should be advised.

Complications

Malignancy [63]

An association between malabsorption and lymphoma has been recognized since the 1930s, but uncertainty existed as to whether the malabsorption was primary or secondary. It is now clear that coeliac disease is a premalignant condition [55]. The main malignancy is the small bowel lymphoma, most commonly malignant histiocytosis, which appears to be of T-cell rather than histiocyte origin [36, 37, 48]. Carcinoma of the gastrointestinal tract also appears to be commoner in the coeliac patient, especially in the pharynx and oesophagus [34]. Adenocarcinoma of the small bowel, an exceedingly rare tumour, has also been described in coeliac disease. There is an 80-fold increased risk of this tumour in coeliacs [63].

The incidence of malignancy in adult coeliac disease is approximately 8%. Lymphoma usually presents after the age of 50 as a progressive illness, accompanied by fever, rashes, worsening bowel symptoms and failure to respond to gluten withdrawal. Haemorrhage, severe abdominal pain, perforation or obstruction are frequent features. Diagnosis is difficult without laparotomy, when diffuse or multiple lesions are found. Surgical resection is rarely possible and medical treatment with radiotherapy or chemotherapy is disappointing, though successful treatment has been reported using chemotherapy. Clinical deterioration is rapid, death usually occurring within a year.

Preventive treatment should offer the best hope, but reports are conflicting. In one study a gluten-free diet did not appear to prevent malignancy and a persistently flat biopsy, or suboptimal response to treatment conferred no increased risk of malignancy [34]. On the other hand in dermatitis herpetiformis a gluten-free diet did appear to be protective against malignancy [43]. It is possible that the benefits of a gluten-free diet will only be fully realized if it is started in infancy. Clarification of this issue is crucial because malignancy is at present the major indication for recommending a lifelong gluten-free diet.

Benign ulceration and strictures

These arc well-documented, but rare complications occurring in treated and untreated coeliac patients [5]. Their importance lies in the high associated mortality (75%) and the similarity of their presentation to lymphoma, with pain, profound weight loss, anorexia, perforation and bleeding. Laparotomy is essential to differentiate the two; while the prognosis for lymphoma is extremely poor, resection of the stricture or ulcer may be curative. The histology of the lesion is non-specific.

Diagnosis and investigations

Clinical awareness of the possibility of coeliac disease and its diverse modes of presentation is all important. Once the suspicion is there, only one investigation will confirm or refute that suspicion—the jejunal biopsy. None of the large number of small intestinal function tests are diagnostic and few are of real practical value. Apart from making the diagnosis, further investigations are needed to look for deficiencies, to assess nutritional status and to exclude other diagnoses.

Radiology

Small bowel meal

This will provide strong support for the diagnosis of coeliac disease, but is perhaps more valuable in excluding other disorders with which it might be confused, especially

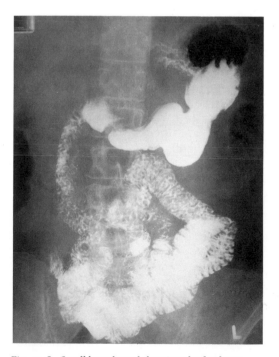

Fig. 42.8. Small bowel meal showing the feathery appearance of the normal jejunal mucosa.

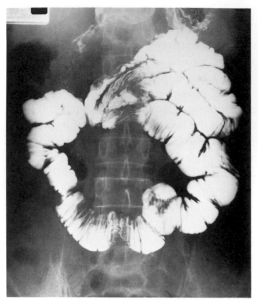

Fig. 42.9. Small bowel meal in untreated coeliac disease showing replacement of the normal feathery appearance by rather featureless loops of bowel showing transverse barring.

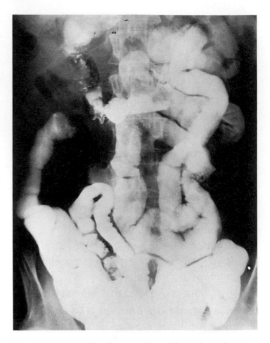

Fig. 42.10. Grossly abnormal small bowel meal in a severely ill patient with unresponsive coeliac disease. The whole small intestine is tubular and featureless.

Crohn's disease and small bowel diverticula. Appearances are abnormal in 90% of coeliac patients, showing a malabsorptive pattern which is, however, quite non-specific. The normal fine feathery appearance of the mucosa (Fig. 42.8) is replaced by a coarse mucosal pattern of broad barring (Fig. 42.9) which may be lost, leaving a featureless tubular appearance (Fig. 42.10) as the disease becomes more severe. The bowel wall is thickened and occasionally the lumen is distended. Changes are maximal in the jejunum, but spread distally with increasing severity of the disease.

Skeletal X-rays

These may show of osteomalacia, but normal bones do not exclude this diagnosis.

Histology

Jejunal histology is the corner-stone of the diagnosis and has already been described. Biopsy technique has been considered in Chapter 41.

Whether a conventional suction capsule or an endoscope is used for the biopsy, jejunal juice should be collected at the same time as the biopsy and both examined straight away—the juice for *Giardia lamblia* and the biopsy for villus morphology.

Haematology

There are no specific haematological tests for coeliac disease. However, anaemia, the commonest presentation, will be picked up on a full blood count, which frequently provides the clue to the diagnosis (see Chapter 6).

Serum iron, iron binding capacity, folic acid and vitamin B_{12} should be measured.

Iron and folic acid are usually low, but B_{12} is frequently normal; indeed a low vitamin B_{12} justifies a Schilling test to exclude pernicious anaemia. Immunoglobulin measurements may demonstrate an isolated IgA deficiency found in 2% of coeliac patients, but more commonly raised IgA and low IgM concentrations are found. Rarely the prothrombin time is prolonged due to vitamin K malabsorption.

Biochemistry

The extent to which biochemical tests are needed depends on the state of the patient. An ill patient needs full assessment: urea and electrolytes may be abnormal, serum albumin is usually low and calcium and alkaline phosphatase concentrations may suggest osteomalacia. Two function tests have stood the test of time because of their relative simplicity and reliability, making them appropriate for any general hospital. A faecal fat estimation will demonstrate fat malabsorption though will not differentiate between a pancreatic and intestinal cause. The D-Xylose absorption test complements the fat analysis providing information about mucosal function. Both tests have their practical problems and shortcomings and these need to be considered in performing the tests and interpreting the results (see Chapter 41). Either test may be normal in 20% of coeliac patients but it is unusual for both to be normal.

In the presence of diarrhoea the stool should be examined for bacteria and parasites.

Response to gluten withdrawal

By definition the diagnosis in coeliac disease can only be confirmed if full clinical and histological recovery occurs following gluten withdrawal. This is, therefore, the ultimate test.

In children a third biopsy after gluten challenge is sometimes recommended to avoid possible confusion with cows' milk or soya protein sensitivity.

Differential diagnosis

Coeliac disease may present in widely diverse ways and the differential diagnosis is correspondingly extensive and varied. Where weight loss and diarrhoea dominate the picture there is need to consider the following.

Crohn's disease

Small bowel Crohn's disease is perhaps the most important alternative diagnosis. Abdominal pain and localized tenderness are frequent features of Crohn's disease, but rarely occur in uncomplicated coeliac disease. Active Crohn's disease is usually reflected by an elevated ESR or C-reactive protein, both of which are unusual in coeliac disease.

Pancreatic disease

Steatorrhoea and weight loss may be gross, but mucosal structure and function are normal.

Giardia lamblia *infestation*

Giardial infestation may mimic coeliac disease clinically and histologically (see Chapter 43). A history of foreign travel or homosexuality provides a clue. The demonstration of motile trophozoites in jejunal juice or cysts in the stool differentiate the two, though occasionally giardial infection may occur in coeliac disease especially when associated with IgA deficiency. Although mucosal abnormalities occur, a truly flat mucosa is rare.

Tropical sprue

A careful history will point to the likelihood of this diagnosis. B_{12} deficiency is the rule by definition, being uncommon in coeliac disease and a flat mucosa is rare (see Chapter 43).

Anorexia nervosa

Weight loss may strongly suggest malabsorption, but blood parameters of malabsorption are usually normal, diarrhoea is not a feature and the mucosa is normal (see Chapter 68).

Thyrotoxicosis

Weight loss and diarrhoea, frequent features of hyperthyroidism, suggest malabsorption but are usually accompanied by the characteristic physical signs suggesting the diagnosis. However, these conditions may rarely occur together.

Whipple's disease

Pyrexia, arthritis and lymphadenopathy accompanying malabsorption in men suggests this rare disease whose diagnosis is confirmed by its unique jejunal histology (see Chapter 47). The dramatic response to antibiotics in this previously fatal disease makes awareness of its diagnosis all the more important.

Although a wide variety of conditions are associated with changes in jejunal morphology (Table 42.3), sub-total villous atrophy is virtually diagnostic of adult coeliac disease in temperate climates and differentiates it from the above conditions.

Treatment

Gluten withdrawal

The treatment of coeliac disease is complete withdrawal of gluten from the diet, following which 85% of adults and all children will make a full recovery. Symptoms recover rapidly in days and weeks, but histological recovery may take a year or longer. Some patients do not respond and these are considered later.

Gluten withdrawal for life?

Changing to a gluten-free diet is a major undertaking and should never be embarked upon without a definite diagnosis. This having been achieved, the probable protection against malignancy and the avoidance of deficiency states at present provides justification to advise a life-long diet. There is good evidence that without treatment relapse may occur unexpectedly at any time.

Deficiency states

While awaiting the response to the diet it is reasonable to treat existing deficiencies appropriately to speed recovery.

The gluten-free diet

This means avoidance of wheat, rye, barley and all products made from their flour. The situation regarding oats has been discussed earlier but, to be on the safe side when initiating treatment, it seems sensible to exclude oats as well.

Time is essential to explain fully the nature of the problem to the newly diagnosed patient, emphasizing that complete recovery can be expected with diet alone, provided the diet is adhered to strictly and for life. It is not reasonable, however, to frighten the patient into complying by threats of malignancy. Symptomatic patients usually have no problem, their dramatic improvement providing the incentive to stick to the diet. The difficulties arise where symptoms are minimal—where, for example, the diagnosis has resulted from a chance blood count. Here major changes in diet for life may be hard to accept. To add to the problem, gluten sensitivity varies greatly. Some patients relapse rapidly after a minor dietary indiscretion, while others can break their diet for long periods without apparent harm. It should not be forgotten that for a single person or a poor cook the demands of the diet are daunting.

Clearly, expert and helpful dietary advice is crucial and should be available whenever required. British patients need to know what is available on a National Health Service prescription and should be informed about the Coeliac Society which, among its many functions, disseminates useful information about changes and advances in dietary measures (see Appendix).

Follow-up

Once the diet is established and fully understood, deficiencies have been corrected and clinical recovery has occurred, follow-up need only be yearly. At these visits, besides clinical assessment, it is sensible to check the following as additional measures of remission: full blood count, vitamin B_{12}, folic acid, iron, calcium, alkaline phosphatase and albumin.

Failure to respond to treatment

Two groups fall into this category—those who respond initially and later relapse and those who never respond. In both groups the essential prerequisite is to confirm compliance to the diet. Of new patients with flat biopsies, approximately 15% never respond to gluten withdrawal and by definition are not strictly coeliacs, but for practical reasons are considered as part of the coeliac

spectrum. Relapse following an initial response to diet is rare.

The disease in non-responders is usually more severe and extends to involve the whole small bowel, which appears featureless and tubular radiologically. The mucosa is atrophic with marked inflammatory cell infiltrate and loss of paneth cells. Patients are often severely ill with multiple nutritional deficiencies. Prednisolone is the best treatment in conjunction with a gluten-free diet. The initial dose is prednisolone 40–60 mg a day to induce a remission, reducing to the minimal dose necessary to maintain that remission. Initial response is often good, but prednisolone has to be continued with the accompanying problems of its unwanted effects.

Twenty-five per cent of such patients pursue a remorseless downhill course and die. Where steroids have failed, azathioprine and cyclophosphamide have been tried with occasional success. In a recent study it was possible to wean three patients off steroids after introduction of azathioprine 2 mg/kg/day. All showed striking symptomatic and histological improvement [61]. Some of these patients may require parenteral nutrition as a life-long treatment.

Apparent failure to respond may be due to the development of ulceration or malignancy, or rarely to concurrent pancreatic exocrine failure due to idiopathic pancreatic atrophy. Exocrine pancreatic supplements may help. A low fat diet and pancreatic supplements are required in addition to gluten withdrawal. The prognosis of these patients is especially poor [18].

Course and prognosis

The adage 'once a coeliac, always a coeliac' seems to hold true. Although sensitivity to gluten varies considerably and some coeliacs can revert to normal diets for long periods without apparent harm, relapse almost invariably occurs sooner or later.

Childhood coeliac disease frequently becomes quiescent in adolescence and young people may stray from their diets. However, almost all relapse at some stage in later life. Of 57 young adults diagnosed as having coeliac disease who had returned to a normal diet only 14 were well with no evidence of deficiency or recurrence [58].

When correctly diagnosed and treated, the prognosis for coeliac disease is excellent, and there is no evidence that life expectation is diminished. However, if symptoms are severe and unrecognized, coeliac disease may be fatal. Complications are rare but carry a grave prognosis when they occur.

Appendix

In the United Kingdom the following food preparations are prescribable for the treatment of coeliac disease on the FP 10 form. Prescriptions must be marked 'as per ACBS' (Advisory Committee on Borderline Substances).

Biscuits

Aproten semi-sweet Biscuits, Gluten-Free & Low Protein
Bi-Aglut Gluten-free Biscuits
Farley's Gluten-free Biscuits
Glutenex
Rite-Diet Gluten-free Biscuits—Sweet (plain) and Savoury
Rite-Diet Low Protein Cream-filled Wafers
Rite-Diet Gluten-free Digestive Biscuits
Verkade Gluten-free Biscuits

Bread

Juvela Gluten-free loaf
Rite-Diet Gluten-free Bread with Soya Bran (tinned)
Rite-Diet Gluten-free Bread (white, tinned)

Flour

Aproten Gluten-free Flour
Juvela Gluten-free Mix: Juvela Low Protein Mix
Rite-Diet White Bread Mix: Rite-Diet Brown Bread Mix
Rite-Diet Gluten-free Flour Mix
Rite-Diet Low Protein Flour Mix
Tritamyl Flour
Trufree Bread Mix with Rice Bran
Trufree Cantabread Mix: Trufree Self-raising Flour

Pasta

Aglutella Gentili—Macaroni, Semolina, Spaghetti and Spaghetti rings
Aproten—Anellini (rings); Ditalini (sticks); Rigatini (Noodles); Tagliatelle (Spaghetti)
Rite-Diet Macaroni

Rusks

Aproten Crispbread
GF Crackers

Addresses of Suppliers

Aproten Products	Carlo Erba (UK) Ltd 28–30 Great Peter Street London SW1
Rite-Diet Products	Welfare Foods (Stockport) Ltd 63–65 Higher Hillgate Stockport Cheshire
Tritamyl Gluten-free Flour	Procea Ltd Alexandra Road Dublin
Farley's Gluten-free Biscuits	Farley Infant Food Ltd Plymouth

GF Products GF Dietary Supplies Ltd
Lowther Road
Stanmore
Middlesex

Useful information

The   Coeliac PO Box No 181
Society London NW2 2QY

The Coeliac Society office provides the following information on request:

UK Holiday Holiday   accommodation
Lists where a gluten free diet can be obtained.

Holidays Helpful information is provided about most European
Abroad countries, together with useful phrases in the appropriate languages.

Insurance A list of companies giving
Companies fair terms for coeliac patients

Coeliac Hand- A comprehensive list of
book Food gluten-free manufactured
List products, updated six monthly.

References

1 ANAND BS, TRUELOVE SC. Coeliac disease: an Arthus-type reacton. In: Truelove SC, Lee E, eds. *Topics in gastroenterology 5.* Oxford: Blackwell Scientific Publications, 1977:339–346.
2 ANDERSON CM, BURKE V. Coeliac disease. In: Anderson CM, Burke V, eds. *Paediatric gastroenterology.* Oxford: Blackwell Scientific Publications, 1975: 175–197.
3 ASQUITH P, HAENEY MR. Immunology of the gastrointestinal tract. In: Asquith P, ed. Edinburgh: Churchill Livingstone, 1978:66–94.
4 BAKLIEN K, BRANDTZAEG P, FAUSA O. Immunoglobulins in jejunal mucosa and serum from patients with adult coeliac disease. *Scand J Gastroenterol* 1977;12:149–159.
5 BAYLESS TM, BAER A, YARDLEY JH, HENDRIX TR. Intestinal ulceration, flat mucosa and malabsorption. In: McNicholl B, McCarthy CG, Fottrell PF,

eds. *Perspectives in coeliac disease.* Lancaster: MTP Press, 1977:311–312.
6 BESTERMAN HS, SARSON DL, JOHNSTON DI, et al. Gut-hormone profile in coeliac disease. *Lancet* 1978;i:785.
7 BRAMBLE MG, ZUCOLOTO S, WRIGHT NA, RECORD CO. Acute gluten challenge in treated adult coeliac disease: a morphometric and enzymatic study. *Gut* 1985;26:169–174.
8 CACCIARI E, SALARDI S, LAZZARI R, et al. Short stature and celiac disease—a relationship to consider even in patients with no gastrointestinal tract symptoms. *J Pediatr* 1983;103:708–711.
9 CICLITIRA PJ, EVANS DJ, FAGG NLK, LENNOX ES, DOWLING RH. Clinical testing of gliadin fractions in coeliac patients. *Clin Sci* 1984;66:357–364.
10 COLE SG, KAGNOFF MF. Celiac disease. *Ann Rev Nutr* 1985; 5:241–266.
11 COOKE WT. Neurological manifestations of malabsorption. In: Vinken PJ, Bruyn GW, eds. *Handbook of clinical neurology. Vol 28: Metabolic and deficiency diseases of the nervous system, part II.* Amsterdam: North Holland Pub Co, 1976:225–241.
12 CORAZZA GR, FRISONI M, VAIRA D, GASBARRINI G. Effect of gluten free diet on splenic hypofunction of adult coeliac disease. *Gut* 1983;24:228–230.
13 CORAZZA GR, LAZZARI R, FRISONI M, COLLINA A, GASBARRINI G. Splenic function in childhood coeliac disease. *Gut* 1982;23:415–416.
14 CORNELL HJ, ROLLES CJ. Further evidence of a primary mucosal defect in coeliac disease. In vitro mucosal digestion studies in coeliac patients in remission, their relatives and control subjects. *Gut* 1978;19:253–259.
15 CORNELL HJ, TOWNLEY RRW. Investigations of possible intestinal peptides on rat liver lysosomes in relation to the pathogenesis of coeliac disease. *Clin Chim Acta* 1973;49:181–187.
16 CORNELL HJ, TOWNLEY RRW. Investigation of possible intestinal peptidase deficiency in coeliac disease. *Clin Chim Acta* 1973;43:113–125.
17 CREAMER B. Malabsorption. In: Creamer B, ed. *The small intestine.* London: Heinemann (William) Ltd, 1974:71–72.
18 CREAMER B. Coeliac disease. In: Creamer B, ed. *The small intestine.* London: Heinemann (William) Ltd, 1974:109.
19 DAWSON AM, KUMAR PJ. Coeliac disease. In: Booth CC, Neale G, eds. *Disorders of the small intestine.* Oxford: Blackwell Scientific Publications, 1986: 153 178.
20 DELAMARRE J, CAPRON J-P, JOLY J-P, et al. Gallbladder inertia in celiac disease: ultrasonographic demonstraton. *Dig Dis Sci* 1984;29:876–877.
21 DICKE WK. *Coeliac disease: investigation of harmful effects of certain types of cereal on patients with coeliac disease.* (Univ. of Utrecht, Doctoral thesis 1950).
22 DIMAGNO EP, GO WVL, SUMMERSKILL WJH. Im-

paired cholecystokinin-pancreozymin, secretion, intraluminal dilution and maldigestion of fat in-sprue. *Gastroenterology* 1972;**63**:25–32.

23 DOUGLAS JG, GILLON J, LOGAN RFA, GRANT IWB, CROMPTON GK. Sarcoidosis and coeliac disease: an association? *Lancet* 1984;**ii**:13–14.

24 EDITORIAL Coeliac disease in the elderly. *Lancet* 1984;**i**:775–776.

25 FALCHUK ZM, ROGENTINE GN, STROBER W. Predominance of histocompatibility antigen HLA8 in patients with gluten sensitive enteropathy. *J Clin Invest* 1972;**15**:1602–1605.

26 FARTHING MJG, EDWARDS CRW, REES LH, DAWSON AM. Male gonadal function in coeliac disease. Sexual dysfunction, infertility and semen quality, *Gut* 1982;**23**:608–614.

27 FARTHING MJG, REES LH, EDWARDS CRW, BYFIELD PGH, HIMSWORTH RL, DAWSON AM. Thyroid hormones and the regulation of thyroid function in man with coeliac disease. *Clin Endocrinol (Oxf)* 1982;**16**:525–535.

28 FARTHING MJG, REES LH, EDWARDS CRW, DAWSON AM. Male gonadal function in coeliac disease: 2 sex hormone. *Gut* 1983;**24**:127–135.

29 FERGUSON A, MCCLURE JP, MACDONALD TT, HOLDEN RJ. Cell-mediated immunity to gliadin within the small intestinal mucosa in coeliac disease. *Lancet* 1975);**i**:895–897.

30 FINELLI PF, MCENTEE WJ, AMBLER M, KOSTENBAUM D. Adult coeliac disease presenting as cerebellar syndrome. *Neurology (Minneap)* 1980;**30**:245–249.

31 FRAZER AC. Discussion on some problems of steatorrhoea and reduced stature. *Proc R Soc Med* 1956;**49**:1009–1013.

32 FRY L, SEAH PP, RICHES DJ, HOFFBRAND AV. Clearance of skin lesions in dermatitis herpetiformis after gluten withdrawal. *Lancet* 1973;**i**:288–291.

33 GENT AE, CREAMER B. Faecal fat, appetite and weight loss in the coeliac syndrome. *Lancet* 1963;**i**:1063–1064.

34 HOLMES GKT, STOKES PL, SORAHAN TM, PRIOR P, WATERHOUSE JAH, COOKE WT. Coeliac disease, gluten free diet and malignancy. *Gut* 1976;**17**:612–619.

35 HOWDLE PD, CICLITIRA PJ, SIMPSON FG, LOSOWSKY MS. Are all gliadins toxic in coeliac disease?—an in vitro study of α, β, γ, and ω gliadins. *Scand J Gastroenterol* 1984;**19**:41–47.

36 ISAACSON PG, O'CONNOR NTJ, SPENCER J, *et al.* Malignant histocytosis of the intestine: a T-cell lymphoma. *Lancet* 1985;**ii**:688–681.

37 ISAACSON PG, WRIGHT DH. Intestinal lymphoma associated with malabsorption. *Lancet* 1978;**i**:64–70.

38 KHUFFASH FA, BARAKAT MH, MAJEED HA, WHITE AG, BESEDA AJ. Coeliac disease in monozygotic twin girls—synchronous presentation. *Gut* 1984; **25**:1009–1012.

39 KINNEY HC, BURGER PC, HURWITZ BJ, HIJMANS JC, GRANT JP. Degeneration of the central nervous system associated with coeliac disease. *J Neurol Sci* 1982;**53**:9–22.

40 KITIS G, HOLMES GKT, COOPER BT, THOMPSON H, ALLAN RN. Association of coeliac disease and inflammatory bowel disease. *Gut* 1980;**21**:636–641.

41 KUMAR PJ. The enigma of celiac disease. *Gastroenterology* 1985;**89**:214–216.

42 LAZZARI R, VOLTA U, BIANCHI FB, COLLINA A, PISI E. R. Reticulin antibodies: markers of celiac disease in children on a normal diet and on gluten challenge. *J Pediatr Gastroenterol Nutr* 1984;**3**:516–522.

43 LEONARD JN, TUCKER WFG, FRY JS, *et al.* Increased incidence of malignancy in dermatitis herpetiformis. *Br. Med J* 1983;**1**:16–18.

44 LEVENSON SD, AUSTIN RK, DIETLER MD, KASARDA DD, KAGNOFF MF. Specificity of antigliadin antibody in celiac disease. *Gastroenterology* 1985; **89**:1–5.

45 LOEB PM, STROBER W, FALCHUK ZM, LASTER L. Incorporation of L-leucine-^{14}C into immunoglobulins by jejunal biopsies of patients with coeliac sprue and other gastrointestinal diseases. *J Clin Invest* 1971;**50**:569–572.

46 LOGAN RFA, RIFKIND EA, BUSUTTIL A, GILMOUR HM, FERGUSON A. Prevalence and 'incidence' of celiac disease in Edinburgh and the Lothian region of Scotland. *Gastroenterology* 1986;**90**:3.

47 LOGAN RFA, TUCKER G, RIFKIND EA, HEADING RC, FERGUSON A. Changes in clinical features of coeliac disease in adults in Edinburgh and the Lothians 1960–79. *Br Med J* 1983;**1**:95–97.

48 LOUGHRAN TP, KADIN ME, DEEG HJ. T-cell intestinal lymphoma associated with celiac sprue. *Ann Intern Med* 1986;**104**:44–47

49 MCCONNELL RB. Membership of the Coeliac Society of the United Kingdom. In: McConnell RB, ed. *The genetics of coeliac disease.* Lancaster: MTP Press, 1981:65–69.

50 MCCREA WM. The inheritance of coeliac disease. In: Booth CC, Dowling RH, eds. *Coeliac disease.* London: Churchill Livingstone, 1970:55–61.

51 MÄKI M, HÄLLSTRÖM O, HUUPPONEN T, VESIKARI T, VISAKORPI JK. Increased prevalence of coeliac disease in diabetes. *Arch Dis Child* 1984;**59**:739–742.

52 MARKS J, SHUSTER S, WATSON AJ. Small bowel changes in dermatitis herpetiformis. *Lancet* 1966;**ii**:1280–1282.

53 MORRIS JS, AJDUKIEWICZ AB, READ AE. Coeliac infertility: an indication for dietary gluten restriction. *Lancet* 1970;**i**:213–214.

54 MYLOTTE M, EGAN-MITCHELL B, MCARTHY CF, MCNICHOLL B. Incidence of coeliac disease in the west of Ireland. *Br Med J* 1973;**1**:703–705.

55 NEILSEN OH, JACONSEN O, PEDERSEN ER, *et al.* Nontropical sprue. Malignant disease and mortality rate. *Scand J Gastroenterol* 1985;**20**:13–18.

56 PALLIS CR, LEWIS PD. Neurological complications of coeliac disease and tropical sprue. In: Walton J, ed. *The neurology of gastrointestinal disease.* Philadelphia: WB Saunders Co, 1974:138–156.

57 PENA AS, MANN DL, HAGUE NE, *et al.* Genetic basis of gluten sensitive enteropathy. *Gastroenterology* 1978;75:230–235.

58 SHELDON W. Prognosis in early adult life of coeliac children treated with a gluten free diet. *Br Med J* 1969;2:401–404.

59 SHINER M. Ultrastructural changes suggestive of immune reactions in the jejunal mucosa of coeliac children following gluten challenge. *Gut* 1973;14:1–12.

60 SIMPSON FG, FIELD HP, HOWDLE PD, ROBERTSON DAF, LOSOWSKY MS. Leucocyte migration inhibition test in coeliac disease—a re-appraisal. *Gut* 1983;24:311–317.

61 SINCLAIR TS, KUMAR PJ, DAWSON AM. Azathioprine responsive villous atrophy. *Gut* 1983;24:A494.

62 SINCLAIR TS, OHANNESIAN AD, JONES D, *et al.* Which gliadin fraction is toxic? *Gut* 1983; cf324:A492.

63 SWINSON CM, SLAVIN A, COLES EC, BOOTH CC. Coeliac disease and malignancy. *Lancet* 1984;i:111–115.

64 UNSWORTH DJ, LEONARD JN, PAYNE AW, FRY L, HOLBOROW DJ. IgA in dermatitis herpetiformis skin is dimeric. *Lancet* 1982;i:478–479.

65 VANDERSCHUEREN-LODEWEYCKX M, WOLTER R, MOLLA A, EGGERMONT E, EECKEL SR. Plasma growth hormone in coeliac disease. *Helv Paediatr Acta* 1973;28:349–357.

66 VERKASALO MA. Adherence of gliadin fractions to lymphocytes in coeliac disease. *Lancet* 1982;i:1384–1386.

67 VISAKORPI JK. An international enquiry concerning the diagnostic criteria of coeliac disease. *Acta Paediatr Scand* 1970;59:463–464.

68 WALSH CH, COOPER BT, WRIGHT AD, MALINS JM, COOKE WT. Diabetes mellitus and coeliac disease: a clinical study. *Q J Med* 1978;185:89–100.

Chapter 43
Tropical Diseases of the Small Intestine

G. C. COOK

Tropical diseases involving the small intestine are of major importance in the practice of medicine in the tropics; travel has made them increasingly important in the West [4].

Cholera [12]

Cholera is the archetypal disease in the context of small intestinal diarrhoea [12]. The causative organism—the *Vibrio cholerae*—is not invasive and exerts its effect through an enterotoxin. Untreated, clinical disease has a 20–80% mortality rate. With modern oral rehydration regimens that figure should be less than 1%. When it occurs, death is a result of dehydration, vascular collapse and renal failure.

Historically, cholera was not confined to tropical countries and involved many temperate areas including northern Europe. In London an epidemic in 1854 was traced to contaminated water from the Broad Street pump. When the handle of that pump was removed by John Snow a rapid decline in the incidence of new cases of disease was recorded [73].

Epidemiology

The disease is endemic in India, Pakistan, Bangladesh, Afghanistan and in many other countries in Southeast Asia [55]. In recent years minor epidemics in the Middle East and Africa have occurred, but have generally been localized [6, 31]. Cholera is endemic along the Gulf Coast of the United States [59]. The condition is closely associated with poverty, overcrowding and low socio-economic status. There is probably a genetic predisposition—blood group O is associated with a higher infection rate than group A. Although in former times cholera spread by population movements such as the annual Hadj to Mecca, instances of outbreaks involving air travellers have now been recorded. The disease tends to affect young people more often than the elderly.

Aetiology

Classical cholera is caused by *V. cholerae* which is now localized to the Indian subcontinent—especially the deltas of the Ganges and Brahmaputra rivers. Elsewhere, the *El tor* biotype, which originated in Indonesia around 1960, has been responsible for most epidemics. The bioecology of the organism is unclear—the habitat of the organism between epidemics may be in river estuaries [54]. In the case of a related organism, *V. parahaemolyticus*, a seasonal appearance has been observed associated with the cyclic appearance of zooplankton in the water column. Each biotype of cholera contains three serotypes—Inaba, Ogawa and Hikojima. The vibrios are curved, Gram-negative, flagellated rods approximately 2 μm in length. Following ingestion, often in seafood [31], gastric acid destroys the vibrios; in anacidity—caused by gastrectomy or smoking *Cannabis indica*, for example, the disease is more common and more virulent. The organisms multiply within the small intestinal lumen and do

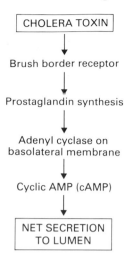

CHOLERA TOXIN

↓

Brush border receptor

↓

Prostaglandin synthesis

↓

Adenyl cyclase on
basolateral membrane

↓

Cyclic AMP (cAMP)

↓

NET SECRETION
TO LUMEN

Fig. 43.1. Mechanism of cholera enterotoxin action on the enterocyte leading to massive net luminal secretion.

not invade the mucosa or enter the portal circulation.

An enterotoxin which adheres tightly to the enterocyte is secreted; the enterotoxin increases the concentration of adenyl cyclase and subsequently cyclic adenosine monophosphate (cAMP) (Fig. 43.1). Cholera toxin has a molecular weight of 60,000, an optimal pH of 8.0 and is inactivated at 60°C. As cAMP accumulates in the enterocytes a massive net secretion into the lumen occurs [68, 84]. When colonic absorptive capacity is overwhelmed, torrential diarrhoea results (see Chapter 4).

Despite its non-invasiveness, *V. cholerae* does induce serum bactericidal and agglutinating antibodies at low concentration.

Pathology

Histologically the small intestinal mucosa is intact. Light and electron microscopy are normal. Following circulatory collapse resulting from gross dehydration, renal tubular necrosis may be demonstrated.

Clinical features

There are no prodromal symptoms. The incubation period is from a few hours to five days. The disease is similar whichever biotype is involved, but there is a wide spectrum of severity. A higher proportion of patients are asymptomatic when the *El tor* biotype is responsible. Onset is sudden— mild diarrhoea rapidly gives way to the passage of large volumes of opalescent fluid— the classical 'rice-water' stools. Up to 24 l of fluid containing a high concentration of vibrios may be passed in 24 hours. Vomiting of similar fluid is a later feature. Thirst, muscle cramps, hoarseness and anuria follow. Clinical signs of severe dehydration are present often by 24 hours after onset in untreated cases. The body temperature is normal or mildly elevated. Circulatory failure and acute renal failure follow. Confusion, disorientation and hypoglycaemic convulsions may also occur. The mortality rate is dependent on the degree of dehydration. Protection is short-lived. A carrier state lasting a few weeks can occur and gall bladder foci have been identified.

Investigations

Vibrios are easily identified in stool specimens; material should be transported to the laboratory in alkaline peptone water (pH 9.0). For accurate serological identification of *V. cholerae*, rigid criteria are necessary [24]. With classical cholera, organisms are present during the incubation period and for up to five days after an attack; in the *El tor* variety, the vibrios can persist for weeks or months.

Biochemically, stools are isotonic with a protein concentration of approximately 10 g/l; pH is around 7.5; typical electrolyte concentrations are Na^+ 139, K^+ 24, Cl^- 106 and HCO_3^- 48 mmol/l. Stools contain a high concentration of immunoglobulin A. Serum immunoglobulins A and M are elevated, the former most markedly in patients with an *El tor* infection. In *in vitro* animal studies, cholera toxin enhances IgA secretion from crypt epithelium to ileal lumen [40].

Serum electrolyte, urea and creatinine concentrations depend on the state and severity of the disease. Excessive potassium loss exacerbates the metabolic acidosis. Urine is concentrated, but its composition also depends on the state and severity of the disease.

Differential diagnosis

Diagnosis is usually straightforward. However, all other causes of small intestinal diarrhoea (with and without vomiting) of acute onset should be considered—travellers' diarrhoea, *Escherichia coli*, staphyloccal, *Clostridium welchii*, (*perfringens*), *C. botulinum*, campylobacter, and viral causes for example, rotavirus, Norwalk agent, etc. *Salmonella* spp and *Shigella* spp should also be considered. *Vibrio parahaemolyticus* (often conveyed by infected raw seafood) and other non-cholera vibrios can also produce similar disease. Rarely *Plasmodium falciparum* malaria can present with severe diarrhoea. Food poisoning caused by toxic agents is a further differential diagnosis.

Prevention

Basic sanitation and public health procedures must be improved [43]. Sterility of water supplies is of paramount importance. Vaccination with dead vibrios gives limited protection—0.5 and 1.0 ml vaccine should be given at an interval of one week and an 0.5 ml booster given every six months. Vaccination was frequently demanded by health authorities before entry to a country. However, the 26th assembly of the World Health Organization (WHO) [86] recommended that cholera vaccination should not be compulsory in any country, because of its limited public health value. Overall

vaccines are disappointing, but do offer a degree of protection to individual travellers who are at special risk, for example, those living in close proximity to overcrowded, infected populations. Contacts of proven cases should be vaccinated; all faeces and bedlinen should be destroyed.

Treatment

Treatment has been revolutionized by the introduction of **oral rehydration regimes** [50]. The enterocyte Na-glucose carrier system is not affected by cAMP, and thus glucose (or glycine)-stimulated membrane, transport takes place normally. Oral solutions should contain:

Sodium chloride	3.5 g
Sodium bicarbonate	2.5 g
Potassium chloride	1.5 g
Glucose	20.0 g

made up to 1 litre. Sachets of pre-prepared glucose/electrolyte solutions can be obtained commercially (for example UNICEF 15-611-00 and Dioralyte (Armour, England)). It is impossible in a previously fit person to overload the circulation by the oral route. The quantity of ingested fluid should be regulated by stool loss which is best measured two-hourly. Rehydration should be accomplished within 48 hours. In unsophisticated situations sucrose is often more easily obtainable than glucose; it seems to give good results although, if severe mucosal damage pre-exists, the sucrase concentration is likely to be depressed and rehydration less readily obtained. **Cereal based electrolyte solutions** have also given satisfactory results [57].

In severe cases, **intravenous fluids** may be necessary for initial rehydration; a widely used composition is:

Sodium chloride	5.0 g
Sodium bicarbonate	4.0 g
Potassium chloride	1.0 g

made up to 1 litre. Degree of rehydration should be assessed on clinical grounds; in a case of average severity in a 50 kg subject, 5 litres should be given (the first litre within 10 minutes).

Aspirin and chlorpromazine have been advocated because they inhibit prostaglandin production and thus the effect of cholera toxin on the enterocyte [66].

Analgesics may be necessary for severe muscle cramps. Intravenous calcium gluconate may be given for tetany.

Tetracycline, 1 g daily for five days, shortens the duration of diarrhoea and also clears the stool of vibrios in the case of the *El tor* biotype. If given, tetracycline should be started several hours after rehydration therapy has begun. However, there is clear evidence that the *El tor* vibrio rapidly develops resistance not only to tetracycline, but also several other antibiotics and it is doubtful whether it should be used in an epidemic.

Prognosis

If cholera is adequately treated there should be no mortality and complete recovery occurs. However, a suggestion has been made that such patients might be predisposed to α-chain disease [1] (see p. 655).

Other acute infective conditions

Until very recently the cause of the vast majority of acute infective conditions involving the small intestine in the tropics was unknown. During the last few years several agents have been identified, although in some cases their true significance is still unknown [47]. Advances in virology have shown that several viruses, especially the rotavirus, are of immense importance in acute diarrhoeal disease—especially in infants from six months to three years [12] (see Chapter 47).

With all of the infections, the vicious combination of gastroenteritis and malnutrition is of paramount importance, espe-

cially in children in developing Third World countries. Malnutrition probably renders the intestinal mucosa more vulnerable to infection.

The small intestine is protected against bacterial infection by gastric acid [18] and by intestinal motility; if either or both of those mechanisms are compromised, increased bacterial proliferation occurs. Low serum iron, extremely common in most Third World populations, also exerts a protective effect against some bacterial infections.

With most infections there is some mucosal invasion: few infections with exception of some *E. coli* and cholera, produce their effects through an enterotoxin alone. Consequently the brush border and its enzymes are often affected [12]. Disaccharidase deficiencies are discussed in Chapters 47 and 77.

Travellers' diarrhoea [14]

Undoubtedly the most common acute infection of the gastrointestinal tract in the context of tropical exposure is travellers' diarrhoea (Basrah belly, Casablanca crud, Delhi belly, Emporiatric diarrhoea, Gyppi tummy, G.I. trots, Ho Chi Minhs, Hong Kong dog, Montezuma's revenge, Simla trots, Rangoon runs, Turista, etc.) [76]. It occurs sporadically and also in epidemics. Although there are several known causative agents, including rotavirus and in a minority *Salmonella* spp and *Shigella* spp, the usual agents are 'foreign' serotypes of *Escherichia coli* which are enterotoxigenic (27, 36, 56, 71, 80). The pathogenesis is similar to that in cholera.

Clinically, there is sudden onset of diarrhoea with nausea, vomiting and abdominal colic. Fever is unusual. Untreated, the disease is self-limiting, lasting from one to three days.

In a straightforward case, investigation is not needed [32]. However, stool samples should be examined if there is any suggestion that a more pathogenic organism is the cause (for example, prolonged symptoms or bloody diarrhoea).

The differential diagnosis is from all other causes of infective diarrhoea of acute onset (see section on cholera, p. 640).

Prevention can be partly accomplished with antibiotics [26]. Neomycin, doxycycline, trimethoprim (either alone, or combined with sulfamethoxazole) and Streptotriad (streptomycin 65 mg, sulphadiazine 100 mg and sulphathiazole 100 mg) have all been used successfully [27]. However, many causative organisms are resistant to several antibiotics and widespread use of antibiotics prophylactically encourages further resistant strains. Routine antibiotic prophylaxis is thus not indicated; it should be reserved for specific cases, for example airline pilots, politicians or businessmen. 'Vioform' and 'Enterovioform' are potentially toxic and should not be used. The mainstay of prophylaxis should be common sense methods of avoiding infection—care taken to sterilize drinking water, milk, fruit and vegetables. Shellfish and ice cream should be viewed with particular suspicion [81].

For treatment of an attack, oral rehydration, as in a cholera infection, is important and, co-trimoxazole (trimethoprim 160 mg plus sulfamethoxazole 800 mg twice daily for 5 days), trimethoprim 200 mg twice daily for 5 days, bicozamycin 500 mg 6-hourly for 3 days and other antibiotics are of value [28, 30]. Diphenoxylate, loperamide or codeine phosphate may be used symptomatically; however, by slowing peristalsis they probably encourage intraluminal bacterial proliferation [33].

Other causes of bacterial food poisoning [47]

The lay term 'food poisoning' covers any gastrointestinal disturbance causally related to a contaminated dietary constituent, which might be a bacterial, viral, or parasitic, or even an organic or inorganic toxin, and also food intolerances and allergies. In this section those causes associated with bacterial contamination of foodstuffs are considered. Their action results from toxin-producing and invasive properties.

Aetiology

In epidemic infantile enteritis and also in adults certain serotypes of *Escherichia coli* are responsible for symptoms in the same way as they are in travellers' diarrhoea. The two enterotoxins produced by the organism are classified as 'heat-labile' (LT) and 'heat-stable' (ST); the former is more likely to produce diarrhoea in children by activating adenyl cyclase in the same way as *Vibrio cholerae* (see Chapter 77). Many are antibiotic resistant [39]. Genes coding for enterotoxin production and antibiotic resistance are frequently transferred together; widespread use of antibiotics will thus increase the prevalence of enterotoxigenic strains.

Staphylococcal food poisoning consists of an acute illness usually with vomiting, but no fever. The incubation period is from one to eight hours and recovery normally occurs in 24–48 hours. It frequently occurs in groups of people who have eaten a contaminated meal. The heat-stable enterotoxin of *Staphylococcus aureus* is usually transmitted through contaminated meat and dairy or bakery produce. Fatal cases have been recorded, but are rare.

Rewarmed or cold cooked meat dishes are usually responsible for *Clostridium welchii* food poisoning. Enteropathogenic strains produce an enterotoxin. Diarrhoea is usually more prominent than vomiting. Fever is unusual. The incubation period is usually 8–16 hours and recovery occurs in one to four days. Of greater importance is *C. botulinum*, which grows readily in tinned and vacuum-packed foods which have been badly prepared. An exotoxin which blocks neuromuscular function is absorbed from the upper small intestine. Neurological signs—diplopia, dysphagia, dysphonia—predominate; respiratory and pharyngeal paralysis are important complications. Vomiting is often present. Incubation is from 24–96 hours and there is a high mortality rate. *C. botulinum* has been implicated as one of the causes of the sudden infant death syndrome [74].

Campylobacter enteritis has recently been shown to be common in children and adults, in the West and Third World [2, 78]. This is a large group of vibrio-like organisms, with several serotypes. There is good evidence that reservoirs of infection exist in many animal species including dogs and birds. Water is also a source of infection. The incubation period is 2–10 days. Diarrhoea and vomiting are usual and there may be a fever. Colonic involvement also occurs and dysentery may result (see Chapter 57).

Food poisoning by *Vibrio parahaemolyticus* and other non-*Cholera vibrios*, *Salmonella* spp and *Shigella* spp present as mild forms of the diseases associated with the more virulent organisms with which they are related (see also Chapter 57). In many cases the illnesses are indistinguishable from travellers' diarrhoea [12]. In fact, *V. parahaemolyticus* is the major cause of travellers' diarrhoea in Bangkok [75].

Anthrax involving the small intestine resulting from poorly cooked meat from infected cattle, sheep or goats is occasionally responsible for food poisoning in the Third World. The resulting enteritis may be severe and resembles **enteritis necroticans** (see below).

Management

Bacteriological examination of faeces and food should always be carried out. Treatment of bacterial food poisoning should be firstly by fluid replacement as in cholera [10]. Antibiotics should be avoided except in severely ill patients. Symptomatic treatment is similar to that used in cholera (see above). In severe *Campylobacter* infections erythromycin 500 mg 6-hourly for 7 days should be given; if septicaemia is present gentamicin is the therapeutic agent of choice. In *C. botulinum* infections, trivalent botulinus antitoxin should be given and the neurological complications treated on their merits; other people who may have eaten the same food should be contacted urgently.

Enteritis necroticans

This acute small intestinal infection also known as 'pig-bel' disease, is caused by the B toxin of heat sensitive type C strains of *C. welchii*; it is a much more severe illness than food poisoning caused by that organism. It has been reported from a number of tropical countries, most notably Papua New Guinea, but also Uganda, Thailand and Singapore [12]. A similar disease, termed 'Darmbrand' was recognized in Germany at the end of the second World War.

Although adults may be affected, children are more severely involved, with a substantial mortality rate. In Papua New Guinea, the disease is most common in the Highlands and has been associated with pig feasts at which partly cooked meat is handled under unhygienic conditions and eaten over subsequent weeks. The disease seems to have some association with malnutrition and it has been suggested that a low concentration of digestive proteases in the small intestinal lumen may allow the clostridial toxin to cause the disease. Severity of the disease varies from acute diarrhoea to a severe dysenteric-like illness with extensive necrosis of the small and to a lesser extent large intestine. Vomiting, abdominal distension, dehydration, toxaemia and shock are serious complications. The disease should be differentiated from other causes of food poisoning, amoebic colitis, intestinal obstruction, peritonitis, pancreatitis, hepatic abscess, mesenteric adenitis and sickle-cell crisis. Gaseous distension and fluid levels may be visible on a straight abdominal radiograph; a neutrophil leukocytosis is usual.

Specific immunization in population groups likely to be affected against type C *C. welchii* has been shown to give significant protection. Treatment of the disease is initially with fluid replacement; gastric suction may be necessary. Chloramphenicol and tetracycline should be given. Type-C gas-gangrene serum should also be given. If there is no improvement, a laparotomy is indicated; resection of necrotic intestine may be necessary [49]. Mortality rate is up to 80%. Long-term sequelae include strictures, fistulae and a malabsorption state [12].

Malabsorption in the tropics [12]

Small intestinal morphology in a developing country differs from that in a temperate area. Finger-shaped villi are very unusual and leaves and ridges dominate the dissecting microscopic appearance (*tropical enteropathy*). The likely cause is luminal contamination with viruses, bacteria and to a lesser extent parasites. Changes are more severe in people from low socio-economic groups. That situation is the norm for people in Third World countries and it does not seem to be a predisposing factor in post-infective tropical malabsorption [12] which is associated with mild absorptive changes (subclinical malabsorption) affecting xylose and B_{12}. However, clinical steatorrhoea is very unusual in tropical countries, perhaps as a result of low dietary fat intake. Although the diminished absorptive area resulting from tropical enteropathy accounts for some of this mild malabsorption, other factors such as folate deficiency and systemic bacterial infections are clearly related to it. Owing to the vast functional reserve of the small intestine and increasing recognition that the colon has the capacity to absorb considerable amounts of protein and carbohydrate (as volatile fatty acids), the nutritional importance of subclinical malabsorption is unclear.

Table 43.1. Major causes of malabsorption in a tropical environment.

Digestive disorders	
Pancreatic	Chronic calcific pancreatitis
Bile salt deficiency	Acute and chronic liver disease
	Ileal tuberculosis
	Trauma to ileum
Absorptive disorders	
Short bowel syndrome	Trauma or surgery
Bacterial colonization of small intestine	Post-infective tropical malabsorption (tropical sprue)
	Severe Kwashiorkor
	Blind loop syndrome (Chapter 44)
Viral and bacterial infections	Viral hepatitis, measles, rotavirus
	Ileocaecal tuberculosis
	Pig-bel disease
Parasitic infections	*Giardia lamblia*, *Strongyloides stercoralis*, *Capillaria philippinensis*, coccidia, cryptosporidium, Kala-azar, acute *Plasmodium falciparum* malaria
Lymphomas	
Venous and lymphatic obstruction	Right-sided endomyocardial fibrosis, constrictive pericarditis, idiopathic tropical cardiomyopathy, filariasis
Isolated malabsorption	
Hypolactasia	Primary (genetic) or secondary to diseases under *absorptive disorders*

Table 43.1 summarizes the major causes of overt malabsorption in tropical countries, but it must be emphasized that all causes of malabsorption in temperate areas (including gluten-induced enteropathy) must also be considered, for many of them also exist in the tropics. The best known condition has for long been known as 'tropical sprue', [11] but post-infective tropical malabsorption may be a better name [15].

Post-infective tropical malabsorption—tropical sprue [12, 15]

Epidemiology

The disease is usually one of young adults, but it is unusual in childhood. The sex ratio seems to be equal. Although most cases are associated with tropical exposure, a minority appear in people who have always lived in sub-tropical or even temperate climates [58]. It may be endemic or epidemic (in South India) [5]. The geographical distribution is of great interest (Fig. 43.2). Although common in the Indian subcontinent, Southeast Asia and the central Americas, post-infective tropical malabsorption is very unusual in the continent of Africa. Reports from Lagos (Nigeria), Durban (South Africa) and Harare (Zimbabwe) suggest that the disease probably exists there, but is less severe than in many patients reported from Asia [12].

There seems little doubt that the overall incidence correlates geographically to some extent with the incidence of underlying acute diarrhoeal disease.

Aetiology [15]

Genetic factors might be important. Some individuals seem to be predisposed and suffer repeated attacks. No ethnic group is exempt; Europeans and Asians in Africa rarely get the disease, but they do in Asia. Africans living in Africa, or Asia seem to be less protected.

The pathophysiology is still not clear and it may well be that it is different, or at least has different triggering mechanisms, in different geographical locations. Most cases clearly start with an acute diarrhoeal attack. In most the attack probably constitutes travellers' diarrhoea, although in some dysentery may be present. Persisting bacterial overgrowth within the small intestinal lumen has been demonstrated conclusively [82]. *Klebsiella pneumoniae, Enterobacter cloacae* and *Escherichia coli* are the predominant bacteria. Adherence of bacteria to enterocytes might be important. The reason for persisting colonization after an acute diarrhoeal episode in a small minority of people is unknown. However, demonstration of delayed small intestinal transit and its correlation with a high circulating plasma enteroglucagon concentra-

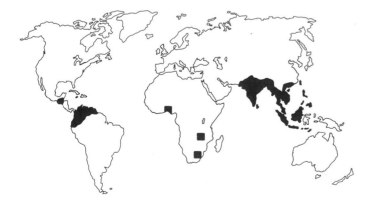

Fig. 43.2. Geographical distribution of post-infective tropical malabsorption (tropical sprue) showing areas principally affected by the disease.

tion may be relevant [7]. It is possible enteroglucagon (which probably has trophic
properties) is liberated in response to mucosal injury—especially in the ileal region
where the most severe changes in post-infective tropical malabsorption exist—and
that it slows small intestinal transit [12].
Whether such a sequence of events
accounts for all cases of tropical malabsorption is unknown; there might even be a
number of syndromes under one umbrella
diagnosis. Fig. 43.3 summarizes the possible pathogenesis: as the disease progresses, the serum folate concentration decreases and that might be an exacerbating
factor in preventing mucosal repair. The
role of the colon in post-infective tropical
malabsorption has recently been studied;
abnormal absorptive function is clearly of
importance [67]. There is no evidence that
immunological factors are of any importance in the pathophysiology of this disease
[70].

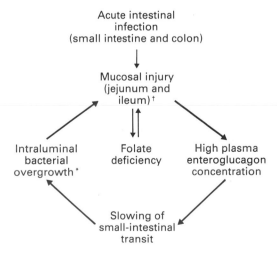

* Decreased by oral
  tetracyline
† Improved by oral folic acid

Fig. 43.3. Hypothetical explanation of the
pathophysiology of post-infective tropical
malabsorption (tropical sprue).

Pathology

As the disease progresses **partial villous
atrophy** occurs, but it is unusual to find a
flat jejunal mucosa. The changes do not
correlate well with the severity of malabsorption. At post-mortem, there is gross
emaciation with loss of subcutaneous
tissue; the bone-marrow shows megaloblastic erythropoiesis and the myocardium
brown pigmentation.

Clinical features

The dominant feature is persisting diarrhoea after an acute gastrointestinal infection. The stools become bulky, pale and
fatty. These symptoms are often made
worse by milk because of secondary hypolactasia [16]. Weight loss is progressive and
is worsened by anorexia. Anaemia, hypoproteinaemia, oedema, glossitis and occasionally vitamin A deficiency follow.
Aphthous ulceration, although common in
most old reports of tropical sprue is now
unusual [11]. Tiredness is common. In
children, in whom tropical malabsorption is
unusual, growth failure—affecting weight
more than height—is common. Untreated,
the disease has an appreciable mortality
after several months duration.

Investigation

Folate deficient megaloblastic anaemia is
progressive and is usually apparent some
four to six months after onset. Tests of small
intestinal mucosal absorption—xylose,
three-day faecal fat, Schilling test—are abnormal. Serum folate and red blood cell B_{12}
concentrations are diminished late in the
disease; B_{12} depletion is largely a result of
luminal bacterial activity. In a severely ill
patient the transaminases may be elevated
and hypoalbuminaemia is usual. Hypogammaglobulinaemia has occasionally
been documented. Microbiology of luminal

fluid reveals bacterial colonization (see Chapter 44). Intestinal parasites should be excluded by stool examination, the string-test (see below) and jejunal biopsy. No immunological abnormalities have been reported. Histological abnormalities consisting of a semi-flat mucosa and lymphatic infiltration have been described—they are more marked in the ileum than jejunum. A barium follow-through shows dilated loops of small intestine with clumping of barium.

Differential diagnosis

This involves all causes of malabsorption associated with tropical exposure (Table 43.1), as well as all the causes in a temperate climate.

Prevention

Avoidance of acute gastrointestinal infection in a tropical country is probably relevant. Drugs that slow small intestinal transit (diphenoxylate, codeine phosphate and loperamide) seem to be best avoided for they might encourage luminal bacterial overgrowth.

Treatment

A good diet is important. Tetracycline 250 mg three times a day for four weeks decreases the small intestinal bacterial flora and may break a vicious cycle (Fig. 43.3). Folic acid 5 mg three times a day for four weeks repletes folate stores and encourages mucosal regeneration. Diarrhoea and stool weight decrease and biochemical tests of absorption return towards normal. If intestinal parasites have been demonstrated they should be treated on their merits. Lactose intolerance may continue to be a problem for several weeks or months until enterocyte regeneration is complete, hence a milk-free diet may help symptomatic recovery.

Properly treated, there should be no mortality, although recurrences may occasionally happen.

Salmonellosis—typhoid fever

Typhoid fever is the most severe illness caused by the *Salmonella* organisms, which consist of three main species—*Salmonella typhi*, *S. enteritidis* (*S. paratyphi A* and *S. typhimurium* are examples) and *S. cholerasuis*. Systemic illnesses result, but the brunt of the insult falls on the ileum; the lymphoid aggregations (Peyer's patches) are primarily involved. Severity of disease seems to vary in different areas; sickle-cell trait probably increases susceptibility.

Epidemiology

The disease is endemic in most tropical countries. Epidemics also occur, usually due to contamination of water supplies, but also due to infected food—milk, poultry, shellfish and watercress. Each year approximately 200 patients in England and Wales have typhoid fever [64]. *S. paratyphi* infections are usually caused by contaminated food. Carriers excrete the organisms for long periods; organisms usually survive in the gallbladder and urinary tract. The disease is more common following gastrectomy. Peak incidence is between 10 and 35 years. It is a notifiable infectious illness—contacts should be kept under surveillance for three weeks.

Aetiology

The causative organisms are Gram-negative, actively motile bacilli. They grow between 4 and 36°C and are killed by rapid boiling and exposure to 60°C for 15 min. They are invasive and do not produce an enterotoxin. They thus resemble colonic rather than small intestinal organisms (see Chapter 57). Following ingestion, multiplication takes place in the second part of the duodenum—where bile forms a good culture medium. Following a septicaemia and widespread organ involvement, the organisms produce severe ileal disease including ulcers in the Peyer's patches. Although the ileum receives the brunt of the attack, lesions as high as the jejunum and in the ascending colon are reported.

Pathology

In the intestine changes can be divided into four stages—hyperaemia, necrosis, ulceration and healing; they correspond roughly to the chronological stages of the disease in weeks. Ulcers are oval (up to 3 or 4 cm in length) lying on the long axis of the ileum. Although usually separate, they may become confluent. Edges are soft, raised and undermined; the floor contains necrotic greenish-black slough. Scarring is minimal and healing is not followed by fibrosis or stricture formation. During the septicaemic phase, all organs can be involved, and pneumonia, lung abscess, myocarditis, pericarditis, parotitis, arthritis, periostitis, osteomyelitis, spondylitis, meningitis, orchitis, peripheral neuropathy, cholecystitis and thrombophlebitis are all recognized complications. Additional complications include hepatocellular jaundice, toxic nephrosis, haemolytic-uraemic syndrome and neuropsychiatric manifestations [12]. The disease tends to be worse in patients with sickle cell disease.

Clinical features [46]

The incubation period is from five to 21 days—usually between 10 and 14 days. Onset is insidious, with a temperature rising in 'step-ladder' fashion over four or five days. There is usually a relative bradycardia which is of great diagnostic value [77]. General constitutional symptoms are prominent. Constipation is usual, although diarrhoea occasionally occurs. At the end of the first week a rash, consisting of 'rosespots', may be seen over the trunk. Soft splenomegaly is often present during the second week. Diarrhoea of small intestinal type is usual although faeces may contain blood. If untreated, severe toxaemia, coma and death may supervene in the third week. Haemorrhage or perforation usually occur in the third week [8, 9]. Relapse one or two weeks later is possible. Paratyphoid fever and other *Salmonella* infections are usually of lesser severity, have a shorter mean incubation period and fewer complications.

Investigations

During the first week blood cultures and more importantly bone marrow culture yield the highest positivity rates [42, 72]. Stool and urine cultures are often positive in the second week. A leucopenia with a relative lymphocytosis is common. Serology is of limited value especially in a tropical setting; previous typhoid immunization should be taken into account when interpreting results. Serology is often positive in the presence of chronic liver disease—probably due to impaired sequestration of antigens by Kupffer cells. Liver function tests are frequently abnormal. Abdominal radiography may show gas under the diaphragm if perforation has occurred.

Differential diagnosis

All causes of disturbed gastrointestinal function (including perforation and haemorrhage) and all causes of pyrexia of undetermined origin [48] should be considered. Apart from the history and major physical findings, a relative bradycardia is valuable in diagnosis.

Prevention

Partial protection is provided by monovalent TAB vaccine. It should be boosted every three years. New oral vaccines are undergoing clinical trials [19]. Basic precautions with drinking water and food (especially fresh fruit and vegetables) as in travellers' diarrhoea are of greater importance [23].

Treatment [19]

The best antibiotic is chloramphenicol —4 g daily for two weeks for an adult [37]. The patient's response is usually dramatic and the temperature falls to normal three to five days after starting treatment. Bone marrow depression due to chloramphenicol, although extremely uncommon, has been reported. Co-trimoxazole 2 tablets twice daily for 14 days and ampicillin 500 mg four times daily for 14 days are also effective. However, resistance to all three agents, especially chloramphenicol, is now common —especially in Third World countries. Schistosomal infections should be treated before an antibiotic is given in the acute disease.

Haemorrhage is treated by blood transfusion. Perforation should probably be treated surgically [8, 9]. However, conservative management is often recommended—with either regime mortality rates are high.

Six negative stool and three negative urine cultures are required ideally before a patient can be declared to be free of the disease. In the carrier state, amoxycillin 2 g three times a day for 28 days gives good results.

Chronic bacterial infections [56, 67]

By far the most common is tuberculosis of the ileocaecal region (Chapter 47). However, the small intestine can be mildly involved in leprosy, [13].

Small intestinal parasites

Many parasites—protozoa, nematodes, trematodes and cestodes, inhabit the human small intestine [21]. Some are pathogenic and can cause severe disease, particularly *Giardia lamblia* and *Ankylostoma duodenale*. However, the spectrum is broad and moderately heavy infection can be present without clinical manifestations [12, 16]. While some parasites exert their pathogenic effect by ingesting the blood of their host, others prevent absorption of dietary nutrients. In both cases nutritional status, so often on a knife-edge in Third World populations, is made worse.

Parasites not associated with malabsorption

Hookworm (Ankylostoma duodenale *and* Necator americanus)

These helminthic infections are very common in Third World countries [86], but only heavy infections are important—iron deficiency anaemia and hypoalbuminaemia. The life cycles are complex: following entry through intact skin—usually bare feet, the larvae traverse the lungs and the adults emerge in the proximal jejunum. It has been estimated that a single *A. duodenale* can withdraw 0.2 ml and a *N. americanus* 0.05 ml blood daily—if 100 worms are present the blood loss is substantial.

Diagnosis is by finding ova in the faeces, or adult worms in the duodenal or jejunal fluid. There may be a peripheral eosinophilia during the invasive stage.

Treatment is aimed first at correcting the anaemia with either oral or injectable iron; in exceptional circumstances blood transfusion is necessary, but overloading the circulation must be carefully avoided. Several agents are used in treatment—albendazole 400 mg single dose, bephenium hydroxynaphthoate (Alcopar) 5 g orally on three consecutive days, or tetrachlorethylene

0.12 ml per kg (max dose 5 ml) which is far cheaper. Pyrantel embonate, mebendazole (Vermox—100 mg twice daily for three consecutive days), or levamisole (Ketrax) also give satisfactory results.

Roundworm (Ascaris lumbricoides)

This is also a very common infection in Third World countries [29, 86]. Ova do not require tropical conditions to survive and are ingested before the larvae emerge (unlike hookworm). Following a complex cycle, adults (up to 40 cm in length) are produced in the jejunal lumen. Most patients are asymptomatic. Major gastrointestinal complications are due to intestinal obstruction, usually in children, or obstruction in the common bile duct, pancreatic duct, appendix and other diverticula.

Demonstration of ova in faeces is the usual method of diagnosis, although adult worms are occasionally passed *per rectum*. Adult worms are occasionally outlined during barium meal examinations.

Treatment is with one of the piperazine compounds; 75 mg/kg (maximum dose 4 g) usually gives a satisfactory cure. Albendazole or mebendazole in the same dose regimes as for hookworm disease also give good results. Other agents used for hookworm disease are also usually effective.

Other nematode infections [51]

Ternidens diminutus, Gnathostoma spinigerum, Trichinella spiralis and *Trichostrongylus orientalis* may also be present, but rarely cause gastrointestinal symptoms [12].

Fasciolopsiasis (Fasciolopsis buski *infection*)

This large fleshy trematode, together with related species is relatively common in Southeast Asia and the Indian subcontinent. While mild gastrointestinal symptoms are common, serious complications are rare, unless infection is heavy. Ova and occasionally flukes may be found in stool samples. Treatment is with praziquantel 25 mg/kg orally, repeated the same day.

Other trematode infections

Schistosomiasis (*S. mansoni* and *S. japonicum*) and paragonimiasis occasionally affect the small intestine. Treatment is with praziquantel 50 mg/kg as one oral dose for an adult.

Tapeworm infections

It is most unusual for these infections to produce intestinal disease. The longest are *Taenia solium* (pork tapeworm) and *T. saginata* (beef tapeworm) which can reach a length of 10 metres. Smaller worms are *Hymenolepis nana* and *H. diminuta* and *Depanidotaemia laceolata*. The fish (*Diphyllobothrium latum*) and dog (*Dipylidium caninum*) tapeworms can also affect man.

The importance of *T. solium* infections is that cysticercosis is an important complication. Cysticerci may lodge anywhere in the body, but the most common areas are brain and skeletal muscle [60].

Diagnosis is by finding segments of the worms or ova in stool samples; calcified cysticerci can be visualized in radiographs of muscle masses, such as the thighs. Treatment is with mepacrine hydrochloride (Quinacrine); a total of 1 g is given, after an overnight fast, down an intraduodenal tube. Chlorpromazine or phenobarbitone should be given to prevent vomiting. Niclosamide (Yomesan) 1 g given twice one hour apart for an adult [62, 69] mebendazole and recently, praziquantel 10 mg/kg as a single oral dose have also been used.

Protozoal infections

Acute *Plasmodium falciparum* malaria is often associated with small intestinal symptoms, including diarrhoea. The mode of action is presumably through an effect of the parasites on mesenteric arterioles. Small intestinal involvement has also been recorded in visceral leishmaniasis (**Kala-azar**).

Parasites associated with malabsorption [20]

Giardiasis (G. lamblia) [35]

This infection caused by the flagellated protozoan *Giardia lamblia* can cause severe gastrointestinal symptoms which may resemble tropical malabsorption (tropical sprue). However, it may also be present without producing any symptoms whatsoever [79].

The condition is not confined to the tropics, but occurs often in epidemics the world over. It is probably the commonest parasitic infection in the UK. Infection is usually through contaminated drinking water and travellers are especially affected [40, 41]. Male homosexuals are infected by the faecal–oral route (see Chapter 57).

The method by which *G. lamblia* causes intestinal disease is unclear [3]. Bacterial overgrowth, as in tropical malabsorption (tropical sprue), is also present. As the parasite descends the gastrointestinal tract it encysts.

Clinical presentation is with acute diarrhoea and excessive flatus after a mean incubation period of approximately two weeks. If malabsorption complicates the picture, bulky, pale, offensive stools and weight loss also occur. Symptoms may persist for several months.

Trophozoites of *G. lamblia* (Fig. 43.4) can be identified in jejunal fluid, in peroral small intestinal biopsies, or by the string-test (see below) [37]. Appearance of trophozoites in

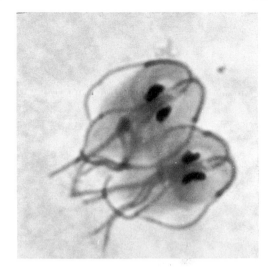

Fig. 43.4. Trophozoites of *Giardia lamblia* in jejunal fluid.

the stool is erratic and cysts are found more frequently. An enzyme-linked immunosorbent assay (ELISA) for the detection of *Giardia* antigen in the faeces has been described [38]. Malabsorption of varying degree can be demonstrated as in tropical malabsorption.

Treatment is with metronidazole 2 g daily on three consecutive days or tinidazole in a single dose of 2 g [21]. Alcohol should be avoided during treatment as nausea, confusion and psychoses are occasionally troublesome if that rule is not obeyed. Mepacrine is an alternative drug.

Strongyloidiasis (S. stercoralis)

Although present throughout tropical countries, infections are most common in Southeast Asia and West Africa. As with *G. lamblia*, although some infections are associated with malabsorption, many are asymptomatic.

Infection is usually due to larvae penetrating intact human skin, although it is occasionally by mouth. Following a complex life cycle, the ova reach the proximal small intestine where they can be found in

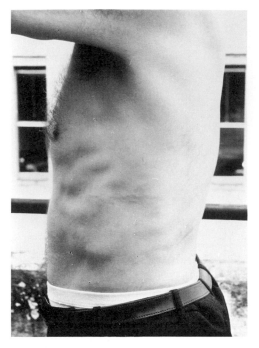

Fig. 43.5. Larva migrans rash caused by *Strongyloides stercoralis* on the trunk of a 64-year-old man who had been a prisoner-or-war in South-east Asia during the Second World War.

syndrome in which larvae are present throughout the body is a serious and sometimes fatal complication.

Mild abdominal symptoms may begin several weeks after infection, and malabsorption is a complication. However, in many patients a recurrent skin eruption on the abdomen, back and buttocks is the only clinical abnormality (Fig. 43.5). Respiratory symptoms also occur during the migratory phase.

The best diagnostic technique is the string-test (or 'entero-test'. A gelatin capsule to which a nylon line is attached is swallowed after an overnight fast; after 3–4 hours the line is withdrawn and the mucus adherent to the distal end is examined for parasites on a microscope slide. Occasionally larvae are present in stool samples (Fig. 43.6). Serological tests for filariasis are often positive—due to cross-reaction with the antigen. A transient eosinophilia (often gross) is common.

Treatment is with thiabendazole (Mintezol) 25 mg/kg twice daily (maximum dose 3 g daily) for three days. Mebendazole has also been used with good effect but is probably inferior to thiabendazole.

the mucosa or crypts. Because auto-infection can occur due to re-entry of larvae around the anal region, infection may persist for several decades [34]. In immunosuppressed individuals a hyperinfection

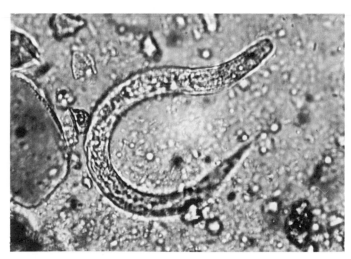

Fig. 43.6. Larva of *Strongyloides stercoralis* in faecal specimen.

S. fülleborni

S. fülleborni gives rise to malabsorption in Zambia and Papua New Guinea. Children are usually affected more severely than adults.

Capillaria philippinensis

This nematode has been clearly associated with diarrhoea and malabsorption in the northern Philippines and Thailand. Epidemics have been recorded. It is contracted by eating various species of marine fish. Thiabendazole and mebendazole have both been used therapeutically but in long courses— the former 12.5 mg/kg twice daily for 30 days, and the latter 100 mg four times a day for 20 days.

Protozoa

Isospora belli, Sarcocystis hominis and *Cryptosporidium* [22, 80] have been incriminated in diarrhoea and malabsorption, especially in immunosuppressed individuals (see Chapter 57). They seem to be more common in tropical compared with temperate areas [48]. Cysts may be found in faecal samples, but they are usually scanty.

Treatment is unnecessary for healthy patients, but spiramycin has given encouraging results in some immunosupressed patients, including those with AIDS [65].

Alpha-chain disease (Mediterranean lymphoma)

Diffuse lympho-plasmacytic proliferation is sometimes associated with alpha heavy chains in the serum and other biological fluids [12, 49].

The disease occurs over much of the tropics, but is especially common in the Middle East and northern and southern Africa [1]. It affects particularly young adults of low socio-economic groups. It affects both sexes equally.

Aetiology is unknown. It has been suggested that chronic infections and genetic influences are important [49]. Chronic diarrhoea in infancy and immune abnormalities have also been postulated. Alpha-chain disease usually involves the upper jejunum, where bacterial infections are common. Exposure to the enterotoxin of *Vibrio cholerae* may be important [1].

Small intestinal biopsy shows that lympho-plasmacytic proliferation is usually limited to the lamina propria [68], and although enterocytes are intact, villous atrophy is often present. In advanced disease immature plasma cells cross the muscularis mucosa. Mesenteric lymph gland involvement is common, but involvement of major abdominal organs is late. Multicentric tumour masses are present later.

The patient presents with chronic diarrhoea, abdominal pain, severe malabsorption, finger clubbing and, late in the disease, small intestinal obstruction.

Alpha-chains can be detected in the sera of most patients. Hypoalbuminaemia and a raised serum alkaline phosphatase concentration are common. Immunoglobulins IgG and IgM are usually diminished. Radiologically, the upper small intestine can be shown to have an abnormal mucosa.

Treatment is with tetracycline. If started early, prognosis is relatively good. Cytotoxic agents have also been used.

References

1 AL-SALEEM TI. Evidence of acquired immune deficiencies in Mediterranean lymphoma. A possible aetiological link. *Lancet* 1978;ii:709–712.
2 ANONYMOUS. Campylobacter enteritis. *Lancet* 1982;ii:1437–1438.
3 ANONYMOUS. Battles against giardia in gut mucosa. *Lancet* 1982;ii:527–528.
4 ARCHAMPONG EQ. Tropical diseases of the small bowel. *World J Surg* 1985;9:887–896.
5 BAKER SJ. Idiopathic small intestinal disease in the tropics. In: Chandra RK, ed. *Critical reviews in tropical medicine.* New York. 1. Plenum Publishing Co. 1982:197–245.
6 BARUA D, BURROWS W. In: Barua D, Burrows W,

eds. *Cholera.* Philadelphia, London, Toronto: WB Saunders, 1974.

7 BESTERMAN HS, COOK GC, SARSON DL, *et al.* Gut hormones in tropical malabsorption. *Br Med J* 1979;2:1252–1255.

8 BITAR R, TARPLEY J. Intestinal perforation in typhoid fever: a historical and state-of-the-art review. *Rev Infect Dis* 1985;7:257–271.

9 BUTLER T, KNIGHT J, NATH SK, SPEELMAN P, ROY SK, AZAD MAK. Typhoid fever complicated by intestinal perforation: a persisting fatal disease requiring surgical management. *Rev Infect Dis* 1985;7:244–256.

10 CARPENTER CCJ. Oral rehydration. Is it as good as parenteral therapy? *New Engl J Med* 1982; 306:1103–1104.

11 COOK GC. Tropical sprue: implications of Manson's concept. *J Roy Coll Phys* 1978;12:329–349.

12 COOK GC. *Tropical gastroenterology.* Oxford, New York, Delhi: Oxford, 1980.

13 COOK GC. Xylose absorption in Papua New Guineans with leprosy. *Acta Tropica* 1982;39:91–96.

14 COOK GC. Travellers' diarrhoea—an insoluble problem. *Gut* 1983;24:1105–1108.

15 COOK GC. Aetiology and pathogenesis of postinfective tropical malabsorption (tropical sprue). *Lancet* 1984;i:721–723.

16 COOK GC. Hypolactasia: geographical distribution, diagnosis, and practical significance. In: Chandra RK, ed. *Critical reviews in tropical medicine, 2.* New York, London: Plenum Press, 1984:117–139

17 COOK GC. Parasitic infection. In: Booth CC, Neale, G. eds. *Disorders of the small intestine.* Oxford: Blackwell Scientific Publications, 1985:283–298.

18 COOK GC. Infective gastroenteritis and its relationship to reduced gastric acidity. *Scand J Gastroent* 1985;20(Suppl 11): 17–23.

19 COOK GC. Management of typhoid. *Trop Doctor* 1985;15154–159.

20 COOK GC. Intestinal parasitic infections. *Curr Opinion Gastroent* 1986;2:118–124.

21 DAVIDSON RA. Issues in clinical parasitology: the treatment of giardiasis. *Am J Gastroenterol* 1984;79:256–261.

22 DEG PC, DUNN JC, FEDERMAN M. Infections caused by intestinal protozoa. *Pathol Annu* 1985;20:463–505.

23 DICK G, GALBRAITH NS, GORTON D. Typhoid vaccine, for whom? *Lancet* 1982;i:970–971.

24 DONOVAN TJ, FURNISS AL. Quality of antisera used in the diagnosis of cholera. *Lancet* 1982;ii:866–868.

25 DUPONT HL. Cryptosporidiosis and the healthy host. *New Engl J Med* 1985;312:1319–1320.

26 DUPONT HL, ERICSSON CD, JOHNSON PC. Chemotherapy and chemoprophylaxis of travelers' diarrhea. *Ann Intern Med* 1985;102:260–261.

27 DUPONT HL, GALINDO E, EVANS DG, CABADA FJ, SULLIVAN P, EVANS DJ. Prevention of travelers' diar-

rhea with trimethoprim-sulfamethoxazole and trimethoprim alone. *Gastroenterology* 1983;84:75–80.

28 DUPONT HL, REVES RR, GALINDO E, SULLIVAN PS, WOOD LV, MENDIOLA JG. Treatment of travelers' diarrhoea with trimethoprim-sulfamethoxazole and with trimethoprim alone. *New Engl J Med* 1982;307:841–844.

29 EDITORIAL. Ascaris infections. *Lancet* 1985;ii:1284.

30 ERICSSON CD, DUPONT HL, SULLIVAN P, GALINDO E, EVANS DG, EVANS DJ. Bicozamycin, a poorly absorbable antibiotic, effectively treats travelers' diarrhea. *Ann Intern Med* 1983;98:20–25.

31 FEACHEM RG. Environmental aspects of cholera epidemiology. 1. A review of selected reports of endemic and epidemic situations during 1961–1980. *Trop Dis Bull* 1981;78:675–698.

32 GEDDES AM. 'I have been back from holiday for a week and still have diarrhoea'. *Br Med J* 1983;287:513.

33 GERTLER S, PRESSMAN J, CARTWRIGHT C, DHARMSATHAPHORN K. Management of acute diarrhoea. *J Clin Gastroenterol* 1983;5:523–534.

34 GILL GV, BELL DR. Longstanding tropical infections amongst former war prisoners of the Japanese. *Lancet* 1982;i:958–959.

35 GILLON J. Giardiasis: review of epidemiology, pathogenetic mechanisms and host responses. *Q J Med* 1984;53:29–39.

36 GORBACH SL. Travelers' diarrhea. *New Engl J Med* 1982;307:881–883.

37 GORDTS B, RETORÉ P, CANRANEL S, HEMELHOF W, RAHMAN M, BUTZLER JP. Routine culture of *Giardia lamblia* trophozoites from human duodenal aspirates. *Lancet* 1984;ii:137–138.

38 GREEN EL, MILES MA, WARHURST DC. Immunodiagnostic detection of gardia antigen in faeces by a rapid visual enzyme-linked immunosorbent assay. *Lancet* 1985;ii:691–693.

39 GROSS RJ, WARD LR, THRELFALL EJ, KING H, ROWE B. Drug resistance among infantile entropathogenic *Escherichia coli* strains isolated in the United Kingdom. *Br Med J* 1982;285:472–473.

40 HAMILTON SR, KEREN DF, BOITNOTT JK, ROBERTSON SM, YARDLEY JH. Enhancement by cholera toxin of IgA secretion from intestinal crypt epithelium. *Gut* 1980;21:365–369.

41 HERZOG C, GEDDES AM. Chloramphenicol in the treatment of enteric fever. *Trans R Soc Trop Med Hyg* 1982;76:848–849.

42 HOFFMAN SL, PUNJABI NH, ROCKHILL RC, SUTOMO A, RIVAI AR, PULUNGSIH SP. Duodenal string-capsule culture compared with bone marrow, blood and rectal swab cultures for diagnosing typhoid and paratyphoid fever. *J Infect Dis* 1984;149:157–161.

43 HOLMBERG SD, HARRIS JR, KAY DE, *et al.* Foodborne transmission of cholera in Micronesian households. *Lancet* 1984;i:325–328.

44 JOKIPII AMM, HEMILA M, JOKIPII L. Prospective study of acquisition of cryptosporidium, giardia lamblia, and gastrointestinal illness. *Lancet* 1985;ii:487–489.

45 JOKIPII L, POHJOLA S, JOKIPII AMM. Cryptosporidiosis associated with traveling and giardiasis *Gastroenterology* 1985;89:838–842.

46 KLOTZ SA, JORGENSEN JH, BUCKWOLD FJ, CRAVEN PC. Typhoid fever: an epidemic with remarkably few clinical signs and symptoms. *Arch Intern Med* 1984;144:533–537

47 LAMBERT HP. Infections of the gastrointestinal tract. *Clin Gastroenterol* 1979;8:549–838.

48 LARSON EB, FEATHERSTONE HJ, PETERSDORF RG. Fever of undetermined origin: diagnosis and follow up of 105 cases, 1970–1980. *Medicine* (Baltimore), 1982;61:269–292.

49 LEWIN KJ, KAHN LB, NOVIS BH. Primary intestinal lymphoma of 'western' and 'Mediterranean' type, alpha chain disease and massive plasma cell infiltration. *Cancer* (NY), 1976;38:2511–2528.

50 MAHALANABIS D. Oral rehydration therapy. In: Chandra RK, ed. *Critical reviews in tropical medicine 2*. New York, London: Plenum Press, 1984:77–91.

51 MARKELL EK. Intestinal nematode infections. *Pediatr Clin North Am* 1985;32:971–986.

52 MATHAN MM, VENKATESAN S, GEORGE R, MATHEW M, MATHAN VI. Cryptosporidium and diarrhoea in Southern Indian children. *Lancet* 1985;ii:1172–1175.

53 MILLAR JS. The surgical treatment of enteritis necroticans. *Br J Surg* 1981;68:481–482.

54 MILLER CJ, DRASAR BS, FEACHEM RG. Cholera and estuarine salinity in Calcutta and London. *Lancet* 1982;i:1216–1218.

55 MILLER CJ, FEACHEM RG, DRASAR BS. Cholera epidemiology in developed and developing countries: new thoughts on transmission, seasonality and control. *Lancet* 1985;i:261–263.

56 MERSON MH, MORRIS GK, SACK DA, *et al*. Travelers' diarrhoea in Mexico. A prospective study of physicians and family members attending a congress. *New Engl J Med* 1976;294:1299–1305.

57 MOLLA AM, SARKER SA, HOSSAIN M, MOLLA A, GREENOUGH WB. Rice-powder electrolyte solution as oral therapy in diarrhoea due to Vibrio cholerae and Escherichia coli. *Lancet* 1982;i:1317–1319.

58 MONTGOMERY RD. CHESNER IM. Post-infective malabsorption in the temperate zone. *Trans R Soc Trop Med Hyg.* 1985;79:322–327.

59 MORRIS JG, BLACK RE. Cholera and other vibrioses in the United States. *New Engl J Med* 1985;312:343–350.

60 NASH TE, NEVA FA. Recent advances in the diagnosis and treatment of cerebral cysticercosis. *New Engl J Med* 1984;311:1492–1496.

61 PALMER KR, PATIL DH, BASRA NGS, RIORDAN JF, SILK DBA. Abdominal tuberculosis in urban Britain—a common disease. *Gut* 1985;26:1296–1305.

62 PEARSON RD, HEWLETT EL. Niclosamide therapy for tapeworm infections. *Ann Intern Med* 1982;102:550–551.

63 PHILLIPS RA. Water and electrolyte losses in cholera. *Fedn Proc Fedn Am Socs Exp Biol* 1964;23:705–712.

64 PHLS COMMUNICABLE DISEASE SURVEILLANCE CENTRE. Typhoid fever, England and Wales, 1978–82. *Br Med J* 1983;287:1205.

65 PORTNOY D, WHITESIDE ME, BUCKLEY E, MACLEOD CL. Treatment of intestinal cryptosporidiosis with spiramycin. *Ann Intern Med* 1984;101:202–204.

66 RABBANI GH, GREENOUGH WB, HOLMGREN J, KIRKWOOD B. Controlled trial of chlorpromazine as antisecretory agent in patients with cholera hydrated intravenously. *Br Med J* 1982;284:1361–1364.

67 RAMAKRISHNA BS, MATHAN VI. Water and electrolyte absorption by the colon in tropical sprue. *Gut* 1982;23:843–846.

68 RAMBAUD JC, SELIGMANN M. Alpha-chain disease. *Clin Gastroenterol* 1976;5:341–358.

69 RICHARDS F, SCHANTZ PM. Treatment of *Taenia solium* infections. *Lancet* 1985;i:1264–1265.

70 ROSS IN, MATHAN VI. Immunological changes in tropical sprue. *Q J Med* 1981;50:435–449.

71 ROWE B, TAYLOR J, BETTELHEIM KA. An investigation of travellers' diarrhoea. *Lancet* 1970;i:1–5.

72 SCHOFIELD PF. Abdominal tuberculosis. *Gut* 1985;26:1275–1278.

73 SNOW J. *On the mode of communication of cholera*. 2nd ed. Churchill, London, 1855.

74 SONNABEND OAR, SONNABEND WFF, KRECH U, MOLZ G, SIGRIST T. Continuous microbiological and pathological study of 70 sudden and unexpected infant deaths toxigenic intestinal *Clostridium botulinum* infection in 9 cases of sudden infant death syndrome. *Lancet* 1985;i:237–241.

75 SRIRATANABAN A, REINPRAYOON S. *Vibrio parahaemolyticus*: a major cause of travelers' diarrhea in Bangkok. *Am J Trop Med Hyg* 1982;31:128–130.

76 STEFFEN R, VAN DER LINDE F, GYR K, SCHÄR M. Epidemiology of diarrhea in travelers. *JAMA* 1983;249:1176–1180.

77 SVENUNGSSON B. Typhoid fever in a Swedish hospital for infectious disease—20-year review. *J Infect* 1982;5:139–150.

78 SYMONDS J. Campylobacter enteritis in the community. *Br Med J* 1983;286:243–244.

79 SYMPOSIUM ON GIARDIASIS. *Trans R Soc Trop Med Hyg* 1980;74:427–448.

80 TAYLOR DN, ECHEVERRIA P, BLASER MJ, *et al*. Polymicrobial aetiology of travellers' diarrhoea. *Lancet* 1985;i:381–383.

81 TAYLOR WR, SCHELL WL, WELLS JG, *et al*. A foodborne outbreak of enterotoxigenic *Escherichia coli* diarrhea. *New Engl J Med* 1982;306:1093–1095.

82 TOMKINS A. Tropical malabsorption: recent con-

cepts in pathogenesis and nutritional significance. *Clin Sci* 1981;**60**:131–137.

83 TOMKINS A, BOOTH CC. Tropical Sprue. In: Booth CC, Neale G, eds *Disorders of the small intestine.* Oxford Blackwell Scientific Publications 1985:311–332.

84 TURNBERG LA. Intestinal transport of salt and water. *Clin Sci* 1978;**54**:337–348.

85 WOLFSON JS, RICHTER JM, WALDRON MA, WEBER DJ, McCARTHY DM, HOPKINS CC. Cryptosporidiosis in immunocompetent patients. *New Engl J Med* 1985;**312**:1278–1282.

86 WHO. Intestinal protozoan and helminthic infections. *Techn Rep Ser* **666** Geneva: WHO, 1981.

Chapter 44
Bacterial Contamination of the Small Intestine

O. F. W. JAMES

The association between upper small intestinal diverticula and a characteristic group of symptoms and laboratory data, together with the abnormal growth of bacteria in this region, was established in the 1950's and 1960's [2,4]. Bacterial contamination of the small intestine can occur not only in the presence of diverticula, but also in association with many other structural abnormalities; it may also occur without any detectable structural change [9, 34]. To complicate matters, structural abnormalities may occur without detectable bacterial contamination and bacterial contamination of the upper small bowel may be present without symptoms or abnormal laboratory findings. The term 'bacterial contamination syndrome' used in this chapter implies clinical and/or biochemical evidence of ill health. Alternative terms include the blind loop syndrome, the stagnant loop syndrome and the bacterial overgrowth syndrome.

Occurrence

Small bowel diverticula

Most duodenal, jejunal and ileal diverticula are said to be acquired; they are commonest in the upper jejunum and lie along the mesenteric border in relation to the arterial blood supply, with an average diameter of 1–4 cm. The diverticula are often thin-walled and consist only of mucosa and serosa. Despite this, rupture of small intestinal diverticula is very rare. It seems probable that diverticula are true herniations of the intestinal mucosa and may arise as a result of raised intraluminal pressure in the small intestine. Small bowel diverticula have been noted in 0.3–1.4% of necropsies and their occurrence increases with increasing age [22]. One careful post-mortem study suggested that they were detectable in up to 4.6% of elderly individuals [28]. Sex distribution is equal. Not all individuals with small intestinal diverticula suffer detectable clinical or biochemical abnormalities. This is particularly true of a solitary diverticulum in the duodenum [4], although many well-documented cases are recorded of severe bacterial contamination syndrome in such patients. A single diverticulum may also be associated with biliary tract disease.

Bacterial contamination syndrome

Precise figures are not available, but the syndrome occurring with, or without a structural abnormality may be commoner than previously realized, particularly in the elderly [21] and in relation to previous gastric surgery or Crohn's disease [32].

Pathophysiology

Bacteriology

Normal flora

The normal duodenum and jejunum contain no more than 10^3–10^4 organisms/ml aspirated juice. These are normally Gram-positive organisms—acid resistant *Staphylococci, Streptococci, Lactobacilli* and fungi— which are presumably contaminants from mouth and food. A few coliform organisms may be present, but strict anaerobes are absent. In the distal ileum there are increasing numbers of faecal organisms—anaerobes and coliforms [6].

Abnormal flora

Although early reports drew attention to the presence of obligate anaerobic organisms in the bacterial contamination syndrome—*Bacteroides, Veillonella, Clostridia* and *Bifidobacteria*—it is increasingly recognized that a variety of other bacteria with widely differing metabolic requirements (notably *Escherichia coli* and *Klebsiella* species) may also be associated with the clinical disorder [10]. It is the wide variety of potentially pathogenic organisms that produces the broad spectrum of clinical and biochemical features of the syndrome and contributes to the lack of completely reliable screening tests, and the difficulties of subsequent effective antibiotic treatment.

Causes of bacterial contamination—failure of normal regulatory factors

Several mechanisms exist to control the bacterial flora of the normal upper small intestine and failure of one or more of these may predispose to bacterial contamination. Suitable conditions obtain for a profuse growth of organisms and a consequent bacterial contamination syndrome if, in addition to one of these factors, a blind-loop or sump exists.

Gastric acidity normally destroys most bacteria before they enter the duodenum so that anacidity, either naturally occurring or following gastric surgery, allows bacteria to enter the duodenum or jejunum. Normal bile salt concentrations within the small intestinal lumen may also discourage bacterial proliferation. Immunoglobulin dificiency, leading to poor antibody formation against bacterially-derived antigens, has been shown to predispose to bacterial contamination of the small intestine particularly in association with anacidity. Moreover, patients with hypogammaglobulinaemia are often also anacidic [18].

Probably the most important factor normally inhibiting bacterial growth in this region is the mechanical cleaning action of normal small intestinal peristalsis. Some patients with the bacterial contamination syndrome, but no obvious anatomical sump for bacteria have been shown to have impaired jejunal peristalsis [38] and the importance of normal peristaltic activity is emphasized by the occurrence of bacterial contamination in association with scleroderma, diabetic neuropathy and intestinal pseudo-obstruction. Part of the reason for the occurrence of small intestinal bacterial contamination following gastric surgery, even without the creation of a blind loop, may be the denervation of the small intestine by unselective vagotomy.

Table 44.1. Underlying causes of bacterial contamination syndrome.

Failure of regulatory factors	Anatomical blind loop
Anacidity	*Duodenojejunal diverticula*
Pernicious anaemia	
Vagotomy	*Post-surgical loops*
Old age	Bilroth II anastomosis
Antisecretory drugs	Enteroenteric
	anastgomosis
Abnormal motility	*Fistulae*
Systemic sclerosis	Enterocolic
Autonomic neuropathy	Gastrocolic
Whipple's disease	
Amyloidosis	*Distal obstruction*
Intestinal pseudo-	Crohn's disease
obstruction	Carcinoid tumour
Surgical denervation	Other small bowel
	tumours
Immunological failure	Tuberculosis
Hypogammaglobulinaemia	Radiation enteritis
Other	
Tropical sprue	
Malnutrition	
Cholangitis + ? liver	
disease	

Establishment of a blind loop

In addition to a failure of one or more regulatory factors inhibiting bacterial proliferation, an area of stasis where such growth may take place is also necessary in the small intestine for the establishment of the bacterial contamination syndrome. The most important causes are listed in Table 44.1.

Mechanisms of damage

The mucosa

There may be no microscopic changes in a small intestinal biopsy from a patient with the bacterial contamination syndrome, but this can be due to sampling error, as subtotal villus atrophy may be patchy [1]. A slight non-specific inflammatory cell infiltrate in the lamina propria and submucosa is probably the typical finding [7]. Electron microscope studies in rats show widespread damage to enterocyte mitochondria and to the smooth and rough endoplasmic reticulum [37].

This injury to the small intestinal epithelium may be directly caused by the bacteria or produced indirectly by secondary bile acids. Proteases secreted by some species of *Bacteroides* markedly inhibit human brush border enzymes, including sucrase and maltase [30]. Heat-stable and heat-labile toxins are produced not only by acute dysenteric organisms such as *Vibrio cholera*, but also by *E. coli* and *Klebsiella* [10, 27]. Such toxins could produce diarrhoea and malaise in the bacterial contamination syndrome. Other, as yet unidentified toxic bacterial products may also be important. Direct damage of the small intestinal mucosa may also be caused by the secondary bile acids—deoxycholic and lithocholic. These arise from dehydroxylation of primary bile acids (cholic and chenodeoxycholic) by the bacteria inappropriately sited

in the upper small bowel. Secondary bile acids may inhibit enzymes in the epithelial cells [11].

Luminal damage

Some, but not all of the pathogenic bacteria found in the bacterial contamination syndrome are able to break the amide bond linking the bile acids to their glycine or taurine conjugates [35]. As only conjugated bile acids form satisfactory micelles and thus promote normal fat absorption, bacterial deconjugation may be important in the pathogenesis of the disease. However, it should be noted that many patients have a severe illness associated with small bowel bacterial contamination by organisms incapable of deconjugation.

Metabolic consequences of bacterial contamination

Steatorrhoea

Steatorrhoea is the best known effect, although it is not universal. Electron microscopy of a jejunal biopsy taken during a fatty meal in a patient with small intestinal bacterial contamination shows a decreased number of fat particles in the absorptive cells. There is also a suggestion of impaired transport of chylomicrons out of the epithelium into the lamina propria [1]. Although bacteria may cause deconjugation of bile salts in the jejunum, the remaining conjugated bile salts form normal micelles with free fatty acids in the aqueous phase of the jejunal contents. Bacteria also act on the dietary unsaturated fatty acids to produce long-chain hydroxy fatty acids [17], one of which is ricinoleic acid—the active ingredient of castor oil. Donaldson [5] has suggested that these hydroxylated fatty acids may stimulate colonic secretion of water and electrolytes, thus producing diarrhoea without severe steatorrhoea. The bacterial species that make up the jejunal flora in a particular patient may thus determine whether steatorrhoea (high bile salt deconjugation activity ± mucosal damage) or diarrhoea (high conversion of unsaturated fatty acids to long-chain fatty acids) predominates.

Severe protein malnutrition

Severe protein malnutrition, occasionally equivalent to Kwashiorkor, may occur [25]. Several factors cause protein malnutrition—catabolism of ingested protein by the gut flora may occur. Enteric bacteria may decarboxylate dietary tryptophan to form tryptamine—intestinal monoamine oxidases convert tryptamine to indoleacetic acid, which is excreted in the urine. In addition, some organisms may split a side chain off tryptophan to form indole, which is converted by intestinal and hepatic enzymes to indican and excreted in the urine. This was the basis of the now abandoned urinary indican test for bacterial contamination. The net result of these two bacterial actions is the absorption of 'unuseable' dietary nitrogen. Indican excretion in some instances may show that over 60% of dietary tryptophan has been metabolized by bacteria in this way.

Protein synthesis may be decreased. Decreased albumin and fibrinogen synthesis and decreased plasma essential amino acids in the presence of increased urea excretion have been observed in patients with bacterial contamination [16, 39]. This suggests nitrogen may be absorbed in a form not available for synthesis into body protein. Some organisms may deaminate the luminal amino acids producing ammonia. In addition, mucosal damage may itself cause diminished transport of amino acids and peptides.

Inanition may inhibit appetite and thus lower protein intake. In many patients with tropical sprue malnutrition itself may pre-

dispose to small intestinal bacterial contamination thus producing further protein malabsorption [10]. Endogenous enteric protein loss (protein losing enteropathy) is rare in the bacterial contamination syndrome.

Carbohydrate

Bacteria may metabolize the sugar D-xylose in the lumen of the gut. For this reason the conventional xylose absorption test cannot distinguish small intestinal mucosal disease from bacterial contamination, in which less D-xylose is available for absorption. Mucosal damage to metabolically-active saccharide transport systems has already been discussed.

Low vitamin B_{12} absorption

Low vitamin B_{12} absorption, even in the presence of adequate intrinsic factor, is an important feature of many patients with small intestinal bacteral contamination. Some, but not all bacterial species bind ingested vitamin B_{12} and prevent its absorption. This binding may occur in competition for binding sites with intrinsic factor, but also occurs when the B_{12} is already bound to intrinsic factor, presumably because the organisms possess particularly avid binding sites for the vitamin [33].

Folic acid

Some strains of *E. coli* found in the bacterial contamination syndrome synthesize considerable quantities of folate, absorbed as 5-methyl-tetrahydrofolic acid; thus some patients may have serum folate concentrations above the normal range [14]. The diagnosis of small intestinal bacterial contamination syndrome should be suspected in a patient with macrocytosis, low serum B_{12}, an abnormal Schilling test in the presence of intrinsic factor, who also has a high serum folate, but in practice this combination is relatively rare. Furthermore many patients with a documented growth of coliform organisms in the small intestinal juice have normal serum folates, and a few with well documented bacterial contamination have low serum folate concentrations [4].

Other vitamins

Despite malabsorption of fat, deficiency of fat soluble vitamins is rare. Although low serum β-carotene concentrations are not uncommon in these patients, night blindness is an extremely rare symptom [18]. Vitamin K deficiency causing an overt clotting disturbance is also very uncommon. Metabolic bone disease is commoner— particularly in the elderly. Patients may present with bone pain or pathological fractures [31]. Encephalopathy associated with nicotinic acid deficiency has also been described, possibly because some enteric bacteria are known to metabolize this vitamin [36].

Clinical features

The classical stagnant, or blind loop syndrome was thought to be a fairly rare disorder, occurring usually in association with small intestinal diverticula or following gastric surgery. The main features were diarrhoea—typically steatorrhoea, weight loss, macrocytic anaemia and general malaise. However, bacterial contamination of the small bowel should be suspected not only in middle-aged patients with symptoms of painless steatorrhoea, but also in elderly individuals with general malaise and physical deterioration, bone pain, or hypoproteinaemia—even constipation does not exclude the diagnosis. Patients who had gastric surgery many years earlier are at particular risk—30–40% of such patients may have a metabolic myopathy, or a peripheral neuropathy, or sometimes subacute combined degeneration of the spinal cord. Bacterial contamination should also be remembered in scleroderma and Crohn's disease. In one series 25% of patients with Crohn's disease had small intestinal bacterial contamination, even those with radiological abnormalities distant from the upper small intestine [32].

Investigations and diagnosis

The haematological and biochemical measurements which are helpful in the assessment of the bacterial contamination syndrome are listed in Tables 44.2 and 44.3. Having suspected bacterial contamination, a barium follow-through is the most important investigation—searching for a blind loop or sump (Fig. 44.1). The important problem is whether one of the metabolic features of the bacteria abnormally resident in the upper small bowel can be used to provide a diagnostic or a reliable screening test for the disease, without the need for small intestinal intubation or technically sophisticated anaerobic bacterial cultures.

Excretion of urinary indican

The tryptophanase activities of bacteria are unfortunately very variable and differences are common, even among strains of the same species. Moreover excretion of indican is influenced by dietary and endogenous sources of tryptophan, intraluminal pH of the gut and hepatic and renal impairment. For these reasons the measurement of urinary indican excretion has little or no value in the diagnosis of small intestinal bacterial contamination [12, 23].

Measurement of intestinal volatile fatty acid

Because some of the anaerobic organisms which colonize the small intestine can pro-

Table 44.2. Investigation of the contaminated bowel syndrome.

Test	Comment
Haematology/biochemistry	
Blood count and film	Anaemia frequent
	Macrocytosis frequent
	Dimorphic film may be seen
Serum proteins	Low serum albumin concentration frequent (hypogammaglobulinaemia may be underlying cause)
Bone chemistry	Calcium may be low; alkaline phosphatase high
Serum B_{12}	Often low
Serum folate, red cell folate	Sometimes raised, occasionally low
Serum iron	Sometimes low
Serum β-carotene	Often low
Radiology	
Plain abdominal X-ray	May show fluid levels in diverticula
Ba examination of duodenum and jejunum	The most important investigation. Duodenal, duodenojejunal or jejunal diverticula seen. Dilated segments of small bowel, distal obstruction or a blind loop from previous gastric surgery may be identified.
Breath tests	
^{14}C-glycocholic acid	Probably most widely used. May give false negative result. May be performed in four hours on sick patients. Very well tolerated.
^{14}C-D-xylose test	Promising idea, but needs considerable verification.
Hydrogen breath test (after oral glucose load)	Non-invasive, no need for isotopes. Some false negatives, needs further evaluation.
Faecal fat excretion/^{14}C Triolein breath test	One of these should be done, if possible.
Urinary indican excretion	Of little value. Should not be used.
Test involving small bowel aspiration	
Bacteriology	If available, this is best. Bacteriology should be quantitative. Mouth organisms should be discounted. A growth of 10^6 organisms/ml aspirate is minimum for diagnosis.
Unconjugated bile acid, or Volatile fatty acid measurement in intestinal juice.	Research procedures needing special gas/liquid chromatography equipment.

Table 44.3. Practical diagnosis of bacterial contamination.

History—note particularly associated disease/previous surgery, likely to be associated with bacterial contamination.

Screening—haematology and biochemistry.

Radiology—of upper small intestine.

If radiology shows a blind loop, or sump (for example, diverticula) then do jejunal aspirate with quantitative aerobic and anaerobic cultures, if possible. If quantitative bacteriology not available, do a screening breath test.
If radiology shows no blind loop or sump, then consider differential diagnoses—coeliac disease, chronic pancreatitis, inflammatory bowel disease, giardiasis.
Do endoscopic duodenal biopsy (to exclude some of the above), with aspiration of juice for bacteriology; $\pm$ screening breath test.

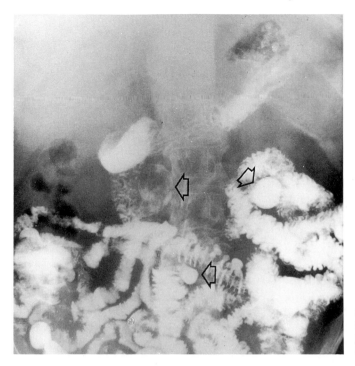

Fig. 44.1. Small intestinal contrast study in a patient with jejunal diverticulosis. Arrows indicate diverticula.

duce volatile fatty acids (acetate, butyrate and proprionate) by fermentation, this reaction has been explored as a test for bacterial contamination. A sample of small intestinal contents is analysed for the presence of volatile fatty acids by gas liquid chromatography [3]. As this involves duodenal intubation and specialized laboratory techniques, the test has not found widespread use. Moreover not all bacteria are capable of carrying out the reaction, so that false negative results are not uncommon.

Breath tests

Three major breath test methods have been proposed for screening patients with possible bacterial contaminations. The ^{14}C-glycocholic acid breath test uses the ability of bacteria in the upper small intestine to deconjugate the ^{14}C-labelled glycine from cholic acid after an oral dose. ^{14}C-glycine is then metabolized and excreted as $^{14}CO_2$ and its specific activity is measured in the exhaled breath [15]. Unfortunately not all bacterial species that cause the bacterial contamination syndrome perform this deconjugation reaction, so that there is a false negative rate of up to 30%. Ileal disease or resection with intestinal hurry, may lead to bacterial deconjugation of bile salts by the normal colonic flora, thus producing a falsely abnormal indication of possible upper small intestinal deconjugation [20]. This second pitfall may be overcome by measurements of faecal ^{14}C-specific activity. This is because absent faecal ^{14}C activity during the test period confirms an intact enterohepatic circulation, suggesting that breath $^{14}CO_2$-specific activity arises from bacterial action in the small bowel. Faecal collections complicate the test considerably, however.

Since bacteria may destroy D-xylose in the lumen of the gut, a ^{14}C-D-xylose breath test has been suggested in which D-xylose with 1 μCi of ^{14}C-labelled D-xylose is given by mouth; breath $^{14}CO_2$ specific activity is recorded 30 and 60 minutes after administration [20]. It is claimed that a clear distinction between bacterial contamination and other causes of malabsorption is possible, but this needs further verification.

A further breath test is based on the principle that while reactions producing hydrogen (H_2) do not occur in human metabolism, most bacteria ferment carbohydrate to produce H_2, which is absorbed through the gut wall and subsequently exhaled [5]. Thus measurements of H_2 content of end-expired air for four hours after a 50 g oral glucose load in patients with bacterial contamination of the small bowel produced no false positives, although a number of false negative tests were recorded [24], again indicating the heterogeneity of the colonizing bacteria. When a ^{14}C-glycocholic acid breath test was also used, only one of twelve patients with culture-proven small intestinal contamination was missed.

Breath tests are thus not infallible screening test for bacterial contamination. If positive, each of these tests suggests the presence of bacteria in the small bowel; a negative test does not exclude the diagnosis.

Aspiration of intestinal juice

Culture of abnormal bacterial flora from small intestinal juice is the only way to make a confident diagnosis. Intestinal juice is aspirated through a radio-opaque plastic tube passed into the jejunum or near to the site of presumed bacterial contamination (diverticulum or blind loop), under radiological control. This may be time-consuming. An alternative is to use a soft sterile tube passed through the biopsy channel of an endoscope, but some workers [13] have found that endoscopic aspiration does not provide reliable samples for bacterial culture. Care must be taken not to inject air into the small intestine during the procedure. Whichever aspiration method is used, the specimen must be transferred promptly to an anaerobic chamber or placed in anaerobic pre-reduced transport medium before culture in strictly anaerobic media [8].

Treatment

The general principles that are used for the treatment of any disease causing malabsorption or malnutrition apply. Any co-existing disorder should be treated, if possible. For example, distal Crohn's disease, an enteric fistula or distal obstruction should be dealt with medically or surgically, as appropriate.

A number of broad-spectrum antibiotics have been used to eliminate bacterial contamination. No antibiotic is completely satisfactory. Tetracycline, lincomycin or clindamycin have proved effective most often (but the latter pair carry a risk of causing another enteric disease—pseudomembranous colitis). Metronidazole is not often effective, despite its apparent suitability in treating anaerobic bacterial flora. Antibiotics should probably be continued for a long period—possibly for life—because bacterial contamination, sometimes more resistant to treatment, may recur after stopping the drugs. After an initial daily dose of tetracycline 750 mg for four weeks, a maintenance dose of 250 mg daily seems effective in most patients. The ^{14}C-glycocholic acid breath test is not very useful in assessing the effectiveness of treatment. The test almost always becomes negative within a few days of starting antibiotics, but this is not an indication for stopping the treatment.

Appropriate nutritional support should also be given. Deficiencies of vitamin B_{12}, folic acid or fat-soluble vitamins should be treated by replacement. If patients are hypoproteinaemic a high protein diet is appropriate. Many patients, particularly the elderly, have poor appetites during the phase of recovery and should be encouraged to eat. A low-fat diet may be helpful during the initial weeks, if steatorrhoea or diarrhoea is a major problem, until bacterial contamination has been eliminated. It should be stressed that full recovery from small intestinal bacterial contamination may take weeks or months.

References

1 AMENT ME, SHIMODA SS, SAUNDERS DR, RUBIN E. Pathogenesis of steatorrhoea in three cases of small intestinal stasis syndrome. *Gastroenterology* 1972;**63**:728–747.

2 BADENOCH J, BEDFORD PD, EVANS JR. Massive diverticulosis of the small intestine with steatorrhoea and megaloblastic anaemia. *Q J Med* 1955;**24**:321–330.

3 CHERNOV AJ, DOE WF, GOMPERTZ D. Intrajejunal volatile fatty acids in the stagnant loop syndrome. *Gut* 1972;**13**:103–106.

4 COOKE WT, COX EV, FONE DJ, MEYNELL MJ, GADDIE R. The clinical and metabolic significance of jejunal diverticula. *Gut* 1963;**4**:115–131.

5 DONALDSON RM. Small bowel bacterial overgrowth. *Adv Intern Med* 1970;**16**:191–212.

6 DRASAR BS, SHINER M, McLEOD GM. Studies of the intestinal flora I. *Gastroenterology* 1969;**56**:71–79.

7 GOLDSTEIN F. Mechanism of malabsorption and malnutrition in the bacterial overgrowth syndrome. *Gastroenterology* 1971;**61**:780–784.

8 GORBACH SL, NAHAS L, LERNER PI, WEINSTEIN L. Studies of intestinal microflora. *Gastroenterology* 1967;**53**:845–855.

9 GRACEY M. The contaminated small bowel syndrome: pathogenesis, diagnosis and treatment. *Am J Clin Nutr* 1979;**32**:234–243.

10 GRACEY MS. Nutrition, bacteria and the gut. *Br Med Bull* 1981;**37**:71–75.

11 GRACEY M, HOUGHTON M, THOMAS J. Deoxycholate depresses small intestinal enzyme activity. *Gut* 1975;**16**:53–56.

12 HAMILTON JD, DYER NH, DAWSON AM, *et al.* Assessment and significance of bacterial overgrowth in the small bowel. *Q J Med* 1970;**39**:265–285.

13 HAMILTON I, WORMSLEY B, SHOESMITH W, AXON ATR. Endoscopic aspiration of duodenal juice in the diagnosis of small bowel bacterial contamination. *Endoscopy* 1982;**14**:89–91.

14 HOFFBRAND A, TABAQCHALI S, BOOTH CC, MOLLIN D. Small intestinal bacterial flora and folate status in gastrointestinal disorders. *Gut* 1971;**12**:27–33.

15 JAMES OFW, AGNEW JE, BOUCHIER IAD. Assessment of the ^{14}C-glycocholic acid breath test. *Br Med J* 1973;**3**:191–195.

16 JONES EA, GRAIGIE A, TAVILL AS, FRANGLEN G, ROSENOER VM. Protein metabolism in the intestinal stagnant loop syndrome. *Gut* 1968;**9**:466–469.

17 KIM YS, SPRITZ N. Hydroxyacid excretion in stea-

torrhoea of pancreatic and non-pancreatic origin. *New Engl J Med* 1968;**279**:1424–1426.

18 KING CE, TOSKES PP. Small intestinal bacterial overgrowth. *Gastroenterology* 1979;**76**:1035–1055.

19 KING CE, TOSKES PP, SPIVEY JC, LORENZ E, WELKOS S. Detection of small intestinal bacterial overgrowth by means of a ^{14}C-D-xylose breath test. *Gastroenterology* 1979;**77**:75–82.

20 LAUTERBERG BH, NEWCOMER AD, HOFMANN AF. Clinical value of the bile acid breath test. *Mayo Clin Proc* 1978;**53**:227–233.

21 McEVOY A, DUTTON J, JAMES OFW. Bacterial contamination of the small intestine is an important cause of occult malabsorption in the elderly. *Br Med J* 1983;**287**:789–793.

22 MORSON BC, DAWSON IMP. In: *Gastrointestinal Pathology*, 2nd ed. Oxford: Blackwell Scientific Publications, 1979:366.

23 MAYER PJ, BEEJKEN WL. The role of urinary indican as a predictor of bacterial colonization in the human jejunum. *Am J Dig Dis* 1975;**20**:1003–1010.

24 METZ G, GASSULL MA, DRASAR BS, JENKINS DJA, BLENDIS LM. Breath-hydrogen test for small intestinal bacterial colonisation. *Lancet* 1976;**i**:668–669.

25 NEALE, G, ANTCLIFF, AE, WELBOURN RS, *et al.* Protein malnutrition. *Q J Med* 1967; **36**: 469–494

26 NEALE G, GOMPERTZ D, SCHONSBY H, TABAQCHALI S, BOOTH CC. The metabolic and nutritional consequences of bacterial overgrowth in the small intestine. *Am J Clin Nutr* 1972;**25**:1409–1417.

27 NETER E. Enteropathogenicity: recent developments. *Klin Wochenschr* 1982;**60**:699–701.

28 NOER T. Non-meckelian diverticula of the small bowel. The incidence in an autopsy material. *Acta Clin Scand* 1960;**120**:175–179.

29 PEARCE VR. The importance of duodenal diverticula in the elderly. *Postgrad Med J* 1980;**56**:777–780.

30 RIEPE SP, GOLDSTEIN J, ALPERS DH. Effect of secreted bacteroides proteases on human intestinal brush border hydrolases. *J Clin Invest* 1980;**66**:315–322.

31 ROBERTS SH, JAMES OFW, JARVIS EH. Bacterial overgrowth syndrome without 'blind loop': a cause for malnutrition in the elderly. *Lancet* 1977;**ii**:1193–1195.

32 RUTGEERTS P, GHOOSE Y, VANTRAPPEN G, EYSSEN H. Ileal dysfunction and bacterial overgrowth in patients with Crohn's disease. *Eur J Clin Invest* 1981;**11**:199–206.

33 SCHJONSBY H, DRASAR B, TABAQCHALI S, BOOTH CC. Uptake of vitamin B12 by intestinal bacteria in the stagnant loop syndrome. *Scand J Gastroenterol* 1973;**8**:41–47.

34 TABAQCHALI S, BOOTH CC. Bacterial overgrowth. In: Booth CC, Neale G, eds. *Disorders of the small intestine.* Oxford: Blackwell Scientific Publications, 1986:249–269.

35 TABAQCHALI S, HATZIOANNON J, BOOTH CC. Bile salt deconjugation and steatorrhoea in patients with the stagnant loop syndrome. *Lancet* 1968;ii:12–16.

36 TABAQCHALI S, PALLIS C. Reversible nicotinamide deficiency encephalopathy in a patient with jejunal diverticulosis. *Gut* 1970;11:1024–1026.

37 TOSKES KP, GIANNELLA RA, JERVIS HR, ROUT WR, TAKEUCHI A. Small intestinal mucosal injury and the experimental blind loop syndrome. *Gastroenterology* 1975;68:1193–1203.

38 VANTRAPPEN G, JANSSENS J, HELLEMANS J, GHOOS Y. The inter-digestive motor complex of normal subjects and patients with bacterial overgrowth of the small intestine. *J Clin Invest* 1977;59:1158–1166.

39 YAP SH, HAFKENSCHEID JM, VAN TONGEREN JHM, TRIJBELS JMF. Rate of synthesis of albumin in relation to serum levels of essential amino acids in patients with bacterial overgrowth of the small bowel. *Eur J Clin Invest* 1974;4:279–284.

Chapter 45
Intestinal Fistulae

M. B. CLAGUE

An intestinal fistula is an abnormal communication between any part of the gastrointestinal tract and either the body surface or another portion of the gastrointestinal tract, or other hollow viscus. Such fistulae may be produced deliberately as a therapeutic measure on a temporary or permanent basis (for example: feeding gastrostomy, jejunoileal bypass for obesity, colostomy), or may arise as the result of trauma or some pathological process within the thoracic, abdominal or pelvic cavities. All intestinal fistulae can give rise to similar problems and similar principles of management apply to them all. Therapeutic fistulae rarely produce problems if constructed correctly, but pathological fistulae with the uncontrolled leakage of intestinal contents and often an underlying disease, can give rise to life threatening complications [19].

From a practical and prognostic aspect intestinal fistulae can be considered as being either external or internal. External fistulae may be of high (draining more than 200 ml daily) or low output. Internal fistulae may involve the bowel alone (for example gastro-colic) or implicate other organs (for example vesico-colic). Arterio-enteric fistulae give rise to special problems and will not be considered further here. Usually only one but on occasions multiple fistulae may exist, such as perineal fistulae in Crohn's disease. Fistulae in association with cancer often involve several viscera.

Incidence and pathophysiology

The incidence, geographical distribution and population affected by intestinal fistulae are determined largely by the disposition and prevalence of the underlying causes. Some of the commoner aetiological factors of non-therapeutic intestinal fistulae are shown in Table 45.1. In the emergent countries, infections still account for most

Table 45.1. Causes of non-therapeutic intestinal fistulae

Congenital

Developmental errors (for example tracheo-oesophageal fistula)

Acquired

Benign

Inflammatory
    Acute —Appendicitis
              —Diverticulitis
    Chronic—Tuberculosis
              —Crohn's disease

Traumatic
    External   —Penetrating (for example stab wound)
                —Blunt (for example crush injury)
    Operative —Anastomotic leak/suture line
                —Inadvertent damage
    Irradiation
    Blast injury
    Foreign body (for example gallstone)

Ulcerative
    Peptic ulceration
Benign intestinal neoplasm

Malignant

Gastrointestinal

Extra-intestinal (for example bladder)

fistulae, while in developed countries surgically-induced lesions predominate [6, 9, 23]. Many factors might account for these differences—better hygiene and availability of anti-microbial agents, improved nutrition, early awareness of disease with improved access to medical and surgical facilities, wider use of surgical procedures and the development of technology enabling surgical procedures on ill and debilitated patients. Most gastroenterologists will encounter only a few cases annually, but despite relatively small numbers, the patients can consume a disproportionately large amount of nursing and medical resources.

The initial event in the formation of most intestinal fistulae is a leak of gastrointestinal content into the peritoneal cavity. If this leak is not localized, then generalized peritonitis will supervene and the individual will succumb to sepsis if surgery is not undertaken. However, if localization by omentum, or adhesion to adjacent tissues has taken place, an abscess may develop with the potential of rupturing into an adjacent hollow viscus or onto the skin surface. Under such circumstances the fistula will be lined by early granulation tissue which may mature either into a more fibrous tract and even become lined by migrating mucosa, or close off. A tumour may penetrate directly and a fistula form, the tract often containing neoplastic cells. If abscess formation has been an intermediate step in the development of the fistula, then spontaneous drainage is frequently inadequate or the tract may become occluded by debris, producing the systemic manifestations of a loculated collection of infected material.

Clinical features

The clinical features are determined by the type of fistula and its underlying cause. Although most external fistulae are obvious, slowly developing lesions in association with chronic disease may not be so readily discernable. In most cases the underlying cause of the fistula is also clinically manifest.

Postoperative gastrointestinal anastomoses may leak and be completely asymptomatic, even when intestinal contents are apparent in drainage tubes. On other occasions, a patient several days following surgery will have a mild pyrexia, vague abdominal pain and a persistent ileus. Symptoms and signs worsen and erythema may develop in the wound, or a few drops exude from a previous drainage site. Removal of some sutures to facilitate drainage of what was initially thought to be a wound infection will produce a variable flow of fluid which, over the ensuing days, will characterize the secretions as those arising from some part of the gastrointestinal tract. Features such as colour, smell, consistency and effect on surrounding unprotected skin are helpful (Fig. 45.1). A swinging pyrexia suggests an undrained pocket of secretions or an abscess.

External fistulae arising from a disease process within the abdomen are often preceded by symptoms that suggest the pathology. An elderly individual with recent change in bowel habit and weight loss before development of a fistula should be suspected to harbour a large bowel neoplasm, while a young underweight adult with episodic right-sided or lower abdominal pain probably has Crohn's disease. An abscess in relation to the abdominal cavity, that is to say in the abdominal wall, groin, perineum, perianal or ischiorectal spaces, that fails to heal after surgical drainage or spontaneous rupture, should be suspected as being fistulous and probably secondary to Crohn's disease, even if intestinal contents cannot be recognized as draining. *Per vaginam* passage of flatus or a faeculent discharge may be the only symptom of a fistulous tract from the gastrointestinal tract into the vagina.

Internal fistulae are usually more difficult

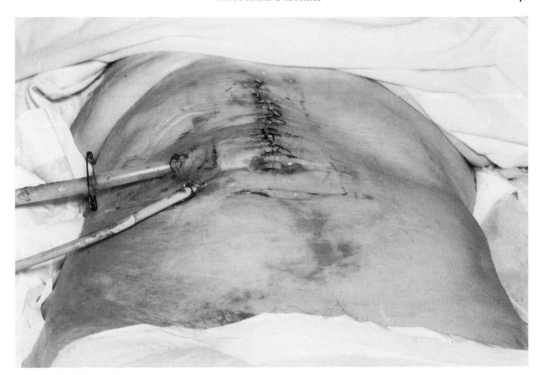

Fig. 45.1. The abdomen of a patient with uncontrolled leakage around a catheter placed into the duodenal stump after a Billroth I procedure for a bleeding gastric ulcer. Note the skin excoriation around the catheter and drainage tubes, extending suprapubically because of the use of an absorbent dressing.

to diagnose on clinical criteria alone and often the diagnosis is not realized. Fistulation to the urinary tract produces symptoms of urinary tract infection and a characteristic pneumaturia. A gastrocolic fistula is characterized by foul smelling eructations, faeculent vomiting and diarrhoea. Enteroenteric fistulae involving other parts of the gastrointestinal tract are often less dramatic and may simply present with diarrhoea, weight loss and the features of malabsorption. Examination of the abdomen may reveal a mass, tenderness, or some thickening at the site of the internal fistula.

The complications of intestinal fistulae are listed in Table 45.2 and, although when fully developed their presence is clinically obvious, thorough clinical investigation is imperative for their early detection.

Table 45.2. Complications of intestinal fistulae.

Fluid and electrolyte losses
Dehydration
Hyponatraemia
Hypokalaemia
Acid-base imbalance
Trace element deficiency

Sepsis
Hepatic failure
Renal failure

Skin excoriation
Tissue autodigestion

Malnutrition
Delayed healing
Predisposition to invasion by secondary pathogens
Respiratory failure
Cardiac failure

Haemorrhage

Investigations

Investigations can be divided into two phases—the initial confirmation of a fistula and investigations for the early signs of complications, and the final delineation of the tract, its origin and detection of any underlying disease.

If an enterocutaneous fistula cannot be verified simply by the nature of the fluid draining from it, then examination of the fluid itself may be helpful. Fluid from the small intestine can be confused with peritoneal exudate, but determination of its amylase concentration in the absence of acute pancreatitis will show its true nature. Similarly, instillation of a marker dye into the upper or lower gastrointestinal tract may be helpful and, by the timing of its appearance, give some idea of its level.

Baseline laboratory investigations must include a blood count, estimation of electrolytes, plasma proteins and trace elements, as well as assessment of hepatic and renal function. Arterial blood gases may be necessary to exclude acid-base imbalance related to fluid losses, poor renal function or sepsis. Laboratory monitoring often has to be repeated at frequent intervals in the early stages.

Fluid appearing from any wound and drainage sites should be sent for bacteriological examination and blood cultures taken in the septic patient. Efforts must be made to collect as much of the fluid as possible so that an accurate assessment of its volume and electrolyte content may be made. In an extremely ill patient monitoring of central venous pressure and other parameters of cardiac function may facilitate resuscitation. Once stabilized, attempts should be made to locate any intra-abdominal collection. Localized exploratory procedures may have to be undertaken as the only means of ascertaining the existence of such collections in the early stage, although computed tomography [11,17], ultrasound [13] or later,[76] Gallium scanning [12] can assist in their location and facilitate the appropriate drainage procedure.

Once the patient is non-septic, rehydrated and the fistulous tract has become established, then radiology should be undertaken to define the fistula and determine if any pathology exists that precludes its closure. In the case of an external fistula the most satisfactory examination is usually a fistulagram—the placing of a fine bore catheter into the fistula with injection of a water-soluble contrast medium into the tract (Fig. 45.2). This will define the course of the fistula and usually the site from which it

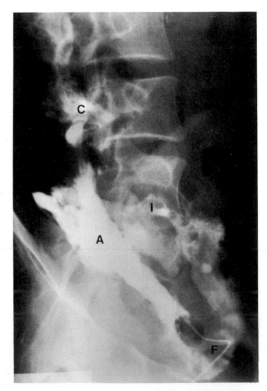

Fig. 45.2. Fistulagram with a fine-bore catheter (F) placed into the external opening in the right groin and showing contrast filling an abscess cavity on the right pelvic wall (A) and communicating with an abnormal terminal ileum (I) or the caecum (C) containing gas and some residual barium from a previous barium enema. The primary pathology was Crohn's disease.

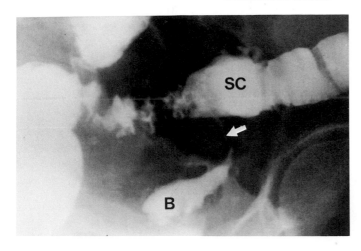

Fig. 45.3. Barium enema showing a fistula (arrowed) between the sigmoid colon (SC) and bladder (B). Note the narrowed area of diverticular disease distal to the fistula which precluded its closure.

arises. Even if a good demonstration is obtained, radiology of the entire gastro-intestinal tract and certainly that part distal to the opening of the fistula into the bowel is imperative to ascertain whether disease or obstruction of the distal bowel is present (Fig. 45.3). Some external fistulae are readily demonstrated by such X-rays without recourse to fistulagrams (Fig. 45.4).

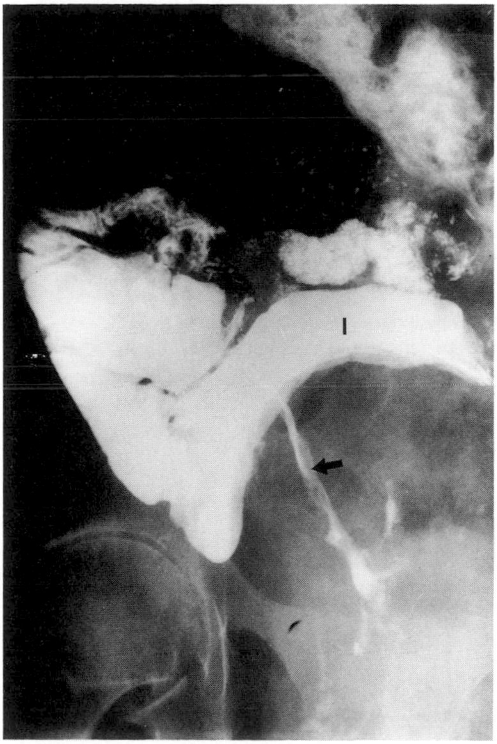

Internal fistulae may be suspected on plain radiographs, where air is present in organs in which it is normally absent (for examples, the biliary tree and urinary tract) and can be confirmed by contrast radiology of the bowel and appropriate systems (Fig. 45.5). Small fistulae may be difficult to demonstrate even radiologically and endoscopy of the upper or lower gastrointestinal tract or the bladder may be necessary to reveal the pathology.

Differential diagnosis

External fistulae that arise following surgery can be mistaken in the early stages for a wound infection or peritoneal exudate. Intestinal fistulae involving the urinary system are often diagnosed at first as simple urinary tract infections, and enteroenteric lesions must be distinguished from the commoner causes of the symptoms that are present.

Fig. 45.4. Barium follow through showing a fistulous connection (arrowed) between a diseased terminal ileum (I) and the perineum. Probable Crohn's disease.

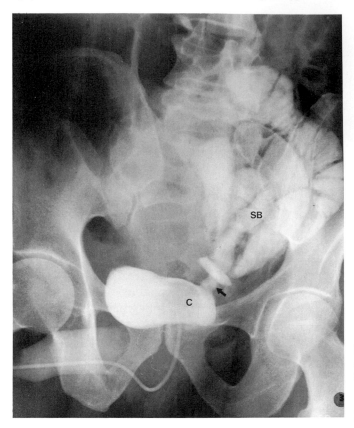

Fig. 45.5. A cystogram with a catheter (C) in the bladder showing an internal fistula (arrowed) between the bladder and the small bowel (SB) in a patient with a bladder tumour.

Medical management

Acute

An overall plan of management is given in Table 45.3. The initial treatment of fistulae is predominantly medical and focused on the problems that arise from complications. Intravenous therapy should replace fluid, electrolytes, proteins and blood to restore and prevent deterioration in the haemodynamic status of the patient. Antibiotics should be administered after samples have been collected for bacterial culture. A regimen that covers most of the normal bowel flora should be used—for example ampicillin 500 mg IV six-hourly, metronidazole 400 mg IV 12-hourly and gentamycin 40 mg IV eight-hourly, or a broad-spectrum cephalosporin. A careful assessment should

Table 45.3. Summary of the management of intestinal fistulae.

Diagnosis of fistula
Baseline laboratory investigations
Intravenous therapy—simple hospital support
—intensive therapy unit
Control of sepsis   —investigation
—surgical drainage
—antibotics
Protection of skin/collection of fluid losses
Nutritional support —parenteral
—enteral
Delineation of fistula/associated disease
Definitive surgical management

be made of the role of any specific infective agent, such as *Mycobacterium tuberculosis*, in the aetiology of the fistula and the regimen modified appropriately. The possibility of secondary overgrowth with yeast or *Sta-phylococci* must be borne in mind. Ino-trophic agents such as dopamine may be needed in the critically ill and patients may require respiratory support.

With an enterocutaneous fistula steps should be taken to protect the skin from excoriation, especially if a high output fis-tula exists. Various barrier creams, Karaya gum and powder, p-site and ion-exchange resins have all been advocated and should be used. Antisecretory agents such as H_2-histamine receptor antagonists and anti-cholinergics may assist in decreasing fluid loss and excoriation. An ostomy bag or some form of suction drainage with a soft catheter placed into or over the fistula is preferable to an absorbent dressing. Care and attention in applying the dressing, as well as the frequency with which it is changed, will be well rewarded. Therapy must also be started to control the primary disease if present.

Intermediate

When sepsis, dehydration and skin excor-iation have been brought under control, attention should be turned to correcting an-aemia and providing nutrition [1]. This can be provided enterally [3, 22] or parenterally [8, 14, 21] although the latter is advocated in the early stages of problematic fistulae as it will more effectively reduce intestinal se-cretions [24] and minimize contamination. In low output or distal internal fistulae this can be replaced after a few days by a slowly introduced low residue enteral or elemental feed [5, 18]. If symptoms recur, parenteral feeding should be re-established. In a few high fistulae a feeding tube can be inserted, or an ostomy created, distal to the fistula, but total parenteral nutrition can prove a much safer procedure [8, 14, 21].

Chronic

Treatment may not only improve the nutri-tional status of the patient but, providing none of the criteria exist that preclude closure of the fistula (Table 45.3), sponta-neous closure of the tract may occur. Symp-tomatic control with conservative measures is required for therapeutic and many pathological fistulae associated with inoper-able malignancies and inflammatory bowel disease, and patients with enteroenteric fis-tulae may only need intermittent courses of antibiotics to prevent bacterial overgrowth in the blind-loop.

Surgical treatment

Acute

The early surgical management of fistulae consists principally of techniques to control sepsis. This may be done simply using local procedures involving widening of the open-ing of the fistula, incision of abscesses and the placement of soft drainage tubes into tracts or abscess cavities. Alternatively a full laparotomy with peritoneal lavage, drainage of collections and attempts at re-pair of the fistula, exteriorization, or resec-tion of the involved segment of bowel, or diversionary procedures may be the only feasible way to control infection. The de-cision to operate and the procedure under-taken should be governed by the general state of the patient, rather than local prob-lems which can often be surmounted by good medical care. Critically ill patients with poor tissues tolerate major surgical procedures badly and the minimum opera-tive technique that can control the imme-diate problem is recommended. A high out-put fistula in a patient who is apyrexial is not an indication for urgent surgery. A patient with a rectovaginal fistula and pel-vic abscess is best managed by drainage of the abscess and a defunctioning colostomy.

A patient with a swinging pyrexia and multiple small bowel fistulae may need a full laparotomy. A resection with primary anastomosis may be the only method of controlling sepsis. Thought should be given to the placement of sump drains to facilitate control of any subsequent anastomotic leak.

Definitive

Many external fistulae will close spontaneously within a month [2, 16]. If a fistula fails to do so, or during investigations a feature is revealed which would prevent it doing so (Table 45.4), then the patient should be rendered as fit as possible and

Table 45.4. Factors decreasing the likelihood of spontaneous closure of an intestinal fistula.

Distal obstruction
Foreign body in tract
Epithelialization of tract
Sepsis
Neoplasia associated with tract
Active inflammatory disease of bowel
Radiation injury
Impaired vascularity
Tracts > 2 cm in diameter and < 2 cm long
Intestinal mucosa at external drainage site

undergo surgery. The fistulous tract and any associated disease should be resected and the bowel repaired where possible. A temporary diversionary procedure or exteriorization of the bowel ends may be required for large bowel lesions.

Where lesions are irresectable (for example inoperable tumour), a by-pass procedure or proximal ostomy can improve the quality of life. If complete resection is inadvisable, as in perianal fistula, then simple curettage of the tract, local excision or interposition of other tissue can minimize symptoms.

Prognosis

Twenty years ago the mortality from intestinal fistulae was 43–45% [4, 6] and this figure was even higher when high output enterocutaneous fistulae alone were considered. Mortality has now fallen to approximately 17%, the improvement being attributed to improved control of sepsis [16, 20] and provision of nutritional support [1, 10]. Fistulae that arise postoperatively have a high rate of spontaneous closure [2, 16] while multiple fistulae may persist despite multiple attempts at closure [7]. The ultimate prognosis of the patient is dependent on eradication of any underlying pathology. Despite these advances, patients with intestinal fistulae provide a challenge to nearly every department of a hospital with good results being the reward for a lot of effort, good resources and team-work [15].

References

1 ANONYMOUS. Nutritional management of enterocutaneous fistulas. *Lancet* 1979;**ii**:507–508.
2 BLACKETT RL, HILL GL. Postoperative external small bowel fistulas: a study of a consecutive series of patients treated with intravenous hyperalimentation. *Br J Surg* 1978;**65**:775–778.
3 BURY KD, STEPHENS RV, RANDALL HT. Use of a chemically defined, liquid elemental diet for nutritional management of fistulae of the alimentary tract. *Am J Surg* 1971;**121**:174–181.
4 CHAPMAN R, FORAN R, DUNPHY JE. Management of intestinal fistulas. *Am J Surg* 1964;**108**:157–164.
5 DIETEL M. Nutritional management of external gastrointestinal fistulas. *Can J Surg* 1976;**19**:505–511.
6 EDMUNDS LH, JR, WILLIAMS GM, WELCH CE. External fistulas arising from the gastrointestinal tract. *Ann Surg* 1960;**152**:445–471.
7 FISCHER JE. The management of high out-put intestinal fistulas. *Adv Surg* 1975;**9**:139–176.
8 GRAHAM JA. Conservative treatment of gastrointestinal fistulas. *Surg Gynaecol Obstet* 1977;**144**:512–514.
9 HALVERSEN RC, HOGLE HH, RICHARDS RC. Gastric and small bowel fistulas. *Am J Surg* 1969;**118**:968–972.
10 KAMINSKY VM, DEITEL M. Nutritional support in the management of external fistulas of the alimentary tract. *Br J Surg* 1975;**62**:100–103.
11 KOEHLER PR, KNOCHEL JQ. Computed tomography in the evaluation of abdominal abscesses. *Am J Surg* 1980;**140**:675–678.

12 KOROBKIN M, CALLEN P, FILLY RA. Comparison of computed tomography, ultrasonography and gallium-67 scanning in the evaluation of suspected abdominal abscess. *Radiology* 1978;**129**:89–93.

13 MacERLEAN DP, OWENS AP, HOURIHANE JB. Ultrasound guided percutaneous abdominal abscess drainage. *Br J Radiol* 1981;**54**:394–97.

14 MacFAYDEN BV JR, DUDRICK SJ, RUBERG RL. Management of gastrointestinal fistulas with parenteral hyperalimentation. *Surgery* 1973;**74**:100–105.

15 MacINTYRE PB, RITCHIE JK, HAWLEY PR, BARTRAM CI, LENNARD-JONES JE. Management of enterocutaneous fistulas: a review of 132 cases. *Br J Surg* 1984;**71**:293–296.

16 REBER HA, ROBERTS C, WAY LW, DUNPHY JE. Management of external gastrointestinal fistulas. *Ann Surg.* 1978;**188**:460–467.

17 ROBISON JG, POLLOCK TW. Computed tomography in the diagnosis and localization of intraabdominal abscesses. *Am J Surg* 1980;**140**:783–786.

18 ROCCHIO MA, Mocha CJ, HAAS KF, RANDALL HT. Use of chemically defined diets in the management of patients with high output gastrointestinal cutaneous fistulas. *Am J Surg* 1974;**127**:148–156.

19 SANSONI B, IRVING M. Small bowel fistulas. *World J Surg* 1985;**9**:897–903.

20 SOETERS PB, EBEID AM, FISCHER JE. Review of 404 patients with gastrointestinal fistulas. Impact of parenteral nutrition. *Ann Surg* 1979;**190**:189–202.

21 THOMAS RJS, ROSALION A. The use of parenteral nutrition in the management of external gastrointestinal tract fistulae. *Aust NZ J Surg* 1978;**48**:535–539.

22 VOITK AJ, ECHAVE V, BROWN RA, McARDLE RA, GURD FN. Elemental diet in the treatment of fistulas of the alimentary tract. *Surg Gynaecol Obstet* 1973;**137**:68–72.

23 WEST JP, RING EM, MILLER RE, BURKS WP. A study of the causes and treatment of external post operative intestinal fistulas. *Surg Gynaecol Obstet* 1961;**113**:490–486.

24 WOLFE BM, KELTNER RM, WILLIAM VL. Intestinal fistula output in regular elemental and intravenous alimentation. *Am J Surg* 1972;**124**:803–806.

Chapter 46
Consequences of Small Intestinal Resection

G.E. GRIFFIN & T.C. NORTHFIELD

Resection of short segments of intestine is a common surgical procedure which usually has no chronic sequelae, unless the ileum, the active transport site for bile acids and vitamin B_{12}, is removed. If more than 50% of the small intestine is resected serious nutritional fluid and electrolyte deficiencies, which can be life-threatening, may occur. Collectively these problems and the associated diarrhoea are known as the short bowel syndrome [3].

Aetiology

Several distinct intestinal disease processes give rise to the need for small intestinal resection. The commonest acute cause is mesenteric vascular occlusion. Other causes are shown in Table 46.1.

Table 46.1. Causes of small intestinal resection.

Vascular	Mesenteric vascular occlusion
	Mechanical obstruction with mesenteric infarction
	Vasculitis
Inflammatory	Regional enteritis
	Radiation injury
Neoplastic	Lymphoma or carcinoma
	Gardner's syndrome
Traumatic	

Prognostic guidelines

Prognostic guidelines (Table 46.2) are based on the extent and level of resection and on the capacity for intestinal adaptation.

Table 46.2. Prognostic guidelines after extensive intestinal resection.

Extent of resection
Site of resection
Intestinal adaptation
Retention of ileocaecal sphincter
Retention of colon (especially the ascending colon)

Extent of resection

The length of the normal small intestine varies between individuals, but it is generally in the region of 4 metres. There is considerable absorptive reserve capacity, so that most patients tolerate a resection of up to 50% of their small intestine and still maintain adequate nutrition on oral intake. When more than 50% of the small intestine is resected, malabsorption and compromised nutritional status may follow [22]. Long-term survival has been recorded in patients with as little as 15–45 cm of jejunum, in addition to a normal duodenum and colon [26].

Site of resection

Assessment of resection should take into account the specific absorptive functions of the terminal ileum and assumes the presence of normal duodenal and colonic function. Resection of relatively small amounts of distal ileum (50–80 cm) may result in malabsorption of vitamin B_{12} and of bile acids. Compromised nutritional status following extensive small intestinal resection is usually not associated with fluid and electrolyte problems. However, when small intestinal resection is combined with colonic resection, fluid and electrolyte homeostasis often become a serious problem [14]. The sodium and water absorptive capacity of the colon decreases distally, so that retention of the ascending colon is a good prognostic feature. Retention of the ileocaecal valve is also a good prognostic indicator due to slowing of intestinal transit and decreased contamination of the remaining small intestine by colonic organisms.

Intestinal adaptation

Intestinal adaptation is the morphological and functional change of the residual intestine, so that absorption is increased per unit length. Following removal of the ileum in animals the remaining intestine undergoes mucosal hyperplasia. The villous height increases and this is associated with an increase in the height and number of enterocytes [23]. It is thought that humoral factors, as well as local luminal stimulation are involved in adaptation of the shortened gut [25]. A similar increase in height of villous epithelial cells has been documented after 75% resection in humans and enhanced segmental glucose and sodium absorption has been shown [6]. The adaptive capacity of the small intestine remaining after extensive resection differs according to the level of resection. The ileum adapts to

a greater extent than the jejunum, so that preservation of the ileum is a good prognostic point. It is thought that intestinal adaptation may take up to one year to be complete. In addition, there is evidence from animal experiments that the colon possesses adaptive capacity in terms of sodium and water absorption following massive small intestinal resection.

Pathophysiology

Ileal resection (Table 46.3)

Even if only a short segment is removed resection of the ileum is important, because it is the only part of the small intestine where vitamin B_{12} and bile acids are absorbed. The consequences of vitamin B_{12} malabsorption may take years to develop, because normal body stores may be sufficient to last for about four years. The consequences of bile acid malabsorption, on the other hand, are immediate. A relatively mild degree of ileal malabsorption of bile acids causes watery diarrhoea. This is because dihydroxy bile acids cause fluid and electrolyte secretion from the colonic mucosa if they are present in solution in the colonic lumen at a concentration greater than 3 mmol/l [16]. The mechanism involved has not been elucidated. Apart from bile acid malabsorption, the other factor in-

Table 46.3. Ileal resection.

Problem	Mechanism	Treatment
Diarrhoea	Increased colonic bile acids conc. stimulates Na^+ and H_2O secretion	Cholestyramine (4 g with each meal)
Steatorrhoea	Low jejunal bile acid conc. decreases fat solubilization	Low fat diet (30 g/day) $\pm$ cimetidine (400 mg $\frac{1}{2}$ hr before meals) or ranitidine (150 mg twice daily)
Vitamin B_{12} deficiency	B_{12} malabsorption	Hydroxocobalamin 1000 μg i.m. every 2 months
Gallstones	Decreased bile acid pool size	Cholecystectomy
Renal oxalate stones	Fatty acids saponify Ca^{++} allowing colonic oxalate absorption	Low fat diet, low dietary oxalate $\pm$ calcium carbonate orally (2.5 g tds)

fluencing aqueous phase bile acid concentration is intraluminal colonic pH. If pH falls below 6, unconjugated bile acids precipitate out of solution [15]. Intraluminal pH may be lower following extensive resections, because of fermentation of the unabsorbed food by bacteria.

Following large ileal resections the problem of watery diarrhoea is compounded by steatorrhoea. This is because the degree of bile acid malabsorption exceeds the capacity of the liver to compensate by increasing bile acid synthesis. Experiments in the rhesus monkey have shown that an interruption of more than 20% in the enterohepatic

circulation of bile acids causes decreased bile acid secretion and therefore an increase in faecal fat excretion [7]. This situation can be critically influenced in humans by the fact that not all of the bile acid is in solution in the upper jejunal lumen. Glycine-conjugated bile acids precipitate out of solution if the pH falls below 5 and upper jejunal contents following ileal resection are often at a pH below this critical value [18]. Fat absorption under these circumstances is also affected by transit rate and by the amount of small intestinal mucosa available for absorption. Fatty acids also cause colonic water and electrolyte

Table 46.4. Massive intestinal resection.

Phase	Problem	Mechanism	Treatment
Acute	Massive GI fluid loss	Gastric hypersecretion + unknown	i.v. supplementation H_2-receptor antagonist
	Malnutrition	No oral intake	Total parenteral nutrition
Adaptive	Diarrhoea and steatorrhoea Malnutrition	Hyperosmolar drinks; lack of absorptive capacity; rapid transit	Gradual introduction of solid food or isotonic liquid feeds. Avoidance of hyperosmolar drinks
			H_2-receptor antagonist antimotility agent
Chronic	Diarrhoea and steatorrhoea	Lack of absorptive capacity	Small frequent meals, resection diet (Table 46.6), cimetidine
	Diarrhoea alone	Increased colonic bile acid conc. stimulates Na^+ and H_2O secretion	Cholestyramine
	Malnutrition	Lack of absorptive capacity	Resection diet; parenteral vitamin supplements; home parenteral nutrition
	Fluid and electrolyte deficiency	Lack of absorptive capacity; absence of colon decreases Na^+ absorption	Oral isotonic glucose electrolyte solution Parenteral $MgSO_4$ (24 mmol/day) Oral metabolic mineral mixture
	Hyperoxaluria	See Table 46.3	Low fat diet (30 g); low dietary oxalate; oral calcium carbonate (2.5 g tds)

secretion [1], so that steatorrhoea is usually accompanied by diarrhoea. Bile acid malabsorption in excess of the liver's ability to compensate by increased synthesis causes a smaller bile acid pool size, thus predisposing to gallstone formation.

Urinary hyperoxaluria may cause renal oxalate stones. It is now appreciated that these can complicate steatorrhoea due to any cause, because unabsorbed fatty acids combine with calcium, leaving oxalate free for absorption. It is thought that this oxalate would normally be sequestered in the gut lumen with calcium and then excreted in the stool.

Massive intestinal resection (Table 46.4)

Acute phase

The production of a large stool or stoma output in the early postoperative phase is not clearly understood. One factor is gastric hypersecretion of acid [17]. This rapidly declines, but may take up to two months to return to normal. It is thought that the hypersecretion may be related to hypergastrinaemia [24].

Adaptive phase

When feeding is recommenced the presence of osmotically active particles in the gut lumen induces flux across the intestinal mucosa. When hypertonic solutions are present in the lumen there is a rapid flow of fluid from the extravascular compartment into the gut lumen until isotonicity is achieved. The presence of food in the lumen induces gastric, pancreatic and biliary secretion, and these may all play a part in the production of diarrhoea.

Chronic phase

When adaptation is complete, diarrhoea continues as a result of malabsorption of bile and fatty acids. This secretory component is compounded by the osmotic forces mentioned above. In addition, if there is associated colonic resection, sodium balance becomes critical, as the colonic capacity to absorb sodium is lost.

Clinical features

Ileal resection

The immediate effect of ileal resection is to cause diarrhoea and/or steatorrhoea, once oral feeding is restarted. Resections of 50–100 cm of ileum tend to cause diarrhoea, while resections of more than 100 cm cause steatorrhoea [13] (Fig. 46.1). Vitamin B_{12}

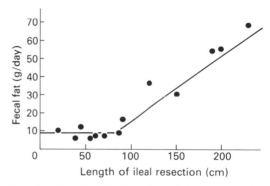

Fig. 46.1. Length of ileal resection related to faecal fat excretion ([13] reproduced with permission from *New Engl J Med.*)

deficiency is unlikely to develop for several years after ileal resection in the presence of adequate vitamin B_{12} stores. There is an increased incidence of cholesterol gallstones following ileal resection and also a propensity for oxalate renal stones to develop.

Massive small intestinal resection

Acute phase

In the acute phase the main problem is that of severe negative fluid and electrolyte balance due to massive loss from the residual alimentary tract. This loss may be in the order of 12 l/day initially, and maintenance of fluid and electrolyte balance is crucial at this stage.

Adaptive phase

This phase starts with oral feeding and may last up to two years. The stool volume and stoma output will progressively decrease over this period. Careful weaning onto a solid diet is required.

Chronic phase

When adaptation is complete and the diet has been optimized (see treatment section), a more or less constant stool volume or stoma output will be achieved. This will probably be in the region of 1.5–4 l/day [10].

Investigations

Ileal resection

It is important to determine whether the predominant problem is one of diarrhoea or steatorrhoea. If this is not obvious from the history, then three or five day stool collection should be done, preferably as an inpatient and on a defined fat intake of 70–100 g/day in order to determine faecal wet weight and faecal fat excretion. Diarrhoea is defined as a faecal wet weight in excess of 200 g/day and steatorrhoea as a faecal fat excretion in excess of 18 mmol/24 h. It is important to carry out a Schilling test of vitamin B_{12} absorption in the presence of intrinsic factor; measurements of serum B_{12} concentrations will give falsely reassuring values until vitamin B_{12} stores are depleted, a long time later.

Bile acid malabsorption gives rise to an abnormal ^{14}C-glycocholate bile acid breath test, because unabsorbed bile acids spill over into the colon where they are decon-

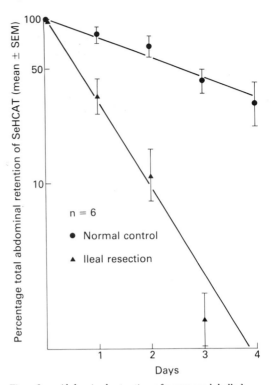

Fig. 46.2. Abdominal retention of a gamma labelled bile acid (SeHCAT) in patients with ileal resection and normal subjects (n = 6 for both groups) (unpublished observations: Ferraris, Jazrawi and Northfield, 1982).

jugated [8]. It may not be clear on clinical grounds whether the problem is one of jejunal bacterial overgrowth, or one of bile acid malabsorption. Tests can be used to distinguish these possibilities. One method is to measure ^{14}C radioactivity in the stools, but this is a research procedure requiring a combustion chamber. The best prospect for a clinical test of bile acid absorption lies in the recent development of a gamma labelled bile acid (^{75}selenium labelled homocholic acid conjugated with taurine—^{75}SeHCAT). Bile acid malabsorption can be detected following oral administration of this labelled bile acid, either by measuring faecal radioactivity using a large volume gamma counter [21], or by measuring abdominal radioactivity on successive days using a gamma camera (Fig. 46.2). More accurate measurements can be made by scanning the gall bladder alone, because this is independent of colonic retention of ⁷⁵SeHCAT[8].

Massive small intestinal resection

Acute phase

Careful monitoring of fluid and electrolyte status is crucial. Urinary and stool (or stoma) volumes should be carefully measured and balance achieved by giving appropriate volumes of intravenous fluid. Measurement of urinary sodium excretion gives a simple and accurate estimate of intravenous sodium requirements. Oliguria will be present and urinary sodium absent, if the volume of intravenous saline is inadequate [11]. This is because the kidney is able to respond homeostatically to the antidiuretic hormone and aldosterone secreted as a result of the metabolic derangement, but the jejunum is unresponsive and the colon has limited capacity.

Adaptive phase

The nutritional status of the patient should be assessed, in addition to continued monitoring of the fluid and electrolyte balance.

Chronic phase

When the chronic phase has been reached, the alimentary tract anatomy should be recorded with a barium meal and follow-through (Fig. 46.3). This may show strictures requiring further surgery. The functional capacity of the tract should be assessed from faecal fat excretion on a defined fat intake and from a glucose tolerance test (Figure 46.4). If high stoma output and oliguria are features of this chronic phase, admission to hospital and a careful assessment of fluid and electrolyte balance are important [11].

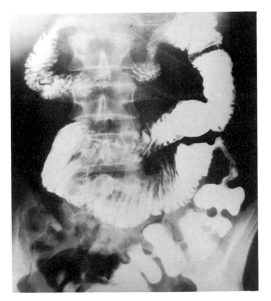

Fig. 46.3. Barium meal and follow-through examination on a patient with 45 cm of jejunum anastomosed to the descending colon one year after resection. Note the widened jejunum and the prominent jejunal folds typical of intestinal adaptation.

When stool output is stable, the nutritional status of the patient becomes the major problem (see Chapter 78). Methods used to assess nutrition are controversial and some maintain that general physical examination by an experienced clinician is as good as quantitative assessment [2]. However, in order to record recovery, measurement of the following simple indices is recommended—body weight, plasma albumin, haemoglobin, mid-arm circumference and skinfold thickness. In addition, clinical photographs of the patient at monthly intervals have proved useful. In centres with specialized facilities, plasma concentrations of retinol binding protein, thyroid binding prealbumin and total body potassium have been used as indices of protein nutrition.

Vitamin and essential fatty acid deficiency may take years to develop. The serum, or whole body measurement of these substances is costly and difficult to

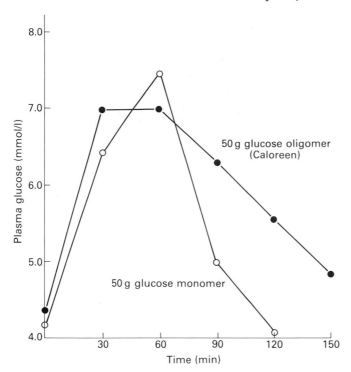

Fig. 46.4. Glucose tolerance tests in a patient with 50 cm of jejunum ending in a jejunostomy one year after resection. 50 g of glucose monomer were ingested fasting and the following day the test was repeated using 50 g glucose oligomer. Similar curves indicate adequate hydrolysis and absorption of the oligosaccharide.

obtain in most centres, and therefore it is recommended that prophylactic treatment is given. The readily available investigations should be done at regular intervals, and include estimation of vitamin B_{12}, folic acid, zinc and magnesium.

Treatment

Ileal resection (Table 46.3)

As diarrhoea is due to the presence of excess bile acids in solution in the colonic lumen, the logical treatment is to use a bile acid binding agent. An anion exchange resin such as cholestyramine 1–3 g with each meal is usually effective for bile acid-induced diarrhoea [13]. The taste is unpleasant and the patient should experiment with different flavoured drinks in order to determine the best way of taking the sachets, or alternatively incorporate the granules in a fruit-flavoured jelly.

Cholestyramine exacerbates the problem in patients with steatorrhoea, because it binds bile acids in the jejunum, thus further decreasing aqueous phase bile acid concentration. A low fat diet, for example, 30 g fat/day (Table 46.5) is the mainstay of treatment. Apart from restricting the choice of food, this diet has no undesirable effects and general nutrition is well maintained. In patients with severe steatorrhoea which does not respond to fat restriction alone, cimetidine can be given in a dose of 400 mg half an hour before each main meal [16]. This decreases acid-mediated bile acid precipitation in the jejunum, improving micellar solubilization and thus absorption of fat [9].

If vitamin B_{12} malabsorption is demonstrated by Schilling test, it is important to give prophylactic vitamin B_{12} therapy: hydroxocobalamin 1000 μg intramuscularly every two months. If this is not started early, the risk of gradual development of vitamin B_{12} deficiency may be forgotten until complications have developed.

Table 46.5. General advice for a low fat diet.*

Dairy products	Skimmed milk, cheese with low fat content (< 17%)
Vegetables	Any fresh, frozen or cooled vegetables without added fat
Fruits	Any fresh (except avocado), canned, frozen or dried
Meat	Lean, well trimmed meat (particularly poultry, liver and fish)
Bread and cereals	All kinds except high fat (such as sponge cake). Try to eat bread without margarine or butter
Fats	Low fat margarine or oil with high concentration of polyunsaturated fats
Avoid	Nuts, olives, peanut butter, coconut Conventional cooking methods with no added fat are the best ways to prepare meat

* Reproduced by permission of Dr H. Andersson, Department of Clinical Nutrition, University of Göteborg.

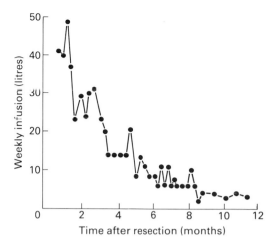

Fig. 46.5. The intravenous fluid requirement of a patient following intestinal resection for mesenteric vascular occlusion. 45 cm of jejunum was anastomosed to the sigmoid colon (see Fig. 46.3).

Massive small intestinal resection (Table 46.4)

Acute phase

Maintenance of fluid and electrolyte balance is crucial during this phase, based on careful balance studies. In addition, total parenteral nutrition should be started early and monitored metabolically (see Chapter 78). The intravenous fluid requirement of a patient with 45 cm of jejunum anastomosed to the sigmoid colon is shown in Fig. 46.5.

Adaptive phase

The stimulus of luminal food is most important to promote intestinal adaptation. In animal models, the small intestine and pancreas atrophy in the absence of intraluminal stimuli despite adequate intravenous nutrition. The introduction of oral food must be gradual, and attention paid to its composition.

The key to enteral feeding is the avoidance of hyperosmolar solutions by providing solid food, or a liquid diet in the form of isosmolar solutions (see Chapter 78). Drinks of high osmolality (for example, Hycal-3,200 mosmol/kg) should be strictly avoided, because the high osmotic load in the lumen of the intestinal remnant causes severe diarrhoea. The effect of inadvertent administration of Hycal 0.5 l/day to a patient with 45 cm jejunum anastomosed to the sigmoid colon is shown in Fig. 46.6. Isosmolar solutions can be delivered by fine-bore nasogastric tube, or as sipping solutions and have the advantage of supplying trace elements and vitamins in addition to calories and protein.

Mucosal hydrolysis of oligosaccharides, for example Caloreen (Roussel Limited), may be adequate in these patients (Fig. 46.4). Such compounds can be used with great benefit, as their osmotic load is considerably less than that of their monomer. For example, Caloreen solutions have only 20% of the osmotic load of solutions

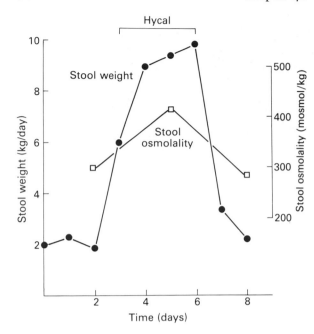

Fig. 46.6. The effect of inadvertent administration of 500 ml Hycal (3,200 mosmol/kg) per day on stool output and osmolality in a patient with 45 cm jejunum anastomosed to the sigmoid colon (see Fig. 46.3).

containing the same amount of glucose monomer.

The relative lack of lactase in these patients demands avoidance of dietary lactose. This can be achieved by using a lactose-free milk substitute (such as Coffeemate), or by digesting lactose in the milk bottle by adding a sachet of commercially available lactase (Lactaid, Granose Food Limited). Formal lactose tolerance tests should be done on these patients about one year after resection when they have reached the chronic phase, in order to determine the necessity for a lactose-free diet—this is a restricting diet which should not be given unnecessarily.

The amount of fat in the diet is usually maintained at 30 g/day, because unabsorbed fatty acids increase fluid and electrolyte loss in the stool, and also increase faecal excretion of calcium and magnesium. The nutritional gain of decreasing the oral fat intake from 100 g to 30 g/day in a patient with 15 cm of jejunum anastomosed to the transverse colon is shown in Fig. 46.7. Cimetidine has been shown to im-

prove nutrient absorption in a patient with 33 cm of jejunum [4]. Medium chain triglycerides (MCT) are absorbed directly through the mucosa and transported into the portal circulation. The substitution of between 50% and 75% of total oral fat intake with MCT has been shown to be an effective way of diminishing faecal loss of water and sodium and improving nutrition. However, oral MCT is unpalatable and there are few suitable preparations containing MCT. The most useful of these is Trisorbon (BDH Pharmaceuticals Ltd), which also contains vitamins and oligosarccharides. Alternatively Liquigen (Scientific Hospital Supplies), an MCT-water emulsion, can be used.

The well-established use of low fat diets has been challenged by a study demonstrating that the use of high fat diets (in excess of 100 g/day) may increase nutritional status without increasing diarrhoea [20]. The rationale behind this is that a fixed percentage of ingested fat is absorbed. Therefore, raising the fat load increases the absolute amount absorbed and enhances the nutri-

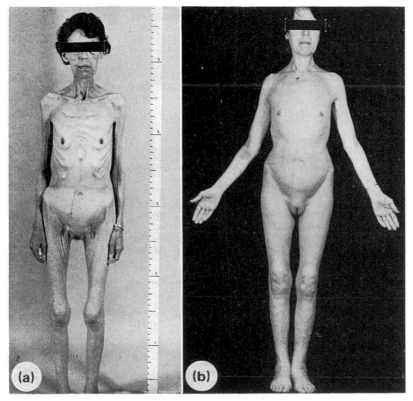

Fig. 46.7. The nutritional effect of reducing dietary fat from *ad libitum* (left) to 30 g daily (right) in a patient with 15 cm of jejunum anastomosed to mid transverse colon. The photographs were taken five months apart [5].

tional state. The combination of cimetidine or ranitidine with this high fat diet should be helpful.

Chronic phase

Intestinal adaptation will be complete after about one year. If an adequate nutritional status has not been attained by this time home total parenteral nutrition should be considered. Fortunately this is a rare occurrence, although patients have been maintained for longer than eight years on this system.

In the chronic phase, when intestinal adaptation is complete, nutritional and fluid and electrolyte deficiencies may still become apparent. The 'resection diet' (see Tables 46.5 and 46.6) has to be maintained, but this alone may be insufficient even with added table salt to maintain adequate salt and water balance, particularly in patients who have little or no colonic absorptive function. Under these circumstances maintenance of fluid and electrolyte balance can be achieved by using glucose/electrolyte solutions based on those used in the treatment of cholera [11].

Even when adequate protein and calorie intake is maintained in these patients, negative magnesium, calcium and trace element balance may exist. The only form of magnesium suitable for treatment is oral or intravenous magnesium sulphate, 24 mmol/day. Calcium balance can be promoted by giving parenteral vitamin D

Table 46.6. An example of a diet for patients after intestinal resection.

Intake per day		Meal pattern	
Skimmed milk*	800 ml	*Breakfast*	
Low fat spread	40 g	Weetabix + milk	
Wholemeal bread	5 slices	Sugar	10 g
Weetabix	2 biscuits	Wholemeal bread	1 slice
Sugar	35 g	Jam	5 g
Jam	5 g	*Mid morning*	
Fruit yoghurt	150 g	Fruit yoghurt	
Chicken	90 g	*Lunch*	
Potato	120 g	Chicken	90 g
Apple	100 g	Potato	120 g
Cottage cheese	50 g	Vegetable	
Rice	20 g	Stewed fruit	
Bournvita	10 g	*Evening*	
Liquigen†	50 ml	Cottage cheese	50 g
		Wholemeal bread	2 slices
		Salad/veg	
		Milk pudding (rice)	
		Wholemeal bread	2 slices
		Bedtime	
		Bournvita drink	

This diet provides 90 g protein with 30 g fat and a total of 2000 kcal. Vitamin supplements, essential fatty acids and trace elements can be added as described in the text. Hyperosmolar solutions are avoided. Extra calories can be given in the form of Caloreen in milk drinks. Table salt to a maximum of 6 g per day can be tolerated if sodium balance is a problem.
* Lactose free if necessary. † Liquigen is added to 300 ml milk for palatability.
(Kindly reproduced by permission of Ms S. Day, dietitian, St George's Hospital).

(100,000 units/month) and added calcium carbonate in the diet (up to 7.5 g/day) which also helps to prevent hyperoxaluria. Trace elements can be supplied orally in the form of Metabolic Mineral mixture (Hospitals Supply Ltd.), or intravenously in the form of Addamel. Essential fatty acid deficiency may become a problem, and manifests initially as a red scaly rash; this can be prevented by rubbing sunflower seed oil into the skin (20 ml/week) or monthly infusions of 500 ml 20% Intralipid. Water soluble and fat soluble vitamin deficiencies may develop. These can be avoided using injected Parentrovite and intravenous Vitilipid dissolved in Intralipid.

Surgical treatment

Reversed loops have been suggested as a mechanical means of delaying transit in the remaining intestine. However, this procedure has been discontinued in view of its small beneficial effect in the face of a large operative risk.

References

1 AMMON HV, PHILLIPS SF. Inhibition of colonic water and electrolyte absorption by fatty acids in man. *Gastroenterology* 1973;**65**:744–749.
2 BAKER JP, DETSKY AS, WESSON DE, *et al.* Nutritional assessment, a comparison of clinical judgment and objective measurements. *N Engl J Med* 1982; **306:** 969–972.
3 BOOTH CC. Intestinal resection and bypass. In: Booth CC, Neale G, eds. *Disorders of the small intestine.* Oxford: Blackwell Scientific Publications, 1986:101–117.
4 CORTOT A, FLEMING CR, MALAGELADA JR. Improved nutrient absorption after cimetidine in short bowel syndrome with gastric hypersecretion. *New Engl J Med* 1979;**300**:79–80.
5 DOWLING RH. The complication and medical treatment of small bowel resection. In: . *Treatment of*

small bowel disease symposium, Nice 1972. Basel: Karger, 1973:102.

6 DOWLING RH. Intestinal adaptations. *N Engl J Med* 1973;**288**:520–521.

7 DOWLING RH, MACK E, SMALL DM, PICOTT J. Effects of controlled interruption of the enterohepatic circulation of bile salts by biliary diversion and by ileal resection on bile salt secretion, synthesis and pool size in the Rhesus monkey. *J Clin Invest* 1970;**49**:232–242.

8 FERRARIS J, JAZRAWI R, BRIDGES C, NORTHFIELD TC. Use of a γ-labelled amino acid (^{75}SeHCAT) as a test of ileal function: methods of improving accuracy. *Gastroenterology* 1986;**20**:1129–1136.

9 FITZPATRICK WJF, ZENTLER MUNRO PL, NORTHFIELD TC. Ileal resection: effect of cimetidine and taurine on intrajejunal bile acid precipitation and lipid solubilization. *Gut* 1986;**27**:66–72.

10 FROMM H, HOFMANN, AF. Breath test for altered bile-acid metabolism. *Lancet* 1971;621–625.

11 GRIFFIN GE, FAGAN E, HODGSON HJF, CHADWICK VS. Enteral therapy in the management of massive gut resection complicated by chronic fluid and electrolyte depletion. *Dig Dis Sci* 1982;**27**:902–908.

12 HILL GL. Massive enterectomy: indications and management. *World J Surg* 1985;**9**:833–841.

13 HOFMANN AF, POLEY RJ. Cholestyramine treatment of diarrhoea associated with ileal resection. *N Engl J Med* 1969;**281**:854–858.

14 LADEFOGED K, ØLGAARD K. Fluid and electrolyte absorption and renin-angiotensin-aldesterone axis in patients with severe short bowel syndrome. *Scand J Gastroenterol* 1979;**14**:729–735.

15 MCJUNKIN B, AMIN P, FROMM H. The role of fecal pH in the mechanism of diarrhoea in bile acid malabsorption. *Gastroenterology* 1981;**80**:1454–1464.

16 MEKHIJIAN MS, PHILLIPS SF, HOFMANN AF. Colonic secretion of water and electrolytes induced by bile acids. Perfusion studies in man. *J Clin Invest* 1971;**50**:1569–1577.

17 MURPHY PJ, KING DR, DUBOIS A. Treatment of gastric hypersecretion with cimetidine in the short bowel syndrome. *N Engl J Med* 1979;**300**:80–81.

18 NORTHFIELD TC, ZENTLER-MUNRO PL, FITZPATRICK WJF. Treatment of pancreatic and ileectomy steatorrhoea. In: Baron JH, ed. *Cimetidine in the 80s*. Edinburgh: Churchill Livingstone, 1981. 208–214.

19 SCHWARTZ MZ, MAEDA K. Short bowel syndrome in infants and children. *Pediatr Clin North Am* 1985;**32**:1265–1279.

20 SIMKO V, MCCARROLL AM, GOODMAN S, WAESNER RE, KELLEY RE. High-fat diet in a short bowel syndrome: intestinal absorption and gastroenteropancreatic hormone responses. *Dig Dis Sci* 1980;**25**:333–339.

21 THAYSEN EH, ORHOLM M, ARNFRED T, CARL J, RØDBRO P. Assessment of ileal function by abdominal counting of the retention of a gamma emitting bile acid analogue. *Gut* 1982;**23**:862–865.

22 WESER E. The management of patients after small bowel resection. *Gastroenterology* 1976;**71**:146–150.

23 WESER E, HERNANDEZ MH. Studies of small bowel adaptation after intestinal resection in the rat. *Gastroenterology* 1971;**60**:69–75.

24 WILLIAMS NS, EVANS P, KING RFGJ. Gastric acid secretion and gastrin production in the short bowel syndrome. *Gut* 1985;**26**:914–919.

25 WILLIAMSON RCN, BUCHHOLTZ TW, MALT RA. Humoral stimulation of cell proliferation in small bowel after transection and resection in rats. *Gastroenterology* 1978;**75**:249–254.

26 WINAWER SJ, ZAMCHECK N. Pathophysiology of small intestinal resection in man. In: Glass GBJ, ed. *Progress in gastroenterology 1*. New York: Grune & Stratton, 1968;334–346.

Chapter 47
Other Diseases of the Small Intestine

G. E. SLADEN

Acquired primary alactasia

This term refers to the common post-weaning phenomenon of relative or absolute loss of the intestinal mucosal enzyme lactase, which is responsible for hydrolysing lactose into its constituent monosaccharides (glucose and galactose) before absorption by the enterocyte. This variable form of mild milk intolerance must be distinguished from other forms of milk sensitivity, especially those related to milk protein allergy. The rare congenital deficiencies of sugar transport that cause infantile and childhood diarrhoea are also distinct from acquired primary alactasia. Finally, relative lack of mucosal lactase can occur in any diffuse small intestinal mucosal disease, and is reversible if the disease can be treated effectively. This secondary phenomenon will not be considered further here, although it is an important cause of milk intolerance.

Prevalence

Gradual loss of intestinal lactase in the years after weaning from breast milk is normal in many parts of the world, especially in much of Africa, South America, South India and along the Mediterranean littoral. By contrast, North Europeans and people derived from the North West regions of India and the former Aryan civilizations of the near East mostly retain intestinal lactase into adult life and are able to drink large amounts of milk without symptoms. Epidemiological studies have shown that in much of Northern Europe and among North American whites, the prevalence of alactasia is between 5 and 15%. In southern Mediterranean countries, southern states of India and parts of Africa, the prevalence figures are between 75 and 100%. There are other regions with intermediate prevalence figures [16, 55, 57, 97].

Aetiology and pathology

The geographic distribution shows that lactase is retained in races and tribes derived from the cattle rearing nomads of the Aryan plains of the Middle and near East. It is presumed either that this represents an evolutionary response to the continuous consumption of cows' milk over many generations, or that in some way the rearing of cattle for milk was selected only by those who could tolerate milk in adult life. There is no scientific evidence that the enzyme is inducible by continued lactose ingestion [29].

Characteristically the intestinal mucosa is quite normal by light and electron microscopy. In this way the disorder is distinguished (if necessary) from secondary acquired alactasia. Undigested lactose produces abdominal symptoms by its capacity to retain water in the small intestine and to accelerate transit of intestinal contents into the colon, where bacterial fermentation produces gas and lactic acid. The greater the load of lactose, the shorter the intestinal transit time and the worse the symptoms [97].

Clinical features

The symptoms are abdominal rumbles, distension, excess flatus and variable watery diarrhoea. The subjects are otherwise fit and most affected people recognize their inability to drink large amounts of milk at an early age without seeking medical advice. The symptoms are very variable in their severity and surveys have revealed many alactasic subjects who are unaware of the problem. However, nearly all alactasics will experience symptoms with 50 g loads of lactose (equivalent to 1 litre of milk) and most will respond to 25 g. Only a minority respond symptomatically to 12 g lactose (1 glass of milk), or less [1, 29, 38]. It is not surprising, therefore, that in spite of the prevalence of this disorder it is seldom a major clinical problem, at least in healthy adults who can simply drink less milk.

The variable symptomatic tolerance of varying loads of lactose (or milk) is difficult to understand, but must be related to differing intestinal motility patterns and perhaps to different bacterial activity in the colon. There is evidence that the colon can adapt to the continued ingestion of unabsorbed sugar [76].

There are usually no clinical consequences of either the syndrome or the restriction of milk intake, although attention has been drawn to the relatively low calcium intake which may result and the possible implication in the development of osteoporosis in later life [69].

Investigations

The simple clinical assessment of the effects of milk withdrawal may suggest the diagnosis, but it is usually helpful to confirm this in view of many types of milk intolerance and the need to clarify the extent to which the restriction should be advised.

The 50 g lactose tolerance test is regarded as normal if the maximal rise of blood glucose over a period of 2–3 h is greater than 1.1 mmol/l (20 mg/100 ml) and if no symptoms are produced. The more recently introduced lactose breath H_2 test avoids the use of venepuncture and will usually be abnormal with lower loads of lactose (for example, 25 g). A rise of breath H_2 by more than 20 ppm within the first 2 h is usually taken to be abnormal [107]. Theoretically, a positive test should be followed by a similar test with the same total dose of 50% galactose and 50% glucose to exclude other intestinal transport problems. In practice, this is seldom necessary, but if there is any serious possibility of a major mucosal abnormality (especially coeliac disease) then a jejunal biopsy should be undertaken. The definitive test is the measurement of lactase activity in histologically normal jejunal mucosa [29], but this is rarely needed in practice.

Management

Restriction of milk intake is all that is required. Small quantities are usually well tolerated and there is no need to avoid milk entirely. Butter, cheese and yoghurt contain little or no lactose. Patients should be encouraged to drink milk within limits of tolerance in order to maintain a reasonable calcium intake. Various lactose-free milks are available commercially and contain normal amounts of calcium [72, 77].

Implications for feeding programmes in the underdeveloped world

Milk is the major source of nutrition in many of the feeding programmes throughout the world and, in many areas, lactase levels will be low for genetic reasons and will be further lowered by recurrent gut infections [60]. This has encouraged the development of lactose-free milks, but there are problems with cost and palatability. It seems that relatively small amounts of milk taken at intervals through the day in order to supplement traditional foods will be tolerated by most children [11].

Abdominal tuberculosis

Tuberculosis (TB) can affect any part of the gastrointestinal tract from mouth to anus. The most frequently affected sites are the ileum, proximal colon and peritoneum. The oesophagus [23] and pancreas [92] are very rarely involved. The condition is now uncommon in the indigenous populations in developed parts of the world as a result of the eradication of bovine tuberculosis and the decline of pulmonary tuberculosis in the last three decades. However, it is still found in emergent countries, and in immigrants in the West from emergent areas [71, 83].

Epidemiology

Abdominal tuberculosis affects both sexes at any age. In the United Kingdom it has been reported most frequently in immigrants, especially from the Indian subcontinent [58]. As with other forms of TB, it should also be considered in the deprived, malnourished and alcoholic sections of the community.

In England 2289 cases of non-respiratory tuberculosis were notified in 1980, compared with 6368 cases of respiratory disease. The decline of non-respiratory disease in the last 20 years has been much less impressive than that of respiratory disease [39]. Compared with respiratory cases, patients with non-respiratory TB tend to be younger adults and this probably reflects the fact that most of them are immigrants. The quoted mortality rate is 4.6%. Separate figures for abdominal tuberculosis are not available [14].

Aetiology

The human strain of *Mycobacterium tuberculosis* is considered to be responsible for the disease in all parts of the world where cattle are free of disease and where milk is pasteurized prior to consumption.

There is no known genetic predisposition to acquiring the infection. Its remarkable prevalence in certain racial groups is presumably environmental.

The organism gains access to the gut from the lumen, following the ingestion of sputum (or infected milk), although it is not always possible to demonstrate simultaneously active pulmonary disease. The long latent period of infection is well-known. Once the organism has penetrated the full thickness of the gut wall it can spread widely through the peritoneal fluid. Haematogenous spread is probably not common. The final result depends on the complex interplay between the load and virulence of the organisms, and the immune resistance of the host. Resistance is in part related to cell-mediated immunity, and this depends on the general health and nutritional status of the individual.

Pathology

Intestinal TB is a submucosal disease involving primarily the Peyer's patches, lymphoid follicles and the draining lymph nodes. Eventual destruction of muscle and mucosa occurs with thickening of the gut wall, mucosal ulceration and later stricture formation [68]. Serosal involvement encourages the development of adhesions to other loops of bowel and to the abdominal wall, with the formation of palpable masses. In comparison with Crohn's disease, fistulation appears to be rare. A mainly serosal infection can produce scattered white nodules (tubercles) throughout the visceral and parietal peritoneum, often with ascites.

Histologically, the characteristic lesion is

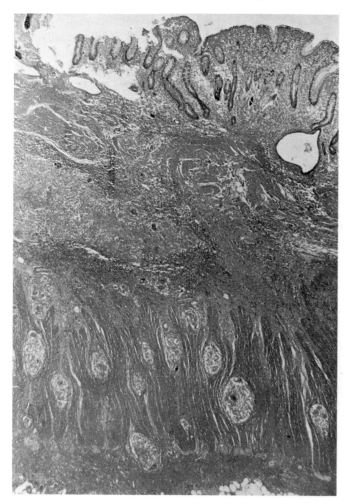

Fig. 47.1. Intestinal tuberculosis. Histopathology of the distal ileum showing transmural inflammation, granulomata and giant cells. H & E stain ([70] with permission of the authors and the *Br Med J*).

the giant cell granuloma with necrosis (caseation) and it is the caseation which particularly distinguishes this lesion from the now much commoner Crohn's disease. Careful use of the Ziehl-Neelsen and auramine stains should reveal the organism in active cases, especially in the area of caseation (Fig. 47.1).

Clinical presentation

The illness is usually subacute, measured in months, although an acute onset is well-recognized [58]. The symptoms are non-specific with malaise, anorexia, abdominal pain, diarrhoea and weight loss. The only distinctive signs are the presence of a tender mass, especially in the right iliac fossa, and ascites. It is interesting that patients tend to have either localized gut disease or ascites, but seldom both [89]. The ascites is rarely 'doughy' in spite of this time-honoured description, which probably applies to long-neglected cases of low virulence. The main complication is intestinal obstruction—bleeding and perforation are very unusual. Active pulmonary disease is found in fewer than 50% of cases, although reports differ in this respect [48, 88]. The association of TB with elderly males, alcoholism and poor nutrition applies more to respiratory, than to non-respiratory disease [14].

Investigations

These patients have moderate degrees of anaemia, leucocytosis and hypoalbuminaemia. Ascitic fluid has a high protein content (> 25 g/litre) and a characteristic excess of lymphocytes. The fluid seldom reveals the organisms on microscopy but culture is positive in about 70% of patients [89].

The radiological changes seen on barium studies are usually most conspicuous in the ileocaecal region and are those of irregular narrowing and ulceration, but they are not distinctive (Fig. 47.2 and Fig. 47.3). Colonoscopy may reveal irregular, thickened lesions with narrowing of the lumen or ulceration [8, 31]. The chest X-ray is normal in 50% of patients. The tuberculin test is positive in 50–80%. The only certain way of making the diagnosis is to see the organism in histopathological material or to grow it on culture. Surgery has usually been needed for this purpose in the past, but colonoscopy may now prove to be helpful. Closed, open and laparoscopic peritoneal biopsy techniques have been described and are safe, provided loops of bowel are not obviously matted together [18, 59, 109].

Differential diagnosis

The main contender is obviously Crohn's disease. Every attempt should be made to consider and exclude TB in all cases of

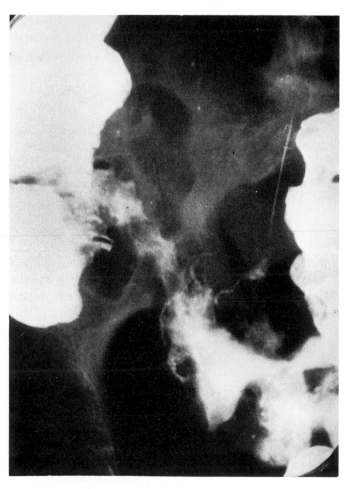

Fig. 47.2. Barium follow-through radiograph showing typical ileocaecal tuberculosis with irregular stricturing of the ileum and caecum ([70] with permission of the authors and the *Br Med J*).

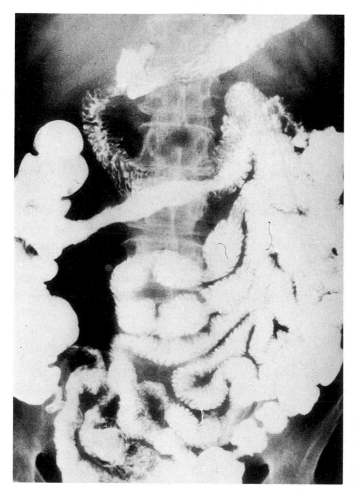

Fig. 47.3. Intestinal tuberculosis. Tuberculous stricture in the transverse colon with sparing of the ileocaecal region ([70] with permission of the authors and the *Br Med J*).

ileocaecal Crohn's disease, especially in immigrants and before starting corticosteroid therapy. Strong pointers to Crohn's disease are characteristic perianal lesions, extraintestinal manifestations of the disease, distinctive histological abnormalities in biopsies from macroscopically normal rectum and a negative tuberculin test. If serious doubt remains and the disease is localized radiologically, then surgical excision for diagnostic and therapeutic purposes should be favoured. If corticosteroid therapy seems necessary, then antituberculosis drugs should be used in addition.

Masses in the RIF may be produced by caecal carcinoma, ileal carcinoid tumour or lymphoma, and rarely chronic infection with amoebiasis or actinomycosis.

The other main differential diagnosis is that of ascites, of which the causes are numerous and careful examination of the fluid for malignant cells, other organisms, protein and amylase is required in all patients.

Medical treatment

Antituberculosis drugs should be started as soon as the diagnosis is confirmed, or if it is strongly suspected. A favourable clinical response to these drugs may prove to be the only way to confirm a presumed diagnosis.

An appropriate programme is rifampicin and isoniazid plus either ethambutol or streptomycin for two months, followed by rifampicin and isoniazid for seven more months—nine months' treatment in all [41]. Response to treatment is rapid and should be apparent within days. Treatment with isoniazid 300 mg and rifampicin 600 mg daily for one month, followed by isoniazid 900 mg and rifampicin 600 mg thrice weekly for a further eight months is also reported to be successful [24].

Supportive treatment may be necessary until the drugs are effective and includes blood transfusion, correction of electrolyte imbalance and enteral or parenteral nutrition, according to need.

Surgical treatment

Apart from the need for diagnostic specimens, surgery should be restricted to the treatment of complications that fail to respond to drugs, or which threaten life acutely. These include stenotic narrowing sufficient to produce obstructive pain or frank obstruction (Fig. 47.4) and, rarely,

bleeding or perforation. Excision and end-to-end anastomosis are preferred, as in the comparable operations for Crohn's disease.

Prognosis

Prognosis is excellent, provided that the organisms are sensitive to the drugs, that the patient complies with the prolonged treatment and that any mechanical complications can be dealt with surgically. Complete cure should be anticipated.

Long-term follow-up and the assessment of family and other contacts should be undertaken by chest physicians and the community physician as appropriate. All patients with tuberculosis in the United Kingdom must be notified to the appropriate health officer.

Whipple's disease

This rare cause of malabsorption can affect many parts of the body. It is considered to be a chronic infection by an unidentified agent, which is sensitive to antibiotics. Formerly it was fatal, but now it can be cured,

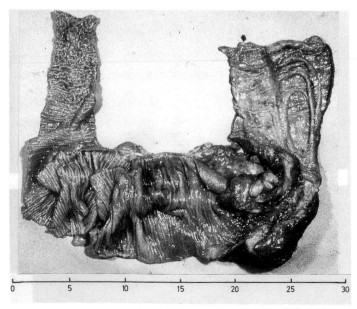

Fig. 47.4. Intestinal tuberculosis. Ileocaecal region resected from a patient with tuberculosis. There is gross thickening and stenosis of distal ileum ([70] with permission of the authors and the *Br Med J*).

although relapses may occur. Hence recognition is important and it has excited an interest out of all proportion to its prevalence in the community.

Epidemiology

The prevalence of Whipple's disease is very low, although several hundred patients have been reported [20,63]. Presumably with increasing recognition many more patients with Whipple's disease are now diagnosed, but not reported. On the other hand, patients with atypical and especially non-intestinal presentations may escape diagnosis in life. The patients are middle-aged or elderly, and almost all are white men. Only four black patients have been described [56].

Aetiology

A *Streptococcus* is believed to be the cause of the disease. Although isolation claims have been made [13], it has not proved possible to culture the organism consistently. Fluorescent antibody techniques applied to tissue have suggested that the organism is a *Streptococcus* with a characteristic set of antigens [7,53]. There is no known immunological deficit in patients who contract Whipple's disease, but a possible link with the HLA-B27 antigen has been suggested [20]. How the infection is acquired remains a mystery.

Pathology

The characteristic lesion is seen on jejunal biopsy material; post-mortem studies have shown that the entire small gut can be affected, often in a patchy way. The villi are swollen and sometimes shortened. The lamina propria of the mucosa is typically full of large macrophages containing much PAS positive material, which represents the bacteria in various stages of degradation (Fig. 47.5). The details of the bacteria have been described in several electron microscopic studies. They are elongated structures with a diffuse outer membrane external to the cell wall. They are found mainly in the lamina propria both within and outside macrophages, but can penetrate the muscularis mucosa and the enterocyte layer [21]. A submucosal variant has been described in one patient, who had been on antituberculosis drugs [56]. The bacteria may also be seen in dilated lymphatics and similar lesions with macrophage accumulation are described in mesenteric and peripheral lymph nodes. The contents are uniformly electron dense, apart from irregular tubular structures in the middle.

A detailed study of the hearts of 19 patients, who had died of Whipple's disease, revealed valvular thickening and deformity and myocardial infiltration by typical macrophages and bacteria in the majority. Cardiac symptoms were said to be present in life in over half, but this is difficult to interpret in middle-aged males [62]. Aortic insufficiency has been described as a presenting symptom [10]. Similar lesions have been seen in the brain at autopsy and on brain biopsies in patients with cerebral variant of the disease [37,45,74].

Clinical features

The typical patient is a middle-aged male with a long history (often of several years) of migratory polyarthritis and a variable malabsorption syndrome with, eventually, anaemia and weight loss. Cerebral symptoms may dominate the clinical picture and precede gut symptoms, but this is unusual [108]. The features are depression, ophthalmoplegias, and hypothalamic disturbances [81]. An acute meningoencephalitis has been described, but in one patient this may have been an allergic phenomenon because it responded promptly to corticosteroids [100]. The usual signs are those of weight

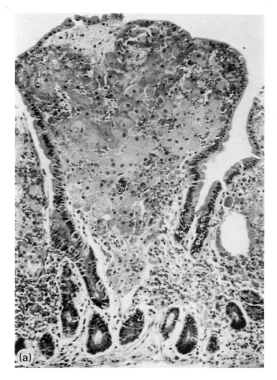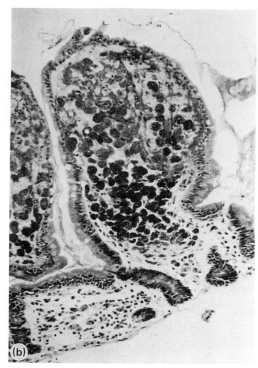

Fig. 47.5. (a) Whipple's disease. Haematoxylin-eosin stain of small intestinal mucosa shows pale macrophages in the lamina propria. The PAS stain (b) shows darkly staining PAS positive material in the macrophages.

loss, anaemia and, often, a non-deforming arthritis. Clubbing and pigmentation may be noted as in other patients with severe malabsorption.

Investigation and diagnosis

The blood abnormalities will be those of any severe malabsorptive state, often with an accompanying protein-losing enteropathy. Barium radiology of the small bowel shows an irregular thickened wall of non-specific appearances. The crucial diagnostic test is the jejunal biopsy and the appearances are quite characteristic. However, patients have been reported with minor or patchy changes missed by conventional biopsy. In the cerebral syndrome, brain biopsy has to be considered and typical macrophages have been identified in cerebrospinal fluid [100] Whipple's disease has to be distin-

guished from all the other causes of malabsorption, but the diagnosis is unlikely to be missed if the periodic acid Schiff (PAS) stain is applied routinely to jejunal biopsy material.

Medical treatment

Antibiotics have revolutionized the treatment of this disease and the outlook is now very good, although the cerebral syndrome may be irreversible on account of structural damage. The usually recommended treatment is oral or intramuscular penicillin and oral tetracycline for two weeks followed by tetracycline alone (1 g daily) for at least six months, according to progress. In cases of antibiotic sensitivity, sulfamethoxazole-trimethoprin has been used successfully and may be the best drug [102]. Chloramphenicol has been used, but it is not a suitable drug for continued treatment and it should probably be reserved for cerebral or meningeal cases, because it penetrates into the CSF effectively [28].

Full supportive therapy may be needed, as in all patients with malabsorption, while awaiting response to antibiotics. Corticosteroids are, in general, not indicated [100].

Prognosis

Prognosis is good and many cures are known. However, the disease can relapse after apparently successful treatment and the patients must be followed-up indefinitely [52] The jejunal biopsy returns to normal within six months of effective therapy and a relapse is diagnosed by repeating this procedure. Permanent cerebral damage can result if the brain is involved. Permanent joint damage is distinctly rare, even in untreated patients.

Ulcerative jejunoileitis [44, 99]

Ulceration of the small intestine is rare, if Crohn's disease is excluded. The ulcers are usually part of a pathological process such as coeliac disease, intestinal lymphoma, Behçet's disease [47] or small vessel disease, especially polyarteritis nodosa. Intestinal ulcers may also be caused by drugs, most notably by enteric-coated potassium chloride tablets [42]. Indomethacin has also been implicated and is known to produce ulceration in the rat small intestine [97].

Primary ulceration of the small intestine may occur as a solitary lesion with an acute presentation [96] or as a diffuse chronic process with malabsorption. The latter can be especially difficult to differentiate from coeliac disease, because peroral jejunal biopsies may show subtotal villous atrophy. However, these patients do not respond to a gluten-free diet and the prognosis is poor [66]. Baer, Byless and Yardley [4] reviewed 47 patients with intestinal ulceration and

malabsorption, but 22 were considered to have coeliac disease (responded to a gluten-free diet) and seven had a small intestinal lymphoma, leaving 18 with unclassifiable ulcerative jejunoileitis.

Clinical features

Clinical features are severe illness, with malaise, fever and malabsorption. Bleeding, perforation and stricture can all complicate the disorder. Small intestinal barium studies show non-specific features of malabsorption, with evidence of scattered focal pathology. Peroral small intestinal biopsy often shows changes suggestive of coeliac disease [4, 66].

Management and course

By definition, these patients do not respond to a gluten-free diet. Corticosteroids may produce temporary improvement, but probably only in a minority [4]. Patients often die from complications of the disease [66]. Surgical treatment is usually needed for the treatment of complications and excision may offer the best hope of survival if the disease is not too extensive.

Eosinophilic gastroenteropathy

Eosinophilic infiltration of the gut is a rare entity which occurs in several forms. A localized form of the disease with single polypoid masses at any point in the gastrointestinal tract should be regarded as part of the spectrum of inflammatory polyps and it has little in common with the more diffuse infiltration associated with systemic illness and peripheral blood eosinophilia which is considered here.

Epidemiology and aetiology

Little is known of the prevalence of this disorder. In 1978, Johnstone and Morson [46] gave a detailed account of 120 cases described in the literature up to that time. It can affect both sexes and all ages. Several reports from Holland, Japan and North America suggest that local outbreaks of the disease are related to infestation with certain nematodes [106].

In many patients the aetiology is unknown, but allergy and parasitic infestations have to be considered. It has been associated with severe multiple allergic states [12], with sensitivities to drugs such as gold [65], with colonic schistosomiasis [40] as well as with nematode infestation. Some patients with polyarteritis nodosa have eosinophilic infiltration of the gut, in addition to widespread small vessel lesions [96].

Pathology

The condition may affect all regions of the gut, but especially the stomach, small intestine and the proximal colon. The lesions may be mainly mucosal, intramural or serosal and can be diffuse or rather localized. The wall is thickened and there are usually small mucosal ulcers. Microscopically there is marked eosinophilic infiltration—especially in the submucosa, with patchy mucosal ulceration, but otherwise retention of the normal mucosal architecture.

Clinical features and diagnosis

These are non-specific, with either obstructive, or malabsorptive symptoms depending on the nature and extent of the mucosal involvement. In diffuse, non-obstructing disease, minor degrees of steatorrhoea and protein-losing enteropathy have been described. Ascites can occur in patients with mainly serosal involvement. Radiological examination of the stomach and small intestine will show patchy or diffuse abnormality of a non-specific nature. Ileocaecal disease may closely resemble Crohn's disease [98]. The peripheral blood eosinophilia is variable, but provides the essential clue. Otherwise the diagnosis depends on histology, which may be obtained from endoscopic or surgical specimens depending on the site of involvement.

In the absence of obstructive symptoms it is arguable whether surgery should be undertaken solely for the purposes of diagnosis, before a trial of corticosteroid therapy.

Management

A careful search for food sensitivity and gut parasites should be undertaken, using, if appropriate, exclusion diets and multiple faecal examinations. The parasite may only be obtained in tissue removed surgically for obstructive reasons [106]. Polyarteritis nodosa should be excluded by muscle biopsy or visceral arteriography, if there is evidence of multisystem disease.

In the absense of any specific cause or need for surgical treatment, severe symptoms justify the use of corticosteroid therapy on an empirical basis and this is usually successful [40, 98]. Favourable response to oral disodium cromoglycate has also been described, with prolonged remission after discontinuing the treatment [33, 65]. The long-term prognosis is difficult to judge but, in the absence of serious multisystem disease such as polyarteritis, appears to be good if a cause can be eliminated, or if the initial response to treatment is satisfactory.

Immunodeficiency and diarrhoea
(see Chapter 57 for AIDS)

The primary immunodeficiency disorders are classified according to whether there is a deficiency of B lymphocytes, of T lymphocytes or a mixed deficiency state. The World Health Organization (WHO) Committee proposed a classification, which is now generally accepted [49, 70] (Table 47.1).

Table 47.1. Simplified World Health Organization classification of primary immunodeficiency syndromes.

Type of immunodeficiency	Incidence of GI disease	Characteristic GI disease
B-cell defects		
Infantile X-linked agammaglobulinaemia (congenital)	Unusual	Malabsorption/diarrhoea (*Giardia lamblia*)— rare. Absence of mucosal plasma cells.
X-linked immunodeficiency with increased IgM	?	GI malignancy, diarrhoea, Candidiasis.
Selective IgA deficiency	5%	Coeliac disease—pernicious anaemia, *Giardia lamblia*.
Secretory IgA deficiency	+	Intestinal candidiasis.
Transient hypergammaglobulinaemia in infancy	+	Diarrhoea.
Variable immunodeficiency (common acquired)	+ + +	Nodular lymphoid hyperplasia, coeliac disease, *Giardia lamblia*, pernicious anaemia, carcinoma of the stomach, colitis, *Campylobacter* diarrhoea.
T-cell defects		
Di George syndrome (thymic hypoplasia: congenital)	(+)	Diarrhoea. Failure to thrive, candidiasis. Mouth or oesophageal ulcers. Diarrhoea.
Combined T- and B-cell defects		
Immunodeficiency with ataxia telangectasia	(+)	B_{12} malabsorption, carcinoma of stomach, malignancy of reticuloendothelial system.
Immunodeficiency with thrombocytopenia and eczema (Wiskott-Aldrich syndrome)	+ + +	Severe diarrhoea ± malabsorption.
Severe combined immunodeficiency autosomal recessive X-linked sporadic	+ + +	Chronic diarrhoea ± malabsorption. Absence of plasma cells.
Cellular immunodeficiency with abnormal immunoglobulin synthesis (Nezelof's syndrome)		Malabsorption, candidiasis.

Diarrhoeal disease is present in many, but not all of these immunodeficiency states. In addition to diarrhoea, these patients may also develop atypical pernicious anaemia with earlier age of onset and absent gastric antibodies, and gastrointestinal malignancy. Diarrhoeal disease in older children and adults is associated particularly with acquired variable immunoglobulin deficiency and less often with selective IgA deficiency. Immunoglobulin deficiency may also be secondary to impaired synthesis, for example in malnutrition, or during immunosuppressive treatment. It may also follow increased loss into the gut in protein-losing enteropathy, especially in intestinal lymphangiectasia [35].

Selective IgA deficiency

This is the commonest immunoglobulin deficiency state and is said to occur in one in 700 of the population [22]. In view of the important protective function of IgA in relation to the gut and the respiratory tract, it is remarkable that most people with this disorder are asymptomatic. Increased mucosal IgM production probably compensates for the IgA deficiency and IgM is secreted into the lumen with attached secretory piece. This increased population of B cells producing IgM may appear as nodular lymphoid hyperplasia of the small intestine.

In a small minority of patients with selective IgA deficiency chronic diarrhoea may be a problem and is usually ascribed to infestation with *Giardia lamblia*, to milk intolerance or to coeliac disease. Coeliac disease is said to be 12 times commoner in selective IgA deficiency than in the normal population [70].

Variable acquired immunoglobulin deficiency

This is a heterogeneous syndrome with prevalence of 10 per million of the population [35] and can be present in childhood, or at any stage of adult life—most patients develop symptoms in the second to fourth decades. The two sexes are equally affected. By contrast the rarer X-linked immunoglobulin deficiency affects boys between the ages of three months and two years [19].

Pathology

The most striking features are the decreased numbers of plasma cells in the lamina propria of the small intestine and the colon and, to a variable extent, the presence of large lymphoid follicles in the submucosa, which can cause macroscopic protrusion of the mucosa into the lumen (Fig. 47.6). This change can be seen throughout the small intestine, when it is called **nodular lymphoid hyperplasia.**

Mucosal abnormalities are variable from mild villous stunting to a flat mucosa indistinguishable from coeliac disease (Fig. 47.7). *Gardia lamblia* trophozoites will often

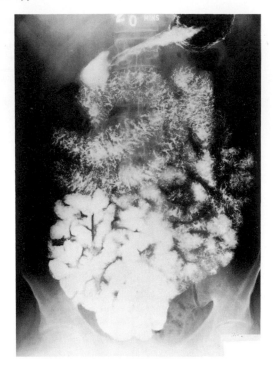

Fig. 47.6. Immunoglobulin deficiency. Barium follow-through examination showing abnormal appearances of the upper small intestine in a patient with immunoglobulin deficiency and giardiasis.

be found in the histological secretion of jejunal mucosa. Other parasites (for example, *Cryptosporidia*) are found much less frequently [90]. It has recently become recognized that *Campylobacter* species is a common cause of chronic diarrhoea in these patients and may be accompanied by histological evidence of colitis. Mycobacterial infections have also been reported [80].

Clinical features

Clinical features may include a past history of upper and lower respiratory infections. Otherwise the usual symptoms are chronic variable diarrhoea or steatorrhoea with weight loss or failure to grow in the more severe cases. There are no distinctive signs, but the patients may be variably malnourished.

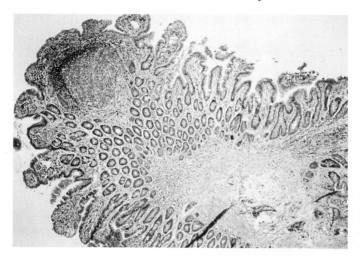

Fig. 47.7. Lymphoid hyperplasia. A large nodule of lymphoid tissue in the submucosa, with local changes of the villous architecture.

Investigations

The critical investigation is the quantitative measurement of blood concentrations of immunoglobulins G, A and M. Small bowel radiology may show the features of nodular lymphoid hyperplasia but is otherwise non-contributory. Jejunal mucosal biopsies and examination of jejunal juice are needed to exclude *Giardia lamblia* infestation and gluten sensitivity. Moderate bacterial overgrowth can often be demonstrated in the juice, but may not be clinically relevant. Vitamin B_{12} malabsorption is frequent and may result from lack of gastric intrinsic factor, from bacterial overgrowth or possibly from ileal mucosal abnormalities. Faecal bacteriology is important to exclude infection with *Campylobacter* species.

Differential diagnosis

More sophisticated studies of B and T cells and their functions will be required if there is doubt about the nature of the immunodeficiency state. The various causes of secondary immunodeficiency must be excluded. Nodular lymphoid hyperplasia has also been described in patients with normal serum immunoglobulins [74, 103].

Treatment

Giardia lamblia infection is eradicated by treatment with metronidazole 400 mg thrice daily for five days, but may recur. Trials of gluten-free diet will be needed, if gross mucosal abnormalities persist after eradication of *Giardia*.

Replacement of immunoglobulin is necessary in all patients who suffer recurrent disabling gut or respiratory infections. Conventionally this is given as intramuscular immunoglobulin injections (25 mg IgG/Kg every 1–2 weeks after high initial loading doses) or, if unwanted effects are troublesome or tolerance is poor, by infusion of fresh plasma (10–15 ml/Kg every 2–3 weeks) [35]. The frequency and dose can be adjusted according to clinical progress and it is recommended that the serum IgG concentration should be maintained above 2 g/l. In view of the many problems with the intramuscular injection of large volumes of relatively impure immunoglobulins, there is much interest in the development of purer preparations for intravenous use [2]. Antibiotics (other than metronidazole) are seldom effective in the treatment of the diarrhoea, although they are often required for the treatment and prevention of respiratory infections.

Prognosis

Prognosis is good and long survival is expected. The major long-term risk is of gastrointestinal malignancy—carcinoma and probably lymphoma—but the magnitude of the risk is unclear [49, 70]. Carcinoma of the stomach is particularly associated with the development of anacidity, which can occur at any early age in these patients [54].

Primary intestinal lymphangiectasia

The lacteals and other lymphatic vessels in the intestinal wall can become distended and leaky as a result of any condition that obstructs their drainage. This may be secondary to malignant disease near the posterior abdominal wall or near the thoracic duct, to constrictive pericarditis, or to rarer fibrotic lesions such as retroperitoneal fibrosis. It may also occur as a result of malrotation of the gut or nodular infiltrative disorders of the gut wall [43]. In the primary condition there is a developmental abnormality of intestinal, and often limb, lymphatics. Primary lymphangiectasia is rare and usually comes to medical attention in childhood, or early adult life. There is very little information available about prevalence or the results of long-term treatment. Both sexes are affected. There is no known genetic predisposition.

Pathology

The intestinal villi are thickened and macroscopically appear white with chyle-like material on the surface. Jejunoscopic appearances are well described by Asakura, Miura, Morishata, *et al.* [3]. Microscopically, the dilated lacteals distort the villi in a very distinctive way and the diagnosis is often apparent on jejunal biopsy (Fig. 47.8). An accumulation of fat droplets can be seen in the enterocytes and in the intercellular spaces, even in the fasting state, reflecting the inability to transport fat away from the intestinal mucosa. Occasionally the jejunal biopsy is normal and the lesion may be patchy [101].

Clinical features

The most striking feature is leg oedema, which may be symmetrical or asymmetrical, and which is caused by impaired lymphatic drainage and by hypoalbuminaemia. Ascites and pleural effusions often occur, but the gut symptoms may be mild.

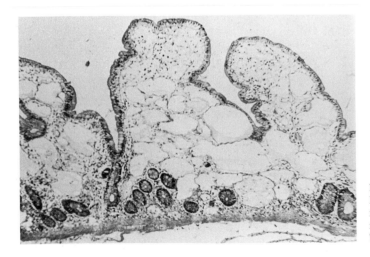

Fig. 47.8. Intestinal lymphangiectasia. The small intestinal villi are filled with numerous wide lymphatics lined by flattened endothelium.

Although many nutrients are absorbed normally, children tend to have impaired growth and development if left untreated [101].

Investigation

The main laboratory features are those of protein-losing enteropathy with low concentrations of albumin, immunoglobulins and lymphocytes, and mild to moderate steatorrhoea. The diagnosis is based on jejunal biopsy and, especially in the older patient, the exclusion of all the various conditions to which lymphangiectasia can be secondary. The protein loss is conventionally documented by the technique of *in vivo* labelling of circulating proteins by $^{51}CrCl_3$ given intravenously. The excretion of isotope is measured in a five day faecal collection—cumulative excretion less than 1% of injected dose in normals. There has been much recent interest in the measurement of faecal α-antitrypsin as a means of avoiding the use of isotopes and, possibly, of such a prolonged collection period. This remains controversial, but recent studies have been hopeful [30, 36, 51].

Differential diagnosis

The numerous causes of protein-losing enteropathy can usually be distinguished fairly readily on clinical or radiological groups. Primary immunoglobulin deficiency should be considered in patients with steatorrhoea and a low serum immunoglobulin concentration. Compared with lymphangiectasia, primary immunodeficiency syndromes are usually associated with much lower concentrations of circulating immunoglobulins, less pronounced protein loss into the gut, more severe steatorrhoea and often, abnormal jejunal biopsies—but without lymphatic distension.

Medical treatment

The essentials of treatment are the restriction of dietary long chain triglycerides and their replacement by medium chain triglycerides. This reduces lymph flow and hence the loss of albumin, immunoglobulins and lymphocytes. The medium chain triglycerides provide a well-absorbed calorie source. Well-being is improved and, in children, satisfactory growth and development can be recorded [101]. However, the biochemical and haematological abnormalities may not be corrected and the patients must be observed for the development of fat soluble vitamin deficiencies (for example, prothrombin time, plasma concentrations of vitamins A and E) with appropriate parenteral replacement. It is not clear from the literature whether essential fatty acids should be prescribed in any formal fashion.

Prognosis

Prognosis appears to be good if adequate treatment is provided. There are case reports of lymphoma and leukaemia developing in patients with lymphangiectasia [50, 104]. This may be related to the abnormal immune responses consequent upon lymphocyte and immunoglobulin depletion [93].

Chronic idiopathic intestinal pseudo-obstruction

The term pseudo-obstruction implies a failure of forward propulsion of gut contents in the absence of mechanical obstruction. Secondary intestinal pseudo-obstruction occurs acutely in the postoperative state (paralytic ileus), or in response to certain drugs, especially those with anticholinergic properties. Acute colonic pseudo-obstruction occurs occasionally in older patients during a serious illness and may need urgent caecostomy to prevent perforation [91].

Chronic secondary intestinal pseudo-obstruction may occur in many diseases, such as progressive systemic sclerosis, hypothyroidism or amyloidosis. It is also seen in primary intestinal conditions, for example in jejunal diverticulosis and possibly in coeliac disease. Secondary pseudo-obstruction is well-reviewed by Faulk, Anuras and Christensen [26]. Patients with chronic idiopathic pseudo-obstruction have abnormalities of gut propulsion in the absence of these well-recognized causes [87].

Epidemiology

Chronic idiopathic pseudo-obstruction is a rare syndrome [32, 87]. The condition is probably under reported, because few patients can be studied in sufficient new detail to warrant publication now that the main clinical features have been described.

Aetiology

Aetiology is unknown, but in many patients there is a family history, suggesting an autosomal dominant type of transmission [27, 86]. Oesophageal motility studies in asymptomatic relatives may suggest such familial associations.

Pathology

The major abnormality is the marked dilation, which can affect all parts of the gut, but especially the duodenum, the rest of the small intestine and/or the colon. The intestinal wall may be thinner or thicker than normal. Marked abnormalities of the muscle fibres have been described [27, 85], while in other patients degeneration of the myenteric plexus has been demonstrated using special histological techniques [84]. Variable abnormality of the small intestinal mucosa does exist, but is probably secondary to the stagnation of luminal contents.

Clinical features

There is chronic, continuous or recurrent abdominal pain and distension, with variable bowel disturbance. If the upper alimentary tract is severely affected there will be dysphagia and/or vomiting. Intestinal involvement may produce steatorrhoea from bacterial overgrowth; constipation can be severe if the colon is involved. Most patients are undernourished as a result of decreased food intake and malabsorption. The main physical signs are variable abdominal distension with a succussion splash and often, scars of previous laparotomies. The course tends to be progressively downhill, with little help from treatment. Impaired micturition has been reported, especially in the familial cases. The bladder is very dilated and ureteric reflux may be a major problem.

Investigations

Investigations may show all the usual features of malabsorption and malnutrition. The main sites of involvement are defined and mechanical obstruction excluded by barium studies (Fig. 47.9). If steatorrhoea is prominent evidence of bacterial overgrowth should be sought.

Cineradiology and manometry of the oesophagus will disclose abnormalities in many of these patients, indicating a widespread lesion even if dysphagia is not a major symptom. Detailed morphological studies require tissue obtained at operation and sophisticated electrical and manometric studies on the small intestine *in vivo* and *in vitro* have been undertaken in a few patients [78, 105]. Chronic idiopathic intestinal pseudo-obstruction has to be distinguished from all kinds of mechanical obstruction, as well as from the various

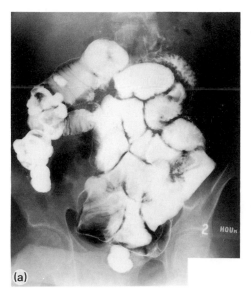
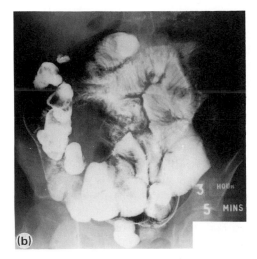

Fig. 47.9. Intestinal pseudo-obstruction showing very slow transit of barium through a dilated small intestine, in the absence of obstruction. (a) two-hour film; (b) three-hour film. The patient had a defunctioning ileostomy and barium from a much earlier enema is present in the ascending colon and rectum.

conditions associated with secondary pseudo-obstruction. Most patients have had at least one laparotomy to exclude mechanical causes.

Treatment

Treatment should be medical if at all possible, because surgery is usually futile. The gut does not respond to cholinergic drugs, or to metoclopramide. Steatorrhoea may improve after treatment with antibiotics, but this is variable. A major concern is the maintenance of nutrition which usually needs a low fat diet, supplemented by high calorie, high protein, and medium chain triglycerides containing liquid feeds. Many patients eventually fail to tolerate adequate oral feeding and may require parenteral nutrition. Surgery may be helpful in patients with marked duodenal obstruction (gastrojejunostomy) or with intractable constipation and colonic dilatation (caecostomy or ileostomy), but it is rarely helpful if the small intestine is involved extensively.

Drugs, alcohol and malabsorption

There are numerous examples of malabsorption induced by drugs. Some are predictable and dose-dependent and others are rare and idiosyncratic. Heavy drinkers often complain of diarrhoea, but severe steatorrhoea in a heavy drinker would suggest pancreatic insufficiency. However, many effects of alcohol on the structure and function of the small intestine have been described [6, 34, 61].

Neomycin induces mild steatorrhoea (< 50 mmol fat/day) when given in a dose of 3 g daily and large doses induce more severe malabsorption. Neomycin is a polybasic compound which precipitates bile salts and fatty acids out of micelles, interfering with the absorption of fat and fat soluble vitamins. It can also damage the small intestinal mucosa and minor, variable abnormalities are described in jejunal mucosal specimens. The drug is prescribed uncommonly now and in smaller doses than formerly.

Cholestyramine is an anion-binding resin that interferes with the re-absorption of bile acids from the ileum and enhances their loss in the faeces. In normal subjects this does not lead to such a loss of bile acids from the enterohepatic circulation that there is any serious malabsorption of fat or fat-soluble vitamins. However, in patients with small intestinal resection or cholestatic liver disease (for whom the drug is often prescribed), steatorrhoea will be aggravated by cholestyramine. There is evidence that the continuous use of cholestyramine in the treatment of primary biliary cirrhosis increases the risk of vitamin D deficiency and frank osteomalacia [15].

Para-amino salicylic acid was commonly associated with unpleasant gastrointestinal unwanted effects including diarrhoea. Case studies have shown modest elevations of faecal fat, impaired vitamin B_{12} absorption and depressed concentrations of serum folate and cholesterol. The mechanism of the malabsorption, which seems to be dose-dependent, is not known. There is no evidence of abnormal jejunal pathology or of interference with micelle formation.

Aluminium hydroxide gels interfere with phosphate absorption and are used in the treatment of hyperphosphataemia in patients with chronic renal failure. Their long-continued use in high dosage for the treatment of peptic ulcer can lead to hypophosphataemia, hypercalciuria and even osteomalacia. It was rare for patients to take the very large doses of antacids required to produce serious phosphate depletion, even in the days when these drugs were the only effective medical treatment for the relief of peptic ulcer symptoms. Aluminium hydroxide also binds bile acids and this may account for its tendency to produce constipation. As with cholestyramine, aluminium salts could lead to steatorrhoea in patients with liver or small gut disease.

Colchicine usually causes diarrhoea when used in short courses in the treatment of acute gout. It interferes with cell division in the mucosal crypts and, in high doses, produces morphological damage to the villi. Chronic ingestion of 0.5–1.0 mg daily is probably without important effects, but at higher dosage malabsorption of fat, xylose and vitamin B_{12} has been described. In a recent study of 12 patients being treated for familial Mediterranean fever with 1–2 mg/day, mild steatorrhoea was found in only three and impaired xylose tolerance in 11, but the jejunal biopsy appearances were normal [25].

Methotrexate interferes with cell division in the intestinal crypts and malabsorption can result. Xylose malabsorption and abnormal mucosal appearances have been described in patients being treated for leukaemia [5, 17, 73]. The effects appear to be cumulative and the interval between treatments is probably important in allowing the mucosa to recover from the effects of each course.

Other drugs

Steatorrhoea has been described in patients taking **tetracycline** [67] and a reversible enteropathy has been ascribed to **methyldopa** [8]. Steatorrhoea and a reversible enteropathy have been described in patients treated with **mefenamic acid** [64]. **Metformin** and **phenformin** interfere with glucose and vitamin B_{12} absorption and the former effect may be relevant to their hypoglycaemic action. Although **laxatives** act mainly on motility and on electrolyte and water transport, steatorrhoea, protein-losing enteropathy and osteomalacia have all been described in chronic laxative abusers [61].

Alcohol in experimental studies in man and animals has shown many adverse effects on mucosal structure, permeability [9] and intestinal transport [6]. Long-term administration of alcohol to normal volunteers interferes with the jejunal absorption of salt and water, with ileal absorption of vitamin B_{12} and possibly with the absorption of folate [34]. Impaired nutrition in chronic alcoholics may aggravate the direct effect of alcohol on absorptive function. Folic acid deficiency in particular is thought to be responsible for some of the morphological abnormalities in jejunal biopsies from chronic alcoholics.

References

1 ANONYMOUS. Lactose malabsorbtion and lactose intolerance. *Lancet* 1979;ii:83–84.

2 ANONYMOUS. Clinical uses of human immunoglobulin. *Lancet* 1983;i:105–106.

3 ASAKURA H, MIURA S, MORISHITA T, et al. Endoscopic and histopathological study on primary and secondary intestinal lymphangectasia. *Dig Dis Sci* 1981;26:312–320.

4 BAER AN, BAYLESS TM, YARDLEY JH. Intestinal ulceration malabsorption syndromes. *Gastroenterology* 1980;79:754–765.

5 BAIRD GM, DOSSETOR JFB. Methotrexate enteropathy. *Lancet* 1981;i:164.

6 BECK IT, DINDA PK. Acute exposure of small intestine to ethanol. Effects on morphology and function. *Dig Dis Sci* 1981;26:817–838.

7 BHAGAVAN BS, HOFKIN GA, COCHRAN BA. Whipple's disease: morphologic and immunofluorescence characterization of bacterial antigens. *Hum Pathol* 1981;12:930–936.

8 BHARGAVA DK, TANDON HD. Ileocaecal tuberculosis diagnosed by colonoscopy and biopsy. *Aust NZ J Surg* 1980;50:583–585.

9 BJARNASON I, WARD K, PETERS TJ. The leaky gut of alcoholism: possible route of entry for toxic compounds. *Lancet* 1984;i:179–181.

10 BOSTWICK DG, BENSCH KG, BURKE JS, et al. Whipple's disease presenting as aortic insufficiency. *New Engl J Med* 1981;305:995–998.

11 BROWN KH, KHATUM M, PARRY L, et al. Nutritional consequences of low dose milk supplements consumed by lactose-malabsorbing children. *Am J Clin Nutr* 1980;33:1054–1063.

12 CALDWELL JH, SHARMA HM, HURTUBISE PE. Eosinophilic gastroenteritis in extreme allergy. *Gastroenterology* 1979;77:560–564.

13 CLANCY RL, TOMKINS WAF, MUCKLE TJ, et al. Isolation and characterisation of an aetiologial agent in Whipple's disease. *Br Med J* 1975;2:569–570.

14 COMMUNICABLE DISEASE STATISTICS. Public Health Laboratory Service HMSO, 1980;33:xv.

15 COMPSTON JE, THOMPSON RPH. Intestinal absorption of 25-hydroxyvitamin D and osteomalacia in primary biliary cirrhosis. *Lancet* 1977;i:721–724.

16 COOK GC. Primary and secondary hypolactase (lactase-deficiency). In: *Tropical gastroenterology*. Oxford: Oxford University Press, 1980:325–339.

17 CRAFT AW, KAY KFM, LAWSON DN, et al. Methotrexate-induced malabsorption in children with acute lymphoblastic leukaemia. *Br Med J* 1977;2:1511–1512.

18 DAS P, SHUKLA HS. Clinical diagnosis of abdominal tuberculosis. *Br J Surg* 1976;63:941–946.

19 DENMAN AM. Immunodeficiency and general medicine. *Br Med J* 1980;281:1376–1378.

20 DOBBINS WO. Is there an immune deficit in Whipple's disease? *Dig Dis Sci* 1981;26:247–252.

21 DOBBINS WO, KAWANISHI H. Bacillary characteristics in Whipple's disease: an electron microscopic study. *Gastroenterology* 1981;80:1468–1475.

22 DOE WF. An overview of intestinal immunity and malabsorption. *Am J Med* 1979;67:1077–1084.

23 DOW CJ. Oesophageal tuberculosis: four cases. *Gut* 1981;22:234–236.

24 DUTT AK, MOERS D, STEAD WW. Short-course chemotherapy for extrapulmonary tuberculosis. *Ann Intern Med* 1986;104:7–12.

25 EHRENFELD M, LEVY M, SHARON P, et al. Gastrointestinal effects of long-term colchicine therapy in patients with recurrent polyserositis. (Familial Mediterranean Fever). *Dig Dis Sci* 1982;27:723–727.

26 FAULK DL, ANURAS S, CHRISTENSEN J. Chronic intestinal pseudoobstruction. *Gastroenterology* 1978;74:922–931.

27 FAULK DL, ANURAS S, GARDNER GD et al. A familial visceral myopathy. *Ann Intern Med* 1978;89:600–606.

28 FELDMAN M, HENDLER RS, MORRISON EB. Acute meningoencephalitis after withdrawal of antibiotics in Whipple's disease. *Ann Intern Med* 1980;93:709–711.

29 FERGUSON A. Diagnosis and treatment of lactose intolerance. *Br Med J* 1981;283:1423–1424.

30 FLORENT C, L'HIRONDEL C, DESMAZURES C, et al. Intestinal clearance of 1-antitrypsin. A sensitive method for the detection of protein-losing enteropathy. *Gastroenterology* 1981;80:777–789.

31 FRANKLIN GO, MOHAPATRA M, PERRILLO RP. Colonic tuberculosis diagnosed by colonoscopic biopsy. *Gastroenterology* 1979;76:362–364.

32 GIBBONS JC, SULLIVAN JF. Chronic idiopathic pseudo-obstructive bowel disease. *Am J Gastroenterol* 1978;70:306–313.

33 GILINSKY NH, KOTTLER RE. Idiopathic obstructive eosinophilic enteritis with raised IgE: response to oral disodium cromoglycate. *Postgrad Med J* 1982;58:239–243.

34 GREEN PHR, TALL AR. Alcohol and malabsorption. *Am J Med* 1979;67:1066–1076.

35 HAENEY M. Defects in specific immunity: antibody deficiency. Hospital Update 1983;9:54–71,203–209.

36 HAENEY MR, FIELDS J, CARTER RA, et al. Is faecal 1-antitrypsin excretion a reliable screening test for protein-losing enteropathy? Lancet 1979;ii:1161–1162.

37 HALPERIN JJ, LANDIS DMD, KLEINMAN GM. Whipple's disease of the nervous system. Neurology 1982;32:612–617.

38 HAVERBERG L, KWON PH, SCRIMSHAW NS. Comparative tolerance of adolescents of differing ethnic backgrounds to lactose-containing and lactose-free dairy drinks. I. Initial experience with a double-blind procedure. Am J Clin Nutr 1980;33:17–21.

39 HEALTH AND PERSONAL SOCIAL SERVICES STATISTICS FOR ENGLAND. Department of Health and Social Security. HMSO, 1982:127.

40 HESDORFER CS, ZIADY F. Eosinophilic gastroenteritis—a complication of schistosomiasis and peripheral eosinophilia? S Afr Med J 1982; 61:591–593.

41 HORNE N. Tuberculosis. Medicine (International) 1982;21:978–983.

42 HYSON EA, BURRELL M, TOFFLER R. Drug-induced gastrointestinal disorders. In: Meyers MA, Ghatremani GG, eds. Iatrogenic gastrointestinal complications. New York: Springer Verlag, 1981:4–6.

43 IIDA F, WADA R, SATO A, et al. Clinico-pathological consideration of protein-losing enteropathy due to lymphangectasia of the intestine. Surg Gynecol Obstet 1980;151:391–395.

44 Jewell DP. Ulcerative enteritis. Br Med J 1983;287:1740–1741.

45 JOHNSON L, DIAMOND I. Cerebral Whipple's disease. Am J Clin Path 1980;74:486–490.

46 JOHNSTONE JM, MORSON BC. Eosinophilic gastroenteritis. Histopathology 1973;2:335–348.

47 KASAHARA Y, TANAKA S, NISHINO M, et al. Intestinal involvement in Behçet's disease: Review of 136 surgical cases in the Japanese literature. Dis Colon Rectum 1981;24:103–106.

48 KASULKE RJ, ANDERSON WJ, GUPTA SK, et al. Primary tuberculous enterocolitis. Report of three cases and a review of the literature. Arch Surg 1981;116:110–113.

49 KATZ AJ, ROSEN FS. Gastrointestinal complications of immunodeficiency syndromes. Ciba Foundation Symposium 1977;46:243–261.

50 KAY AJ, LILLEYMAN JS. Is intestinal lymphangectasia a pre-leukaemic condition? Clin Lab Haemat 1981;3:365–367.

51 KEANEY NP, KELLEHER J. Faecal excretion of 1-antitrypsin in protein-losing enteropathy. Lancet 1980;i:711.

52 KEINATH RD, MERRELL DE, VLIETSTRA R, DOBBINS WO. Antibiotic treatment and relapse in Whipple's disease: long-term follow-up of 88 patients. Gastroenterology 1985;88:1867–73.

53 KEREN DF, WEISBURGER WR, YARDLEY JH et al. Whipple's disease: demonstration by immunofluorescence of similar bacterial antigens in macrophages from three cases. Johns Hopkins Med J 1976;139:51–59.

54 KINLEN LJ, WEBSTER ADM, BIRD AG, et al. Prospective study of cancer in patients with hypogammaglobulinaemia. Lancet 1985;i:263–265.

55 KRETCHMER N. The geography and biology of lactose digestion and malabsorption. Postgrad Med J 1977;53(suppl):65–70.

56 KUHAJDA FP, BELITSOS NJ, KEREN DF, et al. A submucosal variant of Whipple's disease. Gastroenterology 1982;82:46–50.

57 LADAS S, PAPANIKOS J, ARAPAKIS G. Lactose malabsorption in Greek adults: correlation of small bowel transit time with the severity of lactose intolerance. Gut 1982;23:968–973.

58 LAMBRIANIDES AL, ACKROYD N, SHOREY BA. Abdominal tuberculosis. Br J Surg 1980;67:887–889.

59 LEVINE H. Needle biopsy diagnosis of tuberculosis peritonitis. Amer Rev Resp Dis 1968;97:889–894.

60 LISKER R, AGUILAR L, LARES I, et al. Double blind study of milk intolerance in a group of rural and urban children. Am J Clin Nutr 1980;33:1049–1053.

61 LONGSTRETH GF, NEWCOMER AD. Drug-induced malabsorption. Mayo Clin Proc 1975;50:284–293.

62 McALISTER HA, FENDOGLIO JJ. Cardiac involvement in Whipple's disease. Circulation 1975;52:152–156.

63 MAIZEL H, RUFFIN JM, DOBBINS WO. Whipple's disease: a review of 19 patients from one hospital and a review of the literature since 1950. Medicine (Baltimore) 1970;49:175–205.

64 MARKS JS, GLEESON MH. Steatorrhoea complicating therapy with mefanemic acid. Br Med J 1975;4:442.

65 MARTIN OM, GOLDMAN JA, GILLIAM J, et al. Gold induced eosinophilic enterocolitis: response to oral cromolyn sodium. Gastroenterology 1981; 80:1567–1570.

66 MILLS PR, BROWN IL, WATKINSON G. Idiopathic chronic ulcerative enteritis. Report of five cases and review of the literature. Q J Med 1980; 49:133–149.

67 MITCHELL TH, STAMP TCB, JENKINS MV. Steatorrhoea after tetracycline. Br Med J 1982;285:780.

68 MORSON BC, DAWSON IMP. In: Gastrointestinal pathology. Oxford: Blackwell Scientific Publications, 1979:275–279.

69 NEWCOMER AD, HODGSON SF, McGILL DB, THOMAS PJ. Lactase deficiency: prevalence in osteomalacia. Ann Intern Med 1978;89:218–220.

70 OCHS HD, AMENT ME. Gastrointestinal tract and

immunodeficiency. In: Ferguson A, MacSween RNM, eds. *Immunological aspects of the liver and gastrointestinal tract.* Boston: MTP Press Ltd, 1976:83–120.

71 PALMER KR, PATIL DH, BASRAN GS, RIORDAN JF, SILK DBA. Abdominal tuberculosis in urban Britain—a common disease. *Gut* 1985;26:1296–1305.

72 PAYNE DL, WELSH JD, MANION CV, *et al.* Effectiveness of milk products in dietary management of lactose malabsorption. *Am J Clin Nutr* 1981; 34:2711–2715.

73 PINKERTON CR, GLASGOW JFT. Methotrexate enteropathy? *Lancet* 1981;i:996.

74 POLLOCK S, LEWIS PD, KENDALL B. Whipple's disease confined to the nervous system. *J Neurol Neurosurg Psychiatry* 1981;44:1104–1109.

75 RAMBAUD JC, DESAINT-LOUVENT P, MARTI R, *et al.* Diffuse follicular lymphoid hyperplasia of the small intestine without primary immunoglobulin deficiency. *Am J Med* 1982;73:125–132.

76 RANSOME-KUTI O. Lactose intolerance—a review. *Postgrad Med J* 1977;53:73–83.

77 REASONER J, MACULAN TP, RAND AG, *et al.* Clinical studies with low lactose milk. *Am J Clin Nutr* 1981;34:54–60.

78 ROSS IN, ASQUITH P. Primary immune deficiency. In: Asquith P, ed. *Immunology of the gastrointestinal tract.* Edinburgh, London, New York: Churchill Livingstone, 1979:152–182.

79 SARNA SK, DANIEL EE, WATERFALL WE, *et al.* Postoperative gastrointestinal electrical and mechanical activities in a patient with idiopathic intestinal pseudoobstruction. *Gastroenterology* 1978;74:112–120.

80 SCOTT-GILLAN J, URMACHER C, WEST R, SHIKE M. Disseminated *Microbacterium avium-intracellulare* infection in acquired immunodeficiency-syndrome mimicking Whipple's disease. *Gastroenterology* 1983;85:1187–1191.

81 SCHMITT BP, RICHARDSON H, SMITH E, *et al.* Encephalopathy complicating Whipple's disease. Failure to respond to antibiotics. *Ann Intern Med* 1981;94:51–52.

82 SCHNEERSON JM, GAZZARD BG. Reversible malabsorption caused by methyldopa. *Br Med J* 1977;2:1456–1457.

83 SCHOFIELD PF. Abdominal tuberculosis. *Gut* 1985;26:1265–1278.

84 SCHUFFLER MD, JONAK Z. Chronic idiopathic intestinal pseudoobstruction caused by a degenerative disorder of the myenteric plexus: the use of Smith's method to define the neuropathology. *Gastroenterology* 1982;82:476–486.

85 SCHUFFLER MD, LOWE MC, BILL AH. Studies of idiopathic intestinal pseudoobstruction. I. Hereditary hollow visceral myopathy: clinical and pathological studies. *Gastroenterology* 1977; 73:327–338.

86 SCHUFFLER MD, POPE CE. Studies of idiopathic intestinal pseudoobstruction. II. Hereditary hollow visceral myopathy: family studies. *Gastroenterology* 1977;73:339–334.

87 SCHUFFLER MD, ROHRMANN CA, CHAFFEE RF, *et al.* Chronic intestinal pseudoobstruction. A report of 27 cases and review of the literature. *Medicine* 1981;60:173–196.

88 SEGAL I, TIM LO, MIRWIS J, *et al.* Pitfalls in the diagnosis of gastrointestinal tuberculosis. *Am J Gastroenterol* 1981;75:30–35.

89 SHERMAN S, ROHWEDDER JJ, RAVIKRISHNAN KP, *et al.* Tuberculosis enteritis and peritonitis. Report of 36 hospital cases. *Arch Intern Med* 1980; 140:506–558.

90 SLOPER KS, DOURMASHKIN RR, BIRD, *et al.* Chronic malabsorption due to cryptosporidiosis in a child with immunoglobulin deficiency. *Gut* 1982;23:80–82.

91 SOREIDA O, BJERKESET T, FOSSDAL JE. Pseudoobstruction of the colon (Ogilvie's syndrome). A genuine clinical condition? Review of the literature (1948–1975) and report of five cases. *Dis Colon Rectum* 1977;20:487–491.

92 STAMBLER JB, KLIBANER MI, BLISS CM, *et al.* Tuberculosis abscess of the pancreas. *Gastroenterology* 1982;83:922–925.

93 STROBER W, WOCHNER RD, CARBONE PP, *et al.* Intestinal lymphangectasia. A protein-losing enteropathy with hypogammaglobulinaemia, lymphocytopenia and impaired homograft rejection. *J. Clin Invest* 1967;46:1643–1656.

94 STRODEL WE, ECKHAUSER FE, SIMMONS JL. Primary ulceration of the ileum. *Dis Colon Rectum* 1981;24:183–186.

95 STURGES HF, KRONE CL. Ulceration and stricture of the jejunum in a patient on long-term indomethacin therapy. *Am J Gastroenterol* 1973; 59:162–169.

96 SUEN KC, BURTON JD. The spectrum of eosinophilic infiltration of the gastrointestinal tract and its relationship to other disorders of angiitis and granulomatosis. *Hum Pathol* 1979;10:31–43.

97 TANDON RK, JOSHI YK, SINGH DS, *et al.* Lactose intolerance in North and South Indians. *Am J Clin Nutr* 1981;34:943–946.

98 TEDESCO FJ, HUCKABY CB, HAMBY-ALLEN M, *et al.* Eosinophilic ileocolitis. Expanding spectrum of eosinophilic gastroenteritis. *Dig Dis Sci* 1981; 26:943–948.

99 THOMAS WEG, WILLIAMSON RCN. Enteric ulceration and its complications. *World J Surg* 1985; 9:876–886.

100 THOMPSON DG, LEDINGHAM JM, HOWARD AJ, *et al.* Meningitis in Whipple's disease. *Br Med J* 1978;2: 14–15.

101 TIFT WL, LLoyd JK. Intestinal lymphangectasia. Long term results with MCT diet. *Arch Dis Child* 1975;50:269–276.

102 Viteri AL, Green JF, Chandler JB. Whipple's disease: successful response to sulfamethoxazole-trimethoprin. *Am J Gastroenterol* 1981;**75**:309–310.

103 Ward H, Jalan KN, Mitra TK, *et al*. Small intestinal nodular lymphoid hyperplasia in patients with giardiasis and normal serum immunoglobulins. *Gut* 1983;**24**:120–126.

104 Ward M, Le Roux A, Small WP, *et al*. Malignant lymphoma and extensive viral wart formation in a patient with intestinal lymphangectasia and lymphocyte depletion. *Postgrad Med J* 1977;**53**:753–757.

105 Waterfall WE, Cameron GS, Sarna SK, *et al*. Disorganised electrical activity in a child with intestinal pseudo-obstruction. *Gut* 1981;**22**:77–83.

106 Watt IA, McLean NR, Girdwood RWA, *et al*. Eosinophilic gastroenteritis associated with a larval anisakine nematode. *Lancet* 1979;**ii**:893–894.

107 Welsh JD, Payne DLaV, Manion C, *et al*. Interval sampling of breath hydrogen (H$_2$) as an index of lactose malabsorption in lactase-deficient subjects. *Dig Dis Sci* 1981;**26**:681–685.

108 Winfield J, Dourmashkin RR, Gumpel JM. Diagnostic pitfalls in Whipple's disease. *Roy Soc Med* 1979;**72**:859–863.

109 Wolfe JHN, Behn AR, Jackson BT. Tuberculosis peritonitis and role of diagnostic laparoscopy. *Lancet* 1979;**i**:852–853.

Chapter 48
Cancer of the Small Intestine

R. C. N. WILLIAMSON

Enteric neoplasms are surprisingly uncommon. Primary tumours of the small intestine are found in about 0.5% of autopsies and symptomatic lesions are rarer still. The small bowel makes up 80–90% of the luminal surface area of the entire alimentary canal, but only provides 1–2% of alimentary cancers [29]. Specifically, the small intestine seems resistant to primary epithelial neoplasia by comparison with the oesophagus, stomach and colorectum, where carcinoma is 100 times as frequent. Together with the relative inaccessibility of the small bowel to investigation, this rarity undoubtedly delays the diagnosis of enteric cancer and contributes to its poor overall prognosis. Management might be improved if clinicians were to consider the diagnosis more readily in patients with obscure but persistent gastrointestinal symptoms.

Pathology (Table 48.1)

Small bowel tumours have an equal sex distribution and generally develop between the fifth and seventh decades. The main histological types are listed in Table 48.1. Quite common incidental findings at operation or autopsy, benign neoplasms and hamartomas occasionally give rise to symptoms. Thus a submucous lipoma (usually in the ileum) or a Peutz-Jeghers hamartoma (jejunum) can undergo intussusception, causing episodes of intermittent small bowel obstruction. Angiomas and benign ulcerating tumours may present with overt or occult haemorrhage.

Mucosal adenomas display tubular, papillary (villous) and mixed (tubulovillous) patterns, like their colorectal counterparts. Villous adenomas form a larger proportion (40%) of the total than in the large intestine (10%), [21]. Adenomas have a strong predilection for the duodenum, particularly the descending limb, where they may involve the ampulla of Vater. Adenomas can also arise from Brunner's glands in the duodenum.

Benign tumours may contain a single cell type or mixtures of stromal and epithelial

Table 48.1. Histological types of small bowel tumour.

Hamartomas	Benign neoplasms	'Intermediate' neoplasms	Primary malignant neoplasms	Secondary malignant neoplasms
Peutz-Jeghers polyp	Lipoma	Smooth muscle tumours	Adenocarcinoma	Secondary carcinoma
Ectopic pancreas	Adenoma	Carcinoid	Lymphoma	Lymphoma
Vascular malformations	Fibroma, etc.	Villous adenoma	Sarcomas	Melanoma
Neurofibromatosis		Gastrinoma		

elements—for example, fibromyoma or fibroadenoma. Neurofibromas can be solitary or occur as part of Von Recklinghausen's disease. Two types of apudoma affect the small intestine—the ileum is the commonest site for a malignant carcinoid, and the duodenum is the commonest extrapancreatic site for a gastrinoma (see Chapters 39 and 40). Fibrosarcoma and angiosarcoma are exceedingly rare [26]. In patients with acquired immune deficiency syndrome (AIDS) Kaposi's sarcoma may affect the small bowel [8]. The rest of this chapter will concentrate on the major types of enteric neoplasm—adenocarcinoma, lymphoma, smooth muscle tumours and secondary cancers.

Aetiology

There is good evidence to support an adenoma-carcinoma sequence in the small intestine, as well as the large intestine. Villous adenomas seem particularly liable to malignant transformation and duodenal carcinoma is reported in Gardner's syndrome. Reviewing 51 cases of mucosal adenoma, Perzin and Bridge [21] found 33 patients with evidence of carcinomatous change somewhere in the lesion and another five in which the adenoma was found incidentally in a specimen that contained a separate adenocarcinoma. All but nine of the 51 tumours arose in the duodenum, which may explain why 'inch for inch' the duodenum has the highest incidence of small bowel carcinoma [15]. In 1050 cases

of primary enteric carcinoma collected from the world literature, 40% were duodenal, 38% jejunal and 22% ileal [24]. This upper small bowel predominance is unique to carcinoma; carcinomas induced in rats by azoxymethane show a similarly strong affinity for the duodenum and upper jejunum [29]. Direct irradiation of the small intestine will also induce experimental carcinoma, but there is no evidence in man that radiotherapy causes cancer of the small bowel (as opposed to the large bowel).

The association between long-standing Crohn's disease and carcinoma of the small intestine (Table 48.2) is far stronger than mere coincidence—over 60 patients with this combination have been described since 1956 [7, 11]. Most Crohn's carcinomas affect the ileum—the usual site for enteritis, but the most resistant portion of the alimentary tract to epithelial cancer. Since about a third of cases affect bypassed loops of bowel, bacterial infection may play an aetiological role as well as chronic granulomatous inflammation. Patients with regional enteritis probably have a hundred-fold increase in the risk of developing small bowel cancer [7, 12].

Patients with long-standing coeliac disease have an increased risk of gut malignancy, particularly jejunal lymphoma, but also carcinoma of the jejunum, duodenum and oesophagus [4]. These patients have an abnormal immune system and increased crypt-cell proliferation, as in ulcerative colitis. Although the jejunal hamartomas in Peutz-Jeghers syndrome have no particular

Table 48.2. Aetiological associations with small bowel cancer.

Duodenal carcinoma	Jejunal carcinoma	Ileal carcinoma	Lymphoma
Adenoma, especially villous	Coeliac disease	Crohn's disease	Coeliac disease
Gardner's syndrome	(Crohn's disease)	Rare tumours of Meckel's diverticulum	Alpha chain disease
(Coeliac disease)			
(Peutz-Jeghers syndrome)			

tendency to neoplastic change, there may be an increased risk of gastric and duodenal carcinoma in this condition [23].

Carcinoma, lymphoma and especially carcinoids of the small intestine tend to be multiple. They are associated with cancers elsewhere in the intestine, or at other sites in the body in over 20% of cases [29]. Once the normal immunity of the small bowel to cancer is overcome, multiple tumours might be anticipated.

The relative sterility and fluidity of chyme, its short transit time and the rapid turnover of enteric epithelium are all suggested explanations for the rarity of small bowel cancer. None of these account for the strikingly unequal distribution of adenoma and adenocarcinoma. Ileal resistance to neoplasia may therefore reflect a local protective mechanism, possibly immunological in nature and related to the high mucosal content of IgA [18].

Diagnosis

Investigation of the small intestine is considered in detail in Chapter 41. Some tumours can present acutely with perforation (primary lymphoma) or obstruction (carcinoma) and thus preclude much investigation apart from plain abdominal X-rays. More often episodic vomiting and abdominal colic, weight loss, anaemia, or perhaps jaundice or abdominal mass may raise the possibility of small bowel disease, especially if oesophagogastric and colorectal investigations are negative. In particular, iron-deficiency anaemia should alert the clinician to an enteric lesion.

An increasing appreciation of the frequency with which adenomatous and other polyps of the stomach and duodenum occur in familial polyposis coli [22] suggests that upper gastrointestinal endoscopy should be a routine investigation in polyposis patients.

Besides lying within range of an upper gastrointestinal endoscope, most duodenal tumours should be apparent on a conventional barium meal examination (Fig. 48.1(a) and Fig. 48.2(a)); hypotonic duodenography may improve visualization. Occasionally lesions in the distal ileum can be seen on a barium enema or colonoscopy. In between these points satisfactory radiological examination of the jejunoileum can be more difficult and demanding. Barium follow-through examination may show single or multiple strictures and dilated loops of bowel. Delivering the contrast material directly into the duodenum by means of a nasoenteric tube ('small bowel enema') improves the chances of detecting a small tumour.

A bleeding duodenal tumour should be diagnosed endoscopically [25]. If a jejunoileal tumour (angioma, leiomyoma) is actively bleeding, it can be localized by selective superior mesenteric arteriography [6]. Modern radionuclide scanning techniques after *in vivo* labelling of red blood cells offer the prospect of timing the angiogram correctly [20]. Serial scans of the abdomen are obtained after intravenous injection of stannous chloride followed by technetium (^{99m}Tc). Injection of ^{99m}Tc alone may depict a Meckel's diverticulum containing ectopic gastric mucosa. Bleeding may also result from jejunal diverticulosis, mesenteric varices, telangiectasia and angiodysplasia of the small bowel (see Chapter 32 for discussion of small intestinal bleeding).

Adenocarcinoma [22]

Duodenal carcinoma

The 25 cm of the duodenal loop contain the highest concentration of adenocarcinomas in the small bowel. Two-thirds of these tumours present with epigastric pain, sometimes aggravated by eating and often accompanied by vomiting and weight loss (Fig. 48.1) [17, 29]. A similar proportion

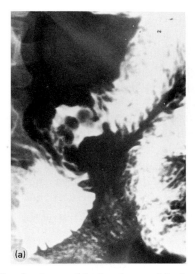
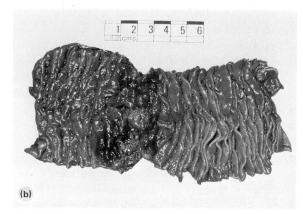

(a)   (b)

Fig. 48.1. Carcinoma of the fourth part of the duodenum. A 58-year-old woman presented with upper abdominal pain and episodes of profuse vomiting, suggestive of gastric outlet obstruction. Barium meal examination (a) shows a filling defect just proximal to the duodenojejunal flexure. Palliative resection with end-to-end duodenojejunostomy was performed in the presence of quite extensive lymph-node spread. The resection specimen (b) shows an annular carcinoma. Postoperative radiotherapy was given, but she died of carcinomatosis nine months later.

cause occult haemorrhage and anaemia (Fig. 48.2); haematemesis and melaena are unusual. Carcinomas are most prevalent in the second part of the duodenum, and jaundice may develop in 20–30% of patients overall. Jaundice is not inevitable even if the tumour surrounds the papilla (Fig. 48.2(b)). Duodenal carcinomas are seldom large enough to be palpable *per abdomen*, though hepatomegaly or even ascites may be found if there is secondary spread.

Duodenal tumours are the most accessible to radiological and endoscopic diagnosis, including direct biopsy. The differential diagnosis includes duodenal ulceration with or without gastric outlet obstruction. Primary carcinoma should be distinguished from cancers involving the duodenum by direct invasion or discrete metastasis [27]. Carcinoma arising in a villous adenoma or a diverticulum of the duodenum may also cause confusion [2].

Complete resection offers the only prospect of cure. Partial pancreatoduodenec-tomy (Whipple's operation) is indicated where possible, that is to say in 50–80% of cases. An irresectable tumour should be bypassed by gastroenterostomy and choledo-chojejunostomy if jaundice is present or imminent. Local excision may suffice for an adenomatous polyp with malignant change, if the stalk is free of invasive tumour. Radiotherapy and chemotherapy are of unproven benefit in duodenal carcinomas (Fig. 48.1 and Fig. 48.2). Five-year survival rates seldom exceed 15–20% [18].

Jejunoileal carcinoma

Most of these lie within 50 cm of the ligament of Treitz. Unlike the duodenum, where carcinomas constitute at least 80% of malignancies, the jejunum and ileum have approximately equal numbers of carcinomas, carcinoids and sarcomas (including lymphoma) [1]. Carcinoma of the jejunum presents with subacute intestinal obstruction (Fig. 48.3) and/or chronic in-

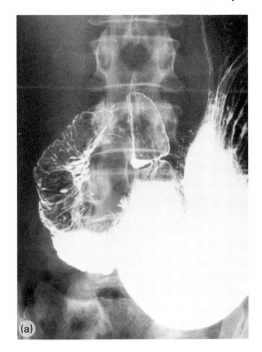
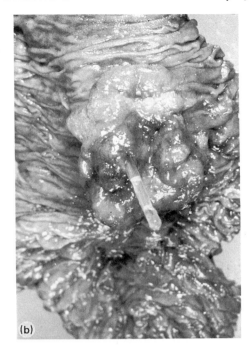

Fig. 48.2. Periampullary carcinoma of the duodenum in a woman of 56 years with iron-deficiency anaemia (Hb 9 g/dl). Endoscopy suggested carcinoma of the ampulla, but liver function tests were entirely normal. Barium meal examination (a) shows a polypoid tumour of the descending duodenum. The lesion was removed by partial pancreatoduodenectomy, though tiny hepatic metastases were seen. A photograph of the operative specimen (b) shows a catheter emerging from the papilla. The hepatic artery was cannulated at operation and a four-day course of 5-fluorouracil (750 mg/day) was given by this route, starting 12 days later. She died 15 months postoperatively.

testinal blood loss, as the tumour tends to be annular and ulcerating. Patients may develop diarrhoea, weight loss and a palpable mass. Perforation and peritonitis are uncommon complications of jejunal carcinoma but may be slightly commoner with ileal carcinoma [29]. Most carcinomas of the ileum occur in association with chronic granulomatous enteritis (see below). Nearly every type of small bowel tumour including carcinoma has been reported in Meckel's diverticulum [28].

Jejunoileal neoplasms should be differentiated from other causes of ulceration and stricture, such as ulcerative jejunitis (in coeliac disease), Crohn's disease, radiation enteritis and nonspecific ulceration. Hamartomas, enteroliths, foreign bodies, inflammatory pseudotumours, endometrioma and a invaginated Meckel's diverticulum can all produce filling defects on barium follow-through examination.

Resection with end-to-end anastomosis is nearly always possible in carcinoma of the jejunum and ileum, but the presence of nodal metastases (Fig. 48.3) often reduces this from a curative to a palliative procedure. Occasionally only a bypass operation is feasible. A search should be made at operation for other primary tumours of the intestinal tract. The overall five-year survival rate of 20–30% is a little better than for duodenal carcinoma. Survival approaches 50% in the absence of overt metastases [3, 29].

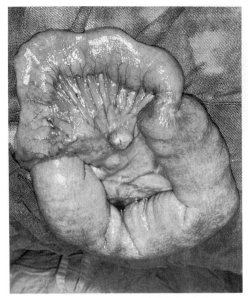

Fig. 48.3. Obstructing carcinoma of the upper jejunum. A man of 75 with no previous history of indigestion developed symptoms suggestive of pyloric stenosis. On examination there was upper abdominal distension, visible peristalsis and a succussion splash. Barium studies revealed a normal stomach but distended loops of proximal jejunum. The operative photograph shows obvious disparity in size between proximal obstructed and distal collapsed loops of jejunum, with a large nodal metastasis. The tumour was resected with end-to-end anastomosis.

Crohn's carcinoma

Originally described by Ginzburg, *et al.* in 1956 [9], this tumour can now be regarded as a distinct entity [7, 11]. Carcinomas arise exclusively in segments of bowel that show evidence of long-standing Crohn's disease. The mean interval between diagnosing regional enteritis and enteric cancer is 18 years. The ileum is involved in nearly 70% of patients and the jejunum in the remainder. These proportions are the reverse of those seen with 'ordinary' carcinoma of the small bowel. Crohn's carcinomas develop some 18 years earlier than usual (47 versus 65 years) and there is a male predominance of about 70%, compared with 50–55% for ordinary carcinoma. Prognosis is very poor, survival for even three years

being exceptional. Death occurs at a mean of eight months after diagnosis. The symptoms of carcinoma are confused with those of the underlying disease and cancers affecting bypassed loops (about 30%) are particularly difficult to diagnose. Cancer may not even be suspected at operation. The histological pattern is often one of diffuse and extensive carcinomatous infiltration, with adjacent areas of epithelial dysplasia.

Lymphoma

Primary

Like carcinomas, primary lymphomas of the small intestine tend to be annular, ulcerating lesions, which are sometimes multiple. Unlike carcinomas, they are randomly distributed through the bowel. They have generally been classified as reticulum cell sarcomas, though lymphocytic lymphoma, Hodgkin's disease and plasmacytoma have also been described in isolated intestinal lesions. The association of lymphoma with coeliac disease is described below and with alpha chain disease in Chapter 43. The mean age at diagnosis of an intestinal lymphoma is about 60 years, irrespective of previous malabsorption.

Obstructive symptoms are about as common in intestinal lymphoma as they are in adenocarcinoma (60–70%), and bleeding is only slightly less common (50%); pain and vomiting are accompanied by anorexia and weight loss. However, lymphomas are more likely to perforate than carcinomas (30%) or become palpable *per abdomen* (40%) [29]. Metastasis occurs to regional lymph nodes and sometimes to the peritoneum.

Primary lymphoma can usually be resected, even if nodal metastases are left behind; otherwise bypass should be undertaken to circumvent obstruction. Lymphomas are more likely than carcinomas to respond to radiotherapy and chemotherapy, but their overall five-year survival rate in some series (15–20%) is almost equally depressing [2, 29].

In coeliac disease

Some association between steatorrhoea and intestinal lymphoma had been recognized long before Gough and colleagues at Bristol suggested in 1962 that coeliac disease could be a premalignant condition [10]. The increased incidence of enteric lymphoma in patients with villous atrophy and crypt hyperplasia has since been shown to be statistically significant [4]. Ulcerative jejunitis may precede the development of frank neoplasia. The ultimate cancer is thought to be a type of malignant histiocytosis [13, 14].

Initial symptoms, often insidious, are weakness, loss of weight, nausea and diarrhoea. Physical signs include fever, anaemia, lymphadenopathy, clubbing, abdominal distension, oedema and skin pigmentation. The diagnosis should always be suspected in coeliac patients whose clinical condition progressively deteriorates despite strict supervision of a gluten-free diet. Malignant cells are seldom observed in peroral jejunal biopsies and radiology is often unrewarding, so that diagnostic laparotomy may be indicated at this stage [4]. Later, obstruction, bleeding or acute perforation can supervene. Treatment includes local resection of the tumour, irradiation, corticosteroids and cytotoxic drugs. As in Crohn's carcinoma of the small bowel, the prognosis is extremely poor.

In other conditions

Malignant lymphoma of the small intestine has been reported in association with diffuse nodular lymphoid hyperplasia [19] and alpha chain disease.

Smooth muscle tumours

Leiomyoma and leiomyosarcoma are included in this description, as histological differentiation between the two can be difficult. Apparently benign lesions are capable of metastasis, while those with an alarming degree of nuclear pleomorphism and mitotic activity may pursue an indolent clinical course. The tumours comprise relatively circumscribed whorls of smooth muscle that lack a proper capsule; variable degrees of hyalinization may be seen [30]. Smooth muscle tumours are equally distributed through the small intestine.

As smooth muscle tumours enlarge, they tend to expand the serosal aspect of the

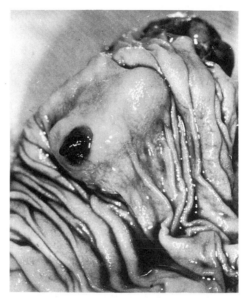

Fig. 48.4. Leiomyoma of the upper jejunum presenting with massive bleeding. Fresh clot can be seen in an ulcer crater on the mucosal aspect of the bowel. Several hours after admission to hospital with severe pain in the chest and upper abdomen, a 55-year-old man passed 1200 ml of reddish blood per rectum and became shocked. Oesophagogastroduodenoscopy was normal and emergency laparotomy was undertaken; after limited jejunectomy the patient made an uneventful recovery. Histological examination showed a smooth muscle tumour with no features to suggest malignancy (photograph courtesy of Mr R. G. Hughes, FRCS).

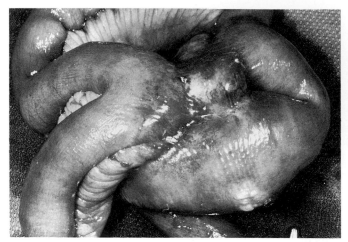

Fig. 48.5. Leiomyosarcoma of the upper jejunum involving two adjacent loops of bowel. A woman aged 64 years developed intermittent abdominal colic and progressive weight loss. A 10 cm tumour was palpable in the left hypochondrium. Barium follow-through examination showed displacement and some dilatation of the small bowel, and a tentative diagnosis of lymphoma was reached. Enlarged lymph nodes were noted at laparotomy, but these were also removed. She developed multiple hepatic metastases and died 15 months after operation.

bowel, but may stretch and even ulcerate the mucosa. The bleeding that ensues can be sudden and severe (Fig. 48.4). Haemorrhage is the commonest presentation, occurring in at least half the patients. Others develop subacute intestinal obstruction, perforation or a palpable mass (Fig. 48.5). A large tumour suggests, but does not necessarily imply, overt malignant change.

Excluding carcinoid, leiomyosarcoma is the third commonest enteric cancer after carcinoma and lymphoma. The tumour spreads to involve adjacent structures and mesenteric nodes, thence by lymphatic or haematogenous routes to the liver (Fig. 48.5). Extra-abdominal metastasis is unusual. Treatment is by resection alone, where feasible, because smooth muscle tumours are resistant to radiotherapy. From limited data it appears that the five-year survival rate (for sarcoma) is about 30%.

Secondary cancer

Carcinoma

The small intestine may be involved in one of two ways. Primary carcinomas of certain organs, including breast, stomach, large intestine and pancreas, may undergo transcoelomic metastasis, causing *carcinomatosis peritonei* and malignant ascites. Small bowel obstruction may need side-to-side bypass between a distended loop and a collapsed loop of intestine. Alternatively, the bowel may be directly invaded from an adjacent organ. Thus cancer of the pancreatic head, hepatic flexure or right kidney can involve the second and third parts of the duodenum, cancer of the pancreatic neck can involve the duodenojejunal flexure and cancer of the left colon can involve contiguous loops of jejunum or ileum. Obstructive features predominate, but bleeding or fistulation sometimes occur. With colonic cancer it is often possible to resect the involved loop of small bowel *en bloc*, but with pancreatic cancer gastroenterostomy is normally indicated.

Lymphoma

The small bowel may become involved in any generalized lymphoma. An unusual example is illustrated in Fig. 48.6.

Melanoma

Metastatic deposits of melanoma in the small intestine are found at autopsy in half the patients dying of disseminated disease

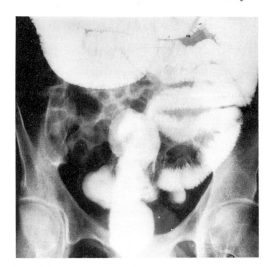

Fig. 48.6. Barium follow-through examination showing an ileosigmoid fistula in a case of Hodgkin's lymphoma. The patient was a man of 26 years who presented with weight loss, fever and gross cervical adenopathy; lymph node biopsy revealed lymphocyte-depleted Hodgkin's disease. He responded well to combination chemotherapy but developed intractable diarrhoea. Operation was carefully timed between courses of cytotoxic drugs. There were two separate fistulas between the distal ileum and lower sigmoid colon. Ileocaecal and rectosigmoid resection were carried out with immediate reconstruction. There were no postoperative problems, but he died of disseminated disease nine months later.

[5]. Perhaps their anergic state impairs the normal immunological protection of the bowel against neoplasia [18]. Acute complications of metastatic melanoma rarely develop, but operation becomes necessary for intestinal obstruction, bleeding or perforation [16]. Melanoma of the small intestine may sometimes cause occult haemorrhage and anaemia (Fig. 48.7).

References

1 ARTHAUD JB, GUINEE VF. Jejunal and ileal adenocarcinoma. Epidemiological considerations. *Am J Gastroenterol* 1979;**72**:638–646.
2 AWRICH AE, IRISH CE, VETTO RM, FLETCHER WS. A twenty-five year experience with primary malignant tumors of the small intestine. *Surg Gyneco Obstet* 1980;**151**:9–14.
3 BRIDGE MF, PERZIN KH. Primary adenocarcinoma of the jejunum and ileum. A clinicopathologic study. *Cancer* 1975;**36**:1876–1887.
4 COOPER BT, HOLMES GKT, FERGUSON R, COOKE WT. Celiac disease and malignancy. *Medicine* 1980;**59**:249–261.
5 DAS GUPTA TK, BRASFIELD RD. Metastatic melanoma of the gastrointestinal tract. *Arch Surg* 1964;**88**:969–973.
6 FORBES W StC, NOLAN DJ, FLETCHER EWL, LEE E. Small bowel melaena: 2 cases diagnosed by angiography. *Br J Surg* 1978;**65**:168–170.
7 FRESKO D, LAZARUS SS, DOTAN J, REINGOLD M. Early presentation of carcinoma of the small bowel in Crohn's disease ('Crohn's carcinoma'). Case reports and review of the literature. *Gastroenterology* 1982;**82**:783–789.
8 FRIEDMAN SL, WRIGHT TL, ALTMAN DF. Gastrointestinal Kaposi's sarcoma in patients with acquired immunodeficiency syndrome. Endoscopic and autopsy findings. *Gastroenterology* 1985;**89**:102–108.
9 GINZBURG L, SCHNEIDER KM, DREIZIN DH, LEVINSON

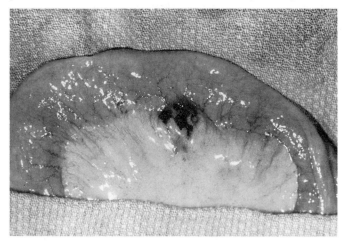

Fig. 48.7. Deposit of malignant melanoma invading the mesenteric border of the mid small bowel. A woman of 54 years presented with a palpable gall bladder, anaemia and guiac-positive stools. Several deposits of melanoma were encountered in the abdominal cavity, with the primary lesion unusually situated in the gall bladder. Two intestinal lesions were locally excised. She died four months later.

C. Carcinoma of the jejunum occurring in a case of regional enteritis. *Surgery* 1956;**39**:347–351.

10 GOUGH KR, READ AE, NAISH JM. Intestinal reticulosis as a complication of idiopathic steatorrhoea. *Gut* 1962;**3**:232–239.

11 HAWKER PC, GYDE SN, THOMPSON H, ALLAN RN. Adenocarcinoma of the small intestine complicating Crohn's disease. *Gut* 1982;**23**:188–193.

12 HOFFMAN JP, TAFT DA, WHEELIS RF, WALKER JH. Adenocarcinoma in regional enteritis of the small intestine. *Arch Surg* 1977;**112**:606–611.

13 ISAACSON PG, O'CONNOR NTJ, SPENCER J, et al. Malignant histiocytosis of the intestine: a T-cell lymphoma. *Lancet* 1985;**ii**:688–691.

14 ISAACSON PG, WRIGHT DH. Intestinal lymphoma associated with malabsorption.

15 JEFFERSON G. Carcinoma of the suprapapillary duodenum causally associated with pre-existing simple ulcer. Report of a case and an appendix of 30 collected cases. *Br J Surg* 1916;**4**:209–226.

16 KLAUSNER JM, SKORNICK Y, LELCUK S, BARATZ M, MERHAV A. Acute complications of metastatic melanoma to the gastrointestinal tract. *Br J Surg* 1982;**69**:195–196.

17 LILLEMOE K, IMBEMBO AL. Malignant neoplasms of the duodenum. *Surg Gynecol Obstet* 1980; **150**:822–826.

18 LOWENFELS AB. Why are small-bowel tumours so rare? *Lancet* 1973;**i**:24–26.

19 MATUCHANSKY C, TOUCHARD G, LEMAIRE M, et al. Malignant lymphoma of the small bowel associated with diffuse nodular lymphoid hyperplasia. *N Engl J Med* 1985;**313**:166–171.

20 MCKUSICK KA, FROELICH J, CALLAHAN RJ, WINZELBERG GG, STRAUSS HW. ^{99m}Tc red blood cells for detection of gastrointestinal bleeding: experience with 80 patients. *Am J Roentgenol* 1981; **137**:1113–1118.

21 PERZIN KH, BRIDGE MF. Adenomas of the small intestine: a clinicopathologic review of 51 cases and a study of their relationship to carcinoma. *Cancer* 1981;**48**:799–819.

22 RANZI T, CASTAGNONE D, VELIO P, BIANCHI P, POLLI EE. Gastric and duodenal polyps in familial polyposis coli. *Gut* 1981;**22**:363–367.

23 REID JD. Intestinal carcinoma in the Peutz–Jeghers syndrome. *JAMA* 1974;**229**:833–834.

24 REINER MA. Primary malignant neoplasms of the small bowel. *Mt Sinai J Med (NY)* 1976;**43**:274–280.

25 SHARON P, STALNIKOVICZ R, RACHMILEWITZ D. Endoscopic diagnosis of duodenal neoplasms causing upper gastrointestinal bleeding. *J Clin Gastroenterol* 1982;**4**:35–38.

26 SLAVIN G. Tumours and tumour-like conditions. In: Booth CC, Neale G, eds. *Disorders of the small intestine.* Oxford: Blackwell Scientific Publications, 1986:363–375.

27 VEEN HF, OSCARSON JEA, MALT RA. Alien cancers of the duodenum. *Surg Gynecol Obstet* 1976; **143**:39–42.

28 WEINSTEIN EC, DOCKERTY MB, WAUGH JM. Collective review. Neoplasms of Meckel's diverticulum. *Int Abstr Surg* 1963;**116**:103–111.

29 WILLIAMSON RCN, WELCH CE, MALT RA. Adenocarcinoma and lymphoma of the small intestine. Distribution and etiologic associations. *Ann Surg* 1983;**197**:172–178.

30 WILSON JM, MELVIN DB, GRAY G, THORBJARNARSON B. Benign small bowel tumor. *Ann Surg* 1975;**181**:247–250.

SECTION IX

INFLAMMATORY BOWEL DISEASE

Chapter 49
Clinical Features of Ulcerative Colitis

J. F. FIELDING

It has long been known that many micro-organisms may be associated with ulcerative inflammation of the colon. In the latter half of the last century it became clear that cases of colitis occurred in the absence of recognizable infective agents, and the condition became known as idiopathic ulcerative colitis. While one or two cases of what we now call post-dysenteric ulcerative colitis may have been described by Leach in 1866 [38], the first accurate description of the disease was not until 1909 at a meeting of the Section of Medicine of the Royal Society of Medicine [4]. White had described the condition in 1888 [68] but most of his 11 cases were what we now describe as Crohn's disease, as were the earlier descriptions by Wilks [70], Allchin [3] and many others [24]. Even the reference of Crohn [15] to a case of ulcerative colitis in 1865 is more likely to also refer to a patient with Crohn's disease.

Epidemiology [42]

Prevalence

Accurate prevalence and incidence figures are only available from Northwestern Europe, the United States of America and Israel. The impression has been formed that these are the areas where the disease is most common, an impression that is now accepted medical belief but may not be valid.

In Bristol an ingenious 'guesstimate' predicted that, because each colitic was on

Table 49.1. Ulcerative colitis prevalence rates.

Population	Year	Prevalence (per 10^5 population)
Oxford, U.K. [21]	1960	79.9
Rochester, U.S.A. [62]	1964	87.0
Tel-Aviv, Israel [29]	1970	37.4
Copenhagen, Denmark [7]	1978	117.0

average admitted to hospital once in 12 years, there would be 12 patients with the disease in the population for each new patient admitted in one year [37]. From Oxford this approach was shown, by one of the best ulcerative colitis epidemiological studies yet performed, to be remarkably accurate [21].

Prevalence rates are shown in Table 49.1; the rates in Europe and America are similar, and roughly double that recorded in Israel. The Israeli figures are of further interest, as Ashkenazi Jews of European/American origin have a higher prevalence than Israeli-born Jews, or African or Asian Jews (Table 49.2). The need for careful analysis is highlighted by the crude prevalence rate of Ashkenazi Jews in Israel which suggests a rate similar to their fellow Ashkenazims in America; the figure corrected for the population-at-risk gives a much truer comparison.

Incidence

Incidence rates for ulcerative colitis are summarized in Table 49.3. Lower incidence rates in Europe and America tend to come from studies based on hospital admission,

Table 49.2. Ulcerative colitis prevalence rates in Tel-Aviv Jews [29].

Birthplace of subgroup	Crude prevalence (per 10^5 population)	*Corrected prevalence (per 10^5 population)
European/North America	51.5	37.3
Israel	18.7	25.8
Africa	24.1	18.9
Asia	25.5	18.5

* Corrected for standardized population

and it has been shown that up to 22% of patients may not be hospitalized [65]. It seems likely that a greater proportion of patients with mild distal disease do not receive hospital admission. Early work reported a two-fold increase in incidence in the decade prior to 1960 [30]; this may have been due to not only a genuine increase but also an apparent increase caused by greater awareness of the condition. Most recent evidence suggests that, at least in the areas of high incidence, the rate has remained similar over the last two decades. There is suggestive evidence that both within Europe [50] and America [1, 44], the incidence rate of ulcerative colitis is higher amongst Jews than the rest of the population.

The risk amongst recent migrant populations to the United Kingdom has not been analysed sufficiently to determine incidence rates, but clinical experience would suggest

Table 49.3. Ulcerative colitis annual incidence rates.

Population	Years of survey	Incidence (per 10^5 population)
Oxford, U.K. [21]	1951–1960	6.5
	1951–1954	4.9
	1957–1960	8.9
Baltimore, U.S.A. [43]	1960–1963	4.6
Norway [30]	1946–1950	1.1
	1951–1955	1.7
	1956–1960	2.3
	1961–1969	3.2
Copenhagen, Denmark [7, 8]	1961–1966	7.3
	1962–1978	8.1
Tel-Aviv, Israel [29]	1961–1970	3.7
Malmo, Sweden [9]	1970	6.4
Multi-centre, U.S.A. [27]	1973 white males	5.5
	white females	5.9
	non-white males	5.7
	non-white females	5.5
Northeastern Scotland [65]	1967–1976	11.3
Cardiff [46]	1968–1977	7.2

they are much less frequently affected by ulcerative colitis than their Caucasian fellow-citizens. However, the incidence rate for ulcerative proctocolitis is the same for whites and non-whites in America [27]. It is of further interest that in New Zealand, a country with a low overall incidence rate, Maoris have a rate only one-twentieth that of their English-descended fellow-countrymen [69].

Sex ratio

Earlier major United Kingdom and European series showed a predominance of females. However, in Copenhagen the female to male ratio of 1.5 to 1 from 1962 to 1969 had fallen significantly to 1.1 to 1 between 1970 and 1978. Moreover, a re-

ulcerative colitis, but it is rare for the disease to begin in the first decade of life or over the age of 80 years. Depending on the method of analysis, most large series show that half the patients present either between 15 and 35, or between 20 and 40, years. Thus 52% of patients in Oxford presented between the ages of 20 and 40 years [20].

The majority of large series show a secondary peak of onset of symptoms in older patients, usually in their sixth or seventh decades (Fig. 49.1). The significance of the secondary peak may be realized more fully when it is related to the population at risk (Table 49.5). Much of the secondary peak relates to proctitis, which may represent a different disease process to idiopathic proctocolitis.

Table 49.4. Sex ratios in ulcerative colitis.

Country	Series	Females	Males	F/M ratio
United Kingdom	Oxford [20]	373	251	1.5:1
United Kingdom	Birmingham [32]	409	267	1.5:1
United Kingdom	Aberdeen [65]	260	274	0.9:1
Denmark	Copenhagen [34]	441	342	1.3:1
United States of America	Chicago [57]	414	470	0.9:1
Israel	Tel-Aviv [28]	244	260	0.9:1

cent United Kingdom series, and those from the United States and Israel, show no such predominance of females (Table 49.4).

Age

Age may be expressed as age at onset of symptoms or age at diagnosis; the former is biologically more accurate, the latter more objective. As the mean duration of symptoms from onset to diagnosis is of the order of one year, in epidemiological terms either figure may be taken.

All age groups are at risk of developing

Aetiology [2]

Genetics

With a prevalence rate for ulcerative colitis of around $100/10^5$, it has been estimated that the familial incidence of the disease would be of the order of 1% [39]. A much higher familial incidence has been found. In the Cleveland study [22] there was a 15.8% incidence of inflammatory bowel disease amongst immediate family members of the 316 ulcerative colitis propositi—four father/son; eight father/daughter; 10

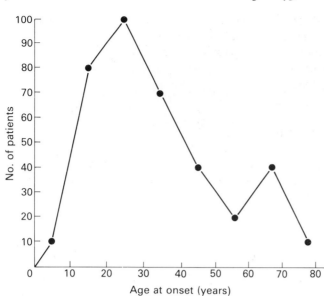

Fig. 49.1. Distribution of typical age at onset for ulcerative colitis [27, 32].

Table 49.5. Age at onset of ulcerative colitis—peak incidence related to population at risk.

Study	Group	Peak (yrs)	Incidence (per 10^5 population)
Baltimore, U.S.A. 1973 [27]	White males	20–29	8.7
		70–79	23.4
	White females	30–39	12.4
		70–79	18.0

mother/son; nine mother/daughter; and 19 sibling/sibling. Moreover, it became apparent that inflammatory bowel disease is more common when the propositus has Crohn's disease than when the propositus has ulcerative colitis (Table 49.6). In mon-ozygotic twins concordance nearly always occurs in Crohn's disease, whereas discordance occurs in over half with ulcerative colitis.

This type of data has been interpreted as evidence that genes at several loci are in-

Table 49.6. Familial inflammatory bowel disease.

Location of study	Diagnosis in propositus	Positive inflammatory bowel disease in family	
		Proportion	Percentage
Liverpool, U.K. [39]	Ulcerative colitis	7/103	6.9
	Crohn's disease	11/39	28.2
Cleveland, U.S.A. [22]	Ulcerative colitis	93/316	29.4
	Crohn's disease	187/522	35.8

volved in the hereditary predisposition to inflammatory bowel disease. Fewer relevant genes are required for the expression of ulcerative colitis, whereas a more complete genotype leads to the development of Crohn's disease. Moreover, the familial associations of Crohn's disease with ulcerative colitis have been taken to more probably reflect a shared genetic background, than necessarily implying differing manifestations of a fundamentally similar disease.

No genetic markers are available for ulcerative colitis. ABO blood group distributions do not differ from those of control populations. HLA-A and B antigen studies have given conflicting results, but there is no strong association of ulcerative colitis with any particular antigen [14]. One HLA study showed a significant association between HLA-BW35 and ulcerative colitis in 60 Israeli patients [17]; it has been suggested that this gene may be related with persistence of circulating immune complexes [58], which have been associated with many of the remote manifestations of ulcerative colitis. The same Israeli study showed that HLA-AW24 was associated with early onset severe disease. Recent HLA-DR2 studies have given conflicting results—one study suggests that the presence of this antigen lessens the risk of ulcerative colitis [11], but another reports an increased risk [5].

Another significant association is the high frequency of HLA-B in patients with either ulcerative colitis or Crohn's disease, and ankylosing spondylitis. Two-thirds of inflammatory bowel disease HLA-B27 positive patients have ankylosing spondylitis compared with only 5% of HLA-B27 positive people in the general population. Inflammatory bowel disease thus appears as a potent initiating or potentiating factor in the development of ankylosing spondylitis [41]. However, as the incidence of HLA-B27 is higher in patients with ankylosing spondylitis without overt inflammatory bowel disease than in those with inflammatory bowel disease, it is likely that they are associated diseases.

Environmental factors

Infective agents

Because of the similarity of ulcerative colitis with the colitides of dysentery and other infective agents a causative organism has been sought for ulcerative colitis (see Chapter 57). From the early excitement engendered by Bargen's 'dyplococcus' [6]—through bacterial, protozoan, fungal, viral and chlamydial searches—all have failed to discover a causative organism. This failure to find an organism does not exclude antigenic determinants from one or more of these agents immunologically triggering the disease in a susceptible host or influencing pathoperpetuation in a diseased host. For example, there is a report from a small series of patients which suggests that cytomegalovirus infection in a diseased patient may increase the risk of toxic megocolon [13].

Psychosocial factors

There is no convincing evidence that patients with ulcerative colitis are subjected to excess life events prior to the onset of disease [45]. The effects of coping on bowel function have not been studied in a group of persons yet to develop ulcerative colitis, compared with controls who do not subsequently develop the disease. Until this unlikely study is performed, it is conjectural to draw conclusions concerning psychosocial stress and ulcerative colitis. Moreover, it must be remembered that patients may have symptoms of irritable bowel syndrome superimposed on quiescent colitis. Most reports show that urban dwellers are more at risk of developing ulcerative colitis than their country cousins. Smoking appears to protect against the development of ulcerative colitis [33] but this unexplained finding in no way justifies advising patients or persons at risk to partake of the habit.

Dietary factors [36]

The recognition of ulcerative colitis followed shortly after the widespread use of milled flour. Countries who ingest high fibre diets are still believed to have low incidence rates for ulcerative colitis, although sound scientific data is lacking. This aspect requires further study, particularly the short- and long-term qualitative, quantitative and durational effects of different dietary fibre intakes on the bacteria-mucosal cell interface.

At one time ulcerative colitis was regarded as an allergic reaction to milk. It is now recognized that some of these patients were really suffering from hypolactasia, which is probably no more prevalent in colitics than in non-colitics. However, colitics with hypolactasia tend to have more persistant attacks of colitis [51]. A further small minority, perhaps 5% of colitics, can be shown to have a flare-up of their disease after the ingestion of milk, and to benefit from its withdrawal.

Pathophysiology

Water and electrolytes

The daily faecal weight in patients with ulcerative colitis is roughly double the upper limit of normal. When the disease is confined to the rectum, with or without sigmoid involvement, the daily faecal weight is at the upper limit of normal [60].

In patients with proctitis the potassium-to-sodium ratio in stools is virtually normal or slightly elevated [60]; when elevated this is due to increased potassium loss, probably in association with mucus, rather than decreased sodium absorption.

The majority of *in vivo* evidence favours a primary defect in the absorption of sodium, chloride and water in extensive ulcerative colitis [52]. These results are supported by *in vitro* studies which have shown no change in serosal to mucosa fluxes of sodium or chloride. Thus, although there is evidence for increased prostaglandin synthesis in active colitis, the absence of enhanced secretion of sodium and chloride must question the significance of their role in the diarrhoea of active colitis [19, 53]. Whole body potassium loss may be largely related to urinary losses due to secondary hyperaldosteronism.

Immunology

While no one doubts an immunological input into at least the pathogenesis and perpetuative of ulcerative colitis, the area is still very much in the hands of the research worker with no clinical implications. Moreover, there is much conflicting evidence and what follows is a consensus view.

Majority evidence suggests that the humoral immune response in ulcerative colitis is normal. Cell mediated immunity is probably also normal, as anergic responses rarely persist after bowel resection and are not present in first degree relatives; observed abnormalities are probably secondary rather than primary phenomena.

Ulcerative colitics, as a group, have higher serum IgG concentrations than controls; there is some evidence that patients with higher IgG concentrations have a better prognosis. Serum IgM concentration may go up post-surgery, but this is probably a response to bacterial or tissue antigen release at the time of operation.

Circulating antibodies against various alimentary tract antigens (such as colon epithelial component, intestinal bacteria and polysaccharide antigen from germ-free rat faeces), have been detected in ulcerative colitics' serum; they have been interpreted as being secondary to a damaged mucosa rather than being disease-specific.

It has been claimed that disease-specific antigens have been detected in the colonic mucosa of patients using purified colitis colon tissue-bound IgG. It is not known whether the proteins recognized by this antibody come from bacteria, or from colonic epithelial cells that become antigenic either after a primary assault or bacterial incorporation [48].

Demonstration of complement in the basement membrane of colitics' colonic epithelium may be taken as supportive evidence for immune complex deposition in the mucosa. Monocytes (both locally and peripherally) may be stimulated by such immune complexes, explaining the increased prostaglandin synthesis that occurs in active ulcerative colitis.

The report of a spontaneous colitis in cotton-top tamarins may speed experimental understanding of ulcerative colitis [40]. Many of the extraintestinal manifestations of ulcerative colitis probably occur as a consequence of circulating immune-complexes.

Pathology

Ulcerative colitis is a non-specific inflammatory disease, predominantly mucosal, extending proximally from the anal region to a varying degree. It may be confined to the rectum—so called **proctitis**; involve the rectum and sigmoid colon—**proctosigmoiditis**; extend towards and to the splenic flexure—**left-sided colitis**; or beyond the splenic flexure to the transverse colon—**sub-total colitis**; or involve the entire colon—**total or universal colitis.** The change from abnormal to normal mucosa may be abrupt or gradual. There is a tendency for the disease to extend proximally with the passage of time. The clinical impression is that the more extensive the disease initially, and the less clear-cut the separation between ab-

normal and normal mucosa, the more likely it is that the process will extend.

Macroscopic appearances

The presence of excoriated anal skin with possibly an anal fissure may be the first evidence of pathology noted by the clinician. Rarely a perianal or ischiorectal abscess may also be present; perianal disease makes Crohn's disease the far more likely diagnosis.

A granular mucosa may be felt on rectal examination and there may be blood on the withdrawn glove. If the disease is active, rigid sigmoidoscopy will confirm the presence of a granular haemorrhagic mucosa; in severe disease there will be blood, pus and mucus coming from the colon into the rectum. When the disease is confined to the rectum, the macroscopic extent of the disease may be determined by rigid sigmoidoscopy. Accurate determination of the extent of the other forms of the disease requires the use of a flexible sigmoidoscope in proctosigmoiditis or a colonoscope. Radiology tends to underestimate the extent of disease.

When the disease becomes inactive the rectal mucosa returns towards normal but it is rare for a normal vessel pattern or a normal light reflex from the mucosa to return. Moreover, the experienced eye will usually detect a degree of fine granularity. Inflammatory polyps, even if covered with epithelium or strictures, may provide evidence of previous disease.

It is now recognized that colonic shortening of long-standing disease is due to a muscle abnormality, rather than fibrosis. It may best be described as a form of muscle contracture of the muscularis propria. A similar contracture of the muscularis mucosae may account for the benign strictures that occur in ulcerative colitis.

Microscopic appearances

Microscopically it is possible to divide the disease into active colitis, resolving colitis, and colitis in remission.

In **active colitis** there is dilatation of the capillary blood supply to the mucous membrane with intermucosal haemorrhages, epithelial cell necrosis and reduction in the goblet cell population. There is a lymphocyte, plasma cell and polymorphonuclear cell infiltration of the lamina propria. The latter also collect within the epithelial crypts forming crypt abscesses. The changes are confined to the mucosa but, if ulceration is also present, the submucosa may be infiltrated with chronic inflammatory cells.

Resolving colitis is recognized by the diminution of the cellular infiltration of the lamina propria and the restoration of the goblet cell population.

Colitis in remission is characterized by shortening of the crypts, with a gap between the base of the crypts and the muscularis mucosae. There is also a loss of parallelism and branching of the tubules. There may be focal collections of chronic inflammatory cells. The epithelium may be hyperplastic and muscularis mucosa thickened.

Precancerous (dysplastic) changes occur in patients with long-standing total or sub-total colitis. The changes consist of increased epithelial cell nuclear size, nuclear crowding, loss of nuclear polarity and variable mucin depletion. The recognition of such changes, although difficult to assess especially in the presence of inflammation, has an important role in patient management (Table 49.7) as the optimal timing of surgery may considerably reduce the risk of cancer in long-standing ulcerative colitis [54, 55]. Scanning electron microscopy may help to detect the present of dysplasia [64]. Dysplastic tissue tends to have fewer cells per unit area, fewer microvilli per unit

Table 49.7. Dysplasia and patient management (adapted from [55]).

Rectal biopsy classification for dysplastic changes	Clinical management
Negative	Continue surveillance.
Indefinite	
Probably negative	Continue surveillance.
Probably positive	Follow-up biopsy within six months.
Positive	
Low grade	Follow-up biopsy within three months; if low grade persists or mass lesion also present proceed to panproctocolectomy.
High grade	Panproctocolectomy.

area and a decreased proportion of microvilli with a normal width. Other aids in the diagnosis of dysplasia (such as carcino-embryonic antigen, staining for sulphated mucopolysaccharides, unusual lectins such as peanut agglutinin, and DNA content of epithelial cells) are as yet of unproven value [55].

Clinical features

Symptoms

The patient will usually present with both intestinal and systemic symptoms. The patient with mild disease may only have intestinal symptoms, and rarely the patient may only present with extra-intestinal manifestations. Symptoms may be of insidious or abrupt origin, and vary from mild to severe. As a rule, the more extensive the disease the more severe the symptoms, but total colitis may have minimal symptoms and patients with proctosigmoiditis severe symptoms. When patients first present some 25% will have a proctitis or proctosigmoiditis, 50% left-sided disease, and 25% a total colitis.

The classical triad of abdominal symptoms in ulcerative colitis are rectal bleeding, diarrhoea and abdominal pain.

The **rectal bleeding** is usually mixed with a liquid stool. A formed stool, coated with blood, suggests proctitis or other rectal pathology.

The large majority of patients present with **diarrhoea,** and its severity is a guide to the extent of involved colon. A small minority of patients, usually older, complain of constipation. They often have either a proctosigmoiditis or left-sided disease with faecal stasis in the proximal normal colon. When these people have active disease they may complain of both diarrhoea (in reality, the passage of blood, mucus and pus) and constipation due to the infrequent passage of small, formed stools. Moreover, when these patients have abdominal pain it is often related to the distended normal colon. Whether the active disease area acts as an 'obstruction', or whether there is reflex 'protective' stasis in the normal colon, is unknown.

Abdominal pain is rarely severe in proctocolitis. It is usually no more than a mild suprapubic ache or crampy pain, relieved by defecation. Persistant severe pain only occurs in extensive disease, and it must always raise the possibility of a present or impending toxic megacolon.

Systemic symptoms consist of fever, anorexia, weight loss, lack of energy and lassitude. Symptoms relating to the skin, eye or joint manifestations of inflammatory bowel disease may also be present.

Signs

Signs vary with the severity of the colitis. They include evidence of weight loss, pyrexia, tachycardia, anaemia and very rarely finger clubbing. Most frequently, examination of the abdomen is normal apart from the evidence of weight loss. There may be slight tenderness over the colon, usually in the left iliac fossa. Rarely, in patients with faecal stasis, a mass may be felt in the right iliac fossa; this mass is often no longer palpable following the passage of solid stools. Bowel sounds may be normal or increased in frequency. A distended abdomen with diminished or absent bowel sounds indicates impending or present toxic dilatation. Examination of the perianal region may reveal a fissure or small tag, but rarely any evidence of sepsis. Digital insertion into the rectum may be associated with the escape of blood, mucus or pus. The mucosa may have a granular feel and there may be fresh blood on the withdrawn finger glove.

Definition of severity

In a classic study some twenty years ago [20] the attacks of ulcerative colitis were defined as mild, moderately severe or severe. These definitions have stood the test of time with regard to prognosis, both in relation to the attack itself and also in the long-term (Table 50.1). A **mild attack** is defined as fewer than four bowel motions per day with no more than small amounts of macroscopic blood in the stool; no fever; no tachycardia; anaemia not severe, and the ESR not raised above 30 mm/1st hour. A **moderately severe attack** lies between a mild and a severe attack. A **severe attack** consists of six or more motions per day with macroscopic blood on the stools; a mean evening temperature of more than 37.5°C, or a temperature of more than 37.8°C on at least two days out of four; a tachycardia with the pulse rate more than 90 beats per minute; a haemoglobin of less than 75% (10.5 g/dl), and an ESR of more than 30 mm/1st hour.

Clinical course

Short-term

The results for the patients first attending the Radcliffe Infirmary, Oxford, between

1953 and 1962 still probably provide the best available short-term results [20]. Of 354 patients presenting with their first attack of ulcerative colitis, 16 (5.4%) died, 304 (85.9%) went into complete remission, 29 (8.2%) improved, two (0.6%) remained unchanged, and three (0.8%) had a colectomy. Eight (50%) of the deaths were due to uncomplicated ulcerative colitis—five of these after emergency surgery. Five deaths were due to complications of the colitis (perforation or massive haemorrhage); one death was related to carcinoma and two to unrelated diseases. Eleven (26.8%) of the 41 patients with a severe attack died; two (2.4%) of 83 with a moderately severe attack, but only one (0.4%) of 227 with a mild attack. Patients over 60 years of age had an increased risk of death.

Long-term

In the same Oxford study, 8% of patients were dead within one year of presentation in their first attack. The observed risk of mortality continued to be significantly greater than the expected mortality throughout the entire period of follow-up; 40% had died within 20 years. In the majority of the survivors, the disease pursued a course of relapses and remissions; a minority had a chronic, continuous form of the disease. Some were symptom-free for a few years after their first attack, but only 4% remained symptom-free after 15 years of follow-up. Over 95% of patients led a normal or near-normal life between attacks.

However, the long-term figures relate to hospital patients diagnosed before 1942 and the outlook is much better today. Indeed, two recent reports [34, 65] show that long-term survival is almost identical to that of the general population. Only those with a severe first attack and men over the age of 40 at diagnosis had an increased mortality risk. Moreover, for the latter group the increased risk was only marginal

and within the first two years of diagnosis. Some half to two-thirds of patients may expect to be symptom-free in any one year. The capacity for work is no different from non-colitics. However, 97% will have had a relapse within 10 years and 99% within 18 years.

Fertility and pregnancy in ulcerative colitis

Fertility is normal in females with ulcerative colitis and pregnancy does not adversely affect colitis (see Chapter 50). The risk of deterioration in colitis is minimized by the patient awaiting pregnancy until the disease is inactive. Similarly ulcerative colitis does not adversely affect pregnancy as some 85% of such pregnancies lead to the birth of a normal full-term infant, a figure similar to that for the general population [23]. The chances of a normal full-term infant are improved if the pregnancy begins when the disease is inactive [71]. Post-ileostomy pregnancies also have a normal outcome as far as the foetus is concerned; occasionally there are minor episodes of intestinal obstruction during pregnancy but these usually respond to medical measures.

Fertility in the male colitic may be adversely affected by either medical or surgical therapy. Sulphasalazine oligospermia is reversible [49]; the risk of impotence should be taken into consideration when planning an elective panproctocolectomy, although a sperm bank is an added insurance against post-surgical impotence.

Complications of ulcerative colitis

Local complications

Toxic megacolon

The aetiology of toxic megacolon is unknown, but there is the disturbing suspicion that faults of commission (the use of opiates or anticholinergic agents or barium enema examination) or omission (prolonged hypokalaemia) in severe disease may at least partly contribute to the risk of toxic megacolon. One may be lulled into a false sense of patient improvement by diminution in stool frequency with the onset of toxic dilatation, but the deterioration in the patient's general state of health, together with the abdominal signs, should alert the physician to the true diagnosis.

Colonic perforation

Colonic perforation usually complicates toxic megacolon, but it may occur in its absence. The classic signs of perforation may be masked by treatment with a high dose of corticosteroids but, again, the sudden deterioration in the well-being of a patient, even in the absence of abdominal signs, will alert the clinician to the possibility of perforation.

Massive haemorrhage

Massive haemorrhage from the colon is rare and presents no diagnostic difficulty.

Carcinoma of the colon

The true risk of carcinoma of the colon in ulcerative colitis is difficult to determine. However, the risk is small in patients in the 10 years following diagnosis. Thereafter there is a significant increase in cancer risk for those patients with total colitis, so that the cumulative risk for these patients after 20 years of active disease lies somewhere between 20% and 40%. The risks seem similar for children and adults, when account is taken of the greater proportion of children with total colitis. These figures are based on hospital patients and the risk of cancer may be much less overall. Hendricksen, Kreiner and Binder [34] suggest an accumulative risk at 10 years of 0.8%, at 15 years of 1.1% and at 18 years of 1.4%. Moreover, they showed no difference

in the risk of those with total colitis. The prognosis for carcinoma complicating ulcerative colitis is the same as for carcinoma in the non-colitic [56].

Remote complications

Skin disease

Some 5% of patients have symptomatic skin lesions. The most common lesions are erythema nodosum and pyoderma gangrenosum; the latter may be precipitated by trauma [25]. Less common lesions include papulonecrotic lesions and ulcerative erythematous plaques.

Eye lesions

Symptomatic eye lesions occur in 5% of patients. They include episcleritis (Fig. 49.2), iritis and rarely, blepharo-keratitis, interstitial keratitis, choroiditis and scleromalacia perforans.

Oral lesions

Apthous ulceration occurs in about 10% of patients. Rarer lesions include ulcers analogous to pyoderma gangrenosum of the skin, pyostomatitis vegetans and haemorrhagic ulcers of the oral mucosa.

Arthritis

Apart from the association with ankylosing spondylitis, some 20–25% of ulcerative colitics develop a peripheral rheumatoid-type of arthralgia or arthritis. It is not as symmetrical as true rheumatoid arthritis and is much less chronic; episodes of pain last only from a few days to one to two weeks, and are followed by resolution. Attacks are nearly always concurrent with active bowel disease and erythema nodosum may also be present.

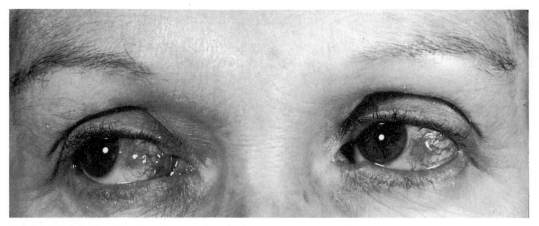

Fig. 49.2. Episcleritis with chemosis in a patient with ulcerative colitis.

Thromboembolic disease

This is rare, usually affecting pulmonary or cerebral vessels. The cause is unknown; thrombocytosis has been a suggested contributary factor.

Liver and biliary tract disease [18, 63, 66]

Only 1–2% of colitics have significant liver disease. Fatty infiltration and pericholangitis are found in up to 50% of liver biopsy specimens but are of no major clinical significance. Chronic active hepatitis and cirrhosis may occur even in the absence of previous blood transfusions. Drug-associated liver disease may also occur.

Two serious biliary tract diseases may occur but these are fortunately rare. They are sclerosing cholangitis (which may be an associated disease rather than a complication) [12] and carcinoma of the bile duct. The onset of painless cholestatic jaundice in an ulcerative colitic is an ominous sign.

Renal disease

Ureteric calculi, due to chronic mild dehydration, may occur in post-ileostomy patients. Rarely secondary amyloidosis may affect the kidneys, and very rarely glome-rulonephritis may occur, possibly due to the deposition of immune-complexes.

Investigations

Endoscopy

Sigmoidoscopy, with rectal mucosal biopsy, confirms the diagnosis in the vast majority of patients (Table 50.2). Repeat sigmoidoscopy may be undertaken to evaluate progress and to assess response to treatment. Rectal sparing is unusual in typical ulcerative colitis, but successful local treatment with rectal steroids may cause improvement in sigmoidoscopic appearances, despite continuing proximal disease activity. If the symptoms are inappropriate for the sigmoidoscopic appearance, colonoscopy may be required to assess the more proximal bowel.

Colonoscopy accurately assesses the proximal limit of colonic disease, usually detecting more extensive disease than a barium enema. It enables multiple biopsies to be taken throughout the colon, especially from areas of suspicion such as strictures or polyps.

Radiology

A **supine plain X-ray of the abdomen** may on occasion strongly suggest the diagnosis of ulcerative colitis. Either a continuously involved ahaustral tubular gas-filled left colon or less frequently, a gas-filled shortened entire colon, are strongly suggestive of the diagnosis. There may be evidence of faecal stasis in the right colon, especially in patients with left-sided disease. Occasionally the gas-filling may be sufficient to outline mucosal irregularities caused by pseudopolyps, particularly in the presence of toxic megacolon.

The radiological diagnosis of toxic megacolon has been variously defined as dilatation of the mid-transverse colon to a diameter greater than 5, 6 or 7 cm. It is more important to remember that, although toxic dilatation most frequently involves the transverse colon, it may involve any part of the colon and, instead of relying on a tape measure diagnosis, one should heed the change in calibre of the lumen in conjunction with the toxic clinical state. A patient admitted to hospital with acute colitis often needs daily supine X-ray films to assess changes in the colonic dilatation and gas pattern.

A **barium enema examination** may be by either a single-contrast barium sulphate mixture or by double-contrast barium-air examination. The double-contrast method is superior for the detection of early changes, hence it more accurately assesses the extent of the disease. A single-contrast examination probably underestimates the extent of the disease. The practical point is that disease extending to the mid-transverse colon by single-contrast examination should be assumed to be universal disease. In the individual patient this may be confirmed or refuted by colonoscopy or a double-contrast study.

A barium enema examination should not be undertaken in an acutely ill patient. There is no therapeutic advantage in knowing the extent of the disease at that point in time and the examination may increase the risk of the patient developing toxic magacolon.

Typically the X-ray changes of ulcerative colitis extend proximally from the left side to a varying degree; they are continuous and symmetrical. Moreover, the severity of the changes either remains the same or diminishes from left to right.

The early changes seen in double-contrast films are punctate ulcers on an oedematous mucosa often producing a finely granular appearance. Single-contrast films reveal a fuzziness of the bowel margins due to the fine ulceration, which is usually shallow. A double lining of the lumen is caused by different densities of barium mixing with a combination of oedema, mucus, exudate and blood. Moreover, the central column of barium may be less clear than normal, with either a ground glass or a granular appearance, caused by its admixture with secretions into the lumen.

Later the mucosa becomes nodular due to inflammatory polyps and pseudopolyps, together with the continuation of varying degrees of inflammatory change. Collarstud ulceration occasionally occurs, probably related to confluence of ulceration within the wall. In the chronic stage the lumen becomes narrow, the wall becomes more rigid, the haustral markings are lost and the bowel shortens (Fig. 49.3).

Lateral films of the pelvis should always be taken. They allow a more accurate assessment of rectal involvement by examination of the mucosa, luminal edge, rectal distensibility and the size of the retrorectal space. The latter may be increased in acute disease, but it is virtually always increased in chronic disease.

Examination of the ileum should always be attempted during barium enema examination. In some 10% of patients with ulcerative colitis features of so-called 'back wash

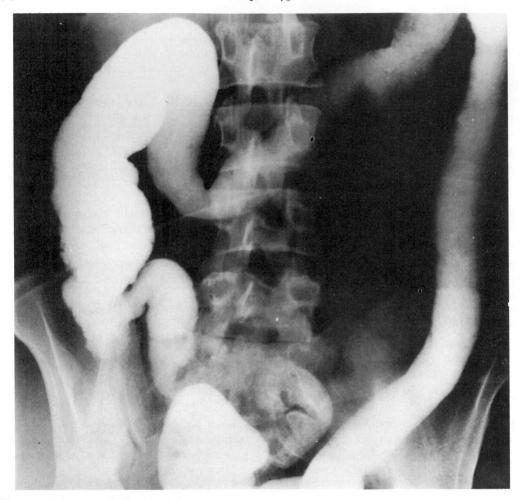

Fig. 49.3. Total colitis with backwash ileitis.

ileitis' may be seen. When this exists the ileum is of normal or increased calibre and, apart from indirect evidence of increased secretions (double contour or haziness of barium) there are no other abnormalities— particularly no evidence of ulcerative disease (Fig. 49.3).

Although benign strictures may occur in ulcerative colitis, radiological 'benign' strictures must always be regarded as malignant until proven otherwise. This may be done endoscopically with multiple biopsies, or by histology following excision. Carcinoma of the colon complicating ulcerative

colitis may on occasion appear like carcinoma in a non-colitic. However, it is more common for the radiological appearance to be much more subtle in colitics. It may be no more than a narrowed segment, perhaps with an eccentric lumen. Obvious mucosal irregularities and tapered margins, if present, remove diagnostic doubt but such ease of diagnosis is rarely present. A high index of suspicion of all persistent asymmetries or irregularities is required. Fortunately, the diagnostic burden has transferred from the radiologist to the endoscopist and pathologist.

Computerized tomography

Computerized tomography can occasionally help in the differentiation of ulcerative from Crohn's colitis. In ulcerative colitis there is a lesser degree of thickening, it is inhomogeneous as distinct from homogeneous in Crohn's colitis and there is a 'target' (as in archery) rectum [31]. Computerized tomography seems an extravagant way to diagnose toxic megacolon [10].

Isotope studies

Labelled leucocytes [2] or technetium 99 m labelled sucralfate [16] may be used to identify diseased colon non-invasively.

Laboratory investigations

Patients with colitis have many reasons for abnormalities in either haematological or biochemical laboratory investigations, summarized in Table 49.8. The common abnormalities are iron-deficiency anaemia, an elevated white cell count and ESR, and a low serum albumin.

All patients with colitis should have some stool samples examined at initial diagnosis, and at the start of each relapse, to exclude the infectious causes of colonic inflammation.

Differential diagnosis

As idiopathic or non-specific ulcerative colitis was so described to separate it from the **infectious colitides,** it is imperative to exclude a specific cause for the patients proctitis or proctocolitis. Those that may need to be excluded are listed in Table 49.9 (see Chapter 57). A few points of practical importance—amoebiasis may precede or coexist with ulcerative colitis and the diagnosis and treatment of the former does not necessarily exclude the latter. Similarly, so-called ulcerative post-dysenteric colitis is

Table 49.8. Laboratory studies in ulcerative colitis.

Test	Possible reasons for abnormal result
Haemoglobin	Blood loss, drug effect
White cell count	Inflammation, infection, drug effect
Platelet count	Disease activity, drug effect
ESR	Disease activity
Urea	State of hydration, renal disease, liver disease
Sodium	Diarrhoea
Potassium	Sodium loss, diarrhoea
Seromucoids, Orosomucoids, C reactive protein	Disease activity
Serum albumin	Loss from GI tract, impaired synthesis
Alkaline phosphatase	Intra-abdominal sepsis, pericholangitis, cholestatic liver disease
Bilirubin	Drug effect, blood transfusion, liver disease
Alanine and asparatate transaminase	Liver disease (drugs, transfusion, viruses, disease-related)
Prothrombin time	Liver disease
Serum folate	Drug effect
Serum iron and TIBC	Disease activity, iron deficiency

almost certainly ulcerative colitis preceded, or revealed, by bacillary dysentery. The finding of *Clostridium difficile* toxin in the stool of ulcerative colitis patients in no way lessens the diagnostic probability of ulcerative colitis. Although tuberculous colitis is seen rarely today, and usually occurs in the presence of cavitating pulmonary disease, the possibility of its presence must be borne in mind, particularly in ethnically-predisposed individuals.

The major problem in the differential diagnosis is the separation of **Crohn's colitis** from ulcerative colitis [35]. The main points of differentiation are summarized in Table

Table 49.9. Specific infections that may simulate, or coexist with or precede ulcerative colitis.

Bacterial	*Salmonella*
	Shigella
	Mycobacterium tuberculosis
	Staphlococcus
	Gonococcus
	Campylobacter
	Clostridium difficile
Viral	Enteroviruses
	Cytomegalovirus
	Herpes virus
Spirochaetal	*Treponema pallidium*
Chlamydial	Lymphogranuloma venereum
Protozoal	*Entamoeba histolytica*
	Balantidium coli
Metazoal	*Shistosoma mansoni*
Mycotic	Histoplasma capsulatum

49.10. It must be remembered that while differentiation is relatively easy in the majority, it may not be initially possible in some 15–20% of patients. It is unfortunate that the patients who are difficult to diagnose clinically are often difficult to separate on radiological and histological criteria. Most patients in whom it is not possible to make an initial definitive diagnosis turn out to have granulomatous colitis on long-term follow-up.

In **cathartic colon** a history of purgative abuse may or may not be ascertained. The addition of sodium bicarbonate may turn the stool pink in those patients who have been abusing a phenolphthalein-containing purgatives and one may find 'melanosis' coli in those who have abused

Table 49.10. Features of differentiation of ulcerative from Crohn's colitis.

	Feature	Ulcerative colitis	Crohn's colitis
History	Diarrhoea	Bloody diarrhoea	Diarrhoea with or without blood
Examination	Clubbing	Rare	Common
	Abdominal mass	Very Rare	Common
	Colour of perineum	Pink	Violaceous
	Large fleshy tags	Absent	Uncommon
	Multiple fistulae	Absent	Uncommon
Sigmoidoscopy	'Normal' rectal mucosa	Absent	Present in half the patients
Radiology	Small bowel disease	Backwash ileitis	Common
	Continuity	Continuous	Discontinuous
	Symmetry	Symmetrical	Asymmetrical
	Ulceration	Shallow	Deep
	Fistulae	Absent	Occur
	Distribution	Decreasing from left to right	Areas of relative or absolute sparing distal to macroscopic disease
Histology	Distribution	Mucosal (and submucosal)	Submucosal and mucosal
		Diffuse	Focal
	Goblet cell population in active phase	Depleted	Not depleted
	Length of tubules in chronic disease	Diminished	Normal
	Diagnostic	None	Granulomata, giant cells

anthroquinone-containing purgatives. The latter change may be noted on histology even if not detected at proctosigmoidoscopy. The radiological findings are those of a long ahaustral colon, rather than the short ahaustral colon in ulcerative colitis (see Chapter 4).

The **pseudomembranous colitis** should be suspected both from the clinical setting (debilitating disease or antibiotic use) together with the typical sigmoidoscopic findings of yellow-white plaques or pseudomembranes on a hyperaemic mucosa. There are also typical microscopic findings (see Chapter 59).

Ischaemic colitis is usually found in an older age group and there is often evidence of ischaemic disease elsewhere. When it occurs in patients under the age of fifty years there is nearly always an obvious precipitating factor, for example, the contraceptive pill, diabetes mellitus or previous abdominal surgery (see Chapter 69).

Diverticulitis will readily be differentiated by the normal rectal mucosa on proctosigmoidoscopy and positive radiological findings. Other causes of local bleeding such as haemorrhoids, a rectal polyp or carcinoma, should readily be differentiated by the history and examination, supported by the appropriate proctosigmoidoscopic and radiological findings.

A history of radiation therapy, and evidence of telangiectasia as well as the inflammatory changes on endoscopy, enable a diagnosis of **post-radiation colitis** to be made (see Chapter 70).

The **irritable bowel syndrome** should be readily distinguished in the large majority of patients by the history, examination, and also by normal laboratory findings. However, the two conditions may coexist.

The **colonic solitary ulcer** syndromes are discussed below.

Behçet's syndrome will be differentiated by its orogenital ulceration. The oral component is far less intermittent than the aphthous ulceration that may occur in ulcerative colitis and involvement of the colon is predominantly right-sided (see Chapter 74).

Collagen disorders such as scleroderma or polyarteritis nodosum will nearly always have typical features outside the gastrointestinal tract.

Solitary ulcers of the large intestine

Solitary ulcers of the large intestine are rare. The terminology is not entirely satisfactory as, although there is typically only one ulcer, there may be multiple ulcers or, at least in the rectum, no ulceration at all! While non-specific solitary ulceration may involve any part of the large intestine, three distinct anatomico-clinical syndromes are recognized.

Solitary caecal or ascending colon ulcer

Patients usually present with right iliac fossa pain and nausea. There may be a preceding history of constipation. A history of blood *per rectum* is extremely rare. The patient may be pyrexial but no mass is felt in the right lower abdomen. There may be a leukocytosis. Perforation with peritonitis is not uncommon. Appendicitis is the usual clinical diagnosis with the correct diagnosis being made at laparotomy. Occasionally the diagnosis is made colonoscopically.

The aetiology is unknown. There are no controlled studies to determine the correct management—local surgical excision is probably advisable, because of the risk of perforation. If a conservative approach is preferred, it is mandatory to perform multiple biopsies to exclude an ulcerating carcinoma.

Solitary sigmoid colon ulcer

This usually presents as recurrent rectal bleeding, constipation and a dull lower abdominal ache. The clinical diagnosis is usually acute diverticulitis. Rigid sigmoidoscopy may reveal blood coming from above but no ulceration is seen; the diagnosis may be made using a flexible instrument. However, it is far more commonly made at surgery as there is a high incidence of perforation.

The aetiology is unknown. Surgical excision is the treatment of choice, often enforced by perforation.

Solitary rectal ulcer [26, 59]

This is the most commonly recognized type of discrete large bowel ulceration. The patient is usually a young adult with a slightly greater chance of being female. The passage of mucus *per rectum* and mild rectal bleeding are the major presenting symptoms. Enquiry will usually reveal an alteration of bowel habit which may be diarrhoea (as defined by the patient), constipation or alternating diarrhoea and constipation. Anorectal or left iliac fossa pain may also be present. The patient may have difficulty in initiating defecation and this may be associated with digital insertion. There may be a feeling of incomplete evacuation.

Rigid sigmoidoscopy usually reveals a single ulcer on the anterior rectal wall between 6 and 13 cm from the anal margin. There may be multiple ulcers or no ulceration but a discreet area of erythema. The ulcers often have a flat margin and a clear yellow or white base. The scope should be slowly withdrawn and the patient asked to strain; this usually reveals a degree of rectal prolapse.

Solitary rectal ulcers have a characteristic histology; fibrous obliteration of the lamina propria with distortion of the muscularis mucosa and extension of the muscle fibres into the lamina propria, together with regenerative changes in the crypt epithelium [26].

The aetiology is uncertain, but the ulceration may be due to rectal prolapse with failure of relaxation of the pubo-rectalis during straining with consequent rectal prolapse [59]. Patients should be put on a high fibre diet and advised to avoid straining at stool. Faecal bulking agents may be added as required. Conventional treatment has unfortunately proved unsatisfactory with the disease pursuing a protracted and symptomatic course.

Two new surgical approaches, transabdominal rectopexy [61] and prolapse repair [67], have been followed by good short-term results.

References

1 ACHESON ED. The distribution of ulcerative colitis and regional enteritis in United States Veterans with particular reference to the Jewish religion. *Gut* 1960;1:291–293.
2 ALLAN RN, HODGSON HJF. Inflammatory bowel disease. In: Pounder RE, ed. *Recent advances in gastroenterology*—6. Edinburgh: Churchill Livingstone, 1986: 310–326.
3 ALLCHIN WH. Case of acute extensive ulceration of the colon. *Trans Path Soc Lond* 1885;36:199–202.
4 ALLCHIN WH. Ulcerative colitis. *Proc R Soc Med* 1909;2:66–156.
5 ASAKURA H, TSUCHIYA M, AISO S, *et al.* Association of the human lymphocyte—DR 2 antigen with Japanese ulcerative colitis. *Gastroenterology* 1982;82:413–418.
6 BARGEN JA. Experimental studies on etiology of chronic ulcerative colitis. *J Am Med Assoc* 1924;83:332–336.
7 BINDER V, BOTH H, HANSON PK, HENDRICKSEN C, KREINER S, TROP-PEDERSEN K. Incidence and prevalence of ulcerative colitis and Crohn's disease in the county of Copenhagen 1962–1978. *Gastroenterology* 1982;83:563–568.
8 BONNEVIE O, RIIS P, ANTHONISEN P. An epidemiological study of ulcerative colitis in Copenhagen County. *Scand J Gastroenterol* 1968;3:432–436.
9 BRAHME F, LINDSTROM C, WENCKHERT A. Crohn's disease in a defined population. *Gastroenterology* 1975;69:342–351.
10 BRAWNER SD, TISHLER JMA, RUBIN E, LUNA RF. Computerised tomographic demonstration of toxic megacolon: report of a case. *Comput Radiol* 1983;7:279–281.
11 BURNHAM WR, GELSTHORPE K, LANGMAN MJS. HLA-D related antigens in inflammatory bowel disease. In: Pena AS, Weterman IT, Booth CC, Strober W, eds. *Recent advances in Crohn's disease*. The Hague: Martinus Nijhoff, 1981:192–196.

12 CHAPMAN RWG, ARBORGH BAM, RHODES JM. *et al.* Primary sclerosing cholangitis: a review of its clinical features, cholangiography and hepatic histology. *Gut* 1980;21:870–877.

13 COOPER HS, RAFFENSPERGER EC, JONES L, FITTS WT. Cytomegalovirus inclusions in patients with ulcerative colitis and toxic dilatation requiring colonic resection. *Gastroenterology* 1977;72:1253–1256.

14 COTTONE M, BUNCE M, TAYLOR CJ, TING A, JEWELL DP. Ulcerative colitis and HLA phenotype. *Gut* 1985;26:952–954.

15 CROHN BB. An historic note on ulcerative colitis. *Gastroenterology* 1962;42:366–367.

16 DAWSON DJ, KHAN AN, MILLER V, RATCLIFFE JF, SHREEVE DR. Detection of inflammatory bowel disease in adults and children: evaluation of a new isotopic technique. *Br Med J* 1985;291:1227–1230.

17 DELPRE G, KADISH V, GAZIT E, JOSHUA H, ZAHIR R. HLA antigens in ulcerative colitis and Crohn's disease in Israel. *Gastroenterology* 1980;78:1452–1457.

18 DEW MJ, THOMPSON H, ALLAN RN. The spectrum of hepatic dysfunction in inflammatory bowel disease. *QJ Med.* 1979;48:113–135.

19 DONOWITZ M. Arachidonic acid metabolites and their role in inflammatory bowel disease: an update requiring addition of a pathway. *Gastroenterology* 1985;88:580–587.

20 EDWARDS FC, TRUELOVE SC. The course and prognosis of ulcerative colitis. *Gut* 1963;4:299–315.

21 EVANS JG, ACHESON ED. An epidemiological study of ulcerative colitis and regional enteritis in the Oxford area. *Gut* 1965;6:311–324.

22 FARMER RG, MICHENER WM, MORTIMER EA. Studies of family history among patients with inflammatory bowel disease. *Clin Gastroenterol* 1980;9(2):271–278.

23 FIELDING JF. Inflammatory bowel disease and pregnancy. *Br J Hosp Med* 1976;15:45–57.

24 FIELDING JF. Crohn's disease in London in the latter half of the nineteenth century. *Ir J Med Sci* 1984;153:214–220.

25 FINKEL SI, JANOWITZ HD. Trauma and the pyoderma gangrenosum of inflammatory bowel disease. *Gut* 1981;22:410–412.

26 FORD MJ, ANDERSON JR, GILMOUR HM, HOLT S, SIRCUS W, HEADING RC. Clinical spectrum of 'solitary ulcer' of the rectum. *Gastroenterology* 1983;84:1533–1540.

27 GARLAND CF, LILIENFELD AM, MENDELOFF AI, MARKOWITZ JA, TERRELL KB, GARLAND FC. Incidence rates of ulcerative colitis and Crohn's disease in fifteen areas of the United States. *Gastroenterology* 1981;81:1115–1124.

28 GILAT T, LILOS P, ZEMISHLANY Z, Riback J, BENAROYA Y. Ulcerative colitis in the Jewish population of Tel-Aviv Jafo. III Clinical course. *Gastroenterology* 1976;70:14–19.

29 GILAT T, RIBAK J, BENAROYA Y, ZEMISHLANY Z, WEISSMAN I. Ulcerative colitis in the Jewish population in Tel-Aviv Jafo. I Epidemiology. *Gastroenterology* 1974;66:335–342.

30 GJONE E, MYREN J. Colitis ulcerosa i Norge. *Nord Med* 1964;71:143–145.

31 GORE RM, MARN CH, KIRBY DF, VOGELZANG RL, NEIMEN HL. CT findings in ulcerative granulomatous and indeterminate colitis. *Am J Rad* 1984;143:279–284.

32 GYDE S, PRIOR P, DEW MJ, SAUNDERS V, WATERHOUSE JAH, ALLAN RN. Mortality in ulcerative colitis. *Gastroenterology* 1982;83:36–43.

33 HARRIES AD, BAIRD A, RHODES J. Non smoking: a feature of ulcerative colitis. *Brit Med J* 1982;284:706.

34 HENDRIKSEN C, KREINER S, BINDER V. Long term prognosis in ulcerative colitis—based on results from a regional patient group from the County of Copenhagen. *Gut* 1985;26:158–163.

35 HOLDSTOCK G, SAVAGE D, HARMAN M, WRIGHT R. An investigation into the validity of the present classification of inflammatory bowel disease. *Q J Med* 1985;214:183–190.

36 HODGSON HJF. Inflammatory bowel disease and food intolerance. *J Roy Coll Phys London* 1986;20:45–48.

37 HOUGHTON EAW, NAISH JM. Familial ulcerative colitis and regional ileitis. *Gastroenterologica* 1958;89:65–74.

38 LEACH H. Two cases of ulceration of the large intestine as a consequence of chronic and scorbutic dysentry. *Trans Path Soc Lond* 1866;17:134.

39 LEWKONIA RM, MCCONNELL RB. Familial inflammatory bowel disease—heredity or environment? *Gut* 1976;17:235–243.

40 MADARA JL, PODOLSKY DK, KING NW, SEHGAL PK, MOORE R, WINTER HS. Characterisation of spontaneous colitis in cotton-top tamarins (sanguinus oedipus) and its response to sulfasalazine. *Gastroenterology* 1985;88:13–19.

41 MCCONNELL RB. Genetics and inflammatory bowel disease. In: Rachmilewitz D, ed. *Inflammatory bowel disorders.* The Hague: Martinus Nijhoff, 1982:152–560.

42 MAYBERRY JF. Some aspects of epidemiology of ulcerative colitis. *Gut* 1985;26:968–974.

43 MONK M, MENDELOFF AI, SIEGAL CI, LILIENFIELD A. An epidemiological study of ulcerative colitis and regional enteritis among adults in Baltimore. I. Hospital incidence and prevalence 1960–1963. *Gastroenterology* 1967;53:198–210.

44 MONK M, MENDELOFF AI, SIEGAL CI, LILIENFELD A. An epidemiological study of ulcerative colitis and regional enteritis among adults in Baltimore. II. Social and dermographic factors. *Gastroenterology* 1969;56:847–857.

45 MONK M, MENDELOFF AI, SIEGAL CI, LILIENFELD A. An epidemiological study of ulcerative colitis and regional enteritis among adults in Baltimore. III. Psychological and possible stress precipitating factors. *J Chronic Dis* 1970;22:565–578.

46 MORRIS T, RHODES J. Incidence of ulcerative colitis

in the Cardiff region 1968–1977. *Gut* 1984;**25**: 846–848.

47 MYREN J, GJONE E, HERTZBERG JN, RYGVOLD O, SEMB LS, FRETHEIM B. Epidemiology of ulcerative colitis and Crohn's disease in Norway. *Scand J Gastroenterol* 1971;**6**:511–514.

48 NAGAI T, DAS KM. Demonstration of an assay for specific cytolytic antibody in sera from patients with ulcerative colitis. *Gastroenterology* 1950;**16**: 1507–1512.

49 O'MORAIN C, SMETHURST P, DORE CJ, LEVI AJ. Reversible male infertility due to sulphasalazine: studies in man and rat. *Gut* 1984;**25**:1078–1084.

50 PAULLEY JW. Ulcerative colitis. A study of 173 cases. *Gastroenterology* 1950;**16**:566–576.

51 PENA AS, TRUELOVE SC. Hypolactasia and ulcerative colitis. *Gastroenterology* 1973;**66**:400–407.

52 PHILLIPS SF. Pathogenesis of diarrhoea in inflammatory bowel disease. In: Rachmilewitz D, ed *Inflammatory bowel diseases*. The Hague: Martinus Nijhoff, 1982:190–203.

53 RAMPTON DS, HAWKEY CJ. Prostaglandins and ulcerative colitis. *Gut* 1984;**25**:1399–1413.

54 RANSOHOFF DF, RIDDELL RH, LEVIN B. Ulcerative colitis and colonic cancer. Problems in assessing the diagnostic usefulness of mucosal dysplasia. *Dis Colon Rectum* 1985;**28**:383–388.

55 RIDDELL RH. Dysplasia and cancer in ulcerative colitis: a soluble problem? *Scand J Gastroenterol* [*suppl*] 1984;**104**:137–149.

56 RITCHIE J, HAWLEY PR, LENNARD-JONES J. Prognosis of carcinoma in ulcerative colitis. *Gut* 1981;**22**: 752–755.

57 ROGERS BHG, CLARK LM, KIRSNER JB. The epidemiologic demographic characteristics of inflammatory bowel disease. An analysis of a computerized file of 1400 patients. *J. Chronic Dis* 1971;**24**: 743–773.

58 ROSSEN RG. HLA and disease: a postulated role for HLA in gastrointestinal diseases. *Gastroenterology* 1980;**78**:1629–1631.

59 RUTTER KRP, RIDDELL RH. The solitary ulcer syndrome of the rectum. *Clin Gastroenterol* 1975;**4**:505–530.

60 SCHILLI R, BREUER RI, KLEIN F, et al. Comparison of the composition of faecal fluid in Crohn's disease and ulcerative colitis. *Gut* 1982;**23**:326–332.

61 SCHWEIGER M, ALEXANDER-WILLIAMS J. Solitary ulcer syndrome of the rectum. Its association with occult rectal prolapse. *Lancet* 1977;**1**:170.

62 SEDLACK RE, NOBREGA FT, KURLAND L, SAUER WG. Inflammatory colon disease in Rochester Minnesota 1935–64. *Gastroenterology* 1972;**62**:935–941.

63 SHERLOCK S. Primary sclerosing cholangitis. *Diseases of the liver and biliary system*. 7th ed. Oxford: Blackwell Scientific Publications, 1985:245–250

64 SHIELDS HM, BATES ML, GOLDMAN H, et al. Scanning electron microscopic appearance of chronic ulcerative colitis with and without dyspasia. *Gastroenterology* 1985;**89**:62–72.

65 SINCLAIR TS, BRUNT PW, MOWAT NAG. Non specific proctocolitis in northeastern Scotland: a community study. *Gastroenterology* 1983;**85**:1–11.

66 WEE A, LUDWIG J. Pericholangitis in chronic ulcerative colitis: primary sclerosing cholangitis of the small bile ducts? *Ann Int Med* 1985;**102**:581–587.

67 WHITE CM, FINDLAY JM, PRICE JJ. The occult rectal prolapse syndrome. *Br J Surg* 1980;**67**:528–530.

68 WHITE WH. On simple ulcerative colitis and other rare intestinal disorders. *Guys Hosp Rep* 1888;**21**: 469–474.

69 WIGLEY RD, MACLAURIN BP. A study of ulcerative colitis in New Zealand showing a low incidence in Maoris. *Br Med J* 1962;**2**:228–231.

70 WILKS S. Morbid appearances in the intestine of Miss Bankes. *Lond Med Gazette* 1859;**2**:264–265.

71 WILLOUGHBY CP, TRUELOVE SC. Ulcerative colitis and pregnancy. *Gut* 1980;**21**:469–474.

Chapter 50
The Medical Management of Ulcerative Colitis

J.J. MISIEWICZ & A.S. MEE

Ulcerative colitis is a chronic disorder characterized by relapses and remissions; a small minority of patients have continuous symptoms. Three main aspects of management need to be considered: the treatment of acute attacks, the maintenance of remission and attention to the long-term risk of colonic carcinoma [33]. Special considerations include the problems of ulcerative colitis in pregnancy and the extraintestinal complications such as arthritis, pyoderma gangrenosum and sclerosing cholangitis.

Unlike Crohn's disease, the treatment of ulcerative colitis is simplified by the close correlation between symptoms and the activity of colonic inflammation [25]. The almost invariable involvement of the rectum allows sigmoidoscopic visualization and histological assessment of the diseased bowel.

Management of the acute attack

It is useful to classify severity of disease by simple clinical and laboratory criteria as mild, moderate or severe (Table 50.1), because such assessment has bearings on the outcome of an attack [57] and treatment varies accordingly.

Investigations

Sigmoidoscopy

This is an essential part of the routine assessment of any patient with bowel symptoms. Although the appearances in ulcerative colitis are non-specific, they are sufficiently characteristic to allow a confident provisional diagnosis. However, variation between observers is appreciable [4] and a system of grading (Table 50.2) may

Table 50.1. Classification of disease activity (adapted with permission from [57]).

	Mild	Moderate	Severe
Bowel frequency	$\leqslant 4$ daily	4–6	6 daily
Blood in stool	$\pm$	+	++
Temperature	Normal	Intermediate between mild and severe	$> 37.8°C$ on 2 days out of 4
Pulse rate	Normal		> 90 beats per minute
Haemoglobin	$> 75\%$		$\leqslant 75\%$
Sedimentation rate (mm in hour)	< 30 mm		> 30 mm

Table 50.2. Sigmoidoscopic grading of rectal mucosal appearances in ulcerative colitis.

Grade I	Normal mucosa
Grade II	Hyperaemic mucosa
Grade III	Bleeding on light contact or spontaneously
Grade IV	Severe changes with an excess of mucus, pus, mucosal haemorrhage and occasional ulceration

lead to less disagreement and be useful for follow-up [23].

Laboratory tests

Although these are generally unhelpful in the diagnosis of an acute episode, haemoglobin concentration, white cell count and erythrocyte sedimentation rate (ESR) provide additional important information about the severity of an attack. Iron deficiency anaemia and a raised ESR are usually present in severe acute disease. Hypoalbuminaemia is also common in this situation and correlates with the clinical outcome. Of patients admitted with acute colitis who have a serum albumin of 20 g/l or less, 60% will need surgery [5].

Examination of the stools

Examination and culture of a fresh stool specimen is mandatory during an initial attack and during every relapse of ulcerative colitis. A number of infections can resemble ulcerative colitis clinically, sigmoidoscopically and radiologically. *Shigella*, *Salmonella* and *Campylobacter* species are all capable of producing a similar picture, although abdominal pain is more prominent in the infectious colitides. *Escherichia coli* serotype 0157:H7 can cause an acute haemorrhagic colitis in previously healthy adults and children.

A fresh, warm stool should be examined for amoebae, if amoebic colitis is suspected clinically. Amoebic colitis rarely occurs in patients who have spent all their lives in

the United Kingdom. The sigmoidoscopic appearances, while characteristically showing punched-out, discrete ulcers with relatively normal intervening mucosa, can mimic the mucosal appearances of ulcerative colitis in 10–15% of cases. The role of *Clostridium difficile* is uncertain. Although the organism, or its toxin, is often present in the stools of patients with ulcerative colitis, there does not appear to be any relationship between its presence and the degree of disease activity [13, 19].

The infectious colitides are described in Chapter 57.

Rectal mucosal biopsy

This is conveniently done at the initial sigmoidoscopy and the biopsy is best taken below the peritoneal reflection to minimize any risk of perforation. It has been widely taught that biopsies should be avoided in severely active disease and for one week prior to barium enema. There is, however, little evidence to substantiate either view and, providing small mucosal biopsy forceps are used that do not injure the muscularis propria, the risks of perforation are minimal and have been overemphasized [22]. It is probably sensible to wait for a day between a biopsy and radiological examination of the colon. The histological appearances of rectal biopsy are usually available within 24 hours and may be particularly helpful in differentiating ulcerative colitis from infectious colitides such as those due to *Salmonella* [8] or *Campylobacter*. Although an inflammatory cell infiltrate and crypt abscess formation is common to both forms of colitis, gland distortion and goblet cell depletion is uncommon with infection.

Radiology

A plain abdominal radiograph is necessary in every patient with acute severe symptoms. An empty anhaustral colonic gas pattern with an irregular mucosal outline due to ulceration and soft tissue projections ('mucosal islands') within the colonic lumen due to sloughing of the surface epithelium, are features highly suggestive of severe colitis. The presence of dilated colon (>5.5 cm diameter) in a severely ill patient with tachycardia, pyrexia, abdominal tenderness and diminished bowel sounds confirms the presence of a toxic megacolon (Fig. 50.1), while free air under the diaphragm indicates colonic perforation. A useful impression of the extent of the disease may be obtained from the distribution of faecal shadows, as faeces are absent from

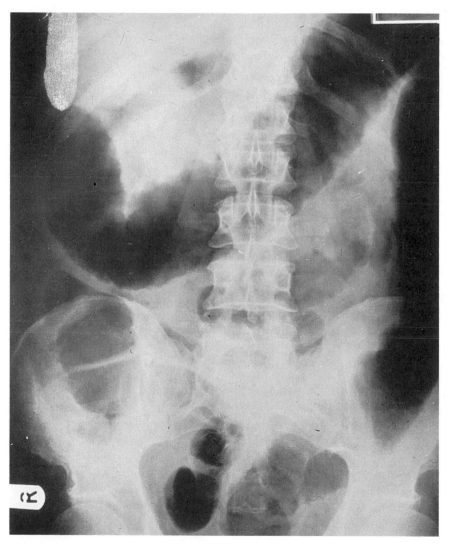

Fig. 50.1. Toxic megacolon—the whole colon is gas-filled and dilated.

inflamed segments of the bowel. Faecal loading is unlikely to occur with infectious colitides which usually affect the entire colon; this may be helpful in distinguishing sub-total, left-sided or distal colitis from infection.

A double-contrast barium enema should be done in all patients with mild or moderately-severe first attacks to confirm the diagnosis and to determine the extent of the disease. The colon in more active colitis should be prepared for radiology without laxatives, using instead a clear liquid diet and cleansing enemas. The radiologist must be told of the provisional diagnosis and the use of a balloon catheter in the rectum during the X-ray is best avoided. With these precautions, the investigation is safe in active ulcerative colitis not complicated by toxic megacolon. The extent of the disease does not necessarily correlate with severity or symptoms and is, therefore, no guide to immediate management. Repeated barium studies during subsequent relapses are unnecessary, except where sigmoidoscopy in a patient previously shown to have only proctitis no longer shows a clearly defined upper limit to the inflammation, thus suggesting extension of the disease.

Air-contrast barium studies are unhelpful in the immediate management of patients with an acute severe attack of colitis, because sigmoidoscopy with biopsy and a plain abdominal radiograph will usually give enough information for a diagnosis to be made and treatment to be started. The barium examination is therefore best deferred until there is clinical improvement.

Colonoscopy

The role of colonoscopy in ulcerative colitis continues to be evaluated. Aside from its undoubted importance in the long-term management of the disease, in the short-term it is generally of limited value. Even though colonoscopy and biopsy show that barium studies underestimate the extent of colitis [60], a precise knowledge of extent of disease is not needed for the immediate treatment of an acute attack. Colonoscopy may be helpful in distinguishing ulcerative colitis from Crohn's disease, or in the rare cases of ulcerative colitis with normal sigmoidoscopic appearances, but even then the rectal biopsy is usually abnormal [16]. Colonoscopy is also useful for evaluating suspicious appearances on barium enema—for example, strictures or filling defects. It is contraindicated in the presence of severely active disease because of the risk of perforation.

General principles of management

At present there is no cure for ulcerative colitis short of colectomy. It is therefore essential that the patient has confidence in, and develops a close rapport with the doctor. The nature of the disease must be explained to the patient and spouse, or relatives. This is especially important because repeated visits to the clinic and long-term surveillance are necessary for management of the condition. Similarly, patients must be able to contact and be seen by their doctor as soon as a relapse occurs, because delay in diagnosis and starting treatment increases the risk of progression to a severe episode of colitis (Fig. 53.1).

Diet

There is no evidence that foods cause ulcerative colitis and changing the diet will not cure the disease, although one of the first questions often asked by the patient is how it should be altered. In general a normal diet should be advised and the former advocacy of low residue diets abandoned. A small number of patients with ulcerative colitis also have hypolactasia; such patients will benefit from a lactose-free diet, which will lessen bowel looseness, but have no effect on the colitis [44, 49].

In addition there may be a group of patients who are not obviously hypolactasic, but who appear to benefit from a milk free diet, with better control of the symptoms and diminished frequency of relapses [64]. Although this approach has generally only limited value, it may be worth a trial in problem patients.

Treatment of an acute attack

The drugs most useful in the treatment of an acute attack are oral steroids and steroid enemas. Sulphasalazine either orally, or rectally, is of only secondary importance in this situation, because it is less effective than steroids in controlling active disease [55]. Its primary role is to maintain the disease in remission.

Diarrhoea in patients with ulcerative colitis implies active disease and must be treated as such. The use of antidiarrhoeal drugs such as opiates, or anticholinergics, produces only a small decrease in frequency of defaecation and may be associated with the development of a toxic megacolon, or proximal faecal retention. Non-specific antidiarrhoeal agents therefore have no place in the routine management of ulcerative colitis. As the symptoms of either total colitis or proctosigmoiditis may be equally troublesome, activity of the disease is of more importance than its extent in planning the treatment of an acute episode.

Proctitis

Proctitis is inflammation confined to the rectum with an upper limit to the inflammatory changes visible at sigmoidoscopy. This type of disease is often troublesome, but not dangerous, as only 5–10% of patients progress to more extensive involvement of the colon. In this situation steroids administered locally as suppositories, ene-

mas, or foam are usually successful in inducing remission, while sulphasalazine should be given concurrently as a maintenance agent. Continuing troublesome symptoms may require a course of oral steroids, for example, prednisolone 20 mg daily. If these measures fail, uncontrolled observations suggest that sulphasalazine enemas, or suppositories [42], acetarsol suppositories [7] or oral disodium cromoglycate [46] may all be tried with benefit in some patients. It has to be admitted however, that some patients with proctitis respond very poorly to treatment.

Mild attacks

A patient with a mild attack of ulcerative colitis (Table 50.1) can usually be treated in Outpatients. Local and systemic steroids are beneficial [32, 53]. Rectally administered steroids, either in aqueous form or as a foam, do not spread further than the proximal sigmoid colon [17] and, depending on the formulation, have a predominantly local action [31] with only 40% of a 20 mg rectal dose of prednisolone-21-phosphate absorbed [30]. Oral and local steroids have approximately equal efficacy in patients with predominantly left-sided disease [38]. Prednisolone metasulphobenzoate enemas provide topical treatment without systemic absorption [36].

In patients with more extensive colitis even mild attacks should not be managed with local steroids alone, and oral prednisolone 20–40 mg daily should be prescribed in addition. There is some evidence to suggest that the use of both routes of administration enhances the therapeutic effect and that rectal steroids help to relieve the discomfort of tenesmus. Oral prednisolone 40 mg daily may be better than 20 mg daily [3]. The steroids should be maintained at the initial dosage until symptoms and sigmoidoscopic appearances improve, before tapering off over the subsequent 3–4 weeks.

Table 50.3. Standard treatment for attacks of ulcerative colitis.

Drug	Proctitis	Mild	Moderate
Oral prednisolone (daily)	20 mg (optional)	20–40 mg	40 mg
Steroid enemas	Once or twice daily	Once or twice daily	Twice daily
Steroid suppositories	For minor symptoms only	–	–
Oral sulphasalazine	1 g b.d.	1 g b.d.	1 g b.d.

A reluctance to use oral steroids in doses of 40 mg daily even for short periods of time is probably misplaced, as the incidence of unwanted effects following one month's use at this dose is minimal, although glucose tolerance may be impaired [32]. Enteric coated sulphasalazine 1 g twice daily should be given concurrently (Table 50.3).

Moderate attacks

Patients in this group do not have serious systemic symptoms (Table 50.1), but may nevertheless have abdominal discomfort, tenesmus and marked diarrhoea. They do not necessarily require admission to hospital, but in general they benefit from bed rest and are able to retain rectal enemas for longer if these are given under nursing supervision. These patients should be treated with oral prednisolone 40 mg daily, twice daily steroid enemas and sulphasalazine 1 g twice daily (Table 50.3). Failure to go into remission as an outpatient is an indication for inpatient treatment.

Severe attacks

These patients are unwell with systemic symptoms of pyrexia, nausea, anorexia and vomiting, tachycardia and abdominal discomfort. Their appearance frequently belies their clinical state. Patients in this group must be regarded as a medical emergency requiring immediate admission to hospital.

Pulse rate, blood pressure and temperature need to be recorded four-hourly. Daily, or in very ill patients twice daily, examination of the patient with particular reference to the presence of signs of peritonism (rebound tenderness), bowel sounds and abdominal girth is necessary; liver dullness should be percussed regularly to detect occult colonic perforation. A plain abdominal radiograph should be done on admission, and repeated and inspected daily if the colon is dilated (see Fig. 50.1). Increasing colonic diameter, or the appearance of mucosal islands on the radiographs are danger signs, while a sudden increase in pyrexia or the pulse rate may indicate colonic perforation. A stool chart recording the daily number of evacuations is helpful. Ideally the clinical management should be shared jointly by the medical and surgical teams, with daily discussion of the patient. An intravenous, or central feeding line, should be set up and where appropriate, fluid, nutritional and vitamin deficiencies corrected (see Chapter 78).

The 'Oxford regimen' consisting of five days of intensive intravenous therapy for the treatment of severe attacks has proved effective in inducing remission in approximately 70% of patients [20, 54]. It has been modified by substituting metronidazole for tetracycline, although recent controlled data on the use of antibiotics in ulcerative colitis suggest that they do not affect the outcome [13]. The regimen is shown in Table 50.4. At the end of five days 60% of patients are in remission, 15% improved, and 25% are unchanged or have deteriorated and therefore need colectomy [56]. Higher rates of remission (approaching 90%) are reached if the intravenous regi-

Table 50.4. Intensive treatment of severe acute attacks of ulcerative colitis.

Nil by mouth.
Fluid and electrolyte replacement iv and/or parenteral nutrition.
Vitamin and K^+ supplements.
Blood transfusion if necessary haemoglobin > 12 gldl).
Intravenous metronidazole 500 mg × 3/24 hours.
Intravenous prednisolone-21-phosphate 64 mg/24 hours in divided doses.
Rectal hydrocortisone 100 mg in 100 ml saline twice daily.

men is used for mild, or moderate attacks of colitis, but the oral route is satisfactory for most patients in this category [27].

The course of severe attacks does not appear to be altered by parenteral nutrition and bowel rest [12]. Patients who have improved after five days, but have not gone into remission (particularly those with a relapse of established disease rather than a first attack), may be helped by the addition of azathioprine 2 mg/kg body weight/day [56]—although there are no controlled data to support this. Those patients who have gone into remission at five days should receive oral steroids and sulphasalazine. The dose of steroids is gradually tapered off over the subsequent six weeks. A suggested regimen is a week each at 40, 30, 20, 15, 10 and 5 mg, although individual preferences vary.

Patients who fail to go into remission, and those who develop complications such as haemorrhage or a toxic megacolon during the acute attack, will need urgent colectomy. The decision to defer operation on a patient who is clinically toxic and has a dilated colon requires a strong nerve and fine judgement. Abdominal pain and localized or rebound tenderness may denote impending perforation. However, the instigation of the 'Oxford regimen', close surveillance by a physician and a surgeon, and a significant improvement in toxic features and colon size on plain abdominal radiograph over the ensuing 24 hours may enable surgery to be avoided. The mortality of severe colitis has been substantially decreased by early surgical intervention.

Maintenance of remission

Ulcerative colitis is mostly a disease of relapse and remission, although some patients have a chronic continuous form of the disease. Corticosteroids do not prevent relapses. However sulphasalazine 2 g daily is significantly effective in maintaining remission (Fig. 50.2) [39]. The chances of relapse when not taking sulphasalazine are approximately four times as great, and the remission inducing effect remains even after five years, or longer on the drug [14].

The usual dose is sulphasalazine 2 g daily. Higher doses are slightly more effective, but at the expense of an increased incidence of unwanted effects [1]. The drug can be conveniently given as 1 g twice daily after meals. The enteric coated form is as effective as the non-coated tablet, and its use may lower the incidence of gastric irritation. Other unwanted effects of sulphasalazine include hypersensitivity rashes, fever, haemolytic anaemia and reversible male infertility due to oligospermia [35,43].

Sulphasalazine consists of 5-aminosalicylic acid linked to sulphapyridine by an azo bond [43,51]. This bond is split by the action of colonic bacteria into the active salicylic acid moiety and the inactive sulphapyridine carrier molecule, which is responsible for the more common unwanted effects of headache and gastrointestinal intolerance. Other formulations of the active moiety have been recently developed. These appear to be as effective as the original compound, but lack its unwanted effects,

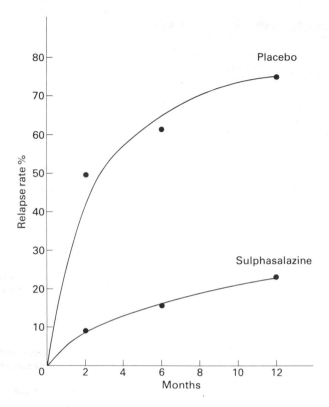

Fig. 50.2. Cumulative percentage relapse in ulcerative colitis on sulphasalazine or on placebo (adapted from [39]).

and include an acrylic resin coated compound [11] and disodium azodisalicylate: two salicylate molecules linked by an azo bond [61]. These new formulations are designed to introduce 5-aminosalicylic acid (mesalazine) into the colon, but they await full clinical evaluation [10, 43, 50].

Disodium cromoglycate has been advocated for maintaining remission, but controlled trials show it to be markedly inferior to sulphasalazine [62].

Immunosuppressive drugs

Experience with the use of immunosuppressives in ulcerative colitis has been limited to azathioprine, and also, to a lesser extent, with its metabolite 6-mercaptopurine. There is no evidence to suggest that either drug is capable of inducing remission either alone or in combination with steroids. However, uncontrolled studies suggest that 6-mercaptopurine may occasionally be useful in maintaining remission in patients with chronic ulcerative colitis not responding to steroids and sulphasalazine [29], while controlled studies in small numbers of patients using azathioprine in conjunction with steroids indicate that it has a steroid-sparing effect [47], decreases the relapse rate in established disease [54] and significantly reduces activity of the disease during a six-month period of treatment [28].

In general, azathioprine is not used routinely in the management of ulcerative colitis, but is given to patients who do not respond to steroids and/or sulphasalazine.

Management of extra-intestinal complications

Acute extra-intestinal complications such as arthropathy, iritis and erythema nodosum settle rapidly with control of the accompanying active colonic inflammation, although spondylitis is unaffected even by removal of the diseased bowel. Pyoderma gangrenosum usually follows the same course as the colitis. A few patients, often those with long standing pyoderma, may even fail to respond to colectomy [52].

Fatty infiltration of the liver is related to severity of the disease and parallels the course of the bowel inflammation. Chronic active hepatitis and cirrhosis are not affected by treatment of the colonic disease. Sclerosing cholangitis may progress even after total colectomy [6, 58] while cholangiocarcinomas can arise several years after surgical removal of the colon.

Management of ulcerative colitis in pregnancy

Except for a small group of women with severely active disease, the chances of a full-term pregnancy and delivery of a live healthy infant are no different in women with ulcerative colitis than in the normal population [15, 18, 63]. There is therefore no indication to advise termination of pregnancy in these patients—either during an initial attack, or a relapse. Neither does the use of corticosteroids, or sulphasalazine appear to have any deleterious effect on the foetus. Sulphapyridine does pass to the mother's milk, but in such a small amount that kernicterus is no hazard [26]. Attacks of colitis occurring during pregnancy should therefore be treated in the usual way [40].

Long-term management— carcinoma of the colon (see

Chapter 64)

It has been appreciated for many years that chronic ulcerative colitis is associated with an increased incidence of cancer developing in the affected bowel [2] and that this in-

creased risk is nil for the first five years of the disease, minimal for the following five years, and then increases in each decade thereafter [24, 37, 45].

The risk is greatest in patients with radiologically extensive colitis—that is, involving the colon to the hepatic flexure or more proximally. The start of the excessive risk period appears to be delayed by a decade in patients whose disease started distal to the mid-transverse colon [21]. The risk in patients with distal colitis appears to be minimal. All these studies are based on radiological assessment of the extent of colitis, which underestimates the histopathological extent of disease [60]. Colitis starting at a young age is now thought not to be a significant risk factor, the increased incidence in this group of patients being a reflection of the longer period of available follow-up. Neither does the degree of disease activity over the years influence the likelihood of developing a cancer.

The degree of risk attached to an individual patient remains controversial [59] because of the type of statistical analyses used, differing referral patterns to specialist centres that have done the studies, and different proportions of patients undergoing proctocolectomy who are thus removed from the cohort. Numbers of patients followed up for long periods are small, so that one case of cancer detected, or missed can affect the results appreciably. Nevertheless the risk is substantial (Fig. 50.3) and may be as high as 35% after 25–30 years of follow-up [9].

Management initially depended on repeated barium enemas after 10 years or more of colitis in the hope of detecting an early carcinoma (Fig. 50.4), or on prophylactic proctocolectomy which many patients with quiescent disease found difficult to accept. Two factors have now altered the management of this problem, although considerable difficulties still exist. The first was recognition that a combina-

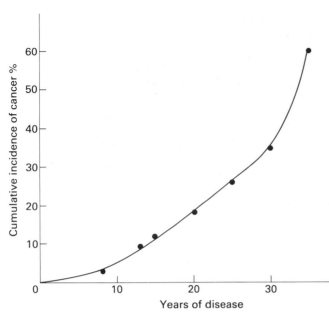

Fig. 50.3. Cancer risk in ulcerative colitis.

tion of histological and cytological abnormalities, termed epithelial dysplasia, indicated that the colonic epithelium had entered a neoplastic phase. The second is colonoscopy.

It was suggested at first that moderate or severe **epithelial dysplasia on a rectal biopsy** was associated with a considerable likelihood of a carcinoma elsewhere in the colon [41]. Such biopsies are easily obtained and obviate the need for repeated barium enemas which have a low diagnostic yield in this situation, because the carcinomas which develop are frequently plaque-like and do not protrude into the lumen. Unfortunately epithelial dysplasia is patchy, may only be present proximal to the rectum and grading into mild, moderate or severe is difficult, particularly if the colitis is active. For these reasons **full colonoscopy**, with endoscopic biopsies at 10 cm intervals and from any suspicious lesions—especially from plaque-like or nodular areas of mucosa, is now advocated [65]. This is a considerable undertaking for the colonoscopist and the histopathologist. It is important to realize that colonoscopic biopsies are small, may

be difficult to orientate and that nodular lesions may have a dysplastic surface concealing an underlying carcinoma.

It has been suggested therefore that patients with long-standing, extensive, or total ulcerative colitis, but no evidence of dysplasia, should undergo **colonoscopic surveillance** at two-yearly intervals, while patients with mild dysplasia need examination at six-monthly to yearly intervals. The presence of moderate to severe dysplasia in a patient with quiescent disease is an indication for removal of the affected colon as the chances of finding a carcinoma in the resected specimen are high, particularly when nodular lesions have been discovered at colonoscopy [34, 41]. Nevertheless, despite this policy, patients still present with established neoplasms, while others with biopsies showing severe dysplasia preoperatively may have no evidence of dysplasia in the resected specimen. Carcinoma can occur in patients whose biopsies show only mild dysplasia [34, 41].

At the present therefore, despite the most careful follow-up of patients with long-standing extensive colitis, the detection of a

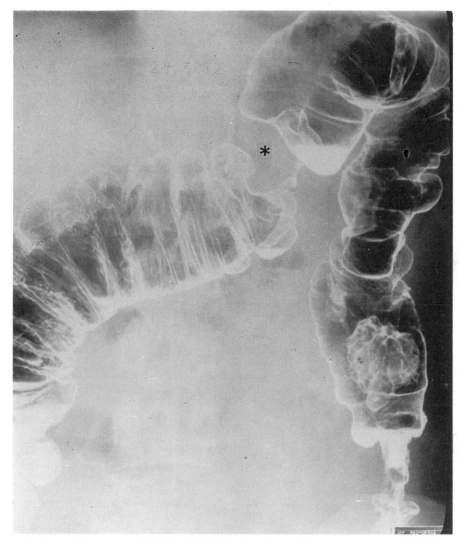

Fig. 50.4. Carcinoma of transverse colon in a patient with ulcerative colitis.

complicating carcinoma cannot be guaranteed and a definitive follow-up surveillance policy has not been finally worked out [48].

References

1 AZAD KHAN AK, HOWES DT, PIRIS J, TRUELOVE SC. Optimum dose of sulphasalazine for maintenance treatment in ulcerative colitis. *Gut* 1980;21:232–240.

2 BARGEN JA. Chronic ulcerative colitis associated with malignant disease. *Arch Surg* 1928;17:561–576.

3 BARON JH, CONNELL AM, KANAGHINIS TG, LENNARD-JONES JE, JONES FA. Outpatient treatment of ulcerative colitis: comparison between three doses of oral prednisolone. *Br Med J* 1962;ii:441–443.

4 BARON JH, CONNELL AM, LENNARD-JONES JE. Variation between observers in describing mucosal appearances in proctocolitis. *Br Med J* 1964;i:89–92.

5 BUCKELL NA, LENNARD-JONES JE, HERNANDEZ MA, KOHN J, RICHES PG, WADSWORTH J. Measurement of serum proteins during attacks of ulcerative colitis as a guide to patient management. *Gut* 1979;20:22–27.

6 CHAPMAN RWG, MARBORGH BA, RHODES JM, *et al.*

Primary sclerosing cholangitis; a review of its clinical features, cholangiography and hepatic histology. *Gut* 1980;**21**:870–877.

7 CONNELL AM, LENNARD-JONES JE, MISIEWICZ JJ, BARON JH, JONES FA. Comparison of acetarsol and prednisolone-21-phosphate suppositories in the treatment of idiopathic proctitis. *Lancet* 1965; i:238–239.

8 DAY DW, MANDAL BK, MORSON BC. The rectal biopsy appearances in salmonella colitis. *Histopathology* 1978;**2**:117–131.

9 DEVROEDE G. Risk of cancer in inflammatory bowel disease. In: Winawar S, Schottenfeld D, Sherlock P, eds. *Colorectal cancer: prevention, epidemiology and screening.* New York: Raven Press, 1980:325–334.

10 DEW MJ, EVANS BK, RHODES J. 5-amino salicylic acid for the treatment of inflammatory bowel disease. *Gastroenterology* 1984;**87**:480–481.

11 DEW MJ, HUGHES P, HARRIES AD, WILLIAMS G, EVANS BK, RHODES J. Maintenance of remission in ulcerative colitis with oral preparation of 5-aminosalicylic acid. *Br Med J* 1982;**285**:1012.

12 DICKINSON RJ, ASHTON MG, AXON ATR, SMITH RC, YEUNG CK, HILL GL. Controlled trial of intravenous hyperalimentation and total bowel rest as an adjunct to the routine therapy of acute colitis. *Gastroenterology* 1980;**79**:1199–1204.

13 DICKINSON RJ, O'CONNOR HJ, PINDER I, HAMILTON I, JOHNSON D, AXON ATR. Double blind controlled trial of oral vancomycin as adjunctive treatment in acute exacerbations of idiopathic colitis. *Gut* 1985;**26**:1380–1384.

14 DISSANAYAKE AS, TRUELOVE SC. A controlled therapeutic trial of long-term maintenance treatment of ulcerative colitis with sulphasalazine (Salazopyrin). *Gut* 1973;**14**:923–926.

15 DONALDSON RM. Management of medical problems in pregnancy—inflammatory bowel disease. *N Engl J Med* 1985;**312**:1616–1618.

16 ELLIOT PR, WILLIAMS CB, LENNARD-JONES JE, et al. Colonoscopic diagnosis of minimal change colitis in patients with a normal sigmoidoscopy and normal air-contrast barium enema. *Lancet* 1982; i:650–651.

17 FARTHING MJG, RUTLAND MD, CLARK ML. Retrograde spread of hydrocortisone containing foam given intrarectally in ulcerative colitis. *Br Med J* 1979;**2**:822–824.

18 FIELDING JF. Pregnancy and inflammatory bowel disease. *J Clin Gastroenterol* 1983;**5**:107–108.

19 GREENFIELD C, AGUILAR RAMIREZ JR, POUNDER RE, et al. *Clostridium difficile* and inflammatory bowel disease. *Gut* 1983;**24**:713–717.

20 GREENSTEIN AJ, SACHAR DB, GIBAS A, et al. Outcome of toxic dilatation in ulcerative and Crohn's colitis. *J Clin Gastroenterol* 1985;**7**:137–144.

21 GREENSTEIN AJ, SACHAR DB, SMITH H, PUCILLO A, et al. Cancer in universal and left sided colitis:

factors determining risk. *Gastroenterology* 1979; **77**:290–294.

22 HARNED RK, CONSIGNY PM, COOPER NB, WILLIAMS SM, WOLTJEN AJ. Barium enema examination following biopsy of the rectum or colon. *Radiology* 1982;**145**:11–16.

23 HEATLEY RV, CALCRAFT BJ, RHODES J, OWEN E, EVANS BK. Disodium cromoglycate in the treatment of chronic proctitis. *Gut* 1975;**16**:559–563.

24 HENDRIKSEN C, KREINER S, BINDER V. Long-term prognosis in ulcerative colitis—based on results from a regional patient group from the County of Copenhagen. *Gut* 1985;**26**:158–163.

25 HODGSON HJF. Assessment of drug therapy in inflammatory bowel disease. *Br J Clin Pharmacol* 1982;**14**:159–170.

26 JARNEROT G, INTO-MALMBERG MB. Sulphasalazine treatment during breast feeding. *Scand J Gastroenterol* 1979;**14**:869–871.

27 JARNEROT G, ROLNY P, SANDBERG-GERTZEN. Intensive intravenous treatment of ulcerative colitis. *Gastroenterology* 1985;**89**:1005–1013.

28 KIRK AP, LENNARD-JONES JE. Controlled trial of azathioprine in chronic ulcerative colitis. *Br Med J* 1982;**284**:1291–1292.

29 KORELITZ BI, GLASS JL, WISCH N. Long-term immunosuppressive therapy of ulcerative colitis. *Am J Dig Dis* 1973;**18**:317–322.

30 LEE DAH, TAYLOR M, JAMES VHT, WALKER G. Plasma prednisolone levels and adrenocortical responsiveness after administration of prednisolone-21-phosphate as a retention enema. *Gut* 1979;**20**:349–355.

31 LEE DAH, TAYLOR M, JAMES VHT, WALKER G. Rectally administered prednisolone-evidence for a predominantly local action. *Gut* 1980;**21**:215–218.

32 LENNARD-JONES JE. Towards optimal use of corticosteroids in ulcerative colitis and Crohn's disease. *Gut* 1983;**24**:177–181.

33 LENNARD-JONES JE. Medical treatment of ulcerative colitis. *Postgrad Med J* 1984;**60**:797–802.

34 LENNARD-JONES JE, MORSON BC, RITCHIE JK, WILLIAMS CB. Cancer surveillance in ulcerative colitis, experience over 15 years. *Lancet* 1983;ii:149–152.

35 LEVI AJ, FISHER AM, HUGHES L, HENDRY WF. Male infertility due to sulphasalazine. *Lancet* 1979;ii:276–278.

36 McINTYRE PB, MACRAE FA, BERGHOUSE L, ENGLISH J, LENNARD-JONES JE. Therapeutic benefits from poorly absorbed prednisolone enema in distal colitis. *Gut* 1985;**26**:822–824.

37 McMANUS JP. Malignant problem in colitis. *Gastroenterology* 1982;**83**:1142–1143.

38 MISIEWICZ JJ, CONNELL AM, LENNARD-JONES JE, AVERY JONES F. Comparison of oral and rectal steroids in the treatment of proctocolitis. *Proc R Soc Med* 1964;**57**:561–562.

39 MISIEWICZ JJ, LENNARD-JONES JE, CONNELL AM, BARON JH, JONES FA. Controlled trial of sulphasalazine in maintenance therapy for ulcerative colitis. *Lancet* 1965;i:185–188.

40 MOGADAM M, DOBBINS WO, KORELITZ BI, AHMED SW. Pregnancy in inflammatory bowel disease. effect of sulfasalazine and corticosteroids on fetal outcome. *Gastroenterology* 1981;80:72–76.

41 MORSON BC, PANG LSC. Rectal biopsy as an aid to cancer control in ulcerative colitis. *Gut* 1967;8:423–434.

42 PALMER KR, GOEPEL JR, HOLDSWORTH CD. Sulphasalazine retention enemas in ulcerative colitis: a double blind trial. *Br Med J* 1981;282:1571–1573.

43 PEPPERCORN M. Sulphasalazine. Pharmacology, clinical use, toxicity and related new drug development. *Ann Intern Med* 1984;101:377–386.

44 PENA AS, TRUELOVE SC. Hypolactasia and ulcerative colitis. *Gastroenterology* 1973;64:400–404.

45 RITCHIE JK, HANLEY PR, LENNARD-JONES JH. Prognosis of carcinoma in ulcerative colitis. *Gut* 1981;22:752–755.

46 ROSEKRANS PCM, MEIJER CJLM, VAN DER WAL AM, LINDEMAN J. Allergic proctitis, a clinical and immunopathological entity. *Gut* 1980;21:1017–1023.

47 ROSENBERG JL, WALL AJ, LEVIN B, BINDER HJ, KIRSNER JB. A controlled trial of azathioprine in the management of chronic ulcerative colitis. *Gastroenterology* 1975;69:96–99.

48 ROSENSTOCK E, FARMER RG, PETRAS R, SIVAK MV JR, RANKIN GB, SULLIVAN BH. Surveillance for colonic carcinoma in ulcerative colitis. *Gastroenterology* 1985;89:1342–1346.

49 SCIARRELTA G, GIACOBAZZI G, VERRI A, ZANIRATO P, GARUTI G, MALAGUTI P. Hydrogen breath test quantification and clinical correlation of lactose malabsorption in adult irritable bowel syndrome and ulcerative colitis. *Dig Dis Sci* 1984; 29:1098–1104.

50 SELBY WS, BARR GD, IRELAND A, MASON CH, JEWELL DP. Olsalazine in active ulcerative colitis. *Br Med J* 1985;291:1373–1375.

51 TAFFET SL, DAS KM. Sulphasalazine: adverse effects and desensitization. *Dig Dis Sci* 1983;28:833–842.

52 TALANSKY AL, MEYERS S, GREENSTEIN AJ, JANOWITZ HD. Does intestinal resection heal the pyoderma gangrenosum of inflammatory bowel disease? *J Clin Gastroenterol* 1983;5:207–210.

53 TRUELOVE SC. Systemic and local corticosteroid therapy in ulcerative colitis. *Br Med J* 1960;1:464–467.

54 TRUELOVE SC, JEWELL DP. Intensive intravenous regimen for severe attacks of ulcerative colitis. *Lancet* 1974;i:1067–1070.

55 TRUELOVE SC, WATKINSON G, DRAPER G. Comparison of corticosteroid and sulphasalazine therapy in ulcerative colitis. *Br Med J* 1962;ii:1708–1711.

56 TRUELOVE SC, WILLOUGHBY CP, LEE EG, KETTLEWELL MGW. Further experience in the treatment of severe attacks of ulcerative colitis. *Lancet* 1978;ii:1086–1088.

57 TRUELOVE SC, WITTS LJ. Cortisone in ulcerative colitis, final report on a therapeutic trial. *Br Med J* 1955;2:1041–1048.

58 WEISNER RH, LA RUSSO NF. Clinicopathological features of the syndrome of primary sclerosing cholangitis. *Gastroenterology* 1980;79:200–206.

59 WHELAN G. Cancer risk in ulcerative colitis: why are results in the literature so varied? *Clin Gastroenterol* 1980;9:469–476.

60 WILLIAMS CB, WAYE JD. Colonoscopy in inflammatory bowel disease. *Clin Gastroenterol* 1978;7:701–717.

61 WILLOUGHBY CP, ARONSON JK, AGBACK H, BODIN NO, TRUELOVE SC. Distribution and metabolism in healthy volunteers of disodium azodisalicylate, a potential therapeutic agent for ulcerative colitis. *Gut* 1982;23:1081–1087.

62 WILLOUGHBY CP, HEYWORTH MF, PIRIS J, TRUELOVE SC. Comparison of disodium cromoglycate and sulphasalazine as maintenance therapy for ulcerative colitis. *Lancet* 1979;i:119–122.

63 WILLOUGHBY CP, TRUELOVE SC. Ulcerative colitis and pregnancy. *Gut* 1980;21:469–474.

64 WRIGHT R, TRUELOVE SC. A controlled trial of various diets in ulcerative colitis. *Br Med J* 1965;2:138–141.

65 YARDLEY JH, BAYLESS TM, DIAMOND MP. Cancer in ulcerative colitis. *Gastroenterology* 1979; 76:221–225.

Chapter 51
Surgery of Ulcerative Colitis

M.M. HENRY

The excision of a severely ulcerated large intestine can rapidly restore a seriously debilitated patient to normal health. In the majority of patients this is achieved at the expense of a stoma. Since many patients consider that an ileostomy imposes unacceptable limitations, there have been developments to avoid either the ileostomy or its bag [17, 29, 43] (see Chapter 55).

The number of patients afflicted by ulcerative colitis who eventually require surgical treatment varies according to the treatment policy of specific units and perhaps to some extent according to local variations in disease behaviour. In Leeds 36.3% of colitics required surgery [41], whereas the corresponding proportion treated surgically at the Mayo Clinic was only 16.7% [42].

Appendicostomy, followed by irrigation of the inflamed colon with saline, was the first operative procedure to be advocated for ulcerative colitis. Ileostomy, with excision of the large intestine as a secondary procedure, was introduced in the 1930s. Colectomy with ileostomy formation, as a one-stage procedure, was advocated in the 1950s [8] and it has remained the standard procedure for the elective surgical treatment of ulcerative colitis [25].

Indications

Elective surgery

Chronic persistent disease and invalidism

Patients who have persistent and disabling symptoms probably constitute the majority who undergo elective surgery for ulcerative colitis. Such patients are more likely to have extensive disease, rather than disease limited to the distal colon. If elective colectomy is being considered, the extent of disease should, ideally, be assessed by colonoscopy. Persistent anaemia, diarrhoea, hypoproteinaemia and weight loss, which are refractory to medical management, would be important factors militating towards a surgical cure of the colitis.

Local complications

Rarely the presence of anal complications, such as fistula or fissure, may require local surgery – for example, the laying open of a fistula tract. Very uncommonly formal rectal excision may be required in order to control symptoms. It is a general principle that, wherever possible, anal lesions should be managed with the minimum of surgical interference in the belief that they will resolve when the underlying rectal disease has been controlled medically [9].

Systemic complications

The course of the majority of the systemic complications of colitis are related to the activity of the colonic disease. Colectomy usually leads to a prolonged remission in patients with a peripheral arthropathy [5] and skin or eye lesions but it is less likely to induce a remission in patients with sacroiliitis and ankylosing spondylitis [13]. A colectomy does not affect the progress of sclerosing cholangitis, which even can arise for the first time after colonic resection [6].

Malignancy and the risk of development of malignancy

The development of an area of malignant change represents one of the few absolute indications for surgery in ulcerative colitis (see Chapter 50). The decision to subject a patient, who may be relatively symptom-free, to surgery on the basis of possible malignancy developing at a later date is not usually straight-forward. The histological criteria should provide an indication for colectomy only if the dysplasia is severe, is consistent in more than one biopsy obtained at different sites or sequentially, and is present in the absence of marked inflammation [21, 26].

Prevention of growth retardation

The younger patient is at risk of physical retardation partly as a direct response to the disease and partly as a result of its treatment with steroids. In this age group surgery, therefore, may need to be considered for less active disease than in the adult colitic.

Emergency surgery

Acute fulminating colitis or toxic megacolon

Acute fulminating colitis is relatively uncommon hence in most hospitals only one operation for acute colitis is performed each year [36]. The timing of surgery is of key importance, balancing the risk of imminent colonic perforation with the possibility of an unnecessary colectomy. The clinical decision to operate is one requiring considerable expertise—if the colon has already perforated before the patient reaches the operating theatre, morbidity and mortality are greatly increased—two-thirds die [36].

In a retrospective study of 181 admissions with acute colitis at St Mark's Hospital, London [22], it was found that a patient with a bowel frequency of less than eight on the first day after admission and a temperature of 38°C or less had a high probability of responding to medical treatment. Conversely, a patient with a higher bowel frequency *and* a higher temperature had a four-in-five chance of failing to respond to drug therapy with a consequent need for operation. After the first day in hospital a sustained fever, despite vigorous treatment, was equally serious—a patient with a maximum temperature greater than 38°C on the fourth day had only a one-in-eight chance of avoiding surgery. The appearance of colonic dilation or mucosal islands was also an indication for surgery. Other important clinical features, often seen in these patients who later needed a colectomy, included a low serum albumin, abdominal tenderness, and oral candidiasis.

Massive haemorrhage

Major haemorrhage is an unusual indication for colectomy in colitis. Twenty-one of 624 patients with colitis required surgery for this reason in a series from Oxford [10] whereas in Leeds it was an indication for colectomy in only one of 465 patients [41].

Preoperative preparation

Nutrition

Weight loss of between 18 and 62% has been reported in patients with ulcerative colitis [40]. Severe nutritional problems can be expected when an acute exacerbation is superimposed on a chronic debilitated state (see Chapter 78). Such problems have been implicated in high infection rates, increased morbidity and mortality with surgery, and depressed wound healing. It might be expected that improvement in nutritional status, by total parenteral nutrition prior to surgery, would be attended by safer surgery and a less complicated recovery. Such a role for parenteral nutrition has yet to be proven adequately [12, 34]. However, it is important to correct anaemia and electrolyte imbalances preoperatively.

Bowel preparation

The source of infective complications is largely the bacteria of the colonic flora. Surgery of the colon in most centres is preceded by attempts to minimize bacterial contamination by a combination of mechanical preparation to expel faeces and preoperative antibacterial chemotherapy. Mechanical preparation might be contra-indicated if there is deep ulceration of the colon, when there is a risk of perforation, or in patients with an obstructing carcinoma. Vigorous purgation of colitics with enemas is probably inadvisable, one of the oral preparations (mannitol, magnesium sulphate or whole gut irrigation) being preferable.

Antibiotics

The role of preoperative antibiotics in colon surgery is now well-established. Metronidazole has been demonstrated to be extremely effective against anaerobic bacteria present in the faeces [14]. This drug is usually combined with either a cephalosporin or an aminoglycoside to counter Gram-negative aerobic organisms. To ensure high tissue concentrations at the time of contamination during surgery, the drugs should be administered approximately one hour preoperatively. Some surgeons also use local antibiotics at the time of operation.

Ileostomy counselling

The consequence of surgery for the majority of these patients is an ileostomy (see Chapter 55). Extensive preoperative counselling is of fundamental importance. This should be provided not only by medical and nursing staff, but in addition by a trained stoma nurse and where possible by a representative of an ostomy association.

Emergency surgery

Preoperative preparation of the acutely ill patient is likely to be minimal. Where time permits, anaemia and electrolyte deficiencies should be corrected prior to surgery. Although a mechanical preparation is not usually indicated prophylactic antibiotics should be employed, particularly as these patients are prone to septicaemia.

Elective operations

Pan proctocolectomy with ileostomy

This is the standard elective procedure practised in most centres dealing with ulcerative colitis. A one-stage operation has now largely replaced earlier attempts at excisional surgery in several phases. The single step procedure may confer advantages since all the diseased bowel capable of toxin absorption and excess protein loss is excised.

The risk of sexual problems arising from surgical damage to the autonomic nerves and plexuses in the pelvis can be reduced by inter-sphincteric dissection and excision of the rectum [23]. The surgeon must ensure that the blood supply to the ileostomy is adequate (see Chapter 55). Inflammatory changes in the skin surrounding the stoma have been greatly reduced following the adoption of the spout ileostomy [5].

Colectomy with ileorectal anastomosis

The procedure of excision of diseased colon and anastomosis of terminal ileum to the rectum was popularized by Aylett [1] using a two-staged procedure—since the majority of anastomoses were defunctioned by a loop ileostomy which was closed after an interval of several weeks.

A clear attraction lies in the avoidance of a life-long stoma. However, this may be achieved at the expense of some residual active disease in the rectum, such that symptoms persist albeit to a lesser degree. An additional disadvantage is that the operation leaves rectal epithelium with an established potential for undergoing malignant change. Finally, there will be a poor functional result if the rectal capacity has been diminished by chronic disease—to some extent this problem can be excluded by preoperative study of rectal capacity using either a contrast proctogram or physiological methods [11].

Because of the potential to develop carcinoma in the retained rectum, patients treated by this operation must be followed-up meticulously with sigmoidoscopy and biopsy at frequent intervals [30].

Ileostomy with continent intra-abdominal pouch (Kock's procedure)

The provision of an abdominal stoma that does not discharge faecal contents spontaneously, but alternatively may be evacuated at will of the patient, is an attractive concept. Kock [18] has been able to achieve this in many patients by creating a pouch from two loops of small bowel, establishing continence by intussuscepting the distal segment of small bowel into the pouch to create a nipple valve. The pouch is emptied by the patient who inserts a catheter through the valve (see Chapter 55).

Ileal reservoir and ileo-anal anastomosis (Parks' procedure)

Parks and Nicholls [31] introduced a development of the Kock operation whereby an abdominal stoma is avoided altogether. A reservoir is created from three segments of terminal ileum, leaving a segment of approximately 8 cm distal to the pouch [4, 28]. This small length of ileum is sutured to the anal canal. A small cuff of rectum, dissected free of its mucosa, is preserved. Since disease activity in colitis is restricted to the mucosa, all the diseased bowel is eliminated. Furthermore, the pelvic floor musculature is undisturbed, which conserves many of the sensory and reflex motor mechanisms responsible for establishing faecal continence (see Chapter 55). An ileal reservoir can also be constructed as a J pouch [37].

Urgent operations in acute colitis

Sub-total colectomy with ileostomy

The greater part of the severely diseased colon is excised leaving a defunctioned stump of rectum, the proximal end of which is established as a stoma in the lower abdomen. In this manner the seriously ill patient is not subjected to the additional stress of a rectal excision. Rectal preservation provides the possibility of a subsequent ileorectal anastomosis in those patients in whom the rectum may only be mildly inflamed or in whom the disease is rendered quiescent by a combination of medical treatment and defunctioning of the rectum. Alternatively, these patients can be considered for a Kock's or Parks' procedure.

Diverting ileostomy and decompression colostomy

Turnbull and his colleagues [39] introduced the concept of treating seriously ill colitics by ileostomy and decompression colostomy in the belief that by performing a lesser procedure the operative morbidity and mortality could be reduced. Some success has also been claimed for a method that involves the establishment of a double-barrelled ileostomy, using the distal loop to irrigate the inflamed colon with hydrocortisone solution [16, 38].

Results and complications

There has been a steady improvement in the safety of surgery in ulcerative colitis. The objective assessment of morbidity and mortality in many series is not always clear since emergency and elective procedures are often considered collectively, in spite of the fact that the former is associated with substantially higher complication rates.

In a study of 294 patients with ulcerative colitis treated surgically within one hospital region during 1967–1972 [36] it was found that the overall mortality for elective surgery was 2.1%. When surgery was performed on the severely ill patient, however, the mortality rate rose to 37.6%. In the emergency group mortality was found to be 66.7% if colonic perforation occurred preoperatively. In addition, age was closely related to mortality in this group. The mortality ranged from 0% in those aged less than 20 years to 76.9% in 70- to 80-year-olds.

Similarly, the incidence of complications

Table 51.1. Complications associated with colectomy and spout ileostomy for ulcerative colitis.

Early
Haemorrhage
Intra-peritoneal sepsis
Pelvic abscess
Small bowel obstruction
Wound infection
Stomal ischaemia/gangrene

Late
Ileostomy dysfunction
Delayed perineal wound healing
Abdominal wound dehiscence
Parastomal herniation
Prolapsed stoma
Stomal fistula
Local dermatitis
Small bowel obstruction
Psychosexual
Electrolyte disorders
Ileostomy stenosis

---

was found to be closely related to urgency with rates of 19% and 31% in elective and emergency cases, respectively. The major complications include intra-abdominal sepsis, intestinal obstruction, pulmonary complications, deep vein thrombosis and wound dehiscence (Table 51.1). The re-operation rate for small bowel obstruction was 13%, and 8% of standard spout ileostomies needed reconstruction [35]. Failure of primary healing of the perineal wound is common in patients with ulcerative colitis—healing within the first six months of surgery occurred in only 51% of patients [35].

Specific complications

Ileorectal anastomosis

The functional results in terms of frequency of bowel action and continence are difficult to ascertain since this information has not been provided in detail by published series. In Aylett's series [1] the mortality for elective surgery was 2.7% and 14 of his 300 patients were described as failures. Failure was ascribed to faecal incontinence in three patients and to the development of a rectal stricture in a further two patients.

Of greater concern is the incidence of malignancy in the rectal stump, which occurred in three patients at the initial follow-up [1]. More recently Baker and his colleagues [2] have examined the long-term results in 374 patients treated with ileorectal anastomosis by Aylett—61% of the patients in this study were followed up for more than 10 years after their surgery. Nineteen patients (5.1%) subsequently underwent rectal excision for persistent rectal disease. A further 22 patients (5.9%) underwent attempted rectal excision following the development of carcinoma in the rectal stump, four of whom were inoperable. In 14 of the 18 operable patients the tumour was a poorly differentiated adenocarcinoma.

Intra-abdominal (Kock) pouch (see Chapter 55)

Whereas there initially was a high incidence of complications with poor functional results, there has been a steady improvement in recent years. The incorporation of a nipple valve has greatly improved function, with a claimed continence rate of 97% [19]. The success rates have not been so high in other centres—continence was achieved in 70% at the Mayo Clinic [3] and in 74% in Leeds [15].

The price of a continent ostomy has been that many of these patients have required frequent operations and revisions to obtain a satisfactory final result. The revision rate in Kock's group was initially 54%, but it has more recently been reduced to 32% by techniques designed to improve stability of the nipple valve.

Other complications such as fistulation and reservoir leakage occur in approximately 8% of patients and a similar percentage develop small bowel obstruction. Other complications reported include valve necrosis, development of previously undiagnosed Crohn's disease, reservoir haemorrhage, volvulus of the reservoir, malabsorption and bacterial overgrowth within the reservoir [7]. Kock [19] initially reported seven deaths out of 280 patients treated with a pouch, although in his most recent series of 152 patients there were no deaths [20]. Goligher [15] reported no deaths in a series of 62 patients and Madigan [24] reported one death in 19 patients.

Ileal reservoir and ileo-anal anastomosis (see Chapter 55)

In the first 21 patients treated by this operation there were no deaths and in only one patient did an abdominal ileostomy have to be re-established [32]. The patient was unable to cope psychologically with self-catheterization; the rest were pleased with their pouches, 50% of which could be evacuated spontaneously and 50% were evacuated with a catheter *per annum* at a mean frequency of 3.8 times per 24-hour period. The majority were fully continent, but two patients described some leakage of mucus which necessitated wearing a pad. Three patients developed small bowel obstruction, and a further three patients developed a pelvic abscess.

In a detailed metabolic study of 14 of these patients [27], haemoglobin, plasma proteins, and vitamin B_{12} absorption were found to be normal. Five patients, were found to have low serum iron concentration and two patients had a low serum folate concentration. Histological abnormalities were observed, but such abnormalities have been observed in patients with Kock ileostomies [33]. Neither small intestinal bacterial overgrowth nor malabsorption were present in any of the patients.

Diverting loop ileostomy

The results from a limited surgical approach in acute colitis have been largely disappointing. Truelove and his colleagues [38] found that only a temporary benefit occurred in many patients and in several the disease persisted unabated. In Turnbull's series [39] eight of 42 patients required colectomy soon after the local procedure and four patients remained toxic in spite of the defunctioning. A further 13 patients developed re-activation of their disease.

Overall comments

The reported results indicate that surgery in ulcerative colitis is safe and relatively complication-free when performed electively on the patient in remission. The results are less satisfactory in the acutely ill colitic, and are very poor if the colon has perforated preoperatively. The management of the acutely ill colitic and the prevention of perforation are of paramount importance.

There will almost certainly be a continuing tendency to offer more colitics a form of 'continent' operation. Before considering such an offer it is important to be absolutely certain that the correct diagnosis is not Crohn's disease. Secondly, such procedures should probably be limited to the fit patient in remission.

The advent of the Parks' procedure with its avoidance of an abdominal wall stoma may, if the long-term results are favourable, eventually replace the Kock operation. It is important to emphasize the need for more experience. For the time being both procedures will probably only be performed in certain specialized centres.

An ileorectal anastomosis represents a satisfactory alternative for those patients with quiescent rectal disease. It would appear that approximately 6% of these patients are at risk of developing malignant change in the rectal stump, but many would consider that the benefits outweigh this small risk. The operation should probably be restricted to those who are unlikely to default on regular follow-up. All patients with an ileorectal anastomosis for ulcerative colitis should be subjected to full clinical examination and proctoscopy at six-monthly intervals.

Finally, the majority of patients with a spout ileostomy are satisfied with their operation. The principal problem, that of dermatitis affecting the skin surrounding the stoma, has been greatly reduced with the advent of the spout, and with advances in stoma management and appliances. Normal social, working and sexual functions are possible for the majority of ileostomists.

References

1 AYLETT SO. A hundred cases of diffuse ulcerative colitis treated by total colectomy and ileo-rectal anastomosis. *Br Med J* 1966;1:1001–1005.

2 BAKER WNW, GLASS RE, RITCHIE JK, et al. Cancer of the rectum following colectomy and ileo-rectal anastomosis for ulcerative colitis. *Br J Surg* 1978;65:862–868.

3 BEAHRS OH. Use of ileal reservoir following proctocolectomy. *Surg Gynec Obstet* 1975;141:363–366.

4 BECKER JM, HILLARD AE, MANN FA, KESTENBERG A, NELSON JA. Functional assessment after colectomy, mucosal proctectomy, and endorectal ileo-anal pull-through. *World J Surg* 1985;9:598–605.

5 BROOKE BN. The management of an ileostomy including its complications. *Lancet* 1952;ii:102–104.

6 CHAPMAN RWG, MARBROUGH BA, RHODES JM, et al. Primary sclerosing cholangitis; a review of its clinical features, cholangiography and hepatic histology. *Gut* 1980;21:870–877.

7 CRANLEY B. The Kock reservoir ileostomy: a review of its development, problems and role in modern surgical practice. *Br J Surg* 1983;70:94–99.

8 CRILE G, THOMAS CY. Treatment of acute toxic ulcerative colitis by ileostomy and simultaneous colectomy. *Gastroenterology* 1951;19:58–68.

9 DE DOMBAL FT, WATTS JM, WATKINSON G, et al. The incidence and management of anorectal abscess, fistula and fissure, occurring in patients with ulcerative colitis. *Dis Colon Rectum* 1966;9:201–206.

10 EDWARDS FC, TRUELOVE SC. The course and prognosis of ulcerative colitis. Part III Complications. *Gut* 1964;5:1–15.

11 FARTHING MJG, LENNARD-JONES JE. Sensibility of the rectum to distension and the anorectal distension reflex in ulcerative colitis. *Gut* 1978;19:64–69.

12 FAZIO VW, KODNER I, JAGELMAN DG, et al. Parenteral nutrition as primary or adjunctive treatment. *Dis Colon Rectum* 1976;19:574–578.

13 FERNANDEZ-HERLIHY L. The articular manifestations of chronic ulcerative colitis. An analysis of 555 cases. *N Engl J Med* 1959;261:259–263.

14 GOLDRING J, SCOTT A, McNAUGHT W, et al. Prophylactic oral antimicrobial agents in elective colonic surgery. *Lancet* 1975;ii:997–999.

15 GOLIGHER JC. *Surgery of the anus, rectum and colon.* 4th edn. London: Bailliere Tindall, 1980:809.

16 HARPER PH, TRUELOVE SC, LEE ECG, KETTLEWELL MGW, JEWELL DP. Split ileostomy and ileocolostomy for Crohn's disease and ulcerative colitis. *Gut* 1983;24:106–113.

17 HULTEN L. The continent ileostomy (Kock's pouch) versus the restorative proctocolectomy (pelvic pouch). *World J Surg* 1985;9:952–959.

18 KOCK NG. Intraabdominal reservoir in patients with permanent ileostomy. *Arch Surg* 1969;99:223–231.

19 KOCK NG, MYRVOLD HE, NILSSON LO, et al. Progress report on the continent ileostomy. *World J Surg* 1980;4:143–148.

20 KOCK NG, MYRVOLD HE, NILSSON LO, et al. Conti-

nent ileostomy: an account of 314 patients. *Acta Chir Scand* 1981;**147**:67–72.

21 LENNARD-JONES JE, MORSON BC, RITCHIE JK, *et al.* Cancer in colitis: assessment of the individual risk by clinical and histological criteria. *Gastroenterology* 1977;**73**:1280–1289.

22 LENNARD-JONES JE, RITCHIE JK, HILDER W, *et al.* Assessment of severity in colitis: a preliminary study. *Gut* 1975;**16**:579–584.

23 LYTTLE JA, PARKS AG. Intersphincteric excision of the rectum. *Br J Surg* 1977;**64**:413–416.

24 MADIGAN MR. The continent ileostomy and the isolated ileal bladder. *Ann R Coll Surg Engl* 1976;**58**:62–69.

25 MOROWITZ DA, KIRSNER JB. Ileostomy in ulcerative colitis. A questionnaire study of 1803 patients. *Am J Surg* 1981;**141**:370–378.

26 MORSON BC, PANG LSC. Rectal biopsy as an aid to cancer control in ulcerative colitis. *Gut* 1967;**8**:423–424.

27 NICHOLLS J, BELLEVEAU P, NEILL M, *et al.* Restorative proctocolectomy with ileal reservoir: a pathophysiological assessment. *Gut* 1981;**22**:462–468.

28 NICHOLLS J, PESCATORI M, MOTSON RW, PEZIM ME. Restorative proctocolectomy with a three loop ileal reservoir for ulcerative colitis and functional adenomatous polyposis. *Ann Surg* 1984;**199**:383–388.

29 NICHOLLS RJ, PEZIM ME. Restorative proctocolectomy with ileal reservoir for ulcerative colitis and familial adenomatous polyposis: a comparison of three reservoir designs. *Br J Surg* 1985;**72**:470–474.

30 OAKLEY J, LAVERY IC, FAZIO VW, JAGELMAN DG, WEAKLEY FL, EASLEY K. The fate of the rectal stump after subtotal colectomy for ulcerative colitis. *Dis Colon Rectum* 1985;**28**:394–396.

31 PARKS AG, NICHOLLS RJ. Proctocolectomy without ileostomy for ulcerative colitis. *Br Med J* 1978;**2**:85–88.

32 PARKS AG, NICHOLLS RJ, BELLEVEAU P. Proctocolectomy with ileal reservoir and anal anastomosis. *Br J Surg* 1980;**67**:533–538.

33 PHILIPSON B, BRANDBERG A, JAGENBURG R, *et al.* Mucosal morphology, bacteriology and absorption in intra-abdominal ileostomy reservoir. *Scand J Gastroenterol* 1975;**10**:145–153.

34 REILLY J, RYAN JA, STROLE W, *et al.* Hyperalimentation in inflammatory bowel disease. *Am J Surg* 1976;**131**:192–200.

35 RITCHIE JK. Ulcerative colitis treated by ileostomy and excisional surgery: 15 years experience at St Mark's Hospital. *Br J Surg* 1972;**59**:345–351.

36 RITCHIE JK. Results of surgery for inflammatory bowel disease: a further survey of one hospital region. *Br Med J* 1974;**1**:264–268.

37 TAYLOR BM, BEART RW, DOZOIS RR, KELLY WA, WOLFF BG, ILSTRUP DM. The endorectal ileal pouch—anal anastomosis. *Dis Colon Rectum* 1984;**27**:347–350.

38 TRUELOVE SC, ELLIS II, WEBSTER CU. Place of a double-barrelled ileostomy in ulcerative colitis and Crohn's disease of the colon: a preliminary report. *Br Med J* 1965;**1**:150–153.

39 TURNBULL RB, HAWK WA, WEAKLEY FL. Surgical treatment of toxic megacolon: ileostomy and colostomy to prepare patients for colectomy. *Am J Surg* 1971;**122**:325–331.

40 WALL AJ, KIRSNER JM. Ulcerative colitis and Crohn's disease of the colon: symptoms, signs and laboratory aspects. In: Kirsner JB, Shorter RG, eds. *Inflammatory bowel disease.* Philadelphia: Lea and Febiger, 1975:101–108.

41 WATTS JM, DE DOMBAL FT, GOLIGHER JC. The early results of surgery for ulcerative colitis. *Br J Surg* 1966;**53**:1005–1014.

42 WAUGH JM, PECK DA, BEAHRS OH, *et al.* Surgical management of chronic ulcerative colitis. *Arch Surg* 1964;**88**:556–569.

43 WILLIAMS NS, JOHNSTON D. The current status of mucosal proctectomy and ileo-anal anastomosis in the surgical treatment of ulcerative colitis and adenomatous polyposis. *Br J Surg* 1985;**72**:159–168.

Chapter 52
Clinical Features of Crohn's Disease

J. RHODES, A.D. HARRIES, J.F. MAYBERRY & M.J. DEW

In 1932 Crohn, Ginzburg and Oppenheimer described 14 young adults with chronic inflammatory disease of the ileum, in several of them associated with fibrotic stenosis of the gut and multiple fistulae [16]. There had been a few previous reports of the condition, including one by Dalziel from Glasgow in 1913 [18], but following Crohn's report the disease became widely recognized.

Crohn's disease may affect any part of the gastrointestinal tract from the lips to the anal margin, although ileocolonic disease is still the commonest presentation. In the last 50 years this obscure condition has become relatively common and has aroused great interest because, although it produces considerable morbidity, the cause remains unknown and treatment, which is not curative, is empirical [1, 24].

Although typical clinical features are well-recognized the diagnosis is often delayed for months, or even years, as a patient may simply complain of weight loss, malaise, anorexia or recurrent fever. It is a diagnosis that should be considered particularly in young adults during the second and third decades, if bowel symptoms are associated with systemic disturbance.

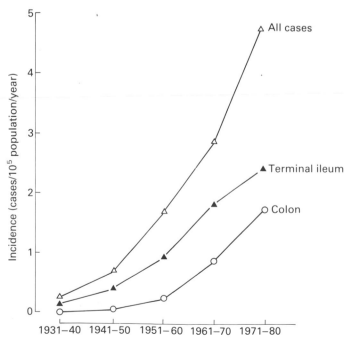

Fig. 52.1. Incidence of Crohn's disease in Cardiff between 1931 and 1980. The mean incidence in each decade is recorded for the total number of cases.

766

Epidemiology

Prevalence

Crohn's disease is most common in North America and northern Europe; it is emerging in southern Europe and is relatively uncommon in other areas of the world. The highest prevalence has been reported from Scandinavia with figures of $54/10^5$ and $75/10^5$ of the population [8, 43], while in Britain high figures are $26/10^5$ and $56/10^5$ [73, 81]. It is more common in urban compared with rural communities although in most instances this difference is not great, particularly where the overall prevalence is high.

Incidence trends

There has been a marked rise in incidence, particularly during the last two decades, that cannot be accounted for by increased awareness of the disease and its differentiation from ulcerative colitis (Fig. 52.1). Some of the current high figures are from South Wales ($4.9/10^5$/year; [72]), Blackpool ($6.1/10^5$/year; [59]) and Gothenburg in southern Sweden ($6.3/10^5$/year; [53]). The incid-

ence varies considerably in different parts of Britain with figures of 2.1 in Aberdeen, 3.1 in Nottingham and 5.3 in North Tees. Some studies suggest that the rise in incidence may have reached a plateau.

Race

Figures from North America and Europe suggest that the prevalence is higher than expected in Jewish populations, although in Tel Aviv there is a low prevalence in the Jewish population [91].

Sex ratio

The condition is marginally more common in females, with male-to-female ratios as high as 1 to 1.6. In some series the figures are almost equal.

Age

The disease is most commonly diagnosed in young patients between the ages of 15 and 40 years (Fig. 52.2). Fewer patients are diagnosed in older age groups, but age specific incidence figures for each decade of life show a rise in incidence for patients

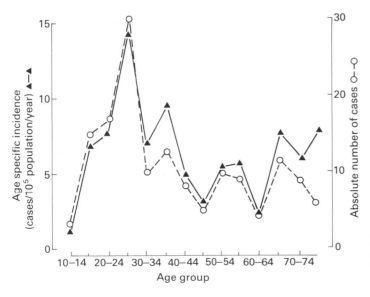

Fig. 52.2. Age-specific incidence and absolute numbers of Crohn's disease for the decade 1971 to 1980 in Cardiff.

around the age of 70 years [28]. Although some series show a preponderance of colonic disease in older patients, population based studies have not shown major differences in the site of disease with respect to age [72].

Aetiology

Most disease is the outcome of interrelationship of genetic and environmental factors, and information about aetiology may be obtained from several fields. For example, epidemiological work may identify causative factors or those subjects who are susceptible to the disease.

With regard to Crohn's disease, much attention has been directed towards the role of immunological mechanisms and the relative lack of progress in ascertaining causative factors may be partly due to this preoccupation with one aspect.

Genetic factors

About 10% of patients have a first degree relative with the disease; siblings are affected 30 times more often than the general population [74, 107]. There are a few reports of twins with the disease, but no consistent HLA association has been found. The increased risk among relatives is not enough to suggest a simple Mendelian pattern of inheritance [44, 89].

Two interesting associations are with ankylosing spondylitis and with atopy. Patients with ankylosing spondylitis have a ninefold greater prevalence of Crohn's disease than would be expected by chance. This is linked with the tissue type HLA-B27 [62]. Although it is not clear whether patients with Crohn's disease are more likely to develop atopic disease, they appear to come from families with an increased prevalence of atopic conditions [87]. Both ankylosing spondylitis and atopy have an inherited basis which lends further support

to a genetic role that increases susceptibility of some people to the disease.

Environmental factors

The possible role of diet has been examined with particular interest in milk, fibre and sugar. Anecdotes suggest that some patients improve with a milk-free diet but there are no formal studies.

Conflicting data have been produced on fibre consumption in Crohn's patients with no consistent relationship established. However, studies from Germany, Britain, Sweden and Israel, a total of 13 altogether, all show a high intake of refined carbohydrates by patients with Crohn's disease compared with controls, with significant

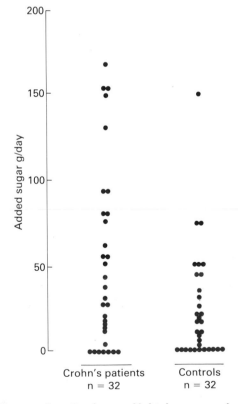

Fig. 52.3. Quantity of sugar added to beverages and cereals in 32 newly-diagnosed patients with Crohn's disease compared with matched controls (adapted with permission from [75]).

differences in most reports [51, 69, 75] (Fig. 52.3). Where sugar intake was estimated at the time of diagnosis it was especially high. The refined carbohydrate may take the form of pastries, confectionery, or sugar added to beverages and cereals. This is one of the few consistently positive findings in patients with Crohn's disease, but its significance in relation to aetiology or treatment remains unresolved [102].

No evidence suggests that Crohn's disease is infectious. Nottingham patients were interviewed for evidence of clustering in time or space, but no evidence was found for person-to-person transmission [81, 82, 87]. These results are supported by studies on nurses and doctors who would be at increased risk from the disease if it were moderately infectious.

Patients with Crohn's disease are significantly more likely to be smokers than are controls, the association being stronger for smoking habit before the onset of disease than for current smoking habit [99]. There is an increased risk of Crohn's disease in oral contraceptive users [61].

Infective agents

Ileocaecal disease occurs in animals and is produced by a variety of organisms. The pathological changes however, although often similar to Crohn's disease, are not identical [71]. Porcine intestinal adenomatosis, sometimes referred to as Crohn's disease, is caused by *Campylobacter sputorum*, subspecies *mucosalis*, but this has not been implicated in man [58]. Attempts to transmit human Crohn's disease to animals has produced inconsistent results and no viruses have been isolated regularly [7, 9]. Pathological similarities between Crohn's disease and tuberculosis have focused attention on *Mycobacteria*, in particular *M. kansasii*, but again there is no consistent evidence that this organism has an aetiological role in the disease [12, 100].

Recent studies from Rotterdam have shown that patients with Crohn's disease have higher faecal counts of anaerobic Gram-negative rods and Gram-positive coccoid rods belonging to the subspecies *Eubacterium* and *Peptostreptococcus*. Patients with Crohn's disease have agglutinins to these bacteria more often than controls or patients with ulcerative colitis. In a survey of 1,000 sera from 17 centres around the world [106] 59% of patients with Crohn's disease showed positive agglutination with these bacteria, compared with 29% in ulcerative colitis and 8% of controls. Results are compatible with the finding that patients with Crohn's disease produce antibodies to a wide range of food and microbial antigens, including bovine serum albumin, gluten, maize, *Bacteroides* and *Escherichia coli*.

Immunology

Humoral immune responses are normal in patients with Crohn's disease but cell mediated immune function may be defective; support for this is that some patients have impaired skin hypersensitivity, a reduction in circulating T lymphocytes and a poor lymphocytic response to non-specific mitogens [93]. Many patients, however, have normal cell mediated immunity, and it is probable that the observed defects are a consequence of the disease itself, medical therapy or even malnutrition rather than a primary phenomenon. There is evidence that the number of T cell lymphocytes in Crohn's disease increases towards normal with improvement in nutritional status; this phenomenon is well-recognized in the tropics among patients with malnutrition. Immune complexes have also been found in the sera of patients with active Crohn's disease and particularly in those with extraintestinal manifestations. The role of these complexes in the pathogenesis of Crohn's disease is not known [101].

Pathology

Clinical features are related to the site and pathology of intestinal disease. Ileocolonic disease is most common, accounting for two-thirds of the cases, but in about 20% inflammation appears limited to the colon. The remainder consists chiefly of patients with ileal disease alone or proximal small bowel involvement [29].

Classical features include chronic inflammation involving all layers of the bowel wall, often associated with granulomas and deep fissuring ulceration. The condition is often discontinuous with clearly demarcated, inflamed areas separated by normal bowel. The resected specimen often shows thickening of the bowel wall with a narrow lumen, which accounts for both obstructive symptoms and dilated gut proximal to the stricture; submucosal fibrosis is largely responsible for the narrow lumen. Mucosal ulcers may be superficial or deep and the coincidence of fissures with transmural inflammation involving the serosa leads to adhesions, inflammatory masses with mesenteric abscesses and fistulae with adjacent organs (Table 52.1). The serosa is often

Table 52.1. Relationship between pathological and clinical features.

Pathological features	Clinical features
1. Thickened bowel wall Submucosal fibrosis Narrow lumen + strictures	1. Obstructive symptoms Proximal bowel distension
2. Transmural fissures Serosal inflammation	2. Adhesions Inflammatory masses Abscesses Fistulae to adherent bowel, skin or other organs

opaque and fibrosis extends into the adjacent mesentery, which contains enlarged fleshy lymph nodes and dilated lymphatics (Fig. 52.4) [84].

The transmural inflammation may be continuous or in the form of multiple lymphoid aggregates. Giant cell 'sarcoid-like' granulomas are diagnostic but are only found in 60% of patients. Granulomas are commonly adjacent to the serosa. Discrete 'aphthoid-like' ulcers overlying lymphoid follicles are often seen in apparently normal mucosa at some distance from obvious disease. Despite mucosal inflammation, the epithelial glandular pattern is usually

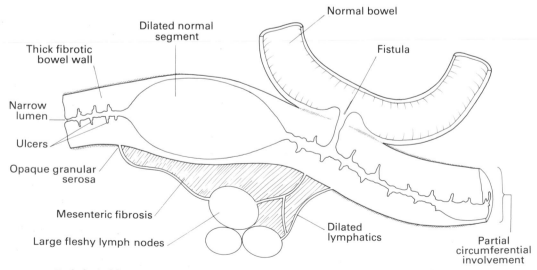

Fig. 52.4. Pathological features in a resected specimen showing common features in Crohn's disease.

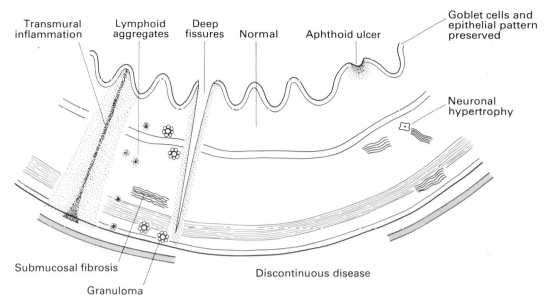

Fig. 52.5. Histological features in Crohn's disease.

well-preserved with normal populations of goblet cells in the colon (Fig. 52.5). In the small intestine 'pseudo pyloric metaplasia' is found in about one-third of patients with long-standing inflammation. Hypertrophied nerve fibres in both the submucosa and mysenteric plexus also occur in areas of inflammation.

Clinical features

Presenting clinical features

It is not easy to give a simple account of the major clinical features in Crohn's disease due to considerable variation in the site, extent and severity of disease at the time of presentation.

In keeping with a basic pathology of chronic inflammation, patients usually complain of **ill health**, a feeling of lassitude and they may have **recurrent fever**. Common features relating to intestinal involvement are abdominal pain, anorexia, nausea, diarrhoea, and often, abdominal tenderness (Table 52.2). In many instances

Table 52.2. Presenting symptoms in 161 patients with Crohn's disease (reproduced with permission from [26]).

Symptoms	Overall incidence	
Pain	139	(87%)
Diarrhoea	106	(66%)
Weight loss	88	(55%)
Anorexia	60	(37%)
Fever	59	(36%)
Vomiting	56	(35%)
Lassitude	51	(32%)
Nausea	48	(30%)
Acute abdomen	41	(25%)
Nutritional disturbance	39	(24%)
Fistula	24	(15%)
Miscellaneous	50	(31%)

the most striking feature is **weight loss**, which is largely due to anorexia causing inadequate food consumption. Although a chronic inflammatory condition, the severity of the initial presentation varies greatly—it may take the form of a fulminant colitis complicated by toxic dilatation, or as a relatively benign condition. Some patients with extensive small bowel disease present because of gradual weight loss, but have scarcely any symptoms despite the extent of disease.

Patients with terminal ileal disease usually complain of **abdominal pain**, localized to the right iliac fossa and associated with a palpable tender mass in this region. Other features such as recurrent fever, anorexia and weight loss depend on the extent and severity of the inflammatory disease. Children developing the illness before puberty may have **retarded growth** and sexual

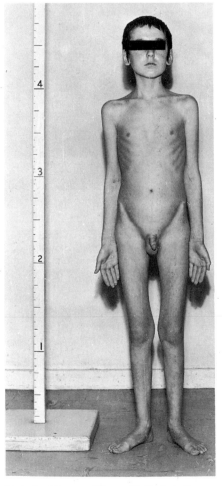

Fig. 52.6. An 18-year-old boy with Crohn's disease limited to a short segment in the terminal ileum. The patient is of short stature with poor physical and sexual development. After resection of the diseased bowel, within one year he grew six inches, gained 10 kg and underwent normal sexual maturation.

development (Fig. 52.6) and, if the disease cannot be treated adequately, the consequences are life-long after fusion of the epiphyses. Resection of localized ileal disease or adequate medical treatment may be followed by a growth spurt enabling the patient to catch up with his peers. Attacks of abdominal pain are largely due to obstruction of the narrowed gut and severe bouts may be complicated by abdominal distension and recurrent vomiting.

Diarrhoea is not usually a very distressing feature although this depends on the severity of colonic involvement. Patients with severe rectal and anal disease may have urgency with faecal incontinence. Urgency is caused by the reduced rectal capacity and an inflamed rectal mucosa.

Major **abdominal findings** in ill patients are abdominal distension, tenderness, and in some patients a firm, palpable inflammatory mass.

It is particularly important to be able to identify **anal and rectal pathology** on which the clinical diagnosis of Crohn's disease is often based. Anal features are especially common with ileocolonic disease but are not common with isolated small bowel involvement. The most distressing feature of anal disease is sepsis from secondary abscesses and perianal fistulae. In the presence of active disease the perianal skin appears 'bluish' and three or more oedematous, pink, fleshy tags may protrude from the anal margin, often with superficial ulceration on the inner surface extending into the anal canal (Fig. 52.7). Superficial fissures with deep, undermined edges, causing little pain, may be present and later heal with a bridge of epithelium. Deep cavitating ulcers, which are usually very painful, in the anal canal, are associated with muscle spasm in the acute phase and form the basis for perianal abscesses that discharge subcutaneously around the anus and may track forwards to involve the genitalia. Healing of these ulcers is often with fibrosis

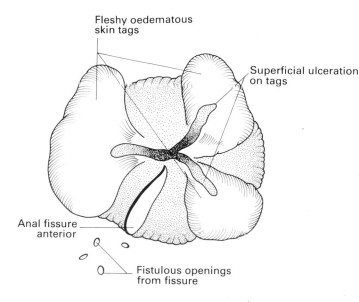

Fleshy oedematous
skin tags

Superficial ulceration
on tags

Anal fissure
anterior

Fistulous openings
from fissure

Fig. 52.7. Some of the anal
features of Crohn's disease. Three
large fleshy skin tags protrude
from the anal margin with linear
ulceration on their inner aspect.
There is a superficial anal fissure,
with undermined edges and more
peripheral fistulous openings.

and stricture formation in the anal canal. Deep cavitating ulcers also affect the lower rectal mucosa producing similar results (Table 52.3). The rectal mucosa is often spared in Crohn's disease, despite severe anal involvement, feeling normal on digital examination. However, with severe rectal disease the mucosa is thickened—it feels diffusely nodular and irregular.

Sigmoidoscopic examination may be quite normal or reveal minimal involvement of the mucosa with oedema and loss of the vascular pattern. Aphthoid-like ulcers are a characteristic feature when present. They are surrounded by a rim of erythematous mucosa and separated by apparently normal mucosa. Inflamed mucosa is often indistinguishable from ulcerative colitis, but with severe change it may be very irregular and ulcerated with a mucopurulent exudate. Deep linear ulcers with undermined edges are not easy to identify because of distortion in the narrowed rectum. In one study of over 1,000 patients, sigmoidoscopic abnormalities were seen in 34% of all patients and 51% of those with colonic involvement [77].

Local complications

Episodes of **intestinal obstruction** are probably the commonest local complication in Crohn's disease. Minor bouts resolve spontaneously or with an increased dose of steroids, but surgery is usually considered with more severe attacks. Intestinal obstruction is sometimes a surgical emergency caused by an over-distended gut becoming gangrenous or perforating. Obstruction may be due to a simple stricture of an inflammatory mass in which adherent loops of inflamed bowel envelope an abscess. **Perforations**, which are contained locally and produce an abscess, are not uncommon in

Table 52.3. Anal and rectal lesions in Crohn's disease (reproduced with permission from [49]).

Associated with active disease
Anal oedematous tags ± ulceration
Anal indolent fissures
Cavitating anal canal ± perianal abscess and fistulae
Deep rectal ulcers ± perirectal abscess and fistulae

Secondary lesions
Skin tags
Anal and rectal strictures
Epithelialized fistulae

patients with very active disease, but free
perforations into the abdominal cavity are
unusual and may be overlooked initially
because of the dampening effect of steroids
on symptoms [9].

Massive rectal bleeding occurs from time
to time, particularly in colonic disease, but
sometimes in patients who only have ileal
involvement. The bleeding, however, is
usually more gradual from inflamed mucosa and is responsible for iron deficiency
anaemia.

Abscesses and fistulae

Intra-abdominal abscesses associated with
active disease often begin as mesenteric
abscesses that adhere to adjacent organs
and then discharge their contents through
fistulae. The ramifications and interconnec-
tions between fistulous tracts are sometimes
very bewildering and those that eventually
open to the skin may follow a long, tortuous course. Almost all persistent enterocutaneous fistulae connect with an abscess
alongside the gut and persist because of inadequate drainage and the communication
with gut contents (Fig. 52.8).

Fistulae sometimes communicate with
the bladder producing recurrent urinary
tract infection, or in the pelvis they may
penetrate the vaginal wall. Abscesses in the
right iliac fossa may involve the psoas

sheath, the patient fixing the affected hip in
a flexed position. Although occurring at
any time they are seen most often during
very active phases of the disease and particularly in the post-operative period after
surgical resections (Fig. 52.9). For this
reason it is often prudent, although not always possible, to delay surgery until the
acute phase has been subdued with medical
treatment.

Liver abscesses in Crohn's disease are
rare and often fatal [34].

Gastrointestinal malignancy

The risk of developing adenocarcinoma of
the gut in Crohn's disease is increased, but
estimates are based on either small figures
or selected populations [33, 35, 36, 97,
105]. As in ulcerative colitis, the risk probably increases with long-standing disease
and this may be particularly relevant in
patients after by-pass surgery or with a retained rectal stump. Adenocarcinoma of the
small bowel occurs in Crohn's disease and
is of particular significance because the
tumour is rare in the general population.

Systemic illness associated with active Crohn's disease (see Fig. 52.12).

Several systemic illnesses occur in Crohn's
disease, some of them related to active

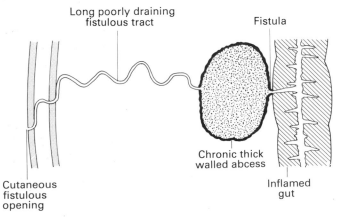

Long poorly draining
fistulous tract

Fistula

Chronic thick
walled abcess

Cutaneous
fistulous
opening

Inflamed
gut

Fig. 52.8. Relationship between
enterocutaneous fistulae and
intra-abdominal abscesses in
patients with Crohn's disease.

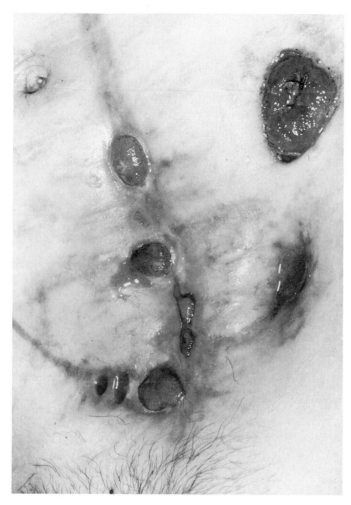

Fig. 52.9. Multiple enterocutaneous fistulae opening through and around a recent laparotomy scar in a patient who had resection of a tight stricture in the sigmoid colon. A colostomy is shown in the right upper part of the illustration.

disease, while others appear to run a relatively independent course (Table 52.4). Features associated with activity include finger clubbing, skin, mouth and eye involvement, as well as large joint arthritis. Although the features may occur with Crohn's disease at any site, involvement of the skin, mouth, eyes and large joints is more closely related to ileocolitis. Patients with any one of these features have a greater risk of developing others [88].

Finger clubbing assessed by measurement of the hyponychial angle occurs with active disease in about 40% of patients and often regresses after surgical resection, only to return with recurrent disease [53].

Erythema nodosum occurs with exacerbations in some patients. Deep, **punched-out skin ulcers**, particularly below the knee, are less common; they appear to be associated with a localized vasculitis. A rare but distressing complication is **pyoderma gangrenosum**, in which necrotic ulcers extend rapidly to destroy considerable areas of skin.

Oral aphthous ulcers are most common but gross oedema of the buccal mucosa or lips, associated with deep linear fissures or ulcers, also occurs (see Chapter 7). This disfiguring lesion may be the only manifestation of the disease and in some patients occurs in conjunction with fleshy anal skin tags [109].

Table 52.4. Systemic illness and Crohn's disease.

Transient systemic illness associated with active disease	
Skin	Erythema nodosum, deep ulcers below the knees or rarely pyoderma gangrenosum (extending gangrenous ulceration).
Mouth	Aphthous ulcers, linear ulcers or fissures on buccal mucosa of the cheeks or lips.
Joints	Acute transient sero-negative arthritis of large joints—knees and ankles.
Eyes	Conjunctivitis, uveitis, iritis.
Vascular	Deep venous thrombosis, arterial occlusions in limbs.
Finger clubbing	Active disease, resolving after intestinal resection and returning with recurrence.

Systemic illness that persists and appears unrelated to the activity of Crohn's disease	
Joints	Ankylosing spondylitis, sacroiliitis (related to HLA-B27).
Liver	Cirrhosis. Pericholangitis, sclerosing cholangitis.
Renal tract	Renal stones (uric acid, calcium, oxalate), entero-vesical fistulae, right hydronephrosis, renal amyloid.

Patients may develop a **'red eye'** due to conjunctivitis. Other eye lesions include iritis or uveitis [55].

The **acute arthritis** which occurs in some patients with active disease is non-erosive and not unlike that encountered in rheumatic fever, causing pain and swelling with a predilection for involvement of knee and ankle joints.

Vascular problems occur in association with active disease and at times of surgery. These may be venous thromboses or arterial occlusions, particularly of limb vessels. Their cause is not fully understood but contributory factors include dehydration, weight loss, thrombocytosis and steroid treatment.

Systemic illness unrelated to the activity of Crohn's disease

The prevalence of **ankylosing spondylitis** is nine times that expected in the general population. Many other patients have radiological evidence of sacroiliitis and simply complain of low back pain from time to time [66]. Patients with these problems usually have HLA type B27 tissue antigens. Some patients suffer from a **sero-negative arthritis** involving peripheral joints and this also runs a course that is independent of bowel disease activity.

Significant **liver disease** is infrequent in Crohn's disease although liver histology at the time of surgery often shows fatty change, pericholangitis or portal triaditis. In pericholangitis, the inflammatory cell infiltrate involves the portal tracts with pseudo bile duct proliferation and occasional granulomas [21]. There is little evidence that these changes are progressive—they probably improve after resection of bowel disease and are of little consequence. Cirrhosis rarely complicates Crohn's disease, and it is difficult to know whether the risk of this condition is greater than in the normal population. Sclerosing cholangitis is an uncommon complication occurring less often in Crohn's disease than in ulcerative colitis [21]. Medical treatment has little effect on this condition which pursues a relentless course over many years, with episodes of cholestasis leading to secondary biliary cirrhosis.

Renal complications of Crohn's disease include urolithiasis [32]. Uric acid stones are more common particularly in patients with an ileostomy who pass more concentrated urine with lower urinary pH. During treatment with steroids calcium is mobilized and excreted in increased amounts, causing recurrent calculi in some patients. A third factor emphasized in recent years is the role of increased colonic oxalate absorption in patients with steatorrhoea [11]. Hydrone-

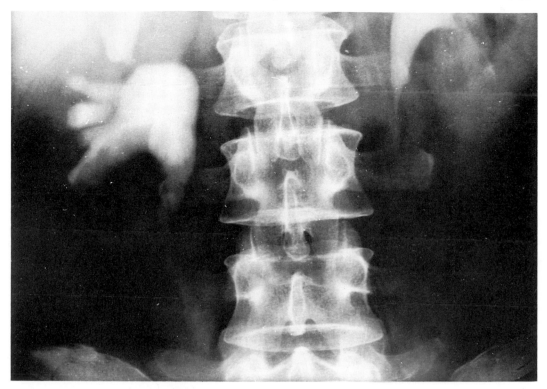

Fig. 52.10. Radiograph showing right-sided hydronephrosis due to extrinsic ureteric compression by an inflammatory mass of Crohn's disease at the pelvic brim.

phrosis, particularly right-sided, may be due to extrinsic ureteric obstruction from an inflammatory mass at the pelvic rim (Fig. 52.10). Enterovesical fistulae can cause serious problems with recurrent urinary tract infection. Occasionally patients have been described with nephrotic syndrome due to renal amyloidosis, but this is rare.

Consequences of extensive ileal resection

Many patients with Crohn's disease have complications which are more closely related to the consequences of surgery than the inflammatory process itself. The incidence of these complications is related to the extent of surgical resections [79]. Severe problems can arise in patients with little remaining bowel (Fig. 52.11).

Table 52.5. Mechanisms responsible for diarrhoea after small bowel resection.

Cathartic effect of bile salts on colon causing mucosal loss of salt and water.

Reduced fluid absorption by shortened small bowel.

Fat malabsorption and steatorrhoea.

Recurrent inflammatory bowel disease.

Diarrhoea is probably the commonest and most troublesome complication. Removal of part of the ileum with the right colon is followed by diarrhoea which usually becomes less severe with the passage of time—the improvement is probably due to a compensatory increase of fluid absorption by the remaining colon. Four factors contribute to the diarrhoea (Table 52.5). Bile salts, normally absorbed in the terminal ileum, are lost in excessive amounts into the colon where they have a

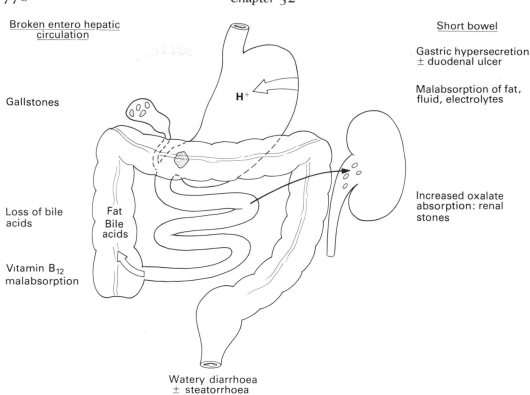

Broken entero hepatic
circulation

Short bowel

Gastric hypersecretion
± duodenal ulcer

Gallstones

Malabsorption of fat,
fluid, electrolytes

H⁺

Loss of bile
acids

Fat
Bile
acids

Increased oxalate
absorption: renal
stones

Vitamin B₁₂
malabsorption

Watery diarrhoea
± steatorrhoea

Fig. 52.11. Clinical consequences of extensive ileal resection in Crohn's disease.

cathartic effect causing excessive loss of salt and water [76]. Substantial loss of small intestine decreases the absorptive area and consequently more fluid pours into the colon. Malabsorption of fat contributes to diarrhoea by producing steatorrhoea—this tends to occur when more than 100 cm of ileum are removed and is partly due to inadequate concentrations of bile acids in the gut lumen because of excessive loss and bacterial deconjugation [46]. Patients without a colon and only short lengths of small intestine live precariously on the brink of dehydration because of enormous fluid losses.

Gastric acid hypersecretion, complicated by duodenal ulceration, may occur with extensive small bowel resection and is associated with increased concentrations of serum gastrin. Occasionally, acid secretion

is very high and of the order usually encountered in patients with the Zollinger-Ellison syndrome [31].

Removal of the terminal ileum breaks the entero-hepatic circulation causing excessive loss of bile acids and vitamin D [5, 46]. This loss greatly reduces the bile salt pool, increasing the lithogenic potential of bile (Fig. 52.11). **Gallstones** have been reported in 32% of patients after ileal resection, which is about three times the expected figure [42]. Twenty-five hydroxy vitamin D is lost by the same mechanism increasing the risk of **osteomalacia** [22, 37]. **Vitamin B₁₂ malabsorption** occurs simply because the ileal absorption site for this vitamin is removed. The incidence of **renal stones** is probably increased, and excessive oxalate absorption accounts for some of the stones. Calcium normally binds to oxalate in the

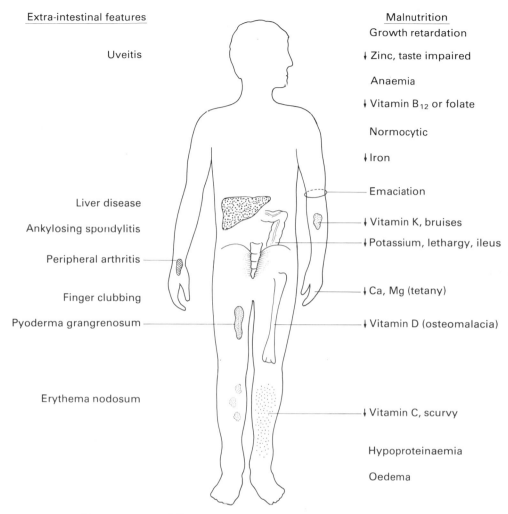

Extra-intestinal features

Uveitis

Liver disease

Ankylosing spondylitis

Peripheral arthritis

Finger clubbing

Pyoderma grangrenosum

Erythema nodosum

Malnutrition
Growth retardation

↓ Zinc, taste impaired

Anaemia

↓ Vitamin B$_{12}$ or folate

Normocytic

↓ Iron

Emaciation

↓ Vitamin K, bruises

↓ Potassium, lethargy, ileus

↓ Ca, Mg (tetany)

↓ Vitamin D (osteomalacia)

↓ Vitamin C, scurvy

Hypoproteinaemia

Oedema

Fig. 52.12. Some of the extra-intestinal illnesses and features of malnutrition found in patients with Crohn's disease.

intestinal lumen but with steatorrhoea the calcium forms soaps, leaving oxalate free for systemic absorption [11].

Nutritional deficiencies in Crohn's disease

For many patients the nutritional consequences of Crohn's disease are severe [39]. Patients eat less because food produces symptoms. Malabsorption is a major factor after extensive small bowel resection and continued inflammation with enteric loss of nutrients plays a part (Fig. 52.11).

Anaemia

Anaemia, which occurs in up to 70% of patients, is often hypochromic, but the peripheral blood film appearances, serum iron and transferrin saturation may be abnormal due to chronic inflammation [25]. This leads to over-diagnosis of iron deficiency, but measurements of serum ferritin as an index of iron stores partly overcome the problem. Values less than $15\,\mu g/l$ always indicate iron depletion although in Crohn's disease concentrations up to $50\,\mu g/l$ may be associated with iron deficiency. Macrocytosis may be due to folate or B_{12} deficiency, or the effects of sulphasalazine producing mild haemolysis, or impaired folate absorption (see Chapter 6).

Hypoproteinaemia

Hypoproteinaemia is generally attributed to gastrointestinal protein loss [6]. The serum albumin reflects the long-term protein nutritional status but the serum prealbumin, which is easily measured by radial immunodiffusion, shows rapid changes in the protein status because of its shorter half-life of two days.

Deficiency of fat-soluble vitamins

Deficiency of fat-soluble vitamins is not uncommon. Abnormal prothrombin times may be found in 30% of patients, particularly with steatorrhoea, and may be responsible in some patients for haematuria or gastrointestinal bleeding. Low plasma vitamin A is often found with hypoproteinaemia but it does not necessarily indicate vitamin A deficiency—in this situation dark adaptation tests are useful to identify those who are truly vitamin A deficient and require supplements [65].

Vitamins B and C

Pellagra due to malabsorption of nicotinic acid has been reported. Although scurvy is rare, patients have low values for leucocyte ascorbic acid and consequently have subclinical vitamin C deficiency [50].

Zinc

A low serum zinc may be found in 40% of patients, but it may not reflect true zinc deficiency since it is closely correlated with serum proteins [63]. Features of the deficiency, however, have been reported and include classical acrodermatitis with impaired taste acuity; the reported association of zinc deficiency with growth retardation must be regarded as speculative [98].

Electrolytes

Hyponatraemia is uncommon but occurs with severe diarrhoea. Hypokalaemia always indicates potassium depletion but the latter may occur with normal plasma concentrations and is sometimes responsible for non-specific symptoms. Similarly, a low magnesium always indicates magnesium deficiency although serum concentrations alone will lead to under-diagnosis. Serum and urinary measurements of magnesium show that more than 80% of patients with severe disease have problems [64].

Osteomalacia

Vitamin D deficiency measured by 25-hydroxy-cholecalciferol is very common in patients with Crohn's disease [22, 37]. It is probably the result of an interrupted entero-hepatic circulation and loss of protein-bound metabolites from inflamed mucosa [5]. Osteomalacia probably occurs in up to 30% of patients but is not always indicated by reduced concentrations of 25-hydroxy-cholecalciferol [13]. Elevated concentrations of either alkaline phosphatase of bony origin, or serum parathormone, are indirect indicators of osteomalacia associated with vitamin D deficiency. For many patients whose vitamin D status is precarious, serum concentrations are normal during summer months, but may fall during winter. True hypocalcaemia is not common although plasma concentrations are often decreased in association with hypoalbuminaemia. A correction for the reduced serum albumin usually gives values in the normal range (for every 6 g of albumin required to bring the patient's value up to 40 g/l, an additional 0.1 mmol/l should be added to the patient's plasma calcium concentration).

Surgery, recurrence and mortality

It is impossible to predict the course of Crohn's disease in an individual patient [56]. Extensive disease may coexist with minimal symptoms for long periods. There may be recurrence of disease activity after many years of apparently normal health.

Need for surgery

The diagnosis is often delayed after initial symptoms—in the National Cooperative Crohn's Disease Study (NCCDS) the average delay was 35 months [78]. The cumulative probability of surgery in these patients was 78% after 20 years (Fig. 52.13) [78]. The interval from initial symptoms to the first operation was shortest for patients with ileocolitis, longer for those with only small bowel involvement and longest for those

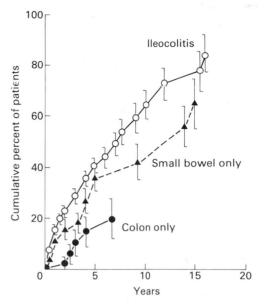

Fig. 52.14. The cumulative probability of abdominal surgery after onset of symptoms for patients with ileocolitis, small-bowel-only, or colon-only involvement. The three curves are statistically significantly different from each other (with permission from [77]).

with colonic disease (Fig. 52.14) [78]. The cumulative probability of surgery in patients presenting to St Mark's Hospital, London, with symptoms lasting less than six months was 17% at one year, and 37% at 10 years—half the operations for chronic symptoms and half for emergencies [27].

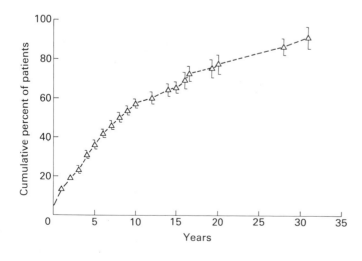

Fig. 52.13. The cumulative probability of abdominal surgery after onset of symptoms for the entire group of patients randomized in the NCCDS (adapted with permission from [78]).

Recurrence after surgery

The course of the disease after surgery is again unpredictable, but after a variable interval recurrence is usual [30, 31]. Recurrence rates vary and are affected by the definition of recurrence, differences between groups and the site of disease. Crohn and Yarnis [17] followed 542 patients for up to 25 years and only 51 of these remained well. Cook [14] reported a figure of 45% recurrence at two years, 68% at five years, and 78% at 10 years in a group of patients receiving both medical and surgical treatment. Lennard-Jones and Stalder [60] used actuarial methods to calculate that one-third of all patients had a symptomatic relapse within five years of the surgical resection of the terminal ileum, and 50% after 10 years. Another large study which involved 168 patients from Leeds [20], showed an overall recurrence rate of 34% in patients seen between 1939 and 1968. The recurrence rate was less in patients with involvement mainly of the large rather than small bowel; it was affected by age, with higher rates in children and adolescents, and lower rates over the age of 60 years. The National Cooperative Crohn's Disease Study showed that a second operation was most common after by-pass surgery and those patients who required two operations appeared to be more likely to require a third [78]. A U.S. study showed that recurrence was more likely if there was an internal fistula or perianal disease as an indicator for surgery [108].

Mortality

Although the natural history in any group of patients is modified by both medical and surgical treatment, as far as mortality is concerned, longitudinal studies show no improvement in spite of 'advances' in treatment, although morbidity has almost certainly been reduced [30, 92]. The overall

Table 52.6. The standardized mortality ratio (SMR) for Crohn's patients with a high mortality risk. The expected mortality for the general population corresponds to an SMR of 1. (Reproduced with permission from [70]).

	SMR
Age at the time of diagnosis 10–19 years	11
Age at the time of diagnosis 20–29 years	3
Extensive disease with simultaneous involvement of several sites	2.9
During first $2\frac{1}{2}$ years after diagnosis	3.8
14 years after the diagnosis	3.2

mortality in Crohn's disease is twice that of the rest of the population but certain groups of patients carry a much higher risk [70]. Young patients diagnosed before the age of 20 years are 11 times more likely to die than their peers. Patients with extensive disease, particularly affecting the small bowel, also have an increased risk of death (Table 52.6). The survival figures from the time of diagnosis show a greatly increased mortality in the first three years (Fig. 52.15), followed by a relatively stable period until, at 14 years, mortality again

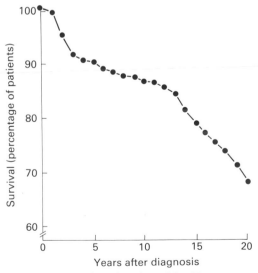

Fig. 52.15. Survival rate based on a life table estimate from 219 patients with Crohn's disease identified in Cardiff between 1934 and 1976 (adapted with permission from [70]).

Table 52.7. Investigations in Crohn's disease.

Object	Major investigations
Initial diagnosis, recurrent disease, extent of disease.	Radiology, endoscopy and histology.
Disease activity.	Clinical features, serum orosomucoids, C-reactive protein, platelets.
Nutritional status and deficiencies.	Anthropometric, haematological and biochemical measurements.

increases. Early deaths are probably related to severe extensive disease, but the increased mortality after 14 years may be due to consequences of recurrent surgery, impaired nutrition or even steroid treatment. In one series the patients given steroids, who probably had more severe disease, had twice the mortality risk of other patients [86].

Investigations

Investigation may be to establish a diagnosis or the presence of recurrent disease (Table 52.7). Diagnosis usually depends on a combination of clinical, radiological and pathological features since there is no specific diagnostic test. Colonoscopy is of additional value to assess the extent of disease and establish the nature of colonic strictures and polyps.

Radiology

The upper bowel is usually examined by a conventional barium meal followed through the small intestine, and the colon by double-contrast barium enema. In some centres the small bowel enema is becoming popular as it gives much clearer mucosal detail. Some of the radiological features are shown in Fig. 52.16. Single or multiple narrowed segments of bowel with ulcerated mucosa are common in the small intestine. Secondary dilatation of gut often occurs proximal to the narrowed segment and duodenal strictures may cause obstruction with gastric dilatation and delayed gastric emptying. In the presence of multiple small bowel strictures, intervening bowel may dilate into irregular pouches or form 'saccular pseudo diverticula' (Fig. 52.17) [67]. The mucosa in narrowed bowel may contain deep 'rose thorn' ulcers with fistulous connections between adherent loops; fistulae and sinuses are most often seen in the terminal ileum communicating with the sigmoid colon, caecum or bladder. Ulceration may be shallow or associated with a 'cobble-stone' appearance (Fig. 52.18). Polyps are not uncommon in areas of inflamed

Bowel wall changes

Strictures

Dilation

Asymmetrical disease

Pseudodiverticula

Puckered distorted caecum

Ileal stricture

Fistula

Anal fistula

Mucosal changes

Aphthoid ulcers
Rose thorn ulcers
Oedematous valvulae conniventes
Linear ulcers

Cobblestoning

Inflammatory polyps

Rectal sparing

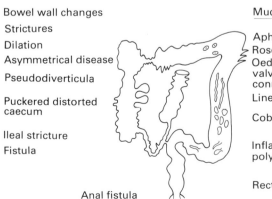

Fig. 52.16. Major radiological features in the small bowel and colon in patients with Crohn's disease.

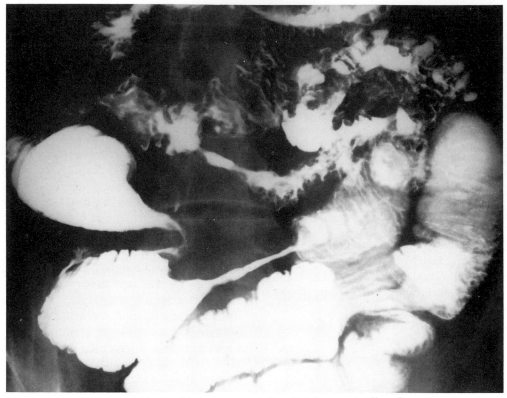

Fig. 52.17. Multiple strictures in the small intestine separated by dilated segments of bowel.

colon (Fig. 52.19). Involved bowel without a strictured lumen may show distortion of the valvulae conniventes due to oedema and lymphoid hyperplasia [68].

Crohn's disease of the colon may appear similar to ulcerative colitis in all respects, but valuable features that help to distinguish between them are discrete 'aphthoid ulcers' surrounded by a halo of oedema, and asymmetrical involvement of the bowel wall (Fig. 52.20). Skip lesions with predominantly right-sided involvement, rectal 'sparing', strictures and fissures are all common findings. Older patients may have coincidental diverticular disease with Crohn's disease producing considerable distortion of the sigmoid colon [94].

The oral administration of sucralfate labelled with technetium 99^M may, in the future, be used as a screening test for Crohn's and ulcerative colitis [19].

Histology

Whenever possible the diagnosis should be confirmed by histology because small bowel and colonic lesions may be wrongly labelled Crohn's disease. Some may turn out to be adenocarcinoma, lymphoma, tuberculosis, or other lesions with radiological appearances that mimic Crohn's disease (Table 52.10). Failure to adhere to such a policy leads to misdiagnosis.

Rectal biopsies

Rectal biopsies are used most often to establish the initial diagnosis, but in many patients they are of only limited value. The histology is invariably abnormal in the presence of sigmoidoscopic changes, but it may be abnormal when the rectum appears normal and this possibility increases with

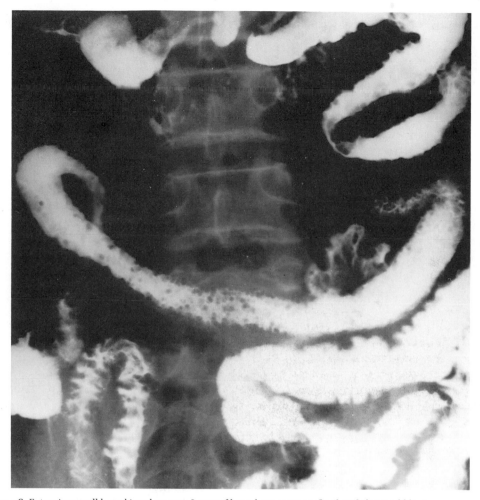

Fig. 52.18. Extensive small bowel involvement. Loops of bowel are narrow, fixed and show cobble-stone mucosa.

colonic lesions close to the rectum. With ileal involvement alone, rectal histology is abnormal in up to 20% of patients. To establish the diagnosis with rectal changes the major distinction is from ulcerative colitis (Fig. 52.21). Features that suggest Crohn's disease include the presence of granulomas, patchy mucosal inflammation and disproportionate inflammation in the submucosa. Goblet cells and glandular architecture are usually well preserved and crypt abscesses tend to be scanty. These features contrast with the uniformly heavy lymphocytic infiltration which is limited to the mucosa in ulcerative colitis [84]. Repeated biopsies give some indication of response to treatment and are used to identify dysplastic changes which may occur with long-standing inflammatory disease.

Fleshy anal tags

Fleshy anal tags are usually associated with Crohn's disease. Two-thirds of these show granulomas where the tag has a fleshy pink oedematous appearance [49], but 'cosmetic' surgery to the anus should be avoided in Crohn's disease.

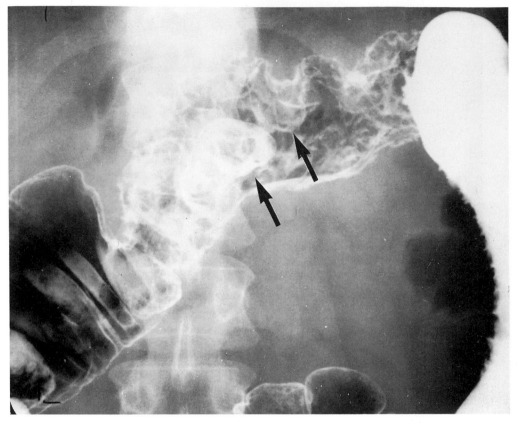

Fig. 52.19. Crohn's disease of the transverse and descending colon. Arrows identify polyps in the inflamed segment of colon which has a distorted mucosal pattern. The transition to normal transverse colon is abrupt. 'Rose thorn ulcers' are seen in the descending colon.

Colonic or jejunal biopsies

Multiple colonic biopsies give some indication of the extent of disease, but they tend to be very small and for this reason contain granulomas less often. Jejunal biopsies are not usually taken to establish the diagnosis but in the presence of jejunal disease with oedematous mucosa they show quite marked abnormalities. A patchy lymphocytic infiltrate of the mucosa, which may be very heavy in places, is often found with considerable disruption of the normal architecture. Villi are often distorted or stunted and the changes may be mistaken for coeliac disease.

Disease activity

It is often of value to measure activity of the inflammatory disease, either to assess response to treatment or to evaluate recurrent symptoms, particularly in patients who have previously undergone surgery [45]. Many indices have been proposed, based on clinical or laboratory values or both. A simple practical one is based on five clinical variables which are general well-being, abdominal pain, diarrhoea, presence of an abdominal mass, intestinal or systemic complications [41] (Table 53.4)—a score of five or more indicates active disease.

Because abdominal pain and diarrhoea

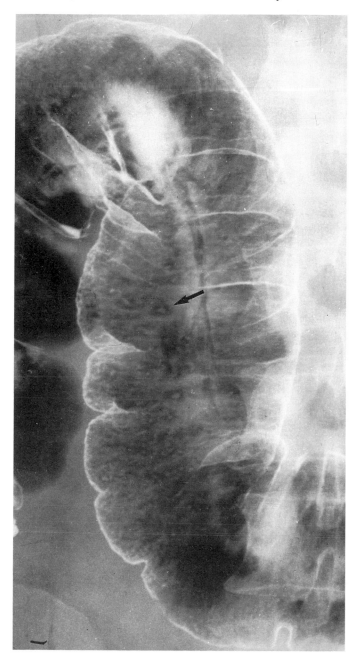

Fig. 52.20. Multiple aphthoid ulcers in the colon of a patient with Crohn's disease showing a central collection of barium surrounded by a halo of radio translucency (with permission from [104]).

may not be related to disease activity, the clinical index should be supplemented with one or more laboratory parameters. Serum orosomucoids or C-reactive protein are acute phase reactants that correlate well with clinical disease activity [2, 45, 85].

Faecal α_1-antitrypsin concentration rises with increased disease activity [80]. Where these cannot be measured the sedimentation rate, albumin concentration and platelet count are useful. There is a particularly good correlation between the

Ulcerative colitis	Features	Crohn's

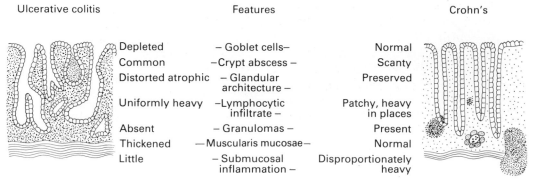

Ulcerative colitis		Crohn's
Depleted	– Goblet cells–	Normal
Common	–Crypt abscess –	Scanty
Distorted atrophic	– Glandular architecture –	Preserved
Uniformly heavy	–Lymphocytic infiltrate –	Patchy, heavy in places
Absent	– Granulomas –	Present
Thickened	—Muscularis mucosae—	Normal
Little	– Submucosal inflammation –	Disproportionately heavy

Fig. 52.21. Histological features in the rectal biopsy that help distinguish between ulcerative colitis and Crohn's disease.

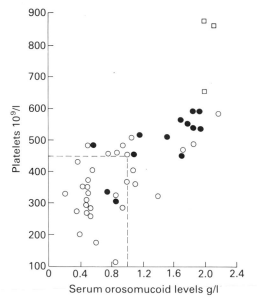

Fig. 52.22. The platelet count and serum orosomucoids in patients with Crohn's disease. Broken lines indicate the upper normal limit. ○ = patients with inactive disease; ● = active disease; □ = very active disease (according to Harvey and Bradshaw's Clinical Index [41]).

platelet count, orosomucoids and clinical activity (Fig. 52.22) [38].

Nutritional status and deficiencies

Since long-term malnutrition is a major problem for many patients, a simple assessment of nutritional status is important. About 70% experience excessive weight loss

and up to 30% of children show impaired linear growth and sexual maturation [48]. Most clinicians rely on regular measurements of body weight and height to follow the overall effect on nutrition; in children these should be plotted on percentile charts to follow progress (Fig. 52.23).

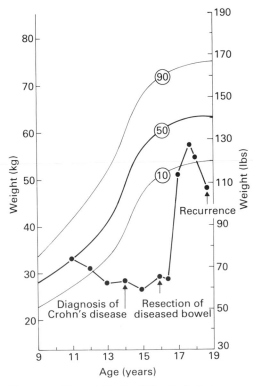

Fig. 52.23. The weight of a child with Crohn's disease plotted on a percentile chart.

Additional assessments of body composition are provided by 'nutritional anthropometry' which involves measurements of height, weight, mid-arm circumference, skin-fold thickness and derived mid-arm muscle circumference (see Chapter 78). Mid-arm muscle circumference and skin-fold thickness reflect respectively skeletal muscle mass and adipose tissue stores and are therefore an index of protein and calories reserves [96]. Reference standards are available for these measurements and the deviation of individual patients from the norm can be calculated easily.

In practice the mid-arm circumference is particularly useful. This is taken mid-way between the acromion and olecranon process; mean measurements from men and women are 29.3 cm and 28.5 cm respectively [52]. Patients with values below 90% of these figures (less than 26.4 cm in men and 25.7 cm in women) may appear well clinically, yet they have a high prevalence of nutritional deficiencies and should be identified and investigated more fully. Similar measurements have been used successfully in the tropics to identify malnourished patients whose weight may be misleadingly high because of oedema [103].

Clinical attempts to predict those most likely to have deficiencies are of limited value, but they are particularly common in

Table 52.8. Patients with high prevalence of nutritional deficiencies.

Mid-arm circumference (Less than 26.4 cm in men, or 25.7 cm in women)
Active disease
Post-operative recurrent disease
Extensive involvement
Previous extensive surgical resections

certain groups—patients with active disease, post-operative recurrent disease, extensive involvement or previous extensive surgical resections [15, 26] (Table 52.8). The value of the mid-arm circumference in identifying those patients who are likely to have nutritional problems is illustrated in Fig. 52.24. Patients with 'thin arms' had a high prevalence of reduced albumin concentrations and similar results are obtained from measurements of haemoglobin, serum ferritin and vitamin D concentration.

Differential diagnosis

There is often difficulty with the diagnosis of Crohn's disease and long delays are common, particularly in children and young adults [26]. In one series although a third of patients were correctly diagnosed within a year, one out of seven patients were not diagnosed until at least 10 years had elapsed after the onset of symptoms. Con-

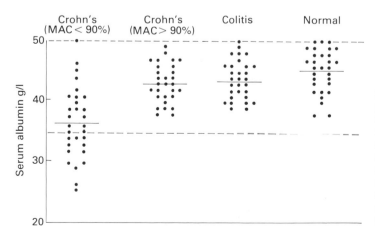

Fig. 52.24. Serum albumin in patients with Crohn's disease, ulcerative colitis and normals. Patients with Crohn's disease are divided into those with a mid-arm circumference (MAC) less than and greater than 90% of the norm. The group with 'thin arms' contained many with a low serum albumin (adapted with permission from [40]).

fusion with the diagnosis also occurs when the label 'Crohn's disease' is given too readily to patients with features of the condition, who are later shown to have another pathology [41]. An increased awareness of diagnostic difficulties in this area will probably reduce errors (Table 52.9).

The protean manifestations of Crohn's disease mean that clinical grounds can only suggest a diagnosis which requires confirmation by adequate radiology and histology—with stool cultures to exclude infection. A barium meal that only examines as far as the duodenum may cause delay for those patients with small bowel disease, who must wait for the clinician to request a barium examination of the small intestine. The unfortunate diagnostic label of 'irritable bowel syndrome' is given too often to young patients with recurrent abdominal

Table 52.9. Conditions that may give the same clinical features as Crohn's disease and cause difficulty in diagnosis.

Anorexia	Anorexia nervosa
	Gastrointestinal malignancy
Abdominal pain	Irritable bowel syndrome
	Small bowel adhesions
	Peptic ulcer
	Gallstones
	Diverticular disease
Diarrhoea	Irritable bowel syndrome
	Infective diarrhoea
	Diverticular disease
	Ulcerative colitis or ischaemic colitis with bleeding
	Coeliac disease
Abdominal mass in right iliac fossa	Appendix abscess
	Gynaecological disease (ovarian tumours or cysts)
	Carcinoma caecum (in elderly)
	Ileocaecal tuberculosis
	Amoeboma
Perianal ulceration	Malignancy
	Behçet's syndrome
	Lymphogranuloma venereum
	Tuberculosis
Sigmoidoscopic appearances	Ulcerative colitis
	Infective colitis
	Pseudomembranous colitis
	Venereal proctitis
	Radiation proctitis

pain and diarrhoea. It may give clinicians a sense of security but it causes diagnostic delay.

Radiological features play a major part in diagnosis but problems arise when the diagnosis is not substantiated by histological confirmation (Table 52.10). In diffuse small bowel disease, a jejunal biopsy can cause

Table 52.10. Conditions that may give the same radiological features as Crohn's disease.

Diffuse small bowel disease	Coeliac disease
	Lymphoma
	Fungi (rarely)
Terminal ileal disease	Ileocaecal tuberculosis
	Lymphoma
	Carcinoma of the caecum
Total colonic involvement	Cathartic colon
	Ulcerative colitis
	Pseudomembranous colitis
	Infectious colitis
	Schistosomiasis with polyps
Isolated or multiple colonic strictures	Neoplasm
Distal colonic disease	Ulcerative colitis
	Ischaemic colitis

confusion because of severe distortion in morphology due to chronic inflammatory cell infiltration. Some of the pathological features in conditions that may be confused with Crohn's colitis are summarized in Table 52.11. Although the features in some of these conditions may be distinctive, difficulties in their interpretation are not uncommon.

Terminal ileal disease is rarely due to tuberculosis in the Western hemisphere but this is not the case in developing countries where it is a common clinical problem. Crohn's disease and intestinal tuberculosis may mimic each other in their clinical, radiological and histological manifestations—with small bowel strictures or an ileocaecal mass as the more common features [95]. A laparoscopy or laparotomy, with biopsies including mesenteric lymph nodes, may be

Table 52.11. Conditions that may show similar pathological features to Crohn's disease on biopsy.

Infective colitis	Infiltrate chiefly polymorphonuclear with minimal chronic inflammatory cell content of lamina propria.
	Pathogenic organisms often seen (*Entamoeba histolytica* and *Schistosoma*).
	Crypt architecture preserved.
Ischaemia	Fibrosis of mucosa and submucosa.
	Haemosiderin laden macrophages in wall of ischaemic bowel.
	Selective necrosis of surface epithelium.
Pseudomembranous colitis	Focal eruptions of mucus, fibrin and polymorphs in areas of pseudomembrane.
Solitary ulcer syndrome	Fibrosis in lamina propria, smooth muscle fibres grow between crypts from thickened muscularis mucosa.
Tuberculosis	Caseating granulomas.
	Circumferential ulceration.

required to establish the diagnosis that should always be considered in patients from Asia and Africa. Rarely the clinical situation may justify a trial of anti-tuberculous treatment.

Severe gastrointestinal infections due to *Salmonella, Shigella, Campylobacter* [57], *Clostridium difficile* [4], cryptosporidiosis [23, 110], or amoebiasis may pose problems by producing severe diarrhoea with proctitis which may resemble inflammatory bowel disease (see Chapter 57). These infections occasionally affect patients with Crohn's disease and may cause confusion in the management. Stools should always be cultured from patients with diarrhoea to exclude pathogenic organisms. *Entamoeba histolytica* should be considered in patients who have been abroad. A diagnosis of amoebiasis can be made from stool specimens, rectal biopsy and serological tests which are positive in 70% of patients with invasive disease.

Ischaemic colitis presents as an acute event, usually in patients over 50 years of age, with blood loss initially and acute cramping pains. Radiological changes often show a segmental colitis limited to the splenic flexure or recto-sigmoid region with 'oedematous thumb prints' distorting the bowel lumen in the acute phase, progressing in severe cases to strictures (see Chapter 72). Differentiation from Crohn's disease may be difficult but the clinical picture and appearance of biopsies are helpful.

Venereal proctitis due to the *Gonococcus, Chlamydia trachomatis* or *Herpes* virus is a diagnosis made in most clinics (see Chapter 57). Homosexual males presenting with proctitis should have specimens taken to culture these organisms. This involves close cooperation with a bacteriologist who will immediately 'plate' the specimens on appropriate culture mediums. *Chlamydia* produces lymphogranuloma venereum and has been reported in large series of Jamaican patients who developed proctitis, rectal strictures and perianal fistulae [3].

Acknowledgements

The authors are grateful for help and advice from Professor L.E. Hughes, Professor K.T. Evans and Dr Geraint Williams respectively from the University Departments of Surgery, Radiology and Pathology at the University of Wales College of Medicine. We are also grateful for help from the Department of Medical Illustration.

References

1 ALLAN RN, HODGSON HJF. Inflammatory bowel disease. In: Pounder RE, ed. *Recent advances in gastroenterology-6*, 1986. Edinburgh: Churchill Livingstone, 1986: 310–326.

2 ANDRE C, DESCOS L, LANDAIS P, FERMANIAN J. Assessment of appropriate laboratory measurements to supplement the Crohn's disease activity index. *Gut* 1981;22:571–574.

3 ANNAMUNTHODO H. Rectal lymphogranuloma in Jamaica. *Dis Colon Rectum* 1961;4:17–26.

4 BARTLETT JG, MOON N, CHANG TW, TAYLOR N, ONDERDONF AB. The role of *Clostridium difficile* in antibiotic-associated pseudomembranous colitis. *Gastroenterology* 1978;75:778–782.

5 BATCHELOR AJ, WATSON G, COMPSTON JE. Changes in plasma half-life and clearance of 3H-25-hydroxyvitamin D3 in patients with intestinal malabsorption. *Gut* 1982;23:1068–1071.

6 BEEKEN WL, BUSCH HJ, SYLVESTER DL. Intestinal protein loss in Crohn's disease. *Gastroenterology* 1972;62:207–215.

7 BOLTON PM, OWEN E, HEATLEY RV, JONES-WILLIAMS W, HUGHES LE. Negative findings in laboratory animals for transmissible agent in Crohn's disease. *Lancet* 1973;ii:1122–1124.

8 BRAHME F, LINDSTROM C, WENCKERT A. Crohn's disease in a defined population. An epidemiological study of incidence, prevalence, mortality and secular trends in the city of Malmo, Sweden. *Gastroenterology* 1975;69:324–351.

9 BUNDRED NJ, DIXON JM, LUMSDEN AB, GILMOUR HM, DAVIES GC. Free perforation in Crohn's colitis. A ten-year review. *Dis Colon Rectum* 1985;28:35–37.

10 CAVE DR, MITCHELL DN, BROOKE BN. Experimental animal studies of the aetiology and pathogenesis of Crohn's disease. *Gastroenterology* 1975;69:618–624.

11 CHADWICK VS, MODHA K, DOWLING RH. Mechanism for hyperoxaluria in patients with ileal dysfunction. *N Engl J Med* 1973;289:172–176.

12 CHIODINI RJ, VAN KRUININGEN HJ, THAYER WR, MARKAL RS, COUTU JA. Possible role of mycobacteria in inflammatory bowel disease. *Dig Dis Sci* 1984;29:1073–1079.

13 COMPSTON JE, HORTON LW, AYERS AB, TIGHE JR, CREAMER B. Osteomalacia after small intestinal resection. *Lancet* 1978;i:9–12.

14 COOKE WT. Nutritional and metabolic factors in the aetiology and treatment of regional ileitis. *Ann R Coll Surg Engl* 1955;17:137–158.

15 COOKE WT, SWAN CHJ. Diffuse jejuno-ileitis of Crohn's disease. *Q J Med* 1974;43:583–601.

16 CROHN BB, GINZBURG L, OPPENHEIMER GD. Regional ileitis; a pathological and clinical entity. *JAMA* 1932;99:1323–1329.

17 CROHN BB, YARNIS H. *Regional ileitis*. New York: Grune and Stratton, 1958.

18 DALZIEL TK. Chronic interstitial enteritis. *Br Med J* 1913;2:1068–1070.

19 DAWSON DJ, KHAN AN, MILLER V, RATCLIFFE JF, SHREEVE DR. Detection of inflammatory bowel disease in adults and children: evaluation of a new isotopic technique. *Br Med J* 1985;291:1227–1230.

20 DE DOMBAL FT, BURTON I, GOLIGHER JC. Recurrence of Crohn's disease after primary excisional surgery. *Gut* 1971;12:519–527.

21 DEW MJ, THOMPSON H, ALLAN RW. The spectrum of hepatic dysfunction in inflammatory bowel disease. *Q J Med* 1979;48:113–135.

22 DIBBLE JB, SHERIDAN P, LOSOWSKY MS. A survey of vitamin D deficiency in gastrointestinal and liver disorders. *Q J Med* 1984;53:119–134.

23 DuPONT HL. Cryptosporidiosis and the healthy host. *N Engl J Med* 1985;312:1319–1320.

24 DWORKEN HJ. Crohn's disease. *Ann Intern Med* 1984;101:258–260.

25 DYER NH, CHILD JA, MOLLIN DL, DAWSON AM. Anaemia in Crohn's disease. *Q J Med* 1972;41:419–436.

26 DYER NH, DAWSON AM. Malnutrition and malabsorption in Crohn's disease with reference to the effect of surgery. *Br J Surg* 1970;60:134–140.

27 ELLIOT PR, RITCHIE JK, LENNARD-JONES JE. Prognosis of colonic Crohn's disease. *Br Med J* 1985;291:178.

28 FABRICIUS PJ, GYDE AN, SHOULDER P, et al. Crohn's disease in the elderly. *Gut* 1985;26:461–465.

29 FARMER R, HAWK W, TURNBULL R. Clinical pattern in Crohn's disease: a statistical study of 615 cases. *Gastroenterology* 1975;68:627–635.

30 FARMER RG, WHELAN G, FAZIO VW. Longterm follow up of patients with Crohn's disease. *Gastroenterology* 1985;88:1818–1825.

31 FREDERICK PL, SIZER JS, OSBORNE MP. Relation of massive bowel resection to gastric secretion. *N Engl J Med* 1965;272:509–514.

32 GELZAYD EA, BREUER RI, KIRSNER JB. Nephrolithiasis in inflammatory bowel disease. *Am J Dig Dis* 1968;13:1927–1934.

33 GLOTZER DJ. The risk of cancer in Crohn's disease. *Gastroenterology* 1985;89:438–411.

34 GREENSTEIN AJ, BACHAR DB, LOWENTHAL D, GOLDOFSKY E, AUFSES AH. Pyogenic liver abscess in Crohn's disease. *Q J Med* 1985;220:505–518.

35 GYDE SN, PRIOR P, MACARTNEY JC, THOMPSON H, WATERHOUSE JAM, ALLAN RN. Malignancy in Crohn's disease. *Gut* 1980;21:1024–1029.

36 HAMILTON SR. Colorectal carcinoma in patients with Crohn's disease. *Gastroenterology* 1985;89:398–407.

37 HARRIES AD, BROWN R, HEATLEY RV, WILLIAMS LA, WOODHEAD S, RHODES J. Vitamin D status in

Crohn's disease: association with nutrition and disease activity. *Gut* 1985;**26**:1197–1203.

38 HARRIES AD, FITZSIMONS E, FIFIELD R, DEW MJ, RHODES J. A simple measure of activity in Crohn's disease. *Br Med J* 1983;**286**:1476.

39 HARRIES AD, HEATLEY RV. Nutritional disturbances in Crohn's disease. *Postgrad Med J* 1983;**59**:690–697.

40 HARRIES AD, JONES L, HEATLEY RV, RHODES J, FITZSIMONS E. Mid-arm circumference as a simple means of identifying malnutrition in Crohn's disease. *Br Med J* 1982;**285**:1317–1318.

41 HARVEY RF, BRADSHAW JM. A simple index of Crohn's disease activity. *Lancet* 1980;**i**:514.

42 HEATON KW, READ AE. Gallstones in patients with disorders of the terminal ileum and disturbed bile salt metabolism. *Br Med J* 1969;**3**:494–496.

43 HELLERS GKG. Crohn's disease in Stockholm County 1955–1974. *Acta Chir Scand* 1979; [Suppl] 490.

44 HERSHFIELD NB. Crohn's disease in a mother, father and son. *Can Med Assoc J* 1984;**131**:1190–1193.

45 HODGSON HJF. Assessment of drug therapy in inflammatory bowel disease. *Br J Clin Pharmacol* 1982;**14**:159–170.

46 HOFMANN AF, POLEY JR. Role of bile acid malabsorption in pathogenesis of diarrhoea and steatorrhoea in patients with ileal resection. 1. Response to cholestyramine or replacement of dietary long chain triglyceride by medium chain triglyceride. *Gastroenterology* 1972;**62**:918–938.

47 HOLDSTOCK G, SAVAGE D, HARMAN M, WRIGHT R. An investigation into the validity of the present classification of inflammatory bowel disease. *Q J Med* 1985;**214**:183–190.

48 HOMER DR, GRAND RJ, COLODNY AH. Growth, course and prognosis after surgery for Crohn's disease in children and adolescents. *Pediatrics* 1977;**59**:717–725.

49 HUGHES LE. Surgical pathology and management of anorectal Crohn's disease. *J R Soc Med* 1978;**71**:644–651.

50 HUGHES RG, WILLIAMS N. Leucocyte ascorbic acid in Crohn's disease. *Digestion* 1978;**17**:272–274.

51 JARNEROT G, JARNMARK I, NILSSON K. Sugar consumption in Crohn's disease, ulcerative colitis and irritable bowel syndrome. *Scand J Gastroenterol* 1982;**17**:352.

52 JELLIFFE DB. The assessment of the nutritional status of the community. *WHO Monograph Series No 53 (Geneva)* 1966.

53 KEWENTER J, HULTEN L, KOCK NG. The relationship and epidemiology of acute terminal ileitis and Crohn's disease. *Gut* 1974;**15**:801–804.

54 KITIS G, THOMPSON H, ALLAN RN. Finger clubbing in inflammatory bowel disease: its prevalence and pathogenesis. *Br Med J* 1979;**2**:825–828.

55 KNOX DL, SCHACHAT AP, MUSTONEN E. Primary, secondary and coincidental ocular complications of Crohn's disease. *Ophthalmology* 1984;**91**:163–173.

56 KRAUSE U, EJERBLAD S, BERGMAN L. Crohn's disease. A long-term study of the clinical course in 186 patients. *Scand J Gastroenterol* 1985;**20**:516–524.

57 LAMBERT JR, TISCHLER M, KARMALI MA, NEWMAN A. *Campylobacter* ileocolitis: an inflammatory bowel disease. *Can Med Assoc J* 1979;**121**:1377–1379.

58 LAWSON GHK, ROWLAND AC, WOODING P. The characterisation of *Campylobacter sputorum* subspecies *Mucosalis*. *Res Vet Sci* 1975;**18**:121–126.

59 LEE FI, COSTELLO FT. Crohn's disease in Blackpool—incidence and prevalence 1968–80. *Gut* 1985;**26**:274–278.

60 LENNARD-JONES JE, STALDER GA. Prognosis after resection of chronic regional ileitis. *Gut* 1967;**8**:332–336.

61 LESKO SM, KAUFMAN DW, ROSENBERG L, *et al*. Evidence of an increased risk of Crohn's disease in oral contraceptive users. *Gastroenterology* 1985;**89**:1046–1049.

62 McBRIDE JA, KING MJ, BAIKIE AG, CREAN GP, SIRCUS W. Ankylosing spondylitis and chronic inflammatory diseases of the intestine. *Br Med J* 1963;**2**:483–486.

63 McCLAIN C, SOUTOR C, ZIEVE L. Zinc deficiency: a complication of Crohn's disease. *Gastroenterology* 1980;**78**:272–279.

64 MAIN ANH, MORGAN RJ, RUSSELL RI, *et al*. Magnesium deficiency in chronic inflammatory bowel disease and requirements during intravenous nutrition. *JPEN* 1981;**5**:15–19.

65 MAIN ANH, MILLS PR, RUSSELL RI, *et al*. Vitamin A deficiency in Crohn's disease. *Gut* 1983;**24**:1169–1175.

66 MALLAS EG, MACKINTOSH P, ASQUITH P, COOKE WT. Histocompatability antigens in inflammatory bowel disease; their clinical significance and their association with arthropathy with special reference to HLA-B7 (W27). *Gut* 1976;**17**:906–910.

67 MARSHAK RK. Granulomatous disease of the intestinal tract (Crohn's disease). *Radiology* 1975;**114**:3.

68 MARSHAK RH, LINDNER AE. *Radiology of the small intestine*. Philadelphia: WB. Saunders Co., 1976.

69 MARTINI GA, BRANDES JW. Increased consumption of refined carbohydrates in patients with Crohn's disease. *Klin Wochenschr* 1976;**54**:367–371.

70 MAYBERRY JF, NEWCOMBE RG, RHODES J. Mortality in Crohn's disease. *Q J Med* 1980;**49**:63–68.

71 MAYBERRY JF, RHODES J, HEATLEY RV. Infections which cause ileocolic disease in animals: are they relevant to Crohn's disease? *Gastroenterology* 1980;**78**:1080–1084.

72 MAYBERRY J, RHODES J, HUGHES LE. Incidence of
    Crohn's disease in Cardiff between 1934 and
    1977. *Gut* 1979;**20**:602–608.

73 MAYBERRY JF, RHODES J, NEWCOMBE RG. Crohn's
    disease in Wales 1967–76; an epidemiological
    survey based on hospital admissions. *Postgrad
    Med J* 1980;**56**:336–341.

74 MAYBERRY JF, RHODES J, NEWCOMBE RG. Familial
    prevalence of inflammatory bowel disease in re-
    latives of patients with Crohn's disease. *Br Med J*
    1980;**1**:84.

75 MAYBERRY JF, RHODES J, ALLAN R, *et al.* Diet in
    Crohn's disease. Two studies of current and pre-
    vious habits in newly diagnosed patients. *Dig Dis
    Sci* 1981;**26**:444–448.

76 MEKHJIAN H, PHILLIPS SF, HOFMANN AF. Colonic
    secretion of water and electrolytes induced by bile
    acids. Perfusion studies in man. *J Clin Invest*
    1971;**50**:1569–1577.

77 MEKHJIAN HS, SWITZ DN, MELNYK CS, RANKIN GB,
    BROOKS RK. National Cooperative Crohn's Disease
    Study: clinical features and natural history of
    Crohn's disease. *Gastroenterology* 1979;**77**:898–
    906.

78 MEKHJIAN HS, SWITZ DM, WATTS DH, DEREN JJ,
    KATON RM, BEMAN FM. National Cooperative
    Crohn's Disease Study: factors determining re-
    currence of Crohn's disease after surgery. *Gas-
    troenterology* 1979;**77**:907–913.

79 MERRICK MV, EASTWOOD MA, FORD MJ. Is bile acid
    malabsorbtion underdiagnosed? An evaluation of
    the accuracy of diagnosis by measurement of
    SeHCAT retention. *Br Med J* 1985;**290**:668.

80 MEYERS S, WOLKE A, FIELD SP, FEUER EJ, JOHNSON
    JW, JANOWITZ HD. Fecal α_1-antitrypsin measure-
    ment: an indicator of Crohn's disease activity.
    Gastroenterology 1985;**89**:13–18.

81 MILLER DS, KEIGHLEY AC, LANGMAN MJS. Chang-
    ing patterns in epidemiology of Crohn's disease.
    Lancet 1974;**2**:691–693.

82 MILLER DS, KEIGHLEY A, SMITH PG, HUGHES
    AO, LANGMAN MJS. Crohn's disease in Notting-
    ham: a search for time-space clustering. *Gut*
    1975;**16**:454–457.

83 MILLER DS, KEIGHLEY A, SMITH PG, HUGHES AO,
    LANGMAN MJS. A case control method for seeking
    evidence of contagion in Crohn's disease. *Gas-
    troenterology* 1976;**71**:385–387.

84 MORSON BC, DAWSON IMP. *Gastrointestinal pathol-
    ogy*. 2nd ed. Oxford: Blackwell Scientific Publica-
    tions, 1979:295–306.

85 PETTIT SH, HOLBROOK IB, IRVING MH. Comparison
    of clinical scores and acute phase proteins in the
    assessment of acute Crohn's disease. *Br J Surg*
    1985;**72**:1013–1016.

86 PRIOR P, FIELDING J, WATERHOUSE JA, COOKE WT.
    Mortality in Crohn's disease. *Lancet*
    1970;**i**:1135–1137.

87 PUGH SM, RHODES J, MAYBERRY JF, ROBERTS DL,

88 HEATLEY RV, NEWCOMBE RG. Atopic disease in ul-
    cerative colitis and Crohn's disease. *Clin Allergy*
    1979;**9**:221–223.

88 RANKIN GB, WATTS HD, MELNYK CS, KELLEY ML.
    National Cooperative Crohn's Disease Study: ex-
    traintestinal manifestations and perianal compli-
    cations. *Gastroenterology* 1979;**77**:914–920.

89 RHODES JM, MARSHALL T, HAMER JD, ALLAN RN.
    Crohn's disease in two married couples. *Gut*
    1985;**26**:1086–1087.

90 RHODES J, ROSE J. Crohn's disease in the elderly.
    Br Med J 1985;**291**:1149–1150.

91 ROZEN P, ZONIS J, YEKUTIEL P, GILAT T. Crohn's
    disease in the Jewish population of Tel-Aviv-Yafo.
    Gastroenterology 1979;**76**:25–30.

92 SACHAR DB. Crohn's disease in Cleveland: a matter
    of life and death. *Gastroenterology* 1985;**88**:1996–
    2002.

93 SACHAR DB, TAUB RN, RAMACHANDAR K, *et al.* T
    and B lymphocytes and cutaneous anergy in in-
    flammatory bowel disease. *Ann NY Acad Sci*
    1976;**278**:565–573.

94 SCHMIDT CT, LENNARD-JONES JE, MORSON BC,
    YOUNG AC. Crohn's disease of the colon and its
    distinction from diverticulitis. *Gut* 1968;**9**:7–16.

95 SEGAL I, OU TIM L, HAMILTON DG, MANNELL A.
    LEE ECG, ed *Crohn's Workshop: A global assessment
    of Crohn's disease*. New York: Heyden, 1981.

96 SHENKIN A, STEELE LW. Clinical and laboratory
    assessment of nutritional status. *Proc Nutr Soc*
    1978;**37**:95–103.

97 SHORTER RG. Risks of intestinal cancer in Crohn's
    disease. *Dis Colon Rectum* 1983;**26**:686–689.

98 SOLOMONS NW, ROSENFIELD RL, JACOB RA, SAND-
    STEAD HH. Growth retardation of zinc nutrition.
    Pediatr Res 1976;**10**:923–927.

99 SOMERVILLE KW, LOGAN RFA, EDMOND M, LANG-
    MAN MJS. Smoking and Crohn's disease. *Br Med
    J* 1984;**289**:954–956.

100 THAYER WR, COUTU JA, CHIODINI RJ, VAN KRUIN-
    INGEN HJ, MARKAL RS. Possible role of mycobac-
    teria in inflammatory bowel disease. *Dig Dis Sci*
    1984;**29**:1080–1085.

101 THOMAS HC, JEWELL DP. *Clinical gastrointestinal
    immunology*. Oxford: Blackwell Scientific Publica-
    tions, 1979.

102 THORTON JR, EMMETT PM, HEATON KW. Smoking,
    sugar and inflammatory bowel disease. *Br Med J*
    1985;**290**:1786–1787.

103 TROWBRIDGE GL. Clinical and biochemical char-
    acteristics associated with anthropometric nutri-
    tional categories. *Am J Clin Nutr* 1979;**32**:758–
    766.

104 VANDENBROUCKE J, BODART P, DIVE L, LENS E, VAN-
    TRAPPEN G. L'ileocolite granulomateuse. *Etude
    clinique et radiologique*. VII Congres International
    de Gastro-Enterologie Bruxelles, 1964;**1**:451–
    481.

105 WEEDON DD, SHORTER RG, ILSTRUP DM, HUIZENGA

KA, TAYLOR WF. Crohn's disease and cancer. *N Engl J Med* 1973;**289**:1099–1103.

106 WENSINCK F, VAN DE MERWE JP, MAYBERRY JF. An international study of agglutinins to *Eubacterium Peptostreptococcus* and *Coprococcus* species in Crohn's disease, ulcerative colitis and control subjects. *Digestion* 1983;**27**:63–69.

107 WETERMAN IT, PENA AS. Familial incidence of Crohn's disease in the Netherlands and a review of the literature. *Gastroenterology* 1984;**86**:449–452.

108 WHELAN G, FARMER RG, FAZIO VW, COORMASTIC. M Recurrence after surgery in Crohn's disease. *Gastroenterology* 1985;**88**:1826–1833.

109 WIESENFELD D, FERGUSON MM, MITCHELL DN, *et al.* Oro-facial granulomatosis—a clinical and pathological analysis. *Q J Med* 1985;**54**:101–113.

110 WOLFSON JS, RICHTER JM, WALDRUN MA, *et al.* Cryptosporidia in immunocompetent patients. *N Engl J Med* 1985;**312**:1278–1282.

Chapter 53
Medical Management of Crohn's Disease

R. E. POUNDER

The doctor and his patient with Crohn's disease need a confident and trusting relationship when faced with a chronic illness that has no known cause and for which there is no cure, an illness characterized by relapse and remission and an illness that may affect any part of the gastrointestinal tract.

Despite the problems of managing Crohn's disease, there is no doubt that an experienced physician, working in close collaboration with a similarly interested surgeon, can provide a high standard of care that minimizes ill health. Crohn's disease remains a sufficiently rare and long-term problem that the patient is best cared for by a physician with a special interest in the condition.

The physician's approach

The physician must be *optimistic*. Although the occasional patient has a disastrous downhill course, the great majority of patients spend little time in hospital, enjoy reasonable health and are able to enjoy normal daily activities. It is important that the physician provides optimistic and enthusiastic support for the patient [16].

The physician should impart an air of '*informed confidence*' that, although the cause of Crohn's disease is unknown and there is no cure, it is usually possible to suppress inflammation, treat infection, deal with mechanical complications, relieve symptoms and maintain nutrition.

The physician should be *available* to deal quickly with any relapse or complication. Early help certainly reassures the patient,

DEPARTMENT OF
GASTROENTEROLOGY
XXXXXXXXX HOSPITAL
XXXXXX

INFLAMMATORY BOWEL
DISEASE

If you suffer a relapse of your inflammatory bowel disease you should phone

Dr XXXXXXXX's secretary

(XX XXX XXXX extension XXX)

who will arrange an urgent appointment.

This emergency service is only for your bowel condition — you must contact your family doctor about all other medical problems.

Phone from 9 a.m. to 5 p.m. (Monday to Friday) and be ready to tell the secretary

— your name
— your hospital number
— a telephone number, if possible
— that you have been given this card.

Fig. 53.1. Card issued to every patient with inflammatory bowel disease.

and it should provide better results. Hospital doctors are often protected by bureaucracy, and should make their services available to respond promptly to any call for help from a patient with inflammatory bowel disease (Fig. 53.1).

The physician should be *problem orientated*, clearly identifying the present problem, to work out whether symptoms are due to a functional abnormality or a struc-

Table 53.1. Classification of problems in Crohn's according to abnormalities of function or structure.

Function	Structure
Absorption/secretion/ exudation	Obstruction
	Perforation
Primary inflammation	Abscess
Secondary bacterial infection	Fistula
	Tissue destruction
Systemic illnesses related to Crohn's disease	Short gut
	Anal sphincter
Malnutrition	Perianal disease
Anxiety/depression	

tural problem (Table 53.1). The physician should remember that even when the patient is free from infection or inflammation, he or she may suffer from long-term nutritional problems due to an extensively damaged gut.

The physician should be *cautious*—better the sins of omission than commission [36]. The surgeons have become more cautious in recent years (see Chapter 54) realizing that they are not aiming to cure a patient with Crohn's disease, but rather they deal with each problem one by one. Similarly, the physician has potent drugs and the availability of long-term parenteral feeding—providing hazards that may outweigh potential benefits.

Finally, the physician must *collaborate* with a surgeon who has a particular interest in Crohn's disease. Although the need for emergency surgery in Crohn's disease is often clear-cut, the indications for elective surgery are much more difficult to define (see Chapter 54) and need considerable understanding between physician and surgeon.

Nutritional treatment [40, 45, 56]

Diet [58]

Patients usually ask for an appropriate diet and are often disappointed when they are told that no decisive change is needed.

Stricture diet

Patients with small intestinal strictures must avoid foods that may cause bolus obstruction. The list (Table 53.2) contains

Table 53.2. Foods that may cause bolus obstruction if there is an intestinal stricture.

Segments of any citrus fruit
Sweet corn
Coleslaw or uncooked vegetables
Raw fruits, unless chewed thoroughly
Nuts
Popcorn
Tough or gristly meat

foods that are not digested and pass essentially unchanged through the small bowel. The patients do not need to eat a low fibre diet [39], but they must avoid lumps of fibre; they can tolerate bran and properly chewed fruits (but they must never swallow segments of citrus fruits). Similarly, tablets that pass intact to the colon (the commonest examples being Slow-K, Navidrex-K Slow-sodium and Asacol) should not be given to patients who have strictures.

Refined carbohydrate

Although patients with Crohn's disease often have a high prediagnosis intake of refined carbohydrate [69], there is no evidence that avoidance of such carbohydrate is associated with clinical improvement. Indeed, as undernutrition is often a problem in Crohn's disease, a low carbohydrate diet could deny the patient helpful, palatable calories. The early report that a diet of unrefined carbohydrate, rich in dietary fibre, decreased the need for hospital admission [25] is being retested by a larger clinical trial.

Milk

There is no convincing evidence that every patient with Crohn's disease should avoid milk. Alactasia is rarely a problem unless something else is wrong with the gut—thus the Crohn's patient with alactasia may notice less diarrhoea if milk intake is moderated. If diarrhoea is a problem, alactasia can be identified by a lactose-hydrogen breath test—if positive a short trial of a low milk intake can be tried and abandoned if there is no rapid benefit. Avoidance of milk does not influence the inflammatory process.

Elemental diets

There has been one report of a controlled trial comparing prednisolone (0.75 mg/kg.day) with an elemental diet (Vivonex) for the early treatment of patients with newly diagnosed Crohn's disease [48]. The Vivonex supplied 150–250 kJ (40–60 kcal)/kg body weight and nitrogen 8–12 g/day. At one and four months both groups of patients had shown similar improvement assessed by clinical score, weight and laboratory values. That such an elemental diet—chemically defined and potentially antigen-free—should rest an inflamed bowel is an attractive idea. However, the palatability of such a diet is so poor that most patients will not tolerate it except when fed by a naso-enteric tube. The combination of an elemental diet plus framycetin, colistin, and nystatin had a similar effect to prednisolone 0.5 mg/kg.day [61].

Food idiosyncrasy

There have been enthusiastic reports that patients with Crohn's disease usually respond to exclusion diets [2, 31, 76]. Such patients have been prescribed an initial extremely restricted diet, followed by reintroduction of a normal diet, food by food. Such diets cannot be recommended as conventional management of Crohn's disease.

Supplementary oral feeding

Poor appetite with an inadequate nutritional intake can be a major problem, especially in children with Crohn's disease. The idea of supplementary feeding using a proprietary polymeric and predigested liquid diet has been tested successfully [23].

Ideally, the nutritional support should be taken as a drink, and it may be necessary for the patient to tolerate an overnight intragastric infusion of a liquid diet, using a fine bore tube.

Parenteral feeding

Parenteral feeding (Fig. 53.2) may be needed during a fulminating episode of inflammation or infection, when there is a small bowel ileus due to subacute obstruction or after surgery, or when a short gut is left after surgical resection [5, 46, 66].

Details of enteral and parenteral feeding are discussed in Chapter 78.

Nutritional deficiences

The identification and treatment of specific nutritional deficiencies can be extremely rewarding, providing the Crohn's disease patient with a decisive and predictable benefit (Fig. 53.3) [22].

Iron

The assessment of iron deficiency is difficult in Crohn's disease—the serum iron and total iron binding capacity will often show a chronic disease pattern and hence overestimate iron deficiency. Even serum ferritin

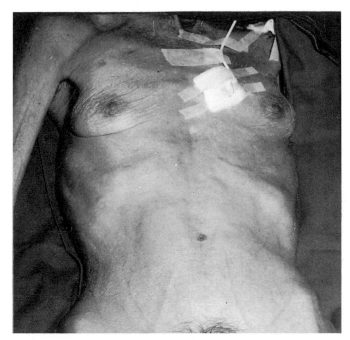

Fig. 53.2. Parenteral feeding for a cachectic patient with small intestinal Crohn's disease.

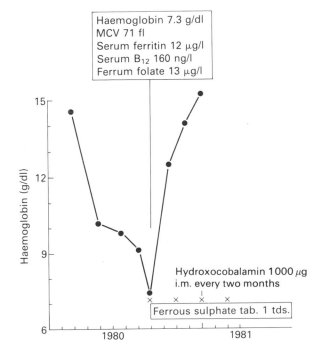

Haemoglobin 7.3 g/dl
MCV 71 fl
Serum ferritin 12 μg/l
Serum B_{12} 160 ng/l
Ferrum folate 13 μg/l

Hydroxocobalamin 1000 μg i.m. every two months

Ferrous sulphate tab. 1 tds.

Fig. 53.3. The response of a 28-year-old woman with Crohn's disease to iron and B_{12} supplements. She received no other treatment.

can be unreliable, but patients who are anaemic with a serum ferritin less than $15\,\mu g/l$ should always receive iron supplements. A bone marrow provides the most accurate information about iron stores and iron utilization (see Chapter 6). Ferrous sulphate tablets (one tablet, three times a day) should be given until the anaemia is corrected, and then for a further three months to replete iron stores.

Vitamin B₁₂

Vitamin B$_{12}$

Vitamin B$_{12}$ deficiency is relatively common in Crohn's disease—especially after ileal resection. If the serum B$_{12}$ concentration is low (less than $160\,pmol/l$), the patient should be advised to receive an intramuscular injection of hydroxocobalamin $1000\,\mu g$ every two months for life. The patient can conveniently keep a box of ampoules in the $+4C°$ part of the home refrigerator.

Folic acid

Folic acid deficiency may affect up to one-third of patients—if detected the patient should receive folic acid 5 mg daily by mouth. Such patients should also receive vitamin B$_{12}$ injections, for fear of allowing neurological complications of B$_{12}$ deficiency by masking its more obvious haematological changes.

Sodium and potassium

Except in the acutely ill patient or the ileostomist with residual small bowel disease, sodium chloride deficiency is rarely a problem (see Chapter 56). Hypokalaemia is more common and is aggravated by corticosteroid therapy. An effervescent or liquid potassium chloride supplement should be used, to avoid either enteric ulceration or bolus obstruction by tablets.

Calcium and fat-soluble vitamins

Osteomalacia is relatively common [11]. In everyday clinical practice, the plasma alkaline phosphatase can be used as a screening test. If elevated, isoenzymes should be checked to exclude an hepatic origin of the abnormality, the serum 25 OH vitamin D and parathormone concentrations measured and a bone biopsy considered.

Vitamin D deficiency is common in patients with active Crohn's disease, even if they have not had any bowel resection [11]. Biochemical osteomalacia should respond to calcium with vitamin D—one tablet, three times a day. Symptomatic osteomalacia is best treated with calciferol injection 100,000 units i.m. monthly (one-third of an ampoule) with an oral calcium supplement. One alpha hydroxycholecalciferol should only be used under expert supervision, for fear of profound hypercalcaemia due to overdosage.

Vitamin A, E and K deficiencies are liable to develop if the patient has long-term steatorrhoea [42, 77]. Monthly injections of vitamin A (100,000 units i.m.) and vitamin K (10 mg i.m.) may be supplemented by oral vitamin E (alpha tocopharyl acetate 3–15 mg daily).

Zinc

Zinc deficiency probably does occur in patients with severe small intestinal Crohn's disease, but it is difficult to measure this deficiency [50]. Serum zinc concentration is related to the serum albumin concentration; hence it is not surprising that many patients with Crohn's disease have a low serum zinc. Poorly nourished patients with Crohn's disease may benefit from zinc sulphate 220 mg daily after a meal; it should not be taken at the same time as iron supplements, as zinc and iron compete for absorption by the small bowel.

Multivitamin supplements may also help

malnourished patients. Overt niacin, thiamine or vitamin C deficiency is extremely rare, but the disadvantages of multivitamin supplementation are few.

Anti-inflammatory drugs and immunosuppressives

Corticosteroids accumulate in inflamed tissue and produce a dose-related inhibition of all the phenomena of chronic inflammation, Prednisone is hydroxylated to prednisolone in the liver and, as prednisolone has a lesser mineralocorticoid effect than cortisone, it is the preferred corticosteroid for systemic treatment.

Prednisolone has many well-known side-effects, although patients with Crohn's disease seem relatively spared from problems compared with, for example, patients who have either rheumatoid arthritis or asthma [37]. This may be surprising as a low serum albumin could result in an increase of non-protein bound prednisolone, which theoretically would increase the metabolic activity of the drug. Prednisolone may be incompletely absorbed by some patients with small bowel Crohn's disease [64].

There are only a few controlled trials of corticosteroids for Crohn's disease [36]. Prednisolone 0.25–0.75 mg/kg body weight.-day (maximum 60 mg/day) over four months was shown to be superior to placebo for patients with ileal or ileo-colonic Crohn's disease (Fig. 53.4) but was only equivalent to placebo in patients with colonic disease [67].

Three trials surprisingly have failed to show that corticosteroids are of benefit as maintenance treatment for Crohn's disease [65, 69]. However in practice, prednisolone 30–60 mg/day is given to patients with acute Crohn's disease to settle a relapse of inflammation, having excluded possible infection. The prednisolone is rapidly decreased to 20–30 mg/day as soon as there is clinical improvement and then gradually withdrawn over the next six to eight weeks. The decrease of dose should be very slow below 12.5 mg/day—patients often appear to relapse if the drug is withdrawn abruptly.

Despite the evidence of clinical trials that suggest that prednisolone is of no benefit as maintenance treatment, there are many patients with Crohn's disease who relapse as the prednisolone is withdrawn—some

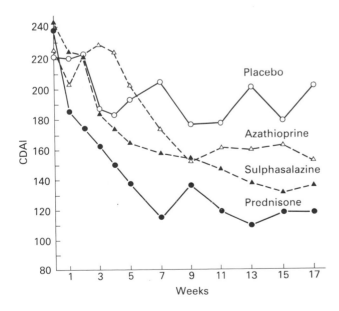

Fig. 53.4. Crohn's disease activity index in 295 patients with active Crohn's disease in a multicentre trial [67].

can be kept in good health taking only prednisolone 6–8 mg/day but promptly relapse as the drug is withdrawn further. Others relapse when the dose drops below 15 mg/day. In the former group there are three therapeutic possibilities—firstly, continue with prednisolone 6–8 mg/day as maintenance treatment (side-effects are rare in any patient taking that dose of prednisolone); secondly, prescribe prednisolone 12–16 mg/day on alternate days (which may lessen the side-effects of corticosteroid therapy); thirdly, add azathioprine for its prednisolone-sparing effect [38]. For those patients who relapse on higher doses of steroids only the latter two strategies are possible, as long-term treatment with more than 10 mg/day of prednisolone is generally unacceptable.

For those patients with inflammatory, rather than infective, Crohn's disease of the anus and rectum, topical corticosteroids may be helpful either as prednisolone suppositories (5 mg), prednisolone 21 phosphate enemata (20 mg in 100 ml water), or as hydrocortisone foam (10%).

Sulphasalazine

Sulphasalazine is the mainstay of maintenance treatment in ulcerative colitis (see Chapter 50) [51, 68]. Similarly, it is probably of benefit in patients with active Crohn's disease, if it involves the colon, but it is probably ineffective for patients who have disease confined to the small bowel [43, 67, 70]. Sulphasalazine (maximum 2.5 g/day) also failed to decrease the relapse rate in patients with inactive Crohn's disease, followed for one to two years [67]. Similarly, sulphasalazine failed to protect against relapse of Crohn's disease after surgical resection [67, 72].

Sulphasalazine's mode of action remains unclear—it is thought to remain intact until its azo-link is broken by enteric bacteria, which releases sulphapiridine and 5 amino salicylic acid into the gut lumen [51]. It is thought that the drug's beneficial effect is due to the anti-inflammatory activity of the 5 amino salicylic acid. Unless there is bacterial contamination of the small bowel, there will be no conversion of sulphasalazine into free 5 amino salicylic acid within the small bowel lumen—perhaps explaining the overall lack of effect in small bowel Crohn's disease.

In practice, sulphasalazine (1 g two to three times a day in divided doses taken after meals) can be given to all the patients with Crohn's disease affecting the colon and, as the drug is relatively harmless, it should be tried in patients with ileal Crohn's disease. The side-effects of sulphasalazine are discussed in Chapter 50 [51, 68].

Azathioprine and 6-mercaptopurine

6-mercaptopurine is a purine antagonist which interferes with nucleic acid synthesis, acting as an immunosuppressive agent. Azathioprine is largely converted to 6-mercaptopurine by the liver. The catabolism of both these drugs requires xanthine oxidase, and concurrent administration of allopurinol will delay excretion of either immunosuppressive, increasing toxicity. The antibiotic trimethoprim also affects nucleic acid synthesis, and should not be co-administered with either 6-mercaptopurine or azathioprine.

The main side-effect of either 6-mercaptopurine or azathioprine is dose-related bone marrow depression; patients should have their full blood count measured at least once a month, perhaps more frequently in the early weeks of treatment. At the start of treatment they should be warned of the symptoms of agranulocytosis, and should be told to stop the immunosuppressive if they develop such symptoms until a white cell count is checked. Occasional patients suffer from pancreatitis, drug-induced fever or nausea. There is some concern that patients receiving long-term immunosuppressive therapy may develop malignancy, due to decreased immunosurveillance of new tumours [34].

The usual dose of azathioprine is 2 mg/ kg body weight.day; the only controlled trial of 6-mercaptopurine started treatment at 1.5 mg/kg.day, thereafter adjusting the dose depending on the white cell and platelet counts [53].

Controlled clinical trials have shown that azathioprine or 6-mercaptopurine are superior to placebo when added to existing corticosteroid therapy in patients with active Crohn's disease [47, 55, 74]. One of the ways of assessing clinical benefit was that patients who received the added immunosuppression tolerated a lower dose of corticosteroid. These results are compatible with the use of azathioprine in most other illnesses—where it is used for its steroid-sparing effect, rather than as a single agent.

When azathioprine was tested as a single agent in patients with active Crohn's disease, it did not appear to be superior to placebo [67]. However, when patients maintained in remission for at least six months on azathioprine 2 mg/kg.day were randomly allocated to continue with the azathioprine or to receive placebo, after one year of follow-up, 5% of the azathioprine-treated patients had relapsed whereas 41% of the placebo-treated patients had become ill [47].

In summary, immunosuppressive drugs do seem to have a role for some patients who have difficult Crohn's disease, where inflammation is only controlled by unacceptably high doses of corticosteroids. Such patients may benefit from azathioprine's or 6-mercaptopurine's prednisolone-sparing effect.

Cyclosporin

Cyclosporin is a potent immunosuppressive agent acting selectively against T-cell mediated immune responses. It is effective as an immunosuppressive when used as a single agent and it has a rapid onset of action, unlike azathioprine which appears to require some months to achieve full activity. A single case report has described a rapid and dramatic response to oral cyclosporin in a patient with active Crohn's disease, who received no other treatment [1]. Controlled studies are awaited.

Antibacterial agents [3]

The role of antibiotics in the medical management of Crohn's disease is uncertain. Surgical drainage is always indicated when there is an intra-abdominal collection of pus. However, it is difficult to assess the extent of the infectious contribution to the inflammation of Crohn's disease [61]. When reviewing the histology of Crohn's disease, observing transmural inflammation and deep fissures, it is difficult to believe that there is no coincidental bacterial invasion of the gut wall.

Without any evidence from controlled trials [70], it is reasonable for all patients with acute inflammation to receive a week's course of metronidazole 400 mg three times a day, as prednisolone is introduced. Such a strategy should also eliminate potential problems due to undetected amoebiasis, giardiasis, or *Clostridium difficile* related colitis.

Antidiarrhoeals, cholestyramine

Antidiarrhoeal drugs such as loperamide, codeine phosphate or diphenoxylate-atropine (Lomotil) should be used cautiously in patients with inflammatory bowel disease. They should not be used to mask inflammation or infection.

However, patients with Crohn's disease—especially after small bowel resection or a right hemicolectomy—may have a degree of diarrhoea that will be helped by the regular use of an antidiarrhoeal or cholestyramine (up to 4 g, three times a day). Cholestyramine may aggravate malabsorption of the fat soluble vitamins, unless given as an enteric coated preparation [28].

Management problems in Crohn's disease

The newly diagnosed patient

The first important step is to make sure the diagnosis is correct (Tables 52.10 and 52.11). A range of investigations should be ordered to provide baseline information about gut structure and function, for comparison in later years. The whole of the gut should be examined radiologically, by barium follow-through from above (or tube enteroclysis) and by double-contrast enema from below. If at all possible, a histological diagnosis should always be achieved—either by rectal biopsy or colonoscopy. If the diagnosis is at all in doubt, a laparotomy should be performed to exclude rarities such as small bowel tuberculosis or lymphoma. In the Third World these conditions are much more common. than Crohn's disease [49, 63]. The minimum investigations required at the time of diagnosis are shown in Table 53.3.

Having made the diagnosis, the patient should receive an optimistic explanation of the disease. There is probably a need for

Table 53.3. Minimum investigations when Crohn's disease is diagnosed.

Full blood picture and ESR.
Biochemistry profile.
Stool culture and examination for parasites.
Histological proof of diagnosis.
Serum B_{12}, folate and ferritin.
Barium follow-through.
Barium enema.

some written explanation of the problem—although most patients are not sufficiently sophisticated to tolerate the remarkably detailed American 'self-help' book (*The Crohn's Disease and Ulcerative Colitis Fact Book* (1983), [4]. Patients should be encouraged to join a self-help group (in the United Kingdom—the National Association for Colitis and Crohn's Disease, 98a London Road, St Albans, Hertfordshire, AL1 INX).

At the time of diagnosis most patients with Crohn's disease should be started on maintenance treatment with sulphasalazine 2–3 g/day in divided doses after meals. Oral prednisolone should be given to control inflammation, aiming to induce remission and then withdraw the drug over a period of six to eight weeks. Nutritional deficiencies should be identified and receive specific treatment—many patients require haematinics at the time of diagnosis. If there are small bowel strictures patients should be told what foods to avoid (Table 53.2).

The major problem with Crohn's disease is that there is no medical strategy to decrease the risk of recurrent disease. Hence, regular follow-up is required and the physician must be available when relapse occurs (see Fig. 53.1).

Out patient follow-up

Any patient found to have Crohn's disease should have indefinite follow-up—the frequency of clinic visits depending upon disease activity. The minimum need is an appointment every six months. Ideally, there should be a joint medical-surgical clinic.

At each visit the patient should be weighed, and perhaps answer a standard questionnaire about disease activity (Table 53.4). A full blood picture, biochemical profile (looking especially at the serum albumin and alkaline phosphatase), and a measurement of an acute phase protein (C-reactive protein or orosomucoid) provides a screen

Table 53.4. Simple clinical index for Crohn's disease (score 0–25) [24].

General well-being	(0 = very well, 1 = slightly below par, 2 = poor, 3 = very poor, 4 = terrible),
Abdominal pain	(0 = none, 1 = mild, 2 = moderate, 3 = severe).
Number of liquid stools yesterday.	
Abdominal mass	(0 = none, 1 = dubious, 2 = definite, 3 = definite and tender).
Complications	(Arthralgia, uveitis, erythema nodosum, aphthous ulcers, pyoderma gangrenosum, anal fissure, abscess—score 1 per item).

against occult infection or nutritional deficiency [52]. Ideally, even the asymptomatic patient should be re-examined, palpating the abdomen for inflammatory masses, and performing a rectal examination with sigmoidoscopy.

Unless surgery is contemplated or the patient is not responding to medical treatment, repeated X-ray examination of the bowel should be avoided. Otherwise there is a tendency for patients with Crohn's disease to receive a substantial life-time hazard from diagnostic irradiation.

Depression may be a particular problem for the patient with Crohn's disease [26].

Is it inflammation or infection?

When a patient relapses with abdominal pain and tenderness, often associated with fever, there can be a major diagnostic dilemma—it is inflammation or infection? The patient should be admitted to hospital but most routine screening tests (white cell count, platelet count, C-reactive protein, stool and blood cultures) will fail to clarify the differential diagnosis [19, 27, 32].

Three new diagnostic aids may help provide evidence of localized pus—ultrasound, CT scanning of the abdomen [18], and indium labelled leucocyte scans [60, 62].

If doubt remains, there are only two options—either a laparotomy or treatment with antibiotics (for example, ampicillin, netilmicin and metronidazole) with simultaneous or later prednisolone. Such a difficult decision requires close collaboration between surgeon and physician.

Subacute intestinal obstruction

The second major medico-surgical diagnostic dilemma is the patient who presents with recurrent subacute obstruction—episodes of colicky abdominal pain, some abdominal distension with borborygmi, usually relieved by a short burst of diarrhoea. This is a particularly common problem in patients who have either disease of the terminal ileum or a history of small bowel resection.

A barium follow-through may show a narrowed loop of bowel, but it will not distinguish active inflammation from residual fibrosis. If the obstruction is due to inflammation the patient will often have a localized tenderness between attacks, and will have an elevated ESR, platelet count or C-reactive protein [27].

If these markers are positive a trial of steroids is justified, to see if the symptoms resolve as the inflammation recedes. All patients with these symptoms should be on a stricture diet (see Table 53.2).

If steroids fail to resolve the symptoms, or if there is no evidence of inflammation, the patient should be explored surgically—perhaps requiring a strictureplasty rather than resection (see Chapter 54).

Perianal sepsis [75]

Despite an horrifying appearance (Fig. 53.5), perianal sepsis in Crohn's disease is often strangely asymptomatic—pain usually indicates abscess formation with pus under pressure.

Surgeons are now relatively reluctant to

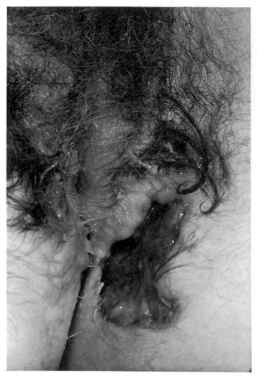

Fig. 53.5. Painless perianal ulceration in Crohn's disease.

operate on perianal Crohn's disease and usually avoid 'cosmetic' operations to tidy-up tags or minor fistulae.

Metronidazole 10–20 mg/kg.day (usually 400 mg three times a day) acts to control anaerobic sepsis and often controls pus formation in the perineum [6, 9]. The disadvantages of the drug are that it causes a metallic taste, has an Antabuse-like reaction with alcohol and, most seriously, can cause a severe peripheral neuropathy characterized by painful parasthesia usually starting in the feet. The latter problem can be severe, and it affected 85% of patients having four to 11 months of continuous treatment with the drug [13].

Perianal inflammation may also be helped by the use of topical corticosteroids—either prednisolone suppositories or hydrocortisone foam.

If sepsis is severe, spreading, or associated with systemic upset, bacteriology swabs and blood cultures should be taken—patients with Crohn's disease are not immune to conventional sepsis with *Staphylococci*, *Streptococci* or *Clostridia*.

Fulminating Crohn's disease [20]

The admission to hospital of a patient profoundly ill with Crohn's disease provides a major diagnostic and management problem. The range of potential complications is so extensive that it is impossible to provide a general management strategy suitable for every patient.

The first priority is to identify all the problems of function and structure (see Table 53.1). How much of the illness is due to inflammation? Is there infection? Is there a surgical problem? Is the patient malnourished? Is there a fistula [17, 29]?

The patient should be observed carefully with daily weights, fluid balance, stool charts and four-hourly nursing observations. Baseline investigations should always include a blood picture and ESR, biochemistry profile, prothrombin time, blood urine and stool cultures, chest and abdominal X-rays, and serum B_{12}, folate and ferritin.

Resuscitation should include rehydration and blood transfusion to maintain a haemoglobin of at least 12 g/dl. If the patient is collapsed and has a history of recent steroid therapy, potential adrenal insufficiency should be covered by immediate intravenous hydrocortisone 200 mg i.v., followed by 100 mg i.v. every eight hours. If infection is suspected it is often necessary to give 'blind antibiotics'—for example, ampicillin 500 mg i.v. six hourly, netilmicin 4–6 mg/kg.day i.v. in three divided doses, and metronidazole 500 mg i.v. eight hourly. If inflammation alone is suspected, prednisolone may be given by mouth if there is no ileus (60 mg/day) or intravenously (prednisolone sodium phosphate 32 mg i.v. 12-hourly). Parenteral feeding should be considered if the patient is malnourished or if no feeding is possible by the enteral route—realizing that such a patient may not only have pre-existing malnutrition, but is also intensely catabolic and may be facing early surgery (see Chapter 78).

Finally, any patient admitted with fulminating Crohn's disease should always be managed jointly by a physician and surgeon—from the time of admission to hospital [17].

Crohn's disease in childhood

Crohn's disease in childhood is essentially the same as in adult life—except that chronic illness will cause growth retardation [8, 21, 41, 59, 73].

Endocrine and metabolic studies have failed to recognize any consistent abnormality in children with Crohn's disease, but recent studies have indicated that inadequate dietary intake is the major cause of growth failure [35]. Numerous approaches have been used to prompt growth by increasing nutritional support—children may need supplementary feeds, naso-enteric feeding, or even parenteral feeding. Attention to the nutritional and growth problems will be focussed by the physician keeping a standard height and weight chart for the child (Fig. 52.23).

Medical treatment is the same as in adults—but corticosteroids are associated with growth retardation. However, children will usually not grow until the disease activity has also been controlled. Hence, the main aims of treatment are to control disease activity and to provide nutritional support. Sulphasalazine is used as in adults, and prednisolone is prescribed sparingly—an alternate day regimen should be used if at all possible. Perianal disease behaves much as in an adult patient with Crohn's disease [44].

The prognosis of children with Crohn's disease is usually good, although it is a disorder of high morbidity and excess mortality—especially if there is diffuse disease of the small intestine [15, 54].

Crohn's disease and pregnancy [12]

Patients who have active Crohn's disease should be advised to delay conception as their disease is likely to remain active during the pregnancy. For patients with inactive disease, however, there appears to be little risk to either the course of the pregnancy or the Crohn's disease itself [7]. If patients require treatment for Crohn's disease during pregnancy, both sulphasalazine and corticosteroids may be prescribed safely [14, 33, 71]. Sulphasalazine may be given late in pregnancy and during breast feeding—there is no risk of kernicterus [30].

References

1 ALLISON MC, POUNDER RE. Cyclosporin for Crohn's disease. *Lancet* 1984;i:1242.

2 ALUN JONES V, DICKINSON RJ, WORKMAN E, WILSON AJ, FREEMAN AH, HUNTER JO. Crohn's disease: maintenance of remission by diet. *Lancet* 1985;ii:177–180.

3 AMBROSE NS, ALLAN RN, KEIGHLEY MRB, *et al.* Antibiotic therapy for treatment in relapse of intestinal Crohn's disease: a prospective randomized study. *Dis Colon Rectum* 1985;28:81–85.

4 BANKS PA, PRESENT DH, STEINER P (eds). *The Crohn's Disease and Ulcerative Colitis Fact Book.* New York: Scribers 1983.

5 BENGOA JM, ROSENBERG IH. Parenteral nutrition therapy in gastrointestinal disease. *Ann Intern Med* 1983;28:363–385.

6 BERSTEIN LH, FRANK MS, BRANDT LJ, BOLEY SJ. Healing perineal Crohn's disease with metronidazole. *Gastroenterology* 1980;79:357–365.

7 BIAOCCO PJ, KORELITZ BI. The influence of inflammatory bowel disease on pregnancy and fetal outome. *J Clin Gastroenterol* 1984;6:211–216.

8 BOOTH IW, HARRIES JT. Inflammatory bowel disease in childhood. *Gut* 1984;25:188–202.

9 BRANDT LJ, BERNSTEIN LH, BOLEY SJ, FRANK MS. Metronidazole therapy for perianal Crohn's disease: a follow-up study. *Gastroenterology* 1982;83:383–387.

10 COOKE WT, MALLAS E, PRIOR P, ALLAN RN. Crohn's disease: course, treatment and long-term prognosis. *Q J Med* 1980;195:363–384.

11 DIBBLE JB, SHERIDAN P. LOSOWSKY MS. A survey of vitamin D deficiency in gastrointestinal and liver disorders. *Q J Med* 1984;**53**:119–134.

12 DONALDSON RM. Management of medical problems in pregnancy—inflammatory bowel disease. *N Engl J Med* 1985;**312**:1616–1618.

13 DUFFY LF, DAUM F, FISHER SE, *et al.* Peripheral neuropathy in Crohn's disease patients treated with metronidazole. *Gastroenterology* 1985;**88**:681–684.

14 FIELDING JF. Pregnancy and inflammatory bowel disease. *J Clin Gastroenterol* 1983;**5**:107–108.

15 GAZZARD BG. Long-term prognosis of Crohn's disease with onset in childhood and adolescence. *Gut* 1984;**25**:325–328.

16 GAZZARD BG, PRICE HL, LIBBY GW, DAWSON AM. The social toll of Crohn's disease. *Br Med J* 1978;**2**:1117–1119.

17 GLASS RE, RITCHIE JK, LENNARD-JONES JE, HAWLEY PR, TODD IP. Internal fistulas in Crohn's disease. *Dis Colon Rectum* 1985;**28**:557–561.

18 GORE RM, COHEN MI, VOGELZANG RL, HARVEY MD, NEIMAN L, TSANG T-K. Value of computed tomography in the detection of complications of Crohn's disease. *Dig Dis Sci* 1985;**30**:701–709.

19 GREENSTEIN AJ, BACHAR DB, LOWENTHAL D, GOLDOFSKY E, AUFSES AH. Pyogenic liver abscess in Crohn's disease. *Q J Med* 1985;**220**:505–518.

20 GREENSTEIN AJ, SACHAR DB, GIBAS A, *et al.* Outcome of toxic dilatation in ulcerative and Crohn's colitis. *J Clin Gastroenterol* 1985;**7**:137–144.

21 GRYBOWSKI JD, SPIRO HM. Long-term prognosis in Crohn's disease in children. *Gastroenterology* 1978;**74**:807–813.

22 HARRIES AD, HEATLEY RV. Nutritional disturbances in Crohn's disease. *Postgrad Med J* 1983;**59**:690–697.

23 HARRIES AD *et al.* Controlled trial of supplemental oral nutrition in Crohn's disease. *Lancet* 1983;**i**:887–890.

24 HARVEY RF, BRADSHAW JM. A simple index of Crohn's disease activity. *Lancet* 1980;**i**:514.

25 HEATON KW, THORNTON JR, EMMETT PM. Treatment of Crohn's disease with an unrefined-carbohydrate, fibre-rich diet. *Br Med J* 1979;**2**:764–766.

26 HELZER JE, CHAMMAS S, NORLAND CC, STILLINGS WA, ALPERS DH. A study of the association between Crohn's disease and psychiatric illness. *Gastroenterology* 1984;**86**:324–330.

27 HODGSON HJF. Assessment of drug therapy in inflammatory bowel disease. *Br J Clin Pharmacol* 1982;**14**:159–170.

28 JACOBSEN O, HOJGAARD L, MOLLER EH, *et al.* Effect of enterocoated cholestyramine on bowel habit after ileal resection: a double blind crossover study. *Br Med J* 1985;**290**:1315–1318.

29 JACOBSON IM, SCHAPIRO RH, WARSHAW AL. Gastric and duodenal fistulas in Crohn's disease. *Gastroenterology* 1985;**89**:1347–1352.

30 JARNEROT G, INTO-MALMBERG MB. Sulphasalazine treatment during breast feeding. *Scand J Gastroenterol* 1979;**14**:896–872.

31 JONES VA, DICKINSON RJ, WORKMAN E, WILSON AJ, FREEMAN AH, HUNTER JO. Crohn's disease: maintenance of remission by diet. *Lancet* 1985;**ii**:177–179.

32 JOSEPH AEA. Imaging of abdominal abscesses. *Br Med J* 1985;**291**:1446–1447.

33 KHOSLA R, WILLOUGHBY CP. Jewell DP. Crohn's disease and pregnancy. *Gut* 1984;**25**:52–56.

34 KINLEN LJ, SHEIL AGR, PETO J, DOLL R. Collaborative United Kingdom-Australasian study of cancer in patients treated with immunosuppressive drugs. *Br Med J* 1979;**2**:1461–1466.

35 KIRSCHNER BS, KLICH JR, KALMAN SS, DE PAVARO MV, ROSENBERG NH. Reversal of growth retardation in Crohn's disease with therapy emphasising oral nutritional restitution. *Gastroenterology* 1981;**80**:10–15.

36 LEADING ARTICLE. Conservative measures in Crohn's disease. *Lancet* 1983;**ii**:831–832.

37 LENNARD-JONES JE. Toward optimal use of corticosteroids in ulcerative colitis and Crohn's disease. *Gut* 1983;**24**:177–181.

38 LENNARD-JONES JE, SINGLETON JE. Azathioprine and 6-mercaptopurine have a role in the treatment of Crohn's disease. *Dig Dis Sci* 1981;**26**:364–371.

39 LEVENSTEIN S, PANTERA C, LUZI C, D'UBALDI. Low residue or normal diet in Crohn's disease: a prospective controlled study in Italian patients. *Gut* 1985;**26**:994–998.

40 LEVI AJ. Diet in the management of Crohn's disease. *Gut* 1985;**26**:985–993.

41 MCNEISH, HUGHES CA. Crohn's disease in childhood. In: Allen RN, Keighley MRB, Alexander-Williams J, Hawkins C, eds. *Inflammatory Bowel Diseases*. Edinburgh: Churchill Livingstone, 1983;338–342.

42 MAIN ANH, MILLS PR, RUSSELL RI, *et al.* Vitamin A deficiency in Crohn's disease. *Gut* 1983;**24**:1169–1175.

43 MALCHOW H, EWE K, BRANDES JW, *et al.* European Cooperative Crohn's Disease Study: results of drug treatment. *Gastroenterology* 1984;**86**:249–266.

44 MARKOWITZ J, DAUN F, AIGES H, KAHN E, SILVERBERG M, FISHER SE. Perianal disease in children and adolescents with Crohn's disease. *Gastroenterology* 1984;**86**:829–833.

45 MOTIL KJ, GRAND RJ. Nutritional management of inflammatory bowel disease. *Pediatr Clin North Am* 1985;**32**:447–469.

46 MÜLLER JM *et al.* Total parenteral nutrition as the sole therapy in Crohn's disease—a prospective study. *Br J Surg* 1983;**70**:40–43.

47 O'DONOGHUE DP, DAWSON AM, POWELL-TUCK J, BOWN RL, LENNARD-JONES JE. Double-blind withdrawal trial of azathioprine as maintenance treatment for Crohn's disease. *Lancet* 1978;**ii**:955–957.

48 O'MORAIN C, SEGAL AW, LEVI AJ. Elemental diet as primary treatment of acute Crohn's disease: a controlled trial. *Br Med J* 1984;**288**:1859–1860.

49 PALMER KR, PATIL DH, BASRAN GS, RIORDAN JF, SILK DBA. Abdominal tuberculosis in urban Britain—a common disease. *Gut* 1985;**26**:1296–1305.

50 PENNY WJ, MAYBERRY JF, AGGETT PJ, GILBERT JO, NEWCOMBE RG, RHODES J. Relationship between trace elements, sugar consumption and taste in Crohn's disease. *Gut* 1983;**24**:288–292.

51 PEPPERCORN, M. Sulphasalazine. Pharmacology, clinical use, toxicity and related new drug development. *Ann Intern Med* 1984;**101**:377–386.

52 PETTIT SH, HOLBROOK IB, IRVING MH. Comparison of clinical scores and acute phase proteins in the assessment of acute Crohn's disease. *Br J Surg* 1985;**72**:1013–1016.

53 PRESENT DH, KOVELITZ BI, WISCH N, *et al.* Treatment of Crohn's disease with 6-mercaptopurine: a long-term randomized double blind study. *N Engl J Med* 1980;**302**:981–987.

54 PUNTIS J, MCNEISH AS, ALLAN RN. Long-term prognosis of Crohn's disease with onset in childhood and adolescence. *Gut* 1984;**25**:329–336.

55 RHODES J, BAINTON D, BECK P, CAMPBELL H. Controlled trial of azathioprine in Crohn's disease. *Lancet* 1971;**ii**:1273–1276.

56 RHODES J, ROSE J. Does food affect inflammatory bowel disease? The role of parenteral nutrition, elemental and exclusion diets. *Gut* 1986;**27**:471–474.

57 ROSENBERG IH, BENGOA JM, SITRIN MD. Nutritional aspects of inflammatory bowel disease. *Annu Rev Nutr* 1985;**5**:463–484.

58 ROSENBERG IH, BOWMAN BB. Diet and nutritional therapy in Crohn's disease. In: Allan RN, Keighley MRB, Alexander-Williams J, Hawkins C, eds. *Inflammatory bowel diseases.* Edinburgh: Churchill Livingstone, 1983;434–44.

59 ROSENTHAL S, SNYDER JD, HENDRICKS K, WALTER MA. Growth failure and inflammatory bowel disease. *Paediatrics* 1983;**72**:481–490.

60 SAVERYMUTTU SH, CAMILLERI M, REES H, *et al.* Indium ^{111}-granulocyte scanning in the assessment of disease extent and disease activity in inflammatory bowel disease. *Gastroenterology* 1986;**90**:1121–1128.

61 SAVERYMUTTU S, HODGSON HJF, CHADWICK VS. Controlled trial comparing prednisolone with an elemental diet plus non-absorbable antibiotics in active Crohn's disease. *Gut* 1985;**26**:994–8.

62 SAVERYMUTTU SH, PETERS AM, CROFTON ME, *et al.* ^{111}Indium autologous granulocytes in the detection of inflammatory bowel disease. *Gut* 1985;**26**:955–960.

63 SCHOFIELD PF. Abdominal tuberculosis. *Gut* 1985;**26**:1275–1278.

64 SHAFFER JA, WILLIAMS SE, TURNBERG LA, HOUSTON JB, ROWLAND M. Absorption of prednisolone in patients with Crohn's disease. *Gut* 1983;**24**:182–186.

65 SMITH RC, RHODES J, HEATLEY RV, *et al.* Low dose steroids and clinical relapse in Crohn's disease: a controlled trial. *Gut* 1978;**19**:606–610.

66 STEIGER E, SRP F. Morbidity and mortality related to home parenteral nutrition in patients with gut failure. *Am J Surg* 1983;**145**:102–105.

67 SUMMERS RW, SWITZ DN, SESSIONS JT, *et al.* National cooperative Crohn's disease study: results of drug treatment. *Gastroenterology* 1979;**77**:847–869.

68 TAFFET SL, DAS KM. Sulfasalazine: adverse effects and desensitization. *Dig Dis Sci* 1983;**28**:833–842.

69 THORNTON JR, EMMETT PM, HEATON KW. Diet and Crohn's disease: characteristics of the pre-illness diet. *Br Med J* 1979;**2**:762–764.

70 URSING B, ALM T, BARANY F, *et al.* A comparative study of metronidazole and sulphasalazine for active Crohn's disease: the cooperative Crohn's disease study in Sweden. II Result. *Gastroenterology* 1982;**83**:550–562.

71 VENDER RJ, SPIRO HM. Inflammatory bowel disease and pregnancy. *J Clin Gastroenterol* 1982;**4**:231–249.

72 WENKERT A, KIRSTENSEN M, EKLAND AE, *et al.* The long-term prophylactic effect of salazosulphapyridine (Salazopyrin) in primarily resected patients with Crohn's disease. *Scand J Gastroenterol* 1978;**13**:161–167.

73 WHITTINGTON PF, BARNES HV, BAYLESS TMB. Medical management of Crohn's disease in adolescence. *Gastroenterology* 1977;**72**:1338–1344.

74 WILLOUGHBY JMT, KUMAR PJ, BECKETT J, DAWSON AM. Controlled trial of azathioprine in Crohn's disease. *Lancet* 1971;**ii**:944–947.

75 WOLFF BG, CULP CE, BEART RW, ILSTRUP DM, READY RL. Anorectal Crohn's disease. *Dis Colon Rectum* 1985;**28**:709–711.

76 WORKMAN EM, ALLAN JONES V, WILSON AJ, HUNTER JO. Diet in the management of Crohn's disease. *Hum Nutr Appl Nutr* 1984;**38A**:469–473.

77 WRIGHT JP, MEE AS, PARAFITT A, *et al.* Vitamin A therapy in patients with Crohn's disease. *Gastroenterology* 1985;**88**:512–514.

Chapter 54
Surgical Management of Crohn's Disease

B. N. BROOKE

The original concept of the disease described in 1932 by Crohn, Ginzberg and Oppenheimer [13] was of localized inflammation confined to the terminal ileum. This 'new' condition came into existence as a differential diagnosis, or even a derivative, of ileocaecal tuberculosis. It is hardly surprising therefore that surgery dominated treatment at the outset—limited resection appeared to be all that was required to eradicate the disease, and this could be undertaken with ease and without eliciting the complications experienced following operation for tuberculous disease.

So it was that Crohn and his colleagues were able to state 'Medical treatment is purely palliative and supportive ... but in general the proper approach to complete cure is by surgical resection ...'. Thirty years were to elapse before experience of the progress and the natural history of the disease began to bring about a more guarded approach, and to reveal the expectation of surgical cure to be false. Two observations have brought this about— firstly, the almost inevitable recurrence of the disease following resection; secondly, the realization that the disease is not limited to ileum, nor even to the small bowel generally, but that the whole of the alimentary tract is at risk. Moreover, neither a cause, nor a cure, has yet been found for Crohn's disease.

The surgical stance is now one of reluctance—operation is withheld as a last resort when all else has failed to achieve palliation or support. Within this overriding assumption the indications for surgery are numerous and the range of operations is wide. In general, operation may be undertaken in an emergency, for palliation of symptoms, to excise malignancy, to establish a diagnosis, or for perianal disease [42].

Indications for surgery

Emergency surgery

Free perforation can occur from small or large intestine; it is rare, developing in approximately 2% of hospital series [11, 19]. The perforation usually occurs at a site of chronic but active disease, sometimes in association with distal stenosis. It is not a complication of acute ileitis.

Acute severe **haemorrhage** necessitating urgent operation is rarer (circa 1%). Bleeding may come not only from either the small or large intestine, but also from the stomach. Simple manoeuvres, such as suture for perforation and underrunning of bleeding points, are ineffective. The choice has to be made between resection for small intestinal sites, resection or colectomy for the colon, and in the stomach either wedge excision or pylorectomy depending upon the site of the lesion [52].

Fulminating colitis is rather more common, but it is still quite rare [20, 47]. The X-ray appearances of colonic dilatation calls for emergency primary colectomy. The evidence of predilatation, demonstrable in ulcerative colitis by the presence of mucosal islands to be seen on the straight abdominal X-ray, cannot be guaranteed in Crohn's colitis. Subsequently an elective operation will be required either to restore intestinal continuity and eliminate the ileostomy, if the state of the rectum proves satisfactory, or to remove the rectum if not.

Subacute obstruction due to stenosis from the disease itself is not a reason for emergency operation. The episode will usually subside on bed rest, electrolyte repletion (potassium in particular) and nasogastric suction [48]. Surgery can usually be postponed to an elective period when a more deliberate operation may be performed.

There is however one special circumstance—sometimes a Crohn's patient can return with **complete obstruction** due to an adhesive band formed as a result of an earlier operation. In a patient, therefore, with an abdominal scar a careful history must be taken to differentiate the two conditions. The sudden onset of colic or continuous abdominal pain calls for an immediate laparotomy; when obstruction is due to Crohn's disease recent attacks of colic can almost always be elicited from the history, since the development of stenosis and obstruction are usually gradual.

Elective surgery—palliation of symptoms

Any one of the major symptoms (**diarrhoea, abdominal pain** or **weight loss**) may be a sufficient indication for surgery when the disability caused thereby is intolerable and uncontrolled by medical means. Indeed, any of the protean forms of clinical manifestation of the disease, either singly or in combination, may prove sufficiently disabling to require removal or exclusion of a major area of activity, although exclusion is very much a matter of last resort and is only defensible for duodenal disease by gastroenterostomy or for severe colitis by ileostomy [25].

The yardstick by which the need for surgery is measured in each circumstance, whether it be malabsorption or malnutrition, or anaemia, or intestinal obstruction, can only be the degree of persistent, unrelieved disability; the degree is best judged by the limitation placed on daily life—work and recreation.

There are two added factors in the young—**retardation of growth** or delayed puberty, and **interference with education.** These added considerations may call for resection of, say, a small intestinal lesion at an earlier stage than would be appropriate in an adult, since a child's percentiles of development may never return to normal if maturation arrest is allowed to persist. Loss of educational opportunity may similarly never be regained, so that resection can be justified in order to obtain a breathing-space free from symptoms during the educational period.

Disability arising from **diarrhoea** is not difficult to assess, the frequency of stool and degree of precipitancy being the indicators. Surgical excision, particularly of the terminal ileum and ascending colon is, however, often followed by a tendency to diarrhoea.

It is important to ascertain the exact nature of **abdominal pain**. The commonest type of abdominal pain arises on taking food, which appears to bring about reflex pain from an inflamed ileum; this symptom also accounts for **weight loss** in the early stages because the patient desists from eating in order to avoid the pain or obtain relief. It may be mildly colicky but unlike the obstructive symptom it does not persist. Since bed-rest and codeine phosphate bring about relief, this reflex pain is not an indication for surgery.

Chronic **small bowel obstruction** usually does demand surgical intervention, although obstructive symptoms during a recrudescence can subside in remission and not recur (Fig. 54.1). If there are no markers of active inflammation (the white cell and platelet counts, the ESR, the C-reactive protein being normal) [31, 49] then the ob-

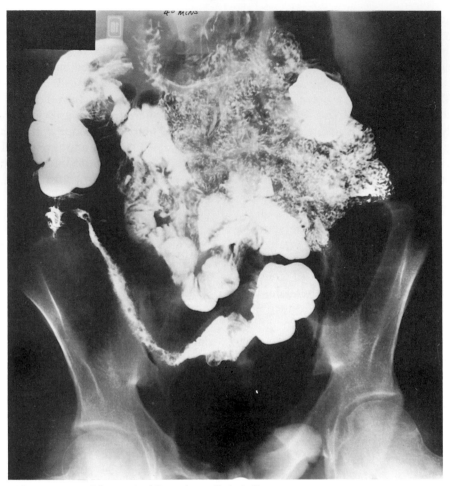

Fig. 54.1. A long stricture of the terminal ileum due to Crohn's disease.

struction is probably mechanical rather than inflammatory, and unlikely to respond to medical treatment (see Chapter 53). Obstructive symptoms should therefore be persistent or recurrent before the decision is made to resect the area of stricture. Obstruction may also complicate a duodenal lesion—usually in the second part—and present with repeated vomiting, when bypass by gastroenterostomy is all that can feasibly be undertaken.

Obstruction may not be confined to the intestine. Due to anatomical juxtaposition, the right ureter is at risk from an ileal lesion. Although the suggested incidence of

25% for ureteric obstruction [7] may be too high, it is certainly sufficiently common to warrant consideration in the routine management of a new patient; to await the symptoms of **obstructive uropathy**—the pain which may be caused by hydronephrosis or pyelonephritis—is to wait too long. The state of the ureter should be ascertained by ultrasound examination (and not by IVP in order to avoid increasing the dosage of investigative X-irradiation) as soon as an ileal lesion has been established. Ultrasound should be repeated at regular two-yearly intervals, for a stricture can develop in the granulation tissue around the ureter, even during a prolonged period of quiescence of the intestinal lesion which initiated the process. At the first hint of ureteric dilatation radiological studies can be undertaken to expose the situation more clearly. Persistent ureteric obstruction is an absolute indication for resection of the ileal lesion together with release of the ureter from its bed of chronic granulation tissue. If surgery is delayed it may prove necessary to excise the ureteric stricture and reimplant the ureter into the bladder.

Yet another cause of abdominal pain necessitating resection is **dyspareunia,** due to pressure during intercourse either through the abdominal wall upon a tender loop, or impingement *per vaginum* upon an ileal lesion in the pelvis [8]. Dyspareunia may also result from the anterior extension of an anal fistula towards the vulva.

Loss of weight may become a predominant indication for operation when the loss is progressive despite all forms of medical treatment, all the more so since this may be due to an undisclosed **enteroenteric fistula.** Enterocutaneous, enteroenteric and enterovesical fistulae develop in up to a quarter of all patients [1,62,63]; they are unlikely to remit either on their own accord or with the inducement of drugs, though an occasional enterocutaneous fistula will close during azathioprine therapy. Not every enteroenteric fistula is necessarily a cause of trouble; nevertheless the demonstration of such fistulae may require resection, particularly when the duodenum becomes involved. Malabsorption due to a diffusely diseased intestine may become compounded by the 'blind-loop' effect.

An enterovesical fistula, nearly always from the ileum but sometimes with the sigmoid included, is an absolute indication for bowel resection with wedge excision of the fistulous orifice in the bladder [13, 44, 50].

Enterocutaneous fistulae are more commonly present after laparotomy and other abdominal surgical manoeuvres in Crohn's

disease [9, 26, 34, 37, 44]. Not infrequently, they present as an abscess pointing on the abdominal wall, necessitating incision if drainage does not occur naturally. It should be borne in mind that any intra-abdominal abscess in association with Crohn's disease will almost certainly form a fistula even though gut contents may not discharge immediately; therefore, it is wise when drainage is undertaken to warn the patient that intestinal contents may be observed subsequently.

Malignancy

It is becoming evident that cancer is an increased hazard of long-standing inflammation whatever the site in the gut [23]. Thus the risk of intestinal cancer is greater in Crohn's patients than in the normal population [24, 58]. In contrast to the situation in ulcerative colitis, this ubiquity defies 'prophylactic' resection or excision. In a group of 440 patients with Crohn's disease there was a twenty-fold increase in malignancy [61]. About a third of the cases occurred in the large bowel, probably reflecting the incidence of Crohn's disease at this site. The association is more marked in excluded loops and at fistula sites [21, 51].

While there is a clear indication to avoid bypass operations, a more positive indication for prophylactic resection or excision is difficult to establish. Nevertheless dysplasia does develop in Crohn's disease as in ulcerative colitis [24, 51], and therefore may be sought in the large intestine in Crohn's colitis in the same way, with the same definite indication for panproctocolectomy on obtaining a positive specimen. The possibility that cancer may develop should be borne in mind when surgical treatment is contemplated for other reasons.

Diagnosis

It is odd that in Crohn's original paper recognition was given to the fact that intestinal lymphoma, lymphosarcoma and intestinal tuberculosis may simulate Crohn's disease, and that differentiation may only be possible on the operating table [13]—yet the need to establish the diagnosis has seldom been proposed as a prime reason for surgical intervention. It may not be possible to establish the diagnosis in any other way—for example, the diagnosis of Crohn's disease in an Asian immigrant, particularly from the Indian continent, should be entertained with scepticism until ileocaecal tuberculosis has been excluded by laparoscopy or laparotomy [56].

In the reverse sense, the abdomen may be opened on a misdiagnosis and what appears to be a Crohn's lesion is found; urgent reassessment as regards to what operation should be undertaken, if any, has then to be made. The example *par excellence* is the discovery of acute ileitis at an emergency operation undertaken for supposed acute appendicitis. This ileitis may be due to Crohn's disease or a specific infection such as *Yersinia enterocolitica*. Yersinial infection is self-limiting or may be brought under control by an antibiotic (see Chapter 57); Crohn's disease is affected in neither way. It is therefore important, in prognostic terms, to establish the diagnosis. The diagnosis of *Yersinia* ileitis can be achieved by culturing the bacteria from the appendix, which should be removed so that half the specimen can be placed in a sterile container for that purpose. In addition antibody titres can be assessed from samples of serum. The fear that 'when ileitis is due to Crohn's disease appendicectomy may lead to fistula' is misconceived; a fistula may develop, as it can after any laparotomy in Crohn's disease, not however from the appendix stump but from disturbance to the lesion itself. If inflammation extends into the caecum, appendicectomy need not and should not be undertaken, since this is a feature of Crohn's disease and not of a yersinial infection or acute appendicitis.

Perianal disease [10, 30, 45, 65]

The surgical approach to perianal disease is more conservative. Because incisions into the perianal skin fail to heal in the presence of active Crohn's disease, excision of fistulae and removal of piles in the form of perianal skin tags must be avoided. Positive indications for surgery are therefore limited to incisions to drain perianal abscesses, and to dilatation of anal strictures.

Anal lesions affect approximately 50% of those with disease limited to the small intestine and 100% of those with rectal involvement [43]. The most common manifestation is slowly **spreading fistulation** with numerous external orifices and a tendency to track forwards exposing new openings *en route*, to involve the base of the scrotum or the vulva. The development of **perianal abscess** heralds a fistula; incision may be required to drain the abscess. If so, the patient should be warned that a persistent discharge will probably ensue; each new orifice presents similarly. Dyspareunia will be experienced by women with abscesses developing in the vicinity of the posterior fornix or in relation to the vagina further anteriorly; usually release of pus will bring relief, sometimes complete, otherwise reliance has to be placed on the use of metronidazole after drainage has been achieved [15].

In association with this common indolent multiple track type of fistula there is a tendency for an **anal stricture** to form at the internal orifice in relation to the anorectal ring. This requires dilation not only because of the difficulty it sometimes causes with effective defecation, but also because it often causes incontinence and soiling—partly through interference with sphincteric action and partly because any fistulous track bypassing the stricture tends to discharge faeces. Initially dilatation has to be performed under general anaesthesia but it can be repeated thereafter in the clinic, using 4% lignocaine jelly at monthly intervals at first, extending to three or six months as seems appropriate.

There is a more acute form of fistulation in which multiple external orifices develop simultaneously; the fistulous tracks are less indurated and present a 'watering can' appearance. Abscesses seldom form or require drainage; this type of perianal disease usually responds well to azathioprine.

Surgery has no place in the two remaining lesions—**perianal skin infiltration** and the **deep anal ulceration** associated with large oedematous skin tags which sometimes resemble anal carcinoma (Fig. 53.5). These ulcers are less painful and disabling than would seem probable at first sight; they are often found in association with severe rectal disease when abscesses may form in the perirectal space which, on discharge in the perineum, form persistent high rectal fistulae. At this stage rectal excision—and possibly total removal of the large bowel—becomes inevitable.

Infiltration of the perianal skin by the disease itself may eventually lead to **widespread ulceration**. In an advanced case the perineum can become denuded of skin, the process spreading even into the groins. This condition demands radical surgery to deflect the faecal stream, probably via an ileostomy associated with colectomy, since widespread metastatic disease that affects the perineum in this way is closely associated with large bowel disease.

Types of operation

It may be taken as a general principle that, when resection becomes inevitable in Crohn's disease, this should be limited. As much intestine as possible must be conserved, not only because function may be impaired throughout the intestine as a result of the disease even in areas not obviously abnormal, but also as further resections may be necessary in the future. For example, where the intestine is affected by skip lesions it is preferable to undertake multiple resections rather than resection of all the lesions together in one piece. In addition anastomoses should be sutured in continuity; the temptation to undertake end-to-side anastomosis should be resisted since this inevitably results in a blind-end thus increasing the liability to malabsorption with steatorrhoea.

By-pass surgery

With the one exception (gastroenterostomy for an active duodenal lesion or a stricture caused thereby) there is no place for the easier option of by-pass, whether by exclusion or in continuity, since recurrence occurs more frequently and sooner after by-pass than resection, soonest after by-pass in continuity [18, 32]. For the rare gastric lesion, pylorectomy or wedge resection may suffice depending upon the site and extent of the lesion, extending to partial gastrectomy if need be.

Fistula

Many enteroenteric fistulae are removed *in toto* within the phlegmonous mass, but not all. An ileo-sigmoid fistula is a not uncommon occurrence resulting from juxtaposition of active ileal lesion with a previously unaffected sigmoid; it poses the problem of whether sigmoid resection is required in addition to ileal resection. The decision must depend upon the degree to which the sigmoid has become incorporated in the active lesion; it is, however, often possible to detach the sigmoid connection, excise the sigmoid opening and resuture the resulting defect. The vesical end of an enterovesical fistula has to be dealt with in this way, the integrity of the bladder suture line being protected by a postoperative indwelling catheter. Gastric or duodenal fistulae usually involve disease in the lower bowel and respond to simple excision [35].

Colectomy

When Crohn's colitis is limited, a resection of the diseased colon alone may be adequate. Often the ileocaecal junction and ascending colon, in part or in whole, will be incorporated in a resection undertaken primarily for ileitis, because the disease frequently spills over from the ileum into the right colon. Similarly, total colitis in which the rectum is spared—a not infrequent occurrence—allows for colectomy and successful ileorectal anastomosis [5].

With rectal involvement the decision to undertake panproctocolectomy and permanent ileostomy is not difficult. When, however, there is marked rectal disease but the colon above is spared except for an area of proximal activity involving the right colon, a difficult choice has to be made between a colostomy with resection of the proximal lesion in order to conserve the normal transverse colon, and ileostomy with panproctocolectomy. It is then helpful to bear in mind that recurrence is likely in the intervening colon, and that the soft stool from a colostomy is more difficult to manage and control than the fluid effluent of an ileostomy.

Ileostomy (see Chapter 55)

Ileostomy alone has a definite place in a sick patient with malnutrition and intra-abdominal complications likely to render removal of the bowel hazardous. Under such circumstances deflection of the faecal stream alone can be life-saving, and in addition can restore the patient ultimately to normal weight.

A 'split' ileostomy, involving a simple loop rather than an end stoma, has been advocated for a particular purpose—to provide a vent for the topical application of steroids to the colon [25, 59]. No evidence is forthcoming that any greater advantage accrues from this than from a simple deflection of the faecal stream by an end ileostomy. The institution of a split ileostomy in order to instil steroids is therefore of doubtful use, moreover, adaptation of an appliance to a loop is less satisfactory.

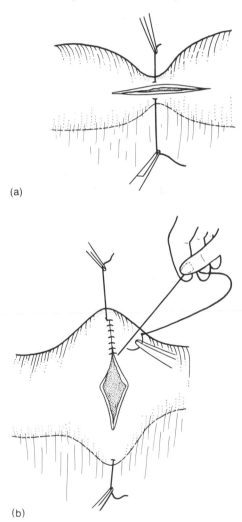

(a)

(b)

Fig. 54.2 Technique of strictureplasty. After cutting through the stricture longitudinally (a), the opening is closed transversely (b).

Strictureplasty (see Fig. 54.2)

An important development is the relief of obstruction by simple division of a short segment stricture in the small bowel and transverse suture–strictureplasty [2, 4, 16, 39]. Lee advocated local bypass around short strictures where disease is still active and where there is thickening of the intestinal wall; he emphasized that the aim of surgical cure of Crohn's disease has gone— surgery is simply to correct a specific complication [38]. Multiple intestinal strictures can be managed by operative dilatation [3].

Complications [27]

There are three surgical complications that are special to Crohn's disease. The formation of an **intestinal fistula** is a particular risk in the immediate postoperative period [9, 17]; this may occur after simple laparotomy without any other procedure. Further surgery may ultimately be required but an expectant attitude should be taken at the outset; azathioprine can be helpful. A review of 114 patients with enterocutaneous fistulae from St Mark's Hospital, London, reported a healing rate of 90.9% and a mortality of 5.3%, using a combined programme of nursing, medical and surgical care [44].

A **persistent perineal sinus** is common after rectal exicision; it can be resistant to treatment with a variety of local applications, to cauterization or to excision of the sinus with surrounding scar tissue [6, 33, 40]. Recently success has been claimed by filling the cavity with a gracilis–cutaneous flap turned up from the thigh after excision of granulations and scar tissue [54].

Recurrent disease may involve a stoma even years after its institution (see Chapter 55). Recurrence at an ileostomy may take the form of ulceration, a granulomatous exuberance, a stricture causing obstruction, or a fistula. Rarely ulceration of the peris-

tomal skin can develop as a manifestation of the disease in the same way that it may affect the perianal area.

Prognosis (also see Chapter 52)

Mortality

The crude mortality related to Crohn's disease is 7% [50]. The mortality risk from all causes in Crohn's disease appears to be increased two- to four-fold compared with matched groups of the general population—an assessment extracted from a review of 382 cases treated in Leeds from 1938 and 1968 [14], 303 in Oxford from 1938–1970 [60] and 513 in Birmingham from 1941–1976 [50]. Certain differences obtain in each group—at Leeds the relative risk of dying tended to increase with age; at Oxford it remained doubled throughout 15 years follow-up—at Birmingham the risk fell with increasing age, the risk of dying being increased twelve-fold under the age of 20.

It is difficult to obtain a clear picture of the relation of surgery to the mortality of the disease and, its risk, this difficulty being compounded by confusion between operative and patient mortality [14]. No specific reference to surgical mortality is forthcoming from Oxford or Birmingham. Of 112 patients under the author's care from 1963 to 1975 in London, 79 had 116 operations: 3 died postoperatively—an operative mortality of 2.6% and a patient mortality of 3.8% [9].

Recurrence

As with mortality, it is difficult to obtain exact figures of recurrence following surgery [12, 55, 64]. This difficulty is partly because recurrence necessitating operation is not always clearly distinguished from symptomatic recurrence. Recurrence rates are a function of the length of follow-up:

Lennard-Jones and Stadler [41] reported cumulative reoperation rates of 16% at five years and 26% at 10; from Aberdeen the relative figures were 30% and 33% respectively [36], with similar figures from Birmingham [29].

In a study from Belgium, recurrence one to 10 years after ileocolonic anastomosis ranged from 72 to 99%—recurrences apparently developing within one year of surgery [53]. The cumulative probability of reoperation is around 80% at 20 years after first and second resections [35]. The recurrence rate remains unaffected by the number of previous resections; it is highest after bypass. After an initial resection chances are even that a further resection will be required within 15 years; a patient first operated upon when 25-years-old may expect two to three further resections during his or her lifetime, usually for recurrences at the anastomosis [29].

The recurrence rate of Crohn's disease at the site of an anastomosis is independent of microscopical disease at the resection margin, hence it is now recommended that surgical resection should be limited to areas of macroscopic disease [28].

References

1 ALEXANDER-WILLIAMS J. Surgery and management of Crohn's disease. *Clin Gastroenterol* 1972;1:469–491.

2 ALEXANDER-WILLIAMS J. The technique of intestinal strictureplasty. *Int J Colorect Dis* 1986;1:54–57.

3 ALEXANDER-WILLIAMS J, ALLAN A, MOREL P, HAWKER PC, DYKES PW, O'CONNOR H. The therapeutic dilatation of enteric strictures due to Crohn's disease. *Ann Roy Coll Surg Engl* 1986;68:95–97.

4 ALEXANDER-WILLIAMS J, HAYNES IG. Conservative operations for Crohn's disease of the small bowel. *World J Surg* 1985;9:945–951.

5 AMBROSE NS, ALEXANDER-WILLIAMS J, KEIGHLEY MRB. Audit of sepsis in operations for inflammatory bowel disease. *Dis Colon Rectum* 1984a;27:602–604.

6 AMBROSE NS, KEIGHLEY MRB, ALEXANDER-WILLIAMS J, ALLAN RN. Clinical impact of colec-

tomy and ileorectal anastomosis in the management of Crohn's disease. *Gut* 1984b;25:223–227.

7 BLOCK GE, ENKER WE, KIRSNER JB. Significance and treatment of occult obstructive uropathy complicating Crohn's disease. *Ann Surg* 1973;178:322–333.

8 BROOKE BN. Dyspareunia; a significant symptom of Crohn's disease. *Lancet* 1979;i:1199.

9 BROOKE BN, CAVE DR, GURRY JF, KING DW. *Crohn's disease.* London: Macmillan, 1977.

10 BUCHMANN P, KEIGHLEY MRB, J, ALLAN RN, THOMPSON H, ALEXANDER-WILLIAMS J. Natural history of perianal Crohn's disease. A 10 year follow-up: a plea for conservation. *Am J Surg* 1980;140:642–644.

11 BUNDRED NJ, DIXON JM, LUMSDEN AB, GILMOUR HM, DAVIES GC. Free perforation in Crohn's colitis: a ten year review. *Dis Colon Rectum* 1985;28:35–37.

12 COOPER JC, WILLIAMS NS. The influence of microscopic disease at the margin of resection on recurrence rates in Crohn's disease. *Ann Roy Coll Surg Eng* 1986;68:23–26.

13 CROHN BB, GINZBURG L, OPPENHEIMER GD. Regional ileitis. *JAMA* 1932;99:1323–1329.

14 DE DOMBAL FT. Results of surgery for Crohn's disease. *Clin Gastroenterol* 1972;1:493–506.

15 DUFFY LF, DAUM F, FISHER SE, *et al.* Peripheral neuropathy in Crohn's disease patients treated with metronidazole. *Gastroenterology* 1985;88:681–684.

16 FAZIO VW, GALANDIUK S. Strictureplasty in diffuse Crohn's jejunoileitis. *Dis Colon Rectum* 1985;28:512–518.

17 GLASS RE, RITCHIE JK, LENNARD-JONES JE, HAWLEY PR, TODD IP. Internal fistulas in Crohn's disease. *Dis Colon Rectum* 1985;28:557–561.

18 GLOTZER DJ. Operation in inflammatory bowel disease: indications and type. *Clin Gastroenterol* 1980;9:371–388.

19 GREENSTEIN AJ, MANN D, SACHAR DB, AUFSES AH JR. Free perforation in Crohn's disease: I. survey of 99 cases. *Am J Gastroenterol* 1985;80:682–689.

20 GREENSTEIN AJ, SACHAR DB, GIBAS A, *et al.* Outcome of toxic dilatation in ulcerative and Crohn's colitis. *J Clin Gastroenterol* 1985;7:137–144.

21 GREENSTEIN AJ, SACHAR D, PUCILLO A. Cancer in Crohn's disease after diversionary surgery. *Am J Surg* 1978;135:86–90.

22 GREENSTEIN AJ, SACHAR DB, TZAKIS A, SHER L, HEIMANN T, AUFSES AH, JR. Course of enterovesical fistulas in Crohn's disease. *Am J Surg* 1984;147:788–792.

23 GYDE SN, PRIOR P, MACARTNEY JC, THOMPSON H, WATERHOUSE JA, ALLAN RN. Malignancy in Crohn's disease. *Gut* 1980;21:1024–1029.

24 HAMILTON SR. Colorectal carcinoma in patients with Crohn's disease. *Gastroenterology* 1985;89:395–407.

25 HARPER PN, TRUELOVE SC, LEE ECG, KETTLEWELL MGW, JEWELL DP. Split ileostomy and ileocolostomy for Crohn's disease of the colon and ulcerative colitis: a 20 year survey. *Gut* 1983;24:106–110.

26 HAWKER PC, GIVEL JC, KEIGHLEY MRB, ALEXANDER-WILLIAMS J, ALLAN RN. Management of enterocutaneous fistulae in Crohn's disease. *Gut* 1983;24:284–287.

27 HEIMANN TM, GREENSTEIN AJ, MECHANIC L, AUFSES AH. Early complications following surgical treatment for Crohn's disease. *Ann Surg* 1985;201:494–498.

28 HEUMAN R, BOERYA B, BOLIN T, SJODAHL R. The influence of disease at the margin of resection on the outcome of Crohn's disease. *Br J Surg* 1983;70:519–521.

29 HIGGINS CS, ALLAN RN. Crohn's disease of the ileum. *Gut* 1980;21:933–940.

30 HOBBIS JH, SCHOFIELD PF. Management of perianal Crohn's disease. *J R Soc Med* 1982;75:414–417.

31 HODGSON HJF. Assessment of drug therapy in inflammatory bowel disease. *Br J Clin Pharmacol* 1982;14:159–170.

32 HOMAN WP, DINEEN P. Comparison of the results of resection, bypass and bypass with exclusion for ileocaecal Crohn's disease. *Ann Surg* 1978; 187:530–535.

33 IRVING AD, LYALL MH. Perineal healing after panproctocolectomy for inflammatory bowel disease. *J R Coll Surg Edinb* 1984;29:313–315.

34 IRVING M. Assessment and management of external fistulas in Crohn's disease. *Br J Surg* 1983;70:233–236.

35 JACOBSON IM, SCHAPIRO RH, WARSHAW AL. Gastric and duodenal fistulas in Crohn's disease. *Gastroenterology* 1985;89:1347–1352.

36 KYLE J. Prognosis after ileal resection for Crohn's disease. *Br J Surg* 1971;58:735–737.

37 LEADING ARTICLE. Enterocutaneous fistulas—encouraging trends. *Lancet* 1984;ii:204–205.

38 LEE ECG. Aim of surgical treatment of Crohn's disease. *Gut* 1984;25:219–222.

39 LEE ECG, PAPAIOANNOU N. Minimal surgery for chronic obstruction in patients with extensive or universal Crohn's disease. *Ann R Coll Surg Engl* 1982;64:229–233.

40 LEICESTER RJ, RITCHIE JK, WADSWORTH J, THOMSON JPS, HAWLEY PR. Sexual function and perineal wound healing after intersphincteric excision of the rectum for inflammatory bowel disease. *Dis Colon Rectum* 1984;27:244–248.

41 LENNARD-JONES JE, STADLER GA. Prognosis after resection of chronic regional ileitis. *Gut* 1967;8:332–336.

42 LINDHANGEN T, EKELUND G, LEANDOER L, HILDELL J, LINDSTROM C, WENCKERT A. Pre-operative and post-operative complications in Crohn's disease with special reference to duration of pre-operative disease history. *Scand J Gastroenterol* 1984; 19:194–203.

43 LOCKHART-MUMMERY HE. Anal lesions of Crohn's disease. *Clin Gastroenterol* 1972;1:377–382.

44 McINTYRE PB, RITCHIE JD, HARLEY PR, BARTRAM CI, LENNARD-JONES JE. Management of enterocutaneous fistula: a review of 132 cases. *Br J Surg* 1984;71:293–296.

45 MARKS CG, RITCHIE JK, LOCKHART-MUMMERY HC. Anal fistulas in Crohn's disease. *Br J Surg* 1981;68:525–527.

46 MEKHIJIAN HS, SWIYZ DM, WATTS HD, DEREN JJ, KATUN RM, BEMAN FM. Factors determining recurrence after surgery. *Gastroenterology* 1979;77:907–913.

47 MORTENSEN NJMC, RITCHIE JK, HAWLEY PR, TODD IP, LENNARD-JONES JE. Surgery of acute Crohn's colitis: results and long-term follow-up. *Br J Surg*, 1984;71:783–784.

48 PALLONE F, BOIRIVANT M, TORSOLI A. Conservative management of acute intestinal obstruction in Crohn's disease. *Lancet* 1984;i:518.

49 PETTIT SH, HOLBROOK IB, IRVING MH. Comparison of clinical scores and acute phase proteins in the assessment of acute Crohn's disease. *Br J Surg* 1985;72:1013–1016.

50 PRIOR P, Gyde S, COOKE WT, WATERHOUSE JAH, ALLAN RN. Mortality in Crohn's disease. *Gastroenterology* 1981;80:307–312.

51 RIDDELL RH. Dysplasia in inflammatory bowel disease. *Clin Gastroenterol* 1980;9:439–458.

52 ROSS TM, FAZIO VW, FARMER RG. Long-term results of surgical treatment for Crohn's disease of the duodenum. *Ann Surg* 1983;197:399–406.

53 RUTGEERTS R, GERBOES K, VANTRAPPEN G, KEREMANS R, Coenegracts JL, COREMANS G. Natural history of recurrent Crohn's disease at the ileocolonic anastomosis after curative surgery. *Gut* 1984;25:665–672.

54 RYAN JA. Gracilis muscle flap for the persistent perineal sinus of inflammatory bowel disease. *Am J Surg* 1984;148:64–70.

55 SACHAR DB. Crohn's disease in Cleveland: a matter of life and death. *Gastroenterology* 1985;88:1996–1997.

56 SCHOFIELD PF. Abdominal tuberculosis. *Gut* 1985;26:1275–1278.

57 SCHRAUT WH, BLOCK GE. Enterovesical fistula complicating Crohn's ileocolitis. *Am J Gastroenterol* 1984;79:186–190.

58 SHORTER RG. Risks of intestinal cancer in Crohn's disease. *Dis Colon Rectum* 1983;26:686–689.

59 TRUELOVE SC, ELLIS H, WEBSTER CU. Place of a double barelled ileostomy in ulcerative colitis and Crohn's disease of the colon. *Br Med J* 1965;1:150–153.

60 TRUELOVE SC, PENA AS. Course and prognosis of Crohn's disease. *Gut* 1976;17:192–201.

61 WEEDON DD, SHORTER RG, ILSTRUP DM, HUIZENGA

KA, TAYLOR WF. Crohn's disease and cancer. *N Engl J Med* 1973;**289**:1099–1103.

62 VAN DONGEN LM, LUBBERS EJC. Fistulas of the bladder in Crohn's disease. *Surg Gynecol Obstet* 1984a;**158**:308–310.

63 VAN DONGEN LM, LUBBERS EJC. Surgical management of ileosigmoid fistulas in Crohn's disease. *Surg Gynecol Obstet* 1984b;**159**:325–327.

64 WHELAN G, FARMER RG, FAZIO VW, GOORMASTIC M. Recurrence after surgery in Crohn's disease. relationship to location of disease (clinical pattern) and surgical indication. *Gastroenterology* 1985; **88**:1826–1833.

65 WOLFF BG, CULP CE, BEART RW, ILSTRUP DM, READY RL. Anorectal Crohn's disease. *Dis Colon Rectum* 1985;**28**:709–711.

Chapter 55
Stomas and Stoma Care

S. A. RAIMES & H. B. DEVLIN

A stoma is an ectopic opening of the bowel onto the anterior abdominal wall. Stomas may be used for enteral feeding, (constructed in the stomach or jejunum) or to divert or allow outflow from the distal bowel. Ileostomy and colostomy are common temporary or permanent stomas in gastrointestinal surgery (see Table 55.1).

A surgeon may perform a stoma to save life, to improve the quality of life, or to facilitate or make safer distal surgery on the colon. Although the surgeon who constructs the stoma may see his role in such simple terms, he or she must remember the mutilation that these operations can effect on the patient's body image [4].

It is the duty of medical staff not only to save the patient's life but also to protect the patient's standard of living [19]. Ostomate care requires a team approach that begins preoperatively and ideally continues until rehabilitation is complete, although

Table 55.1. Indications for gastrointestinal stomas.

Function	Anatomy	Clinical indications
Input stomas (temporary)	Gastrostomy.	Malnutrition, severe catabolic states due to oesophageal obstruction, oesophageal stricture, corrosive burns, carcinoma, trauma, neurologic disorders of swallowing, motor neuron disease, coma.
	Jejunostomy (fine-tube enterostomy).	Jejunostomy is a preferred access after gastrectomy or when access to stomach is limited.
Diversion stomas (temporary)	Pharyngostomy. Oesophagostomy.	To divert swallowed saliva and protect the bronchial tree in neonatal oesophageal atresia and tracheo-oesophageal fistula. In adult oesophageal obstruction to divert saliva from the oesophagus and bronchial tree.
	Ileostomy ('loop' or 'split').	To divert the faecal stream from the colon (e.g. in anorectal Crohn's disease or fistula, etc.).
	Colostomy ('loop' 'transverse', 'sigmoid').	Anorectal agenesis, trauma, distal inflammation or perforation. To 'cover' distal surgical manoeuvres (not recommended). Side-effects of radiation. Relief of left colonic obstruction.
	Temporary end-colostomy with primary excision of colonic lesion.	Diverticular disease. Colon and rectal carcinoma.
Output stomas (permanent)	Ileostomy ('terminal').	Ulcerative colitis. Colorectal Crohn's disease. Ischaemic colitis. Familial polyposis coli. Malignant or premalignant tumour of the colon.
	Colostomy ('terminal', 'iliac').	Rectal carcinoma. Anal carcinoma. Unrepairable anorectal malformations. Severe anorectal injuries

unfortunately this latter goal is often un-obtainable.

The surgeon advises the patient to undergo the operation—it is his or her duty to ensure that the operation is performed correctly and that the postoperative care is adequate. Many junior medical and nursing staff do not understand and have little insight into the problems of stoma care. Yet patients often depend on these staff for their initial support. Hence the surgeon must ensure that all the staff have an adequate basic knowledge of the phsyiology of stomas and the possible complications that may occur. The early postoperative period is when the patient's self-confidence is at its lowest ebb and it may disintegrate altogether if trust is lost.

Epidemiology

There are approximately 100,000 patients with permanent colostomies in Great Britain and about 5,000 new permanent colostomies are constructed each year [3]. This number may be decreasing due to sphincter-saving techniques for low rectal anastomisis, which have reduced the number of abdomino-perineal resections [13, 15].

There are fewer patients with permanent ileostomies—around 10,000 in Great Britain. Each year 200 to 300 new ileostomies are constructed, the majority for ulcerative colitis [5]. The number of ileostomies being constructed has fallen each year since 1975 [8].

Patient counselling

When the surgeon advises any operation he or she must be prepared to describe and discuss the procedure and its consequences. Leaflets and diagrams are often helpful and the ostomy clubs provide well-presented booklets. A stoma care nurse is invaluable—he or she will often be able to visit the patient's home and arrange for the patient to meet an ostomate of the same sex and age for reassurance. The patient's spouse or family should also be counselled.

The ostomy voluntary associations provide excellent 'visitors' who have been trained in counselling. Being ostomates themselves these visitors have a particular insight often not acquired by even the most experienced professionals. The voluntary associations also have particular expertise in handling employment and insurance problems.

Stoma siting and construction

This is most important—a well-sited stoma makes postoperative care easier, but a badly-sited stoma can be a disaster. The site should take into account the patient's shape and also any other disabilities. The stoma should be far enough from bony prominences, natural skin creases and old scars to allow an appliance to be fitted with complete adherence. The stoma site should be checked by the patient wearing the chosen appliance at the proposed site preoperatively.

Stomas must never be brought out through main wound incisions because of the risk of serious sepsis, difficulties in wound management and the risk of herniation. Effectively there are only four really suitable sites for stomas on the anterior abdominal wall—on the flat surface of the rectus muscle above the umbilicus (right or left, either of which is ideal for a temporary colostomy) and on the summit of the infra-umbilical mound of rectus muscle (right or left, both suitable for temporary or permanent ileostomies, but only on the left for a permanent colostomy) (Fig. 55.1).

In making any stoma the surgeon should endeavour to place it so that the emergent gut penetrates through the rectus sheath and muscle in a truly direct and horizontal plane. The stoma should be without any

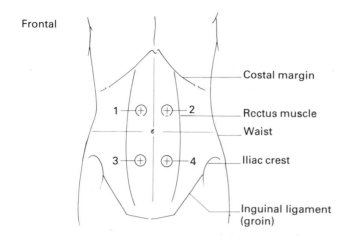

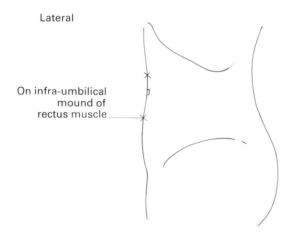

Fig. 55.1. The siting of a stoma. Stomas should be placed away from flexure creases or bony prominences. They should be away from wounds. The stability of the appliance should not be compromised when the patient moves or changes position. Effectively there are four suitable stoma sites over the flat surface of the rectus above or below the umbilicus. The stoma site must be visible to the patient hence, if below the umbilicus, the stoma must be sited on the summit of the infra-umbilical rectal mound.

tension on it ensuring an adequate blood supply; it should be stabilized with a rod or sutures as it passes through the abdominal wall; it should be opened immediately and a good mucocutaneous opposition obtained with interrupted sutures; finally, a transparent appliance should be fitted in theatre. With attention to these operative details the complications of intra-mural stenosis, herniation, retraction and ischaemia should be unknown.

Temporary stomas

Indications (Fig. 55.2)

A temporary stoma may be constructed when the distal bowel is affected by injury, obstruction, perforation or infection.

The common emergency indications include **distal malignancy**, usually a carcinoma of the left colon or rectum; **diverticular disease of the colon; anorectal and left colon injuries**, when exteriorization of a temporary colostomy is almost mandatory

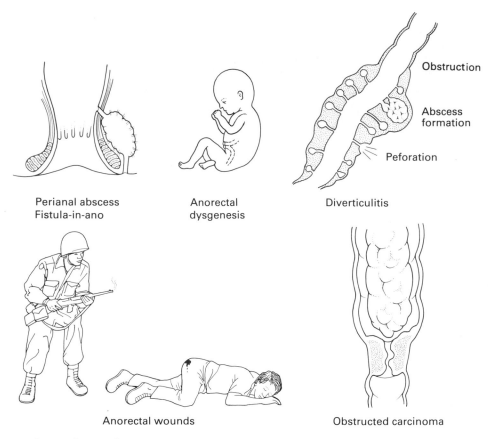

Obstruction

Abscess
formation

Peforation

Perianal abscess
Fistula-in-ano

Anorectal
dysgenesis

Diverticulitis

Anorectal wounds

Obstructed carcinoma

Fig. 55.2. Some indications for a temporary colostomy.

prior to reconstruction [23]; **anorectal suppuration** due to a high extra-spincteric
fistula-in-ano; **severe anorectal Crohn's disease post-radiation stricture; colorectal endometriosis; anorectal dysgenesis** (see Chapter 76); **Hirschsprung's disease** (see Chapter
62).

A temporary stoma may be constructed
as a planned procedure, when an anastomosis is to be constructed distally that will
heal more safely in a defunctioned state (for
example, ileorectal anastomosis for inflammatory bowel disease or a low colorectal
anastomosis for cancer).

Temporary loop colostomy

Construction

This colostomy can be constructed either in
the transverse or the sigmoid colon. The
transverse site is usually preferred as it is
farther from the common sites of large
bowel disease, and thus allows mobilization
of a longer length of colon for reconstruction at subsequent surgery. The transverse
colon can be brought out through the
greater omentum decreasing the risk of
general contamination of the peritoneal
cavity. The stoma is constructed over the
supra-umbilical flat portion of the rectus
muscle as far away as possible from the
laparotomy wound. The stoma is supported
at skin level with a short length of firm

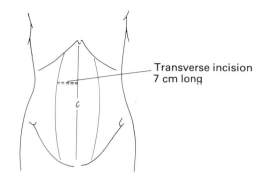

(a)

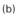

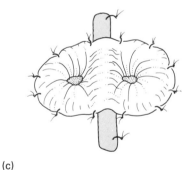

Transverse incision 7 cm long

Loop of colon brought up and supported by rod at skin level

Greater omentum

(b)

(c)

Fig. 55.3. Construction of a temporary colostomy. (a) the ideal site is over the upper right rectus muscle. (b) the spur is raised and supported at skin level by a short length of rubber or plastic tube fixed to the skin. The supporting rod must be as compact as possible to facilitate fixation of the appliance. (c) the spur must be prominent enough to prevent 'carry over' of faeces.

tube. It is important to support the stoma 'spur' at skin level to prevent 'spill over' of faeces (Fig. 55.3), ideally using a very short length of polyethylene or rubber tube that is sutured to the skin on either side. Subcutaneous rods have been used but, while the appliance is easier to fit, the spur is less efficient at preventing spill-over of faeces. A skin bridge can be created using an omega-shaped skin incision. The stoma may be rotated through 180° to make the afferent loop dependent [27]. Some authorities regard the loop colostomy as outmoded, a hangover from the past, which should no longer feature in clinical practice. The loop ileostomy is a preferable technique for defunctioning the colon [31].

Closure

Before closing and returning any temporary stoma to the peritoneal cavity two important requirements must be satisfied. (1) The distal bowel must be patent and the anastomosis, if present, healed. Both can be confirmed by endoscopy or barium contrast studies. Closure of a defunctioning stoma in the presence of distal obstruction of sepsis is dangerous and may lead to a faecal fistula, sepsis and perhaps peritonitis [11, 30]. (2) The stoma must be healthy and its blood flow adequate. Initial postoperative congestion and oedema usually take about 14 days to subside. If the stoma is stenosed or the spur remains oedematous it is probably safer to excise the segment and construct an end-to-end anastomosis [12].

Closure of a loop colostomy does not require a formal laparotomy. An elliptical incision is made just outside the mucocutaneous junction leaving a cuff to which tissue forceps can be applied. The bowel is then freed from all layers down into the peritoneal cavity, the mucocutaneous junction excised, and the bowel edges 'freshened'. Transverse closure is in two layers—the inner layer involving all coats using a continuous absorbable material, and the outer seromuscular layer using interrupted non-absorbable material. Recent impressive results have used a stapling device [25].

The **complications of colostomy closure** are often underestimated. Wound infections are common but the place of prophylactic antibiotics is uncertain. Herniation occurs in up to 5% of patients. Faecal fistulae occur when there is an anastomotic leak due to technical error, ischaemia at the closure site, or if there is distal obstruction or inflammation. A fistula should close spontaneously, but if it persists the distal bowel should be re-investigated. There is a low, but obviously significant, mortality associated with colostomy closure—the main factors are whether the initial operation was an elective procedure or an emergency (in which case mortality is higher), and also the time interval between establishment and closure. Present evidence suggests that closure within 28 days is associated with more problems.

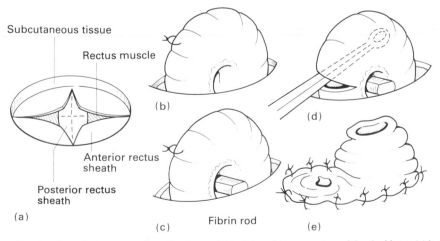

Fig. 55.4. Construction of a temporary loop ileostomy: (a) incision; (b) preparation of the ileal loop; (c) bridge sutured to the anterior rectus sheath; (d) incision in the distal limb; (e) formation of the spout (adapted with permission from [10]).

Temporary loop ileostomy

A temporary ileostomy is constructed on the summit of the infra-umbilical mound of rectus muscle. The afferent loop is everted and the whole contraption supported by an absorbable fibrin rod (Biethium) placed subcutaneously and sutured to the anterior rectus sheath. Thus the skin around the stoma is uncluttered and a standard ileostomy appliance can be fitted easily.

The principles of closure are the same as for the loop colostomy, with the same mandatory preconditions as to safety. After mobilization the spout is everted back and the opening closed with two layers of catgut. To lessen any chance of stenosis at the join, the antimesenteric margin of both the proximal and distal ends of gut are split back about 2 cm and the splayed-open ends anastomosed to widen the effective lumen (Fig. 55.4).

Historically, the stoma was used to defunction distal bowel affected by inflammatory bowel disease or to cover ileorectal and ileo-anal anastomoses after total colectomy. It does, however, provide a small, easily manageable stoma which produces predictable volumes of relatively inoffensive faecal effluent—it is a truly defunctioning stoma. For these reasons and because, using the Biethium rod, it is easy to 'bag', it is the temporary stoma of choice. By comparison, the transverse loop colostomy is difficult to 'bag', it produces loose offensive faeces, and is also prone to prolapse.

Bloch–Paul–Mickulicz operation

Occasionally used in the frail, elderly patient with either obstructing or perforated left colonic lesions, this operation exteriorizes the affected segment by suturing the proximal and distal limbs of the loop to form a double-barrelled colostomy that can be closed without re-opening the abdomen. Although it saves the patient a second laparotomy, it has the disadvantage of not

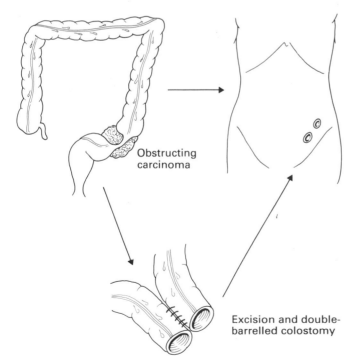

Obstructing carcinoma

Excision and double-barrelled colostomy

Fig. 55.5. Bloch–Paul–Mickulicz operation. Useful in patients with an obstructing sigmoid cancer who are unfit to undergo extensive radical surgery.

provoding adequate mesenteric clearance to be a good cancer operation (Fig. 55.5).

Devine operation

In this procedure primary resection of a left colonic carcinoma is performed; the proximal bowel end is brought out as functional end stoma and the distal end as a mucous fistula (Fig. 55.6). This is a two-stage pro-

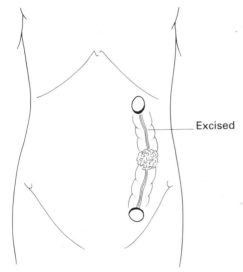

Excised

Fig. 55.6. Devine operation. Double colostomy with primary excision.

cedure with re-anastomosis at a later operation. Recent studies suggest that the results of the two-stage procedure are superior to the formation of a defunctioning colostomy and a later-stage resection and then closure of colostomy (three-stage procedure) [10].

Hartmann operation

A primary resection of an obstructing carcinoma in the upper rectum is performed in this procedure. The proximal end is brought out as a left iliac fossa end colostomy, and the rectum stump is closed. At the second operation continuity can be restored, a

manoeuvre that is considerably easier using a circular stapling device [20].

Caecostomy

This stoma is described only to condemn its use—except in very exceptional circumstances. The caecum should not be exteriorized as it produces large volumes of enzyme-rich faeces that cannot be controlled and cause severe skin problems. A tube caecostomy decompresses rather than defunctions the large bowel, but it is used by some surgeons to protect left-sided anstomoses. It is, however, a considerable nursing problem. There is a danger that the caecum may detach from the anterior abdominal wall leading to faecal peritonitis. Sepsis may develop around the tube and occasionally the resulting fistula, when the tube is removed, fails to close spontaneously.

Permanent stomas

Two permanent stomas are in current use—the permanent ileostomy, usually established in the right lower abdomen, and the permanent colostomy in the lower left abdomen. Indications for these stomas are summarized in Table 55.1.

Attempts have been made to give these stomas continence and reservoir capacities—the Kock pouch (Fig. 55.7) and Parks' pouch (Fig 55.8) have been developed for the ileostomy [17, 20] and the Erlangen magnetic device for the colostomy [1, 9].

The Parks' pouch

The concept of an internal reservoir or pouch as an alternative to the 'lost' colon is attractive, but problems with the continence of the nipple valve and the ever present ectopic anus in the Kock operation led to a search for alternatives. Parks devised an ingenious alternative operation

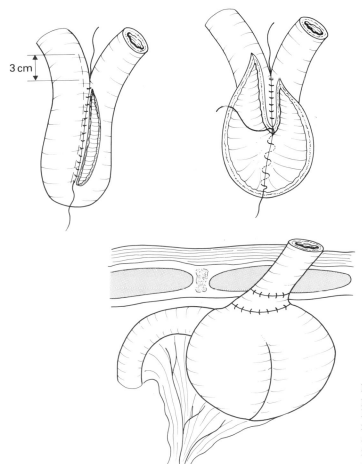

3 cm

Fig. 55.7. The Koch pouch. The pouch is constructed out of a 'U' loop of ileum; the valve is a reversed intussusception of ileum and the stoma is placed inconspicuously in the lower abdomen.

which has given some outstanding results [21] (see Chapter 51).

The operation

As the disease in ulcerative colitis and familial polyposis involves only the mucosa, why not remove the diseased mucosa alone, and leave behind the anal sphincter with its proprioceptive receptors in the perirectal musculature? The mucosa of the rectum, from the dentate line proximally for 8–10 cm, is removed transanally [14]. First saline and adrenaline solution is injected into the submucous layer and then a cylinder of mucosa is dissected out using sharp scissors through an anal retractor. A tripli-

cated pouch is formed of terminal ileum and the distal outflow limb, some 15 cm long in males or 10 cm in females, is threaded down through the intact anorectal musculature and sutured circumferentially to the anal mucosa at the dentate line. A temporary loop ileostomy is raised 'to protect' the pelvic surgery. After two weeks the pouch is tested for soundness by a Gastrografin enema and the ileostomy is closed.

Complications

Initially patients may experience some incontinence but this gradually improves. Other problems are 'cuff' abscesses between the layers in the neo-rectum, stenosis of the

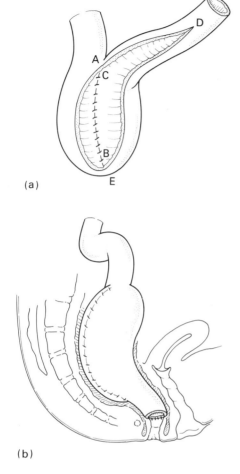

(a)

(b)

Fig. 55.8. The Parks' mucosal proctectomy and ileal pelvic pouch operation. (a) construction of ileal pouch from terminal 50 cm of small intestine B, C, E and the mid-point between D and E are points of folding. ABC is the first fold. The final two folds will be complete when D and E are approximated. (b) appearances of completed operation (adapted with permission from [21]).

ano-ileal anastomosis, and an inability to evacuate naturally. Intermittent catheterization *per anum* is usually satisfactory for the latter problem (see Fig. 55.8).

Results

The results of this procedure, when performed by an experienced team, are most encouraging. At least 50% of patients gain full continence with the ability to evacuate naturally. In those who cannot evacuate naturally, intermittent catheterization is a preferable alternative to an external appliance [17, 22]. The authors' experience with this operation is so favourable that it is felt the rectum should always be retained in patients with ulcerative colitis so that a restorative continent pouch can be constructed by an experienced surgeon at a later date.

The Kock pouch

The conventional ileostomy discharges faecal fluid more or less continuously day and night with peak outputs in the two hours after a meal. This is inconvenient for the patient and necessitates wearing an appliance continuously. In 1969 Kock described an ingenious operation with a reservoir constructed out of ileum and continence achieved by a reversed nipple valve of ileum, which could be intubated to drain it when convenient to the ostomate [16, 18]. Furthermore, because there was no need for a leakproof appliance, the stoma could be placed discretely out of sight in the suprapubic area (see Fig. 55.7) (see Chapter 51).

Operation

The operation can be performed as part of the initial proctocolectomy or as a secondary procedure for the patient with an established ileostomy. To make the pouch, two 15 cm lengths of ileum are joined side-to-side and the valve is made by intussuscepting 5 cm of intestine retrogradely into the lumen of the reservoir. A further 5 cm of intestine is used to counteract the 'outflow' through the abdominal wall. The whole system requires meticulous suturing and fixation to the abdominal parietes, to prevent either the valve undoing itself or the pouch twisting and strangulating.

Complications

The important complications are eversion of the valve leading to incontinence, stenosis of the valve preventing catheterization, sepsis due to suture link leaks and dehiscences and volvulus of the pouch. In the longer term, an enteritis has been described in the pouch, and questions about bile salt and vitamin B_{12} absorption remain unanswered [2, 26].

The operation must not be used in Crohn's disease when the pouch may become involved. It should also be remembered that failure of the operation means the loss of at least 45 cm of valuable terminal ileum.

Ileostomy output

The normal colon receives about 1500 ml per 24 hours through the ileocaecal valve and absorption decreases the water content of the faeces to 100–200 ml. The ileostomate's faecal output is summarized in Table 55.2. Excessive ileostomy output is discussed in Chapter 56.

Water, sodium and potassium

The volume of effluent is on average about 500 ml per day containing four times the normal faecal sodium and about half the normal faecal potassium. Several adaptive mechanisms compensate for these losses including hypertrophy of intestinal villi, and increased aldosterone and ADH secretion.

Although the majority of patients with a normally functioning ileostomy have no clinical evidence of any deficiency, occult deficiencies of water and sodium are probably common, becoming important whenever there is an increased ileostomy output (for example, in the early postoperative period, during gastroenteritis, partial obstruction, and more insidiously when excessive sweating occurs). The only metabolic problem of real significance is salt and water depletion. The symptoms are not always easily recognized but the commonest complaints are loss of appetite, nausea and headaches, and less often, cramps and photophobia.

Decreased urine volume predisposes ileostomates to urinary calculi, the incidence being 0.7–4.3% in British studies. All types of calculi are reported but, with a persistent

Table 55.2. Ileostomy physiology.

	Average daily faecal losses	
	Normal subject	Ileostomate
Faecal sodium	10 mmol	38–40 mmol
Faecal potassium	12 mmol	3–6 mmol
Faecal magnesium	3–3.5 mmol	3.5–4.5 mmol
Faecal calcium	5.5 mmol	7.5–20 mmol
Faecal nitrogen	up to 107 mmol	43–171 mmol
Faecal fat	11–18 mmol	5–13 mmol
Faecal bilirubin	—	118–166 μmol
Faecal stercobilinogen	35–420 μmol	5–52 μmol
Faecal volume	100–150 ml	350–500 ml
	Average daily urine losses	
	Normal subject	Ileostomate
Volume	1500 ml	800–1000 ml
Sodium	110–240 mmol	93 mmol
Potassium	35–90 mmol	114 mmol

bicarbonate loss from the stoma, an acid urine favours uric acid precipitation. Patients should be advised to have a high intake of water. Efforts to alkalinize the urine are rarely successful. Excessive ileostomy fluid loss is best controlled by either codeine phosphate 30 mg or loperamide 2 mg, taken on demand up to six times a day (see Chapter 56).

Calcium and magnesium

Both these cations are lost in increased amounts but only in prolonged high output states are deficiencies clinically evident.

Bile salts

Loss of part or the whole of the terminal ileum may interrupt the enterohepatic circulation of bile salts predisposing to gallstone formation. Up to 25% of ileostomates have radiological evidence of gallstones, about three times that of the equivalent normal population. However, the number requiring cholecystectomy is not increased and an expectant policy is advised. Treatment with bile acids is contra-indicated as they cause severe diarrhoea in ileostomates.

Vitamin B_{12}

Decreased B_{12} absorption is reported in the first 12 months after operation, possibly related to a change in the bowel flora. It does not require treatment and persistent deficiency is only seen in those patients who have extensive resections or disease of the terminal ileum.

Colostomy output

The left colon usually stores faeces, and it has only a small role in fluid absorption. In the absence of a sphincter, the frequency with which the colostomy acts depends upon the motility of the patient's colon. It takes up to three months for an activity pattern to be established and this rarely is the same as the patient's preoperative bowel function. The regularity with which the colostomy functions may vary from one or two actions per day to an almost continuous discharge.

Methods of colostomy control

Natural method

A high fibre diet and the judicious use of laxatives can control the activity of the colostomy to a predictable pattern. When successful the colostomy acts mainly in the morning, the colon being stimulated by a hot drink and breakfast, and less frequently after the evening meal. A quarter to one-third of colostomates have two or fewer motions per day, but up to one-third have more than five motions per day. The natural method requires the wearing of an appliance throughout the day [7].

Irrigation method

Patients often find intermittent colostomy irrigation a practical and convenient method to regulate their colostomy. Performed once every 24–48 hours the colon is stimulated by distension with fluid producing mass emptying. It requires about 30 minutes per irrigation and involves running 1000–1500 ml of warm tap water into the colostomy using a soft rubber tube and a plastic cone-shaped stoma occluder. Once contractions are induced the contents are evacuated through a spout or the large bore tube into the lavatory. Successful patients virtually eliminate wearing an appliance and can wear a protective dressing or a waterproof stoma cap. Flatus and odour are not usually a problem but a deodourizing filter incorporated into the stoma cap is helpful [29]. The risk of perforation is low and is considerably reduced by using a soft plastic cone to introduce the fluid. Success of this method depends very much on patient selection and adequate instruction. Unsuitable patients include the aged, those with disabilities such as blindness or severe arthritis, and those who have colostomies with mechanical problems such as herniation, stenosis, prolapse or recession.

Practical aspects of stoma management

Stoma appliances

An effective appliance must collect the faecal effluent, not leak, prevent odour and protect the peristomal skin. At the same time it should be unobtrusive and relatively simple to use. Two basic designs of appliance are used.

Disposable one-piece appliances incorporate a skin seal or flange and pouch. Although simple to use, repeated changing may traumatize the peristomal skin. Drainable pouches are available but they tend to smell if used and emptied too often.

Two-piece appliances consist of adhesive base plate onto which disposable pouches can be fastened. The base plate, which is hypoallergenic, can be left attached to the skin for long periods.

Appliance adhesives

Skin adherents/protectives based on vegetable gums are used commonly. The first such gum to be introduced in the United Kingdom was karaya in the late 1960s [24]. Many comparable products are now obtainable commercially (for example, Stomahesive, Comfeel and Hollihesive). Strong adhesive tapes should be avoided—they not only cause skin damage but also seal in any leaking effluent under the base plate and prolong skin contact with the irritating fluid.

If a stoma is placed too close to a scar or natural fold, leakage may be a serious problem leading to effluent contact dermatitis and also inevitable embarrassment with loss of confidence. The defect can be filled with Stomahesive paste, or eliminated by creating a platform with silicone polymer that is allowed to set around the stoma. The adhesive plate is then applied over the flattened surface.

A transparent pouch is worn for the first postoperative week so that the new stoma can be observed. After this most patients use an opaque pouch or a cotton cover. The pouch must be of plastic that not only protects against odour but also contains some form of flatus filter so the bag does not inflate and become obtrusive. Once emptied, pouches should be either burned or placed in the dustbin, not flushed away.

Odour prevention

Odour is caused mostly by fermentation of undigested carbohydrates by the colonic bacteria. While it is a particular problem for colostomates, some bacterial colonization occurs in the terminal ileum and ileostomates may also complain of odour. There are three methods of dealing with this problem.

Dietary adjustment

Patients should avoid foods that predispose to excessive flatus formation. While there is individual variation, onions, eggs and beans often cause problems.

Chlorophyll

This is popular, but there is little evidence to support its efficiency.

Appliance

An odour-proof plastic is used that incorporates a filter of activated carbon or charcoal. Some patients put commercially available instillates into the pouch, others place a wide variety of substances into their pouches, the most popular being an aspirin, in the belief that this decreases bacterial fermentation.

Surgical complications

Haemorrhage

Haemorrhage in the early postoperative period is usually due to small mucosal vessels, which can often be controlled by applying an adrenaline-soaked swab over the affected area. Occasionally a vessel in the submucosa or mesentery will need to be exposed, picked up with artery forceps and ligated. Granulation tissue may be responsible for later bleeding, which can be treated by careful painting with silver nitrate. Pyogenic granulomas may be mucosal or at the mucocutaneous junction. They cause frequent bleeding and should be removed. It should be stressed that superficial bleeding is common during cleaning of the stoma and peristomal skin, and it should not be a cause for concern. In colostomates a metachronous malignancy may present as bleeding.

Ischaemia

Ischaemia is uncommon in loop stomas but end-stomas may be affected if the inferior mesenteric artery is ligated high or if branches of the ileocolic artery are ligated too near the bowel. Elderly patients with atherosclerotic vessels are more at risk.

Changes due to ischaemia become evident in the first 48 hours. While duskiness and some swelling of the stomal mucosa is acceptable, further darkening should cause concern. If necrosis is confined to the mucosa the changes will regress after a period of bullous oedema. The bowel will slough if all the layers of the bowel are affected. The stoma should therefore be examined gently and, if the changes extend throughout the thickness of the abdominal wall, a further laparotomy is required to prevent perforation and peritonitis.

If only the distal stoma is affected a conservative approach can be taken—the stoma may slough and be replaced by granulation tissue with later retraction and stenosis. With an ileostomy the functional result will be unsatisfactory and formal reconstruction will be needed. However, a colostomy may be left alone if there is stenosis unless there are obstructive problems.

The spout of an ileostomy may be damaged by a tight appliance flange, leading to stenosis, fistula formation around the base and occasional sloughing of the spout leaving flush stoma. Since the ileostomy is insensitive this process may occur without the patient noticing discomfort.

Ischaemia may also occur when an ileostomy undergoes alternate prolapse and retraction, which can damage small vessels in the terminal ileal mesentery.

Ileostomy obstruction

Ileostomy obstruction may be mechanical but more commonly is due to bolus obstruction by high fibre food or insufficiently chewed food. Citrus fruits and rhubarb are notorious as they are hydrophilic and swell in the intestine. Impaction occurs either at the site of adhesions or more commonly at the point where the ileum penetrates the anterior abdominal wall. Irrigating the ileostomy with warm water, using a soft rubber catheter, often relieves the problem. It is a wise precaution to perform an ileostomy barium enema, once recovery is complete, to exclude prestomal ileitis.

Prolapse

Prolapse of end-stomas is uncommon and is usually associated with inadequate fixation of the mesentery within the abdomen. When the opening in the abdominal wall is too large the stoma will prolapse and retract depending on posture, causing leakage when the stoma lies flush. The stoma can be reconstructed at a local operation mobilizing the stoma down to the peritoneal cavity, excising the excess length and fixing the mesentery to the peritoneum with fine non-absorbable sutures before refashioning the stoma.

Prolapse of a transverse colostomy is common and occurs in around 15% of patients. Curiously the distal loop is more likely to prolapse retrogradely. The only solution is to close the stoma as soon as is thought safe. In the rare patients where closure is not contemplated, the distal loop can be closed and the proximal colon trimmed and fashioned as an end-colostomy.

Retraction

Retraction may occur because of tension on the stoma caused by poor mobilization, secondary to ischaemia, or reversibly in the supine position with a prolapsing stoma.

The retracted colostomy can be observed—refashioning is necessary only if stenosis results. The retracted ileostomy causes considerable problems with leakage, producing skin problems and demoralization. Although a local procedure can be feasible, in most patients a formal laparotomy is needed with mobilization of the mesentery and refashioning of the stoma.

Stenosis

Stenosis of a stoma is usually due to either a tight opening in the abdominal wall or is secondary to ischaemia. Refashioning is usually necessary.

Herniation

Herniation is rare in ileostomies but is common in end-colostomies. Twenty to 25% of patients develop para-colostomy hernias, which are usually small and of little significance. It appears that the extraperitoneal route does not lessen this problem, but it is suggested that a small trephine incision placed through the rectus sheath does decrease the risk.

The complications of a hernia include problems in fitting an appliance and an increased risk of obstruction, not only of faeces in the tortuous large bowel but also when loops of small bowel become adherent within the hernia sac. Herniation also makes colostomy irrigation difficult and potentially dangerous.

A local repair of the hernia can be attempted, reducing the sac and inserting non-absorbable sutures in all layers, but recurrence is likely and a laparotomy with reconstruction of the colostomy is then needed.

Inflammatory problems

Parastomal abscesses may occur when there is breakdown of part of the mucocutaneous suture line or when a haematoma becomes infected. They should be drained and allowed to granulate. Serosal sutures that have been placed too deeply and penetrate the mucosa lead to abscesses and usually a fistula. If superficial they may be laid open and allowed to granulate, but rarely a parastomal fistula enters the bowel within the peritoneal cavity and excision of the affected bowel with formal refashioning will be required. Abscesses, fistulae and stenosis can be manifestations of recurrent Crohn's disease.

Perforation

Perforation is a serious complication with high mortality and morbidity. It may occur during colostomy irrigation, though this risk is small with modern irrigation nozzles. It has also been reported as a complication of colostomy barium enemas. Emergency laparotomy is indicated.

Malignancy

Adenocarcinoma of an ileostomy has been reported but is very rare. Carcinoma developing at a colostomy is relatively common and can occur in one of three ways. Firstly, if the resection line was too close to the carcinoma and the colostomy is involved by spread in mural lymphatics. Secondly, when there is intraperitoneal spread a metastasis may grow adjacent to, and later invade, the stoma. Thirdly, there is a very real risk of a metachronous lesion developing proximal to the resection line in large bowel malignancy. Any change of colostomy habit or bleeding merits serious investigation.

Caput medusae

Ostomates with portal hypertension may develop varices at the skin-to-gut junction around a stoma, and troublesome bleeding may occur from such anastomotic vessels.

Dermatological complications

Two distinct types of dermatitis are seen— effluent and contact dermatitis [6].

Effluent dermatitis

Effluent dermatitis is caused by liquid faeces. It is seen mainly in patients with ileostomies and in those with transverse colostomies. It is less frequent with left (sigmoid) colostomies. The patients usually give a history of problems with their appliance, although in some the inflammation arises after an attack of diarrhoea. A history of recent treatment with broad-spectrum antibiotics should raise the suspicion of a secondary fungal infection (usually *Candida*). Effluent dermatitis has a geographic outline with marked hyperaemia and excoriation.

Contact dermatitis

Contact dermatitis is caused by an allergy to part of the appliance and usually has a clearly delineated 'geometric' outline. Patients often have a history of hypersensitivity or dermatoses, and the reaction is often itchy. Patients with skin problems should be patch tested using the various appliance materials before their operation.

While effluent and contact dermatitis are two separate primary conditions, secondary infection of the damaged skin usually occurs—swabs should be taken before treatment.

Treatment

The inflamed skin must be protected from further damage. It should be cleaned with water and a bland soap and dried carefully (cotton wool should be avoided as adherent strands may be left predisposing to further leakage). The skin should be protected with Stomahesive, Comfeel, or karaya. With effluent dermatitis the leakage point must be identified and the defect built up to allow full contact by the appliance. In severe cases the stoma may need to be refashioned or resited. Thickening the effluent is also helpful. For contact dermatitis the appliance is changed and the patient patch tested. A short course of local corticosteroid cream, such as 0.1% betamethasone is helpful, but its prolonged use should be avoided as skin atrophy and more rarely, systemic absorption can be problems. With super-added fungal infection an antifungal agent can be used either alone or with the steroid preparation. Topical antibiotic preparations are notorious for inducing hypersensitivity reactions and should be avoided except in severe cases where a short course of a preparation containing a corticosteroid, an antifungal agent and an antibiotic such as Tri-adcortyl (Squibb) is justified.

Psychosocial problems

However careful the preoperative counselling, patients are universally shocked to see their stoma and the immediate response is of denial, although this is not usually prolonged. Some patients with denial experience a 'phantom rectum'—a sense of rectal fullness associated with desire to defecate. The patient's own body image is distorted and they may regard themselves as mutilated, fragile and weak. In some patients there are profound feelings of horror, shame, degradation and a fear of rejection by others.

In general ostomates develop a new order of living, with a change in personality characterized by a conscious control of the range and the type of their social participation. There may be a tendency towards regression in thought and behaviour resulting in a restriction in their interests and withdrawal from emotional involvement, while others may be obsessively involved in trying to live a 'normal life'. The elderly in particular may become socially isolated. Depression is common and a proportion will require psychiatric treatment.

Even with the most careful care and support, it is apparent that these patients do not necessarily resume the same quality of life they previously experienced. However, an ileostomy is no barrier to successful return to work in nearly all occupations [28].

Sexual problems

These problems are of two types. Firstly, **anatomical in origin**—either due to distorted pelvic anatomy, adhesion and scarring, or due to damage to the pelvic autonomic nerves. Secondly, **psychosexual in origin**—the emotional responses of the ostomist and their partner can be the greatest sexual problem.

Surveys show that dysfunction is more common after cancer operations, but are evident in up to 30% of ileostomates. Fortunately problems are less common in the younger patient and in those who had normal preoperative sexual function.

Pregnancy for the ileostomate does carry additional risks, notably with displacement of the stoma and more importantly with small bowel obstruction. The symptoms of obstruction may easily be confused with the symptoms of a disordered pregnancy. The obstetrician should view any interruption of ileostomy flow with the highest index of suspicion. Two-thirds of ileostomates can be delivered by the vaginal route.

Useful addresses

Colostomy Welfare Group
38/39 Eccleston Square
London
SW1V 1PB

Ileostomy Association of Great Britain and Ireland
149 Harley Street
London
W1N 2DE.

References

1 ALEXANDER-WILLIAMS J, AMERY AH, *et al.* Magnetic colostomy device. *Br Med J* 1977;1:1269–1270.
2 CRANLEY B. The Kock reservoir ileostomy: a review of its development, problems and role in modern surgical practice. *Br J Surg* 1983;70:94–100.
3 DEVLIN HB. Colostomy. *Ann R Coll Surg Engl* 1973;52:392–408.

4 DEVLIN HB. Stoma therapy review. *Coloproctology* 1982;4:172-176, 250–259, 298–306, 366–374.

5 DEVLIN HB, DATTA D, DELLIPIANI AW. The incidence and prevalence of inflammatory bowel disease in North Tees health district. *World J Surg* 1980;4:183–193.

6 DEVLIN HB, ELCOAT C. Alimentary tract fistula: stomatherapy techniques of management. *World J Surg* 1983;7:489–494.

7 DEVLIN HB, PLANT JA, GRIFFIN M. The aftermath of surgery for anorectal cancer. *Br Med J* 1971;3:413–418.

8 DEVLIN HB, RAIMES SA. Diversion and temporary stomas. In: Devlin HB, ed. *Stoma care today*. Oxford: Medical Education Services, Ltd, 1985:10.

9 FEUSTEL H, HENNIG G. Kontinente kolostomie durch Magnetverschluss. *Deut Med Wschr* 1975;100: 1063–1064.

10 FIELDING LP, STEWART-BROWN S, BLESOVSKY L. Large bowel obstruction caused by cancer. *Br Med J* 1979;2:515–517.

11 FINCH DRA. The results of colostomy closure. *Br J Surg* 1976;63:397–399.

12 FORRESTER DW, SPENCE VA, WALKER WF. Colonic mucosal-submucosal blood flow and the incidence of faecal fistula formation following colostomy closure. *Br J Surg* 1981;68:541–544.

13 FOSTER ME, LEAPER DJ, WILLIAMSON RCN. Changing patterns in colostomy: the Bristol experience. *Br J Surg* 1985;72:142–145.

14 GOLIGHER JC. Eversion technique for distal mucosal protectomy in ulcerative colitis. *Br J Surg* 1984;71:26–28.

15 HEALD RJ. Towards fewer colostomies—the impact of circular stapling devices on the surgery of rectal cancer in a district hospital. *Br J Surg* 1980;67:198–200.

16 JARVINEN HJ, MAKITIE A, SIVULA A. Long-term results of continent ileostomy. *Int J Colorect Dis* 1986;1:40–43.

17 JOHNSTON D, WILLIAMS NS, NEAL DE, AXON ATR. The value of preserving the anal sphincter in operations for ulcerative colitis and polyposis: a review of 22 mucosal proctectomies. *Br J Surg* 1981;12:874–878.

18 KOCK NG, MYRVOLD HE, NILSSON LO, PHILIPSON BM. Continent ileostomy. An account of 314 patients. *Acta Chir Scan* 1981;147:67–72.

19 MacDONALD LD, ANDERSON HR, BENNETT AE *Cancer patients in the community: outcomes of care and quality of survival in rectal cancer*. London: DHSS/HMSO 1982.

20 MITTAL VK, and CORTEZ JA. Hartmann procedure reconstruction with EEA stapler. *Dis Colon Rectum* 1981;24:215–216.

21 PARKS AG, NICHOLLS J. Proctocolectomy without ileostomy for ulcerative colitis. *Br Med J* 1978;2:85–88.

22 PARKS AG, NICHOLLS RJ, BELLIVEAU P. Proctocolectomy with ileal reservoir and anal anastomosis. *Br J Surg* 1980;67:533–538.

23 PARKS TG. Surgical management of injuries of the large intestine. *Proc R Soc Med* 1981;68:725–728.

24 PLANT JA, DEVLIN HB. Ileostomy and its management. *Nurs Times* 1968;711–714.

25 QUILL DS, CONWAY W, PEEL ALG. The staple closure of loop colostomies. *Br J Surg* 1982;69:413–416.

26 SCHJONSBY H, HALVORSEN JF, HOFSTADT T, HOVDENAK N. Stagnant loop syndrome in patients with continent ileostomy (intra-abdominal ileal reservoir). *Gut* 1977;18:795–799.

27 SCHOFIELD PF, CADE D, LAMBERT M. Dependent proximal loop colostomy; does it defunction the distal colon? *Br J Surg* 1980;67:201–202.

28 WHATES PD, IRVING M. Return to work following ileostomy. *Br J Surg* 1984;71:619–22.

29 WILLIAMS NS, JOHNSTON D. Prospective controlled trial comparing colostomy irrigation with 'spontaneous action' method. *Br Med J* 1980;281:107–109.

30 WINKLER MJ, VOLPE PA. Loop transverse colostomy—the case against. *Dis Colon Rectum* 1982;25:321–326.

31 YAJKO RD, NORTON LW, BLOEMENDALE L, EISEMAN B. Morbidity of colostomy closure. *Am J Surg* 1976;132:304–306.

Chapter 56
Ileostomy: Function and Dysfunction

G. E. SLADEN

The physiological consequences of an ileostomy

The main effect of an ileostomy is an increased loss of water, sodium and chloride from the stoma, compared with the very small losses in normal faeces. Figure 56.1 compares the electrolyte composition of ileostomy and faecal fluids.

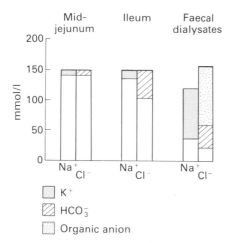

Fig. 56.1. Composite ionograms showing typical composition of fluid sampled at mid-jejunum and ileum and of faecal fluid [34].

Ileostomy fluid volumes in subjects with an intact ileum vary from 400–1000 ml/day [13, 19, 22], compared with normal faecal losses of 80–150 ml/day (Fig. 56.2). Studies of total body water and exchangeable sodium suggest that healthy ileostomists have a chronic mild degree of dehydration and salt depletion [2, 12, 16].

The composition of ileostomy fluid varies little but the level of ileostomy influences

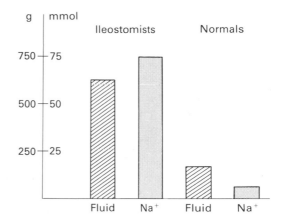

Fig. 56.2. Mean daily output of fluid (g) and sodium (mmol) in ileostomists and normal subjects.

the pH and bicarbonate concentration of ileal fluid. **The pH of ileostomy fluid** is between 7 and 8, very similar to that found in the intact ileum using intubation techniques [21]. The bicarbonate concentration is higher, and that of chloride lower, than is found in plasma. Early reports [19] stated that ileostomy fluid pH is around 6, but this may be caused by bacterial activity *in vitro* during 24 hour collection periods. By contrast, jejunal fluid has a pH of about 6 and a relatively low bicarbonate concentration (Fig. 56.1). Thus the volume and pH of stomal effluent will indicate approximately how much functioning ileum remains. This pH difference is of little clinical significance, because acid-base disturbances are unusual in ileostomy dysfunction.

Salt depletion in an ileostomist produces changes in cation composition, which can be mimicked by exogenously administered 'salt-active' corticosteroids [7]. In severe dehydration, **sodium** concentrations as low as 80 mmol/l and **potassium** as high as 40 mmol/l have been described in ileostomy fluid [6]. In these circumstances, renal conservation of sodium will be intense at the expense of increased potassium losses; serious potassium depletion may occur.

The ingestion of **water** has relatively little effect on ileostomy volume because it is rapidly absorbed from the jejunum [19]. However, the small intestine has a limited capacity to absorb sodium chloride and the ingestion of salt produces marked increases in ileostomy volume [18]. This is important in the oral replacement of salt and water in dehydrated ileostomists. Food in general stimulates ileostomy flow and, empirically, many patients avoid certain items of food, especially fruits, nuts and vegetables [1].

The **major nutrients** are well-absorbed in ileostomists with an intact ileum. Ileal output of fat is similar to that in the faeces of normal subjects [19]. Clinical and laboratory indices of nutritional state are generally normal, but with a tendency to very mild iron deficiency [16]. There is little evidence that calcium or magnesium deficiency occurs in ileostomists and, indeed, loss of these cations in ileostomy fluid tends to be less than that found in normal faeces [38].

Special problems in the ileostomist with Crohn's disease

Crohn's ileostomists produce more ileal effluent than those operated on for ulcerative colitis, even in the absence of overt recurrent disease [22]. They are more likely to be underweight and to have a modest reduction of haemoglobin and serum albumin, and elevation of ESR [16]. Associated ileal resection or overt ileal recurrence will lead to malabsorption of fat, vitamin B_{12} and bile salts in proportion to the length of ileum affected. Loss of more than 25 cm of ileum will produce detectable malabsorp-

tion, which will be gross if as much as 100 cm are resected [29]. Under these circumstances, calcium and magnesium deficiencies may also be observed [9].

Ileal adaptation

It is often stated that ileostomy volumes will decrease with time and that the fluid will thicken. It is difficult to judge this in the first few weeks, until normal eating habits are re-established. Hill [11] considers that adaptation does occur over a period of a year after surgery, except in patients who have had appreciable ileal resection.

The best evidence concerning ileal adaptation is that produced by intubation studies in healthy subjects, in which ileal flow rates in the fasting and fed states have been measured and compared with similar observations in ileostomists [21, 30]. These studies show that the normal ileal fluid has a lower K^+ concentration (4–6 mmol/l) than that found in ileostomists (8–16 mmol/l). The mechanism of this adaptation is unclear, but salt depletion and a chronic aldosterone drive seem to be major influences [11, 16].

Extra-intestinal consequences of ileostomy

Psychological state and sexual function

Most ileostomists have full and satisfying lives, and can indulge in a wide range of active leisure pursuits, although contact sports have to be avoided. The majority probably enjoy normal sexual activities; normal pregnancy can be anticipated [31]. However, there are a number of studies which have shown that many patients experience difficulty with sexual activity related both to psychological and physical disturbances. An important adverse factor in the male is the dissection required in the operation of proctectomy, which can damage the pelvic parasympathetic nerves. That psychological factors may be of greater importance in the majority is suggested by a recent report that sexual difficulties are experienced much less frequently in patients with a continent than a conventional ileostomy [26]. This whole topic is discussed in detail with many references by Young and Shipes [39] and by Kennedy *et al.* [16].

In general, life expectancy in ileostomists with previous ulcerative colitis is considered to be almost the same as that of the general population [31].

Kidney stones

It is generally accepted that kidney stones are more frequent in ileostomists than in healthy controls. Prevalence rates in published series vary from 2–18% in ileostomists compared with 1–4% in the general population of the United Kingdom [16]. Radiolucent renal stones, composed mainly of uric acid, are found most frequently in ileostomists and are ascribed to the passage of relatively small volumes of concentrated urine with lower than normal sodium concentration and of relatively low pH [3]. The solubility of uric acid is much reduced at low pH. Although there has been some disagreement about the low pH of ileostomists' urine [33], there is general agreement that ileostomists should endeavour to maintain as near normal urinary outputs of salt and water as possible. Measures to alkalinize the urine are not normally required.

Oxalate stones are described in patients with Crohn's disease, especially those with steatorrhoea and an intact colon. This is thought to be the result of increased colonic absorption of dietary oxalate leading to 'enteric hyperoxaluria' [4]. If this is correct, Crohn's ileostomists should not be at any extra risk of oxalate stones.

Gallstones

Gallstones occur more commonly in patients with Crohn's disease and small gut resection, owing to loss of bile salts from the enterohepatic circulation [5, 10]. There is some evidence that ileostomists have an increased prevalence of gallstones [16], but the mechanism is obscure. Ileostomists with an intact ileum do not lose bile salts excessively [29].

Disturbed ileostomy function

Ileostomists are liable to all the many causes of **disturbed gut function** that afflict normal subjects. These are usually related to dietary indiscretions or infection, are self-limiting and are only of significance if there is a temporary increased loss of salt and water.

Ileostomists are liable to bouts of abdominal colic, distension, and temporary partial or complete cessation of ileal flow. These **obstructive episodes** may be caused by impaction of a bolus of food, by twisting of loops of ileum caused by adhesions or, in patients with Crohn's disease, by stenosing recurrence. In general, the clinical picture and management are the same as in patients without an ileostomy.

The most serious disturbance is an intermittent or chronic **increase of ileostomy flow.** Fluid loss increases in proportion to the length of ileum diseased or resected [22]. Recurrent disease poses an obvious threat to Crohn's ileostomists. In such patients, radiology and endoscopy can define the presence and extent of recurrent disease, and anti-inflammatory drugs may be effective in suppressing it and reducing ileostomy flow. Surgical excision may be unavoidable if the recurrence is complicated by structure or fistula, but clearly should be as conservative as possible.

Increased fluid loss, with or without obstructive pain, is often ascribed to **chronic** partial **obstruction** at or near the stoma [11]. The obstruction may result from a poorly constructed stoma or may be caused by adhesive peritoneal bands deep to the stoma. These bands may be related to local chronic pockets of sepsis, only apparent at laparotomy. The diagnosis is based on digital, endoscopic and radiological examination; the condition will usually respond to surgical reconstruction of the stoma in well-selected cases. It is not clear why chronic partial obstruction should be accompanied by increased fluid loss, but there is animal evidence that obstructed and distended intestinal loops fail to absorb salt and water normally [11].

A related problem, but now apparently a rare one, is so-called **prestomal ileitis**. This was commoner as a post-operative problem at the time when flush ileostomies were created with the serosa sutured to the skin. These stomas were liable to stenosis caused by inflammation, oedema and later, fibrosis. A severe diarrhoeal state was accompanied by non-specific inflammation and ulceration of the distal ileum. It could only be cured by reconstruction of the stoma and resection of the affected ileal segment. It seems to be rarely, if ever, a problem with the modern everted spout ileostomy, which became popular in the 1950s. Some cases of chronic prestomal ileitis have been described in more recent papers, but they are an ill-defined group [20]. It is obviously important to exclude Crohn's disease (the initial diagnosis may not have been certain) and to deal with a tight or unsatisfactory stoma if present. Topical or systemic steroids have been used, especially if diarrhoea is accompanied by blood and mucus and if general health is impaired. The condition appears to be quite unrelated to so-called 'backwash ileitis' seen on barium enema examinations of some patients with total ulcerative colitis, prior to the creation of an ileostomy.

Treatment of patients with large ileostomy losses

Most acute disturbances of ileostomy function can be treated by **intravenous 0.9% sodium chloride** and, if appropriate, by withholding oral food and fluid. Careful fluid balance records and regular weighing are essential; measurement of urinary sodium provides the best guide to the adequacy of salt replacement.

A chronic modest increase in ileostomy losses can often be controlled by **conventional antidiarrhoeal agents.** Loperamide is probably more effective than codeine phosphate or diphenoxylate and large doses, up to 16 mg/day, may be required [36]. All these drugs can produce colicky abdominal pain and nausea; patients may prefer to tolerate a moderate increase in ileostomy losses. Another concern is that of drug dependence, but it is believed to be less of a problem with loperamide than with codeine phosphate.

Bulking agents, such as methyl cellulose, can increase the viscosity of ileostomy effluent, but tend to increase faecal volume and the total losses of water and salt [23]. There is also the risk of bolus obstruction in patients liable to obstructive episodes. In general, agents of this sort are of very limited value in ileostomy management.

Patients who lose more than 1 litre of fluid daily should deliberately take extra **salt and water.** Kennedy *et al.* [16] recommend one teaspoon of salt (approximately 120 mmol of sodium) and an extra litre of fluid as minimum supplements. Simple guides to these needs include a check on the number of times the bag is emptied per day (approximately 150 ml fluid each time) and the sodium concentration of a 'spot' sample of urine. A urinary sodium of less than 10 mmol/l implies avid salt retention, and the oral intake should be increased (ideally the urinary Na^+/K^+ ratio should exceed 1 [11]).

If the ileal losses are two litres or more, the oral replacement of these large quantities of salt and water poses a major problem. Isotonic saline is unpleasant to drink and is poorly absorbed from the small intestine, so that purgation results. The addition of avidly absorbed nutrient molecules such as sugars and amino acids greatly enhances absorption of water and salt by the small intestine; this has led to the use of **oral rehydration mixtures** for the treatment of cholera and a variety of acute diarrhoeal illnesses, especially in children [32]. This principle has been applied to the long-term management of chronic ileostomy diarrhoea and a variety of solutions has been used successfully (Table 56.1). It must be stressed that these patients may have to drink 2–3 litres or more of these solutions each day to the exclusion of all other forms of fluid. The criteria of success are the maintenance of adequate hydration as judged clinically and of a urinary Na^+ concentration greater than 10 mmol/l. Many such patients have now been described, who formerly would have needed repeated intravenous saline infusions and would have run the additional risk of K^+ depletion [37].

A small number of patients, with very short small intestines, may be unable to maintain adequate hydration in this way and will require intermittent or long-term **parenteral feeding**. In some such patients, reversal of a segment of remaining small bowel has successfully decreased ileostomy losses of fluid and nutrients [28].

The continent ileostomy

There has been much recent interest in surgical methods of avoiding the problems of the conventional ileostomy and its inevitable appliances. These are designed to avoid the need for bags by producing a continent ileostomy with the opening either on the abdominal wall (Kock) or at the anus (Parks) [24].

Apart from the problem of continence, these procedures do not mitigate any of the functional disturbances consequent upon loss of the colon and additional physiological disturbances may be created [15]. However, there is evidence that patients may be much better satisfied by well-functioning

---

Table 56.1. Recommended oral rehydration solutions in treatment of severe diarrhoea and profuse ileostomy losses.

The fluid recommended for upper small intestinal losses reflects the higher chloride and lower bicarbonate concentrations of jejunal compared with ileal fluid (see Fig. 56.1). Caloreen (a glucose polymer) provides additional substrate to promote sodium chloride and water absorption, without imposing a large osmotic load.

The *WHO solution* contains per litre:
Glucose 20 g (approx. 4 heaped 5 ml spoons)
Sodium bicarbonate 2.5 g (less than a level spoon)
Sodium chloride 3.5 g (less than a level spoon)
Potassium chloride 1.5 g (half a level spoon)

	Oral Rehydration Solutions (mmol/l)	
	WHO recommended solution for cholera/gastroenteritis	A solution recommended for high ileostomy/jejunostomy losses [8]
Glucose	111	100
Caloreen	—	20 (18 g/l)
Sodium	90	85
Potassium	20	12
Bicarbonate	30	9
Chloride	80	88

continent ileostomies than by conventional ileostomies, especially in papers written from Kock's own group [17, 26].

In patients with Kock ileostomies faecal volumes are similar to those in patients with conventional ileostomies but, in one study, about one-third of the patients had daily losses of greater than 1 litre [14]. There is a tendency to increased faecal losses of fat and impaired vitamin B_{12} malabsorption, related in part to the inevitable loss of ileal surface area required by the creation of the ileal pouch. However, abnormal bacterial proliferation in the lower small intestine may also contribute to this malabsorption and beneficial effects of metronidazole therapy have been reported [15]. Morphological and histochemical changes in the pouch mucosa have been described, but they are of mild degree and probably lessen with the passage of time [27].

The patients are presumably at risk of chronic salt and water depletion and are liable to form kidney- [35] and, perhaps, gallstones. Isotopic studies using tritiated water and total body potassium showed no evidence of chronic depletion compared with healthy controls [25], but this is difficult to reconcile with the ileostomy and urine volumes and urinary sodium losses reported elsewhere [14].

Useful addresses

1. International Ostomy Association
   General Secretary: Edwin J Ward
   9135 Fordham Street
   Indianapolis
   IN 46268
2. Ileostomy Association of Great Britain and Ireland, Central Office Address:
   Amblehurst House
   Chobham
   Woking
   Surrey GU24 8PZ
   Tel: (09905) 8277

References

1 BINGHAM S, CUMMINGS JH, McNEIL NI. Diet and health of people with an ileostomy. *Br J Nutr* 1982;**47**:399–406.

2 CLARKE AM, CHIRNSIDE A, HILL GL, POPE G, STEWART MK. Chronic dehydration and sodium depletion in patients with established ileostomies. *Lancet* 1967;ii:740–743.

3 CLARKE MA, McKENZIE RG. Ileostomy and the risk of urinary uric acid stones. *Lancet* 1969;ii:395–397.

4 DOBBINS JW, BINDER HJ. Importance of the colon in enteric hyperoxaluria. *N Engl J Med* 1977;**296**: 298–301.

5 DOWLING RH, BELL GD, WHITE J. Lithogenic bile in patients with ileal dysfunction. *Gut* 1972; **13**: 415–420.

6 GALLAGHER ND, HARRISON DD, WYATT JV, SKYRING AP. Sodium conservation by the small intestine in a patient with chronic ileostomy diarrhoea. *Gut* 1969;**10**:202–205.

7 GOULSTON K, HARRISON DD, SKYRING AP. Effect of mineralocorticoids on the sodium/potassium ratio of human ileostomy fluid. *Lancet* 1963;ii:541–542.

8 GRIFFIN GE, FAGAN EF, HODGSON HJ, *et al.* Enteral therapy in the management of massive gut resection complicated by chronic fluid and electrolyte depletion. *Dig Dis Sci* 1982;**27**:902–908.

9 HEATON KW, CLARK CG, GOLIGHER JC. Magnesium deficiency complicating intestinal surgery. *Br J Surg* 1967;**54**:41–45.

10 HEATON KW, READ AE. Gall stones in patients with disorders of the terminal ileum and disturbed bile salt metabolism. *Br Med J* 1969;**3**:494–496.

11 HILL GL. Normal ileostomy physiology. In: *Ileostomy. Surgery, Physiology and Management*. New York: Grune and Stratton, 1976:79–82.

12 HILL GL, GOLIGHER JC, SMITH AH, MAIR WSJ. Long term changes in total body water, total exchangeable sodium and total body potassium before and after ileostomy. *Br J Surg* 1975;**62**:524–527.

13 KANAGHINIS T, LUBRAN M, COGHILL NF. The composition of ileostomy fluid. *Gut* 1963;**4**:322–337.

14 KELLY DG, BRANON ME, PHILLIPS SF, KELLY KA. Diarrhoea after continent ileostomy. *Gut* 1980;**21**:711–716.

15 KELLY DG, PHILLIPS SF, KELLY KA, *et al.* Dysfunction of the continent ileostomy: clinical features and bacteriology. *Gut* 1983;**24**:193–201.

16 KENNEDY HJ, LEE ECG, CLARIDGE G, TRUELOVE SC. The health of subjects living with a permanent ileostomy. *Q J Med* 1982;**51**:341–357.

17 KOCK NG, MYRVOLD HE, NILSSON LO, PHILIPSON BM. Continent ileostomy. An account of 314 patients. *Acta Chir Scand* 1981;**147**:67–72.

18 KRAMER P. The effect of varying sodium loads on the ileal excreta of human ileostomised subjects. *J Clin Invest* 1966;**45**:1710–1718.

19 KRAMER P, KEARNEY MM, INGETFINGER FJ. The effect of specific foods and water loading on the ileal excreta of ileostomised human subjects. *Gastroenterology* 1963;**42**:535–546.

20 KRULL-JONES RP, MORSON B, WILLIAMS R. Prestomal ileitis: clinical and pathological findings in five cases. *Q J Med* 1970;**39**:287–297.

21 LADAS S, ISAACS PET, SLADEN GE. Effects of foods on ileal and ileostomy flows in healthy and ileostomised subjects. *Gut* 1986; in press.

22 MCNEIL NI, BINGHAM S, COLE TJ, *et al.* Diet and health of people with an ileostomy. 2. Ileostomy function and nutritional state. *Br J Nutr* 1982;**47**:407–415.

23 NEWTON CR. The effect of codeine phosphate, lomotil and isogel on ileostomy function. *Gut* 1973;**14**:424–425.

24 NICHOLLS RJ. The continent ileostomy and restorative proctocolectomy with ileal reservoir. *Clin Gastroenterol* 1982;**11**:247–258.

25 NILSSON LO, ANDERSSON H, BOSAEUS I, *et al.* Total body water and total body potassium in patients with continent ileostomies. *Gut* 1982;**23**:589–593.

26 NILSSON LO, KOCK NG, KYLBERG F, *et al.* Sexual adjustment in ileostomy patients before and after conversion to continent ileostomy. *Dis Colon Rectum* 1981;**24**:287–290.

27 NILSSON LO, KOCK NG, LINDGREN I, *et al.* Morphological histochemical changes in the mucosa of the continent ileostomy reservoir 6–10 years after its construction. *Scand J Gastroenterol* 1980;**15**:737–747.

28 PENTLOW BD, EVERETT WG. Intractable ileostomy diarrhoea associated with short small bowel treated by a reversed bowel segment. *Proc R Soc Med* 1976;**69**:360–361.

29 PERCY-ROBB IW, JALAN KN, McMANUS JPA, *et al.* Effects of ileal resection on bile salt metabolism in patients with ileostomy following proctocolectomy. *Clin Sci* 1971;**41**:371–382.

30 PHILLIPS SF, GILLER J. The contribution of the colon to electrolyte and water conservation in man. *J Lab Clin Med* 1973;**81**:733–746.

31 RITCHIE JK. The health of ileostomists. *Gut* 1971;**12**:536–540.

32 SACK RB, PIERCE NF, HIRSCHHORN N. The current status of oral therapy in the treatment of acute diarrhoeal disease. *Am J Clin Nutr* 1978;**31**:2252–2257.

33 SINGER AM, BENNET RC, CARTER NG, *et al.* Blood and urinary changes in patients with ileostomies and ileo-rectal anastomoses. *Br Med J* 1973;**2**:141–143.

34 SLADEN GE. Absorption of fluid and electrolyte in health and disease. In: McColl I, Sladen GE, eds. *Intestinal absorption in man.* New York: Academic Press, 1975:67.

35 STERN H, WILSON DR, MICKLE DAG. Urolithiasis risk factors in continent reservoir ileostomy patients. *Dis Colon Rectum* 1980;**23**:556–558.

36 TYTGAT GN, HUIBREGSTE K. Loperamide and ileostomy output—placebo-controlled double-blind crossover study. *Br Med J* 1975; **2**:667–668.

37 WARD K, MURRAY B, FEIGHERY C, *et al.* Salt-losing ileostomy diarrhoea: long-term treatment with a glucose electrolyte solution. *Gut* 1981;**22**:A864.

38 WRONG OM, EDMONDS CJ, CHADWICK VS. Composition of large bowel contents. In: *The large intestine.* Lancaster: MTP Press Ltd, 1981; 17.

39 YOUNG CH, SHIPES E. Sexual implications of stoma surgery. *Clin Gastroenterol* 1982;**11**:383–396.

Chapter 57
Colonic Infections and Infestations

C. O. RECORD

Colonic infections and infestations are of particular importance in the differential diagnosis of inflammatory bowel disease, as not only may the clinical picture be similar but gastrointestinal infections may complicate and be responsible for an apparent exacerbation of inflammatory bowel disease.

Amoebic dysentery

The term dysentery was used by Hippocrates to indicate a condition characterized by the frequent passage of stools containing blood and mucus and accompanied by painful defaecation. Much of the dysentery in older writings was probably bacterial rather than amoebic, due to absence of liver involvement.

Intestinal amoebiasis is an important cause of diarrhoea and colitis in warm and humid parts of the world, particularly developing countries where sanitation is poor [26, 88]. Sporadic cases also occur in Europe, while in the United States of America intestinal carriage of cysts has been established at about 5% of the population [16]. The disease is transmitted mainly by person-to-person contact or ingestion of infected food or water. Vectors such as pets and insects may also be important and serve as a reservoir of infection. It is one of the pathogens causing proctocolitis in homosexual men [80, 102].

Entamoeba histolytica exists as active motile trophozoites, which are characteristic of amoebic dysentery, or as cysts which are more resistant to environmental stresses and occur in formed stools. Cysts are able to survive outside the body and are responsible for the transmission of infection. The factors responsible for invasion of the colonic mucosa by trophozoites are unknown, but cytolysis secondary to enzyme production and toxin production have both been suggested. Even less well characterized are the factors that are responsible for the transformation of ingested cysts into active trophozoites in the colon. An autopsy series showed that cysts were able to exist in the colonic lumen in the absence of tissue damage, while ulceration was present in some clinically inactive carriers [34]. The pathogenesis of tissue damage does appear however to be closely related to colonic bacterial flora: studies in germ-free guinea pigs have shown that intestinal disease does not develop unless bacteria are also present [94]. The beneficial effects of metronidazole may be partly related to its anti-bacterial action.

Colonic ulceration due to amoebae are classically flask-shaped ulcers, which are narrower at the mucosal surface and wider at the submucosa (Fig. 57.1). The mucosa between ulcerations may be hyperaemic or normal, whereas in bacillary dysentery the colitis is diffuse. Submucosal haemorrhages may develop and in severe cases large areas of mucosa may slough with the passage of mucosal casts. A lymphocytic cellular reaction develops but occasionally granulomas may occur which lead to the formation of tumour-like lesions (amoebomas) or to segmental colonic strictures.

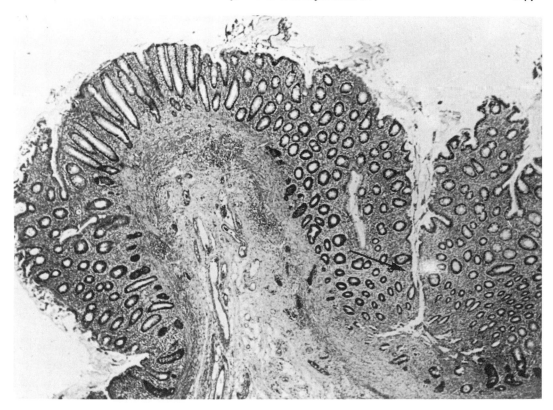

Fig. 57.1. Section through colonic mucosal biopsy, showing penetrating ulcer due to *Entamoeba histolytica*.

Clinical features

Intestinal symptoms closely resemble those of ulcerative colitis and may vary from mild diarrhoea to fulminant bloody diarrhoea. The onset is usually gradual with looseness and abdominal discomfort which may or may not progress. Mild fever and leucocytosis are common but leucocytes are unusual in the stools. A chronic intestinal infection may develop in the absence of specific therapy when intermittent diarrhoea and constipation are associated with vague abdominal discomfort. The presence of cysts in the stool of such patients may not account for their symptoms [88].

Metastatic amoebic infections may occur throughout the body but liver abscess is the most common. Such abscesses may rupture with spread to the lungs, pleura and peri-cardium. Liver abscesses complicate 1–3% of cases and about 40% of these also have concurrent intestinal symptoms. Liver abscesses may present acutely with fever, pain and tenderness over the right upper quadrant or may develop insidiously with the symptoms of a pyrexia of unknown origin. Jaundice occasionally occurs in patients with hepatic abscesses probably due to intrahepatic duct compression.

Amoeboma, perforation, stricture and haemorrhage may all complicate intestinal amoebiasis, as indeed may toxic dilatation. Pseudopolyp formation and 'thumb printing' may be seen radiologically [68].

Diagnosis

Laboratory confirmation of the diagnosis may be achieved in three ways: stool micro-

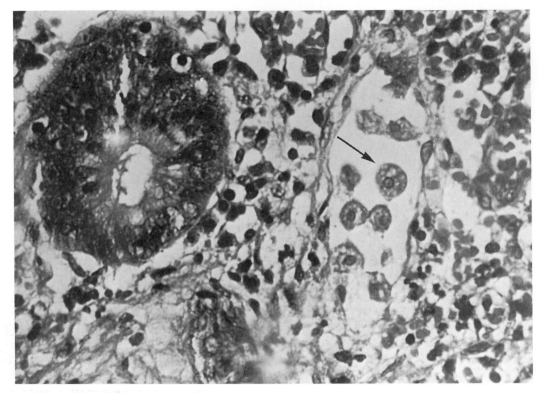

Fig. 57.2. High power view of colonic biopsy from a patient with amoebic dysentery showing amoebae within the lymphatics.

scopy, rectal biopsy (Fig. 57.2) and serology. Only trophozoites are present in the stools of severely ill patients and these can be difficult to find unless fresh specimens are examined (within one hour of passage). Contrast media and anti-diarrhoeal preparations make identification of amoebae impossible, while amoebae disappear from the stool after antibiotic administration [68]. Rectal biopsy can be particularly helpful in diagnosis, amoebae staining as PAS positive particles particularly prominent in the surface exudate. Serological tests are most valuable in patients with extra-intestinal amoebiasis (92–98% positive: [68]) when stool examination for amoebae is frequently negative. Serological tests are also valuable for active intestinal infection and for screening patients with suspected inflammatory bowel disease in order to exclude an amoe-bic aetiology, particularly prior to systemic corticosteroid administration [51]. Non-pathogenic amoebae found in the human stools (such as *Entamoeba hartmanni* and *coli*, *Endolimax nana*, *Iodamoeba butschlii* and *Dientamoeba fragilis*) need to be carefully distinguished from *Entamoeba histolytica* [32].

Therapy

Metronidazole is the drug of first choice for acute invasive amoebic dysentery as it is very effective against vegetative trophozoites both in the intestine and liver; 800 mg tds for 10 days is usually effective. Diloxanide furoate is the drug of first choice in chronic intestinal infections associated with the passage of cysts in the stool; 500 mg tds for 10 days is usually effective [68]. The cardiotoxic drugs emetine and emetine bismuth iodide are now rarely required.

For hepatic abscesses metronidazole alone or in combination with chloroquine (600 mg/day for five days followed by 300 mg/day for 14–21 days) may be used. For large abscesses (containing more than 100 ml pus) aspiration combined with drug therapy speeds resolution. Diloxanide is ineffective for hepatic amoebiasis.

Bacillary dysentery

Bacillary dysentery is due to infection with *Shigella* species and some shigella-like *E. coli*. The virulence of these organisms is due to their invasiveness whereby the infecting strain is capable of penetrating the epithelial lining of the gut. Shigella organisms appear to multiply in the small intestine which secretes water and electrolytes, possibly due to activation of cyclic AMP by shigella toxin. However, the principal manifestations of the disease are due to invasion of the colonic wall with ulceration and the development of dysenteric symptoms. Four principal serogroups are responsible for human disease: *S. dysenteriae*, *S. flexneri*, *S. boydii* and *S. sonnei*.

The disease is spread by person-to-person contact, faecal excretion of the organism continuing for 1–4 weeks in untreated patients. Rare continued excretion for up to one year has been documented [75]. Food and waterborne outbreaks are also recognized while flies appear to harbour pathogenic organisms. Transmission rates within families vary from 60% in those under one year of age to approximately 20% for all ages. The high communicability probably results from the low inoculum necessary to produce human illness [31]. *Shigella* strains remain viable at room temperature for periods up to six months. *Shigella dysenteriae* produces a more severe illness than other strains, the mortality in epidemics in developing countries being about 20%. In the West, *Shigella sonnei* is now the most frequently isolated serogroup [32].

Clinical features

The onset is characterized by fever, abdominal pain and watery diarrhoea. These symptoms are followed after 24–72 hours by the development of the colonic phase when the stools become bloody and mucoid. In severe cases waves of intense cramps and tenesmus are associated with frequent small volume stools containing blood and mucus. In a series of sporadic cases presenting in the United States, the onset was gradual in two-thirds of patients; high fever was present in one-third of patients and moderate fever in a further one-third; the stools of only half of the patients contained blood. By contrast, in a Central American epidemic the onset was abrupt with rapid progression to bloody diarrhoea within 24 hours in 70% of patients [62]. Aseptic meningitis, febrile convulsions, respiratory symptoms and haemolytic uraemic syndrome may all complicate shigellosis. The development of Reiter's syndrome (arthritis, uveitis, conjunctivitis) following shigella infections is a well-recognized complication, associated with HLA B27 positivity [19].

Diagnosis and treatment

The specific diagnosis of shigella infections can only be made by stool culture. Stool microscopy reveals large numbers of polymorphonuclear leucocytes, while on sigmoidoscopy the rectal mucosa appears congested with superficial ulceration. In addition to inflammatory changes and ulceration, rectal histology may show crypt abscesses.

Antibiotic therapy is valuable in reducing the duration of symptoms, shortens the period of post-infection carriage and may thus decrease the spread of infection. However the disease is self-limiting and is usually of only mild severity. For patients requiring specific therapy a five-day course of ampicillin is best, an absorbable antibiotic being required in order to reach organisms within the lamina propria of the gut [47]. However, *Shigella sonnei* strains may be resistant, when co-trimoxazole should be used. Rehydration with oral glucose and electrolyte solutions is an important aspect of therapy, particularly in children.

Salmonellosis

Salmonella gastroenteritis is a common problem in all parts of the world, but particularly in developed countries where dissemination of the organism occurs through mass production and distribution of food. By contrast, typhoid or enteric fever, the most serious salmonella infection, is usually related to reduced economic development and sanitation.

More than 1400 serotypes of salmonella have been identified and virulence depends on their ability to invade endothelial cells. Poultry and domestic livestock [33] are the major non-human reservoir of salmonella infection, but humans are the only important reservoir for the typhoid bacillus (*Salmonella typhi*). Although salmonella infections were thought to involve mainly the small intestine, colonic involvement is now well-recognized [13, 82].

Clinical features

There are three major patterns of salmonella infection: (1) acute gastroenteritis; (2) typhoid (enteric) fever, with septicaemia or localized infection; (3) asymptomatic carrier state. The disease expression depends mainly upon the infecting strain: *S. typhi*, *S. paratyphi* and *S. cholerae suis* characteristically cause systemic features or enteric fever, while other strains lead to acute gastroenteritis without blood stream invasion.

Salmonella gastroenteritis

Clinical symptoms of gastroenteritis such as headache, abdominal pain, fever and diarrhoea develop 8–48 hours after ingestion of contaminated food [13, 23, 99]. Stools are watery and rarely contain blood; stool culture at this stage reveals the responsible organism. Antibiotics are not valuable in the management of salmonella gastroenteritis unless the patient is severely ill or has a salmonella bacteraemia. Treatment of uncomplicated gastroenteritis results in prolonged stool carriage of the pathogen together with the development of *in vivo* resistance to the drug. The resolution of symptoms appears to be similar in antibiotic and non-antibiotic treated groups.

Typhoid fever

The incubation period of typhoid fever averages from 10–20 days (range: 3–56 days) and varies depending on the size of the inoculum. The onset is insidious with mounting fever, vague abdominal pain, headache and cough. In the second week the patient becomes dull and apathetic with sustained fever and abdominal distension. Diarrhoea, splenomegaly and the characteristic rose spots become evident. Rose spots are areas of cutaneous vasculitis which occur mainly on the abdomen. Intestinal haemorrhage and perforation are serious complications, the latter accounting for much of the mortality [63]. The diagnosis of perforation may be difficult because of extreme toxaemia, when the classical signs of perforation are frequently absent. Perforation is best managed surgically with simple closure and peritoneal drainage combined with antibiotic therapy.

Neuropsychiatric complications including delerium, meningism and encephalomyelitis, together with disseminated intravascular coagulation, haemolytic uraemic syndrome, toxic myocarditis, hepatitis, pancreatitis and metastatic salmonella infections particularly in bone, are all recognized [83].

Confirmation of the diagnosis of typhoid fever depends upon isolation of the offending organism from blood, bone marrow, stool or urine. Blood cultures are positive in 80% of patients, particularly during the first week of the illness, while stool cultures are mainly positive during the second and third weeks. Serology can be valuable in the absence of culture facilities, a rising titre of 'O' antibody indicating active infection [83].

The antibiotic most widely used for the treatment of enteric fever is chloramphenicol. With a 14-day course the mortality has been reduced from 20% to below 2%. However, drug-resistant strains are becoming widespread, and for these patients amoxycillin or co-trimoxazole appear to be equally efficacious [83]. Dexamethasone appears to decrease mortality in severely ill patients with disturbed consciousness [52].

Asymptomatic carriers

Carriers of *salmonella typhi* are a major source of endemic and epidemic typhoid fever, and can be a particular hazard in the gastrointestinal investigation unit. The organism is frequently carried in the gallbladder and cholecystectomy may be necessary in patients with gallstones. High-dose antibiotic therapy for up to two months may be necessary to eliminate the organism.

Salmonella infections and ulcerative colitis

Both idiopathic ulcerative colitis and salmonella infections are common diseases and their coexistence may lead to diagnostic and therapeutic difficulties [29]. In a study of 153 patients with ulcerative colitis 5% were shown to have developed a salmonella infection [77]. Both salmonella and ulcerative colitis can lead to bloody diarrhoea, although this is uncommon in the former. Thus the persistence of bloody diarrhoea in a patient with salmonella infection suggests the coexistence of ulcerative colitis. Histological features, including crypt abscesses, are common to both conditions [24] and differentiation on morphological grounds may be difficult. Stool samples should always be cultured at the start of every relapse of inflammatory bowel disease.

Campylobacter infections

Campylobacters have been known to cause infectious infertility and abortions in cattle and sheep for many years but their importance as pathogenic organisms in man was not recognized until the development of selective media for their isolation from stools [73]. Skirrow [109] showed that this organism was present in the stools of 7.1% of British children and adults with acute diarrhoea. Campylobacters are now recognized as world-wide pathogens and their isolation often outnumbers those of salmonella and shigella together [9, 18, 112].

Campylobacter infections in man are thought to be contracted mainly from infected food, particularly poultry, but water-borne [91] and milk-related outbreaks [104] and infection from dogs [8, 33], are also recognized. Campylobacters affect both the small and large intestine, dissemination of the organism being thought to be via blood stream invasion with subsequent localization in the gut, a mechanism similar to that seen in *Salmonella typhi* infections [44]. Evidence for enterotoxin production and local invasion has recently been found [121].

Because of the frequency of isolation of campylobacters many laboratories now routinely culture stools for this organism. Diagnosis can also be confirmed by the demonstration of a rise in a specific antibody, which appears in the blood on about the fifth day [18]. Blood cultures may reveal the organism in the presymptomatic phase of the disease.

Clinical manifestations

The disease consists mainly of a self-limiting attack of acute diarrhoea lasting for a few days. Patients seeking medical attention, with a bacteriologically confirmed diagnosis, present after an average incubation period of 3–5 days. Diarrhoea may be preceded by fever, malaise, headache, myalgia and abdominal pain. Eventually the abdominal pain becomes colicky and is associated with the appearance of diarrhoea. Rectal bleeding frequently follows. The symptoms persist for 1–2 weeks, after which they spontaneously remit. Diagnosis

is by stool culture, the organism persisting in the stool for 2–5 weeks. In children symptoms may mimic an acute abdomen and an unnecessary laparotomy may result. Intussusception has also been considered where rectal bleeding has been prominent in the absence of diarrhoea [18]. Massive lower gastrointestinal haemorrhage [85], a reactive arthritis [7], Reiter's syndrome [119] and Guillain-Barré syndrome [103] may all complicate the infection. Campylobacter infections are one of the causes of proctocolitis in homosexual men [100].

Campylobacter infections need to be differentiated from other infective causes of colitis, histological evidence of inflammation being similar to that seen in salmonella and shigella infections [97]. Campylobacter colitis must also be differentiated from the first manifestation of idiopathic ulcerative colitis, particularly when the course of the former is prolonged. Clinical, sigmoidoscopic and histological features may be

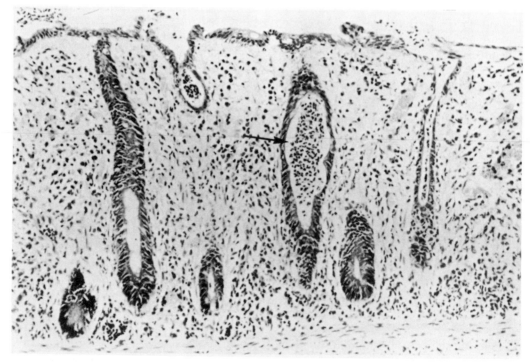

Fig. 57.3. Section through biopsy of rectal mucosa showing crypt abscess due to campylobacter infection [129].

similar in the two conditions including the presence of crypt abscesses [69, 121, 129] (Fig. 57.3).

Treatment

The great majority of campylobacter infections are self-limiting, symptoms resolving before bacteriological diagnosis has been made. Under such circumstances the organism rapidly disappears from the stool and antibiotic treatment is inappropriate. However, a more prolonged illness may ensue and antibiotics may shorten the course of the disease in such patients.

Studies of the *in vitro* sensitivity of campylobacters to antibiotics have shown that erythromycin, tetracycline, chloramphenicol and gentamicin are the most active, but some strains are resistant. Penicillins show little activity, while all but a few isolates are resistant to cephalosporins and lincomycin [120].

Erythromycin has advantages over other antibiotics in that it has a narrow spectrum of activity and low toxicity, while serum concentrations are achieved that should enable the antibiotic to act on organisms in the tissues. A placebo-controlled trial of a five-day course of erythromycin (250 mg, six-hourly) showed rapid eradication of the organism from the stool, but the mean duration of symptoms following initiation of therapy was similar to the two groups [3]. Because some strains are resistant to erythromycin, severely ill septicaemic patients should be treated with a combination of erythromycin plus gentamicin or chloramphenicol.

Yersinia infections

Yersinia are Gram-negative rods previously known as pasteurella. *Yersinia pestis*, the plague bacterium, causes adenitis, sepsis, pneumonitis and meningitis. *Yersinia pseudotuberculosis* has been recognized for many years as a cause of mesenteric adenitis particularly in children, while more recently *Yersinia enterocolitica* has been implicated as a common cause of gastroenteritis [71, 123].

There is considerable overlap between the clinical syndromes caused by each organism, but *Y. pseudotuberculosis* and *Y. enterocolitica* can be distinguished by their biochemical reactions *in vitro* [90]. Yersinia are widely disseminated in birds, pets, livestock and poultry. Person-to-person transmission has been suggested by family and hospital outbreaks, but the major mode of transmission is thought to be by contamination of food or milk and animal excreta. The incubation period ranges from 4–10 days. Yersinia infections cause diarrhoea initially by toxin production—both by activation of cyclic AMP and also by direct cytotoxicity in the ileum and colon. Later invasion of the colonic wall may lead to dysenteric symptoms with blood and pus in the stool.

Clinical symptoms

Acute gastroenteritis is a mild self-limiting illness characterized by diarrhoea (78%), fever (43%) and abdominal pain (84%) [123]. The stool frequency varies from 3–10/day, the motions usually being watery although blood may be present in up to 10% of patients (Fig. 57.4). The enteritis can be more severe and cause ulceration, with perforation and peritonitis.

When periumbilical or right lower quadrant abdominal pain are the principal manifestation, **mesenteric adenitis/terminal ileitis** may be confused with acute appendicitis. However, at laparotomy the appendix is normal while the mesenteric lymph nodes are enlarged. The terminal ileum appears inflamed, thickened and hyperaemic. The disease appears to be self-limiting, but occasionally the persistence of symptoms and surgical findings can mimic

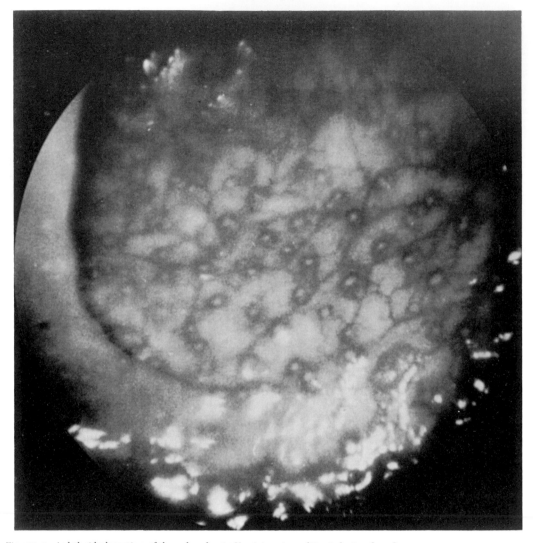

Fig. 57.4. Aphthoid ulceration of the colon due to *Yersinia enterocolitica* infection [122].

Crohn's disease [106]. Yersinia organisms are not causally related to Crohn's disease.

A **septicaemic illness** can result from yersinia infection, particularly in the elderly or immunocompromised. Extraintestinal manifestations of yersinia infections include erythema nodosum and polyarthritis [15].

Diagnosis and treatment

Diagnosis of yersinia infections depends on the isolation of the organism from the stool [28], or blood, or the demonstration of a rising titre of agglutinins to a pathogenic serotype. A titre of 1 in 160 is usually considered significant [90].

In patients with an inflamed terminal ileum radiological features consisting of coarsening of the folds of the terminal ileum associated with nodule formation and ulcers, while endoscopic examination shows small aphthoid ulcers with normal intervening mucosa [122].

Yersinia strains are sensitive to a wide range of antibiotics including chloramphenicol, co-trimoxazole and tetracycline. In severely ill patients, or when symptoms persist, treatment with antibiotics should be given, although prospective studies comparing different antibiotics have not been reported.

Chlamydial infections

Chlamydial infections cause non-specific urethritis, a sexually-transmitted disease. The latter is caused mainly by the D–K serotypes of *C. trachomatis*, while the A–C serotypes cause hyperendemic trachoma in developing countries. Lymphogranuloma venereum (LGV) is a tropical manifestation of the LGV serotypes I–III of *C. trachomatis*, the principal manifestation of which is inguinal adenopathy.

The rectum is commonly affected in women with both chlamydial and gonococcal infections and represents extension of the disease process to adjacent structures [107]. Under such circumstances the rectum is congested and characteristic chlamydial follicles develop [30]. More recently ulcerative proctitis in homesexual men has been attributed to chlamydial infections and needs to be differentiated from episodes of idiopathic ulcerative proctocolitis [10, 76, 101]. Rectal ulcers and granulomas may be present in such patients (Fig. 57.5).

In a prospective study of 171 homosexual men, 96 had symptoms of a proctitis—*C. trachomatis* was isolated from the rectum of 14, LGV serotypes were isolated from three who had severe symptoms and sigmoidoscopic findings suggestive of Crohn's proctitis. There were 11 non-LGV isolations, eight of whom were symptomatic—in this group sigmoidoscopy showed erythema and rectal biopsy scattered polymorphonuclear leucocytes in the lamina propria [101].

The diagnosis of chlamydial infections of the rectum depends on isolation of the organism from the rectum. Alternatively, high-titre microimmunofluorescence antibody titre (1:512), seroconversion, or a four-fold rise in antibody titre can usually be demonstrated in infected patients [101]. Treatment with tetracycline (2 g/day) for 2–3 weeks is usually effective [101].

The gay bowel [35, 36, 55, 124, 127, 128]

It is now clear that male homosexuals frequently suffer from enteric infections, or may be carriers of intestinal pathogens or parasites [4, 27, 102, 108]. For example, in a prospective study of 194 homosexual men from Seattle, one or more intestinal pathogen was found in 80% of the men with gut symptoms, and in 39% of the symptom-free men (Table 57.1). *Herpes simplex* proctitis causes particularly severe rectal pain with tenesmus [41, 105].

There appears to be a specific enteropathy with the acquired immunodeficiency syndrome [67], with usually fatal malabsorption and secretory diarrhoea due to Cryptosporidiosis [95, 111]. It appears that the protozoan parasite Cryptosporidiosis usually causes a self-limiting diarrhoea in healthy subjects [54], but patients with immune deficiency are unable to clear such enteric parasites [86] (see p. 862).

Pseudomembranous colitis and *Clostridium difficile*

Clostridium difficile is a large, Gram-positive obligately anaerobic bacillus which was first described in 1935 by Hall & O'Toole [46]. Subsequent work showed that the organism produced a heat labile toxin *in*

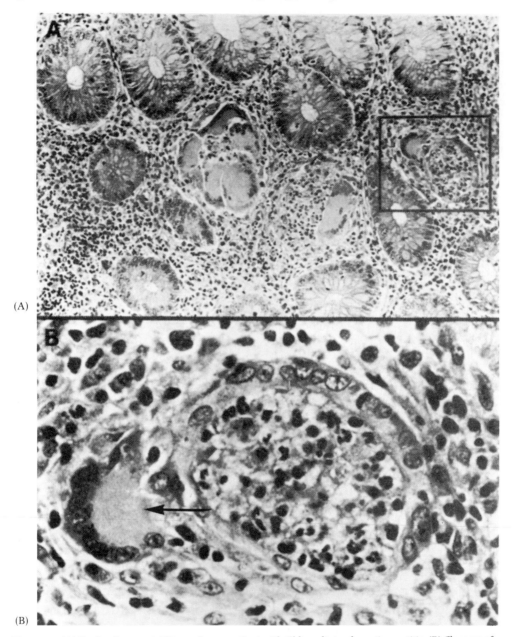

Fig. 57.5. (A) Section from rectal biopsy from a patient with *Chlamydia trachomatis* proctitis. (B) Close-up of boxed section in (A) showing macrophage granulomas with multinucleated giant cells [101].

vitro [110], that different strains of the organism produced a variable amount of toxin, and the toxin was lethal to laboratory animals 3–9 days after intra-dermal or subcutaneous injections [22].

The organism received little attention over the years because of culture difficulties but using a selective medium containing 0.2% para cresol it was possible to isolate the organism from the stools of normal

Table 57.1. Enteric infections in U.S. homosexuals [102].

	Symptomatic	Asymptomatic
No.	119	75
Age (years)	27.0	27.8
Lifetime sexual partners		
median	50	100
(range)	(1 1000)	(2–400)
Rectal swabs		
Neisseria gonorrhoeae	31%	23%
Herpes simplex	19%	4%
Clamydia trachomatis	10%	5%
Treponema pallidum	5%	1%
Stool samples		
E. histolytica	29%	25%
Giardia lamblia	14%	4%
Campylobacter jejununi	7%	3%
Shigella flexneri	3%	1%
C. difficile	3%	1%
Echo virus II	3%	1%

neonates, the vaginal flora of most women, and environmental sources [45].

Interest in *C. difficile* infections was stimulated by the isolation of a toxin from the stools of patients with pseudomembranous colitis [74] and the observation that the toxin could be neutralized by *C. sordelli* antitoxin. Stool culture observations, however, implicated *C. difficile* as the organism responsible for pseudomembranous colitis, and subsequent experiments showed cross reactivity between *C. difficile* and *sordelli* antitoxin. *C. difficile* and its toxin are now thought to be the principal pathogenic factors associated with pseudomembranous colitis [5].

C. difficile infections are also thought to be of importance in antibiotic-associated diarrhoea in the absence of pseudomembrane formation [78] and in cases of sporadic diarrhoea [14].

Pseudomembranous colitis

Pseudomembranous colitis is a term applied to patients with symptoms of a colitis when there is formation of a pseudomembrane (Fig. 57.6). Sigmoidoscopy shows exudative punctate raised plaques with intervening areas of hyperaemic oedematous mucosa, the lesions occurring predominantly in the colon (Fig. 57.7). Histologically there are areas of focal necrosis with polymorphonuclear cells to form a characteristic 'summit' lesion (Fig. 57.8). In more severe cases the surface inflammatory exudate becomes more extensive and forms a typical pseudomembrane, but crypt abscesses are rarely seen [98].

Pseudomembranous colitis has been recognized for many years as an unusual complication of abdominal surgery, colonic obstruction, and as a complication of debilitating diseases. In the early 1950s it was associated with the use of the newly-introduced antibiotics chloramphenicol and tetracycline. More recently pseudomembranous colitis has been linked to lincomycin and clindamycin, a 10% incidence being associated with the latter [116]. It is now recognized as being an important complication of the use of virtually all antibiotics used either alone or in combination.

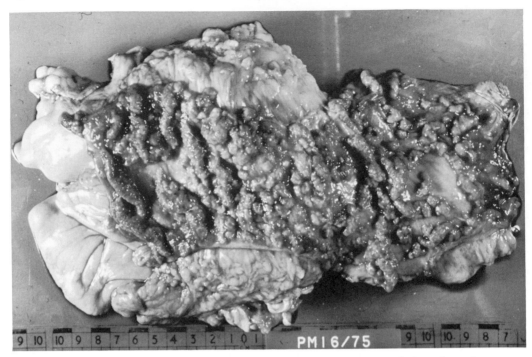

Fig. 57.6. Rectum from a patient dying from pseudomembranous colitis, showing marked pseudomembrane formation.

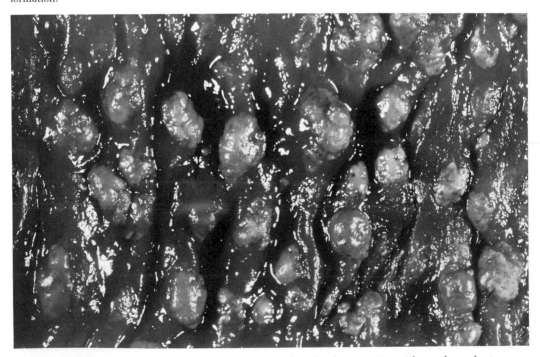

Fig. 57.7. Naked eye appearance of summit lesions affecting the colon from a patient with pseudomembranous colitis.

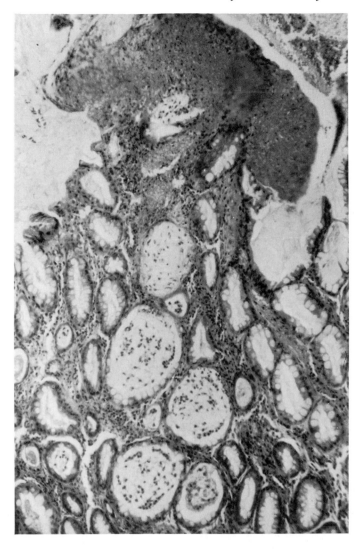

Fig. 57.8. Section through rectal biopsy to show typical summit lesion with pseudomembrane.

Lincomycin/clindamycin and ampicillin/amoxycillin, however, account for 87% of cases [12].

Pathogenesis

C. difficile is normally present in the stools in about 2% of the population [38, 39]. Failure to culture this organism from normal stool may be due to small numbers of organisms present rather than indicate true absence. The precise factors which favour proliferation of *C. difficile* and its toxin in the colon are unknown but coincidental administration of antibiotics is of major importance. However, some cases of pseudomembranous colitis due to *C. difficile*, developing in the absence of antibiotic administration, have been described [53, 93, 125]. Antibiotics were at first thought to favour the growth of resistant strains of *C. difficile*, but it is now known that many strains are quite sensitive to the antibiotic being administered [5]. Proliferation and toxin production by *C. difficile* in the colon are influenced by environmental conditions [5], and, as yet undefined, alteration in intracolonic conditions brought about by antibiotic exposure is most likely to favour toxin production with the development of the disease. *C. difficile* toxin is thought to be directly cytotoxic to colonic epithelial cells.

Clinical features

A spectrum of disease exists from a mild illness, with an increase in bowel frequency and looseness, to severe symptoms with the passage of multiple motions containing blood and associated with marked abdominal pain and tenesmus. Fever is present in the majority of patients, while rebound abdominal tenderness and leucocytosis occur in about one-fifth. The disease may begin during the course of antibiotic administration, usually after 5–10 days of therapy, but in 30% of patients symptoms commence after the antibiotic has been discontinued [114].

In patients developing symptoms during the course of antibiotic administration, discontinuation of antibiotics led to rapid resolution in 4–14 days. There was a 20% mortality, however, in patients developing symptoms after antibiotics had been discontinued or if antibiotics were continued after the onset of the illness [114]. Pseudomembranous colitis can be particularly severe in patients after abdominal surgery, particularly when antibiotics are required for infective complications. A 40% mortality has been recorded in such patients [58]. In a prospective study, 4% of patients having gastrointestinal operations developed *C. difficile* toxin-positive diarrhoea [59]. In general the severity of symptoms correlates with the titre of toxin in the stool [17].

Diagnosis and treatment [43]

Diagnosis of pseudomembranous colitis depends mainly on the demonstration of the typical sigmoidoscopic and histological features. However, since the recognition of *C. difficile* toxin as the aetiological agent in pseudomembranous colitis it has become evident that there are many patients with toxin present in the stool who have normal proctosigmoidoscopic appearances. Such patients may have typical pseudomembranes in the more proximal parts of the colon [115].

Simplified laboratory methods are now available both for the culture of *C. difficile* from stool [1] and also the demonstration of the cytotoxin in stool [37]. Many laboratories are now including such methods in their routine stool screen for patients suspected of infective diarrhoea; in one such series *C. difficile* was the third most common pathogen recovered [56]. The routine screening of stools for *C. difficile* and its toxin has revealed both organism and toxin in a number of patients without bowel symptoms especially infants, where in a special care unit 78% were culture positive and 67% toxin positive [79]. The apparent tolerance of the neonatal bowel to *C. difficile* remains unexplained.

Oral vancomycin (2 g/day) appears to be effective for the treatment of pseudomembranous colitis, treatment being followed by resolution of symptoms, improved sigmoidoscopic appearances and disappearance of *Clostridium difficile* toxin from the stool after 7–10 days of therapy [117, 130]. Oral vancomycin is poorly absorbed and high faecal levels have been recorded. Furthermore virtually all *C. difficile* strains appear to be sensitive. Vancomycin, 500 mg/day in divided doses for five days is also effective [60] but relapse may follow even 17-day courses of therapy [40]. Severe cases may be fatal despite elimination of the organism [50]. Despite its rapid absorption, metronidazole can also be used [92]; it is much cheaper than vancomycin and may be equally effective [113].

Clostridium difficile and inflammatory bowel disease

Exacerbations of inflammatory bowel disease have been associated with the presence of *C. difficile* toxin [42] and symptoms have apparently improved with vancomycin or metronidazole therapy with disappearance of toxin from the stool [11, 118]. In these studies, however, the titre of toxin was not determined. Other groups have not been able to confirm a relationship between *C. difficile* and inflammatory bowel disease [61, 78, 84], *C. difficile* toxin being present only in patients who had received anti-microbials. It thus seems unlikely that *C. difficile* plays an important role in inflammatory bowel disease and when present frequently disappears spontaneously without therapy. Some reports have implicated *C. difficile* in the pathogenesis of neonatal necrotizing enterocolitis, while others have been unable to confirm this [65, 79].

Clostridium difficile and cross infection

There have been several reports of clustering of patients with *C. difficile* colitis and cross infection has been suggested [70]. There seems little doubt that *C. difficile* is exceedingly common in neonatal units and appears to be acquired from environmental sources [2], spores persisting in the environment for more than six months [64]. *C. difficile* is also widespread in adults but whether simple acquisition of the organism alone is sufficient to result in the development of intestinal symptoms is unknown. Nevertheless in units managing severely ill patients, where antibiotics are widely used, it would seem prudent to barrier nurse *C. difficile* infected patients.

Schistosomiasis

Schistosomiasis is a worm infestation that affects more than 200 million people in three continents [25, 81, 96]. Three species are recognized, two of which affect the gastrointestinal tract while the third affects mainly the vesical plexus (*S. haematobium*). *S. mansoni* occurs mainly in the Middle East, Africa and South America while *S. japonicum* occurs in China, Japan and South East Asia.

Schistosomes spend part of their life cycle in a snail intermediate host; cercariae liberated from the snails into fresh water penetrate the human skin and migrate via the blood stream to the lungs and liver. The adult worms reside mainly in the inferior (*S. mansoni*) and superior (*S. japonicum*) mesenteric veins where they produce large numbers of eggs. The majority of eggs are retained in the wall of the intestine and portal vasculature of the liver where they cause a granulomatous reaction, but a proportion penetrate the bowel wall and are passed out of the body in the faeces. On contact with fresh water these release miracidiae which penetrate susceptible snails. The granulomatous reactions produced by the schistosomal eggs leads to fibrosis as the inflammatory reaction subsides and obstruction to venous blood flow. In the liver a presinusoidal block causes portal hypertension.

Clinical syndromes

Cercarial penetration of the skin causes dermatitis known as swimmer's itch. Approximately 40 days after heavy infestation, maturation of the worms with the onset of egg production produces a serum sickness-like syndrome with fever, malaise, eosinophilia, lymphadenopathy and hepatosplenomegaly (Katayama fever). Most patients with chronic infestations are asymptomatic but a proportion show the sequelae of chronic fibro-obstructive disease. Non-specific symptoms are probably no more common than in controls. Rectal bleeding may occur while bowel polyps are also recognized. In rare cases pseudoneoplastic lesions occur, usually in the descending and sigmoid colon. These lesions can obstruct the colonic lumen and consist of fibrotic tissue containing masses of eggs.

Diagnosis and treatment [48]

Diagnosis depends on identification of eggs in stool or rectal biopsy specimens. Egg excretion correlates with the intensity of the infestation. Praziquantel is now the drug of choice for treating schistosomiasis, taken as three doses of 20 mg/kg, four hours apart [87]. Oxamniquine has activity against immature as well as mature worms; a single oral dose of 15–20 mg/kg is effective [96]. Niridazole (25 mg/kg orally for 5–10 days) can also be used [81, 126].

Cryptosporidiosis [21, 49]

The coccidian parasite *Cryptosporidium* has become a fashionable parasite, causing diarrhoea in calves and a fatal illness in immunocompromised patients, particularly those with acquired immunodeficiency syndrome (AIDS) [72]. The parasite infects the enterocytes of the small and large intestine and causes traveller's diarrhoea, often in association with giardiasis [57]. Ingestion of infected water and person-to-person transmission appear to be important [66].

In normal children and adults cryptosporidiosis causes a mild, self-limiting gastroenteritis lasting one to two weeks [49]. About 2% of 3000 diarrhoeal stool samples from the UK, Australia and Finland contained cryptosporidial cysts [72].

In patients with AIDS, enteric infection with cryptosporidia causes severe protracted watery diarrhoea, with profound weight loss. No therapeutic agent has been found that will clear the parasite.

Diagnosis depends on demonstration of the parasite either in intestinal biopsies or in the stool [6, 20].

References

1 AL-JUMAILI IJ, BINT AJ. Simple method of isolation and presumptive identification of *Clostridium difficile*. *Zentralbl Batteriol Mikrobiol Hyg [A]* 1981;**A250**:142–146.

2 AL JUMAILI IJ, SHIBLEY M, LISHMAN A, RECORD CO. Incidence and origin of *Clostridium difficile* in neonates. *J Clin Microbiol* 1984; **19**:77–78.

3 ANDERS BJ, LAUER BA, PAISLEY JW, BARTH RELLER L. Double blind placebo controlled trial of erythromycin for treatment of campylobacter enteritis. *Lancet* 1982;**i**:131–132.

4 BAKER RW, PEPPERCORN MA. Gastrointestinal ailments of homosexual men. *Medicine (NY)* 1982;**61**:390–405.

5 BARTLETT JG. Antibiotic associated colitis. *Clin Gastroenterol* 1979;**8**:783–801.

6 BAXBY D, BLUNDELL N, HART C. The development and performance of a simple, sensitive method for the detection of *Cryptosporidium* oocytes in faeces. *J Hyg (Lond)* 1984; **93**:317–323.

7 BERDEN JHM, MUYTJENS HL, VAN DE PUTTE LBA. Reactive arthritis associated with *Campylobacter jejuni* enteritis. *Br Med J* 1979;**1**:380–381.

8 BLASER M, CRAVENS J, POWERS BW, WANG WL. Campylobacter enteritis associated with canine infection. *Lancet* 1978;**ii**:979–981.

9 BLASER MJ, WELLS JG, FELDMAN RA, POLLARD RA, ALLEN JR. Campylobacter enteritis in the United States. *Am Intern Med* 1983;**98**:360–365.

10 BOLAN RK, SANDS M, SCHACTER J, MINER RC, DREW WL. Lymphogranuloma venereum and acute ulcerative proctitis. *Am J Med* 1982; **72**: 703–706.

11 BOLTON RP, SHERRIFF RJ, READ AE. *Clostridium difficile* associated diarrhoea: a role in inflammatory bowel disease? *Lancet* 1980;**i**:383–384.

12 BORRIELLO SP, LARSON HE. Antibiotic and pseudomembranous colitis. *J Antimicrob Chemother* 1981;**7**:53–62.

13 BOYD JF. Pathology of the alimentary tract in *Salmonella typhimurium* food poisoning. *Gut* 1985; **26**:935–944.

14 BRETTLE RP, POXTON IR, MURDOCH JMcC, BROWN R, BYRNE MD, COLLEE JG. *Clostridium difficile* in association with sporadic diarrhoea. *Br Med J* 1982;**284**:230–233.

15 Br Med J. Polyarthritis and *Yersinia enterocolitica* infection. 1975;**i**:404–405.

16 BROOKE MM. Epidemiology of amoebiasis in the U.S. *JAMA* 1964;**188**:519–521.

17 BURDON DW, GEORGE RH, HOGG G, et al. Faecal toxin and severity of antitoxin associated pseudomembranous colitis. *J Clin Pathol* 1981;**34**:548.

18 BUTZLER JP, SKIRROW MB. Campylobacter enteritis. *Clin Gastroenterol* 1973;**8**:737–765.

19 CALIN A, FRIES JF. An 'experimental' epidemic of Reiter's syndrome revisited. Follow up evidence on genetic and environmental factors. *Ann Intern Med* 1979;**84**:564–566.

20 CASEMORE DP, ARMSTRONG M, SANDS RL. Laboratory diagnosis of cryptosporidiosis. *J Clin Pathol* 1985;**38**:1337–1341.

21 CASEMORE DP, SANDS RL, CURRY A. Cryptosporidium species: a 'new' human pathogen. *J Clin Pathol* 1985;**38**:1321–1336.

22 CHANG T-W, BARTLETT JG, TAYLOR NS. Clostridium difficile toxin. *Pharmacol Ther* 1981;**13**:441–452.

23 COMMUNICABLE DISEASES SURVEILLANCE CENTRE. Food poisoning and salmonella surveillance in England and Wales: 1983. *Br Med J* 1985;**291**:394–396.

24 DAY DW, MANDAL BK, MORSON BC. The rectal biopsy appearance in salmonella colitis. *Histopathology* 1978;**2**:117–131.

25 DE-COCK KM. Human schistosomiasis and its management. *J Infect* 1984;**8**:5–12.

26 DEGIROLAMI PC, DUNN JC, FEDERMAN M. Infections caused by intestinal protozoa. *Pathol Annu* 1985;**20**:463–505.

27 DOBBINS WO, WEINSTEIN WM. Electron microscopy of the intestine and rectum in acquired immunodeficiency syndrome. *Gastroenterology* 1985;**88**:738–749.

28 DORAISWAMY NV, CURRIE ABM, GRAY J, LYNTON MOLL C, MAIR NS. Terminal ileitis: Yersinia enterocolitica isolated from faeces. *Br Med J* 1977;**ii**:23.

29 DRONFIELD MW, FLETCHER J, LANGMAN MJS. Coincident salmonella infections and ulcerative colitis: problems of recognition and management. *Br Med J* 1974;**1**:99–100.

30 DUNLOP EMC. Venereal disease: Chlamydial genital infection and its complications. *Br J Hosp Med* 1983;**29**:6–11.

31 DU PONT HL, HORNICK RB. Clinical approach to infectious diarrhoeas. *Medicine* (*Baltimore*) 1973;**52**:265–270.

32 DU PONT HL, PICKERING LK. *Current topics in infectious diseases*. New York: Plenum, 1980:21–46.

33 ELLIOT DL, TOLLE SW, GOLDBERG L, MILLER JB. Pet-associated illness. *N Engl J Med* 1985;**313**:985–995.

34 FAUST EC. Amebiasis in the New Orleans population as revealed by autopsy examination of accident cases. *Am J Trop Med* 1941;**21**:35–48.

35 FRIEDMAN SL, WRIGHT TL, ALTMAN DF. Gastrointestinal Kaposi's sarcoma in patients with acquired immunodeficiency syndrome. Endoscopic and autopsy findings. *Gastroenterology* 1985;**89**:102–108.

36 GEDDES AM, ELLIS CJ. Infection in immunocompromised patients. *Q J Med* 1985;**216**:5–14.

37 GEORGE RH. A micromethod for detecting toxins in pseudomembranous colitis. Technical methods. *J Clin Pathol* 1979;**32**:303–304.

38 GEORGE RH, SYMONDS JM, DIMOCK F, et al. Identification of Clostridium difficile as a cause of pseudomembranous colitis. *Br Med J* 1978;**1**:695.

39 GEORGE WL, SUTTER VL, FINEGOLD SM. Toxicity and antimicrobial susceptibility of Clostridium difficile, a cause of antimicrobial agent associated colitis. *Curr Microbiol* 1978;**1**:55–58.

40 GEORGE WL, VOLPICELLI NA, STINER DB, et al. Relapse of pseudomembranous colitis after vancomycin therapy. *N Engl J Med* 1979;**29**:414–415.

41 GOODELL SE, QUINN TC, MKRTCHIAN PAC, et al. Herpes simplex virus proctitis in homosexual men. *N Engl J Med* 1983;**308**:868–871.

42 GREENFIELD C, AGUILAR RAMIREZ JR, POUNDER RE, NOONE P. Clostridium difficile and inflammatory bowel disease. *Gut* 1983;**24**:713–718.

43 GROSS MH. Management of antibiotic-associated pseudomembranous colitis. *Clin Pharmacol* 1985;**4**:304–310.

44 GUERRANT RL, LAHITA RG, WINN WC, ROBERTS RB. Campylobacteriosis in man: pathogenic mechanisms and review of 91 bloodstream infections. *Am J Med* 1978;**65**:584–592.

45 HAFIZ S, MCENTEGART MG, MORTON RS, WAITKINS SA. Clostridium difficile in the urogenital tract of males and females. *Lancet* 1975;**i**:420–421.

46 HALL K, O'TOOLE E. Intestinal flora in newborn infants with description of a new pathogenic anaerobe, Bacillus difficilus. *Am J Dis Child* 1935;**49**:390–402.

47 HALTALIN KC, NELSON JD, RING R, SLADOYE M, HINTON LV. Double blind treatment study of shigellosis comparing ampicillin, sulfadiazine and placebo. *J Pediatr* 1967;**70**:970–981.

48 HARRIES AD, WALKER J, FRYATT R, CHIODINI PL, BRYCESON ADM. Schistosomiasis in expatriates returning to Britain from the tropics: a controlled study. *Lancet* 1986;**i**:86–89.

49 HART CA, BAXBY D. Cryptosporidiosis in immunocompetent patients. *N Engl J Med* 1985;**313**:1018–1019.

50 HAWKER PC, HINE KR, BURDON DW, THOMPSON H, KEIGHLEY MRB. Fatal pseudomembranous colitis despite eradication of Clostridium difficile. *Br Med J* 1981;**282**:109–110.

51 HEALY GR, KRAFT SC. The indirect haemagglutination test for amebiasis in patients with inflammatory bowel disease. *Am J Dig Dis* 1972;**103**:17–97.

52 HOFFMAN SL, PUNJABI NH, KUMALA S, et al. Reduction of mortality in chloramphenicol-treated

severe typhoid fever by high dose dexametha-
zone. *N Engl J Med* 1984;**310**:82–87.

53 HOWARD JM, SULLIVAN SN, TROSTER M. Spontaneous pseudomembranous colitis. *Br Med J*
1980;**281**:356.

54 HUNT DA, SHANNON R, PALMER SR, JEPHCOTT AE.
Cryptosporidiosis in an urban community. *Br
Med J* 1984;**289**:814–816.

55 JAFFE HW, DARROW WW, ECHENBERG DF, *et al.*
The acquired immunodeficiency syndrome in a
cohort of homosexual men. *Ann Int Med*
1985;**103**:210–214.

56 JEWKES J, LARSON HE, PRICE AB, SANDERSON
PJ, DAVIES HA. Aetiology of acute diarrhoea in
adults. *Gut* 1981;**22**:388–392.

57 JOKIPII L, POHJOLA S, JOKIPII MM. Cryptosporidiosis associated with travelling and giardiasis.
Gastroenterology 1985;**89**;838–842.

58 KAPPAS A, SHINAGAWA N, ARABI Y, *et al.* Diagnosis of pseudomembranous colitis. *Br Med J*
1978;**i**:675–678.

59 KEIGHLEY MRB, ALEXANDER-WILLIAMS J, ARABI Y,
et al. Diarrhoea and pseudomembranous colitis
after gastrointestinal operations. A prospective
study. *Lancet* 1978;**ii**:1165–1167.

60 KEIGHLEY MRB, BURDON DW, ARABI Y, *et al.*
Randomised controlled trial of vancomycin for
pseudomembranous colitis and post operative
diarrhoea. *Br Med J* 1978;**i**:1167–1169.

61 KEIGHLEY MRB, YOUNGS D, JOHNSON M, ALLAN RN,
BURDON DW. *Clostridium difficile* toxin in acute
diarrhoea complicating inflammatory bowel disease. *Gut* 1982;**23**:410–414.

62 KEUSCH GT. Shigella infections. *Clin Gastroenterol*
1979;**8**:642–662.

63 KHANNA AK, MISRA HK. Typhoid perforation of
the gut. *Postgrad Med J* 1984;**60**:523–525.

64 KIM KH, FEKETY R, BATTS DH, *et al.* Isolation of
Clostridium difficile from the environment and
contacts of patients with antibiotic associated colitis. *J Infect Dis* 1981;**143**:42–49.

65 KLIEGMAN RM & FANAROFF. Necrotizing enterocolitis. *N Engl J Med* 1984;**310**:1093–1102.

66 KOCH LD, PHILIPS DJ, ABER RC, CURRENT WL.
Cryptosporidiosis in hospital personnel. Evidence
for person-to-person transmission. *Ann Int Med*
1985;**102**:593–596.

67 KOTLER DP, GAETZ HP, LANGE M, KLEIN EB, HOLT
PR. Enteropathy associated with the acquired
immunodeficiency syndrome. *Ann Int Med*
1984;**101**:421–428.

68 KROGSTAD DJ, SPENCER HC, HEALY GR. Current
concepts in parasitology: amebiasis. *N Engl J Med*
1978;**298**:262–265.

69 LAMBERT ME, SCHOFIELD PF, IRONSIDE AG, MAN-
DAL BK. Campylobacter colitis. *Br Med J* 1979;**i**:
857–859.

70 LANCET EDITORIAL. Cross infection and *Clostridium
difficile*. *Lancet* 1982;**ii**:476.

71 LANCET EDITORIAL. Yersiniosis today. *Lancet*
1984;**i**:84–85.

72 LANCET EDITORIAL. Cryptosporidiosis. *Lancet*
1984;**i**:492–493.

73 LANCET EDITORIAL. Campylobacter in Ottawa.
Lancet 1985;**ii**:135.

74 LARSON HE, PRICE AB. Pseudomembranous colitis:
presence of clostridial toxin. *Lancet* 1977;**ii**:
1312–1314.

75 LEVINE MM, DU PONT HL, KHODABANDELOW M, *et
al.* Long term shigella carrier state. *N Engl J Med*
1973;**288**:1169–1171.

76 LEVINE JS, SMITH PD, BRUGGE WR. Chronic proctitis in male homosexuals due to lymphogranuloma venereum. *Gastroenterology* 1980;**79**:
563–565.

77 LINDEMAN RJ, WEINSTEIN L, LEVITAN R, *et al.*
Ulcerative colitis and intestinal salmonellosis. *Am
J Med Sci* 1967;**254**:855–861.

78 LISHMAN AH, AL-JUMAILI IJ, RECORD CO. Spectrum of antibiotic associated diarrhoea. *Gut*
1981;**22**:34–37.

79 LISHMAN AH, AL-JUMAILI IJ, EL SHIBLY E, HEY E,
RECORD CO. *Clostridium difficile* isolation in neonates in a special care unit; lack of correlation
with necrotising enterocolitis. *Scand J Gastroenterol* 1984;**19**:441–444.

80 MCMILLAN A, GILMOUR HM, MCNEILLAGE G, SCOTT
GR. Amoebiasis in homosexual men. *Gut*
1984;**25**:356–360.

81 MAHMOUD AA. Current concepts: schistosomiasis.
N Engl J Med 1977;**297**:1329–1331.

82 MANDAL BK, MANI V. Colonic involvement in salmonellosis. *Lancet* 1976;**i**:887–888.

83 MANDAL BK. Typhoid and paratyphoid fever.
Infections of the GI tract. *Clin Gastroenterol*
1979;**8**:715–735.

84 MAYERS S, MAYER L, BOTTONE E, DESMOND E, JAN-
OWITZ HD. Occurrence of *Clostridium difficile* toxin
during the course of inflammatory bowel disease.
Gastroenterology 1981;**80**:697–700.

85 MICHALAK DM, PERRAULT J, GILCHRIST MJ, *et al.*
Campylobacter fetus ss. jejuni a cause of massive
lower gastrointestinal haemorrhage. *Gastroenterology* 1980;**79**:742–745.

86 MODIGLIANI R, BORIES C, LE CHARPENTIER Y, *et al.*
Diarrhoea and malabsorption in acquired immune deficiency syndrome: a study of four cases
with special emphasis on opportunistic protozoan
infestations. *Gut* 1985;**26**:179–187.

87 MOST H. Treatment of parasite infections of
travellers and immigrants. *N Engl J Med*
1984;**310**:298–304.

88 NANDA R, BAVEJA U, ANAND BS. Entamoeba histolytica cyst passers: clinical features and outcome
in untreated subjects. *Lancet* 1984;**ii**:301–304.

89 O'CONNOR HS, AXON ATR. Gastrointestinal
endoscopy: infection and disinfection. *Gut*
1983;**24**:1067–1077.

90 PAFF JR, TRIPLETT DA, SAARI TN. Clinical and laboratory aspects of *Yersinia pseudotuberculosis* infections, with a report of two cases. *Am J Clin Pathol* 1976;66:101–110.

91 PALMER SR, GULLY PR, WHITE JM, *et al.* Water borne outbreak of campylobacter gastroenteritis. *Lancet* 1983;1:287–290.

92 PASHBY NL, BOLTON RP, SHERRIFF RJ. Oral metronidazole in *Clostridium difficile* colitis. *Br J Med* 1979;i:1695–1606.

93 PEIKEN SR, GALDIBINI J, BARTLETT JG. Role of *Clostridium difficile* in a case of non-antibiotic associated pseudomembranous colitis. *Gastroenterology* 1980;79:948–951.

94 PHILLIPS BP, WOLFE PA, REES CW, *et al.* Studies on amoeba bacteria: relationships in amoebiasis: comparative results of intracaecal inoculation of germ free monocontamined and conventional guinea pigs with *Entamoeba histolytica*. *Am J Trop Med* 1955;4:675–692.

95 PORTNOY D, WHITESIDE ME, BUCKLEY E, MacLEOD CL. Treatment of intestinal cryptosporidiosis with spiramycin. *Ann Int Med* 1984;101:202–204.

96 PRATA A. *Schistosomiasis mansoni. Clin Gastroenterol* 1978;7:49–75.

97 PRICE AB, JEWKES J, SANDERSON PJ. Acute diarrhoea: campylobacter colitis and the role of rectal biopsy. *J Clin Pathol* 1979;32:990–997.

98 PRICE AB, DAVIES DR. Pseudomembranous colitis. *J Clin Pathol* 1977;30:1–12.

99 PUBLIC HEALTH LABORATORY SERVICE. Food poisoning and salmonella surveillance in England and Wales, 1982. *Br Med J* 1984;288:306–308.

100 QUINN TC, GOODELL SE, FENNELL C, *et al.* Infections with *Campylobacter jejuni* and *Campylobacter*-like organisms in homosexual men. *Ann Int Med* 1984;101:187–192.

101 QUINN TC, GOODELL SE, MKRTICHIAN E, *et al. Chlamydia trachomatis* proctitis. *N Engl J Med* 1981;305:195–200.

102 QUINN TC, STAMM WE, GOODELL SE, *et al.* The polymicrobial origin of intestinal infections in homosexual men. *N Engl J Med* 1983;309:576–582.

103 RHODES KM, TATTERSFIELD AR. Guillain-Barre syndrome associated with campylobacter infection. *Br Med J* 1982;285:173–174.

104 ROBINSON DA, JONES, DM. Milk-borne *Campylobacter* infection. *Br Med J* 1981;282:1374–1376.

105 SAMARASINGHE PL, OATES JK, MacLENNAN IPB. Herpetic proctitis and sacral radiomyelopathy—a hazard for homosexual men. *Br Med J* 1979;ii:365–366.

106 SAVAGE A, DUNLOP D. Terminal ileitis due to *Yersinia pseudotuberculosis*. *Br Med J* 1976;ii:916–917.

107 SCHACTER J. Confirmatory serodiagnosis of lymphogranuloma venereum proctitis may yield false positive results due to chlamydial infections of the rectum. *J Sexually Transmitted Diseases* 1981;8:26.

108 SCOTT GILLEN J, URMACHER C, WEST R, SHIKE M. Disseminated *Mycobacterum avium-intracellulare* infection in acquired immunodeficiency syndrome mimicking Whipple's disease. *Gastroenterology* 1983;85:1187–1191.

109 SKIRROW MB. Campylobacter enteritis—a 'new' disease. *Br Med J* 1977;ii:9–11.

110 SNYDER ML. Further studies on *Bacillus difficilis*. *J Infect Dis* 1937;60:223–229.

111 SOAVE R, DANNER RL, HONIG CL, *et al.* Cryptosporidiosis in homosexual men. *Ann Int Med* 1984;100:504–511.

112 SYMONDS J. Campylobacter enteritis in the community. *Br Med J* 1983;286:243–244.

113 TEASLEY DG, GERDIG DN, OLSON MM, *et al.* Prospective randomised trial of metronidazole versus vancomycin for *Clostridium difficile* associated diarrhoea and colitis. *Lancet* 1983;ii:1043–1046.

114 TEDESCO FJ. Clindamycin associated colitis: review of the clinical spectrum of 47 cases. *Am J Dig Dis* 1976;21:26–32.

115 TEDESCO FJ. Antibiotic associated pseudomembranous colitis with negative proctosigmoidoscopy examination. *Gastroenterology* 1979;77:295–297.

116 TEDESCO FJ, BARTON RW, ALPERS DH. Clindamycin associated colitis—a prospective study. *Ann Intern Med* 1974;81:429–433.

117 TEDESCO FJ, MARKHAM R, GURWITH M, CHRISTIE D, BARTLETT JG. Oral vancomycin for antibiotic associated pseudomembranous colitis. *Lancet* 1978;ii:226–228.

118 TRNKA YM, LAMONT TJ. Association of *Clostridium difficile* toxin with symptomatic relapse of chronic inflammatory bowel disease. *Gastroenterology* 1981;80:693–696.

119 URMAN JD, ZURIER RB, ROTHFIELD NF. Reiter's syndrome associated with *Campylobacter fetus* infection. *Ann Intern Med* 1977;86:444–445.

120 VANHOFF R, VANDERLINDEN MP, DIERICKX R, LAUWERS S, YOURASSOWSKY E, BUTZLER JP. Susceptibility of *Campylobacter fetus subsp. jejuni* to 29 antimicrobial agents. *Antimicrob Agents Chemother* 1978;14:553–556.

121 VAN SPREEUWEL JP, DUURSMA GC, MEIJER CJLM, BAX R, ROSEKRANS PCM, LINDEMAN J. Campylobacter colitis: histological immunohistochemical and ultrastructural findings. *Gut* 1985;26:945–951.

122 VANTRAPPEN G, AGG HO, PONETTE E, *et al.* Yersinia enteritis and enterocolitis. *Gastroenterology* 1977;72:220–227.

123 VANTRAPPEN G, AGG HO, GEBOES K, PONETTE E. Yersinia enteritis. *Med Clin North Am* 1982;66:639–653.

124 VOLBERDING PA. The clinical spectrum of the ac-

quired immunodeficiency syndrome. *Ann Int Med* 1985;**103**:729–733.

125 WALD A, MENDELOW H, BARTLETT JG. Non-anti-biotic associated pseudomembranous colitis due to toxin producing Clostridia. *Ann Intern Med* 1980;**92**:798–799.

126 WARREN KS. *Schistosomiasis japonica. Clin Gastroenterol* 1978;**7**:77–85.

127 WELLER IVD. Gay gastroenterology. In: Pounder RE, ed. *Recent advances in gastroenterology — 6.* Edinburgh: Churchill Livingstone, 1986:161–180.

128 WELLER IVD. The gay bowel. *Gut* 1985;**26**:869–875.

129 WILLOUGHBY CP, PIRIS J, TRUELOVE SC. Campylobacter colitis. *J Clin Pathol* 1979;**32**:986–989.

130 YOUNG GP, WARD PB, BAYLEY N, *et al.* Antibiotic-associated colitis due to *Clostridium difficile*: double-blind comparison of vancomycin with bacitracin. *Gastroenterology* 1985;**89**:1038–1045.

SECTION X

DISEASES OF THE LARGE INTESTINE

Chapter 58
Investigation of the Colon

R. H. TEAGUE

History

A full history of the patient's complaints will often provide the diagnosis before any examination. Further useful clinical information will be obtained by careful general, abdominal and rectal examination with proctoscopy and sigmoidoscopy where indicated. Radiology, endoscopy and pathological investigations may be required if the diagnosis remains in doubt.

Historical features

A large bowel problem may be indicated by symptoms of anaemia, an obvious history of bleeding, or weight loss. A family history of inflammatory bowel disease, polyposis or colorectal cancer could be important. An assessment of dietary fibre and calorie intake should be obtained. It is also important that a full drug history be taken including questions on past and present use of laxatives, antibiotics, antidepressants and analgesics. In this context it is important to remember that proprietary and herbal medicines, which the patient may not consider as 'drugs', can have profound effects upon the colon.

Other symptoms of colonic disease include pain, a palpable mass, increased borborygmi, abdominal distension and perianal problems such as pruritis, pain on defaecation, or prolapse.

Pain

Colonic pain may be felt at the site of its origin but is more often generalized and colicky in nature. Occasionally it is referred into the upper thighs and perineum, loins, or back and may be present as a constant nagging ache rather than as colic.

Abdominal swelling

The complaint of a palpable abdominal mass is rare but should rapidly direct the clinician to an enlarged organ, tumour or faecal collection. Abdominal swelling may indicate fat, fluid or faeces but more often is due to gaseous distension, in which case it is often worse in the latter part of the day. Borborygmi are a common but non-specific symptom of large bowel malfunction.

Bowel change

A 'change in bowel habit', unrelated to drugs or diet, is always an important symptom of colo-rectal disease. The history should include details of stool frequency, day and night, plus size, shape, consistency and colour of the stool. The presence of excess mucus in the stool, recognized by the patient as increased 'jelly or slime', can be a useful symptom. Other symptoms such as abnormal buoyancy or odour may help to distinguish steatorrhoea from diarrhoea, but are not often observed accurately by the patient.

Rectal bleeding

Anorectal bleeding is one of the most important symptoms in large bowel disease. The character of the bleeding will often give a clue to its possible origin. Dark red bleeding, with or without clots but occurring with defaecation, or separate from the stool, is indicative of a source above the rectum. Bright red bleeding which is seen on the toilet paper, spatters or drips into the lavatory pan, or coats the stool is most probably coming from the anal or lower rectal area. Unfortunately rigid criteria cannot be applied and any patient with rectal bleeding should be investigated carefully as a serious underlying cause may be present in approximately one in eight patients [22].

Anorectal symptoms

Pruritis ani may suggest the presence of haemorrhoids, fissures or minimal anal incontinence. Incontinence is a common and distressing symptom with many causes. It may just be the result of diarrhoea with urgency, excessive mucus secretion or faecal impaction. Patients often complain of a 'lump coming down' on defaecation, which can be caused by haemorrhoids but may be due to a tumour of the rectum or rectal prolapse. Anal pain can often be severe and distressing. Usually local examination reveals an obvious cause such as fissure or thrombosed external haemorrhoid but occasionally an examination under anaesthetic will be required. The length of time the patient spends straining at stool and the symptom of rectal dissatisfaction are seldom mentioned by the patient and require a direct enquiry.

Examination

Abdomen

Abdominal examination in a normal, thin patient often reveals a palpable caecum which gurgles on pressure and a palpable sigmoid colon. In the presence of spasm, or faeces, any part of the colon may be palpable, often with marked local tenderness and a drawing feeling across the abdomen. Colonic neoplasms may be palpable in any area of the abdomen and need to be distinguished from faeces. If doubt exists re-examination after purgation or an enema, should be performed. When abdominal distension is present ascites and enlarged viscera should be sought and eliminated. The groins should be palpated for lymphadenopathy and herniae.

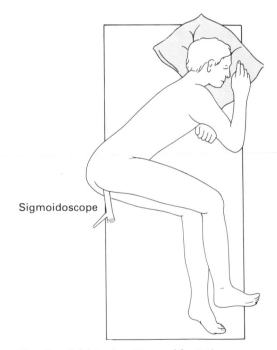

Sigmoidoscope

Fig. 58.1. Left lateral position used for rigid sigmoidoscopy.

Perineum

When the abdominal examination has been completed the patient should be turned onto his or her left side and positioned to lie diagonally across the couch with the legs bent up and the buttocks over the edge of the couch (Fig. 58.1). The anus and perineal area should be examined carefully, with the buttocks spread apart, and the patient should be asked to strain 'as at stool'. These manoeuvres will reveal pathology such as prolapsing haemorrhoids, fissures, fistulae and rectal prolapse and provide evidence on the tone of the anal sphincter. It is also important to palpate the perianal region to detect the presence of induration or tenderness which may suggest infection or a tumour deposit.

Rectal examination

Many patients are being examined rectally for the first time and it is both courteous and kind to give an explanation of what you are about to do. The immortal words 'turn onto your left side' followed by the insertion of a large finger without warning into a previously unviolated rectum are not good enough—they may scar the patient's memory for life.

Following an adequate explanation of what is being done a gloved and well-lubricated finger should be inserted gently into the anal canal. This is best achieved by firm, gentle horizontal pressure on the posterior part of the anal sphincter until relaxation occurs when the finger can easily slide into the canal with the nail uppermost so that the maximal diameter of the finger is in the sagittal plane. After examination of the anal canal and sphincter the finger is inserted into the rectum. The whole of the circumference of the rectum and its contents is then examined by rotating the finger gently around the wall of the rectum—this is helped by the examiner going

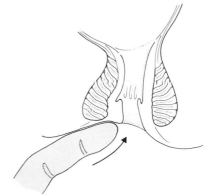

(a) Upward pressure on post-anal area until sphincter relaxes.

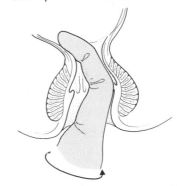

(b) Examine rectum by rotation of hand.

Fig. 58.2. Technique for rectal examination. (a) Firm pressure on posterior part of anal sphincter to induce relaxation of sphincter; (b) Digital examination using rotation of hand to examine all sides of rectum.

down onto his knees (Fig. 58.2). During this the presence and type of faecal matter should be assessed and any polyps, tumours or fistulae should be detected. In males an examination of the prostate gland is carried out at this stage. Finally the finger is withdrawn and the glove inspected for the presence of blood, mucus or melaena stool.

Sigmoidoscopy

In Britain this is usually performed in the left lateral, or Sims' position (Fig. 58.1), but some clinicians prefer to use the 'knee-elbow' position, or a tilting table. If the patient is obese, a pillow placed under the left buttock may make the examination easier.

Initial sigmoidoscopy should be performed on the unprepared bowel. In this way the presence of blood, pus and mucus can be detected and the colour and consistency of any stool present assessed. If the amount of stool present obscures the examination then a simple disposable phosphate enema is all that is necessary to produce evacuation and adequate cleansing.

There are a variety of disposable and non-disposable sigmoidoscopes available of various sizes. The standard Lloyd-Davies, or Welch-Allyn sigmoidoscope with fibreoptic illumination, of 30 cm length is a good instrument for routine use. Many clinicians prefer to use the adolescent-size instrument because it is more comfortable for the patient and easier to pass the recto-sigmoid junction. More specialized sigmoidoscopes are used for operative and paediatric use.

As with rectal examination it is important to give an adequate explanation of the procedure to the patient. Many patients find the air insufflation during sigmoidoscopy distressing as it causes the sensation of imminent incontinence or produces pain.

Technique

With the obturator in position the sigmoidoscope is passed gently through the anal sphincter for a few centimetres into the rectum and the obturator is removed. After insufflation a clear, lumen should be seen ahead of the instrument, if not it should be withdrawn a few centimetres to establish the luminal position. Advance is then carried out only when a clear lumen is visible. In many cases it should be possible to insert the full length of the instrument by carefully manoeuvring it around the flexures. If there is any discomfort at any stage, the instrument should be withdrawn. In this way a careful examination of the rectum

and, in some cases, the lower sigmoid colon should be possible and any polyps, tumours or mucosal inflammatory changes detected. The normal rectal mucosa is pink in colour with the blood vessels clearly visible on its surface ('vascular pattern'). Disturbance of this 'vascular pattern' with contact bleeding is often the first sign of proctitis. As proctitis becomes more severe the mucosa becomes more granular with ulcers, pus and spontaneous bleeding. Small polyps if present can often be removed with the biopsy forceps, but this can be attended by inappropriate haemorrhage. An alternative course of action is to schedule the patient for total colonoscopy when the polyp can easily be removed with the diathermy snare and a search made for other synchronous lesions. Biopsy of larger polyps is inappropriate as it often gives a false indication of the true nature of the lesion. Carcinomas of the rectum and sigmoid colon are usually recognized easily and can be confirmed by biopsy.

Biopsy technique

The purpose of the biopsy forceps is to take a representative sample of mucosa or tissue without incurring a significant risk of perforation or haemorrhage. Tumour biopsy usually presents no problem but mucosal biopsies are better taken from the extra-peritoneal part of the rectum (lower 6 cm) on the posterior wall. Not all forceps supplied with sigmoidoscopes are suitable for mucosal biopsy, the standard Patterson forceps is usually safe and easy to use, although perforation is still possible if insufficient care is taken. The examiner should try to nip off a small piece of mucosa by half-opening the jaws and pressing them lightly against the mucosa in this position. When a small but firm grip has been obtained the mucosa should be removed using a twisting movement. Recently a new variety of forceps has become available that allows single or multiple biopsies to be taken to a virtually constant depth with minimal risk of perforation [17].

After removal of the forceps from the sigmoidoscope the specimen should be eased from the jaw with a needle to avoid damage. Ideally the specimen should be orientated on a glass slide, using a dissecting microscope, with the mucosal surface uppermost. The slide is then placed in 10% formal saline and sent for histological examination. If these precautions are followed, an uncurled specimen is delivered to the histopathologist (Fig. 58.3) thus reducing the risk of tangential sectioning.

Fibreoptic sigmoidoscopy

In recent years it has been recognized that fibreoptic sigmoidoscopy can be an extremely useful diagnostic investigation in

the out-patient clinic [4, 20]. Under these circumstances it may be used as a substitute for rigid sigmoidoscopy although patient preparation is required. Such preparation is relatively straightforward and can be carried out by the out-patient nurse while the clinician is seeing another patient. Adequate cleansing is usually achieved by one or two phosphate disposable enemas. Most patients find the procedure completely acceptable without any sedation—pain should be an indication for abandoning the procedure. Many patients prefer fibreoptic sigmoidoscopy to rigid sigmoidoscopy, although its diagnostic benefit has been questioned [19].

Any colonoscope can be used for this procedure but the shorter (60 cm) instruments are more convenient and have larger biopsy/suction channels, which render aspiration of liquid faeces easier.

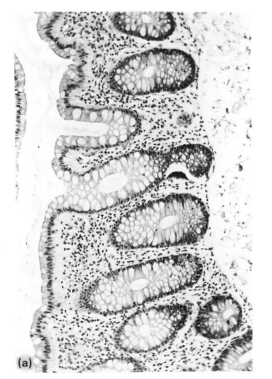 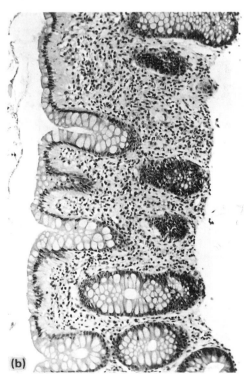

Fig. 58.3. Well orientated rectal biopsies showing full length of glands and surface epithelium. (a) Normal; (b) Showing chronic inflammatory infiltrate.

Technique

The patient is positioned in the left lateral position and the examiner is usually seated. The well-lubricated instrument is inserted either directly into the rectum or alongside the examining finger. Advance is achieved by means of distal tip manipulation and torque applied to the instrument. Provided the usual precautions are taken, such as withdrawal of the instrument when mucosal blanching occurs, then complications should be relatively rare. With practice rapid intubation of the whole of the sigmoid colon with views into the descending colon can be achieved within 10 minutes.

The obvious advantage of fibreoptic sigmoidoscopy is that it allows more of the lower bowel to be examined. This means that in some cases the upper limit of proctosigmoiditis can be defined and tumours or polyps in the lower colon can be detected. Polyps can be removed with a diathermy snare but it should be remembered that the bowel has been incompletely prepared and flammable gas may be present. The risk of an explosion can be removed if carbon dioxide is used and minimized if several air exchanges are carried out before the procedure. Some clinicians prefer to leave the polyps until a 'total' colonoscopy is performed to rule out any other synchronous lesions.

Proctoscopy

During rigid and fibreoptic sigmoidoscopy it can be difficult to examine adequately the middle and lower part of the anal canal. For this reason it is essential to carry out a proctoscopic examination after sigmoidoscopy. The Megan-Morgan proctoscope is favoured by most clinicians, and those proctoscopes that accept a fibreoptic light cable are simple and convenient to use. Proctoscopes are usually of a slightly wider calibre than sigmoidoscopes and the patient should be warned of this fact. Smaller sizes are available for paediatric use or where there is obvious perianal disease.

The well-lubricated proctoscope is inserted into the rectum and the obturator is then removed and the instrument is slowly withdrawn while the anal canal is inspected. It is often useful to repeat the procedure while the patient is straining so that lesions such as haemorrhoids may prolapse into the canal and be clearly visible. Simple surgical procedures such as banding of haemorrhoids, injection, or infra-red photocoagulation can be carried out during proctoscopy.

Radiological investigation (Table 58.1)

Plain abdominal X-ray

A plain abdominal X-ray should always be performed before a barium study is requested, as it can provide valuable information. Perforation, obstruction, sigmoid or caecal volvulus all have their typical radiological appearances. In inflammatory bowel disease the plain film may show an absence of faecal matter in parts of the colon indicating the level of active disease—if the whole colon is empty of faeces 'total colitis' can be presumed. **Toxic dilatation** will be associated with an increased diameter of the colon (normal < 5.5 cm in the transverse colon) and mucosal ulceration with undermined edges may be visible on the plain film. A plain X-ray is also diagnostic of **pneumatosis coli** in which multiple air-filled cysts are seen in the colonic wall.

Barium enema

Barium contrast studies of the large intestine offer a rapid and relatively accurate method for the diagnosis of large bowel disorders [4, 7]. There are few contraindications, but these must include pregnancy,

Table 58.1. Indications and value of different radiological investigations.

Technique	Indication(s)	Value
Plain X-ray	Suspected obstruction	Distribution of colonic gas Distension/colon/small intestine
	Suspected perforation	Free sub-phrenic gas Soft tissue shadow
	Ulcerative colitis/ Crohn's disease	Mucosal surface Toxic dilatation
Barium enema (single/double)	Change bowel habit Diarrhoea Rectal bleeding	Inflammatory bowel disease Colonic polyp(s) Colonic carcinoma Diverticulosis/-itis Fistulae
	Inflammatory bowel disease	Re-assessment Complications
Ultrasound	?Liver metastases Abdominal masses	Site of origin/size Directed biopsy
	Abscesses	Origin/size/site Aspiration/biopsy
CT scan	Abdominal masses	Site/size/biopsy
	Tumour infiltration	Particularly in pelvis
	?Liver metastases	Number/size
Arteriography	GI bleeding	Site in colon
	?Tumour	Abnormal vascularity Hepatic spread

acute inflammatory bowel disease and peritonitis. Cautious radiologists eschew such studies within two weeks of rectal biopsy.

There are two basic techniques for the examination—single- or double-contrast—but variations include the instant enema and the per-oral enema. In all circumstances, except the instant enema, rigorous cleansing of the bowel prior to the examination is mandatory. This is achieved by various combinations of diet, purgation and washouts [13, 16]. The responsibility for adequate preparation must lie with the radiologist and, if inadequate preparation is achieved by the usual method, this should be repeated using a more aggressive technique. All too often the X-ray report reads 'there is no gross lesion present but the presence of faeces prevents the exclusion of polyps or early inflammatory bowel disease'. This is comparable to the physician writing in the notes 'no abnormality on physical examination but the presence of clothes prevented the exclusion of some lesions' [2]. The use of a per-oral washout technique using a non-absorbable sugar such as mannitol will result in adequate bowel cleansing but the rate of passage is unpredictable and, if the enema is carried out too soon, marked dilution of the barium will occur.

Single-contrast enema

In this technique a column of barium is run into the colon under X-ray screening until adequate filling is achieved. Standard views are then taken and the patient is allowed to evacuate the barium. A prone, post-evacuation film is taken to complete the examination. This technique should only be used when a large bowel obstruction is suspected or when looking for fistulae and intussusception. An additional indication is when a water-soluble medium is being used to look for a perforation or anastomotic dehiscence.

Double-contrast enema

This method was first described by Fischer in 1923 [6] and was later refined by the Malmo clinic in Sweden [21]. It involves the introduction of a suitable barium contrast material to partially fill the colon, which is then distended with air to produce a thin film of barium over the mucosal surface of the large intestine. The patient is rotated to ensure an even coating of the mucosa and glucagon (1 mg i.v.) or hyoscine-N-butyl bromide (Buscopan 40 mg i.v.) is given to relax any areas of spasm in the colon. This technique also allows partial filling of the distal ileum with air and barium. Radiographs are taken in many standard positions so that overlying loops of bowel can be viewed separately.

The diagnostic accuracy of a double-contrast barium enema is far superior to that of a single-contrast study and, apart from those indications outlined previously, it should always be used when large bowel pathology beyond the reach of the sigmoidoscope is suspected. With practice it should take no longer than the single contrast technique and should detect lesions as small as a few millimetres in diameter.

Small polyps always represent a challenge to the radiologist as they have to be distinguished from faeces, air bubbles and diverticular disease. When the double-contrast technique is used there is usually no doubt about the diagnosis of a carcinoma of the colon.

A double-contrast enema is mandatory in the differential diagnosis and management of inflammatory bowel disease [12]. In most cases it will establish the exact diagnosis and determine the extent of the disease process and its complications. When total colitis is suspected, an attenuated preparation is advisable, but with limited disease the normal preparation can be used.

Per-oral enema

If adequate demonstration of the caecum and ascending colon is not achieved with the standard double-contrast enema, a per-oral enema may be attempted. Barium is given by mouth, as for a standard barium follow-through examination, and is watched fluoroscopically until it reaches the transverse colon. Metoclopramide (10 mg i.v.) may be used to accelerate the passage of the barium. When the transverse colon is reached, air is introduced rectally and the right colon is outlined; antispasmodics may be used to relax the colon.

Instant enema

This technique is only used on the unprepared patient with ulcerative colitis. It should never be regarded as a substitute for a standard double-contrast enema, but it can be useful in establishing the extent of the disease when this is above the reach of the sigmoidoscope. The technique relies on the fact that solid faeces will not be found in the presence of an inflamed mucosa; it will therefore only identify the extent of the disease. While the risks of carrying out an enema after rectal biopsy have probably been exaggerated, it is wise to delay biopsy if an instant enema is contemplated.

The technique is simple and quick. Barium is run into the colon until solid obstructing faeces are encountered. The colon is then distended with air and at least four films of the left colon are taken. In this way the clinician can obtain an almost instant record of the extent of the disease.

Conclusion

The barium enema remains the investigation of choice to identify pathology beyond the reach of the sigmoidoscope. Complications of a barium enema are extremely rare: **perforation** following rectal biopsy, or immediately proximal to a colostomy stoma, if a distension balloon is used, and during the preparation of an obstructed bowel is the commonest. Other much rarer complications include **extravasation** into the perirectal space or the circulation and **leakage** of contrast from a colonic anastomosis if an enema is performed too soon after surgery.

Computerized tomography and ultrasound

The value of these techniques in colonic disorders is very limited. This applies particularly to ultrasound as the tissue/gas interface of the colonic lumen totally reflects the sound waves so that intraluminal structures are impossible to see. Computerized tomography has proved of most value in detecting tumour spread within the pelvis and in detecting liver metastases. Another role for this examination is in the detection of intra-abdominal abscesses in association with tumours, diverticular disease and after colonic surgery.

Colonoscopy

The first fibreoptic sigmoidoscope was successfully used in 1963 [15], since then there has been a rapid development of the technique and the instruments available for it. Modern instruments allow an experienced colonoscopist to reach the caecum in over 95% of patients, enabling a rapid and comprehensive examination of the lumen of the colon (Table 58.2).

Table 58.2. Indications for colonoscopy.

1 Evaluation of a radiological abnormality.
2 Investigation of persistent large bowel symptoms e.g. bleeding.
3 Inflammatory bowel disease.
  a. Differential diagnosis
  b. Determining extent of disease
  c. Evaluation of strictures
  d. Dysplasia surveillance
  e. Preoperative assessment
4 Therapeutic procedures.
  a. Polypectomy
  b. Control of rectal bleeding
  c. Removal of foreign bodies
5 Postoperative endoscopy.
  a. Inspection of anastomoses
  b. Inspection of by-passed bowel
6 Surveillance.
  a. High risk groups e.g. polyposis
  b. Cancer or polyp follow-up

It is essential for any gastroenterologist carrying out colonoscopy to establish a close working relationship with the radiology department. Colonoscopy and radiology are complementary procedures and poor radiology should never be the indication for colonoscopy. Any films purporting to show a filling defect should always be reviewed by the radiologist before colonoscopy is attempted, as it may be more expedient to carry out a repeat barium enema, with more aggressive preparation, than to perform a colonoscopy.

Contraindications for colonoscopy

There are few contraindications to colonoscopy. Major medical problems, such as a recent myocardial infarction, bronchopneumonia or pulmonary embolism will obviously delay the procedure. In addition colonoscopy must be delayed in severe inflammatory bowel disease, acute diverticulitis and peritonitis. Other contraindications are relative and depend upon the experience of the colonoscopist and the reason for the procedure. There is no doubt that previous pelvic surgery or sepsis, and diverticular disease, can make the examination extremely difficult or impossible. The presence of a stricture can prevent more proximal examination of the bowel, even when a small calibre instrument is used.

Preparation

There are two basic methods—the first comprises a dietary restriction with fluids only for 48 hours, followed by purgation and washouts. Many purgatives can be used, but senna derivatives and castor oil are the most popular. The major drawback to this method is that an adequate washout is essential and total success depends on the enthusiasm of the nurse. The second method consists of the use of oral nonabsorbable hypertonic solutions—the osmotic purge. These agents are normally given after a dietary regimen and are more effective if used with a laxative. Magnesium citrate, mannitol, or sorbitol may be used. If electrosurgery is contemplated after mannitol preparation it is necessary to insufflate the colon with carbon dioxide as bacterial digestion can release a potentially explosive concentration of hydrogen.

Whatever preparation is used, it will not be suitable for every patient and whenever there is a history of severe constipation it is probably wise to give purgatives for three to four days before commencing the routine preparation.

Premedication

Total colonoscopy may be well tolerated without sedation but it is impossible to predict this in advance, so most colonoscopists use sedation. The favourite premedication is a combination of pethidine (25–50 mg) and diazepam (10–30 mg)—this is often given as 'Diazemuls' to prevent venous thrombosis. Midazolam (5–15 mg) is also sometimes used instead of diazepam. If pethidine, or diamorphine is used, the respiratory effects may be rapidly reversed by naloxone (0.4 mg) if respiratory depression occurs.

Providing sufficient sedation is used, even small children will tolerate the procedure well. There is rarely an indication for general anaethesia. On rare occasions hyoscine-N-butylbromide (40 mg) or glucagon (0.5–1 mg) is given intravenously to relieve colonic spasm.

Instruments and techniques

Only a long colonoscope (> 165 cm) will always reach the caecum but, in experienced hands, it may be possible to reach the caecum with shorter instruments. Paediatric colonoscopy has been made easier with the advent of small calibre, highly flexible instruments which will pass easily around the tight loops of a child's colon.

The prerequisite of a complete colonoscopy is the successful negotiation and straightening of the colonic flexures. Most colonoscopists adopt the one-handed technique in which the left hand is used to manipulate the distal tip of the instrument, and the air/water and suction valves. The right hand is used to advance, withdraw and twist the instrument. It cannot be over-emphasized that the essence of a rapid and comfortable colonoscopy is the frequent

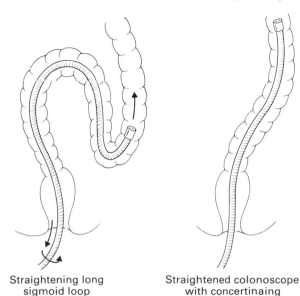

Straightening long
sigmoid loop

Straightened colonoscope
with concertinaing
of sigmoid loop

Fig. 58.4. Diagrammatic demonstration of how withdrawal of the colonoscope with locking of the tip and rotation can straighten a long sigmoid loop.

withdrawal of the instrument to straighten out incipient loops. This can most effectively be done after negotiation of the sigmoid-descending colon flexure or during attempts to reach the hepatic flexure. When loops have been straightened, rapid jiggling movements of the tip will help advance the instrument without reforming the loop.

The second most important aspect of the technique is to be aware of the position of the colonoscope's tip in relation to the bowel lumen at all times. This may be determined by the arrangement of the mucosal folds, with their concavity pointing towards the lumen. If this luminal view is lost, instrument withdrawal will always re-establish its position. As more instrument is inserted the risk of loop formation increases and this should be recognized by a failure of the tip to advance. When looping occurs there is stretching of the control wires so that tip deflection becomes impaired. If X-ray screening is used, it is easy to recognize loop formation. As the endoscopist becomes more experienced, X-ray screening will be used infrequently. The

flexibility of modern instruments means that stiffening devices are rarely, if ever, needed.

During intubation, without X-ray screening, the position of the instrument can be established by landmarks. The spleen may be seen through the colonic wall at the splenic flexure and the liver at the hepatic flexure. In thin patients the position of the tip may be seen by transillumination of the light through the abdominal wall. Unfortunately these features are inconsistent and even experienced operators may not be aware of the exact position until the colonoscope enters the caecum. Fortunately the caecum is easily recognized by the presence of the valve, appendix orifice and the configuration of the folds. Once intubation to the caecum has been achieved it is nearly always possible to negotiate the tip into the terminal ileum, although this may take time. It is unusual to be able to advance the tip for more than 10 to 15 cm along the ileum, but this is usually sufficient to exclude distal ileal Crohn's disease.

Much of the colonic mucosa will have

been seen during intubation, but a more comprehensive and accurate examination is carried out during withdrawal. This is achieved by tip manipulation and twisting movements (using the torque of the shaft). Some areas may require several passes before the endoscopist is satisfied that he or she has not missed disease. There are three regions where a complete circumferential view may be difficult or impossible—the hepatic and splenic flexures, and the descending-sigmoid junction zones.

As in all endoscopic procedures, it pays to be obsessional and blind spots may be eliminated, or kept to a minimum, by repeated passes of the instrument and by changing the position of the patient. Every colonoscopist has had the mortifying experience of seeing pathology, such as polyps, during insertion of the instrument that cannot be found during withdrawal. This has led many colonoscopist's to biopsy the lesion, to make it bleed, or to spray dye onto it so that it can be found again during withdrawal.

Complications

These can be classified into two groups—those that result from the technique itself and those that follow operative procedures performed at the same time. Both groups of complications have been extensively reviewed [14].

Procedure related

Sedation, particularly with benzodiazepines, may cause **respiratory depression** or arrest. Apnoea has been recorded with as little as 2.5 mg of diazepam [9]. Morphine derivatives, used as analgesia, are also potentially hazardous and synergistic with diazepam causing repiratory depression and hypotension.

Bacterial or viral cross-infection via the colonoscope can occur if inadequate sterili-

zation is carried out between patients. There is also a theoretical risk of bacterial endocarditis in patients with pre-existing cardiac disease, although it has not been seen in colonoscopic practice.

Perforation is the commonest complication with an incidence of 0.15% [8]. This may occur at the tip or along the shaft of the instrument when a large loop of colon is being stretched. Distal pneumatic perforation may occur when the wall of the bowel is weakened by a disease process such as diverticulosis, colitis or carcinoma.

Intraluminal haemorrhage is very rare, but minor or severe **intra-abdominal haemorrhage** may be commoner than has been recognized.

Other complications include the **post-colonoscopy distension syndrome** and **volvulus** formation.

Operation related

These are dealt with in greater detail later in the book but include perforation, diathermy accidents and haemorrhage.

Conclusion

Colonoscopy offers a major advance in the diagnosis and treatment of colonic disease, but it is unlikely to supplant double-contrast radiology as the primary investigation in patients with suspected colonic disease. The main reason is the length of time it takes to perform a colonoscopy—only the most expert colonoscopist could expect to compete with the work-rate of a radiologist carrying out double-contrast barium enemas using two screening rooms [2]. The two investigations are therefore complementary.

Anal manometry [11]
(see Chapter 62, Part I)

Pressure changes within the anal canal may be measured with open-tipped, constantly perfused, or balloon-tipped catheters attached to suitable transducers. Non-perfused tubes are rarely used because they are liable to block with faeces.

The resting and maximal 'squeeze' pressures that the patient can exert are measured as the catheter is withdrawn through the anal canal, the maximal resting pressure usually being measured 1.5 cm from the anal verge. This maximum resting pressure is largely the result of internal sphincter tone [3], while the 'squeeze' pressure represents external sphincter function.

Both the resting and squeeze pressure measurements may be used to investigate idiopathic incontinence [1]. Resting pressure may be reduced or absent following surgical procedures, such as anal dilatation, and in incomplete rectal prolapse—but it is not a major factor in the maintenance of continence. This appears to be a function of the external sphincter—in patients with idiopathic incontinence the maximum squeeze pressure is either low, unsustained, or entirely absent. Anal manometry can also be used in assessing the effects of haemorrhoidectomy [18].

A third measure of anal pressure is the recto-sphincteric reflex. In normal individuals, distension of the rectum (usually with 50 ml of air or water) will produce a brief rise in the maximum resting pressure followed by a marked fall, often to below half the resting value. In Hirschsprung's disease this reflex is lost (see Chapter 62). Care must be taken to introduce a sufficient volume of air or fluid to induce this reflex (up to 400–500 ml) in patients who have a chronically distended rectum, otherwise false positive results will be obtained.

Pelvic floor electromyography

The standard electromyographical measurements of pelvic floor musculature employ unipolar concentric needle electrodes inserted into the external sphincter and puborectalis muscles. After five minutes the amplified potential is observed and displayed on an oscilloscope. Unlike skeletal muscle the pelvic floor muscles display electrical activity at rest. This is thought to be a function of a spinal reflex, as it is abolished in patients with tabes dorsalis.

With the electrodes in place a suitably amplified response is observed at rest, after voluntary contraction of the pelvic floor, or during coughing. Many patients with idiopathic incontinence will have reduced activity at rest, and a poor response to contraction and coughing. These electrical abnormalities are non-specific and their main value lies in the ability to detect abnormalities of the muscle ring, due to agenesis or trauma, and to identify the abnormal zone for direct corrective surgery.

More accurate and detailed information can be obtained by measuring the latency of the anal reflex. A unipolar electrode is inserted into the external sphincter and the perianal skin is stimulated by a bipolar surface electrode. The afferent and efferent pathways for this reflex are conducted along the pudendal nerves allowing an accurate measurement of pudendal nerve function [10].

Colonic transit and motility studies

The measurement of colonic transit is normally carried out using nonabsorbable radioactive markers such as Cr^{51}-labelled chromic oxide in various sizes and shapes of plastic pellets. Modern sophisticated measurements employ four or five different-shaped pellets to give an accurate estimate of colonic transit time. Such measurements have contributed greatly to our knowledge of the mechanisms involved in constipation and diarrhoea but are of little diagnostic value.

References

1 BARTOLO DCC, JARRATT JA, READ MG, DONNELLY TC, READ NW. The role of partial denervation of the puborectalis in idiopathic faecal incontinence. *Br J Surg* 1983;**70**:664–667.

2 BECKLEY DE, STEVENSON GW. In: Hunt RH, Waye G, eds. *Colonoscopy: techniques, clinical practice & colour atlas.* Chicago: Year Book Medical Pubs., Inc, 1981:63–64.

3 DUTHIE PL, WATTS JM. Contribution of the external anal sphincter to the pressure zone in the anal canal. *Gut* 1965;**6**:64–68.

4 FARRANDS PA, O'REGAN D, TAYLOR I. An assessment of occult blood testing to determine which patients with large bowel symptoms require urgent investigation. *Br J Surg* 1985;**72**:835–837.

5 FARRANDS PA, VELLACOTT KD, AMAR SS, BALFOUR TW, HARDCASTEL JD. Flexible fibreoptic sigmoidoscopy and double-contrast barium-enema examinations in identification of adenomas and carcinomas of the colon. *Dis Colon Rectum* 1983;**26**:727–729.

6 FISCHER A. A roentgenologic method for examination of the large intestine: combination of contrast material with insufflation with air. *Klin Wochenschr* 1923;**2**:1593.

7 FORK F-TH. Reliability of routine double-contrast examination of the large bowel: a prospective study of 2,590 patients. *Gut* 1983;**24**:672–677.

8 FRUHMORGEN P, DEMLING L. Complication of diagnostic and therapeutic colonoscopy in the Federal Republic of Germany. Results of an enquiry. *Endoscopy* 1979;**2**:146–150.

9 HALL SC, OVASSAPIAN A. Apnoea after intravenous Diazepam therapy. *JAMA* 1977;**238**:1052.

10 HENRY MM, PARKS AG. The investigation of anorectal function. *Hospital Update* Jan. 1980:29–41.

11 HENRY MM, SNOKS SJ, BARNES PRH, SWASH M. Investigation of disorders of the anorectum and colon. *Ann R Coll Surg Engl* 1985;**67**:355–356.

12 LANFER I, HAMILTON JD. The radiological differentiation between ulcerative colitis and granulomatous colitis by double contrast radiology. *Am J Gastroenterol* 1975;**66**:259.

13 LEE JR, FERRANDO JR. Variables in the preparation of the large intestine for double-contrast barium enema examination. *Gut* 1984;**25**:69–72.

14 MACRAE FA, TAN KG, WILLIAMS CB. Towards safer colonoscopy: a report on the complications of 5,000 diagnostic or therapeutic colonoscopies. *Gut* 1983;**24**:376–383.

15 OVERHOLT BF. Description and experience with fibresigmoidoscopes. *Proc Sixth Nat Cancer Conf* (1968). Philadelphia: J.B. Lippincott, 1970:443–446.

16 POCKROS PJ, FOROOZAN P. Golytely lavage versus a standard colonoscopy preparation. Effect on normal colonic mucosal histology. *Gastroenterology* 1985;**88**:545–548.

17 PRESTON DM, LENNARD-JONES JE, BUTT JH, MORSON BC, WILLIAMS CB. New rectal-mucosal biopsy forceps. *Lancet* 1983;**i**:157.

18 READ MG, READ NW, HAYNES WG, DONNELLY TC, JOHNSON AG. A prospective study of the effect of haemorrhoidectomy on sphincter function and faecal continence. *Br J Surg* 1982;**69**:396–398.

19 SPENCER RJ, WOLFF BG, READY RL. Comparison of the rigid sigmoidoscope and the flexible sigmoidoscope in conjunction with colon X-ray for detection of lesions of the colon and rectum. *Dis Colon Rectum* 1983;**26**:653–655.

20 TRAUL DG, DAVIS CB, POLLOCK JC, SCUDMORE HH. Flexible fibreoptic sigmoidoscopy—the Monroe Clinic experience. A prospective study of 5,000 examinations. *Dis Colon Rectum* 1983;**26**:161–166.

21 WELIN S. Results of the Malmo technique of colon examination. *JAMA* 1967;**199**:119–121.

22 WILLIAMS JT, THOMSON JPS. Anorectal bleeding: a study of causes and investigative yields. *Practitioner* 1977;**219**:327–331.

Chapter 59
Appendicitis

M. H. THOMPSON

The recognition of appendicitis as a pathological entity of clinical importance follows the observation 100 years ago that, in cases of typhlitis or perityphlitis, the caecum (thought to be the seat of the disease) was intact and it was the appendix that was diseased [11]. There followed the performance of appendicectomy by Morton and Cutler in Philadelphia and by Toit in London in the 1880s, with a detailed description of the disease and its treatment by McBurney in 1889 [21].

Following these pioneering efforts the disease became more widely recognized and the operation of appendicectomy gained rapid acceptance as the appropriate treatment.

Epidemiology

In 1972 appendicectomy was the third most common operation performed in England and Wales [27]. Since then there has been a fall in the appendicectomy rate [26] which fell by 27% between 1966 and 1978 in England and Wales. Even when adjustment is made for a declining birth rate, a real decrease is still observed (Fig. 59.1).

In parallel with this fall in the United Kingdom, there has been a rise in its incidence in Africa, becoming the commonest cause of emergency admission for abdominal pain in Ibadan [1]. These changes are thought to be related to the fall in dietary fibre intake in Africa and the rise in England [6]. In Zimbabwe and Kenya the disease is still comparatively uncommon in young children, the majority of cases occurring in young adult males who have moved into an urban environment in search of work [12, 23]. Europeans living in the same area have an age pattern for the disease similar to those living in Europe. In South Africa, appendicectomy rates also appeared

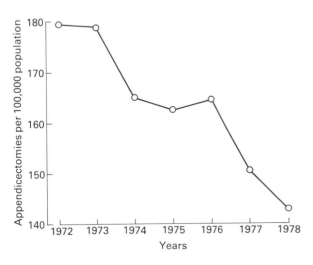

Fig. 59.1. The falling appendicectomy rate (1972–78) (derived from hospital inpatient enquiry data).

to fall with increasing intakes of dietary fibre [33]. A study from Cardiff [35] suggests that people who change from a normal to a high fibre diet have a reduced chance of appendicectomy, especially in the first two decades of life.

Aetiology

It is clear from epidemiological data that the consumption of dietary fibre appears to affect the development of the disease, although this view has been challenged [12]. Access to early medical care may have influenced appendicectomy rates in some series, but it is unlikely to have been a major influence.

It has long been felt that there is a genetic element in appendicitis, as there is an increased incidence of appendicectomy in relatives of children with appendicitis [2]. However, there is also an increased incidence in relatives of females who have had normal appendices removed suggesting that the familial mechanism involves hospital admission for abdominal pain rather than appendicitis.

Emotional factors may also play a part— stressful events may lead to appendicitis [8, 24] although more commonly they result in abdominal pain for which a normal appendix is removed.

Faecaliths (inspissated intestinal contents) or tumours may obstruct the appendix lumen leading to appendicitis.

Pathology

It seems likely that obstruction of the lumen is an important factor in the development of appendicitis. In about two-thirds of patients a faecalith is present, and the inflammation distal to it. The obstructing lesion in the remaining patients is likely to be enlargement of the lymphoid tissue in the lamina propria and submucosa.

Following obstruction, secretion contin-ues in the presence of stasis and appendicitis develops from proliferation of the normal intestinal bacteria. Once infection is established, microvascular changes occur with thrombosis leading to gangrene and perforation. This sequence can occur within 36 hours under experimental conditions [16, 20, 34]. The number of occasions that appendicitis develops and resolves spontaneously is unknown.

The appendix may also be involved in **yersiniasis** and **tuberculosis. Crohn's disease** may also involve the appendix either directly or as part of the commoner ileocaecal disease. Various parasites (including *Oxyuris* and *Enterobius*) are found in the appendix, although they are rarely associated with acute appendicitis.

Generalized peritonitis follows perforation unless the appendix is walled-off by the defence mechanisms of the surrounding intestine, omentum and mesentery, when an abscess results. Pelvic, subdiaphragmatic or subhepatic abscesses ensue if the patient survives a perforation without surgical intervention. Pelvic abscesses may discharge spontaneously via the rectum or vagina but other abscesses will usually require surgical drainage.

The bacteria involved in the inflammatory process are usually those normally found in the bowel—*E. coli*, **anaerobic** *Streptococci*, and *Bacteroides* **species.**

Clinical features

Much recent research confirms the long-standing clinical views concerning the importance of a good history and physical examination in the diagnosis of acute appendicitis (see Chapter 3). Poor history taking, in particular, leads to an unnecessarily low diagnostic rate. The clinical features are therefore very important.

The clinical features of appendicitis vary according to the site of the appendix, particularly as it is the distal part of the appendix which is most often involved. The various sites are shown in Fig. 59.2, representing places where an abnormal appendix can be found (most are pelvic or retrocaecal).

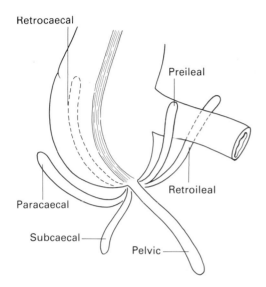

Fig. 59.2. The various positions the appendix may adopt.

Pain

This usually begins in the central abdomen, although not always around the umbilicus. When the parietal peritoneum near the appendix becomes irritated, the pain shifts to the right iliac fossa. From being somewhat intermittent in character, when centrally positioned, the pain generally becomes more constant although its severity can wax and wane. The pain is almost always made worse by movement—ask about pain during the journey to the hospital. A diagnostic feature of a retrocaecal appendicitis may be pain on walking, with the development of a limp due to irritation of the iliacus and posterior abdominal wall muscles. The pain may also be aggravated by micturition or defecation, particularly if the appendix lies in the pelvis.

Anorexia

Anorexia, with nausea and occasionally one or two vomits, is characteristic. Repeated vomiting is unusual, and should alert one to an alternative diagnosis. A good appetite and an ability to eat a meal virtually excludes the diagnosis of appendicitis.

Bowels

A change in bowel habit is rarely important, usually it is only that the patient has not moved his or her bowels on the day of the illness. Severe diarrhoea is uncommon although spurious diarrhoea may be a feature with a pelvic appendicitis.

Micturition

Urinary symptoms are unusual although a pelvic appendix lying on the bladder may cause frequency. A retrocaecal appendicitis may also produce secondary urinary tract inflammation.

Physical signs

The patient with established appendicitis appears unwell with, sometimes, mild facial flushing and a characteristic fetor on the breath. The temperature rises early in the illness to between 37 and 38°C. The pulse rate increases to around 95 beats/minute.

Generally the patient lies still and, if he or she moves around with the pain, an alternative diagnosis should be considered. The degree of respiratory movement of the abdominal muscles depends upon the stage of the disease but, as most patients arrive at hospital when appendicitis has already involved the parietal peritoneum, restriction of movement would be expected. Asking the patient to 'suck in' his or her abdomen often reproduces the pain.

In an established case there is tenderness on palpation over the right iliac fossa, usually maximal at or close to McBurney's point—which is two inches from the anterior superior iliac spine along a line to the umbilicus [21]. If not clear on palpation then gentle percussion may help locate the point of maximal tenderness. The abdominal tenderness is usually accompanied by rigidity and guarding in the right iliac fossa, and tenderness on the right side during rectal examination. It is important to distinguish the anal discomfort of rectal examination from the pelvic pain of appendicitis.

When generalized peritonitis has developed, the physical signs change to board-like abdominal rigidity, absent bowel sounds, and the systemic changes associated with severe sepsis.

Effect of anatomical variations

Variations in the position of the appendix will alter the physical signs of appendicitis. If it is **retrocaecal** maximum tenderness may be paraumbilical or right hypochondrial and rectal tenderness will be absent. Conversely, if the appendix lies **within the pelvis** there may be little or no abdominal tenderness but there will be severe pain on pelvic examination, sometimes associated with a palpable mass. Very occasionally malrotation of the colon will result in an unusually placed caecum so that appendicitis gives rise to very unusual signs. For example, if it lies in the right upper quadrant cholecystitis is usually diagnosed in error.

Appendix mass and abscess

The course of untreated appendicitis depends upon the effectiveness of the local defence mechanisms. Some patients will recover without active treatment. If surgery is delayed the remainder will progress to either generalized peritonitis, if the appendix perforates, or a local abscess if the infection is contained—under these circumstances an appendix mass or abscess will form.

Patients with an appendix mass have usually been ill for four or five days, by which time the inflamed appendix has become walled-off from the general peritoneal cavity by adhesions between the caecum, omentum and surrounding small bowel. This results in the formation of a tender mass in the right iliac fossa by the fifth day.

Appendicitis in special circumstances

In **very young children** the presentation of appendicitis is unusual and can cause diagnostic difficulties. Vomiting, sleeplessness and anorexia are the common features combined with guarding in the right iliac fossa. There may be some difficulty in distinguishing appendicitis from intussusception. However, the combination of screaming attacks, with remission between the attacks, especially if accompanied by blood or mucus in the stool, is much more in favour of the latter diagnosis. This will be supported by the finding of a mass with an 'empty' right lower quadrant on examination. Plain X-ray can occasionally confirm the diagnosis although often a barium enema is required. The latter can be used to reduce the intussusception by hydrostatic pressure. Operation is required if barium reduction is incomplete. At operation the reduction is completed and the source of the intussusception is sought; rarely it may be due to an invaginated appendix. If viability of the bowel is in doubt it should be covered with warm packs and observed. Resection may occasionally be required for local gangrene.

Appendicitis occurs in about 1 in 2000 **pregnant women**, most commonly in the middle trimester and least commonly in the last [3]. The symptoms are usually typical, but the site of tenderness moves upwards as the caecum is displaced by the enlarging

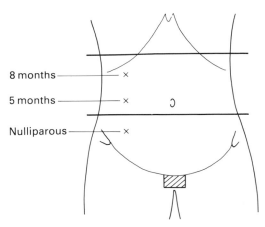

8 months —————— x

5 months —————— x

Nulliparous —————— x

Fig. 59.3. The change in position of the base of the appendix during pregnancy.

uterus. By the fifth month the appendix lies at the level of the umbilicus (Fig. 59.3). The enlarging uterus also prevents the omentum reaching the area of the inflamed appendix so that appendicitis tends to run a more rapid course.

Old people do not respond to appendicitis in the usual way. They become ill and sometimes confused without developing the classical features of the disease [28]. Constipation tends to occur, but tenderness in the right iliac fossa is usually present. Silent perforation with peritonitis is common.

Many of the first appendicectomies were performed because the offending organ was in an **external hernia.** These were usually diagnosed as a strangulated hernia, but, if the appendix is removed, recovery is usual [32].

Investigation

The diagnosis of acute appendicitis requires little help from the laboratory. Although a leucocytosis is often present, it is not universal, so that a normal white count does not exclude appendicitis. Nevertheless, this investigation may provide useful confirmatory information in the difficult case.

Plain abdominal X-rays are unlikely to provide much useful information if a confi-

dent clinical diagnosis can be made. Their major value is in excluding other conditions, such as renal colic, if doubt exists.

Microscopy of the urine may be helpful in excluding a urinary tract infection, although proximity of an inflamed appendix to the ureter or bladder may induce white cell loss into the urine.

Differential diagnosis

Gastroenteritis usually presents with abdominal pain, diarrhoea and vomiting although even with this combination of symptoms it is as well not to dismiss appendicitis without due thought. Generally no history of shifting pain, and an absence of tenderness and guarding in the right iliac fossa, makes appendicitis unlikely.

Mesenteric adenitis provides real diagnostic difficulty in children. If there is a history of a recent upper respiratory infection, cervical lymphadenopathy and a fever of over 38°C, then this diagnosis is more likely.

Distal ileal disease—Acute ileitis, *Yersinia* infection and Crohn's disease may all present as appendicitis in young adults. In patients with Crohn's disease the history may be longer and there may be associated perianal manifestations, but, if the first attack mimics appendicitis, then differentiation may be impossible without an operation (see Chapter 54).

Caecal carcinoma may present as appendicitis if the tumour obstructs the appendix causing frank appendicitis or a perforation produces a local pericolic abscess. The age group for caecal carcinoma is quite different to that of appendicitis and so in older patients the clinician must be aware of this possibility.

A **perforated duodenal ulcer** or, less likely, **gastric ulcer** may present as tenderness in the right iliac fossa because the released intestinal contents track down the right paracolic gutter into this area. The history is that of sudden onset and thereafter unremitting pain, unlike appendicitis which begins gradually and varies in intensity. Plain abdominal X-rays will usually demonstrate gas under the diaphragm.

Cholecystitis can be rather more difficult, as the onset is not as dramatic as a perforation. Particular attention should be paid to a previous dyspeptic history and the site of onset of the pain (which is likely to be either epigastric or right hypochondrial). Tenderness in the right hypochondrium usually develops with a positive Murphy's sign on careful examination.

Meckel's diverticulitis is a rare complication of this congenital embryological remnant [19]. The pain is ill-localized, particularly initially, and the tenderness is more medial. Usually the diagnosis is only made at operation but, if the condition resolves without operation, then investigation by ^{99}Tc pertechnate scan may show a separate uptake of the isotope away from the stomach in the lower abdomen, if the diverticulum contains ectopic gastric mucosa. Uptake of the isotope may be assisted by coincidental pentagastric stimulation.

Diverticulitis—Occasionally the apex of the sigmoid colon may lie in the right iliac fossa and, if it develops diverticulitis, it may mimic acute appendicitis. Usually in such circumstances the tenderness is not localized to the right side.

Salpingitis usually produces pain which is more centrally placed and which radiates towards the external genitalia. Tenderness is usually lower and more towards the mid-line than in appendicitis. There is often an accompanying vaginal discharge.

Ruptured ectopic pregnancy particularly on the right side, can cause diagnostic confusion. It is usually associated with a history of a missed period and a sudden onset of persistent pelvic pain and pelvic tenderness, often accompanied by collapse.

Ruptured follicular cyst or torsion—A ruptured follicular ovarian cyst, in mid-cycle, also causes pain and tenderness in the right iliac fossa. The timing of the attack in relationship to the menstrual cycle, and the absence of gastrointestinal symptoms, help to make the diagnosis. There is also often a history of previous similar attacks.

Torsion of a cyst, which is much less common, can occur at any time. It is usually accompanied by severe pain of sudden onset associated with vomiting and a palpable mass on pelvic examination.

Laparoscopy has emerged as a valuable investigation in the diagnosis of suspected gynaecological problems, sparing around one-third of such patients an operation [7, 18] (Fig. 59.4).

A **urinary tract infection** may mimic appendicitis but should be diagnosed by examination of the urine. If right renal colic is a real possibility, an emergency limited intravenous pyelogram may provide diagnostic information.

Even after all the above possibilities have been considered, the commonest alternative diagnosis of acute lower abdominal pain is that of '**non-specific pain**'. The differentiation of these patients from those with genuine acute appendicitis is dependent more upon the lack of specific diagnostic features than on any characteristics of their own. Anorexia, nausea and vomiting are usually present in acute appendicitis and anyone who is hungry on admission is unlikely to have this condition. Persistent tenderness in the right iliac fossa, persistent pyrexia and anorexia are unusual in patients with non-specific pain. It is the lack of specificity of either symptoms or signs which makes this group so difficult to categorize and diagnose, but it is also in this group that an increasing interest is being taken in the use of the diagnostic laparoscopy.

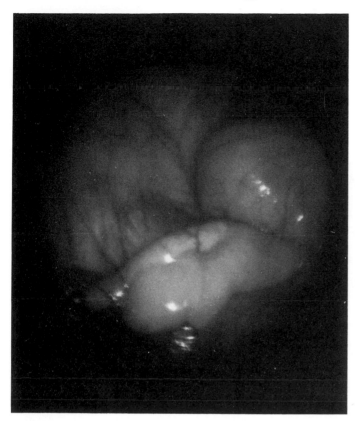

Fig. 59.4. Normal pelvic appendix seen at laparoscopy.

Management

The treatment of appendicitis has remained essentially the same since the condition was first recognized—immediate appendicectomy. Antibiotic therapy has not proved to be an acceptable alternative to this under normal circumstances.

Surgical technique

Through an incision in the right iliac fossa (muscle splitting, muscle cutting or transrectus sheath) the diagnosis is confirmed. The appendix is delivered into the wound, mobilizing the caecum if it is retrocaecal. Its vessels of supply are ligated and divided and the appendix is amputated at its base. The stump may, or may not, be buried by a purse string suture [10]. It is rarely necessary to drain the peritoneum providing adequate peritoneal toilet has been undertaken, the exception being an established abscess cavity.

Metronidazole

Numerous studies have proved the efficacy of pre-, per- and postoperative metronidazole in the prevention of wound infection. Other septic sequelae are also probably reduced by its use. The course of administration need only be very short—an intravenous or suppository dose of 500 mg, given with the anaesthetic premedication, is usually adequate [5, 31].

Problems during surgery

Crohn's disease or distal ileitis may be found (see Chapter 54) when removal of the appendix is reasonably safe. There is a risk of a postoperative faecal fistula, but this appears to be small and can occur even when the appendix has not been removed [14].

If there is localized mesenteric adenitis, then culture of one of the lymph nodes is worthwhile in order to positively establish or refute the diagnosis of *Yersinia*.

When a carcinoma of the caecum is found, either the small gridiron incision should be closed and a separate vertical abdominal incision made, or the original incision should be enlarged by muscle cutting in an oblique direction. In any event, a right hemicolectomy should be performed. Rarely the appendix itself will be found to be the seat of a carcinoma at subsequent histology—if so, it is probably wise to re-operate and perform a right hemicolectomy. A **carcinoid tumour** at the tip of the appendix can be ignored but one at the base should be treated by a limited right hemicolectomy assuming there is no further spread (see Chapter 40).

If an appendix mass has already formed by the time the patient presents then he or she should be restricted to a fluid diet and started on metronidazole (400 mg t.i.d. by mouth). The mass should diminish in size quite quickly. Once settled it is important to differentiate this cause from Crohn's disease or caecal carcinoma by barium radiology. If the diagnosis of an appendix mass is confirmed, caecal carcinoma and Crohn's disease having been excluded, the appendix should be removed some four to six weeks after the mass has resolved [29].

An **appendix abscess** can be more difficult—the patient is often seriously ill with a severe systemic toxaemia. Early surgical drainage is indicated under these circumstances once any dehydration has been corrected. The appendix should be removed if possible, but it may be left for later removal when resection is judged to be difficult or dangerous. The role of metronidazole in the management of an appendix abscess is not clearly established, but it probably aids in the resolution of the inflammatory reaction. Where an abscess has formed, the appendix may have been completely destroyed but this happens rarely [15]. Usually some or all of the appendix may be left. Any remaining part of the appendix may predispose to a recurrent abscess [4], so later appendicectomy is advisable.

Appendicitis in pregnancy [17]

Management of appendicitis during pregnancy depends upon two important factors—firstly, the appendix moves during pregnancy compounding difficulties in diagnosis (see Fig. 59.3); secondly, the normal localizing factors may be absent. The differential diagnosis includes urinary infection, tubal pathology, round ligament pain between the 14th and 22nd weeks and red degeneration of a fibroid.

An obstetrician should be involved from the outset in the management of a pregnant patient. Where a confident diagnosis is made, early appendicectomy is indicated. The greater risk is to allow the appendicitis to progress to peritonitis. In one series, nine out of 24 appendices removed during pregnancy were normal but no maternal complications occurred [25]. Premature delivery may ensue, but if peritonitis occurs, maternal and foetal mortality rises. The only difference in technique is that the incision may need to be made higher than usual, depending on the size of the uterus.

Prevention

From the epidemiological evidence there would appear to be a strong case for a high fibre diet as a prophylactic measure. This is being actively pursued by health educationalists because of its wider health implications. Presumably this dietary change will need to affect children as well as adults if the appendicectomy rate is to fall.

It is doubtful if **chronic appendicitis** exists, and it is equally doubtful whether appendicectomy will cure recurrent attacks of right iliac fossa pain for which no cause exists.

For a long time it has been popular to remove the appendix during other intra-abdominal operations such as cholecystectomy or hysterectomy. The role for such a prophylactic operation is controversial, particularly as many such procedures are performed after the peak incidence for acute appendicitis. However, it has been shown that there is no significant risk attached to this procedure [13, 22, 30]. Appendicectomy should certainly be performed when a patient is explored through a right iliac incision for suspected appendicitis, even if the appendix is normal, to prevent later diagnostic confusion should the patient re-present with right iliac pain.

References

1 AJAD OG. Abdominal emergencies in a tropical African population. *Br J Surg* 1981;**68**:345–347.
2 ANDERSSON N. Is appendicitis familial? *Br Med J* 1979;**2**:697–698.
3 ARANSON M. Appendicitis during pregnancy. Ten year review at Maine Medical Center. *J Maine Med Assn* 1979;**70**:341–344.
4 BEFELER D. Recurrent appendicitis—incidence and prophylaxis. *Arch Surg* 1964;**89**:666–668.
5 BUCKELS JAC, BROOKSTEIN R, BONSER R, BULLEN B, ALEXANDER-WILLIAMS J. A comparison of the prophylactic value of cefotetan and metronidazole in appendectomy. *World J Surg* 1985;**9**:814–818.
6 BURKITT DP. The aetiology of appendicitis. *Br J Surg* 1971;**58**:695–699.
7 CLARKE PJ, HANDS LJ, GOUGH MH, KETTLEWELL MGW. The use of laparoscopy in the management of right iliac fossa pain. *Ann Roy Coll Surg Eng* 1986;**68**:68–69.
8 CREED F. Life events and appendicectomy. *Lancet* 1981;**i**:1381–1385.
9 DEDOMBAL FT, MATHARU SS, STANILAND JR, *et al.* Presentation of cancer to hospital as 'acute abdominal pain'. *Br J Surg* 1980;**67**:413–416.
10 ENGSTROM L, FENYO G. Appendicectomy: assessment of stump invagination versus simple ligation: a prospective, randomised trial. *Br J Surg* 1985;**72**:971–972.

11 FITZ RH. Perforating inflammation of the vermiform appendix; with special reference to its early diagnosis and treatment. *Am J Med Sci* 1886;**92**:321–345.
12 FRIEDLANDER ML, GELFAND M. Acute appendicitis, an urban disease in Africans. *Trop Doct* 1980;**11**:22–23.
13 GOUGH IR, MORRIS MI, PERTNIKOVS EI, MURRAY MR, SMITH MB, BESTMANN MS. Consequences of removal of a 'normal' appendix. *Med J Aust* 1983;**1**:370–372.
14 HELLERS G, EWERTH S, BERGSTRAND O. The incidence of faecal fistula following exploratory laparotomy and appendicectomy in patients with ileo-colic Crohn's disease. *Acta Chir Scand* 1980;**500**(suppl):37–38.
15 HOMANS J, POWERS JH. Appendiceal abscess: treatment of appendix. *N Eng J Med* 1929;**199**:319–321.
16 KING DW, GURRY JF, ELLIS-PEGLER RB, BROOKE BN. A rabbit model of perforated appendicitis with peritonitis. *Br J Surg* 1975;**62**:642–650.
17 LEADER. Appendicitis in pregnancy. *Lancet* 1986;**i**:195–196.
18 LEAPE LL, RAMENOFSKY ML. Laparoscopy for questionable appendicitis: can it reduce the negative appendicectomy rate? *Ann Surg* 1980;**191**:410–413.
19 LEIJONMARCK C-E, BONMAN-SANDELIN K, FRISELL J, RAF L. Meckel's diverticulum in the adult. *Br J Surg* 1986;**73**:146–149.
20 LINDGREN I, AHO AJ. Microangiographic investigations on acute appendicitis. *Acta Chir Scand* 1969;**135**:77.
21 McBURNEY C. Experience with early operative interference in cases of disease of the vermiform appendix. *NY Med J* 1889;**50**:676–684.
22 MULVIHILL S, GOLDTHORN J, WOOLLEY MM. Incidental appendicectomy in infants and children. Risk v rationale. *Arch Surg* 1983;**118**:714–716.
23 OCHOLA-ABILA P. Appendicitis in children and adults at Kenyatta National Hospital Nairobi. *East Afr Med J* 1979;**56**:368–374.
24 PAULLEY JW. Psychosomatic factors in the aetiology of acute appendicitis. *Arch Middlesex Hosp* 1955;**5**:34–41.
25 PUNNONEN R, AHO AJ, GRONROOS M, *et al.* Appendicectomy during pregnancy. *Acta Chir Scand* 1979;**145**:555–558.
26 RAGUVEER-SARAN MK, KEDDIE NC (1980). The falling incidence of appendicitis. *Br J Surg* 1980;**67**:681.
27 REPORT ON THE HOSPITAL IN-PATIENT ENQUIRY. Dept of Health and Social Security and Office of Population Censuses 1972. Acute appendicitis in the over-eighty age group. *Br J Surg* 1985;**72**:245–246.
28 SHERLOCK DJ. Acute appendicitis in the over-sixty age group. *Br J Surg* 1985;**72**:245–246.

29 SKOUBO-KRISTENSEN E, HVID I. The appendiceal mass. Results of conservative management. *Surgery* 1983;**196:**584–587.

30 STROM PR, TURKELSON ML, STONE HH. Safety of incidental appendicectomy. *Am J Surg* 1983;**145:**819–822.

31 TANNER WA, ALI AE, COLLINS PG, FAHY AM, LANE BE, McCORMACK T. Single dose intra-rectal metronidazole as prophylaxis against wound infection following emergency appendicectomy. *Br J Surg* 1980;**67:**809–810.

32 THOMAS WEG, VOWLES KDJ, WILLIAMSON RCN. Appendicitis in external herniae. *Ann Roy Coll Surg Eng* 1982;**64:**121–122.

33 WALKER AR, RICHARDSON BD, WALKER BF, WOOLFORD A. Appendicitis, fibre intake and bowel behaviour in ethnic groups in South Africa. *Postgrad Med J* 1973;**49:**243–249.

34 WANGENSTEEN OH, DENNIS C. Experimental proof of the obstructive origin of appendicitis in man. *Ann Surg* 1939;**110:**629–647.

35 WESLAKE CA, STLEGER AS, BURR ML. Appendicectomy and dietary fibre. *J Hum Nutr* 1980;**34:**267–272.

Chapter 60
Colonic Diverticular Disease

M. EASTWOOD

Diverticula can be found throughout the gastrointestinal tract but are most common in the descending and sigmoid colon. Such diverticula are acquired, their occurrence being influenced by age and environmental factors.

Epidemiology

A distinction needs to be drawn between the occurrence of diverticula and the presence of associated symptoms or complications. Asymptomatic colonic diverticulosis is vastly more common than clinical diverticular disease.

Post-mortem studies show that the prevalence of colonic diverticula increases with age. In Australia diverticular disease is rare under 30 years of age, but occurs in more than 50% of those over 70 years [15]. Barium follow-through studies in volunteers in Oxford gave a similar figure [22]. On the other hand colonic diverticulosis is said to be unknown in African [3] and Asian countries, and right-sided disease predominates in Japan [31].

In Edinburgh 23% of all barium enemas performed during the period 1970–73 demonstrated diverticula. The annual incidence increased with age (0.17 per thousand under 45 years, 1.3 per thousand in those 45–59 years, 3.9 per thousand in those 60–74 years, and 5.7 per thousand in those over 75 years of age [6]. Women were affected more frequently than men.

The incidence of diverticular disease varies with its presentation and the source of information. Series based upon radiology,

surgery or referrals to out-patient clinics all give different results [9]. It is apparent that communities with a low life expectancy, poor hospital facilities and a diet high in dietary fibre have a low incidence of this disease [26]. The opposite also applies— Brodribb and Humphreys [2] showed that those presenting to a surgical unit with diverticular disease had a low dietary fibre intake, and Gear et al. [12] demonstrated that vegetarians had a lower incidence of the disease than omnivorous individuals of a similar age group.

Diverticular disease results in 12.8 hospital admissions per 100,000 population in Aberdeen whereas in Fiji, Lagos and Singapore no more than 0.3 per 100,000 present with this disease [19]. The incidence of the disease varies throughout Scotland and even within different areas of Edinburgh [6].

Diverticular disease is said to be a disease of the twentieth century, as it was not described in nineteenth century medical literature. The descriptive and mortality figures suggest that complicated diverticulitis is being recognized more often.

Aetiology

Symptomatic and asymptomatic diverticulosis must be distinguished from one another. The development of colonic diverticula has been ascribed to a lifelong diet deficient in dietary fibre [13]. Such a diet results in a small stool, the propulsion of which requires high intracolonic pressures. These lead to protrusion of the mucous

893

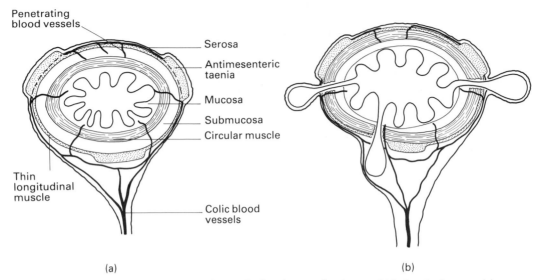

Fig. 60.1. Diagrammatic transverse view of sigmoid colon showing the sites at which diverticula occur. (a) normal; (b) sites of diverticula.

membrane through vulnerable points in the sigmoid and descending colon. Such vulnerable points occur at the site where blood vessels penetrate the colonic wall between the mesenteric border and the lateral taenia coli (Fig. 60.1). This hypothesis is supported by the demonstration of increased intra-colonic pressures in the sigmoid colon of symptomatic patients and by the relief in symptoms that follows an increase in the cereal fibre content of their diet [26].

The distinction between symptomatic and asymptomatic diverticular disease is important, as the improvement that follows the introduction of increased dietary cereal fibre in symptomatic patients does not necessarily imply an aetiological relationship between the two.

It has been shown that the incidence of diverticular disease increases with age; aging has been demonstrated to be associated with a decreased tensile strength of the longitudinal and circular muscle fibres of the colon. The strength to withstand a breaking load is greatest in the rectum, intermediate in the transverse and ascending colon and lowest in the sigmoid and de-

scending colon [9]. This is in accord with the distribution of diverticula. If, in 'in vitro' experiments, the colon is distended by water or air to its bursting point, the rupture tends to occur through the taenia rather than at sites where diverticula occur. When a pressure/volume curve is obtained for colons with and without diverticula, the affected colon is less distensible than the normal. This suggests that there is a structural change throughout the distal colon in association with diverticular disease [9].

Patients with diverticulosis have been shown to have a wide range of stool weight, transit time and colonic motility indices [8].

There appears to be no genetic or racial associations in this condition. Comparisons of Japanese and Africans in their native lands and after migration show that there is a steady increase in the incidence of this disease with adoption of a different life pattern and, possibly, increased longevity.

What is not known is why some diverticula become symptomatic, but it is likely to be multifactorial. It is possible that a modest fibre content, reduced stool weight, constipation and stool stasis with increased con-

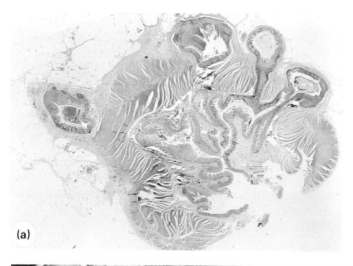

(a)

Fig. 60.2. (a) Histological cross-section of sigmoid colon showing diverticula; (b) external appearance of colon bearing diverticula.

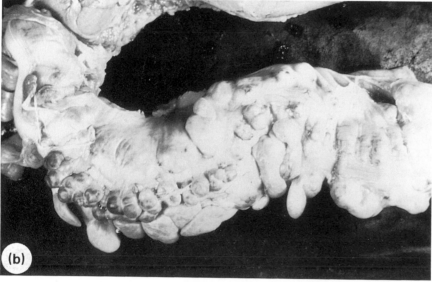

(b)

centrations of spasmogens in the stool (e.g. bile acids, reduced calcium content, an exaggerated hormone response to food) may lead to the onset of the characteristic symptoms [7].

Colonic motility studies have transformed our understanding of this disease and profoundly influenced our management of it. Painter [26] showed that individuals with colonic diverticula had motility patterns similar to the normal but that the segmenting action became more frequent and stronger in response to food, prostigmine and morphine. There is evidence that this exaggerated response is more obvious in symptomatic rather than asymptomatic patients with diverticulosis [26]. A similar motility response in an individual without diverticula would be diagnosed as the **irritable bowel syndrome** (see Chapter 67).

In patients with connective tissue disorders, such as Ehlers-Danlos and Marfan's syndrome, diverticula occur at an unusually young age.

Pathology

Colonic diverticula can occur at any point from the appendix to the rectosigmoid junction. In Eastern and Hawaiian communities they are seen most commonly on the right side of the colon. The increased haustral folds and hypertrophied lymphoid tissue suggest a separate aetiology to that of Western countries [24].

A diverticulum consists of a protrusion of mucous membrane covered with peritoneum occurring where a blood vessel pierces the wall (Fig. 60.1) and communicating with the lumen of the gut by small slit-like apertures (Fig. 60.2). Sometimes a diverticulum protrudes into an appendix epiploica.

The most consistent feature is thickening of the circular muscle fibres and of the taeniae, so that the bowel develops a concertina-like or 'saw tooth' appearance on barium enema (Fig. 60.3). The diverticula occur between the muscle clefts, making the mucosal surface appear trabeculated [24]. Pace [25] has shown that the thickening of circular and longitudinal muscle increases with age while the amount of connective tissue (collagen, elastin and reticular tissue) between the muscle layers decreases with advancing age [9]. Recent studies have shown that the elastin content of the taeniae coli is increased by more than 200% compared with controls in the colons of patients with diverticulosis [32]. This explains the concertina-like corrugation of the circular muscle.

Diverticulitis is relatively uncommon and probably results from inspissation of faeces, often in a solitary diverticulum. As the wall of the diverticulum is thin, there is early involvement of the pericolic fat with a potential for local peritonitis and perforation. The latter may result in general peritonitis, intra-abdominal abscesses, or fistulae to small bowel, bladder, vagina or other viscus. A pericolic abscess consists of pus, faeces and necrotic tissue with a fibrous wall; repeated episodes of diverticulitis may lead to the sigmoid colon being surrounded by fibrous tissue [24].

Inspissated faeces within a diverticulum may cause erosion of the blood vessel at its neck, provoking a major intestinal bleed.

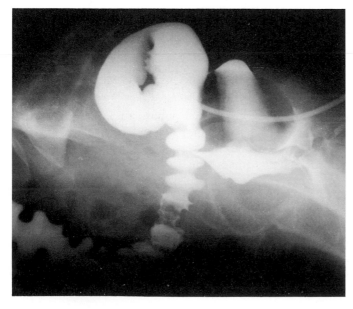

Fig. 60.3. Barium enema showing 'saw tooth' appearance of sigmoid colon. *Note*—Irregular narrowing in centre of sigmoid loop which is difficult to distinguish from a carcinoma. Colonoscopy would be advisable.

Clinical features

Patients may be classified into those who present as an out-patient referral and those with emergency complications. The majority of individuals pass through life unaware of the presence of their colonic diverticula. Symptoms frequently result in only a brief hospital contact, as more than 70% of patients have no further morbidity from their condition—a figure that can be increased by treatment with a high fibre diet [16, 21]. In younger patients, especially men, the disease appears to be more aggressive with a higher complication rate and greater symptoms.

Uncomplicated diverticulosis

There is a poor correlation between symptoms and the extent of colonic involvement. Symptomatic patients may complain of pain which is felt anywhere along the line of the colon, most frequently in the sigmoid or descending colon. The pain is often accompanied by a change of bowel habit with the passage of broken or pellety stools, the passage of which may relieve the symptom. This pain is characteristically steady or colicky and different to the intermittent pain seen in carcinoma or colitis. The passage of blood with an unformed stool is unusual in diverticulosis and should alert one to the possibility of an underlying less benign condition. Many patients also have associated upper abdominal pain which may be due to a coincidental peptic ulcer, biliary disease or hiatus hernia.

Complicated diverticulosis

True **diverticulitis** will present with pain, fever, leucocytosis and a raised ESR. Occasionally an abdominal mass is found if a pericolic abscess has occurred. **Perforation** may present as generalized peritonitis, with air under the diaphragm, or as a late sub-

phrenic or pelvic abscess. **Fistulae** to the bladder will cause severe cystitis and pneumaturia; to the vagina a faecal discharge; and to the small intestine features of diarrhoea and severe malabsorption due to intestinal bacterial colonization. Less common complications include **hydronephrosis** due to ureteral obstruction, and **portal pyaemia with liver abscess** [28]. The complication of **acute bleeding** usually occurs without any other features of diverticulitis, occurring particularly in patients on anticoagulants.

Approximately 10–20% of patients with the complications of diverticulitis eventually require surgical treatment. The mortality rises with age [4].

Because diverticula occur in an aging population other conditions may coexist, notably hiatus hernia and gallstones ('Saint's triad').

Investigations

History and examination

A careful history is essential with particular emphasis upon pain and bowel habits, questioning to identify symptoms of associated complications such as fistulae, abscess formation etc.

On examination a thickened and palpable sigmoid colon or the clinical features of a pericolic abscess may be found. Rectal and sigmoidoscopic examination with occult blood testing is important to exclude a carcinoma.

Radiology

A plain abdominal X-ray may show gas-filled diverticula or less commonly the features of obstruction or perforation.

A double-contrast barium enema is the most important investigation (Fig. 60.4). Early diverticular disease is characterized by a hypermotile segment with a 'saw tooth'

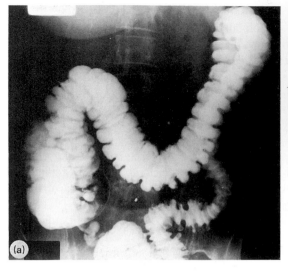
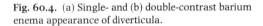
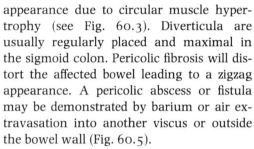
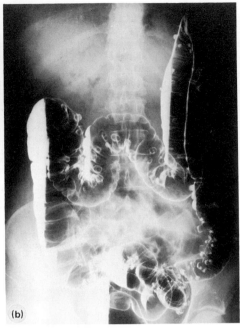

Fig. 60.4. (a) Single- and (b) double-contrast barium enema appearance of diverticula.

appearance due to circular muscle hyper-trophy (see Fig. 60.3). Diverticula are usually regularly placed and maximal in the sigmoid colon. Pericolic fibrosis will distort the affected bowel leading to a zigzag appearance. A pericolic abscess or fistula may be demonstrated by barium or air extravasation into another viscus or outside the bowel wall (Fig. 60.5).

Any unusual appearance should raise the possibility of an underlying carcinoma [5]. Where doubt exists colonoscopy with biopsy must be done to resolve the problem [1] (see Chapter 58). Selective visceral angiography is rarely necessary [11].

Motility studies

While such studies have helped enormously in the understanding of the pathophysiology of this condition [26] they are rarely indicated in its routine investigation or management.

Other studies

Where urological involvement is suspected, urine culture, pyelography and cystoscopy may be indicated. Studies of faecal weight, transit or faecal constituents are of little diagnostic value and are rarely required.

Differential diagnosis

Change of bowel habit

The major differential diagnoses are carcinoma of the colon or rectum and Crohn's colitis.

Bleeding

Carcinoma of the colon, ulcerative colitis, Crohn's disease, ischaemic colitis, and angiodysplasia (see Chapter 32) are the common differential diagnoses.

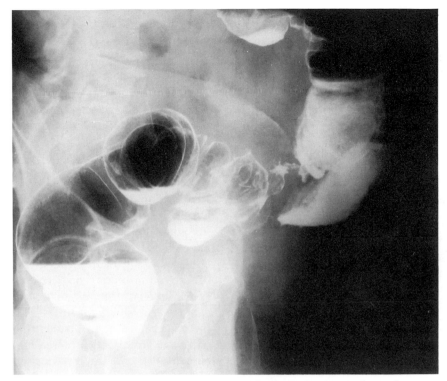

Fig. 60.5. The distortion of the proximal sigmoid colon produced by a pericolic abscess. *Note*—These appearances could be produced by a carcinoma.

Fistulae

Crohn's disease and colonic carcinoma are the most common other causes.

In most of these stituations sigmoidoscopy, biopsy and a barium enema will clarify the diagnosis, but occasionally a colonoscopy or laparotomy will be required.

Prevention

Aging and living in the West on a Western diet are the main contributing factors to the development of diverticulosis [26]. It is possible that changing to a high fibre diet may avoid development of the condition [13]. It is also possible that such a diet may prevent complicated diverticular disease from occurring [16].

Treatment

Medical therapy

The chance finding of asymptomatic diverticulosis requires no treatment, but it may be provident to suggest an increase in the fibre content of the patient's diet.

Pain

Reassurance is important. It should be explained that diverticulosis is part of growing older, and that the tests show no evidence of an underlying cancer. Painter's work [26] has shown the advantages of a high fibre diet with the resultant restoration of a normally-shaped stool. Fibre increases stool bulk in three ways—by water holding [10], proliferation of bacteria [30], and by the products of bacterial fermentation [14].

Cereal bran acts reliably and effectively, but it should be noted that the coarser the fibre the greater is the faecal bulking and unpalatability [17]. Cooking and processing bran improves its taste, but reduces its water-holding capacity—increased amounts are therefore required [33].

Fruit and vegetables produce a modest increase in bulk, in part due to increased bacterial proliferation.

Most patients respond to a high fibre diet [2, 26], even those who have required hospital admission for complications [14, 18]. The most important factor determining therapeutic effect is not the source but the water-holding capacity of the bran [29]. A good clinical response is usually obtained by including two handfuls of bran as a morning cereal, together with an apple and orange per day.

Some patients do not respond to this regimen; under these circumstances it is important to review the original diagnosis. Treatment for an 'irritable bowel' with spasmolytic agents such as propantheline bromide, dicyclomine or mebeverine may help under these circumstances (see Chapter 67). Occasionally symptoms persist and the affected segment may have to be removed surgically.

Diverticulitis

Antibiotic therapy is indicated when there are clinical signs and symptoms of inflammation such as pyrexia, leucocytosis and local or generalized tenderness. The antibiotics usually recommended are metronidazole (for anaerobic organisms) and a wide-spectrum antibiotic such as aminoglycoside (gentamicin or netilmicin) or one of the new generation of cephalosporins (cefotaxime, latamoxef or cefoxitin).

Haemorrhage

Mild haemorrhage is unusual in diverticular disease; it will present as iron-deficiency anaemia and is treated by iron therapy. Massive or persistent bleeding requires the resection of the affected area of the colon (see Chapters 32 and 61).

Prognosis

Diverticular disease of the colon is usually a benign and self-limiting disorder, except in younger patients, particularly males [27]. More than 80% of patients, treated either medically or surgically, remain symptom free and require no further treatment [20]. Surgery is required in a small percentage and is without severe risks, accepting that many of the patients are in the older age-groups [23]. Increasing the fibre content of the diet decreases the incidence of complications to approximately 5% of patients [16].

References

1 BOULOS PB, KARAMANOLIS DG, SALMON P, CLARK GC. Is colonoscopy necessary in diverticular disease? *Lancet* 1984;i:95–96.
2 BRODRIBB AJM, HUMPHREYS DM. Diverticular disease; three studies. *Br Med J* 1976;1:424–30.
3 BURKITT DP, CLEMENTS JL, EATON SB. Prevalence of diverticular disease, hiatus hernia, and pelvic phleboliths in black and white Americans. *Lancet* 1985;ii:880–881.
4 Chambers K, WILSON JMG, SMITH AN, EASTWOOD MA. Diverticular disease of the colon in Scottish Hospitals over a decade. *Health Bull* 1983; 41/1:32–41.
5 CUMMACK DH. *Gastrointestinal X-ray diagnosis.* Edinburgh: E & S Livingstone Ltd, 1969.
6 EASTWOOD MA, SANDERSON J, POCOCK SJ, MITCHELL WD. Variation in the incidence of diverticular disease within the City of Edinburgh. *Gut* 1977;18:571–574.
7 EASTWOOD MA, SMITH AN, BRYDON WG, PRITCHARD J. Comparison of bran, ispaghula and lactulose on colon function in diverticular disease. *Gut* 1978;19:1144–1147.

8 EASTWOOD MA, SMITH AN. *Handbook of Experimental Pharmacology.* Berlin, Heidelberg, New York:Springer-Verlag, 1982.

9 EASTWOOD MA, WATTERS DAK, SMITH AN. *Clinics in Gastroenterology.* London, Philadelphia and Toronto: WB Saunders Company Ltd, 1982.

10 EASTWOOD MA, ROBERTSON JA. *Colon structure and function.* New York: Plenum Medical Book Co, 1983.

11 EISENBERG H, LAUFFER I, SKILLMAN JJ. Arteriographic diagnosis and management of suspected diverticular haemorrhage. Selective angiography with rectal haemorrhage and diverticular disease. *Gastroenterology* 1973;**64**:1091–1100.

12 GEAR JSS, WARE A, FURSDON P, *et al.* Symptomless diverticular disease and intake of dietary fibre. *Lancet* 1979;**i**:511–14.

13 HEATON KW. Diet and diverticulosis—new leads. *Gut* 1985;**26**:541–543.

14 HELLENDOORN EW. *Topics in Dietary Fiber Research.* New York: Plenum Press Ltd, 1978.

15 HUGHES LE. Postmortem survey of diverticular disease of the colon. *Gut* 1969;**10**:336–351.

16 HYLAND JMP, TAYLOR I. Does a high fibre diet prevent the complications of diverticular disease? *Br J Surg* 1980;**67**:77–79.

17 KIRWAN WO, SMITH AN, McCONNELL AA, MITCHELL WD, EASTWOOD MA. Action of different bran preparations on colonic function. *Br Med J* 1974;**4**:187–8.

18 KRUKOWSKI ZH, KORUTH NM, MATHESON NA. Evolving practice in acute diverticulitis. *Br J Surg* 1985;**72**:684–686.

19 KYLE J, ADESOLA AO, TINCKLER LF, DE BEAUX J. Hospital admission rates to major teaching hospitals in Fiji, Singapore, Nigeria, North East Scotland. *Scand J Gastroenterol* 1967;**2**:77–80.

20 LARSON DM, MASTER SS, SPIRO HM. Medical and surgical therapy in diverticular disease. *Gastroenterology* 1976;**71**:734–736.

21 LEAHY AL, ELLIS RM, QUILL DS, PEEL AL. High fibre diet in symptomatic diverticular disease of the colon. *Ann R Coll Surg Eng* 1985;**67**:173–174.

22 MANOUSOS ON, TRUELOVE SC, LUMSDEN K. Prevalence of colonic diverticulosis in general population of the Oxford area. *Br Med J* 1967;**3**:762–63.

23 MITTY WF, BEFELER D, GROSSI C, ROUSSELOT LM. Surgical management of complications of diverticulitis in patients over 70 years of age. *Am J Surg* 1969;**117**:270–76.

24 MORSON BC. *Clinics in Gastroenterology.* London, Philadelphia and Toronto: WB Saunders Company Ltd, 1975.

25 PACE JL. '*A detailed study of the musculature of the human large intestine*'. University of London PhD Thesis, 1966.

26 PAINTER NS. *Diverticular Disease of the Colon.* London: William Heinemann Medical Books Ltd, 1975.

27 PARKS TG. *Clinics in Gastroenterology.* London, Philadelphia and Toronto: WB Saunders Company Ltd, 1975.

28 Small WP, Smith AN. *Clinics in Gastroenterology.* London, Philadelphia and Toronto: WB Saunders Company Ltd, 1975.

29 SMITH AN, DRUMMOND E, EASTWOOD MA. The effect of coarse and fine Canadian Red Spring Wheat and French Soft Wheat Bran on colonic motility in patients with diverticular disease. *Am J Clin Nutr* 1981;**34**:2460–2463.

30 STEPHEN AM, CUMMINGS JH. Mechanisms of action of dietary fibre in the human colon. *Nature* 1980;**284**:283–284.

31 SUGIHARA K, MUTO T, MORIOKA Y, ASANO A, YAMAMOTO T. Diverticular disease of the colon in Japan—a review of 615 cases. *Dis Colon Rectum* 1984;**27**:521–537.

32 WHITEWAY J, MORSON BC. Elastosis in diverticular disease of the sigmoid colon. *Gut* 1985;**26**:258–266.

33 WYMAN JB, HEATON KW, MANNING AP, WICKS ACB. The effect on intestinal transit and the feces of raw and cooked bran in different doses. *Am J Clin Nutr* 1976;**29**:1474–79.

Chapter 61
Surgery for Colonic Diverticular Disease

M. G. W. KETTLEWELL

The role of surgery in diverticular disease of the colon has changed dramatically over the last 10 to 15 years. This coincides with the widespread use of high fibre diets and disillusionment with colonic resection for symptomatic but uncomplicated disease. Although the role of surgery has diminished, its place in management has become more clearly defined. At present the majority of operations are performed for complications of the disease and only a few for symptoms such as abdominal pain or a changed bowel habit.

Types of operation

The choice of operation is wider in diverticular disease than in colonic carcinoma and the role of each procedure is different. Broadly the choice lies between resection, myotomy and colostomy. In some situations a combination of these procedures is useful.

Colonic resection

Sigmoid colectomy is the most frequently used operation for diverticular disease. The technique is similar to that used for carcinoma except that there is no need for a wide resection or for proximal ligation of the inferior mesenteric artery. The resection margins need only be sufficient to fashion a sound anastomosis in a healthy colon. Anastomoses can be made with one or two layers with a range of materials; the use of staples remains a personal choice, as controlled trials have failed to show clear

advantage for any one technique [4, 10, 14]. On occasions where the active disease spreads proximal to the sigmoid colon resection may need to be more extensive.

The advantage of resection, particularly in complicated disease, is that the inflammatory mass or site of perforation is resected, so removing a source of further sepsis [19]. The disadvantages are several— firstly, the operation is often technically difficult because of the pericolic fibrosis and inflammation. This results in a danger of damage to the ureter or iliac vessels and a lengthy operation in an elderly and ill patient. These risks may be further compounded if surgery is being performed as an emergency at night and the surgeon is inexperienced or tired.

Secondly, resection does not treat the primary pathology, merely the complications of the muscle hypertropy and increased luminal pressure. The luminal pressure remains high postoperatively and is only restored towards normal if the patient eats sufficient dietary fibre [31].

Thirdly, resection involves making an anastamosis with a small but definite risk of faecal leakage. If the risk appears high then the anastomosis may be delayed so inflicting a second operation on the patient.

Colomyotomy

Reilly introduced longitudinal myotomy of the circular muscle (Fig. 61.1) for diverticular disease [26, 27]. The theory was that this overcame the raised intraluminal pressure by destroying the action of the hypertrophied circular muscle bundles. Certainly luminal pressure is reduced [30], but this effect is evanescent unless the patient is maintained on a high fibre diet when the pressure remains low. The operation is a simple and effective one for symptomatic disease. It avoids the potential hazards of an anastomosis but a long myotomy down to the mucosa carries a risk of perforation and subsequent faecal leakage [5]. In fact, the morbidity and mortality do not appear to differ from those after resection, although a formal comparative trial has never been made.

The major advantages of this operation are its ease and the rapidity of postoperative recovery. The colon is widened, lengthened and straightened as a result of myotomy [17]. It is particularly useful for patients with abdominal pain and bowel disturbance refractory to medical therapy. Myotomy may also be useful if there is partial obstruction from stenosis or fixed angulation of the

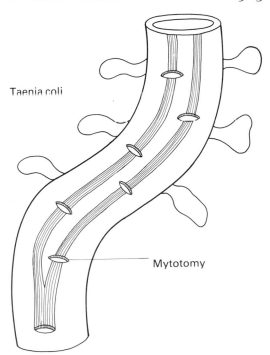

Fig. 61.2. Horizontal myotomy of taeniae coli [17].

colon. It is of no value for sepsis or perforation when resection is the operation of choice.

Faecal diversion

A proximal colostomy, with or without pelvic drainage, has a long tradition in the management of perforated or purulent diverticulitis [13]. It is easy and surgically safe, but it neither removes the inflammatory mass nor the site of perforation. While its simplicity is attractive to young, inexperienced surgeons, its mortality is, in general, greater than that after sigmoid colectomy [13], although the latter requires greater surgical expertise for good results.

Current indications for operation

Most patients with diverticular disease are either asymptomatic or have symptoms that are readily controlled by medical and dietary measures. Surgery is now reserved

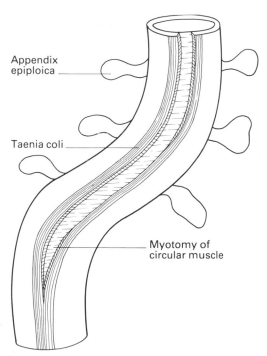

Fig. 61.1. Longitudinal myotomy for diverticulosis as described by Reilly [26].

Table 61.1. Indications for operation.

Sepsis
Recurrent diverticulitis
Perforated diverticulitis
Purulent peritonitis
Faecal peritonitis
Pelvic or paracolic abscess

Colonic obstruction
Inflammatory stricture
Fibrotic stricture
? Malignancy

Fistulae
Colovesical
Colovaginal
Ileocolic

Major Haemorrhage

---

for the few patients who prove refractory to such measures or have serious complications of their disease (Table 61.1) [32].

Symptomatic diverticular disease

Twenty years ago patients with intractable abdominal pain and disordered bowel habit, who failed to respond to a low residue diet and antispasmodics, were offered sigmoid colectomy on the grounds that the symptoms were due to recurrent inflammation rather than disordered colonic physiology. The fashion for colectomy remained such that patients were offered resection not only for current symptoms but also to prevent later complications requiring emergency surgery. This approach was fostered by data showing that the mortality of emergency resection was 14.7% compared to only 1.4% for an elective resection [28]. It was further encouraged by the belief that medical treatment for diverticulitis was no more effective than that for cholecystitis. Nevertheless, it was shown in one study, following up patients who had previously been treated medically that, whereas 25% required readmission, only 7% came to an operation and only 2% died of their disease (all after surgery) although 28% had died

of other causes during the follow-up period [24].

Few patients now require surgery for symptoms alone since most respond to medical management. In those whose symptoms prove resistant to such treatment the choice lies between colomyotomy and sigmoid resection. If there is little inflammation, and there is no suspicion of an underlying malignancy, a myotomy is a satisfactory procedure. Patients usually recover rapidly and can then be maintained permanently on a high fibre diet. Resection is preferable if there is substantial inflammation or a possibility of carcinoma.

Recurrent diverticulitis

It is important to distinguish the minority of patients who suffer from febrile attacks with left iliac peritonism from those described above. These patients usually improve with intravenous fluids and antibiotics. The antibiotics used in such patients are most commonly a combination of ampicillin (500 mg q.i.d.) and metronidazole (400 mg q.i.d.)—provided the patient is not sensitive to penicillin.

If symptoms fail to resolve or they recur, sigmoid colon resection may be required. When it is necessary to resect an acutely inflamed and unprepared colon a Hartmann's operation may be safer than performing a primary anastomosis (Fig. 61.3). Resection with a primary anastomosis is ideal for patients with recurrent diverticulitis when operated on electively following adequate bowel preparation; myotomy has no role in these circumstances.

Diverticular abscess

Acute diverticulitis can lead to a local peritonitis with abscess formation either in the paracolic or pelvic area. The presence of such an abscess will be suspected by clinical signs such as a tender mass or

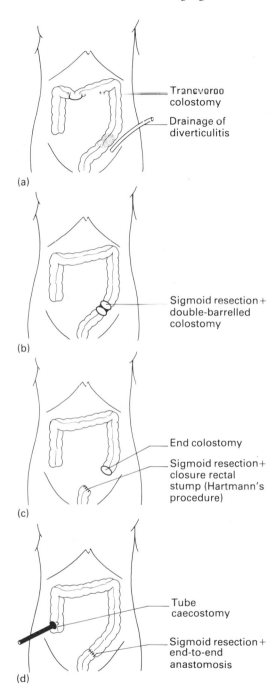

(a)

Transverse colostomy

Drainage of diverticulitis

(b)

Sigmoid resection+ double-barrelled colostomy

(c)

End colostomy

Sigmoid resection+ closure rectal stump (Hartmann's procedure)

(d)

Tube caecostomy

Sigmoid resection+ end-to-end anastomosis

Fig. 61.3. Diagrammatic representation of the choice of procedures available for the management of 'acute perforated diverticulitis'.

constitutional upset. When in doubt the diagnosis can be confirmed by ultrasound, computed tomography, or indium-labelled leucocyte scanning.

It is wise to let such an abscess localize as it then becomes a simple matter to drain the pus either through a small incision over it, or through the vagina or rectum. Drainage can also be achieved by ultrasound- or computed tomography-guided cannulae inserted under local anaesthesia [15]. There is rarely any need to perform a proximal transverse colostomy even if faeces appear in the drainage, as most fistulae will heal spontaneously. If drainage persists, an elective sigmoid colectomy with primary anastomosis can be performed at a later time. Parenteral antibiotics should be reserved for patients who are toxic, frail or elderly and for those with heart-valve lesions. Oral metronidazole and ampicillin usually suffice.

Perforated diverticulitis (Fig. 61.3)

Acute diverticulitis may be complicated by generalized purulent peritonitis, either by direct spread from the inflamed pelvic colon or by rupture of a peridiverticular abscess [20]. The clinical picture is of severe intraperitoneal sepsis with toxaemia, ileus and abdominal pain. Septicaemia may follow. Emergency laparotomy is almost always required, although adequate time must be allowed for adequate rehydration and the administration of a loading dose of antibiotics. Parenteral gentamicin (80 mg i.v.) and metronidazole (500 mg i.v.) are the best first-line antibiotics under these circumstances, although gentamicin can be replaced by netilmicin or a cephalosporin (such as cefurozime, cefotaxime or latamoxef).

If there is doubt about the diagnosis it is important to exclude other causes of an acute abdomen that may not require surgery. These include pelvic inflammatory disease, ureteric calculus, urinary extravasation and even pulmonary embolus. In such circumstances it is worth considering a laparascopic examination before proceeding to laparotomy.

The most widely advocated operation in this condition is peritoneal toilet, closure of the perforation, pelvic drainage, and transverse colostomy (Fig. 61.3) [13]. However, this leaves the phlegmonous colon as a septic focus and the left colon may still be full of faeces. Recovery is slow and mortality is high [6]. The same operation, but without colostomy, appears to fare as well [2]. In addition, between 10 and 20% of colonic perforations thought to be due to diverticulitis are, in fact, associated with a sigmoid colonic carcinoma [6, 22].

For these reasons more radical measures are favoured by experienced surgeons [16, 29, 33]. When a sigmoid colectomy is chosen the alternatives are a Paul-Mikulicz resection (Fig. 61.4), a double-barrelled left iliac fossa colostomy, a Hartmann's procedure with end colostomy (Fig. 61.3c), or a resection with primary anastamosis usually protected by a proximal colostomy or caecostomy [1, 9, 23].

The advantages of a Paul-Mikulicz resection are its relative ease and a simple secondary closure of the colostomy. Its disadvantages are that it is unlikely to be curative if the lesion turns out to be a carcinoma, and the distal end is often short and under considerable tension. In contrast the Hartmann's procedure is safe and effective, although subsequent reconnection may involve a major and difficult operation in elderly patients. Resection with primary anastamosis has its obvious attractions, but carries the risk of leakage. There have been no formal comparisons of these different options but the Hartmann's procedure is the one most popular with experienced surgeons [13].

Faecal peritonitis

Faecal peritonitis is a grave complication with a very high mortality, particularly in the elderly. A diverticulum ruptures, often with little or no surrounding inflammation, liberating quantities of faeces into the peritoneal cavity. This produces rapid and severe shock with septicaemia. Energetic resuscitation is required followed promptly by laparotomy, peritoneal toilet with lavage, and a Hartmann's operation. An alternative procedure, which is simple and safe, is to exteriorize the perforation as a loop colostomy. When there is little inflammation it may be safe to close the perforation, with a patch of appendices epiploica, and drain the pelvis.

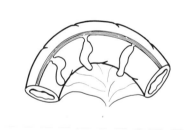

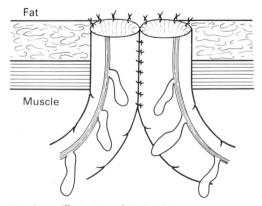

Fig. 61.4. Illustration of Paul-Mikulicz resection with creation of double-barrelled colostomy.

Intestinal obstruction

Recurrent inflammation with fibrosis and muscle hypertrophy can lead to progressive stenosis and colonic obstruction. Occasionally this may present acutely. Conservative management is worthwhile for a partial obstruction, provided a carcinoma can be excluded by barium enema or colonoscopy with biopsy and cytology. With the aid of a stool softener (see Chapter 62) the symptoms may resolve and the stricture gradually dilate. If these measures fail, the bowel should be prepared gently for resection and primary anastamosis. Unduly vigorous preparation will damage the obstructed bowel. It is sometimes possible to relieve the stenosis with a myotomy, which has the advantage of simplicity and safety in an elderly patient [18].

Acute or complete colonic obstruction requires a transverse colostomy with later resection or myotomy, although an alternative employed by some surgeons is resection with a double-barrelled colostomy.

Small bowel obstruction sometimes accompanies acute diverticulitis because the ileum becomes adherent to the inflamed sigmoid colon. The differentiation of small from large bowel obstruction is usually straightforward; the former is treated by laparotomy with division of the adhesions after a short period of rehydration. Small bowel resection is occasionally required to relieve the obstruction.

Fistulae

A colovesical fistula usually presents with recurrent urinary tract infections, associated with pneumaturia or faecuria. Diverticulitis is certainly the commonest cause of such a fistula, although carcinoma and Crohn's colitis should also be considered and excluded.

Fistulae may also occur between the colon and the vagina, ureter, and ileum—these seldom heal spontaneously [13]. An ileal fistula can result in small intestinal bacterial colonization with severe malabsorption and diarrhoea, the other fistulae seldom produce severe constitutional symptoms.

Sigmoid colectomy is undoubtedly the best treatment for a fistula. Most surgeons perform this as a one-stage procedure, after adequate bowel preparation. Colostomy is rarely required. A fistula into the bladder is closed and urethral catheter drainage is continued for about one week.

Haemorrhage

Major haemorrhage is an uncommon but well-recognized complication of diverticular disease (see Chapter 32). It is usually self-limiting, only requiring blood transfusion, but occasionally it is life threatening. The precise reason for the bleeding is not known, but angiographic and colonoscopic studies suggest that many bleeds, attributed to diverticula, are caused by other lesions such as polyps and angiodysplasia [3].

Repeated or minor haemorrhage is seldom caused by diverticula and is more likely to be due to carcinoma or polyps. It is therefore crucial to exclude other sources of bleeding by a double-contrast barium enema followed, if necessary, by colonoscopy. The source of a persistent major haemorrhage must be sought urgently and good selective or super-selective angiography (while bleeding) is required. As the haemorrhage can be from any part of the colon, good localization is an essential prelude to any operation.

Blind colonic resections have a particularly poor record [7, 11], which has led some surgeons to advocate transverse colostomy, to find out from which half of the colon the bleeding is coming before resection at a second-stage operation [25]. Others have felt it safer to perform a total colectomy with ileorectal anastomosis [21]. However, this is a formidable procedure to employ in an elderly patient and, with angiography, should seldom be necessary.

Good angiography enables an accurate and limited resection of the bleeding segment to be carried out and may also allow selective vasopressin or therapeutic embolization, to be used as an alternative to operation [8, 12]. If the bleeding is not too rapid it is worth considering colonoscopy and electrocoagulation or photocoagulation (laser) of the bleeding point, a technique which is sometimes very rewarding if the source of the bleed is a polyp or angiodysplasia. Total colectomy may then be reserved for the rare occasion when all else has failed and the patient's life is threatened.

References

1 ALEXANDER J, KARL RS, SKINNER DB. Results of changing trends in the surgical management of complications of diverticular disease. *Surgery* 1983; **94:**683–690.

2 BARABAS AP. Peritonitis due to diverticular disease of the colon: review of 44 cases. *Proc R Soc Med* 1971;**64:**253–254.

3 BOULOS PB, KARAMANOLIS DG, SALMON PR. Is colonoscopy necessary in diverticular disease? *Lancet* 1984;**i:**95–113.

4 BRENNAN SS, PICKFORD IR, EVANS M, POLLOCK AV. Staples or sutures for colonic anastomoses—a controlled clinical trial. *Br J Surg* 1982;**69:**722–724.

5 DANIEL O. Sigmoid myotomy with peritoneal graft. *Proc R Soc Med* 1969;**62:**811–812.

6 DAWSON JL, HANON I, ROXBURGH RA. Diverticulitis coli complicated by diffuse peritonitis. *Br J Surg* 1965;**52:**354–357.

7 DRAPANAS T, PENNINGTON DG, KAPPELMAN M, LINDSEY ES. Emergency subtotal colectomy: preferred approach to management of massively bleeding diverticular disease. *Ann Surg* 1973;**177:**519–526.

8 EISENBER H, LAUFER I, SKILLMAN JJ. Arteriographic diagnosis and management of suspected colonic hemorrhage. *Gastroenterology* 1973;**64:**1091–1100.

9 ENG K, RANSON JHC, LOCALIO SA. Resection of the perforated segment: a significant advance in treatment of diverticulitis with free perforation of abscess. *Am J Surg* 1977;**133:**67–72.

10 EVERETT WG. A comparison of one layer and two layer techniques for colorectal anastomosis. *Br J Surg* 1975;**62:**135–140.

11 GIANFRANCISCO JA, ABCARIAN H. Pitfalls in the treatment of gastrointestinal bleeding with blind subtotal colectomy. *Dis Colon Rectum* 1982;**25:**441–445.

12 GOLDBERGER LE, BROOKSTEIN JJ. Transcatheter embolization for the treatment of diverticular haemorrhage. *Radiology* 1977;**122:**613–617.

13 GOLIGHER JC. *Surgery of the Anus, Rectum and Colon.* 4th ed. Baillière Tindall, 1980.

14 GOLIGHER JC, LEE, PWG, SIMPKINS KC, LINTOTT DJ. A controlled comparison of one- and two-layer techniques of suture for high and low colorectal anastomoses. *Br J Surg* 1977;**64:**609–614.

15 GRECO RS, KAMATH C, NOSHER JL. Percutaneous drainage of peridiverticular abscess followed by primary sigmoidectomy. *Dis Colon Rectum* 1982;**25:**53–55.

16 GREIF JM, FRIED DO, McSHERRY CK. Surgical treatment of perforated diverticulitis of the sigmoid colon. *Dis Colon Rectum* 1980;**23:**483–487.

17 HODGSON J. Transverse taeniomyotomy: a new surgical approach for diverticular disease. *Ann R Coll Surg Engl* 1974;**55:**80–89.

18 KETTLEWELL MGW, MOLONEY GE. Combined horizontal and longitudinal colomyotomy for diverticular disease: preliminary report. *Dis Colon Rectum* 1977;**20:**24–28.

19 KORUTH NM, HUNTER DC, KRUKOWSKI ZH, MATHESON NA. Immediate resection in emergency large bowel surgery: a 7 year audit. *Br J Surg* 1985;**72:**703–707.

20 KRUKOWSKI ZH, MATHESON NA. Emergency surgery for diverticular disease complicated by generalized and faecal peritonitis: a review. *Br J Surg* 1985;**71:**921–927.

21 McGUIRE HH, HAYNES BW. Massive hemorrhage from diverticulosis of the colon: guidelines for therapy based on bleeding patterns in fifty cases. *Ann Surg* 1972;**175:**847–853.

22 MacLAREN IF. Perforated diverticulitis: a survey of 75 cases. *J R Coll Surg Edinb* 1957;**3:**129–144.

23 MADDEN JL. Primary resection and anastomosis in the treatment of perforated lesions of the colon. *Am Surg* 1965;**31:**781–786.

24 PARKS TG. Natural history of diverticular disease of the colon. a review of 521 cases. *Br Med J* 1969;**4:**639–642.

25 QUINN WC. Gross hemorrhage from presumed diverticular disease of the colon: results of treatment in 103 patients. *Ann Surg* 1961;**153:**851–860.

26 REILLY M. Sigmoid myotomy. *Proc R Soc Med* 1964;**57:**556–557.

27 REILLY M. Sigmoid myotomy. *Br J Surg* 1966;**53:**859–863.

28 RODKEY GV, WELCH CE. Diverticulitis of the colon: evolution in concept and therapy. *Surg Clin North Am* 1965;**45:**1231–1243.

29 SHEPHARD AA, KEIGHLEY MRB. Audit on complicated diverticular disease. *Ann Roy Coll Surg Eng* 1986;**68:**8–10.

30 SMITH AN, ATTISHA RP, BALFOUR T. Clinical and manometric results one year after sigmoid myotomy for diverticular disease. *Br J Surg* 1969;**56:**895–899.

31 SMITH AN, KIRWAN WO, SHARRIFF S. Motility effects of operations performed for diverticular disease. *Proc R Soc Med* 1974;**67**:1041–1043.

32 TAGART RE. Diverticular disease of the colon: clinical aspects. *Br J Surg* 1969;**56**:417–423.

33 UNDERWOOD WJ, MARKS OG. The septic complications of sigmoid diverticular disease. *Br J Surg* 1984;**71**:209–211.

Chapter 62
Constipation and Megacolon

I CHILDREN *by* R. NELSON & J. WAGGET

II ADULTS *by* P. R. H. BARNES & J. E. LENNARD-JONES

I   CHILDREN

Constipation

Constipation in children is a difficult symptom to define as there have been few studies of bowel frequency and stool consistency in children of different ages [81]. When it is defined as the infrequent passage of hard solid faeces it is a common symptom, particularly in children between two and nine years of age. Incomplete emptying of the rectum and colon is a frequent occurence and may lead to faecal incontinence (encopresis).

There are many possible causes of constipation, but the majority are functional.

Organic causes include Hirschsprung's disease and metabolic/endocrine disorders such as hypercalcaemia and hypothyroidism. Other causes tend to vary with the age of the child (Table 62.1).

Almost all children with incontinence have an underlying faecal retention usually detectable on abdominal or rectal examination, but sometimes only at radiology [41]. In severely disorganized and unhygienic families, faecal incontinence may continue beyond infancy into later childhood as a primary disorder of bowel control. Under these circumstances incontinence is not perceived by the child as a disorder [31].

Table 62.1. Aetiological classification of constipation in infancy and childhood.

Abnormal faeces	Cystic Fibrosis	Delay in passage of meconium in the newborn 10% develop intestinal obstruction Minority have constipation/incontinence when older
	Meconium plug syndrome	Premature neonates
	Coeliac disease	Minority have constipation ? Related to depressed gastrointestinal motility and transit
Malformations	Hirschsprung's disease Congenital anal stenosis Spinal cord lesions e.g. spino-bifida	
Metabolic/endocrine	Hypercalcaemia Hypothyroidism Hypopituitarism Renal tubular acidosis Diabetes mellitus/insipidus	Majority idiopathic
Functional (see table 62.2)	Neonatal stress Multiple aetiology	Majority aged 3–9 years

Functional constipation and faecal incontinence

Epidemiology

The incidence of constipation and faecal incontinence is difficult to define, particularly as the age at which a child is expected to be lavatory-trained is subject to cultural variation. A study of almost 10,000 children at school entry revealed encopresis in 1.5% [27]. This problem is five times as common in boys; it tends to decrease in incidence with age, being rare in adolescence.

Aetiology

Many potential aetiological factors have been proposed (Table 62.2). Some children appear to have a natural potential for the development of constipation and its complications [41]. Most children develop constipation around two years of age, during the period of autonomy and potty training, although some show this tendency from early infancy. Psychosocial factors of aetiological importance are found in the majority [27, 52]. These factors vary and a careful history and observation is required to elicit psychological causes. This is of importance as (in some patients) successful treatment will require counselling and other manoeuvres to correct the underlying cause.

In many children there is probably a voluntary reluctance to defecate during the period of toilet training. This leads to progressive faecal retention, with distension of the colon and rectum and loss of sensory or motor function. A vicious circle is thus established—overflow of faeces from the lower colon, with loss of rectal sensation and internal sphincter function can lead to incontinence of loose and semi-liquid faeces with soiling of clothes.

Although encopresis has been associated with retarded neurological or intellectual development, the majority of patients are of normal intelligence.

Table 62.2. Aetiological factors in functional constipation of childhood.

Physiological factors	? Individual difference in intestinal water absorption.	
	? Individual variations in intestinal motility and transit.	
Psychological factors	Child's personality	Obstinate, strong willed, stubborn.
	Parent's personality	Overanxious.
		Obsessional, unrealistic standards of cleanliness and hygiene for the child's age.
	Faulty bowel training	By feckless, inadequate, disorganized parents and families.
		Overemphasis on early bowel training by obsessional parents.
	Negativism	Normal stage of behavioural development from about the age of 18 months.
		Refusal to defecate, eat or sleep may be a child's means of asserting independence.
	Fear	Fear of defecation following harsh toilet training.
		Fear of the toilet, of being flushed down the toilet etc.
		Fear of pain or defecation, large hard stool and previous anal fissure.
	Maintenance of abnormal behaviour	Careful history of behaviour, of family situation and psychological assessment may be needed to discover factors that maintain the behaviour.

Clinical features

Children presenting with severe constipation usually have symptoms dating back to early infancy. The parents may have observed that the child is consciously retaining faeces, sometimes with at least a week between bowel actions.

Children may present at this stage, but more commonly they are referred when regular faecal soiling is present. Denial of this symptom is common and parents may only become aware of the problem by finding hidden, soiled underclothing. Typically the child is unaware that the soiling is occurring as a result of the loss of rectal sensation.

Evidence of psychological causative factors may include:

1. A history of unrealistically early potty training, indicative of the parents' obsession with cleanliness and their premature demands for perfection. Some children are described as being clean by the age of six months, when they are developmentally unready for such demands, being unable to sit unaided.
2. Some toddlers' refusal to defecate may be a manifestation of negativism which the child is unable to express openly [52]. Evidence for this may include other aspects of negative behaviour such as refusal to eat or sleep. Attention to these other behaviour problems may enable the clinician to modify the parent–child relationship that has initiated the bowel problem.
3. It is difficult to evaluate the role that fear of the toilet, or pain on defecation, may play in the aetiology of long-standing constipation. Parents may interpret the child's tearful reactions to toilet training as a manifestation of fear. Many children with constipation do complain of pain on defecation and have a history of rectal bleeding due to anal fissures, but other psychological causes probably produce the primary condition necessary for faecal retention and the eventual passage of a large hard faecal mass.

Some children complain of diarrhoea with incontinence when the underlying problem is that of faecal retention with spurious diarrhoea. Virtually all children with long-standing faecal incontinence have an underlying colonic retention.

Examination

Physical examination may reveal abdominal distension with faecal masses on abdominal palpation. Digital examination of the rectum is most important. If the faecal incontinence and/or diarrhoea is spurious, a large faecal mass will usually be felt within the rectum. The level of the retained faeces does not help in differentiating functional constipation from Hirschsprung's disease. Because of the psychological nature of this problem, physical examination, and particularly rectal palpation, should only be carried out with the child's informed consent. It is vitally important that the clinician and the supportive staff are not perceived by the child as other figures of authority.

Investigations

It is usually fairly easy to distinguish functional from other organic causes of constipation (Table 62.1). Only in conditions such as cystic fibrosis, or malabsorption due to coeliac disease, or cow's milk allergy, is there likely to be faecal retention and eventual incontinence.

Almost all cases of childhood encopresis are associated with previous constipation and faecal retention [6]. A **plain abdominal radiograph** may be needed to demonstrate colonic faecal retention when it is not readily palpable on abdominal or rectal examination.

The most common differential diagnosis is Hirschsprung's disease and several investigations have been developed to identify

Table 62.3. Investigations to differentiate Hirschsprung's disease from functional constipation.

Physical examination	Not normally helpful in differentiating from functional constipation.	
Radiology	Barium enema without bowel preparation using a fine 5 FG rectal catheter:	(a) 'Coning down' of the transition zone between ganglionic and aganglionic bowel. (b) Dysrhythmic bowel contractions and 'saw toothing' of the mucosa may be seen. (c) Will indicate approximately the length of bowel involved.
Rectal biopsy Histology	Biopsy taken 2.5 cm from anal margin.	Histological features are absent ganglion cells with hypertrophied nerve fibres in submucosal nerve plexuses.
Increased mucosal acetylcholinesterase	Detected by—	(a) Histochemical staining (b) Biochemical enzyme assay (c) Staining with monoclonal antineurofilament antibodies.
Anorectal manometry	Characteristic changes in—	(a) Hirschsprung's disease (b) Severe idiopathic constipation (see Figs 62.1 and 62.2)

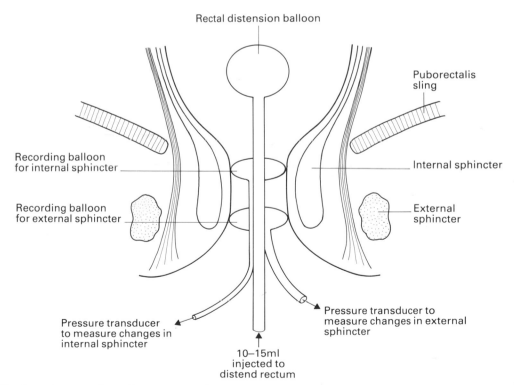

Fig. 62.1. Apparatus for performing anorectal pressure manometry.

this condition (Table 62.3). In ultra-short segment Hirschsprung's disease, constipation and faecal soiling in middle childhood is an uncommon but recognized feature [15]. In most cases of this disease the diagnosis depends upon **rectal biopsy** with histological examination and/or the demonstration of increased acetylcholinesterase activity in the specimen.

Anorectal manometry is a useful screening test in older children with long-standing constipation [40]. In ultra-short Hirschsprung's disease, where only the internal sphincter is involved, manometry may be the only method of investigation which will confirm the diagnosis (see Chapter 58). It is usually performed with a triple lumen catheter and balloon system (Fig. 62.1), although other systems are available [43, 66].

Technique

The distal balloon is placed within the rectum and the two proximal balloons within the anal canal opposite the internal and external sphincters. The proximal balloons are attached to transducers to measure the changes in sphincter tone in response to changes in the volume of the distal rectal balloon. In the normal subject a recto-anal inhibitory internal sphincter reflex can be demonstrated—an increase in rectal distension producing a relaxation of the internal sphincter (Fig. 62.2). In Hirschsprung's disease this recto-anal inhibitory reflex is characteristically absent.

The majority of children with constipation and/or faecal incontinence will show changes on anorectal manometry. These changes include an increase in the

(a) Normal pressure trace

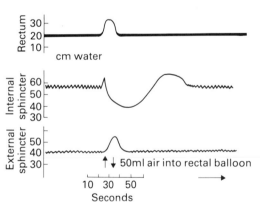

(b) Pressure trace in Hirschsprung's disease

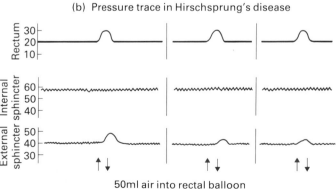

Fig. 62.2. Anorectal manometry pressure tracings. (a) normal, showing typical relaxation of internal sphincter in response to rectal distension. (b) typical trace in Hirschsprung's disease.

threshold pressure for inducing the recto-anal inhibitory sphincter reflex, anal hypertony or an increase in the maximal resting anal pressure, and a decrease in conscious rectal sensitivity [43, 46].

Callaghan and Nixon [12] divided rectal pressure changes into three grades:

1. An **enlarged rectum** where an increased distending volume is required to inhibit the internal anal sphincter.
2. An **expanded rectum** where rectal pressure changes only occur after a very large volume of air is introduced into the rectum.
3. The **inert rectum** where sphincter inhibition only occurs with very large rectal volumes without any conscious rectal sensation.

Medical treatment

Children with constipation and encopresis require a combined therapeutic approach, using counselling to modify any psychological factors and medications to aid faecal evacuation.

Counselling and psychotherapy

As faecal incontinence in children engenders a negative response from parents, other adults and peers, a first priority is to support the child and reduce psychological pressures. Parents should have the mechanical nature of the problem explained to them, particularly the loss of rectal sensation and the mechanism involved in the incontinence. A regular regimen of bowel evacuation should be encouraged, using the gastrocolic reflex after meals as an aid, until normal rectal sensation is restored.

Not infrequently these bowel symptoms are resistant to medication, simple support and advice. Simple behavioural modification techniques, such as star charts, designed to reward and potentiate a response may be helpful [33]. More complicated techniques have been used successfully to discover the family relationships and conditions that reinforce the abnormal behaviour which maintains the bowel problem [32]. Once the parents and family appreciate the family relationships that maintain the bowel disorder they can, with expert help, modify the circumstances that reinforce the bowel problem.

Other forms of psychotherapy have been used including play therapy, allowing the child to be messy and to express his or her aggression, and parental and family psychotherapy [42].

Medication

Because of the sensory changes associated with faecal retention, all patients require medication to empty the rectum and colon. Initially a programme of rectal washouts, with phosphate enemas or bisacodyl suppositories (Dulcolax), may be required to empty the rectum and, in severe cases, this will have to be performed as an in-patient [14, 54]. Any procedure involving rectal intubation should be undertaken with the child's informed consent to avoid the development of a negative reaction to the medical and nursing staff.

Enemas and/or suppositories should only be used in the most severely affected patients, and only until the rectum is empty and not as a form of maintenance. Oral laxatives have been used successfully but may be required for a prolonged period (months or years) until normal rectal sensation and evacuation are restored. The laxative agents employed may be stimulant (senna, danthron etc.), lubricant (liquid paraffin), softening (dioctyl sodium sulphosuccinate), or osmotic (lactulose or magnesium sulphate). Any of these agents may be effective, but they often need to be given in large doses. Controlled trials have shown that large doses of lactulose plus senna, or liquid paraffin, can be highly effective [72].

If our society took a diet high in bran

and roughage the problem of childhood constipation and encopresis would probably be less common. However, introducing a large amount of bran to the diet after the problem has developed is seldom helpful, although it may be advisable once bowel emptying is re-established.

Surgical treatment

Anal dilation, under general anaesthesia, can improve or cure up to 80% of the rare patients resistant to medical treatment [39]. This treatment, or an excisional anorectal myotomy, has been effective in the management of ultra-short Hirschsprung's disease [7].

Prognosis

Like many functional disorders in children, chronic constipation and encopresis can be extremely difficult to treat successfully. Medical treatment needs to continue for many months or years and the patients and their families can easily become disheartened by the apparent lack of progress. Faecal soiling is a particularly important symptom to control because of its psychological impact when others know of it (for example parents, siblings, teachers, peers etc). Despite these difficulties, the problem is usually controlled and rarely persists into adult life. Even the most difficult patients manage to improve their bowel control during or shortly after adolescence.

Hirschsprung's disease

Epidemiology

Congenital aganglionosis of the intestine occurs in approximately 1 in 4,500 live births [51]. It is a familial disease but is not inherited as a simple Mendelian trait.

Pathology

The major feature of Hirschsprung's disease is an absence of ganglion cells in the neural plexus of the intestinal wall associated with hypertrophy of the nerve trunks. This results from a failure of migration of neuroblasts into the gut from the vagal nerve trunks before the twelfth week of foetal life [50].

The loss of ganglion cells extends for a variable distance from the anorectal junction. In about two-thirds of patients the rectum and lower sigmoid colon are involved, but involvement of extremely short segments of the lower rectum or of the whole intestinal tract have been described. Zonal aganglionosis [45] and distal acquired aganglionosis [82] may produce a similar clinical picture; both are extremely rare and may result from later selective damage to the neural plexus. Perfusion experiments in dogs produce similar lesions as those seen in Hirschsprung's disease [49].

The severity of symptoms is not always consistent with the length of the intestinal segment involved and may be related to the number of acetylcholinesterase positive nerve fibres [28]—the concentration of acetylcholine is increased in the distal segment [35].

Clinical features

The clinical picture varies from acute intestinal obstruction in the newborn, to chronic constipation in later life [65]. In the newborn the delayed passage of meconium accompanied by mild abdominal distension should alert the paediatrician that Hirschsprung's disease may be present. Obstruction in the first weeks of life is extremely serious as it is often complicated by an enterocolitis (see Chapter 77), with the added complications of perforation and septicaemia. There is still a high mortality from Hirschsprung's disease at this age.

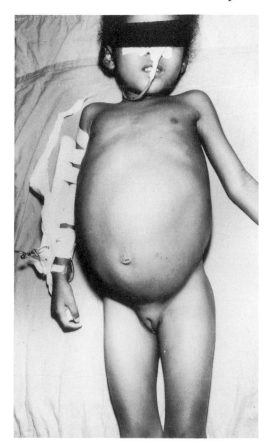

Fig. 62.3. Photograph of massive abdominal distension in a child with Hirschsprung's disease—late presentation.

Chronic constipation, beginning in the first few weeks of life, should arouse suspicion that it is due to this condition. The classical picture—gross abdominal distension, chronic constipation and failure to thrive (Fig. 62.3)—should be rare with a greater awareness of the diagnosis. Severe constipation, without soiling, in otherwise healthy children and adults can be due to ultra-short segment Hirschsprung's disease. Faecal soiling is not usually a feature of this diseases although it has been reported in ultra-short segment disease [15].

Diagnosis

Rectal biopsy

Confirmation of the diagnosis depends on a histopathological demonstration of aganglionosis and hypertrophic nerve fibres in the nerve plexus. This requires a biopsy of sufficient size and depth for the pathologist to see a representative area of at least one nerve plexus. Suction rectal biopsies, obtained with the Great Ormond Street pattern of biopsy forceps or something similar, will often give sufficient information to render a formal strip rectal biopsy unnecessary. Two specimens are usually taken from just above the anorectal junction. One is sent for biochemistry and one for histochemistry

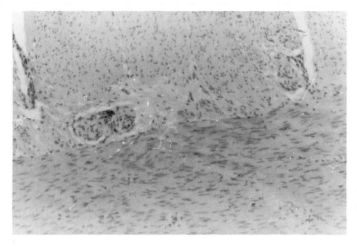

Fig. 62.4. Photomicrograph showing hypertrophied nerve fibres in the inter-muscular plexus in Hirschsprung's disease.

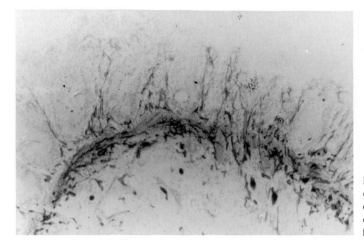

Fig. 62.5. Photomicrograph demonstrating the normal distribution of acetyl cholinesterase staining nerve fibres in a suction rectal biopsy.

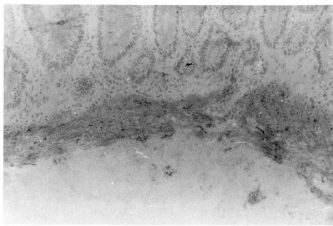

Fig. 62.6. Photomicrograph showing congenital aganglionosis distribution of acetyl cholinesterase staining nerve fibres in suction rectal biopsy.

and histopathology. The increase in acetylcholinesterase staining nerve fibres (Figs. 62.4, 62.5 and 62.6) is reflected in an increased assay of this enzyme [14]. These two estimations correlate well with standard histopathology [19].

Anorectal manometry

Anorectal manometry is a useful screening test in the constipated but otherwise fit young child or adult. The rectosphincteric inhibitory reflex is absent in congenital agangliosis [40]. This test is unreliable in the ill new-born infant because of poor anal tone.

Radiology

Erect and supine abdominal radiographs are useful if the large intestine is obstructed; they will show distended loops of small and large intestine, with fluid levels, consistent with a low intestinal obstruction (Figs. 62.7 and 62.8). Intramural gas indicates enterocolitis and free peritoneal gas, a perforation.

An enema, using a water-soluble contrast medium, will often confirm the diagnosis and provide an indication of the length of involved intestine. A rectal examination should not be performed prior to the X-ray as it may dilate the abnormal segment and destroy important radiological

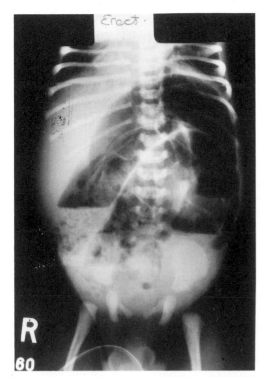

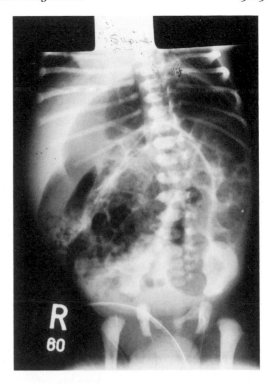

Fig. 62.7. Erect radiograph of a neonate with intestinal obstruction from Hirschsprung's disease.

Fig. 62.8. Supine radiograph of a neonate with intestinal obstruction from Hirschsprung's disease.

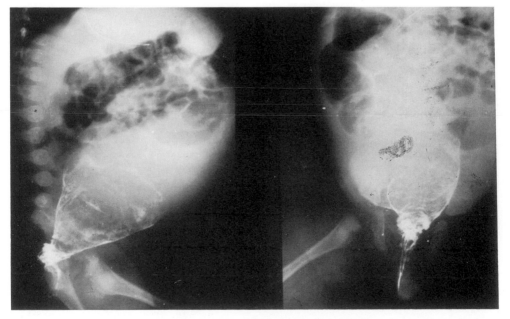

Fig. 62.9. A barium enema (lateral and A.P.) showing typical 'coning down' appearance at transition zone between dilated upper colon and narrow distal segment in Hirschsprung's disease.

features. The medium should be instilled through a fine 5FG catheter under screening control, with the patient in the lateral position. The coning down of the transition zone, saw-toothing of the mucosa and dysrhythmic contraction of the bowel are important positive findings (Fig. 62.9).

Treatment

The treatment of congenital aganglionosis will depend on four main factors:
1. Age of the patient.
2. Length of the involved segment.
3. Severity of symptoms.
4. The presence of enterocolitis.

In the new-born presenting with intestinal obstruction, and in any child or adult presenting with enterocolitis, an initial colostomy is required. The site of the colostomy should be selected as low as possible in the ganglionated segment, using peroperative frozen section biopsies to establish the presence of these ganglia. This is important as the transition zone may be distended by the propulsive power of the normal proximal colon making it difficult for the surgeon to decide where the normal colon ends (Fig. 62.10).

In the child or adult with constipation alone, the dilated bowel can be evacuated with repeated rectal saline washouts and enemas as a first step. The choice of the procedure to follow this will depend upon the length of the involved segment.

Short segment disease with minimal symptoms may respond well to an extended myectomy, performed by removing a strip of rectal wall up to the area where normal ganglion cells commence [67].

Long segment disease may be helped by one of four operations; three are designed to preserve the pelvic nerves and external rectal sphincters when the ganglionated segment of colon is brought down to within a centimetre of the anorectal margin for at least part of its circumference. The fourth operation consists of a combination of an anterior resection of the rectum with an anorectal myectomy [51]. These operations and their modifications are shown in diagrammatic form in Fig. 62.11.

Usually the definitive operation is preceded by a temporary colostomy for a few months, which allows the proximal distended colon to return to its normal calibre. If the colostomy has been performed in the new-born period, the definitive operation is delayed until the child weighs approximately 10 kg, when the pelvis is still shallow but is wide enough to give good access. Usually the child is between 10 months and one year of age; toilet training can usually begin soon after the operation.

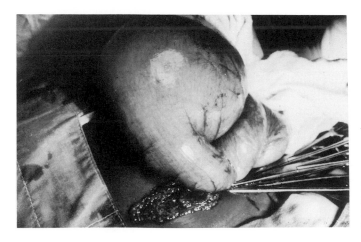

Fig. 62.10. The appearance of the colon at operation. This shows the area at which the colon 'cones down'.

(a) Swenson's procedure

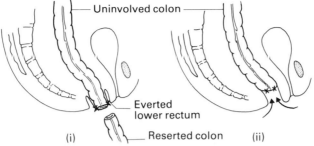

Uninvolved colon

Everted
lower rectum

Reserted colon

(i) (ii)

(b) Duhammel's procedure

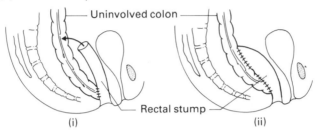

Uninvolved colon

Rectal stump

(i) (ii)

(c) Soave's procedure

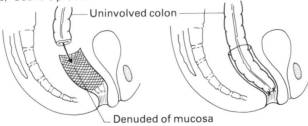

Uninvolved colon

Denuded of mucosa

(d) Anterior resection + myotomy

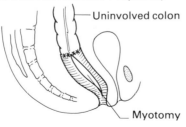

Uninvolved colon

Myotomy

Fig. 62.11. Diagrammatic representation of operations for congenital aganglionosis.

It is sometimes possible to clear the retained faeces with enemas and laxatives in an older child; if the colon can be kept clear for several months it may be possible to perform a one-stage operation. It is essential to have biopsy evidence of ganglion cells in the colon chosen for the new rectum. Postoperative anal dilations are started on the tenth day and continued until the surgeon is satisfied that the suture line is supple and soft.

Postoperative management

Swenson and his colleagues have drawn attention to the pitfalls in the management of this condition; their experience indicates that a few mistakes are the cause of most complications [9]. The commonest mistake is to leave a segment of aganglionic intestine in a position to obstruct the intestine, either at the colostomy site or after the definitive procedure. This should be avoided by careful peroperative biopsy techniques.

Children who have had operations for Hirschsprung's disease appear to be more severely affected by gastroenteritis than normal children of the same age. They may occasionally develop enterocolitis with dilation of the colon and severe fluid and electrolyte loss. The cause of this problem is unclear but may be related to three factors—firstly, the short length of aganglionic segment remaining after the Duhamel and Swenson procedures may be enough to cause an obstruction; secondly, there is a loss of length in the colon; thirdly, the function of the colon and distribution of ganglion cells in the innervated segment may not be entirely normal.

II   ADULTS

Constipation

Constipation is a symptom which has two common meanings—difficult passage of hard stools or infrequent defecation (see Chapter 5). In surveys of the general population, 10% of Britons [76] and 17% of Americans [21] complained of having to often strain at stool; in studies of bowel frequency 1% of Britons [17] and 4% of Americans passed less than two stools per week [21]. Straining at stool is common in Western societies although a bowel frequency of less than one stool every other day is rare, particularly in men. The use of laxatives increases with age, but it is not known whether this is due to a physiological change, or to customs of an earlier era (Table 62.4) [17].

Table 62.4. Causes of constipation.

Classification of constipation in adults.

No structural abnormality
Faulty diet or bowel habit
Pregnancy
Old age or infirmity
'Idiopathic slow transit' in women
A symptom of the 'irritable bowel syndrome' (Chapter 67)

Structural diseases
Anal pain or stenosis
Colonic stricture
Aganglionosis and/or an abnormal myenteric plexus
  Congenital Hirschsprung's disease
  Acquired   Chaga's disease
              East Africa megacolon
              Colonic pseudo-obstruction

A secondary abnormality of the colon
Endocrine or metabolic cause
  Hypothyroidism
  Hypercalcaemia
  Porphyria
Neurological cause
  Damage to sacral outflow or spinal cord
  Central nervous disorder
  Pain induced by straining—for example sciatic nerve compression
Systemic sclerosis and other connective tissue disorders
Psychological diseases
  Depression
  Anorexia nervosa
  Denied bowel habit
Drug side-effects

Constipation without structural abnormality of anus, colon or rectum

Faulty diet or bowel habit (see Chapter 5)

The average stool weight of adults in Britain and America is 100–150 g/day while in Africa and India it is 200–400 g/day [10, 75]. It is not surprising, therefore, that straining at stool is common in Western countries. The addition of poorly absorbed carbohydrate to the diet—in the form of wholemeal bread, fruit, vegetables and bran—increases the daily stool weight and water content, mainly by increasing its content of bacteria [73].

Many patients appear to lose the habit of daily defecation by regularly suppressing the urge to defecate at inconvenient times.

Pregnancy

Reduced bowel frequency with venous congestion and haemorrhoids are common problems during the later weeks of a pregnancy. Such patients should be encouraged to take a high residue diet, but may also require a mild laxative (for example—magnesium hydroxide, lactulose or a senna preparation) as a temporary measure.

Old age

Elderly patients tend to eat less and to be less mobile. Cerebral degeneration may lead to a lack of awareness of the urge to defecate, while immobility or poor social circumstances may prevent access to a toilet. Drug treatment for a systemic disease may lead to secondary constipation.

Spurious diarrhoea may result from faecal retention with overflow, this is easily diagnosed by rectal examination [62, 63]. Treatment of this diarrhoea with constipating agents will exacerbate the situation.

Idiopathic slow transit

This is a disorder of women [64] and is characterized by an apparently normal barium enema and rectal biopsy (except for melanosis coli due to the use of laxatives), associated with a prolonged whole gut transit time. Often the infrequent bowel function begins during adolescence or even childhood. Sometimes it follows an abdominal or pelvic operation. Gynaecological problems, such as irregular menses, difficulty in conception, hysterectomy and ovarian cystectomy tend to be more common among these patients [59].

There are usually several days, or even a week or more, between bowel actions. Some patients only pass a stool after a laxative. An increase in dietary fibre is ineffective and may increase abdominal discomfort and distension. By the time of referral most women have already tried a wide variety of stimulant laxatives with less and less success.

The cause of this disorder is unknown. Preliminary observations of abnormalities in some regulatory peptides and sex hormones have been made but these changes may be secondary [55, 61]. Physiological studies have shown a failure of relaxation of the puborectalis and external anal sphincter on straining [37, 57, 64, 83] although the internal sphincter relaxes normally on rectal distension. Colonic motor activity tends to be normal or reduced.

Irritable bowel syndrome

Constipation with abdominal pain and distension, sometimes associated with episodes of loose stools, is one of the symptoms of this syndrome (see Chapter 67). Although there is often increased motor activity present, the total gut transit time is usually normal.

Structural disease of the colon, rectum or anus

Anal lesions

Surgery for anal atresia in childhood can be followed by constipation with an enlarged rectum in later life (Fig. 62.12). Anal stenosis from any cause, or inelasticity of the anal canal (for example from a Tiersch

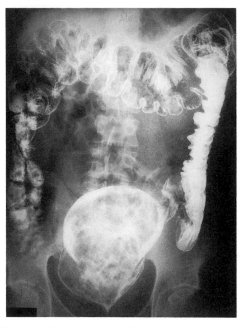

Fig. 62.12. Megarectum in a man aged 24 treated surgically during infancy and childhood for anal atresia.

wire for rectal prolapse), can lead to retention of faeces. Similarly, a painful anal lesion, such as a fissure or after haemorrhoidectomy, can cause the patient to resist the desire to defecate.

Colonic stricture

The recent onset of constipation in an adult should always lead to a full investigation of the large intestine to exclude a stenotic lesion such as a carcinoma.

Aganglionosis and/or myenteric plexus lesion

Hirschsprung's disease is usually diagnosed in infancy or childhood, but a few patients are only recognized in adult life or old age [3, 65, 77]. Such patients usually give a history of infrequent bowel actions since birth accompanied by abdominal distension and the need to use laxatives or enemas regularly. Retained faecal masses can cause stercoral ulceration of the colon with bleeding or perforation. Respiratory failure can result from the greatly distended abdomen pushing up the left hemidiaphragm with a shift of the mediastinum.

The internal anal sphincter response to rectal distension should be tested in all adults presenting with chronic constipation associated with megacolon. Only those with an absent or equivocal inhibition of this sphincter should have a full thickness rectal biopsy.

Chaga's disease: *Trypanosoma cruzi*, transmitted by bites from *Triatominae* insects, causes neuronal damage to cells of the autonomic nervous system. The heart and hollow abdominal viscera are most commonly affected [24, 26]. Megacolon and megaoesophagus (see Chapter 10) often occur together. The dilation develops over many years and is preceded by a phase of aperistalsis. This disease is endemic in tropical South America, particularly Brazil. It has been estimated that 7,000,000 people may be affected [84].

The acute phase is usually seen in children who present with malaise, fever, muscle pain, lymphadenopathy, oedema and hepatosplenomegaly. Megacolon occurs in the chronic phase of the disease—investigation will demonstrate a dilated, aperistaltic segment of bowel, often the sigmoid colon. Constipation, stercoral ulceration, perforation and volvulus can occur. The complement fixation test for *Trypanosoma cruzi* is positive in 95% of patients.

East Africa megacolon, with dilatation and hypertrophy of the sigmoid colon and a liability to volvulus, has been described in male members of certain tribes in Africa. Ganglion cells are present, but some appear abnormal, as does the myenteric plexus [8]. No infectious agent has been identified.

Colonic pseudo-obstruction occurs in some patients with intractable unexplained constipation. Abnormalities of the sub-mucosal and myenteric plexi have been demonstrated by silver staining of thick sections [36, 70]. Interpretation of these changes has proved difficult as some drugs, notably anthracene laxatives, can also cause damage to these plexi. While the changes may be secondary to laxative damage, it is considered that the myenteric degeneration is due to another cause in some patients [23, 36, 66].

Further work is needed on the anatomy of the myenteric plexus and the localization of neurotransmitters and regulatory peptides in patients with unexplained constipation.

Idiopathic megarectum and megacolon

In a series of 90 adult patients with megacolon, only 20 had true Hirschsprung's disease [77]. Idiopathic megacolon occurs equally in both sexes. Its cause is unknown although many believe that it is an acquired condition due to pot refusal during toilet training leading to faecal retention [48, 52]. Some cases may be congenital.

Radiological investigation usually shows a grossly enlarged rectum with proximal colonic distension over a variable distance [60]. When the diagnosis is suspected, X-rays should be performed without previous bowel preparation, using a small quantity of a water-soluble contrast medium to prevent barium impaction. Such X-rays frequently show gross faecal loading in an enlarged rectum and, possibly, colon (Fig. 62.13). Physiological studies show that the

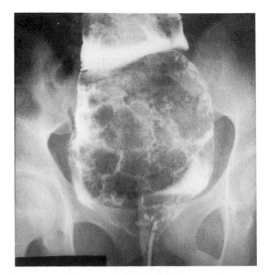

Fig. 62.13. Megarectum and faecal impaction outlined with water-soluble contrast material in girl aged 13 whose main complaint was of faecal soiling.

rectum is enlarged with a greatly decreased or absent sensation of rectal fullness when a balloon is distended in the rectum. Inhibition of internal and external anal sphincters is generally still demonstrable but at an unusually high distending volume [3, 12, 53]. This inhibition may occur before the sensation of rectal fullness, thus explaining the incontinence and soiling often encountered in such patients. These patients, like others with constipation, have difficulty in expelling an inflated balloon from the rectum even though a normally elevated intrarectal pressure is recorded during straining [2].

Adult patients with this condition can be arbitrarily divided into two main subgroups—those who develop constipation, rectal impaction and faecal soiling in childhood, and those who present sporadically in later life with constipation and abdominal pain but no soiling [3]. In both groups the major symptom is constipation with the infrequent passage of stools. The stools passed are hard, large and often block the toilet; painful defecation is common. Unlike patients with Hirschsprung's disease, these patients are in good health and are often unperturbed by their lack of bowel function. In one adult series 7 out of 42 patients were mentally subnormal and two had a personality disorder [38].

Examination often reveals a hard faecal mass rising out of the pelvis and palpable on rectal digital examination just above the anal canal. The anus is often patulous due to inhibition of the sphincters. Faecal soiling of the perianal skin is common and the buttocks may be held tightly together to improve continence.

It is important to exclude 'short segment aganglionosis' by demonstrating the rectosphincteric distension reflex and, if necessary, by a full thickness rectal biopsy. Contrast X-ray examination should include a lateral pelvic view to exclude a narrow distal rectal segment [79].

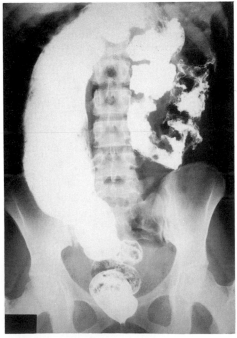

Fig. 62.14. Segmental colonic enlargement with a normal-sized rectum. Note—malrotation of descending colon.

Idiopathic segmental megacolon

A few patients present with an enlarged segment of colon proximal to a normal sized rectum (Fig. 62.14) [38, 74]. In such patients it is essential to exclude aganglionosis of the rectum. This type of megacolon tends to present with an acute sigmoid volvulus. The cause of the condition is unknown and surgical resection specimens often show a thinned colonic wall, in contrast to the hypertrophied wall found in most other forms of megacolon.

Constipation secondary to an abnormality outside the colon

Endocrine and metabolic causes

Bowel symptoms, especially constipation, are common in **hypothyroidism**. Megacolon has been recorded in myxoedematous patients [11, 71]. Histological examination of the colon in this condition has shown the wall to be thickened with myxoedematous infiltration and the mucosa to be atrophic with cystic distension of the crypts and diffuse infiltration by lymphocytes and plasma cells. The megacolon decreases in size as the patient becomes euthyroid on thyroxine treatment.

Hypercalcaemia or acute porphyria can present with constipation.

Neurological causes

Damage to the pelvic parasympathetic nerve supply to the rectum, or of the sacral cord, causes severe constipation usually accompanied by urinary retention. Transection of the spinal cord leads to loss of rectal sensation and automatic defecation [29].

Constipation can also be a problem in **dementia** due to lack of attention to, or awareness of, rectal sensation [80]. Megacolon, with sigmoid volvulus in some patients, has been reported in **Parkinsonism,** but it is unclear as to whether this is due to the disease or to the drug treatment of it [13].

Systemic sclerosis and connective tissue and muscle disorders

Megacolon has occasionally been reported in association with systemic sclerosis, the Ehlers-Danlos syndrome, myotonia dystrophica and Thomson's disease.

Psychological disorders

Constipation may be one of the presenting symptoms of **depression.** Patients with **anorexia nervosa** often develop intractable constipation, presumably due in part to an inadequate diet although other features resemble the idiopathic slow transit form of constipation seen in women on a normal diet (see Chapter 68).

Rarely a patient may deny passage of stool even though studies using radio-opaque non-absorbable markers confirm that defecation has occurred [34]. This unusual psychological disorder may present as intractable constipation; it demonstrates the need for objective evidence of prolonged intestinal transit before surgical treatment is proposed.

Drug side effects

Many drugs influence bowel function either through the central nervous system or through a local action on the colonic musculature (Table 62.5).

A full drug history is extremely important when assessing any patient complaining of the recent onset of constipation.

Table 62.5. Drugs that can cause constipation.

Muscle relaxants
Ganglion blocking agents
Anti-convulsants
Psychotrophic drugs
Monoamine oxidase inhibitors
Barbiturates
Phenothiazines
Benzodiazepines
Tricyclic anti-depressants
Opiate analgesics
Other analgesics—notably codeine derivatives
Aluminium containing antacids
Iron supplements
Diuretics
Cytotoxic drugs

Treatment of constipation

General measures

Although it has never been formally tested, most patients with constipation probably benefit from an increased fluid intake, an increase in physical activity and unhurried visits to the toilet. Neglecting the 'call to stool' is a frequent cause of constipation [1].

Diet

Fibre is the only component of the diet to benefit the constipated patient. It has been used for centuries to treat constipation [20]. There is no universal dose—the required amount is that necessary to produce at least one soft stool daily or on alternate days. The aim should be to double the patient's fibre intake from around 20 g/day to 40 g/day. If there is no response one should look again for an organic cause.

Fibre intake can be increased by—
1. Increasing bread intake to about 200 g (6 slices) per day and changing to 100% wholemeal bread.
2. Eating a wholewheat breakfast cereal, a cereal with added bran, or an oat-based muesli.
3. Increasing fruit and vegetable intake.

4. Eating more legumes such as peas, beans and lentils.

5. Using concentrated fibre foods such as cereal bran or bulk forming laxatives.

The dangers of increasing fibre intake are small. As fibre is fermented in the colon to produce gas, a rapid increase in fibre intake may be associated with abdominal distension, bloating, pain and increased flatus. This can be avoided by a slow build-up in dose. Other complications such as intestinal obstruction or mineral malabsorption are largely theoretical. However, because of the high phytic content of raw bran, one should use fibre with caution in those whose mineral balance is precarious such as in the very young, the elderly and during pregnancy.

Laxatives

Laxatives are a safe, valuable and effective part of the management of the constipated patient. There are five groups of laxatives, each having a different mode of action [18].

Bulk laxatives are a purified form of dietary fibre, acting by retaining fluid in the gut and by stimulation of colonic bacterial activity.

There are three types—those derived from **ispaghula** (a seed mucilage from the Plantago family), **sterculia** (a plant gum), or **methylcellulose.** Tablets of compressed bran are also available.

Bulk laxatives are best given with meals, or mixed with a carbonated drink, starting with 5 g daily and increasing up to 20 g daily. No one preparation is superior so it is worth a constipated patient trying the whole range before moving on to more potent agents.

Stimulants are very effective and widely used. They act by direct stimulation of colonic motor activity. **Senna and sodium picosulphate** require bacterial activation, so their action is reduced by antibiotic therapy. **Bisacodyl and phenolphthalein** have

an enterohepatic circulation. These laxatives can produce abdominal colic, so initially they are best taken as a small dose at night (doses = bisacodyl 5–10 mg; danthron 25–75 mg; Senokot 2–4 tablets).

Faecal softeners (detergents) are mild aperients which are mainly used for patients with haemorrhoids or another anal problem. The detergent properties are said to cause softening of the faecal mass. Their main danger is the possibility that the detergent action may increase the absorption of other drugs'. When used they should be taken throughout the whole day (doses = dioctyl sodium sulphosuccinate 100–200 mg t.i.d., liquid paraffin 10–30 ml t.i.d.).

Dioctyl sodium sulphosuccinate also alters water and electroyte movement across the mucosa with fluid and electrolyte accumulation in the lumen [22].

Salts used as laxatives are all poorly absorbed and act by drawing water into the colon by osmosis (see Chapter 4). They may also release gut hormones (such as cholecystokinin) which stimulate colonic motor activity. The available preparations are mostly magnesium and sodium salts (for example magnesium sulphate, hydroxide, citrate or carbonate; sodium sulphate; sodium–potassium tartrate).

These preparations are undoubtedly laxative and are of most value when used as a single dose to return bowel function to normal on specific occasions, for example after a period of inactivity or after an alteration of life-style or diet. They are also useful in the right-sided constipation of ulcerative colitis. The relative efficacy varies with the osmotic effect of the salt. In general, sulphates are the most potent, magnesium salts being stronger than sodium. On theoretical grounds, magnesium sulphate is the first choice (dose = 5–15 g with 100–200 ml of water, or magnesium sulphate mixture 10–20 ml with water).

Lactulose, a disaccharide of galactose and

fructose, is another effective laxative. It has several actions including an osmotic effect (because it is not absorbed), a fermentation effect, also lowering pH in the caecum. Because it also lowers the ammonia concentration in the colon, by stimulating microbial protein synthesis, it is widely used in hepatic encephalopathy. It is a mild and effective laxative at doses from 15 ml twice daily.

Others—many other laxatives are available including castor oil, bile salts, frangula, rhubarb, podophyllum etc. Often several laxatives are mixed together in a proprietary preparation.

A number of laxatives are available as suppositories or enemas. Enemas are particularly useful as a once-only treatment for constipation, while suppositories can be useful in patients with abnormal anorectal function.

Management of specific problems

Pregnancy

As medications should probably be avoided during pregnancy, these patients are best managed with a high fibre diet (avoiding raw bran), increased fluid intake and bulk laxatives. If these measures fail, lactulose, bisacodyl suppositories, or oral senna are without danger to the foetus or mother.

Old age

Constipation in elderly patients occurs for all the same reasons as in the young and should be managed similarly. However, such patients more often develop faecal impaction leading to incontinence, intestinal obstruction, rectal bleeding, urinary retention and restlessness. Faecal impaction is diagnosed by rectal examination. Initially treatment may involve daily enemas to empty the rectum, this should be followed by large doses of senna to empty the re-

mainder of the colon. Occasionally manual removal of the faecal mass, under a general anaesthetic, will be required. Prevention is best [25].

Idiopathic slow transit constipation

Treatment of this condition is generally unsatisfactory. Osmotic laxatives are ineffective in small doses and produce explosive watery stools, with incontinence, when given in large amounts. Some patients can be managed with large doses of an osmotic or stimulant laxative, or with regular phosphate enemas. Occasionally symptoms are very severe and medical treatment is ineffective. Under these circumstances total colectomy with ileorectal anastomosis may be advised. Partial colectomy is usually ineffective and should not be recommended. Total, or near-total, colectomy is usually satisfactory although mild constipation or liquid stools with incontinence can still be a problem [55].

Hirschsprung's disease

An extended internal sphincterotomy may be adequate treatment for patients with short segment disease. More extensive disease in adults is more difficult to treat as the proximal bowel is often enormously dilated and hypertrophied, and the pelvis is relatively deep. The Duhamel operation (Fig. 62.11b) is prefered although a colostomy may be required in older patients [44, 77]. An alternative procedure is that of anorectal myectomy [30], although experience with this procedure is limited.

Chaga's disease

There is no curative treatment for the type of megacolon found in this disease. Patients with symptoms uncontrolled by medical measures require surgical resection of the dilated, hypertrophied segment of colon.

Idiopathic megacolon and megarectum

Treatment is directed at emptying the rectum and keeping it empty. As a first step disimpaction by enemas, washouts and even manual removal under general anaesthesia may be required. Thereafter the patient must be encouraged to develop a regular daily habit of attempting defecation, even if there is no urge to empty the rectum present. Regular and continuous laxatives are generally needed, otherwise impaction tends to recur. Magnesium sulphate (10–20 ml/day) is often satisfactory but some patients prefer to use lactulose either alone, or with magnesium sulphate. A few patients need to give themselves evacuant suppositories or phosphate enemas at the first sign of impaction. Medical treatment is often successful when the patient understands the problem and adheres to a regular regimen [3].

Surgical treatment is sometimes needed, if medical treatment fails. Sigmoid resection gives unsatisfactory results, unless recurrent volvulus is present. Usually sub-total colectomy with ileorectal or caecorectal anastomosis is required. Results of such operations are unpredictable (particularly in megarectum alone) and recurrent faecal retention in the rectum, or diarrhoea with urgency and incontinence, may occur [3, 5, 38].

Where segmental megacolon fails to respond to medical treatment, resection of the dilated segment, with an end-to-end anastomosis, is often successful.

Neurological causes (including cord injuries)

These patients often have a disturbance of the rectoanal reflex activity and need careful management. They should be encouraged to empty their bowels regularly, even though they may have no sensation of a full rectum.

A high fibre diet does not help these patients, and should be used only with great care. Bowel evacuation can usually be achieved by giving a laxative on alternate nights followed by a suppository, such as bisacodyl (5–10 mg), on the next day. Suppositories are particularly important in patients with lesions above the cauda equina; normal reflex activity is preserved in these patients although consciousness of this is lacking. Occasionally enemas, or digital removal of the faeces, may be needed [1].

References

1 AVERY-JONES F, GODDING EW. *Management of Constipation*. Oxford: Blackwell Scientific Publications, 1972.
2 BARNES PRH, LENNARD-JONES JE. Balloon expulsion from the rectum in constipation of different types. *Gut* 1985;**26**:1049–1052.
3 BARNES PRH, LENNARD-JONES JE, HAWLEY PR, TODD IP. Hirschsprung's disease and idiopathic megacolon in adults and adolescents. *Gut* 1986;**27**:534–541.
4 BARR LC, BOOTH J, FILIPE MI, LAWSON JON. Clinical evaluation of the histochemical diagnosis of Hirschsprung's disease. *Gut* 1985;**26**:393–399.
5 BELLIVEAU P, GOLBERG SM, ROTHENBERGER DA, NIVATVONGS S. Idiopathic acquired megacolon: the value of subtotal colectomy. *Dis Col Rectum* 1982;**25**:117–121.
6 BELLMAN M. Studies on encopresis. *Acta Paediatr Scand Suppl* 1976;**170**.
7 BENTLEY JFR. Post-excisional ano-rectal manometry in management of chronic faecal accumulation. *Arch Dis Child* 1966;**4**:144–147.
8 BOHM GM, SMITH AB. Pathology of an East African megacolon. *Gut* 1966;**7**:662–665.
9 BRENNAN LP, WEITZMAN JJ, SWENSON O. Pitfalls in the management of Hirschsprung's disease. *J Pediatr Surg* 1967;**2**:1–12.
10 BURKITT DP, WALKER ARP, PAINTER NS. Dietary fibre and disease. *JAMA* 1974;**229**:1068–1074.
11 BURRELL M, CRONAN J, MEGNA D, TOFFLER R. Myxoedema megacolon. *Gastrointest Radiol* 1980;**5**:181–186.
12 CALLAGHAN RP, NIXON HH. Megatrectum: physiological observations. *Arch Dis Child* 1964;**39**:153–157.
13 CAPLAN LH, JACOBSON HG, RUBINSTEIN BM, ROTMAN MZ. Megacolon and volvulus in Parkinson's disease. *Radiology* 1965;**85**:73–79.
14 CLAYDEN GS. In condemnation of the suppository in childhood. *Lancet* 1981;**i**:273.

15 CLAYDEN GS, LAWSON JON. Investigation and management of long standing chronic constipation in childhood. *Arch Dis Child* 1976;**51**:918–923.

16 CLEGHORN GJ, STRINGER DA, FORSTNER GG, DURIES PR. Treatment of distal intestinal obstruction syndrome in cystic fibrosis with a balanced intestinal lavage solution. *Lancet* 1986;**1**:8–11.

17 CONNELL AM, HILTON C, IRVINE G, LENNARD-JONES JE, MISIEWICZ JJ. Variation of bowel habit in two population samples. *Br Med J* 1965;**2**:1095–1099.

18 CUMMINGS JH. The use and abuse of laxatives. In Bouchier IAD ed. *Recent Advances in Gastroenterology* London: Academic Press, 1976:124–149.

19 DALE G, BONHAM JR, RILEY WA, WAGGET J. An improved method for the determination of acetylcholinesterase activity in rectal biopsy tissue from patients with Hurschsprung's disease. *Clin Chim Acta* 1977;**77**:407–413.

20 DIMOCK EM. 'The treatment of habitual constipation by the bran method.' Cambridge University, MD Thesis, 1936.

21 DROSSMAN DA, SANDLER RS, McKEE DC, LOVITZ AJ. Bowel patterns among subjects not seeking health care. Use of a questionnaire to identify a population with bowel dysfunction. *Gastroenterology* 1982;**83**:529–534.

22 DONOWITZ, M, BINDER HJ. Effect of dioctyl sodium sufosuccinate on colonic fluid and electrolyte movement. *Gastroenterol* 1974;**69**:941–950

23 DYER NH, DAWSON AM, SMITH B, TODD IP. Obstruction of bowel due to lesion in the myenteric plexus. *Br Med J* 1969;**1**:686–689.

24 EARLAM RJ. Gastrointestinal aspects of Chaga's disease. *Dig Dis Sci* 1972;**17**:559–571.

25 EXTON-SMITH AN. Constipation in geriatrics. In: Jones FA, Godding EW, eds. *Management of Constipation*. Oxford: Blackwell Scientific Publications, 1972.

26 FERREIRA-SANTOS R. Megacolon and megarectum in Chaga's disease. *Proc R Soc Med* 1961;**54**:1047–1053.

27 FRITZ GK, ARMBRUST J. Enuresis and Encopresis. *Psychiatr Clin North Am* 1982;**5**:283–296.

28 GARRETT JR, HOWARD ER, NIXON HH. Autonomic nerves in rectum and colon in Hirschsprung's disease. A cholinesterase and catecholamine histochemical study. *Arch Dis Child* 1969;**44**:406–417.

29 GUTTMAN L. The regulation of rectal function in spinal paraplegia. *Proc R Soc Med* 1958;**52**:86–88.

30 HAMDY MH, SCOBIE WG. Anorectal myectomy in adult Hirschsprung's disease: a report of six cases. *Br J Surg* 1984;**71**:611–613.

31 HERBERT M. *Emotional Problems of Development in Children* London: Academic Press, 1974:159–161.

32 HERBERT M. *Behaviour Treatment of Problem Children—Practical Manual*. London: Academic Press, 1981.

33 HILL P. Behaviour modifications with children. *Br J Hosp Med* 1972;**27**:51–60.

34 HINTON JM, LENNARD-JONES JE. Constipation: definition and classification. *Postgrad Med J* 1968;**44**:720–723.

35 IKAWA H, YOKOYAMA J, MORIKAWA Y, HAYASHI A, KATSUMATA K. A quantitative study of acetylcholine in Hirschsprung's disease. *J Pediatr Surg* 1980;**15**:48–52.

36 KRISHNAMURTHY S, SCHUFFLER MD, ROHRMANN CA, POPE CE. Severe idiopathic constipation is associated with a distinctive abnormality of the colonic myenteric plexus. *Gastroenterology* 1985;**88**:26–34.

37 KUIJPERS HC, BLEIJENBERG G. The spastic pelvic floor syndrome. *Dis Colon Rectum* 1985;**28**:669–672.

38 LANE RHS, TODD IP. Idiopathic megacolon: a review of 42 cases. *Br J Surg* 1977;**6**:305–310.

39 LAWSON JON. Physiological aspects and treatment of severe chronic constipation. *Arch Dis Child* 1974;**49**:245.

40 LAWSON JON, NIXON HH. Anal canal pressures in the diagnosis of Hirschsprung's disease. *J Pediatr Surg* 1967;**2**:544–552.

41 LEVINE MD. Encopresis: its potentiation, evaluation and alleviation. *Pediatr Clin North Am* 1982;**29**:315–330.

42 LEVINE MD, BEHOUR H. Children with encopresis: a descriptive analysis. *Pediatrics* 1975;**56**:412.

43 LOENING-BANCKE VA. Anorectal manometry—Experience with strain gauge pressure transducer for the diagnosis of Hirschsprung's disease. *J Pediatr Surg* 1983;**18**:595–600.

44 McCREADY RA, BEART RW. Adult Hirschsprung's disease: results of surgical treatment at Mayo Clinic. *Dis Colon Rectum* 1980;**23**:401–407.

45 MacIVER AG, WHITEHEAD R. Zonal colonic aganglionosis, a variant of Hirschsprung's disease. *Arch Dis Child* 1972;**47**:233–237.

46 MEUNIER P, MARACHAL JM, DE BEAUJEN MJ. Rectoanal pressures and rectal sensitivity studies in chronic childhood constipation. *Gastroenterology* 1979;**77**:330–336.

47 MINNCHIN S, FISHMAN HC. *Family Therapy Techniques*. Cambridge, Massachusetts: Harvard University Press:1981.

48 NIXON HH. Megarectum in the older child. *Proc R Soc Med* 1967;**60**:3–5.

49 OKAMOTO E, IWASAKI T, KAKUTANI T, UEDA T. Selective destruction of the myenteric plexus: Its relation to Hirschsprung's disease. *J Pediatr Surg* 1967;**2**:444–454.

50 OKAMOTO E, UEDA T. Embryogenesis of intramural ganglia of the gut and its relation to Hirschsprung's disease. *J Pediatr Surg* 1967;**2**:437–443.

51 ORR JD, SCOBIE WG. Presentation and incidence of Hirschsprung's disease. *Br Med J* 1983;**287**:1671.

52 PINKERTON P. Psychogenic megacolon in children: the implications of bowel negativism. *Arch Dis Child* 1958;**33**:371–380.

53 PORTER NH. Megacolon: a physiological study. *Proc R Soc Med* 1961;**54**:1043–1047.

54 POSTUMA R. Whole bowel irrigation in pediatric patients. *J Pediatr Surg* 1982;**17**:350–352.

55 PRESTON DM, ADRIAN TE, CHRISTOFIDES ND, LENNARD-JONES JE, BLOOM SR. Pancreatic polypeptide and motilin response in functional bowel disorders. *Scand J Gastroenterol [Suppl]* 1983;**18**:199–200.

56 PRESTON DM, HAWLEY PR, LENNARD-JONES JE, TODD IP. Results of colectomy for severe idiopathic constipation in women (Arbuthnot Lane's disease). *Br J Surg* 1984;**71**:647–552.

57 PRESTON DM, LENNARD-JONES JE. Is there a pelvic floor disorder in slow-transit constipation. *Gut* 1981;**22**:A890.

58 PRESTON DM, LENNARD-JONES JE. Anismus in chronic constipation. *Dig Dis Sci* 1985;**30**:413–418.

59 PRESTON DM, LENNARD-JONES JE. Severe chronic constipation of young women: 'Idiopathic slow transit constipation'. *Gut* 1986;**27**:41–48.

60 PRESTON DM, LENNARD-JONES JE, THOMAS BM. Towards a radiologic definition of idiopathic megacolon. *Gastrointest Radiol* 1985;**10**:167–169.

61 PRESTON DM, REES LH, LENNARD-JONES JE. Gynaecological disorders and hyperprolactinaemia in chronic constipation. *Gut* 1983;**24**:480A.

62 READ NW, ABOUZEKRY L. Why do patients with faecal impaction have faecal incontinence. *Gut* 1986;**27**:283–287.

63 READ NW, ABOUZEKRY L, READ MG, HOWELL P, OTTEWELL D, DONNELLY TC. Anorectal function in elderly patients with fecal impaction. *Gastroenterology* 1985;**89**:959–966.

64 READ NW, TIMMS JM, BARFIELD LJ, DONNELLY TC, BANNISTER JJ. Impairment of defecation in young women with severe constipation. *Gastroenterology* 1986;**90**:53–60.

65 RICH AJ, LENNARD TWJ, WILSDON JB. Hirschsprung's disease as a cause of chronic constipation in the elderly. *Br J Med* 1983;**287**:1777–1778.

66 ROSENBERG AJ, VELA AR. A new simplified technique for pediatric anorectal manometry. *Pediatrics* 1983;**71**:240–245.

67 SCOBIE WG, MACKINLAY GA. Anorectal myectomy in treatment of ultra-short segment Hirschsprung's disease. *Arch Dis Child* 1977;**52**:713–715.

68 SEIBER WK. Hirschsprung's disease In: Ravitch MM, Welch KJ, Benson CD, ABERDEEN E, RANDOLPH JG, eds. *Pediatric Surgery*. Chicago: Chicago Year Book Medical Publishers Inc, 1979.

69 SMITH B. *The Neuropathology of the Alimentary Tract*. London: Edward Arnold, 1972.

70 SNOOKS SJ, BARNES PRH, SWASH M, HENRY MM. Damage to the innervation of the pelvic floor musculature in chronic constipation. *Gastroenterology* 1985;**89**:977–981.

71 SOLANO FX JR, STARLING RC, LEVEY GS. Myxedema megacolon. *Arch Intern Med* 1985;**145**:231.

72 SONDHEIMER JM, GERVAISE EP. Lubricant versus laxative in the treatment of chronic constipation of children. *J Pediatr Gastroenterol Nutr* 1982; **1**:223–226.

73 STEPHEN AM, CUMMINGS JH. The microbiological contribution to human faecal mass. *J Med Microbiol* 1980;**13**:45–56.

74 SWENSON O, RATHAUSER F. Segmental dilation of the colon: a new entity. *Amer J Surg* 1959; **97**:734–738.

75 TANDON RK, TANDON BN. Stool weights in North Indians. *Lancet* 1975;**ii**:560–561.

76 THOMPSON WG, HEATON KW. Functional bowel disorders in apparently healthy people. *Gastroenterology* 1980;**79**:283–288.

77 TODD IP. Adult Hirschsprung's disease. *Br J Surg* 1971;**64**:561–565.

78 TURNBULL GK, LENNARD-JONES JE, BARTRAM CI. Failure of rectal expulsion as a cause of constipation: why fibre and laxatives sometimes fail. *Lancet* 1986;**1**:767–769.

79 VARMA JS, SMITH AN. Reproducibility of the proctometrogram. *Gut* 1986;**27**:288–292.

80 WATKINS GL, OLIVER GA. Giant megacolon in the insane, further observations on patients treated by subtotal colectomy. *Gastroenterology* 1965; **48**:718–727.

81 WEAVER LT, STEINER H. The bowel habit of young children. *Arch Dis Child* 1984;**59**:649–652.

82 WEINBERG RJ, KLISH WJ, SMALLEY JR, BROWN MR, PUTNAM TC. Acquired distal aganglionosis of the colon. *J Pediat* 1981;**101**:406–409.

83 WOMACK NR, WILLIAMS NS, HOLMFIELD JMH, MORRISON JFB, SIMPKINS KC. New method for the dynamic assessment of anorectal function in constipation. *Br J Surg* 1985;**72**:994–998.

84 WORLD HEALTH ORGANISATION REPORT Chaga's disease: report of a study group. *Technical Report Series 202*. Geneva, World Health Organisation, 1960.

Chapter 63
Colonic Polyps

E. T. SWARBRICK

A polyp is any tumour that projects into the lumen of the intestine. It can be single or multiple, sessile or pedunculated. Colonic polyps are of great importance as many are adenomatous and have the potential for malignant change. Improved radiological techniques and fibreoptic endoscopy have revolutionized the diagnosis and management of polyps.

As macroscopic appearances are deceptive, all polyps must be examined histologically for evidence of malignant change. Subsequent management depends on the histological findings, in the hope that treatment will decrease the death rate from colorectal cancer [9].

Colonic polyps may be subdivided into four major groups—hamartomatous, metaplastic, inflammatory and neoplastic (Table 63.1). While some can be correctly categorized macroscopically, histological diagnosis is essential for correct management [4].

Hamartomatous polyps

A hamartoma is a non-neoplastic tumour composed of an abnormal mixture of tissues often with an excess of one type. Juvenile and Peutz-Jegher polpys are of this type.

Juvenile polyps

These are usually single, although they may be multiple or, rarely, diffuse. They occur at any age and are usually smooth, round, cherry-red, friable and pedunculated; most are small but they can grow up to 2–3 cm in diameter. Histologically, there is a predominance of highly vascular connective tissue, sometimes containing glands, covered by normal epithelium; epithelial cysts may occur. Frequently juvenile polyps ulcerate, become infected and auto-amputate. Their malignant potential is low.

Peutz-Jeghers syndrome

This syndrome is associated with multiple gastrointestinal hamartomatous polyps and buccal pigmentation. The polyps predominate in the upper intestine but can also be found in the colon in 50% of patients. Macroscopically, they look like adenomas, but on histological examination they show tree-like branches of smooth muscle covered by a normal mucin-secreting mucosa. The normal epithelium may be displaced within the polyp causing a mistaken diagnosis of malignant change. These polyps are not malignant but a higher incidence of carcinoma in the adjacent bowel, notably stomach and duodenum, has been reported [24].

Metaplastic polyps

These are the commonest type of polyp found in the colon. They tend to be sessile, covered by healthy, glistening normal mucosa. They are usually small, although occasionally they may be over 1 cm in diameter. Around 75% of adults over 40 years of age have metaplastic polyps, most often in the rectum. Occasionlly the polyps may be so numerous as to suggest the diagnosis of familial polyposis.

Histologically, metaplastic polpys represent an exaggeration of normal differentiation of the mucosa; as such they have no malignant potential.

Inflammatory polyps

These 'pseudo' polyps are found in patients with ulcerative colitis and Crohn's disease (see Chapters 49 and 52). They are usually small, pink, and worm-like but can become rounded and over 1 cm in diameter [30]. Usually at least one severe attack of colitis is required before they occur. These polyps are non-neoplastic and are unrelated to the premalignant change sometimes seen in chronic inflammatory bowel disease [20].

Similar inflammatory polyps may arise in other forms of colitis due to ischaemia, or bacillary, amoebic or schistosomal infection. Schistosomal polyposis can result in severe diarrhoea with fluid, electrolyte and protein loss which may be relieved by endoscopic polypectomy [16].

Adenomas

Colonic adenomas are common, occurring in 40–60% of men and 30–50% of women over 55 years of age [5, 25]. They are found throughout the colon but are more common on the left side [11]. The polyps are multiple in 25% of patients and can recur elsewhere after removal, emphasizing the need for regular supervision of such patients [4, 32]. There are three different

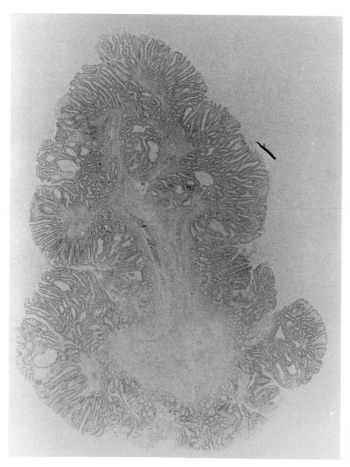

Fig. 63.1. Tubular adenoma. This type constitutes 75% of colonic adenomas.

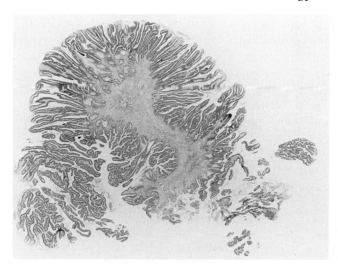

Fig. 63.2. Villous adenoma. This type constitutes 10% of colonic tumours.

histological types—tubular, villous and tubulo-villous.

Approximately 75% of all adenomas are **tubular** in type (Fig. 63.1)—these polyps are usually small, lobular and pedunculated. Around 10% of adenomatous polyps are **villous** adenomas—these polyps are shaggy, velvety and flat and may be large spreading extensively and circumferentially (Fig. 63.2). **Tubulo-villous** polyps (Fig. 63.3) have a mixed histological pattern, and account for 15% of adenomatous polyps.

Many **adenomatous polyps** show dysplasia of their surface epithelium amounting to carcinoma-*in-situ*. However, the terms 'carcinoma' and 'cancer' by definition require invasion of the stalk and muscularis mucosae by malignant cells. This definition is important as it has therapeutic implications.

Evidence for the polyp–cancer sequence is discussed in Chapter 65 [19]; in summary the important facts are:

1. The larger the polyp the more likely is the chance of invasive cancer. In a series of 2,849 adenomas only 1.3% of polyps < 1 cm in diameter showed invasive changes; the incidence was 9.5% in those 1–2 cm, and 45% in those > 2 cm [23].

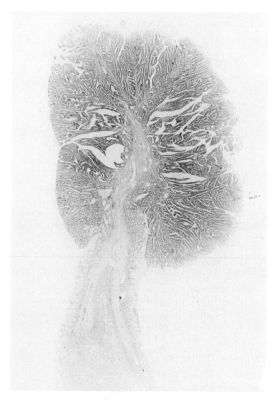

Fig. 63.3. Tubulo-villous adenoma. This type constitutes 15% of colonic adenomas.

2. Many carcinomas contain non-malignant adenomatous tissue adjacent to malignant cells.

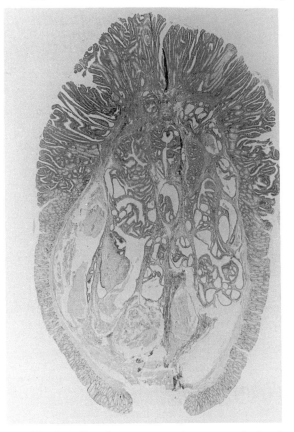

Fig. 63.4. 'Pseudocarcinomatous' invasion by displaced benign adenomatous tissue.

3. Approximately 20% of patients with co-lorectal cancers will either have synchronous or metachronous neoplastic polyps [22].

4. The majority of patients with untreated polyposis coli will develop one or more carcinomas [1].

5. It is rare to find small invasive colonic cancers.

6. Villous polyps are more likely to contain cancer (40%) than tubulo-villous (22%) or tubular polyps (5%).

Studies of patients who have refused surgery for polyps suggest that it usually takes over five years for an adenoma to develop into a carcinoma, and that only about 1:1,000 will transform in this way. It is impossible to predict which ones will do so.

Occasionally 'pseudo-invasion' (Fig. 63.4) is mistaken for true invasion [22].

Other 'polyps'

Lymphoid hyperplasia is not uncommon in the rectum, particularly in children, and can be mistaken for familial polyposis. It is sometimes associated with immunodeficiency syndromes. The polyps are small, smooth, round and contain normal lymphoid cells.

Other rarer tumours may present as polyps (Table 63.1). **Lipomas** are fairly common in the area of the ileocaecal valve and

Table 63.1. Subdivisions of colonic polyps.

Hamartomas
  Juvenile polyps
  Peutz Jeghers syndrome

Metaplastic polyps

Inflammatory polyps

Neoplastic
  adenoma
  lipoma
  leiomyoma
  neuroma
  lymphangioma

Other 'polyps'
  Mucosal tags
  Fatty deposits at ileocaecal valve
  Lymphoid hyperplasia
  Endometriosis
  Pneumatosis coli
  Vascular hamartomas

present as yellowish, soft protrusions that dimple easily with the biopsy forceps; they should not be removed. **Pneumatosis coli** often appears as coarse, nodular, flat domes covered with hyperaemic friable mucosa in the rectum and colon; these deflate when pricked (see Chapter 73). Occasionally **heterotopic tissue** (e.g. pancreatic and gastric 'rests') may form polypoid lesions in the colon.

Clinical features

Most polyps are **asymptomatic** being found incidentally during radiological or endoscopic assessment for gastrointestinal symptoms. The commonest symptom is **rectal bleeding.** Villous papillomas may present with **diarrhoea,** the excessive mucous secretion can cause fluid, protein and electrolyte loss (most notably potassium). Polyps may **intussuscept** causing vague abdominal pain or acute obstruction; it is thought that this process may cause the formation of the stalk in pedunculated polyps.

At physical examination one should look particularly for oral pigmentation and skin lesions (to detect the Peutz-Jeghers syndrome) and sigmoidoscopy should be performed to look for polyps in the lower rectum. Small polyps may be covered with normal-looking mucosa, but larger ones are often dark and lobulated. Polyps can be sessile or pedunculated and covered with mucus; they may also bleed when touched. The macroscopic appearances of different types of polyp are seldom of diagnostic value. Biopsies can also be misleading as they are often unrepresentative [29]; they are rarely deep enough to include the stalk and muscularis mucosae, which must be assessed to detect invasion.

Investigation

Double-contrast barium enema

Double-contrast barium enema remains the corner-stone of colonic investigation and

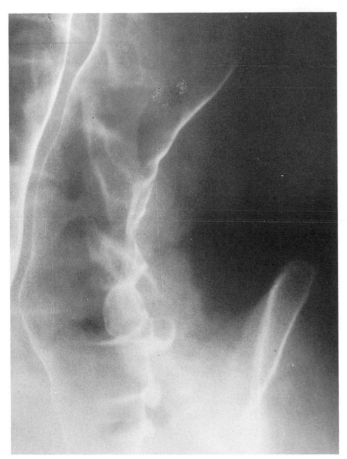

Fig. 63.5. Colonic polyp on a stalk demonstrated by double-contrast barium enema.

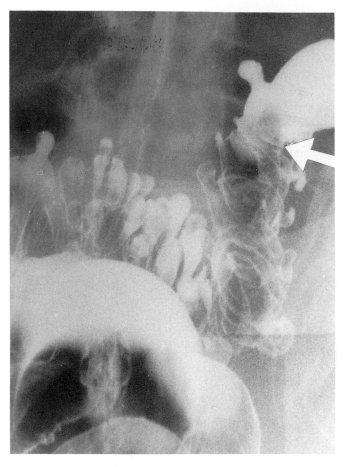

Fig. 63.6. Colonic polyp on a long stalk in the sigmoid colon in the presence of diverticular disease. Note straight line produced by stalk.

can accurately detect even very small polyps. The barium forms lines around the polyps 'like the patch on the inner surface of a bicycle tyre' with a meniscus where the polyp or stalk joins the mucosal wall (Fig. 63.5). When viewed *en face* this meniscus may appear as a target lesion. The straight line of a long stalk is a helpful sign (Fig. 63.6). Large polyps are often seen better during the filling phase of the examination (before air insufflation) (Fig. 63.7). In decubitus radiographs polyps frequently 'hang down', but small blobs of mucus may simulate polyps in this situation. A more difficult problem is to distinguish polyps from diverticula (Fig. 63.8) and only careful screening during the examination and detailed examination of the films will help. It

may be misleading to attribute bleeding to diverticula in this situation and the threshold for colonoscopy should be low [7, 28].

Colonoscopy

Although colonoscopy is more accurate than barium enema, for small lesions, it carries a definite risk of morbidity and mortality (Chapter 58). It is indicated in patients with even one unexplained episode of rectal bleeding; several studies having shown that important lesions can be found in 40% of such patients, even with a normal barium enema. In 10% the lesions will be cancer and in 15%, adenomatous polyps [28, 31].

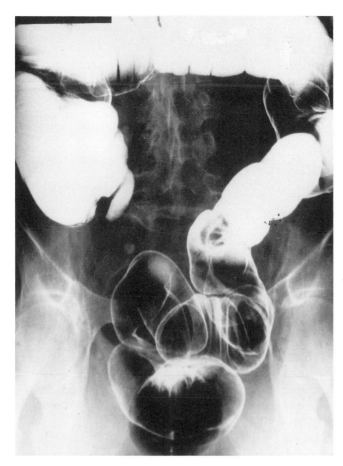

Fig. 63.7. Polyp in sigmoid colon shown as filling defect.

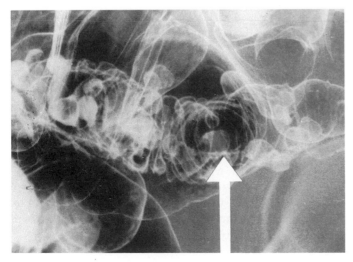

Fig. 63.8. Colonic polyp in sigmoid colon severely affected by diverticular disease.

Colonoscopic polypectomy

The aims of management are to establish a diagnosis, to treat symptoms and to remove malignant or potentially malignant lesions as safely and easily as possible. Colonoscopic polypectomy can achieve these aims for the majority of patients [27].

Technique

Colonoscopic examination of the whole colon is required to ensure that all polyps are detected. Careful attention must be paid to the 'blind areas' at the flexures and within the sigmoid colon. The polypectomist should be familiar with, and experienced at, colonoscopy, as briefly described in Chapter 58 [14, 34].

Once the polyps have been localized a decision needs to be made as to whether they should be removed. Polyps up to 4 cm in diameter on stalks or narrow bases (0.5–1.0 cm across) usually present no difficulty. A loop snare is inserted through the biopsy channel and advanced to the base of the polyp and opened (Fig. 63.9(a)). The loop is manoeuvred over the polyp and tightened, one-third to half-way along the stalk (that is closer to the polyp than the bowel wall) (Fig. 63.9(b)). If the stalk is short the loop should be tightened as close to the polyp as possible (Fig. 63.9(b)). The snare should be tightened until the apex of the polyp becomes cyanosed but not so as to cut through the stalk. Diathermy is then applied using a low setting to coagulate the stalk blood vessels before increasing the current to cut through the tissues. The current should be applied in short bursts (2–3 seconds) to avoid overheating the bowel wall; the operator must take care to avoid touching the bowel in other places to prevent 'contralateral burns' which can result in later perforation. Slight traction on the polyp may avoid this problem.

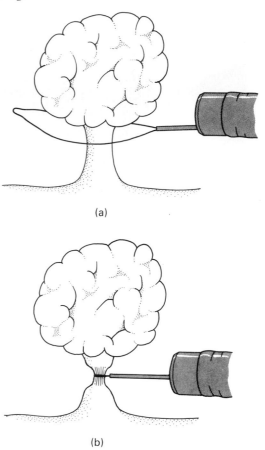

(a)

(b)

Fig. 63.9. Colonoscopic polypectomy. The snare loop is manoeuvred over the polyp head (a) and tightened around the stalk nearer to the polyp than the bowel wall (b).

Small polyps can be removed by the hot biopsy technique (Fig. 63.10 [33]) in which the current is applied through the metal cusps of a modified biopsy forceps. This preserves the biopsy while coagulating the tented base of the pulled up mucosa.

Large polyps (> 2–3 cm) may present problems and the colonoscopist will have to decide whether to remove them piecemeal (Fig. 63.11), perhaps at more than one session, or to refer the patient for surgical excision. The decision usually depends upon the experience of the operator [2, 21].

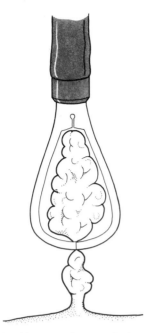

Fig. 63.10. 'Hot' biopsy technique. The biopsy is preserved within the more conductive metal cusps of the forceps. Current is concentrated at the 'tented' false stalk causing coagulation at this point only.

Risks of polypectomy

Colonoscopic polypectomy is potentially hazardous. It is important that the equipment is correct, in good repair and properly assembled, and that all safety precautions are followed. The bowel must be adequately prepared and clean, to reduce the risk of an accumulation of explosive gases within the lumen. Insufflation of CO_2, instead of air, should be used to further reduce the risk of an explosion [15].

Bleeding occurs after 1–2% of polypecto-mies; the risk is related to the width of the stalk [26]. Minor oozing will usually stop but may require irrigation with iced saline containing 5 ml 1:1,000 adrenaline per litre. More dramatic arterial bleeding may be stopped by re-snaring and coagulating the base if feasible, or by coagulating the base with a button coagulator or the snare tip.

Perforation is a rarer complication, related to excessive coagulation of the bowel wall. A 'closed' perforation can also occur which presents with fever and local tenderness without free peritoneal gas. This usually resolves with conservative management, bed rest and antibiotics.

Broad-based polyps

These polyps require surgical removal. The colonoscopist can assist the surgeon by identifying the site of such lesions at the time of operation, or by the injection of sterile indian ink into the polyp base for its subsequent identification. Rectal villous adenomas are usually removed by submucosal dissection (rather than rectal excision) unless there is evidence of malignant change.

Subsequent management

This depends on the histological features of the polyp. It is important to retrieve all excised polyps, even if this means repeated insertion of the colonoscope. Small metaplastic polyps require no further action.

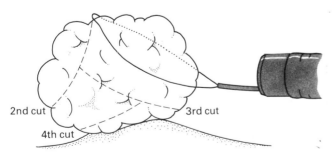

2nd cut
3rd cut
4th cut

Fig. 63.11. Large sessile polyps may be removed 'piece-meal'.

The management of adenomatous polyps depends on the degree of any dysplasia present and whether there is malignant infiltration of the base:

1. **No dysplasia**—repeat colonoscopy in one year to remove any further polyps and if clear repeat every 3–5 years.

2. **Carcinomatous infiltration** into submucosa requires a decision on whether to proceed to colectomy or to observe. This decision depends upon whether the line of resection is clear, and also upon the degree of differentiation of the cancer. Even if the resection line is involved, the wall of the bowel may be clear and a management policy needs to be drawn up in consultation between the clinician, polypectomist and pathologist. Careful follow-up colonoscopy is often appropriate.

Patients with adenomatous polyps require life-long follow-up to prevent the development of further polyps and invasive cancer. The work-load and economic implications of such a policy are daunting. The burden will be a large and continually expanding one.

Familial polyposis coli

The tendency towards colonic malignancy in this condition is well-recognized [1]. It is a genetic disorder with an autosomal dominant pattern of inheritance. Patients presenting with symptoms have a 60–70% chance of already having an established carcinoma while this risk is only 15% in asymptomatic family members.

The only way to avoid cancer of the colon is to remove the large intestine of all affected members of the family. Isolated cases, without a family history, do occur presumably because of a genetic mutation. The children of such patients are at risk to the same degree as those with a strong family history.

In this condition the colon is studded with adenomatous polyps. There are always more than 100 and often many thousands. The polyps vary in size, but most are under 1 cm, and are distributed throughout the colon and rectum. Adenomas may also occur in the stomach, duodenum, and ileum [17]; therefore the upper gastrointestinal tract should be examined.

The average age for the onset of symptoms is 25 years, but polyps can develop in children as young as 4 months or in adults as old as 74 years. Colonoscopic screening of family members usually starts in the early teens (as the risk of a carcinoma is low before this age), but should be continued, by sigmoidoscopic screening, every two years for life. This is because 50% of patients only develop their polyps when over 35 years of age, and in 10% they first appear when the patients are over 50 years old.

Treatment of polyposis coli

This is by total colectomy with (in the United Kingdom) an ileorectal anastomosis. These patients require regular follow-up at annual intervals with repeated sigmoidoscopy and fulguration of any polyps that appear in the rectum. The risk of developing a carcinoma in the rectal stump is approximately 10–15% over 25 years. Because of this some authorities recommend a total proctocolectomy with ileostomy [18] or, more recently, mucosal proctectomy and ileo-anal anastomosis [35]. This should certainly be recommended to any patient who cannot, or is unwilling to, attend for regular review after colectomy.

Gardner's syndrome

This is a familial condition in which adenomatous polyposis of the colon is associated with osteomas, multiple epidermoid cysts and soft-tissue tumours of the skin [8]. There is a familial variation in expression of this syndrome but all show, in addition to an increased incidence of carcinomas of the colon, an increase in other tumours (including tumours of the ampulla of Vater, small intestine, thyroid and adrenal glands). Other lesions include lipomas, fibromas, fibrosarcomas, leiomyomas, desmoid tumours and malignant tumours of the central nervous system.

Cronkhite-Canada syndrome

The Cronkhite-Canada syndrome [3] is a condition where multiple hypertrophic mucosal polyps of the colon and intestinal tract are found in association with alopecia, pigmentation, nail atrophy and watery diarrhoea. The polyps are adenomatous in type and there is an increased risk of malignancy.

Screening programmes for polyps

It has been suggested that if all colonic polyps were removed the mortality from carcinoma of the colon and rectum would fall significantly [9]. Screening programmes designed to test this hypothesis are currently being studied [6, 10, 12, 36]. They are based on the detection of occult bleeding from the intestine and routine sigmoidoscopy/colonoscopy of large populations. At present the cost effectiveness, and patient's acceptability of these programmes, have not justified their widespread introduction. However, screening programmes of those patients 'at risk' are fully justified, although the manpower and economic implications of even such a restricted programme are enormous.

References

1 BUSSEY HJR. Gastrointestinal polyposis. *Gut* 1970;**11**:970–978.
2 CHRISTIE JP. Malignant colon polyps—cure by colonoscopy or colectomy? *Am J Gastroenterol* 1984;**79**:543–547.
3 CRONKHITE LW, CANADA WJ. Generalised gastrointestinal polyposis: an unusual syndrome of polyposis, pigmentation, alopecia and onychotrophia. *N Engl J Med* 1955;**52**:1011–1012.
4 DAY DW, MORSON BC. The polyp problem. In: Hunt RH, Waye J, eds. *Colonoscopy, Techniques Clinical Practice and Colour Atlas.* London: Chapman & Hall, 1981:301–326.
5 EIDE TJ, STALSBERG H. Polyps of the large intestine in northern Norway cancer. *Cancer* 1978;**42**: 2839–2848.
6 FARRANDS PA, GRIFFITHS RL, BRITTON DC. The Frome experiment—value of screening for colorectal cancer. *Lancet* 1981; i:1231–1232.
7 FARRANDS PA. VELLACOTT JD, AMAR SS, BALFOUR TW, HARDCASTLE JD. Flexible fibre optic sigmoidoscopy and double-contrast barium enema examination in the identification of adenomas and carcinomas of the colon. *Dis Colon Rectum* 1983;**26**:725–727.
8 GARDNER EJ, RICHARDS R. Multiple cutaneous and subcutaneous lesions occurring simultaneously with hereditary polyposis and osteomatosis. *Am J Hum Genet* 1953;**5**:139–147.
9 GILBERTSEN VA. Proctosigmoidoscopy & polypectomy in reducing the incidence of rectal cancer. *Cancer* 1974;**34**:936–939.
10 GILBERTSEN VA, McHUGH R, SCHUMAN L, WILLIAMS SE. The earlier detection of colorectal cancers. *Cancer* 1980;**45**:2899–2901.
11 GILLESPIE PE, CHAMBERS TJ, CHAN KW, DORONZO F, MORSON BC, WILLIAMS CB. Colonic adenomas—a colonoscopic survey. *Gut* 1979;**20**:240–245.
12 HARDCASTLE JD, BALFOUR TW, AMAR SS. Screening for symptomless colorectal cancer by testing for occult blood in general practice. *Lancet* 1980;i:791–793.
13 HOFF G, VATN M. Epidemiology of polyps in the rectum and sigmoid colon. Endoscopic evaluation of size and localization of polyps. *Scand J Gastroenterol* 1985;**20**:356–360.
14 HUNT RH, WAYE J, eds. *Colonoscopy: Techniques, Clinical Practice and Colour Atlas.* London: Chapman Hall, 1981.
15 HUSSEIN AMJ, BARTRAM CI, WILLIAMS CB. Carbon dioxide insufflation for more comfortable colonoscopy. *Gastrointest Endosc* 1984;**30**:68–70.
16 HUSSEIN AMT, MEDANY S, ABOU EL MAGD AM, SHERIF SM, WILLIAMS CB. Multiple endoscopic polypectomies for schistosomal polyposis of the colon. *Lancet* 1983;i:673–674.
17 JÄRVINEN H, NYBERG M, PELLTOKALLIO P. Upper gastrointestinal tract polyps in familial adenomatosis coli. *Gut* 1983;**4**:333–339.
18 MOERTEL CG, HILL JR, ADSON MA. Surgical management of multiple polyposis. *Arch Surg* 1970;**100**:521–526.
19 MORSON BC, DAWSON IMP. *Gastrointestinal Pathology.* 2nd ed. Oxford: Blackwell Scientific Publications, 1979.

20 MORSON BC, PANG LSC. Rectal biopsy as an aid to cancer control in ulcerative colitis. *Gut* 1967;8:423–434.

21 MORSON BC, WHITEWAY JE, JONES EA, MACRAE FA, WILLIAMS CB. Histopathology and prognosis of malignant colorectal polyps treated by endoscopic polyrectomy. *Gut* 1984;25:427–444.

22 MUTO T, BUSSEY HJR, MORSON BC. Pseudocarcinomatous invasion of ademonatous polyps of the colon and rectum. *J Clin Path* 1973;26:25–31.

23 MUTO T, BUSSEY HJR, MORSON BC. The evolution of cancer of the colon and rectum. *Cancer* 1975;36:2251–2270.

24 REID JD. Duodenal carcinoma in the Peutz Jeghers syndrome. *Cancer* 1965;18:970–977.

25 RICKERT RR, ANERBACH O, GARFINKEL L, HAMMOND EC, FRASCA JM. Adenomatous polyps of the large bowel; an autopsy study. *Cancer* 1979;43:1847–1857.

26 ROGERS BHG. Complications and hazards of colonoscopy. In Hunt RH, Waye J, eds. *Colonoscopy, techniques, clinical practice and colour atlas.* London: Chapman Hall, 1981.

27 ROGERS BHG, SILVIS SE, NEBEL OT, SUGAWA C, MANDELSTAN P. Complications of fibreoptic colonoscopy and polypectomy. *Gastrointest Endosc* 1975;22:73–75

28 SWARBRICK ET, HUNT RH, FEVRE DI, WILLIAMS CB. Colonoscopy for unexplained rectal bleeding. *Gut* 1976;17:823.

29 TAYLOR EW, THOMPSON H, OATES GD, DORRICOTT NJ, ALEXANDER-WILLIAMS J, KEIGHLEY MRB. Limitations of biopsy in preoperative assessment of villous papilloma. *Dis Colon Rectun* 1981;24:259–262.

30 TEAGUE RH, REID AE. Polyposis in ulcerative colitis. *Gut* 1975;16:792–795.

31 TEDESCO FL, WAYE JD, RASIN JB, MORRIS SJ, GREENWALD RA. Colonoscopic evaluation of rectal bleeding—a study of 304 patients. *Ann Intern Medicine* 1978;89(6):907–909.

32 WEBB WA, McDANIEL L, JONES L. Experience with 1000 colonoscopic polypectomies. *Ann Surg* 1985;201:626–632.

33 WILLIAMS CB. Diathermy-biopsy—a technique for the endoscopic management of small polyps. *Endoscopy* 1973;5:215–218.

34 WILLIAMS CB, COTTON PB. *Practical Gastrointestinal Endoscopy.* 2nd ed. Oxford: Blackwell Scientific Publications, 1982.

35 WILLIAMS NS, JOHNSTON D. The current status of mucosal proctectomy and ileo-anal anastomosis in the surgical treatment of ulcerative colitis and adenomatous polyposis. *Br J Surg* 1985;72:159–168.

36 WINAWAR SJ, ANDREWS M, FLEHINGER B, *et al.* Progress report on controlled trial of fecal occult blood testing for the detection of colorectal neoplasia. *Cancer* 1980;45:2959–2964.

Chapter 64
Clinical Features of Colorectal Cancer

L. P. FIELDING & L. BLESOVSKY

Epidemiology

Over the last 15 years numerous articles have suggested that environmental factors are responsible for the variability in the incidence of colorectal cancer between different communities (Fig. 64.1). In the Western world only bronchial carcinomas are more common. In the United Kingdom there are

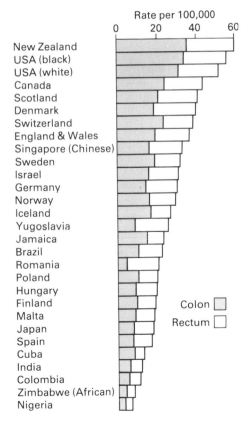

Rate per 100,000

New Zealand
USA (black)
USA (white)
Canada
Scotland
Denmark
Switzerland
England & Wales
Singapore (Chinese)
Sweden
Israel
Germany
Norway
Iceland
Yugoslavia
Jamaica
Brazil
Romania
Poland
Hungary
Finland
Malta
Japan
Spain
Cuba
India
Colombia
Zimbabwe (African)
Nigeria

Colon □
Rectum □

Fig. 64.1. Incidence of colorectal cancer—age-standardized rates per 100,000 males aged 35–64 in 1968–1972 (adapted with permission from [34]).

around 17,000 deaths from colorectal cancer per year—38/100,000 population [39].

Sub-site distribution

While there are variations in the absolute incidence of colorectal cancer within a given population, the relative incidence at different sites is quite stable (Fig. 64.2). There are relatively more sigmoid than right colon tumours in high- versus low-risk populations [13].

Sex incidence

Men are more likely to be affected than women (1.3:1 for colon and 1.5:1 for rectum) although not all reports demonstrate this difference [34]. Women tend to be younger (55.1 years) than men (58.6 years) at diagnosis [20].

In addition women have a better prognosis than men, even after correction for their earlier age at diagnosis [56]. This improved survival appears to depend on whether the woman has had children, nulliparous women behaving like men [56].

Effect of migration

Most studies have shown a rise in incidence when people move from a low- to a high-incidence area—for example Poles who moved to the United States or Australia [98], or far Eastern migrants to Britain [34]. There is also some evidence to suggest that the reverse happens when people move from a high- to a low-incidence area (Fig. 64.3).

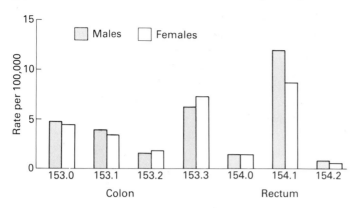

Fig. 64.2. Incidence of colorectal cancer by subsite from Standardized Mortality Cancer Rates—age-standardized rates per 100,000 population aged 35–64 in 1967–1971 (adapted with permission from [34]).

These observations are of considerable interest, the rapid change occurring in migrant populations suggesting that environmental factors are very important in this cancer. While little can be done about genetic or hormonal factors in tumour induction, it may be possible to delay or prevent the occurrence of this disease by identifying the environmental agents.

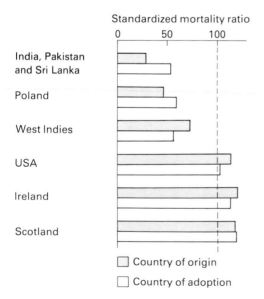

Fig. 64.3. Mortality from colon cancer among male immigrants in England and Wales in 1970–1972 (adapted with permission from [34]).

Aetiology

Genetics

There are two types of inherited polyposis—neoplastic and hamartomatous (see Chapter 63). While the latter (juvenile and Peutz-Jeghers polyposis) have a proven genetic basis, malignancy is uncommon, although greater than in the general population. By contrast, untreated familial polyposis has an exceptionally high incidence of invasive carcinoma [10].

Familial adenomatosis coli

This condition can be divided into 'dense' or 'coarse' types, depending on whether there are more or less than 5,000 polyps present. It affects 1 in 10,000 of the population. Its inheritance pattern is that of an autosomal dominant gene with an 80–94% penetrance [9, 92, 110]—that is nine out of 10 children will be affected.

Three subtypes are described depending on the occurrence and nature of extra-colonic manifestations. These are **familial polyposis coli**; **Gardner's syndrome**—associated with multiple sebaceous and dermoid cysts, bony exostoses and soft tissue tumours (Chapter 63); and **Turcot's syndrome**—associated with malignant central nervous system tumours.

Other extracolonic manifestations

include gastric polyps [108, 109]; duodenal adenomas [112]; and jejunal adenomas [82].

Cancer family syndrome

There are a few families with an unusually high incidence of cancers at different sites—principally colon and endometrium. These tumours develop at a relatively young age with a high incidence of multiple primaries and proximal colonic tumours.

In addition it is important to recognize that the incidence of large bowel cancers, in first degree relatives of those with sporadic colonic tumours, is higher than in the general population. These individuals, therefore, constitute a high risk group for screening programmes [67].

Environmental factors [102]

It is tempting to use the different patterns of dietary intake to explain observed differences in the incidence of colorectal cancer in different communities [8, 23]. The acceptability of this dietary theory is enhanced by the fact that some Clostridial bacteria can produce carcinogenic-like compounds (sterols) from food substances. Bran, and allied substances, have been shown to affect the binding of bile acids and the generation of mutagenic compounds, thus enhancing the dietary theory.

However, there remain diametrically opposed views on the acceptability of this theory [99, 105]. Stemmermann concludes that 'the available evidence does not support a strong role for bowel transit, amount of dietary fat, or intestinal bile salt profile or neutral sterols in human colorectal carcinogenesis'. Thompson, on the other hand, states that 'there is a positive correlation between the incidence of colon cancer and the consumption of fat and animal protein and an inverse relationship with dietary fibre. There is a further positive correlation

with faecal bowel acid concentration and the carriage of bacteria able to degrade bile acids to carcinogenic-like precursors.'

There is no simple explanation for these polarized views, which probably reflect different methods of epidemiological survey and differing statistical analyses.

Pre-existing diseases

Ulcerative colitis

Ulcerative colitis is associated with a 5- to 17-fold increase in the incidence of colorectal cancer over a normal population [44, 69]. The risk increases if the disease starts before 25 years of age or as total colitis, and if symptoms become chronic after the first attack [53]. The tumours are often flat and multiple. They are more often anaplastic than sporadic colonic cancers and are advanced at presentation [59]. The prognosis is comparable for similar histological and Dukes stage tumours [81], but the late presentation and greater anaplasia often results in a worse outcome.

For these reasons there has been anxiety about leaving the diseased colon *in situ* after 10 years. This 10 year figure is arbitrary and based upon the rapid rise in incidence after this time found in retrospective studies [2, 11, 16, 69].

Over the past two decades there has been increased interest in the relationship between epithelial dysplasia in rectal and colonic biopsies and cancer [54, 61, 76, 83, 94]. In the Lennard-Jones study no patient, out of 303 patients with extensive ulcerative colitis, developed a cancer within 10 years of the onset of their disease—the risk of cancer being calculated as 1 in 90 patient years. Mucosal dysplasia was classified by subjective criteria into mild, moderate and severe [76]. The incidence of carcinoma was found to be—1/22 (5%) for 'mild', 4/27 (14%) for 'moderate' and 5/17

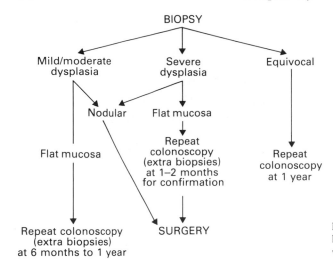

Fig. 64.4. Suggested policy when biopsy reveals dysplasia (adapted with permission from [61]).

(30%) for 'severe' dysplasia. In all groups there were a significant number of patients, who did not undergo surgery, in whom later biopsies showed no dysplasia. This led the authors to recommend a 'flow diagram' policy as outlined in Fig. 64.4.

Out of 175 patients, still attending their clinic in 1980, 119 were still receiving medical treatment, 37 had undergone operation for control of their disease, 19 had undergone resection for moderate or severe dysplasia—in 11 of these an early cancer (Dukes' A or B) was found. Only two had 'failed' the protocol and were found to have advanced tumours at the time of surgery. This low failure rate must be weighed against the known morbidity and mortality rate of elective resection for ulcerative colitis (see Chapter 51).

Although ileorectal anastomosis is a successful operation for ulcerative colitis, the malignant potential remains in the retained rectum [1, 4, 42, 43]. The risks of malignancy with the various 'pouch' procedures, being advocated at present, remains to be determined [86].

Crohn's colitis

It was once thought that Crohn's disease was immune from the risk of colorectal cancer, but over the last 10 years it has been established that cancer does occur although the risk is probably lower than in ulcerative colitis [46, 62, 113].

Barrett's oesophagus

In a review of 65 patients with Barrett's oesophagus it was found that 29 (45%) had colonic tumours—19 benign and 10 malignant [97]. The reason for this association is unknown.

Hormones

Women with endometrial tumours have a two-fold increase in colonic cancers. This suggests a common aetiological factor. Both exogenous oestrogens and low parity are known to be associated with endometrial carcinoma. This led Weiss, Daling and Chow [114] to study hormonal factors in colorectal malignancy. They found that women with one or two children had a 30% reduction, and those with three or more a 50% reduction in the incidence of colonic cancer, when compared with nulliparous controls. No association was found for rectal cancer.

Colonic mucus

Considerable interest in the chemical nature, structure and function of gastrointestinal mucus has occurred during the last 15 years [33]. It has been shown that the mucins in the cells of an adenocarcinoma, and in the transitional cells in its neighbourhood, are abnormal. Histochemical staining demonstrates an increase in sialomucins relative to sulphomucins [29, 31, 58, 65] a change that also occurs in experimentally-induced (dimethylhydrazine) colonic carcinoma [30]. In addition changes were observed in the structure and function of the colonic mucus layer on scanning electronmicroscopy [106]. Similar changes have been observed in human colorectal cancer and colonic polyps.

Immunology

Patients with malignant disease display evidence of depressed immunological competence which is often related to the stage of the disease and the risk of recurrence [25]. A relationship between the absolute lymphocyte count and survival has been demonstrated [111], a low count being associated with a poor overall survival. There is accumulating evidence for an association between advancing stage of the disease and immunodeficiency, although colorectal cancer has also been shown to be associated with immunodeficiency at all stages of the disease [6].

An additional important facet to this is the effect of various therapies upon immunocompetence. Many of these produce immunosuppression, including surgery [7], radiotherapy [100], and chemotherapy [48]. Thus it becomes rational to consider immunotherapy as an attempt to overcome both the immunodepressive effect of treatment and that of the tumour.

Pathology

Adenocarcinoma of the colon is potentially an invasive and metastasizing tumour arising from secretory cells within the acinus of the large bowel mucosa.

Cytological features

Proliferative abnormalities in colonic epithelial cells [63]

A modified epithelial cell proliferative activity is an early abnormal characteristic of the colonic epithelial cells of individuals with a genetic predisposition to colorectal cancer. During progressive stages of abnormal development, the epithelial cells gain an increased ability to proliferate and accumulate in the mucosa. In the normal colon, these cells proliferate in the lower and mid-regions of the colonic crypts (Fig. 64.5) and then migrate to the surface of the mucosa to be extruded. Studies in healthy humans have shown that the colonic mucosa is replaced by new cells every 4–8 days.

Cellular dysplasia

The hallmark of increased malignant risk is cellular dysplasia (cellular atypia) which is characterized by pathological features common to malignant degeneration in all epithelial surfaces. As dysplasia increases there is a greater variation in nuclear size, shape, depth of staining and a decrease in mucin content. Mitotic figures increase in frequency and may be abnormal. There is a progressive loss of cell polarity, the nuclei lose their normal uniform basal position and the glands become irregular and poorly formed, with intraglandular bridging [104]. These changes may be graded as mild,

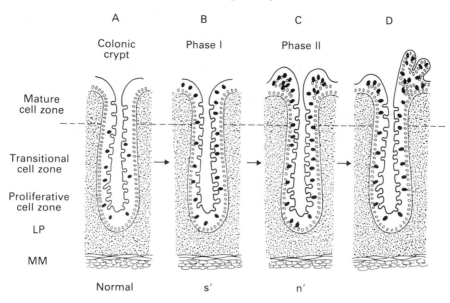

A   B   C   D

Colonic crypt   Phase I   Phase II

Mature cell zone

Transitional cell zone

Proliferative cell zone

LP

MM

Normal   s′   n′

Fig. 64.5. A sequence of events to account for the location of abnormally proliferating colonic epithelial cells before and during the formation of polypoid neoplasms in man. (A) shows location of proliferating and differentiating epithelial cells in normal colonic crypt. Dark cells illustrate thymidine labelling in cells that are synthesizing DNA and preparing to undergo cell division. As cells pass from proliferative zone through the transitional zone, DNA synthesis and mitosis are repressed, and migrating epithelial cells leave the proliferative cell cycle to undergo normal maturation before they reach the surface of the mocosa. (B) shows the development of a Phase I proliferative lesion in colonic epithelial cells as they fail to repress the incorporation of thymidine ^{3}H into DNA (s′) and begin to develop an enhanced ability to proliferate. The mucosa is flat and the number of new cells born equals the number extruded without excess cell accumulation in the mucosa. (C) The development of a Phase 2 proliferative lesion in colonic epthelial cells. The cells incorporate thymidine ^{3}H into DNA and also have developed additional properties that enable them to accumulate in the mucosa as neoplasms begin to form (n′). (D) shows further differentiation of abnormally retained proliferating epithelial cells into pathologically defined neoplastic lesions including adenomatous polyps and villous papillomas (adapted with permission from [64]).

moderate or severe—the latter may resemble areas of infiltrating adenocarcinoma. However, if these changes remain localized above the muscularis mucosae it is a mistake to make a diagnosis of malignancy, which should be made only if dysplastic epithelium is seen invading through this layer.

Adenoma-carcinoma sequence

There is considerable evidence which supports the concept that adenocarcinomas of the colon arise from pre-existing epithelial adenomas—the 'adenoma-carcinoma sequence' [74].

Clearly the majority of adenomas of the large bowel do not progress to carcinoma, but the risk increases with size. In one series polyps of less than 1 cm in diameter had a malignancy rate of 1.3%; those of 1–2 cm a rate of 9.5%; and those over 2 cm a 46% malignancy rate—most of the polyps were < 1 cm (60%) while only 15–20% were over 2 cm in diameter [78]. The malignant potential was further increased by the histological type (tubular with a 5% risk; tubulo-villous with a 22% risk; and villous with a 40% risk) although size seemed to be of greater importance [74].

The histological differentiation of invasive tumours is now usually classified into four types [39]—well, moderately, and poorly differentiated, plus colloid types. These histological gradings correlate with the patient's prognosis, with the colloid type having a relatively poor outcome. There remains considerable confusion amongst pathologists about the features that distinguish well from moderately differentiated tumours and greater standardization is required [5].

Tumour spread

Carcinoma of the large bowel can spread in five ways—by direct tumour invasion of surrounding structures, by extramural lymphatics, by the blood stream, via the peritoneal cavity and by implantation on raw surfaces or suture lines in the bowel.

Once tumour cells have penetrated the muscularis mucosae, infiltration is usually outwards with little longitudinal spread. This feature is of importance because of the small lateral margin of resection that is achieved with a modern sphincter-saving operation. When lymph nodes become involved they are not necessarily along the most direct route between the tumour and the origin of the mesenteric vessel. Therefore a 'fan-shaped' mesenteric resection is advisable, if all local lymph node spread is to be removed. This is of particular importance in rectal tumours where all of the mesorectum should be removed if local recurrence is to be prevented.

Although most tumours spread radially in a progressive manner, lymph node and vascular spread can occur without full thickness invasion of the bowel wall. Indeed this type of skip process can lead to distant metastases (e.g. in the liver) without the local tumour being very advanced or there being overt nodal or venous invasion present. These disorderly types of tumour spread has significance for prognosis [13].

Although the liver is the commonest site for tumour metastases from carcinoma of the colon, secondary lesions can also be found in the lung, bone, adrenals, brain and other sites in 10% of patients at autopsy. Palpable liver metastases are found in 10–15% of patients at the time of operation and 'occult' impalpable liver metastases are probably present in a further 10–15%. Another route of spread is via the peritoneal cavity. This can produce peritoneal plaques of tumour, often causing obstruction.

Rare cases of direct tumour implantation into traumatized tissue have been described, but suture line recurrence is of greater practical importance. This was thought to be due to an inadequate tumour clearance, at the anastamotic site, but it is now clear that an inadequate clearance of the involved mesentery is a more likely explanation. Thus surgical/technical factors are important in the incidence of local recurrence, a factor confirmed by the finding that it is 'surgeon-related' [88].

Clinical features

The following data is based on 4,500 patients included in the Large Bowel Cancer Project (organized by the authors).

Age and sex distribution

The sex incidence was similar overall but varied at different sites (male incidence—right colon 45%, splenic flexure 47%, left colon 47%, rectum 60%).

Seventy-five per cent of tumours presented after 60 years of age with a peak incidence in the eighth decade. Right-sided lesions occurred more commonly in the very young or older age groups (Fig. 64.6).

Predisposing causes

Only 0.8% of the patients had a prior history of ulcerative colitis, and only 0.2% of Crohn's disease, suggesting that these

Chapter 64

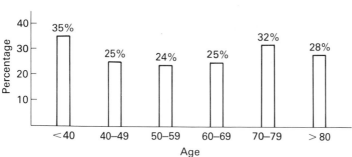

Fig. 64.6. Percentage of patients with 'right sided' colonic tumours.

diseases are only rarely responsible for carcinoma of the colon in the normal population.

Symptoms

It has been shown that the symptoms of large bowel cancer are variable [52]. Symptoms depend on the site of the lesion.

Elective presentation

Symptoms, other than weight loss and anorexia, vary with the site of the tumour. Right-sided lesions may present with occult anaemia, mild diarrhoea, vague abdominal pain, malaise or occasionally, a palpable mass, while left-sided lesions are said to present with a change in bowel habit with increasing constipation, spurious diarrhoea, blood and mucus *per rectum* and increased borborygmi. In distal lesions the symptoms of rectal bleeding, incomplete evacuation and tenesmus are prominent features. Rectal pain is rare unless perirectal invasion has occurred, rectovaginal or rectovesical fistulae suggest considerable local spread.

However, only 40% of patients with colorectal cancer present with these classical features [52].

Emergency presentation

Twenty-nine per cent of the patients in the authors' Large Bowel Cancer Project presented as an emergency—14.1% with obstruction, 2.5% with a perforation (0.8% with both) and 11.5% with a variety of other problems including severe anaemia, profuse blood loss, an abdominal mass, change in bowel habit, jaundice, pericolic abscess or any combination of these. The proportion of patients presenting as an emergency did not differ between University (30.5%) and District General Hospitals (32.3%) with the exception of St Mark's Hospital.

Bowel obstruction [89]

While it is generally thought that left-sided tumours are more likely to obstruct, the authors' studies show (Table 64.1) that it is the splenic flexure lesions that often present with an obstruction.

Table 64.1. Incidence of obstruction by site of tumour.

	Right colon	Splenic flexure	Left colon	Rectum
Total pts	1025	144	1614	1110
No obstruction (n)	806	82	1330	1087
Obstructed (n)	219	62	284	23
	21.4%	43.1%	17.7%	2.1%

Overall Figure—15.1% of 3,893 pts who underwent surgery

Table 64.2. The site and incidence of perforation of the colon in patients included in the Large Bowel Cancer Project ('suspected' includes patients with a pericolic abscess).

	Right colon	Splenic flexure	Left colon	Rectum
Total patients	1025	144	1614	1110
Definite Perforation	55 (5.4%)	12 (8.3%)	83 (5.1%)	13 (1.2%)
Suspected Perforation	58 (5.6%)	4 (2.8%)	88 (5.5%)	20 (1.8%)

Perforations can be classified into three principal types—firstly, a local perforation through the tumour, producing a pericolic abscess; secondly, an intraperitoneal perforation causing generalized peritonitis; and thirdly, a proximal perforation of the colon secondary to distal obstruction. In the Large Bowel Cancer Project 8.6% of 3,893 patients presented with a perforation; about half of these were free perforations into the peritoneal cavity either through the tumour, or proximal to it (Table 64.2).

Differential diagnosis

The variety of symptoms and modes of presentation result in a long list of differential diagnoses (Table 64.3). To aid their consideration the bowel is divided into two basic parts—the right side up to the splenic flexure, and the left side distal to this point.

The prelude to reaching a differential diagnosis is, of course, a careful history, physical examination and appropriate investigations. Sometimes the history indicates a specific diagnosis (for example, rectal bleeding, with a feeling of incomplete evacuation and a change in bowel habit, suggests a rectal carcinoma) but more often it provides only a vague hint of intra-abdominal disease.

The sequence of investigation should be determined by a knowledge of the relative incidence and age spectra of common diseases. For example in a 20-year-old patient, in the United Kingdom, nausea,

vomiting, abdominal pain and a right iliac fossa mass is more likely to be appendicitis, or Crohn's disease than carcinoma. It should also be remembered that 'common things occur commonly', and rare diagnoses should only be considered when these have been excluded.

Some of the common differential diagnoses are listed in Table 64.3. This is not an exhaustive list but it gives an indication of the extent of the problem. Occasionally, when the clinical problem is urgent (for example an obstruction or perforation), the diagnosis may only be made at the time of surgery, after initial resuscitation, when other investigations will only delay definitive treatment.

Prevention of colorectal carcinoma

The term prevention has different meanings at different stages of the disease.

Screening for asymptomatic neoplastic colonic disease [24]

The mainstay of such screening has been faecal occult blood testing [26, 47, 95, 96, 116], but barium enema [93] and fibreoptic sigmoidoscopy [115] have also been used [32].

In occult blood testing studies there is approximately a 1% yield of positive tests with around half such patients having adenomas or carcinomas in the large bowel on investigation. As would be hoped, there

Table 64.3. Differential diagnosis.

Major problem

Right-sided colonic cancer
Pain ± malaise ± anaemia
  Peptic ulcer
  Biliary disease
  Chronic pancreatitis
  Pancreatic cancer
  Crohn's disease
  Diverticular disease

Acute pain or mass
  Appendicitis ± abscess
  Cholecystitis ± empyema
  Perforated duodenal ulcer
  Perforated Crohn's
  Caecal diverticulitis
  Ovarian cyst/torsion/tumour
  Fibroid
  Tubal pregnancy
  Pelvic inflammatory disease

Obstruction
  Adhesions
  Intussception
  Caecal volvulus
  Crohn's disease
  Small bowel tumour

Left-sided lesions
Rectal bleeding
  Haemorrhoids
  Anal fissure
  Ulcerative colitis
  Crohn's colitis
  Ischaemic colitis
  Amoebiasis
  Endometriosis
  Angiodysplasia

Change of bowel habit or obstruction
  Diverticular disease
  Crohn's disease
  Ischaemic colitis
  Irradiation stricture
  Faecal impaction
  Sigmoid volulus
  Pseudo-obstruction

Mass
  Diverticular abscess
  Ovarian cyst/torsion/tumour
  Fibroid
  Crohn's disease

Fistula
  Crohn's disease
  Diverticular disease
  Previous surgery
  Carcinoma uterus/bladder
  Irradiation

is a greater preponderance of Dukes' A and B lesions among these patients than are found in those colons resected on account of symptoms. A scheme for such screening has been proposed by Winawar [116] (Fig. 64.7).

The removal of adenomas at colonoscopy offers the hope of breaking the adenoma-carcinoma sequence [38, 79]. Nevertheless, the cost of detecting such lesions is high, as the overall yield is low in the average population—but may be increased if screening is restricted to a high risk population.

It must be remembered that any mortality from resection of asymptomatic disease may have a profound effect on the overall risk-benefit ratio. Thus controlled studies are mandatory to identify a policy that will

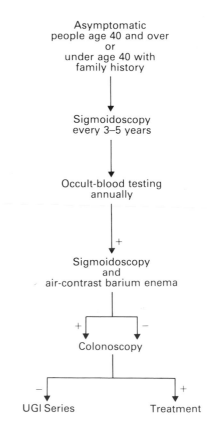

Fig. 64.7. Scheme for screening 'high risk' patients for colorectal cancer.

that will provide the greatest good for the largest number of patients.

Screening in high risk groups

Although occult blood testing seems the best candidate for population screening it needs to be supplemented by fibreoptic sigmoidoscopy and colonoscopy in the follow-up of high risk groups [67]. These include:
1. Ulcerative colitis—those with total disease for over seven years and left-sided disease for over 15 years (see Chapter 50).
2. Patients who have previously undergone treatment for colonic neoplasia (polyp or carcinoma—see Chapter 63).
3. Patients, and relatives, of those with a genetic predisposition to colonic tumour (multiple polyposis syndromes; cancer family syndrome; and Peutz-Jeghers syndrome—see Chapter 63).
4. Women who have had a genital tract or breast cancer.

In such a screening programme it is not only obvious tumours that are sought but also areas of mucosal dysplasia [12].

Prevention of diagnostic delay in symptomatic patients

Delayed diagnosis places an unnecessary burden upon patients who are symptomatic. Often a delay of three months or more is found. Part of this delay is due to the patients themselves, who are often reluctant to seek medical advice through fear or ignorance. The remainder is physician related [52]. However, despite the hope that early diagnosis would yield more patients with curable disease, this does not appear to be the case [52, 68, 90].

A subject that has received less attention is that the earlier diagnosis of symptomatic patients may reduce the proportion presenting as an emergency, thus lowering the overall mortality. It will require a large study to confirm or refute this hypothesis.

Prevention of metastatic disease

Operative technique

There seems to be little doubt that the basic tenets of good cancer surgery are being taught and practised less than in the past, notably *en bloc* resection. Every effort should be made not to breach the tumour surface during the dissection and to remove any organ attached to the tumour *without developing a plane between them*. The patient's long-term survival will depend considerably upon the surgeon's ability to prevent later intra-abdominal recurrence [28, 91].

Turnbull and his colleagues at the Cleveland Clinic [107] described the no-touch isolation technique and suggested that this improved the survival of patients with Dukes' C lesions. They attributed this to entrapment of circulating tumour cells within the specimen, thereby reducing the number of liver metastases. Although this concept is attractive, there are no objective data to support it. In fact it would require a very large trial to test this hypothesis, as it could only influence the results in Dukes' B and C tumours. As there is no increased morbidity associated with this technique, it is recommended as the standard method whenever possible.

Adjuvant chemotherapy

Conventional systemic agents (Chapter 65)

There have been a number of major randomized trials of adjuvant chemotherapy for colorectal cancer [14, 22, 45, 49, 60] but none has shown a significant increase in survival of the treated group. In each study the treated patients fared slightly better than the controls, so a small advantage for the treated group may have been missed through a type II statistical error [35].

The routine use of adjuvant chemotherapy cannot be recommended at present.

Intraportal 5-Fluorouracil (FU) and heparin

Based on evidence that malignant cells can be found in the blood at the time of surgery, a prospective randomized study of intraportal infusion of 5-FU and heparin, in patients undergoing curative resection for carcinoma of the colon, was undertaken [103]. Initial results were encouraging, with a longer tumour-free interval and a reduction in mortality from liver metastases; whether this was due to the 5-FU or the heparin has yet to be determined.

Adjuvant irradiation

Colorectal tumours can respond to irradiation and a number of attempts to use this as an adjuvant treatment in rectal tumours have been made [77, 84]. However, it is likely that the doses used to date have been too low and further studies with higher doses are awaited with interest. A recent study has suggested that a combination of adjuvant irradiation and chemotherapy can reduce the onset of recurrence although survival is unchanged [36].

Removal of aetiological factors— public health issues

The epidemiological and experimental studies suggest that dietary factors (notably high fat/low fibre) are involved in the development of large bowel cancer and it is proposed that altering these dietary factors may prevent the disease [80]. Unfortunately the degree of change may be too drastic to be acceptable; however, there is evidence that the addition of small amounts of certain cancer inhibitors (retinoids, plant steroids and selenite) can reduce experimental cancer by 50% in rats. This suggests that modest changes in the fat/fibre content of the diet, with the addition of such inhibitors, might effectively reduce the incidence of colonic cancer.

Prognosis

The overall prognosis for patients with large bowel tumours has changed little over the last two decades [40]. The prognosis is influenced by a number of factors present at the time of presentation—age, extent of local tumour, histological grade, duration of symptoms, mode of presentation and whether it is possible to remove all tumour at the time of operation [13].

Extent of tumour spread (Fig. 64.8)

There have been many attempts to classify the extent of tumour spread. Probably the best-known is that of Dukes [17], which was originally developed for rectal tumours but later used for colonic tumours as well [36, 117]. All classification systems attempt to relate prognosis to local tumour spread and the presence or absence of lymph node metastases [3, 17, 18, 21, 55, 66, 96].

The systems of classification vary but all assume that there is an orderly progression of the disease from mucosa to local lymph nodes, and to widespread dissemination, and that this progression is directly related to outcome. Although this notion is generally true there are exceptions, for example 15% of tumours skip some of these stages. In addition there are other important factors which must be brought into the computation of prognosis for the individual patient. These include histological differentiation, venous tumour cell invasion, site, patient's age and sex, nature of presentation, and surgical technique [28, 107].

While some of these factors are interrelated, others act independently. Statistical techniques can be used to ascertain the degree of independence and dependence of these factors—in the Large Bowel Cancer Project there were 4,583 patients of whom 2,518 underwent curative resection [87]. Simple log-rank survival analysis revealed that the following factors influenced survi-

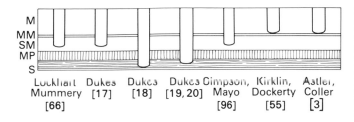

Fig. 64.8. Variation in degree of penetration of colorectal wall, classified as stage A, by different authors. M = mucosa; MM = muscularis mucosa; SM = submucosa; MP = muscularis propria (includes circular and longitudinal layers); S = serosa (adapted with permission from [117]).

Stage B

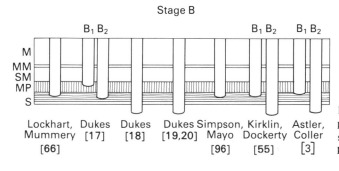

Fig. 64.9. Variation in degree of penetration of colorectal wall, classified as stage B, by different authors (adapted with permission from [117]).

Stage C

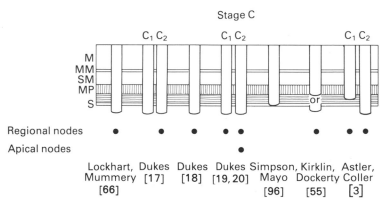

Fig. 64.10. Variation in degree of penetration of colorectal wall, classified as stage C, by different authors (adapted with permission from [117]).

val—depth of tumour penetration through the wall, tumour differentiation, presence or absence of vascular invasion, presence and pattern of lymph node involvement, and age. The five-year age-adjusted figures were:

1. In the absence of lymph node involvement—Dukes' A = 82%; Dukes' B = 65%.

2. Less than four lymph nodes involved = 62%; more than four lymph nodes involved = 21%.

3. Apical lymph node not involved = 46%; apical lymph node involved = 22%.

4. No vascular invasion = 71%; vascular invasion = 48%.

5. Well differentiated tumour = 62%; moderately differentiated = 60%; poorly differentiated = 42%.

Operative technique—anterior resection versus abdomino-perineal

The relative merits, from a prognostic point of view, of these two operative techniques for removal of a rectal tumour have never been tested in a controlled trial. Most studies comparing these two operations have included too few patients for any meaningful comparison of results to be undertaken (type II statistical error).

In the Large Bowel Cancer Project local tumour recurrence was greater after restorative surgery (anterior resection) than after abdomino-perineal resection in a 'similar mix of patients' (17% versus 11%) [88].

Tumour fixity

The tumour is fixed to an adjacent organ (small bowel, bladder, uterus, ovary, stomach, duodenum etc.) in around 10–12% of patients. Under these circumstances the need for *en bloc* resection becomes of paramount importance; failure to perform this will frequently result in local and intraperitoneal recurrence within 12–24 months [27].

Obstruction and perforation

These complications are rare in rectal tumours but account for over a quarter of all patients presenting with colonic tumours (obstruction = 20%; perforation = 7% [41, 57]). For those undergoing curative resection after an obstruction the prognosis is about half that for non-emergency cases (25% versus 50%). Five-year survival after perforation is very low (5–10).

Local treatment of rectal tumours

Small, mobile rectal tumours are the most suitable for irradiation, diathermy, cryotherapy or local excision [71, 72, 73, 85].

Electrocoagulation for advanced rectal lesions provides an overall five-year mortality which is no different to that after abdomino-perineal resection [70].

Group I (operable patients) 72/144 (69%) alive at five years versus 46–55% for abdomino-perineal resection.

Group II (inoperable disease) 14/41 (34%) alive at five years.

Group I + II = 58% alive at five years, compared with 52% after abdomino-perineal resection for all removable tumours.

Other factors

Sex

Women survive longer than men.

Age

While there is doubt as to whether the prognosis is worse if the tumour occurs at a young age, there is no doubt the operative mortality is adversely influenced by age and the general health of the patient.

Length of history

There is evidence that the prognosis is inversely related to the length of the history, except when presentation is as a perforation or obstruction.

Site of growth

Tumours arising at the splenic and hepatic flexures appear to fare worse than do those of other sites, possibly because they more often present as an obstruction, or as an emergency.

Acknowledgements

We wish to gratefully acknowledge the collaboration of the 93 surgeons and 21 pathologists in the Large Bowel Cancer

Project, our associated Research Fellows (Sarah Stewart-Brown, Rosemary Hittinger, Valerie Saunders) and Mrs Joanne Ciarcia, our secretary. We are indebted to the continuing encouragement and support from Professor H. A. F. Dudley, and for financial grants from Down Surgical Limited, the Jessie Williment bequest, the locally organized Research Scheme, North West Thames Regional Health Authority and the Cancer Research Campaign.

References

1 ADSON MA, COOPERMAN AM, FARROW GM. Ileorectostomy for ulcerative disease of the colon. *Arch Surg* 1972;**104**:424–428.

2 ALBRECHTSEN D, BERGAN A, NYGAART K, *et al.* Urgent surgery for ulcerative colitis: early colectomy in 132 patients. *World J Surg* 1981;**5**(4):607–615.

3 ASTLER VB, COLLIER FA. The prognostic significance of direct extension of carcinoma of the colon and rectum. *Ann Surg* 1954;**139**:846–851.

4 AYLETT SO. Ileorectal anastomosis: review. *Proc R Soc Med* 1971;**64**:967–977.

5 BLENKINSOPP K, FIELDING LP, STEWART-BROWN, *et al.* Histopathology reporting in large bowel cancer. *J Clin Path* 1981;**34**:509–513.

6 BOLTON PM, MANDER AM, DAVIDSON JM, *et al.* Cellular immunity in cancer: comparison of delayed hypersentivity skin tests in 3 common cancers. *Br Med J* 1975;**3**:18–20.

7 BOLTON PM, NUGENT M. Does surgery stimulate phagocytes? *Aus NZ J Surg* 1977;**47**:109.

8 BRISTOL JB, EMMETT PM, HEATON KW, WILLIAMSON RCN. Sugar, fat, and risk of colorectal cancer. *Brit Med J* 1985;**291**:1467–1470.

9 BUSSEY HJR. *Familial Polyposis Coli.* Baltimore: Johns Hopkins University Press, 1975.

10 BURTS RW, BISHOP T, CANNON LA, DOWDLE MA, LEE RG, SKOLNICK MH. Dominant inheritance of adenomatous colonic polyps and colorectal cancer. *N Engl J Med* 1985;**312**:1540–1544.

11 BUTT JH, LENNARD-JONES JE, RITCHIE JK. A practical approach to the risk of cancer in inflammatory bowel disease. *Med Clin North Am* 1980;**64**:1203–1220.

12 BUTT JH, KONISHI F, MORSON BC, *et al.* Microscopic lesions in dysplasia and carcinoma complicating ulcerative colitis. *Dig Dis Sci* 1983;**28**(1):18–26.

13 CHAPUIS PH, DENT OF, FISHER R, *et al.* A multivariate analysis of clinical and pathological variables in prognosis after resection of large bowel cancer. *Br J Surg* 1985;**72**:698–702.

14 CORBETT TH, GRISWOLD DP, ROBERTS DVM, *et al.* Evaluation of single agents and combinations of chemotherapeutic agents in mouse colon carcinomas. *Cancer* 1977;**40**:2660–2680.

15 CORREA P, HAENSZEL W. The epidemiology of large bowel cancer. *Cancer Res* 1978;**26**:1–141.

16 DEDOMBAL FT, WATTS JM, WATKINSON G, *et al.* Local complications of ulcerative colitis: stricture pseudopolyposis and carcinoma of the colon and rectum. *Br Med J* 1966;**1**:1442–1447.

17 DUKES CE. The classification of cancer of the rectum. *Br J Surg* 1929;**17**:643–648.

18 DUKES CE. The classification of cancer of the colon. *J Pathol* 1932;**35**:323–332.

19 DUKES CE. Histological grading of rectal cancer. *Proc R Soc Med* 1936;**30**:371.

20 DUKES CE. Cancer of the rectum: an analysis of 1,000 cases. *J Bact* 1940;**50**:527–539.

21 DUKES CE. The spread of rectal cancer and its effect on prognosis. *Br J Cancer* 1958;**12**:309–320.

22 DWIGHT RW, HUMPHREY EW, HIGGINS GA, *et al.* FUDR as an adjuvant to surgery in cancer of the large bowel. *J Surg Oncol* 1973;**5**:243–249.

23 EDITORIAL. Diet and colon cancer. *New Engl J Med* 1985;**313**:1413–1414.

24 EDITORIAL. Screening for colorectal cancer: the issues. *Gastroenterology* 1985;**88**:841–844.

25 EILBER FR, MORTON DL. Impaired immunological reactivity and recurrence following cancer surgery. *Cancer* 1970;**25**:362–367.

26 ELLIOT MS, LEVENSTEIN JH, WRIGHT JP. Faecal occult blood testing in the detection of colorectal cancer. *Br J Surg* 1984;**71**:785–786.

27 ENKER WE. Extent of operations for large bowel cancer. In: *Large Bowel Cancer.* Edinburgh: Churchill Livingstone, 1981:78–93.

28 ENKER WE, LAFFER UTH, BLOCK GE. Enhanced survival of patients with colon and rectal cancer based upon wide anatomic resection. *Ann Surg* 1979;**190**:350–360.

29 FILIPE MI. Value of histochemical reactions for muco-substances in the diagnosis of certain pathological conditions of the colon and rectum. *Gut* 1969;**10**:577–586.

30 FILIPE MI. Mucous secretion in rat colonic mucosa during carcinogenesis induced by dimethylhydrazine. *Br J Cancer* 1975;**32**:60–77.

31 FILIPE MI, BRANFORT AC. Abnormal patterns of muco-secretion in apparently normal mucosa of large intestine with carcinoma. *Cancer* 1974;**34**:282–290.

32 FLETCHER SW, DAUPHINEE WD. Should colorectal carcinoma be sought in periodic health examinations? An approach to the evidence. *Clin Invest Med* 1981;**4**(1):23–31.

33 FORSTNER G, WESLEY A, FORSTNER J. Clinical aspects of gastrointestinal mucus. *Adv Exp Med Biol* 1982;**144**:199–224.

34 FRASER P, ADELSTEIN AM. Colorectal cancer—re-

cent trends. Recent results *Cancer Res* 1982;**83**:1–10.

35 Freiman JA, Chalmers TC, Smith H Jr, *et al.* The importance of beta, the type II error and sample size in the design and interpretation of the randomized control trial. *N Engl J Med* 1978;**299**:690–694.

36 Gabriel WB, Dukes CE, Bussey HJ. Lymphatic spread in cancer of the rectum. *Br J Surg* 1935;**23**:395–413.

37 Gastrointestinal Tumor Study Group. Prolongation of the disease-free interval in surgically treated rectal carcinoma. *N Engl J Med* 1985;**312**:1465–1472.

38 Gilbertson UA, Nelms JM. The prevention of invasive cancer of the rectum. *Cancer* 1978;**41**:1137–1139.

39 Goligher JC. *Surgery of the Anus, Rectum, and Colon.* 4th ed. London: Bailliere Tindall, 1980:375.

40 Goligher JC. *Large Bowel Cancer.* London: Churchill Livingstone, 1981:154–165.

41 Goligher JC, Smiddy FG. The treatment of acute obstruction or perforation with carcinoma of the colon and rectum. *Br J Surg* 1959;**45**:270.

42 Griffen WO, Lillehei RC, Wangensteen OH. Ileoproctostomy in ulcerative colitis: long-term follow-up extending in early cases to more than 20 years. *Surgery* 1963;**53**:705–710.

43 Grundfest SF, Fazio V, Weiss RA, *et al.* The risk of cancer following colectomy and ileorectal anastomosis for extensive mucosal ulcerative colitis. *Ann Surg* 1981;**193**:9–14.

44 Gyde S, Prior P, Waterhouse J, *et al.* A new look at the cancer risk in ulcerative colitis. *Gut* 1981;**22**:A418–A419.

45 Hafstrom L, Domellof RL and the Swedish Gastroentestinal Tumour Adjuvant Therapy Group. A randomized trial of oral 5-fluorouracil versus placebo as adjuvant therapy in colorectal cancer Dukes' B and C: results after 5 years observation time. *Br J Surg* 1985;**72**:138–141.

46 Hamilton SR. Colorectal carcinoma in patients with Crohn's disease. *Gastroenterology* 1985;**89**:398–407.

47 Hardcastle JD, Balfour TW, Amar SS. Screening for symptomless colorectal cancer by testing for occult blood in general practice. *Lancet* 1980;**i**:791–793.

48 Harris J, Sengar T, Stewart T, *et al.* The effect of immunosuppressive chemotherapy on immune function in patients with malignant disease. *Cancer* 1976;**37**:1058.

49 Higgins GA, Humphrey E, Juler GL, *et al.* Adjuvant chemotherapy in the surgical treatment of large bowel cancer. *Cancer* 1976;**38**:1461–1467.

50 Holden WD, Dixon WJ, Kuzma JW. The use of triethylenethiophosphoramide as an adjuvant to the surgical treatment of colorectal carcinoma. *Ann Surg* 1967;**165**:481–503.

51 Jolly KD, Scott JP, MacKinnon MJ, *et al.* Diagnosis and survival in carcinoma of the large bowel. *Aust N Z J Surg* 1982;**52**(1):12–16.

52 Keddie N, Hargreaves A. Symptoms of carcinoma of the colon and rectum. *Lancet* 1968;**ii**:749–750.

53 Kewenter J, Ahlman H, Hulten L. Cancer risk in extensive ulcerative colitis. *Ann Surg* 1978;**188**:824–828.

54 Kewenter J, Hulten L, Ahren C. The occurrence of severe epithelial dysplasia and its bearing on treatment of long standing ulcerative colitis. *Ann Surg* 1982;**195**:209–213.

55 Kirklin JW, Dockerty MB, Waugh JM. The role of peritoneal reflection in the prognosis of carcinoma of the rectum and sigmoid colon. *Surg Gynecol Obstet* 1949;**88**:326–000.

56 Koch M, McPherson TA, Egedahl RD. Effect of sex and reproductive history on the survival of patients with colorectal cancer. *J Chron Dis* 1982;**35**(1):69–72.

57 Koruth NM, Hunter DC, Krukowski ZH, Matheson NA. Immediate resection in emergency large bowel surgery: a 7 year audit. *Br J Surg* 1985;**72**:703–707.

58 Lapertosa G, Fulcheri E, Pietra A. Histochemical study of mucin in the mucosa adjacent to colo-rectal carcinoma associated with solitary or multiple adenomatosis polyps. *Pathologica* 1981;**731025**:467–471.

59 Lavery IC, Chiulli RA, Jagelman D, *et al.* Survival in carcinoma arising in muscosal ulcerative colitis. *Ann Surg* 1982;**195**(4):598–612.

60 Lawrence W Jr, Terz JJ, Horsley S III. Chemotherapy as an adjuvant to surgery for colorectal cancer. *Arch Surg* 1978;**113**:164–168.

61 Lennard-Jones JE, Morson BC, Ritchie JK, *et al.* Cancer surveillance in ulcerative colitis: experience over fifteen years. *Lancet* 1983;**ii**:149–152.

62 Lightdale CJ, Sternberg SS, Posner G, *et al.* Carcinoma complicating Crohn's disease. *Am J Med* 1975;**59**(2):262–268.

63 Lipkin M. Phase 1 and phase 2 proliferation lesions of colonic epithelial cells in diseases leading to colon cancer. *Cancer* 1974;**34**:878–888.

64 Lipkin M. Early identification of population groups at high risk for gastrointestinal cancer. *Colon Carcinog* 1981;**12**:31–46.

65 Listinsky CM, Riddell RH. Patterns of mucin secretion in neoplastic and non-neoplastic diseases of the colon. *Hum Pathol* 1981;**12**(10):923–929.

66 Lockhart-Mummery JP. Cancer and heredity. *Lancet* 1925;**i**:427–429.

67 Lynch HT. Lynch PM. The cancer-family syndrome: a pragmatic basis for syndrome identification. *Dis Colon Rectum* 1979;**22**(2):106–110.

68 McDermott F, Hughes E, Pihe E, *et al.* Symptom duration and survival prospects in carcinoma of the rectum. *Surg Gynecol Obstet* 1981; 153(3):321–326.

69 McDougall IP. The cancer risk in ulcerative colitis. *Lancet* 1964;ii:655–658.

70 Madden J.L. Fulguration of malignant rectal tumors. In: Tard IP, Fielding LP, eds. *Operative Surgery.* Vol. 3. London: Butterworth 1983:404–407.

71 Madden JL, Kandalaft S. Electrocoagulation. A primary and preferred method of treatment for cancer of the rectum. *Ann Surg* 1967;166:413–419.

72 Madden JL, Kandalaft S. Clinical evaluation of electrocoagulation in the treatment of cancer of the rectum. *Am J Surg* 1971;122:347–352.

73 Mason AY. The spectrum of selective surgery. *Proc R Soc Med* 1976;69:237.

74 Morson BC. A polyp cancer sequence in the large bowel. *Proc R Soc Med* 1974;67:451.

75 Morson BC, Day DW. Pathology of adenoma and cancer of the large bowel. London: Churchill Livingstone, 1981.

76 Morson BC, Pang LSG. Rectal biopsy as an aid to cancer control in ulcerative colitis. *Gut* 1967;8:423–434.

77 MRC Working Party. A trial of preoperative radiotherapy in the management of operable rectal cancer. First report of an MRC Working Party. *Br J Surg* 1982;69:509–513.

78 Muto T, Bussey HJR, Morson BC. The evolution of cancer of the colon and rectum. *Cancer* 1975;36:2251–2351.

79 Nagy ND, Fevre DI. Colonic polypectomy, its role in cancer prevention. *Gastroentest Endosc* 1981;27(2):126–136.

80 Nigro ND. A strategy for prevention of cancer of the large bowel. *Dis Colon Rectum* 1982;25: 755–758.

81 Ohman U. Colorectal carcinoma in patients with ulcerative colitis. *Am J Surg* 1982;144(3): 344–349.

82 Ohsato K, Hiida M, Itoh H. Small intestine involvement in familial polyposis diagnosis by operative intestinal fibrescopy: reports of four cases. *Dis Colon Rectum* 1977;20(5):414–420.

83 Otto HF, Grebbers JO. The local immune response in ulcerative colitis. *Pathol Res Pract* 1979;165(4):349–364.

84 Pahlman L, Glimelius B, Graffman S. Pre- versus postoperative radiotherapy in rectal carcinoma: an interim report from a randomized multicentre trial. *Br J Surg* 1985;72:961–966.

85 Papillon J. Endocavitary irradiation in the curative treatment of early rectal cancers. *Dis Colon Rectum* 1974;17:172–180.

86 Parks AG, Nicholls RJ, Belliveau P. Proctocolectomy with ileoreservoir and anal anastamosis. *Br J Surg* 1980;67(8):533–538.

87 Phillips RKS, Hittinger R, Blesovsky L, *et al.* Large bowel cancer—surgical pathology and its relationship to survival. *Br J Surg* 1984; 71:604–610.

88 Phillips RKS, Hittinger R, Blesowsky L, *et al.* Local recurrence after curative surgery for large bowel cancer. *Br J Surg* 1984;71:12–16.

89 Phillips RKS, Hittinger R, Fry JS, Fielding LP. Malignant large bowel obstruction. *Br J Surg* 1985;72:296–302.

90 Polissar L, Sim D, Francis A. Survival of colorectal cancer patients in relation to duration of symptoms and other prognostic factors. *Dis Colon Rectum* 1981;24:364–369.

91 Polk H. Extended resection for selected adenocarcinomas for the large bowel. *Ann Surg* 1972;175:892–899.

92 Reed TE, Neel JV. A genetic study of multiple polyposis of the colon. *Am J Hum Genet* 1955;7:236–263.

93 Ribet A, Escourrow J, Frexinos J. *et al.* Screening for colorectal tumours—result of two year experience. *Cancer Detect Prev* 1980;3:449–461.

94 Riddell RH, Morson BC. Value of sigmoidoscopy and biopsy in detection of carcinoma and pre-malignant change in ulcerative colitis. *Gut* 1979;20:575–580.

95 Simon JB. Occult blood screening for colorectal carcinoma: a critical review. *Gastroenterology* 1985;88:820–837.

96 Simpson WC, Mayo CW. The mural penetration of the carcinoma cell in the colon: anatomic and clinical study. *Surg Gynecol Obstet* 1939;68: 872–877.

97 Sontag SJ, Chejfec G, Stanley MM. Barrett's oesophagus and colonic tumours. *Lancet* 1985;i:946–948.

98 Staszewski J, McCall MG, Stenhouse NS. Cancer mortality in 1962–1966 among migrants to Australia. *Br J Cancer* 1971;25:599–610.

99 Stemmermann GN, Nomura AMY, Mower H, *et al.* Clues (true or false) to the origin of colorectal cancer. In: DeCosse JJ, ed. *Clinical Surgery International.* Vol 1. London: Churchill Livingstone, 1981:1–15.

100 Stjernsward J, Jondal M, Vanky E, *et al.* Lymphopaenia and changes in distribution of human B and T lymphocytes in peripheral blood induced by irradiation for mammary carcinoma. *Lancet* 1972;i:1352.

101 Stuart M, Killingback MJ, Sakkes S, *et al.* Hemoccult II test, routine screening procedure for colorectal neoplasm? *Med J Aust* 1981;1(12): 629–631.

102 Stubbs RS. The aetiology of colorectal cancer. *Br J Surg* 1983;70:313–316.

103 Taylor I. Studies on the treatment and prevention of colorectal liver metastases. *Ann R Coll Surg Engl* 1981;63(4):270–276.

104 THOMPSON JPS, NICHOLS RJ, WILLIAMS CB. In: *Colorectal Disease*. New York: Appleton Century Crofts, 1981.

105 Thompson MJ. In: *Colonic Carcinogenesis*. Boston: MTP Press Ltd, 1982:49–58.

106 TRAYNOR OJ, WOOD CB, COSTA N. Ultrastructural alterations in the colonic mucous layer during carcinogenesis; a scanning electron microscopy study. *Adv Exp Med Biol* 1982;**144**:225–229.

107 TURNBULL RB JR, KYLE K, WATSON FR, *et al*. Cancer of the colon: the influence of the no-touch isolation technique on survival rates. *Ann Surg* 1967;**166**:420–427.

108 UTSUNOMIYA J, IWAMA I, HIRAYAMA R. Familial large bowel cancer. In: Large Bowel Cancer. London: Churchill Livingstone, 1981.

109 UTSUNOMIYA J, MAKI T, HAMAGUCHI A, *et al*. Gastric lesion of familial polyposis of the large intestine. *Cancer* 1974;**34**:745–754.

110 VEALE AMO. *Intestinal Polyposis*. London: Cambridge University Press, 1965.

111 WANEBO HJ, RAO B, ATTIYEH F, *et al*. Immune reactivity in patients with colorectal cancer: assessment of biologic risks by immuno-parameters. *Cancer* 1980;**45**:1254–1263.

112 WATANEBE H, ENJOJI M, YAO T *et al*. Gastric lesions in familial adenomatosis coli. *Fukuoka Acta Medica* 1977;**67(6)**:255–269.

113 WEEDON DD, SHORTER RG, ILSTRUP DM, *et al*. Crohn's disease and cancer. *N Engl J Med* 1973;**289**:1099–1103.

114 WEISS NS, DALING JR, CHOW WH. Incidence of cancer of the large bowel in women in relation to reproductive and hormonal factors. *Cancer Res* 1981;**67**:57–60.

115 WHERRY DC. Screening for colorectal neoplasia in asymptomatic patients using flexible fiberoptic sigmoidoscopy. *Dis Col Rectum* 1981;**24**:521–522.

116 WINAWAR SJ. Prevention screening and early diagnosis in large bowel cancer. In: De Cosse JJ, ed. *Clinical Surgery International*. London: Churchill Livingstone, 1981:46–62.

117 ZINKIN LD. A critical view of the classification and staging of colorectal cancer. *Dis Colon Rectum* 1983;**26**:37–43.

Chapter 65
Management of Colorectal Cancer

G. R. GILES

It is now over 160 years since Reybard, working in Lyon, carried out the first successful colonic resection. Since then the surgical techniques for colorectal cancer have been fully evaluated and have showed little change over the last 25 years. One of the recent developments has been that of sphincter preserving procedures for rectal cancer.

Although the incidence of colorectal cancer is rising, there is little evidence of any improvement in survival. The failure of surgery to significantly alter survival has led to two additional complementary approaches—attempts to diagnose the condition earlier (see Chapter 64) and to develop new methods of treatment.

Tumour spread and its surgical implications

While cancer of the large bowel can spread in a number of ways (Chapter 64) it has a tendency to spread more rapidly in the transverse than in the longitudinal axis, ultimately leading to obstruction of the lumen. The speed with which this occurs is obviously variable but Miles[45] suggested that, in rectal carcinomas, six months was required for the tumour to cover one quadrant and two years to completely encompass the bowel. Initially it was thought that longitudinal spread of colorectal cancer was very extensive; this led surgeons to resect long lengths of bowel. While this approach was easy for colonic tumours it could be very difficult in low rectal tumours; however recent studies have shown that rectal

cancer rarely spreads more than 15–20 mm distal to the lower edge of the tumour. Thus a distal surgical clearance of 5 cm is regarded by most surgeons as satisfactory although Eng [38] is happy to accept only a 3 cm clearance.

Lateral spread can result in infiltration of the serosa and pericolic or perirectal fat. The involvement of the serosa can lead to invasion of other organs, such as the small intestine or the abdominal wall, which may require an *en bloc* excision with the carcinoma for adequate local control. Rectal tumours can invade adjoining organs such as prostate, seminal vesicles, bladder, uterus, vaginal wall, and the lateral pelvic wall structures and lymphatics. Under these circumstances it may be impossible to carry out an adequate wide local excision and pre- or postoperative radiotherapy may be required as additional treatment.

Lymphatic involvement is usually dealt with by carefully isolating and removing the nodes that lie along the mesenteric vessels. While there is no evidence that a careful lymph node dissection affects the prognosis, it can help select those patients who require adjuvant treatment by providing better evidence on the Dukes' stage of the tumour.

The management of polyps

This problem is causing increasing concern as they are often found at fibreoptic colonoscopy (see Chapter 63). While many of these polyps are benign the potential for malignant transformation exists (see

Chapter 64). Although size and histological characteristics can predict the likelihood of malignancy in a polyp, it is good practice to remove every polyp.

What should be done if an excised polyp contains invasive cancer, that is invasion of the basement membrane and lamina propria? Pedunculated polyps, which have carcinoma *in situ* (where the lamina propria is intact), do not require further treatment. Sessile polyps present a greater problem, particularly if the *in situ* changes are at the margin of excision; under these circumstances it seems safer to recommend a colectomy rather than repeated colonoscopies, unless the patient is unfit for operation.

An additional problem arises when a pedunculated polyp contains invasive carcinoma as there may be local lymph invasion, or residual tumour within the base of the polyp. The question is whether colectomy is justified or not. There is no uniformity of opinion on this point. Polypectomy will suffice if the carcinoma is limited to the tip of the polyp, if it is well-differentiated, if there is no lymphatic invasion, and if the pedicle is not invaded [59].

Preoperative preparation for colon cancer surgery

This does not differ significantly from that required for any abdominal operation. In particular a chest X-ray, ECG, full blood count, urea and electrolytes, and liver function tests are all required. A raised alkaline phosphatase may provide suggestive evidence of hepatic metastases. Routine ultrasound, CT or scintiscanning of the liver, to detect metastases, cannot be recommended as the results are unlikely to affect any management decision. Such information is, however, clearly relevant to prognosis in clinical trials.

Intravenous urogram

It is advisable to perform a preoperative intravenous urogram if the carcinoma is situated where it might involve, or removal might threaten, a ureter. This should show whether the ureter is obstructed and whether the opposite kidney is functioning normally. However, it is not required routinely.

Mechanical bowel preparation [2]

There is no doubt that good mechanical cleansing of the colon is of considerable value. Traditionally this is achieved by placing the patient on a liquid or elemental diet for two to three days, followed by the administration of a cathartic (such as magnesium sulphate mixture 5 ml hourly, until diarrhoea occurs, and then 10 ml every four hours for 24 hours) and mechanical washouts with saline, or Veripaque enemas.

An alternative approach is the use of whole-gut irrigation [26]. In this technique a nasogastric tube is passed into the stomach and irrigating fluid (saline with added potassium and sodium bicarbonate at 37°C) is administered at 75 ml per minute. The patient is seated on a commode and within 45 minutes the bowel starts to empty and clear fluid is passed within a further 30 minutes. Usually the irrigation takes two to three hours and 10 to 13 litres of fluid is given. It does provide excellent bowel preparation, but two to three litres of fluid is absorbed, which can be a hazard to elderly patients with cardiac problems.

A modified technique involves the use of mannitol, which can be drunk or passed down a tube, followed by a free fluid intake. This also produces good cleansing but increases the amount of hydrogen in the colon, with an increased risk of an explosion during diathermy; it may also increase the risk of wound infection. An alternative effective method is the use of polyethylene glycol.

Adequate mechanical preparation may not be possible if there is a distal obstructive lesion.

Wound prophylaxis

Mechanical preparation does not remove bacteria from the colon. For this reason many surgeons used to give a non-absorbable antibiotic (for example pthalylsulphathiazole or neomycin) for a few days prior to operation. This approach has been questioned in recent years, as evidence has accumulated that it may increase the resistance of the bacteria in the colon without significantly reducing the risk of late septic complications.

There is now conclusive evidence that the prophylactic use of broad-spectrum antibiotics, *effective against both aerobic and anaerobic organisms*, can significantly reduce the risk of subsequent wound infection [57]. Those most commonly used are a combination of metronidazole and an aminoglycoside or cephalosporin [25]. The first dose should be given with the premedication, or at anaesthetic induction, to achieve an adequate tissue concentration during surgery—it has been shown that antibiotic prophylaxis is less effective if given during or after the operation. Treatment should probably be continued for at least 48 hours after surgery.

Radical excision of colorectal cancer

Radical colonic resection involves excision of the lymph nodes along the major colic vessels of supply. Thus for **carcinoma of the caecum, ascending, or transverse colon** it is necessary to ligate the major feeding artery close to its origin from the superior mesenteric artery. Inevitably this will devascularize a wider area of colon than is strictly necessary solely for the excision of intramural spread.

With **left-sided lesions** the artery of supply is ligated close to the inferior mesenteric artery, or its origin from the aorta If such a radical ligation is performed, the rectum will now only be supplied through the middle and inferior haemorrhoidal arteries; fortunately the rectum and lower sigmoid usually remain viable, allowing retention of up to 12 cm of colon above the peritoneal reflection. Such a radical left hemicolectomy is recommended in the younger patient, without signs of distant spread, to achieve the greatest chance of 'cure', but may not be advisable in elderly, unfit or obese patients as their blood supply may be less effective.

In **rectal carcinoma** the inferior mesenteric artery should be ligated at its origin, and the mesenteric vein at the left colic artery. the marginal artery of the colon is ligated in the mesentery at the junction tween the descending colic and first sigmoid branch of the inferior mesenteric artery (Fig. 65.1). This determines the level at which the bowel is transected for a subsequent end colostomy or an anterior resection anastomosis. For an anterior resection the rectum should, ideally, be divided at least 5 cm beyond the tumour, though a 3 cm margin may suffice with a small, well-differentiated carcinoma. The aim is to reduce the risk of anastomotic recurrence.

In most instances, however, anastomotic recurrence occurs because the tumour has extended into the surrounding pelvirectal tissues, and lateral clearance has been inadequate [54, 55]. Attempts to increase the radical nature of the clearance by deliberately dissecting the lymph nodes along the internal iliac arteries, *en bloc* with the lateral ligaments of the rectum, has not proved to be any more effective. Recurrence can more appropriately be dealt with by pre- or postoperative adjuvant radiotherapy, although a recent report on

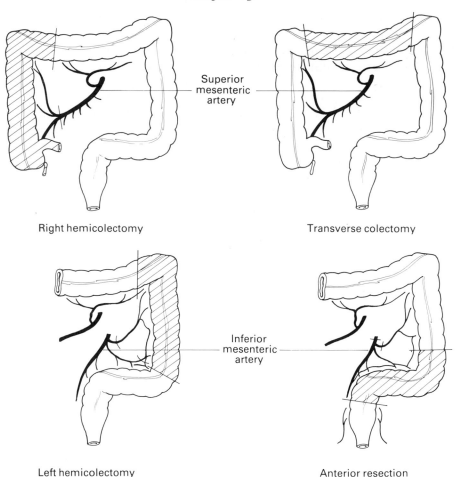

Right hemicolectomy   Transverse colectomy

Left hemicolectomy   Anterior resection

Fig. 65.1. Diagrammatic illustrations of anatomical reasons for amount of colon resected at 'radical' colectomy for lesions in different areas.

preoperative low-dose X-ray therapy has failed to confirm any benefit from such an approach (Second MRC Report 1984).

Establishment of continuity

In most instances this is accomplished by an end-to-end anastomosis, after adequate mobilization of the proximal intestine. Although most surgeons have a personal preference for a particular suture material or technique, there seems to be no major advantage for one technique over another. Anastomotic leakage rates of 1–5% are re-

ported in most series where this has been examined.

Locally advanced cancers

Colonic cancer can involve adjacent organs by direct infiltration. A proportion of these will be clearly inoperable because of local extent or distant metastases; others may only be removed leaving residual disease (a palliative resection). However, in some patients the degree of infiltration is relatively confined so that an *en bloc* resection is feasible. This approach is readily justified if it is only a loop of small intestine, dome of the bladder, or a short length of ureter that is involved; it is probably only palliative if there is direct involvement of pancreas, liver or duodenum.

Carcinoma of the rectum can invade adjacent structures at a relatively early stage. In carefully selected patients, where lymph node invasion is absent, a radical pelvic clearance can give worthwhile results with survival rates of 50% at five years [10, 36]. Even with lymph node involvement, five-year survival can be 20%. This radical approach can also be justified for sigmoid cancers if there is no evidence of distant spread and the surgical team is experienced.

The management of small cancers of the rectum

Carcinomas arising in the lower half of the rectum are occasionally small and mobile on rectal examination. This suggests that the tumour is confined to the mucosa and, if it is accessible, consideration may be given to the use of local excision, regional radiotherapy or electrocoagulation.

Local excision [66]

This can be accomplished through the anal canal or via a trans-sphincteric approach. By this means it is possible to excise a small tumour, with a healthy margin of tissue (at least 0.5 cm all around), with considerable advantages for the elderly.

When the trans-sphincteric approach is used the sphincters can be repaired, by careful suturing, but it is advisable to perform a proximal colostomy until healing is complete. With the trans-anal approach the mucosal wound can be left open—provided it does not occupy more than half of the circumference of the bowel, otherwise some form of mucosal repair is advisable.

The resected specimen should be carefully pinned out on a cork board for later pathological examination. If this reveals submucosal infiltration formal rectal excision should be considered.

Local radiotherapy

This is an alternative approach, particularly the use of endocavity irradiation [50]. A radiation probe is introduced via the anal canal and applied directly to different parts of the surface of the tumour. By this means it is possible to deliver a high dose of radiation (up to 2000 rads/min), and three or four treatments can be given over two months. Clearly, appropriate selection is vital for this treatment. The lesion should be within 10–12 cm of the anal verge, and be small and papillary in type rather than ulcerating or infiltrating. Given these pathological characteristics, and a well differentiated histology, lymph node metastases are unlikely. The best reports describe a five-year survival of 70% [50].

Electrocoagulation

This is an old technique [6, 42] which is ideally suited to the papillary or exophytic (rather than deeply ulcerating) type of tumour. It is important that the technique is carried out expertly and thoroughly.

Ideally the patient should be placed in a jack-knife position with the anal canal held widely open with anal retractors. The exophytic part of the tumour is coagulated with a diathermy needle thrust into it from various angles and at different levels; the coagulated tissue is then scraped away with a diathermy loop until the underlying muscle layer is exposed. In large tumours it may be necessary to repeat the treatment two or three times before satisfactory local control is obtained. Complications include postoperative haemorrhage, often delayed for up to a week, and perforation.

Electrocoagulation is a particularly useful technique in elderly patients provided they can withstand the required operative position. Survival rates of 50% at five years have been reported.

A comparable technique is that of **nitrogen-cryotherapy**. In this technique the tumour is frozen, by means of a nitrogen-cooled cryoprobe to temperatures of $-180°C$, which results in subsequent tissue necrosis. It has been mainly used for the treatment of unresectable rectal lesions but also has a role in the treatment of early rectal carcinomas. Another recent method is that of laser photocoagulation which is particularly useful for extensive villous rectal tumours [4].

Management of established rectal cancer

Abdominoperineal excision of the rectum

The majority of rectal cancers are unsuitable for local treatment and removal of the entire rectum, perirectal tissues and lymphatics, lateral ligaments, levator ani muscles and perianal skin is required for adequate tumour clearance. This type of excision involves the construction of a terminal colostomy, which is usually brought out retroperitoneally, to minimize the risk of small intestinal obstruction around it, in the left iliac fossa (see Chapter 55). This type of resection provides the best chance of avoiding local recurrence and gives survival rates at least equivalent to those achieved with sphincter-saving procedures.

The surgeon has to decide whether the patient will benefit from such a radical procedure if there are distant, or hepatic metastases. In the absence of severe local symptoms one option is to fix the sigmoid colon to the anterior abdominal wall in the left iliac fossa, for later construction of a colostomy if required, and either to do nothing to the local disease or to invite the radiotherapist to give a course of palliative irradiation to the tumour.

Rectal excision with anastomosis (anterior resection)

Tumours situated more than 8–10 cm from the anal verge can be treated by rectal excision and colorectal anastomosis. This procedure has been in use for over twenty years and provides survival results comparable to those for abdominoperineal resection. The anastomosis can be performed with sutures, either one or two layers, but it can be difficult when carried out deep in the pelvis; a covering colostomy is often performed, although the value of this has recently been questioned [13].

Over the last few years a number of developments have occurred that have extended the role of anterior resection. The most widely-used is that of **stapling devices** [40]. These allow more secure end-to-end anastomoses to be performed deep within the pelvis (Fig. 65.2). When using such devices it is necessary to carefully prepare the rectal stump, and distal colon, so that no extraneous tissue is drawn into the anastamosis as the stapling device is applied. It is also important to use the correct anvil size to achieve satisfactory apposition.

Anastomoses at this low level can also be performed using a **pull-through technique** (Cleveland Clinic). In this technique the colon is pulled through the everted rectal stump and anastomosed either five or more days later, or immediately with a circular stapling device. In an alternative **coloanal approach** [52] the rectal stump is denuded of its mucosal lining and the colon is drawn through it and anastomosed to the anal verge (Fig. 65.3) with, on some occasions, the creation of a proximal pouch [35, 51].

The **posterior approach** is a further method for performing a sphincter-saving rectal excision [39]. This involves a posterior incision with, if necessary, excision of a short segment of sacrum, exposing the lower part of the posterior wall of the rectum. Excision of the tumour can then be

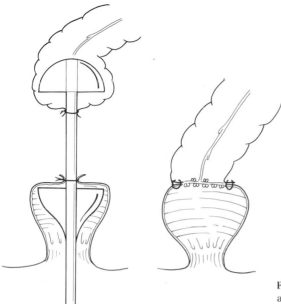

Fig. 65.2. Low colorectal anastomosis performed with circular stapling device.

performed and a coloanal anastamosis made under direct vision—a technique which requires considerable expertise.

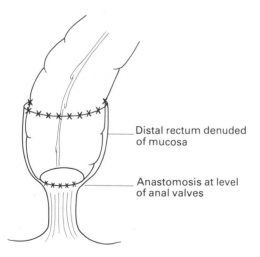

Distal rectum denuded of mucosa

Anastomosis at level of anal valves

Fig. 65.3. Colo-anal anastomosis leaving short segment of lower rectum denuded of mucosal lining (Parks' technique).

Results of sphincter-saving procedures [33]

While there can be no doubt that the results of the standard anterior resection procedure are similar to those of an abdominoperineal resection, the newer sphincter-saving procedures have not been done for a sufficient time to be fully evaluated.

The major argument concerns the risk of local recurrence, some authors claiming a low recurrence rate [68, 69] and others an unacceptably high recurrence rate [29, 40, 62]. Only longer-term review will resolve this controversy and until such results are available the reader is advised to weigh carefully the advantages of preserving the anal sphincter against the possible disadvantage of trying to remove recurrent tumour.

Diagnosis and management of recurrent or inoperable carcinoma

Most patients are kept under regular review after discharge from hospital, however this approach has been criticized as there is little the clinician can do to prevent recurrence, unless adjuvant treatment is given. There is no role for regular X-ray examination of the colon, but sigmoidoscopy, after anterior resection, can detect anastomotic recurrence at an early stage. If the recurrent growth is mobile, an abdominoperineal excision of the rectum offers the possibility of cure. If it is fixed to surrounding tissues it is probably more appropriate to ask a radiotherapist for assistance—after six fractions of irradiation (approximately 3000 rads) it may be feasible to remove the rectum.

A policy of a second-look laparotomy six months after curative resection for colorectal cancer, has been advocated for high-risk patients. Approximately half of the asymptomatic patients have recurrent tumour, but only 10% are helped by further radical surgery [20]. Nevertheless, recourse to laparotomy can be justified if symptoms occur, as completely benign conditions may mimic cancer recurrence—for example strictures, adhesions, internal herniae, and sterile abscesses [11, 12].

Current interest centres around the use of measurements of plasma carcinoembryonic antigen (CEA) concentration in detecting recurrence [15]. In many centres CEA concentrations are measured at monthly intervals; if there is a progressive rise, even if it remains within the normal range, recurrent tumour is likely [3]. It has been suggested that such measurements will give an indication of recurrence 2–18 months ahead of clinical detection. Unfortunately 20–30% of patients with recurrent tumour do not have an elevated CEA and transient rises may be detected in patients who are apparently disease-free. Nevertheless, a 'second-look' laparotomy in those with a rising CEA concentration found localized disease in 41% of such patients [44].

Adjuvant therapy for colorectal cancer [32]

The ultimate purpose of adjuvant therapy (chemo- and/or radiotherapy) is to improve the survival rate, and time, in patients who would otherwise have a poor prognosis. Two difficulties are immediately apparent—firstly, who should be treated, and secondly, do the side-effects of treatment outweigh any gain in survival achieved (see also Chapter 65)? Ideally adjuvant therapy should only be given to those patients who have residual cancer present after operative treatment, unfortunately there is no specific marker which can signal small residues of cancer cells.

Adjuvant chemotherapy should be selected for those patients with disseminated microscopic tumour foci while radiotherapy is appropriate for patients with a localized tumour. The true incidence of distant micrometastases in colorectal cancer remains unknown. There is general agreement that local recurrence remains the major problem, particularly with rectal cancer—for example, of 105 recurrences in 280 patients, 63 were only local, but 15 were both local and distant—that is an overall local recurrence rate of 75% [5]. Similar results were found by Whittaker and Goligher [67] and Olsen, et al. [48]. Features that have been shown to be related to the risk of recurrence include poor Dukes' stage, the presentation as an obstruction or perforation, tumour fixity, and the surgeon performing the procedure [54, 55].

If adjuvant chemotherapy is to be used to destroy distant micro-metastases, it is only applicable to a small number of patients. While local residual disease might be responsive to chemotherapy, it seems probable that malignant cells in scar tissue will have a reduced blood supply and therefore be less accessible to blood-borne agents.

Adjuvant chemotherapy

Early attempts at adjuvant cytotoxic chemotherapy used only single agents such as nitrogen mustard, thiotepa, cyclophosphamide, or 5-fluorouracil. The aim of these early studies was the elimination of circulating cancer cells at the time of operation, rather than treatment of micro-metastases. There was a recognition of the importance of the hepatic bed as a seat for metastatic spread and several workers proposed the direct injection of the cytotoxic agent into the portal venous system to deal with cancer cells displaced during the handling of the primary tumour. Another technique was to instil the agent into the lumen of the bowel allowing time for it to be absorbed via the portal venous system.

A study in 1959 used **nitrogen mustard** in four doses (total 0.4 mg/kg)—one dose injected into the portal vein, a second dose into the peritoneal cavity, and the third and fourth doses given on the first and second postoperative days [47]. Myelotoxicity was a limiting factor. Although the initial report appeared to show an apparent increase in the disease-free interval this was not confirmed on later analysis. This study was important, not only in demonstrating the difficulties of producing a satisfactory adjuvant chemotherapeutic trial, but also in showing that a cytotoxic agent could be given preoperatively without severe postoperative complications.

A subsequent large study used **thiotepa** instead of nitrogen mustard with intraportal injection and a short postoperative course showed no increase in postoperative complications or in the overall survival of the treated versus the non-treated controls [9].

A Veterans group study, using **5-fluorouracil**, gave the drug in two five-day courses—one preoperatively and the second at six to eight weeks after surgery. Three clinical groups were ultimately analysed (curative resection, proven palliative, and clinically palliative). In all groups there was an apparent improvement of survival but this failed to reach statistical significance. This study was extended by a similar trial in which the 5-fluorouracil was given, if possible, up to the nineteenth postoperative month, to patients with colorectal cancers that had involved the lymph nodes or extended locally. Toxicity was reported in 32%, and 10% of these had to discontinue therapy. The conclusion from these two trials was that 5-fluorouracil had produced significant benefit for the patients in the first trial but not for those in the prolonged therapeutic study [27].

An alternative approach used direct installation of the cytotoxic agent *into the lumen of the segment of colon to be resected* [58], aiming to allow the agent to flow along natural and pathologically affected channels, where it might come in contact with cancer cells at a high local concentration. Initially nitrogen mustard was used but this was later replaced by 5-fluorouracil. No significant increase in overall survival occurred although a slight improvement was apparent, particularly in Dukes' C rectal tumours and colonic lesions with serosal involvement [24, 58].

There has been only one trial in which 5-fluorouracil has been said to decrease recurrence (a five-year disease-free rate of 81.6% versus 58.5% for Dukes' B cases and 57.5% versus 24.3% for Dukes' C cases) [37]. Unfortunately this study used historical controls and is therefore considered to be invalid.

5-fluorouracil (1 g with 5,000 units of heparin in 5% dextrose) has also been infused directly *into the portal vein* for seven days postoperatively. This treatment has been associated with a lower incidence of hepatic metastases and an increase in overall survival, particularly in Dukes' B colon cancer [63].

The most recent trend has been to combine 5-fluorouracil with a nitrosourea (Methyl CCNU). Unfortunately early reports are not encouraging [28, 43, 70].

Other trials have added **non-specific immunotherapy**, with BCG given orally [41,49] or intradermally [31]. None of these trials appears to have improved cancer control and, unfortunately, the nitrosourea seems to have significantly added to the toxicity with 60% having severe side-effects and 10% life-threatening toxicity.

There is some evidence that the survival for rectal cancer may be improved by a combination of radiotherapy (4,000–4,400 rads) with 5-fluorouracil (usually 500 mg/m^2.day on the last three days of the irradiation). Again toxicity is a major problem for 60% of the patients, but the underlying trend does suggest an improvement in survival over that of surgery alone or surgery plus chemotherapy [19, 43, 46, 65].

Adjuvant radiotherapy [7]

Radiotherapy should be used to destroy cancer cells which exist in tissues beyond the field of surgical excision. Its use has been confined to rectal tumours because it is possible to precisely locate the primary lesion and local recurrence is quite common (see Chapter 64). Preoperative irradiation could, theoretically, have a beneficial effect by making it less likely that viable cancer cells would be dispersed during surgery, and by destroying small local foci allowing more complete *en bloc* excision. Furthermore, when the bulk of tumour is large and apparently fixed, preoperative radiotherapy may reduce its size and make resection easier. Indeed there have been studies where no tumour could be found in the excised specimen after earlier irradiation.

Preoperative radiotherapy is preferred to postoperative as, in the latter case, the tumour cells may be encased in fibrous tissue and be more radio-resistant. However, giving all patients preoperative radiotherapy means that some patients will receive it unnecessarily. In addition, radiotherapy can also delay wound and anastomotic healing, particularly if the interval between treatment and surgery is under four weeks.

Most studies of preoperative radiotherapy have been uncontrolled or have used historical controls. One American study reported on 720 patients, mainly Dukes' C tumours, and claimed an improved 5-year survival of 55% compared with 45% in historical controls [60]. However, a later study failed to show any difference in survival [61].

Recently a controlled trial has been reported on an adjuvant study using a relatively low dose of preoperative radiotherapy (500 or 2,000 rads)—unfortunately this has failed to show any benefit upon either survival or disease-free interval. A further study using a higher dose-schedule is currently in progress (Second MRC Report 1984).

Postoperative radiotherapy can be used in a more selective manner, but it is not without hazard as loops of small intestine may be fixed in the irradiation field by postoperative adhesions causing radiation enteritis.

In conclusion, there remains considerable interest in the possible role of adjuvant radiotherapy in the management of rectal carcinoma, but one must conclude that, at present, the benefits to be achieved are unproven.

Survival and palliation

Survival times for patients with advanced colorectal cancer are related to the patients' preoperative performance status and whether he or she has lost more than 10% of their weight in the six months prior to operation. These two factors influence survival far more than any treatment regime [34]. Additional, although less strong, factors are the presence of liver or peritoneal metastases. A further factor affecting survival which has recently been identified is whether or not the patient has received a blood transfusion [18].

It is possible to produce an equation which weights these factors to give a fairly accurate estimate of a patients' expected survival [34]. This is of major value in clinical trials, but it may also help the clinician who wants to assess the likely benefit of supportive treatment for an individual patient.

It cannot be claimed that there is strong evidence that either chemotherapy or radiotherapy improves the quality of life or survival for patients with advanced colorectal cancer, although bone pain can be relieved. A sensible compromise can be reached, for the fully informed patient, between the potential side-effects of treatment and the possible benefit of increased length of survival and the patients' feelings that 'something is being done'.

Cytotoxic therapy in advanced colorectal cancer

Most patients with metastatic colorectal cancer are likely to die within a relatively short time. Under these circumstances the clinician may feel that chemotherapy is worth trying. It must be recognized, however, that it is unlikely that currently available cytotoxic regimens will ultimately affect the fatal progression of the patients' disease.

Improved short-term survival can be expected if the metastatic tumour shows an objective reduction in size, in response to

Table 65.1. Criteria used to assess responses to cytotoxic therapy.

Complete response	Complete disappearance of known metastases.
Partial response	A reduction of 50% or more in the size of an indicator lesion. (Product of two maximal perpendicular diameters). No new lesions.
Static response	No change in size of indicator lesion (or <25% increase in product of two diameters).
Progression	Appearance of new lesions or an increase in indicator lesion with product increase of >25%.

cytotoxic treatment (Table 65.1). While detection of an objective response is, inevitably very crude, it is important as it justifies continuing with the treatment. If the deposits increase in size, or there is a continued progressive rise in CEA concentration, then continued treatment is unjustified [15].

It is uncertain whether there is any advantage in changing the cytotoxic drugs when progression of the disease is evident. Table 65.2 lists some of the combinations

Table 65.2. Combination chemotherapy for colorectal cancer.

Regimen	Response rate %	Mean response duration (weeks)	Mean survival (weeks)
Mitomycin C +Methotrexate	15%	16	–
5-FU+Doxorubicin +Mitomycin C	17%	18	–
5-FU+Methyl CCNU+ Mitomycin C	0%	–	–
5-FU+Methyl CCNU	16%	22	43
5-FU+MitomycinC	18%	18	43
Ftorafur+Methyl CCNU	19%	6.5	22

Table 65.3. Various 5-fluorouracil regimens used in colorectal cancer [1].

12.5 mg/kg i.v. × 5 days; then 6 mg/kg i.v. daily until toxicity develops and then 15 mg/kg weekly.

15 mg/kg i.v. *weekly* × 4; then 20 mg/kg weekly.

500 mg i.v. *daily* × 4; then weekly.

15 mg/kg *orally* daily × 6; then weekly.

---

which have been tested in advanced colorectal cancer. In almost all reports, those showing an objective response showed improved survival, but the duration of response was short lived and extended survival uncommon.

If survival is not improved by different drug combinations, is there an optimal delivery regimen for 5-fluorouracil? This drug was developed 25 years ago and is widely used; however its performance is far from impressive—objective responses being seen in only 15–20% of patients treated. Table 65.3 illustrates some of the various 5-fluorouracil regimens that have been used in colorectal cancer [1]. The best results are achieved when the drug is used up to its limit of toxicity.

The treatment of hepatic metastases

The treatment of hepatic metastases from colorectal cancer has attracted a lot of attention recently [64]. Unfortunately much of this work has failed to take into account the natural history of such patients [14]. It is now recognized that several factors influence survival in patients with hepatic metastases—the number and size of the lesions the preoperative 'performance-status' of the patient, the histological features of the tumour, liver function, and the amount of weight lost by the patient [16]. For example, a patient with less than four metastases and a normal 'performance-status' has a median survival of 18–24 months while a patient with more than four lesions, disturbed liver function and more than 10% weight loss will only survive for about six months [21]. It is therefore important to take these facts into account when considering treatment for hepatic metastases.

Hepatic resection has been used for localized metastases from a colorectal tumour. Most studies suggest that survival time is prolonged in patients with solitary metastases [16, 64] although adequate controlled trials have not been performed.

Systemic chemotherapy has been reported using both single and combination therapy. Improved survival and complete or partial remissions have been reported using combined cytotoxic therapy [30, 56], but these studies were not randomized and treatment was associated with significant morbidity. Oral urea has also been used with an associated median survival of 20 months and very little morbidity [8].

Another controversial point is whether the response to treatment can be improved by infusing the cytotoxic agent into the hepatic artery [17]. A prospective randomized trial, comparing intrahepaticarterial infusion with intravenous administration of 5-fluorouracil, has shown a 34% response rate in the former group when compared with a 24% response rate when 5-fluorouracil was given intravenously [23]. Another study [53] used a combination of mitomycin C (15 mg/m^2) and floxurodine (FUDR) (100 mg/m^2) infused into the hepatic artery every 30 days and produced an objective response rate in 83% of patients with a median survival of 16 months.

Radiotherapy has also been investigated in the management of hepatic metastases but, apart from the relief of pain, it has not been shown to be of any benefit in this condition.

Hepatic artery ligation and embolization have been used in the management of hepatic metastases. The rationale for such studies is the observation that most liver metastases derive their major blood supply through the hepatic arterial circulation while the normal liver can withstand interruption of this blood flow. While these techniques are useful in relieving liver pain, they have not been shown to improve survival [64].

References

1 Ansfield FJ, Klotz J, Nealon T, *et al.* A phase II study comparing the clinical utility of 4 regimens of 5-fluorouracil—a preliminary report. *Cancer* 1974;39:34–40.

2 Beck DE, Harford FJ, Di Palma JA. Comparison of cleansing methods in preparation for colonic surgery. *Dis Colon Rectum* 1985;28:491–495.

3 Boey J, Cheung HC, Lai CK, Wong J. A prospective evaluation of serum carcinoembryonic antigen (CEA) levels in the management of colorectal carcinoma. *World J Surg* 1984;8:279–286.

4 Brunetaud JM, Mosquet L, Houcke M, *et al.* Villous adenomas of the rectum. Results of endoscopic treatment with argon and Nd:YAG lasers. *Gastroenterology* 1985;89:832–837.

5 Cass AW, Million RR, Pfaff WW. Patterns of recurrence following surgery alone for adenocarcinoma of the colon and rectum. *Cancer* 1976;37:2861–2865.

6 Crile G, Turnbull RB. The role of electrocoagulation in the treatment of cancer of rectum. *Surg Gynecol Obstet* 1972;135:391–396.

7 Cummings BJ. Adjuvant radiation therapy for rectal adenocarcinoma. *Dis Colon Rectum* 1984;27: 826–836.

8 Danapoulou ED, Danapoulou IE. Eleven years experience of oral urea treatment in liver malignancies. *Clin Oncol.* 1981;7:281–289.

9 Dixon WJ, Longmuir WP, Holden WD. Use of triethylene-thiophosphoramide as an adjuvant to surgical treatment of gastric and colorectal cancer: 10 year follow-up. *Ann Surg* 1971;173: 26–39.

10 Durdey P, Williams NS. The effect of malignant and inflammatory fixation of rectal carcinoma on prognosis after rectal excision. *Br J Surg* 1984;71:787–790.

11 Ellis H. Second-look surgery for suspected recurrences in cancer of the large bowel. *Cancer Treat Rev* 1974;1:205–220.

12 Ellis H. Recurrent cancer of the large bowel (Editorial). *Br Med J* 1984;287:1741–1742.

13 Fielding LP, Stewart-Brown S, Hittinger R, Blesovsky L. Covering stoma for elective anterior resection of the rectum: an outmoded operation? *Am J Surg* 1984;147:524–530.

14 Finan PJ, Marshall RJ, Cooper EH, Giles GR. Factors affecting survival in patients presenting with synchronous hepatic metastases from colorectal cancer: a clinical and computer analysis. *Br J Surg* 1985;72:373–377.

15 Fletcher RH. Carcinoembryonic antigen. *Ann Intern Med* 1986;104:66–73.

16 Fortner JG, Silva JS, Golbey RB, Cox EB, Maclean BJ. Multivariate analysis of a personal series of 247 consecutive patients with liver metastases from colorectal cancer. I. Treatment by hepatic resection. *Ann Surg* 1984;199:317–324.

17 Fortner JG, Silva JS, Cox EB, Golbey RB, Gallowitz H, Maclean BJ. Multivariate analysis of a personal series of 247 consecutive patients with liver metastases from colorectal cancer. II. Treatment by intrahepatic chemotherapy. *Ann Surg* 1984;199:317–324.

18 Foster RS, Costanza MC, Foster JC, Wanner MC, Foster CB. Adverse relationship between blood transfusions and survival after colectomy for colon cancer. *Cancer* 1985;55:1195–1201.

19 Gastrointestinal Tumour Study Group Prolongation of the disease-free interval in surgically treated rectal carcinoma. *N Engl J Med* 1985;312:1465–1472.

20 Gilbertson VA, Wangansteen OH. A summary of 13 years experience with the second-look program. *Surg Gynecol Obstet* 1962;114:438–442.

21 Goslin R, Steele G, Zamchek N, Mayer R, Macintyre J. Factors influencing survival in patients with hepatic metastases from adenocarcinoma of the colon or rectum. *Dis Colon Rectum* 1982;25:749–754.

22 Gottrup F, Diederich P, Sorensen K, Nielsen SV, Ornsholt J, Brandsborg O. Prophylaxis with whole gut irrigaition and antimicrobials in colorectal surgery. A prospective randomised double-blind clinical trial. *Am J Surg* 1985; 149:317—322.

23 Grage TB, Hill GJ, Cornell GN, Frelick RW, Moss SE. Adjuvant chemotherapy in large bowel cancer: demonstration of effectiveness of single agent chemotherapy in a prospectively randomized trial. In: Bonnadona G, Mathe G, Salmon SE, eds. *Recent Results in Cancer Research* Berlin: Springer-Verlag, 1979.

24 Grossi CE, Wolff WI, Nealon TF, Pasternack B, Ginzburg L. Rousselot LM. Intraluminal fluorouracil chemotherapy adjunct to surgical procedures to resectable carcinoma of the colon and rectum. *Surg Gynecol Obstet* 1974;45:549–554.

25 Hares MM, Alexander-Williams J. The effect of bowel preparation on colonic surgery. *World J Surg* 1982;6:175–181.

26 Hewitt J, Reeve J, Rigby J, Cox AG. Whole gut irrigation in preparation for large bowel surgery. *Lancet* 1973;ii:1825–1827.

27 Higgins GA, Lee LG, Dwight RW, Keehn RJ. The

case for adjuvant 5-fluorouracil in colorectal cancer. *Cancer Clin Trials* 1978;1:35–41.

28 HIGGINS GA, AMADEO JH, McELHINNEY J, McCAUGHAN JJ, KEEHN RJ. Efficacy of prolonged intermittent therapy with combined 5-fluorouracil and methyl-CCNU following resection for carcinoma of the large bowel. A Veterans Administration surgical oncology report. *Cancer* 1984;53:1–8.

29 HURST PA, PROUT WG, KELLY JM. Local recurrence after low anterior resection using the staple gun. *Br J Surg* 1982;69:275.

30 KEMENY N, YAYONA A, *et al.* Therapy for metastatic colorectal carcinoma with a combination of methyl CCNU, 5FU, Vincristine and Streptozotocin. *Cancer* 1980;45:44–49.

31 KILLEN JY, HOLYOKE ED, MITTELMAN A. Adjuvant therapy of carcinoma of the colon following clinically curative resection: an interim report from the Gastrointestinal Tumour Study Group (GITSG). In: Salmon SE, Jones SG, eds. *Adjuvant Therapy of Cancer III* New York: Grune & Stratton, 1981;527–537.

32 LANCET LEADER. Adjuvant treatment of carcinoma of the rectum and colon. *Lancet* 1985;ii:367–368.

33 LANCET LEADER. Local recurrence after restorative resection for rectal carcinoma. *Lancet* 1986;i:136.

34 LAVIN P, MITTELMAN A, DOUGLASS H, ENGSTROM P, KLASSEN D. Survival and responses to chemotherapy for advanced colorectal adenocarcinoma. *Cancer* 1980;46:1536–1543.

35 LAZORTHES F, FAGES P, CHIOTASSA P, LEMOZY J, BLOOM E. Resection of the rectum with construction of a colonic reservoir and colo anal anastomisis for carcinoma of the rectum. *Br J Surg* 1986;73:136–138.

36 LEDESMA EJ, BRUNO S, MITTELMAN A. Total pelvic exenteration in colorectal disease. *Ann Surg* 1981;194:701–703.

37 LI MC, ROSS ST. Chemoprophylaxis for patients with colorectal cancer. Prospective study with five year follow-up *JAMA* 1976;235:2825–2828.

38 LOCALIO SA, ENG K. Malignant tumours of the rectum. *Curr Probl Surg* 1975;12:1.

39 LOCALIO SA, GOUGE TH, RANSOME JHC. Abdominosacral resection for carcinoma of the mid-rectum: 10 year experience. *Ann Surg* 1978;188:745–750.

40 McGINN FP, GARTELL PC, CLIFFORD PC, BRUNTON FJ. Staples or sutures for low colorectal anastomoses: a prospective randomized trial. *Br J Surg* 1985;72:603–605.

41 McPHERSON TA, YOUNG D, LIM C, DEWAR G, McMURRAY B, BONE G. Adjuvant chemo-immunotherapy in B2 and colorectal cancer. In: Salmon SG, Jones SG, eds. *Adjuvant Therapy of Cancer II.* New York: Grune & Stratton, 1979;603–612.

42 MADDEN JR, KANDILAFT S. Electrocoagulation in the treatment of cancers of rectum: a continuing study. *Ann Surg* 1971;174:530–565.

43 MANSOUR EG, MacINTYRE JM, JOHNSON J, LERNER HJ, MUGGIA FM. Adjuvant studies in colorectal carcinoma: experience of the Eastern Co-operative Oncology Group (EOG). In: Gerard A, ed. *Progress and Perspectives in the Treatment of Gastrointestinal tumours.* Oxford: Pergamon Press, 1981:68–75.

44 MARTIN EW, JAMES KJ, HURTUBISE PG, CATALAND P, MINTON JP. The use of CEA as an indicator for gastrointestinal tumour recurrence and second-look procedures. *Cancer* 1977;39:440–446.

45 MILES WE *Cancer of the Rectum.* London: Harrison, 1926.

46 MITTELMAN A, HOLYOKE E, THOMAS PRM. Adjuvant chemotherapy and radiotherapy following rectal surgery: an interim report from the Gastrointestinal Tumour Study Group (GITSG). In: Salmon SE, Jones SG, eds. *Adjuvant Therapy for Cancer III* New York: Grune & Stratton 1981: 547–557.

47 MZAREK R, ECONOMU, McDONALD GD, SLAUGHTER CP, COLE WH. Prophylactic and adjuvant use of nitrogen mustard in the surgical treatment of cancer. *Ann Surg* 1959;150:745–755.

48 OLSEN RM, PERERCAVICH MD, MALCOLM MW, WILSON RG. Patterns of recurrence following curative resection of adenocarcinoma of the colon and rectum. *Cancer* 1980;45:2969–2974.

49 PANNETTIERE FJ, HEILBRUN L. Effectiveness of postoperative adjuvant therapy with methyl CCNU plus 5-FU with or without B.C.G. in an attempt to prevent recurrence of Dukes' B2 or C colon cancer. In: Jones SG, Salmon SE, eds. *Adjuvant Therapy of Cancer II.* New York: Grune & Stratton: 1979: 592–602.

50 PAPILLON J. Endocavity irradiation of early rectal cancer for cure: a series of 123 cases. *Proc R Soc Med* 1973;66:1179–1181.

51 PARC RM, TURET E, FRILEUZ P, MOSZKOSKI E, LOYGUE J. Resection and colo-anal anastomosis with colonic reservoir for rectal carcinoma. *Br J Surg* 1986;73:139–141

52 PARKS AG. Trans-anal technique in low rectal anastomosis. *Proc R Soc Med* 1972;65:975–976.

53 PATT YZ, MAVLIGIT GM, CHUANG VIP, *et al.* Percutaneous hepatic arterial infusion (HAI) of Mitomycin C and Floxurodine (FUDR): An effective treatment for metastatic colorectal carcinoma of the liver. *Cancer* 1980;46:261–265.

54 PHILLIPS RKS, HITTINGER R, BLESOVSKY L, FRY JS, FIELDING LP. Local recurrence following 'curative' surgery for large bowel cancer. I The overall picture. *Br J Surg* 1984;71:12–16.

55 PHILLIPS RKS, HITTINGER R, BLESOVSKY L. FRY JS, FIELDING LP. Local recurrence following 'curative' surgery for large bowel cancer. II The rectum and rectosigmoid. *Br J Surg* 1984;71:17–20.

56 RAPAPORT AH, BURLESON RC. Survival of patients treated with systemic fluorouracil for hepatic metastases. *Surg Gynecol Obstet* 1970;130:773–777.

57 ROLAND M, BERGAN T, BJERKERSET T, *et al.* Prophylactic regimens in colorectal surgery; comparisons between metronidazole used alone or with ampicillin for one or three days. *World J Surg* 1985;9:626–632.

58 ROUSSELOT LM, COLE DR, GROSSI CE, CORK AJ, GONZALES DM, PASTERNACK DS. Adjuvant chemotherapy with 5-fluorouracil in surgery for colorectal cancer. *Dis Colon Rectum* 1972;15:169–174.

59 SHATNEY CH, LOBER PH, GILBERTSON WA. The treatment of pedunculated adenomatous polyps with focal cancer. *Surg Gynecol Obstet* 1974;134:844–850.

60 STEARNS MW JR, DEDDISH MR, QUAN SH. Preoperative roentgen therapy for cancer of the rectum. *Surg Gynecol Obstet* 1959;109:225–228.

61 STEARNS MW JR, DEDDISH MR, QUAN SH, LEAMING RH. Preoperative roentgen therapy for carcinoma of the rectum and rectosigmoid. *Surg Gynecol Obstet* 1979;188:584–589.

62 TAGART REB. Restorative rectal resection: an audit of 220 cases. *Br J Surg* 1986;73:70–71.

63 TAYLOR I, MACHIN D, MULLEE M, TROTTER G, COOKE T, WEST C. A randomized controlled trial of adjuvant portal vein cytotoxic perfusion in colorectal cancer. *Br J Surg* 1985;72:359–363.

64 TAYLOR I. Colorectal liver metastases—to treat or not to treat (Review). *Br J Surg* 1985;72:511–516.

65 WASSIF SB. Ten years' experience with a multimodality treatment of advanced stages of rectal cancer. *Cancer* 1983;52:2017–2024.

66 WHITEWAY J, NICHOLLS RJ, MORSON BC. The role of surgical local excision in the treatment of rectal cancer. *Br J Surg* 1985;72:694–697.

67 WHITTAKER M, GOLIGHER JC. The prognosis after surgical treatment for carcinoma of the rectum. *Br J Surg* 1976;63:384–388.

68 WILLIAMS NS, DURDEY P, JOHNSTON D. The outcome following sphincter-saving resection and abdomino-perineal resection for low rectal cancer. *Br J Surg* 1985;72:595–598.

69 WILLIAMS NS, JOHNSTON D. Survival and recurrence after sphincter-saving resections and abdominoperineal resection for carcinoma of the middle third of the rectum. *Br J Surg* 1984;71:278–282.

70 YORKSHIRE GASTROINTESTINAL TUMOUR GROUP Chemotherapy after palliative resection of colorectal cancer. *Br J Surg* 1984;71:283–286.

Chapter 66
Perianal Disease

J. P. S. THOMSON

Of new patients attending a rectal clinic, around 55% will have **haemorrhoids** and 20% a **fissure-in-ano.** The remaining 25% of patients will have a variety of conditions which affect the perianal area including infections, tumours and pelvic floor problems. It is of paramount importance that a correct diagnosis is made before treatment is commenced or a serious problem, such as a tumour or an inflammatory bowel disease, may be missed.

Haemorrhoids

Haemorrhoids are vascular swellings involving the internal or external venous plexi, or both, associated with redundancy of the mucosa or perianal skin.

Epidemiology and aetiology

Haemorrhoids are common in Western countries but rare in some areas such as rural Africa. Both sexes are affected but it is unusual to find them in children, except when associated with a rectal haemangioma.

The aetiology is usually unclear [47]. Frequently there is a strong family history; constipation and straining at stool are often reported. In women the onset of haemorrhoids is associated with pregnancy or an ovarian or uterine swelling. The often quoted association with carcinoma of the rectum is probably not causal, nor are haemorrhoids often present in portal hypertension.

Pathology

Haemorrhoids can occur anywhere around the anal canal. The primary sites are left lateral, right posterior and right anterior (3, 7 and 11 o'clock), probably related to the position of the vessels of supply. Secondary sites lie between these primary sites; infrequently a complete circular involvement occurs.

Clinical features

Symptoms

The traditional classification of haemorrhoids (Table 66.1) only takes into account the symptoms of bleeding and prolapse.

Table 66.1. Traditional classification of haemorrhoids.

First degree	Bleeding
Second degree	Prolapse (with or without bleeding)
Third degree	Prolapse (with or without bleeding) requiring replacement

Bleeding is bright red in colour and often occurs as a spurt of blood after defecation. Prolapse is readily described by patients, but it is important to differentiate haemorrhoidal prolapse from that of other causes. Other symptoms include discomfort or pain, due to stretching of the skin by venous engorgement. This engorgement may take time to disappear or need digital pressure to relieve it, especially if there is a tight sphincter. If the internal component is permanently prolapsed there may be mucous discharge and, if there are perianal skin tags, skin cleaning may be difficult leading to pruritus ani. The symptoms vary considerably from time to time.

Signs

Haemorrhoids may only be detected as vascular swellings at proctoscopy. However, asking the patient to strain when examining the perineum may result in signs akin to those on defecation, allowing an assessment of size to be made (Fig. 66.1). Prolapse

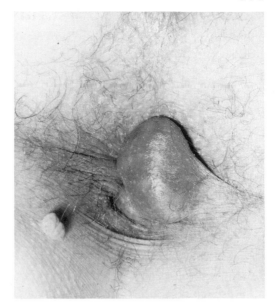

Fig. 66.2. A clotted venous saccule—'perianal haematoma'.

days to resolve. It may involve the external plexus extensively (external haemorrhoidal thrombosis), or locally, a clotted venous

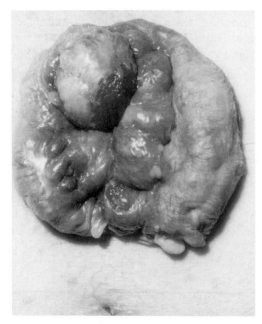

Fig. 66.1. Large intero-external haemorrhoids. In addition to haemorrhoids at the three primary sites there is involvement at the secondary sites as well.

may be seen with reddening of the mucosa (traumatic proctitis) with bleeding and, if longstanding, with whitening or opacification of the mucosa from squamous epithelial change.

Complications

Thrombosis of the venous plexi results in severe pain which can take 10 or more

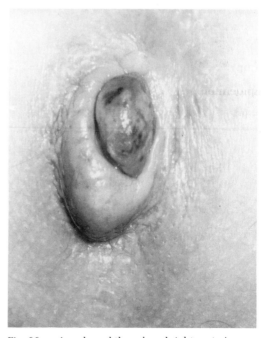

Fig. 66.3. A prolapsed thrombosed right posterior internal haemorrhoid.

saccule—often called a **perianal-haema-toma** [48] (Fig. 66.2), or the internal plexus, when prolapse invariably occurs (Fig. 66.3).

A **fissure** may occasionally complicate a prolapsing haemorrhoid.

Management

General measures

The most important step is exclusion of serious disease by careful and complete examination. Many patients only require reassurance that their symptoms do not herald a serious disease for symptom relief.

Additional measures include advice on a high residue diet, increased fluid intake and appropriate laxatives. If there is a history of straining at stool, attempts should be made to break this habit by the use of suppositories and disposable enemas, as straining can damage the pelvic floor.

Local treatment of uncomplicated haemorrhoids (Table 66.2)

Injection sclerotherapy consists of the injection of about 5 ml of 5% phenol in arachis oil at the anorectal junction of each primary site. When correctly placed, the injection results in a mucosal elevation that has a pearly appearance. Small vessels may be identified. Repeated injections can be given.

It is a simple technique which can be performed on an out-patient basis. The major complications are mucosal ulceration, formation of an oleogranuloma, or prostatitis if the injection is given too deeply.

Infra-red photocoagulation is a recent technique where infra-red light is used to produce a small mucosal burn, which results in mucosal fixation. It is a painless procedure, without the risks of a misplaced injection. The major complication is occasional secondary haemorrhage. Initial short-term results suggest that it is as effective as injection sclerotherapy [2, 3, 42].

Elastic band ligation consists of placement (by a special applicator) of an elastic band around the base of the redundant mucosa of the internal haemorrhoid (Fig. 66.4). After a few days necrosis occurs and the ligated mucosa falls off leaving an ulcer that heals with fixation of the mucosa to the underlying muscle layers. It is usual to treat only one, or at the most two, areas at a session. The procedure may be done on an out-patient basis without anaesthesia.

Complications include severe pain, if sensitive skin is included in the ligation, or rarely, extensive necrosis occurs. Secondary haemorrhage (sometimes up to 21 days later) may occur in a few patients and can be severe enough to require transfusion. Good results, which appear superior to those following injection therapy, have been reported [10, 30].

Cryotherapy which consists of freezing the haemorrhoids with liquid nitrogen ($-180°C$) or nitrous oxide ($-80°C$) has been advocated by some workers [40]. It is only appropriate for internal haemorrhoids and its use remains controversial [24]. While good results have been claimed [49]

Table 66.2. Treatments for haemorrhoids.

Aim of treatment	Technique
Fixation of mucosa	Injection sclerotherapy Infra-red coagulation
Fixation of mucosa and removal of redundant mucosa	Elastic band ligation Cryotherapy
Reduction in sphincter tone	Manual dilatation of the anus Partial internal sphincterotomy
Removal of internal and external venous plexus, together with redundant mucosa and skin	Haemorrhoidectomy

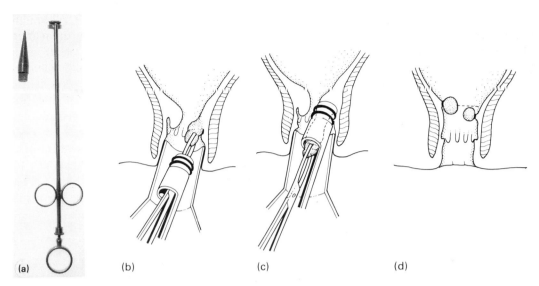

(a)   (b)   (c)   (d)

Fig. 66.4. Method of elastic band application. (a) equipment; (b) haemorrhoid grasped; (c) rubber band application; (d) final banded internal haemorrhoids.

it is associated with some discomfort and a prolonged discharge due to frostbite.

Manual (or maximal) anal dilatation—Forceful anal dilatation, perhaps rupturing the anal internal sphincter, undoubtedly benefits many patients [16]. However it requires general anaesthesia, does not correct prolapse or the external component, and may be followed by disturbances of anal function with incontinence of flatus and, rarely, faeces.

Partial internal sphincterotomy—Lateral sphincterotomy (as used for a fissure) has been adopted by some as a less severe form of anal dilatation. It has not been widely accepted.

The operation of **excisional haemorrhoidectomy** has an evil reputation for postoperative pain, which is greatly exaggerated. For this reason surgeons have sought alternative forms of therapy, even if these are less effective. A well-performed haemorrhoidectomy usually results in a permanent cure. This is especially true in patients with a large symptomatic external component. In addition to removing the three primary haemorrhoids, taking care not to damage

any fibres of the internal or external sphincter, it is also possible to remove secondary haemorrhoidal tissue [28].

Various types of haemorrhoidectomy have been described: the closed technique [11] and the submucosal technique [31] have a reputation for producing less pain, but the ligation and excision technique is still the most-widely used method today. Complications include delayed healing and late stenosis, retention of urine and faeces, and secondary haemorrhage.

Most patients with haemorrhoids are treated adequately by injection sclerotherapy or elastic band ligation. Only 8–10% will require surgical excision.

Thrombosed haemorrhoids

Most surgeons recommend a conservative approach during the acute phase. This includes ice packs or evaporating lotions (for example lead and spirit lotion) to reduce the swelling, bed rest, analgesia and a lubricant laxative. In those patients with severe or continuous pain an anal dilatation or sphincterotomy may be helpful, as may emergency haemorrhoidectomy—although this can be difficult. Attempts to reduce a prolapsed thrombosed haemorrhoid are extremely painful and quite fruitless.

Haemorrhoids in inflammatory bowel disease

It is not uncommon for haemorrhoids and inflammatory bowel disease to co-exist. The treatment of haemorrhoids in patients with ulcerative colitis can be beneficial and safe [18] but perianal surgery, in patients with Crohn's disease, is best avoided as it can be followed by anal ulceration and sepsis.

Fissure

An anal fissure is an ulcer within the anal canal, which may extend as high as the anal valves. It may simply be a breach in the epithelium, or it may be a deep ulcer exposing the internal sphincter fibres with undermining of the edges. There may also be an associated hypertrophied anal papilla or fibrous polyp and skin tag, often referred to as the 'sentinel pile' (Fig. 66.5).

Epidemiology and aetiology

A fissure can occur at any age but is commoner in the young, and in women [25].

Its precise aetiology is unknown, although it is often associated with a tight unyielding distal anal sphincter. It may occur as a complication of large prolapsing haemorrhoids or anal polyps. An anterior fissure may be a complication of labour and can cause problems during the puerperium. Fissuring may also occur in those who practice anal intercourse through local trauma; sexually transmitted disease must also be considered in such patients (see Chapter 57). An apparent fissure may be the result of excoriation due to pruritus ani.

Clinical features

Symptoms

While some fissures are asymptomatic, most patients experience a tearing pain during defecation which can last for an hour or so afterwards, and may be accompanied by bleeding. The bleeding is usually slight and only noted on the toilet paper.

Signs

On inspection a 'sentinel pile' should be readily visible and this should alert the examiner to the possibility of a fissure. The next step should be to gently part the

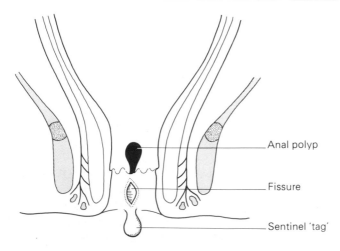

Anal polyp

Fissure

Sentinel 'tag'

Fig. 66.5. Diagram of fissure-in-ano. Note the undermined skin edges, fibrous anal polyp and 'sentinel' tag.

buttocks to stretch the anal area, opening up the anal canal. If a fissure is present it is diagnosed on inspection. Further examination can be done after placing local anaesthetic (10% Amethocaine) on the fissure or by using smaller instruments than usual (e.g. Lloyd-Davies paediatric sigmoidoscope) to diagnose hypertrophied anal papillae, anal polyps and inflammatory bowel disease.

Complications

The intense spasm of the anal sphincter can lead to severe constipation and faecal impaction. Sepsis can also rarely lead to an intersphincteric abscess, or superficial fistula.

Differential diagnosis

While most ulcers seen in this area are simple, there are a number of other causes that need to be considered. These include Crohn's disease, syphilis (primary chancre), herpes simplex, leukaemia, carcinoma and malignant melanoma.

Management

Traditionally the mainstay of treatment has been the passage of an anal dilator, lubricated with local anaesthetic jelly, two or three times a day. Recent work suggests that this instrument achieves little [13, 26]; most patients require operative treatment for permanent cure.

The standard operation is a lateral sphincterotomy. A small incision is made in the right or left lateral positions, and the internal sphincter is divided precisely up to the line of the anal valves. A sentinel pile, or polyp, is removed, with any undermined mucosa along the edge of the fissure, at the same time. Lateral sphincterotomy has replaced dorsal sphincterotomy in all cases except those with an intersphincteric abscess as healing is quicker and soiling is less.

Some surgeons advocate manual dilatation as the treatment of choice for a fissure, but it is illogical to stretch both internal and external sphincters when only division of the distal internal sphincter will suffice. Furthermore published results favour lateral sphincterotomy which gives a cure rate of over 95%. Complications of lateral sphincterotomy are unusual but include sepsis and occasional soiling, especially in females who may preoperatively have had a very tight internal sphincter with dysfunction of the external sphincter.

Proctalgia fugax

Proctalgia fugax is an intensely painful paroxysm of perineal pain usually occurring unexpectedly and waking the patient at night [46]. Little is known of the pathogenesis but some have noted puborectalis spasm in patients examined during the attack. The avoidance of constipation, the use of a mild tranquillizer at night, quinine bisulphate, amyl nitrite or salbutamol [52] may be helpful.

Infections (Table 66.3)

Perianal abscess and fistula

Abscess and fistula are best regarded as being different phases of the same disease process—an abscess presenting in the acute phase and a fistula in the chronic phase.

Most abscesses and fistulae are non-specific—arising from an infection of the anal intersphincteric glands with gut bacteria (for example *Escherichia coli* or *Bacteroides* species), but some have a specific basis—Crohn's disease, tuberculosis, trauma (for example perforation by a foreign body) and, very rarely, malignancy.

Initially the infection involves one anal

Table 66.3. Classification of infections.

Bacterial	Abscess and fistula
	Pilonidal disease
	Hildradenitis suppurativa
	Syphilis
	Erythrasma
Viral	Condylomata acuminata
	Molluscum contagiosum
	Herpes simplex
Fungal	*Candida albicans*
Parasitic	Threadworms
	Lice
	Scabies

gland causing an intersphincteric abscess. This small pea-shaped abscess may remain localized, but usually it spreads either vertically, horizontally or circumferentially, or in any combination.

Vertical spread downwards will result in a perianal abscess and upwards either an intermuscular or supra-levator abscess depending upon which side of the longditudinal muscle of the rectum the infection spreads (Fig. 66.6). **Horizontal spread** across the internal sphincter will result in an opening into the anal canal, usually at the anal valve level, or if across the external sphincter it will produce an ischiorectal abscess (Fig. 66.6). **Circumferential spread** around the anal canal may occur in the intersphincteric or supra-levator spaces, or

from one ischiorectal rectal fossa to the other (Fig. 66.6).

An anal **fistula** has external and internal openings into the anal canal joined by a granulation tissue-lined track of varying complexity depending on the way in which the original infection spread. It is important to recognize, however, that at any one time either the internal or external opening may be closed making diagnosis and management difficult. The most useful physical sign is the presence of induration around the opening.

Classification of fistulae [32]

A superficial fistula is a short subcutaneous track, often formed as a result of epithelial bridging over a fissure. This type is not due to an anal gland infection.

An **intersphincteric fistula** occurs when the infection has been confined to the intersphincteric space (Fig. 66.7). Although there may be a long subcutaneous track leading to the external opening it should be possible to manage the fistula without dividing any of the external sphincter.

A **transsphincteric fistula** occurs when the primary track extends across the external sphincter. However this may not always be at the level of the anal valves (Fig. 66.8), the most frequent site of the internal open-

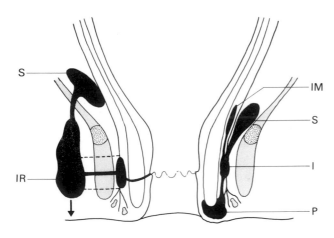

Fig. 66.6. The directions in which abscesses can spread in anal and perianal areas. Arrow indicates direction of spread.
IM = intermuscular abscess;
S = supralevator abscess;
I = intersphincteric abscess;
P = perianal abscess;
IR = ischiorectal abscess.

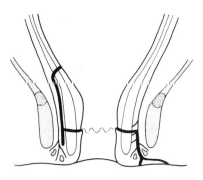

Fig. 66.7. Development of an intersphincteric fistula-in-ano. Note on the left side the track passes across the internal sphincter at level of anal valves and penetrates the circular muscle coat high in the rectum. On the right side a long subcutaneous track has been formed.

ing. It may be either below, or above this level, in which case care must be exercised in management as division of the external sphincter may jeopardize control of flatus and faeces.

A **suprasphincteric fistula** is a very rare form of fistula where the primary track crosses the striated muscle of the pelvic floor above the puborectalis muscle (Fig. 66.9). It results from spread of infection from a supra-levator abscess across the levator ani. It is important to recognize this type, as incontinence will occur if the primary track is laid open.

An **extrasphincteric fistula** can occur

through the injudicious use of a fistula probe but the usual cause is some form of pelvic sepsis. A pelvic abscess secondary to appendicitis, Crohn's disease, or diverticular disease may discharge through the levator ani muscle and present in the perineum, rather than draining direct into the rectum, and lead to this type of fistula.

Management

Abscess

Drainage of abscesses in the perianal and anal region is best carried out in the lithotomy position under general anaesthesia. Sufficient tissue should be excised for adequate drainage but care should be taken to avoid division of the sphincters. Pus should be sent for culture. The isolation of enteric organisms strongly suggests an underlying fistula [14].

If, after the oedema and hyperaemia have subsided, there is continued induration or if there is a history of recurrent abscesses or culture of gut organisms, an examination under anaesthesia should be performed to define the fistula track.

Fistula

The main principles involved in management are definition of the pathoanatomy,

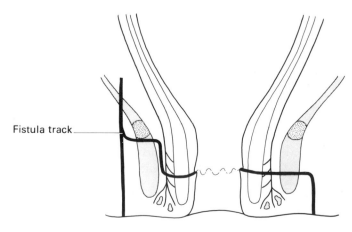

Fistula track

Fig. 66.8. Development of a transsphincteric fistula-in-ano. Note on the left side the track passes across the sphincter above the anal valves and has a supralevator extension.

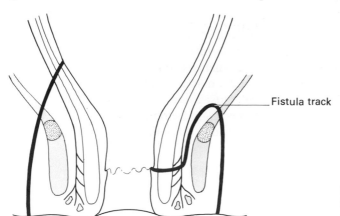

Fistula track

Fig. 66.9. An extrasphincteric fistula is shown on the left and a suprasphincteric on the right.

drainage of the intersphincteric space and primary and secondary tracks, and careful postoperative dressing to encourage healing from within outwards.

With the more complicated fistulae there is still controversy as to the ideal method of management [45].

Failure of a fistula wound to heal may be due to failure to locate all the tracks, poor postoperative dressing, hair growth into the wound, excessive granulation tissue, or an undiagnosed underlying specific cause (for example Crohn's disease or tuberculosis).

Pilonidal disease

A pilonidal sinus usually occurs in the natal cleft but may present close to the posterior margin of the anal opening. It consists of a tuft of hairs buried beneath the skin with an external opening usually in the midline. While most cause pain, some are asymptomatic and found incidentally. If infection occurs a pilonidal abscess will develop, which needs drainage. The simplest method is to lay it open allowing the area to heal by second intention. In the uncomplicated pilonidal sinus excision and primary suture is often used. Some surgeons favour more complicated procedures such as excision and primary suture or other plastic procedures, but the results do not seem to be any better than with the more simple treatment.

Hidradenitis suppurativa

This is an infection of the apocrine sweat glands. It gives rise to multiple small and large subcutaneous abscesses in the perianal, suprapubic and axillary skin areas. It may be associated with Crohn's disease. No specific organism is involved, but anaerobic organisms can be found in the pus [23]. Treatment is difficult. If medical treatment fails to control the disease wide excision of the overlying skin, curettage of the granulation tissue and healing by second intention or skin grafting, may be required.

Syphilis

Primary infection with *Treponema pallidum* may result in an ulcer at the anal margin or in the perianal region (**primary chancre**). During the secondary phase **condylomata lata** may be seen [37].

Erythrasma

This is an infection caused by *Corynebacterium minutissimum*. It is diagnosed by the presence of salmon-pink flourescence in ultraviolet light and is treated by erythromycin. It is a rare cause of pruritus ani.

Viral infections

Condylomata acuminata (warts—Fig. 66.10) are caused by a **papilloma virus**. The distribution of the lesions needs to be carefully defined as treatment will only succeed if all wart tissue is removed. As many as 75% of patients may have additional lesions in the anal canal and rectum.

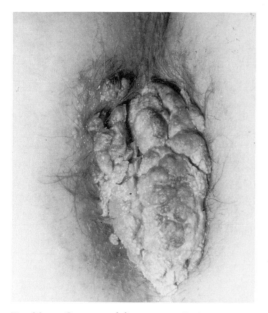

Fig. 66.10. Severe condylomata acuminata.

Treatment methods include destruction of the warts by chemicals [19] (podophyllin, trichloracetic acid); electrocautery or diathermy; cryotherapy or simple excision with scissors [44]. The latter technique is less traumatic to the surrounding normal tissues and when done under general anaesthesia or regional anaesthesia, provides a 75% chance of cure.

Herpes simplex anal ulcerative proctitis, usually in homosexuals, can cause severe pain with marked tenesmus (see Chapter 57).

Fungal infections

Fungal infections should always be considered in any patient with pruritus ani and inflammation of the perianal skin. Diabetic patients are particularly prone to this problem, as are women with fungal vulvovaginitis. The diagnosis is made by detecting fungi in skin scrapings using direct microscopy or by a positive culture on Sabouraud's medium. Topical treatment with an appropriate antifungal agent (nystatin, clotrimazole etc.) is usually effective.

Parasitic infestations

Threadworms (*Enterobius vermicularis*) may cause severe pruritus at night and can be difficult to diagnose. They may be seen on the perianal skin or during sigmoidoscopy on the mucosa of the rectum. Their ova can be detected by microscopic examination of a piece of adhesive tape previously placed on the perianal skin. Piperazine phosphate, given as a single oral dose (4 g) with a sennoside, repeated after 14 days is usually effective treatment. Mebendazole (100 mg) can also be used as a single dose treatment in patients of any age. It is important to treat *all* the members of a family to prevent cross infection.

Lice and scabies can also cause pruritus ani.

Pruritus ani

Pruritus ani is primarily itching in the perianal area, but on many occasions soreness and pain develop from breaches in the epithelium. However it is a symptom and not a disease and a cause must be sought before effective treatment is possible. Some of these causes are listed in Table 66.4.

Table 66.4. The causes of pruritus ani.

Poor hygiene (especially if stool loose)	
Anal pathology	Haemorrhoids
	Fissure
	Fistula
Infections	Bacterial
	Viral
	Fungal
	Parasitic
Primary dermatological problems	Eczema
	Psoriasis
	Atrophic dermatoses
	lichen sclerosis et atrophicus
	lichen planus
	Paget's disease
	Bowen's disease
Reactions to medicine	Allergic contact dermatitis
	lanoline
	local anaesthetics
	neomycin and soframycin
	parabens (preservative)
	Steroid effects
	Broad spectrum antibiotics
Sphincter dysfunction	
Systemic disorders	Obstructive jaundice
	Hodgkin's disease
Dietary excesses	Coffee, cola, chocolate

Assessment (Table 66.5)

History

An accurate history is the first essential. Attention should be paid to any difficulty in achieving complete cleansing after defecation, poor hygiene being probably the commonest cause of the condition [1]. Excessive use of toilet paper or soiling of underwear are clues to this being the cause. Even patients who wash, bathe or shower regularly may fail to clean the perineum satisfactorily. Details of stool consistency may also be relevant as a loose stool may tend to seep out onto the perineal skin during the day. A careful history of the use of creams or ointments is essential as contact sensitivity to the treatment may be responsible for perpetuating the condition.

Examination

Before examining the patient the perineum should be looked at under ultraviolet light to detect erythrasma (very rare) and scrapings should be taken for mycological examination. In female patients this is an opportune time to take a high vaginal swab, also for mycological examination. The patient's urine should be examined for glucose.

A full anorectal and sigmoidoscopic examination is required in all patients. If there is definite skin disease the remainder of the skin should be examined—eczema and psoriasis often occur elsewhere—and a skin biopsy taken. It is only by this means that rare problems (for example Paget's disease Fig. 66.11) will be diagnosed.

Finally, anorectal physiological studies

Table 66.5. The assessment of pruritus ani.

Stage of assessment		Possible factor in production of pruritus
History		Difficulty with cleansing
		Usage of ointments
		Diet
General examination		Systemic disorders
		Generalized skin problems
Rectal examination		
Inspection		Perianal pathology and skin disorders
	Ultra violet light	Erythrasma
	Skin scrapings	Fungal infection
	Wipe with damp cotton wool	Faecal soiling
	Test anal reflex	Sphincter dysfunction
Digital	Assessment of anal tone	Sphincter dysfunction
Sigmoidoscopy		Threadworms
		Loose stool
Proctoscopy		Haemorrhoids
Special Investigations		
	Stool culture	
	Barium enema	Loose stool
	Faecal fat estimation	
	Urine testing	Diabetes (fungal infection)
	Anorectal physiology	Sphincter dysfunction
	Patch testing	Allergic contact dermatitis
	Biopsy	Skin disorders

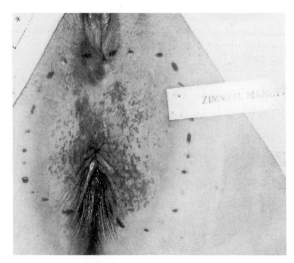

Fig. 66.11. Paget's disease of perianal area showing the line of excision (Mr W.J.L. Harries' patient).

may be useful if anal sphincter dysfunction is suspected (see Table 66.5).

Management

With careful assessment, a cause for pruritus ani should be found in over 90% of patients. In patients with faecal soiling, advice on perianal skin and distal anal canal cleansing using damp cotton wool is often extremely helpful. This may be needed three or four times daily. If the stool is loose a small dose of codeine phosphate or loperamide may be beneficial. The patient should be asked to stop all creams or ointments as these may be causing contact dermatitis. Any severe skin inflammation or excoriation usually responds to a short course of a topical steroid (for example betamethasone 0.1% twice daily for two weeks) but prolonged courses should be avoided. Specific treatments are indicated for established causes.

Premalignant and malignant conditions

Tumours in this region are classified into those of the **anal canal** (above the valves) and those of the **anal margin**. The different types, all of which are rare, are summarized in Table 66.6 [29].

Anal margin tumours

A precise histological diagnosis is essential before deciding treatment. Total excision biopsy may be an effective treatment for a small tumour. **Condylomata acuminata** are best managed by scissor excision (see earlier) but giant condylomata may require excision of the rectum and anal canal. **Bowen's disease**, an *in situ* squamous carcinoma, can be treated by wide excision of the anal skin with or without grafting. It may also respond to topical 5-fluorouracil. **Paget's disease** may be complicated by invasive carcinoma but wide local excision may be adequate treatment (Fig. 66.11).

While small **squamous carcinomas** may respond to local excision, larger tumours may require excision of the rectum [15]. Radiotherapy, either as preoperative treatment or as the sole therapy, has been reported to produce acceptable results [17, 36, 39]. Secondary anal carcinoma will need to be treated at the same time as the primary.

Table 66.6. A classification of anal tumours.

	Anal margin	Anal canal
Benign and premalignant conditions	Condylomata acuminata Giant condyloma Keratoacanthoma Bowen's disease Apocrine gland adenoma Paget's disease (extra mammary)	
Malignant	Squamous cell carcinoma Verrucous carcinoma Secondary carcinoma implantation within haemorrhoidal tissue	Squamous cell carcinoma Basaloid carcinoma Mucoepidermoid carcinoma Adenocarcinoma rectal type anal glands within fistula Malignant melanoma

Anal canal tumours

Provided that they are operable, these tumours are best treated by excision of the rectum and anal canal. The perineal skin has to be excised widely, the ischiorectal fat removed, and the levator ani divided close to the pelvic wall.

Involved lymph nodes should be removed by block dissection, but a routine prophylactic dissection is no longer recommended because of morbidity. Occasionally radiotherapy, either by local implant or external beam, is used as an alternative to operation.

Malignant melanoma of the anus is a rare condition. It may present as a black swelling or ulcerative lesion in this area. Treatment by local excision or radical abdominoperineal resection produces comparable results with approximately a 20% five year survival [9, 50].

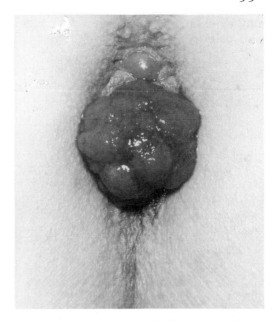

Fig. 66.12. Large pedunculated polyp arising in the sigmoid colon and prolapsing through the anal canal.

Prolapse

Prolapse, by definition, implies that tissue has come through the anus and the patient is conscious of it. As with all symptoms the exact cause must be determined (Table 66.7). If, after careful examination, no

Table 66.7. Causes of prolapse.

Anal canal	Haemorrhoids
	Hypertrophied anal papillae
	Anal (fibro-epithelial) polyps
	Condylomata acuminata
Rectum	Incomplete (mucosal) prolapse
	Complete (full thickness) prolapse
	Polyps—usually sessile adenoma
Colon	Polyp—usually pedunculated adenoma

cause is found then the possibility that it is due to an adenomatous polyp of the sigmoid colon, intussuscepting through the anus (Fig. 66.12), should be considered.

Mucosal prolapse

Mucosal prolapse from the upper anal canal or lower rectum is distinguished from prolapsing haemorrhoids by the absence of an external component, and from a full prolapse by having only two layers (Fig. 66.13) and a good anal sphincter. These patients also complain of a mucus discharge.

Treatment is either by a modified haemorrhoidectomy or a Delorme procedure. In the latter operation the prolapsed mucosa is excised, after submucosal infiltration with adrenaline in saline (1 in 300,000) and the rectal mucosa is then sewn to the anoderm at the level of the anal valves incorporating a small bite of internal sphincter to anchor the suture line.

Complete prolapse

Complete prolapse (Fig. 66.14) can affect any age group and either sex, but there is a marked preponderance in elderly nulli-

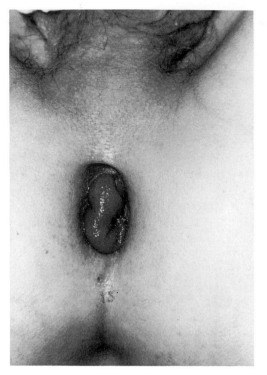

Fig. 66.13. Mucosal or incomplete prolapse.

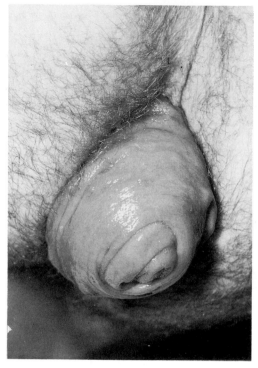

Fig. 66.14. The appearance of a full thickness 'complete prolapse' of the rectum.

parous women. Only about 2% have evidence of neurological disease.

Aetiology

The precise aetiology is unknown but there are many well documented pathoanatomical abnormalities. These are:
1. Intussusception of the rectum, starting at a point about 8 cm above the anus [6].
2. Laxity of the lateral ligaments of the rectum.
3. A very deep rectovaginal or retrovesical peritoneal pouch.
4. Laxity of the pelvic floor musculature and the external anal sphincter. Initially there is a stage of internal intussusception that inhibits the anal sphincter tone (rectosphincteric reflex). Later the full prolapse results in the anal sphincter being kept open with varying degrees of incontinence.
5. Production of traumatic proctitis in the

rectal mucosa, with a distinctive histological appearance showing smooth muscle fibres growing up into the lamina propria. Other causes of proctitis, a clinical descriptive term, are given in Table 66.8.

Table 66.8. Causes of proctitis.

Non-specific	Idiopathic (ulcerative colitis) Crohn's disease
Specific	Bacterial Chlamydial Viral Fungal Parasitic
Traumatic	
Irradiation	
Ischaemic	
Disuse	

Clinical features

If the patient complains of a prolapse then diagnosis is relatively easy, but this is not always the case. Anorectal bleeding, discharge of mucus, increased bowel frequency and incontinence may be the only symptoms. There may also be a long history of straining at stool.

On examination the anus may be patulous, and on straining there is perineal descent and the prolapse may appear. In some patients, however, there may be a good sphincter and it may be necessary for them to strain in the squatting position before the prolapse occurs. Palpation will give some indication of the strength of the pelvic floor and sigmoidoscopy may show 'proctitis' up to approximately 8 cm (Table 66.8).

Management

Control of the prolapse

Many different surgical methods have been used to control complete prolapse [12, 51]. Some form of abdominal rectopexy is the most popular method and two techniques are in common use—in the United Kingdom polyvinyl alcohol sponge (Ivalon, Prosthex) is anchored to the presacral fascia behind the mobilized rectum and this is then wrapped around the rectum over three-quarters of its diameter (Fig. 66.15)

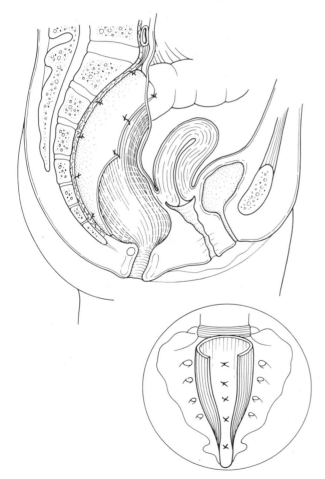

Fig. 66.15. Diagrammatic representation of the technique for abdominal rectopexy using polyvinyl alcohol sponge (Prosthex). Note how the material is fixed to presacral fascia.

994 Chapter 66

to fix it; in the United States mersilene mesh is attached to the front of the upper sacrum encircling the rectum after its complete mobilization. Both techniques give good results with only a 2–3% recurrence rate and an operative mortality of less than 1% [4, 22]. The major complication is sepsis around the implanted foreign material.

Re-education of bowel habit

Not all patients have a problem with defecation. It is important, though, that those who do should be helped to achieve an easy evacuation without straining. Oral laxatives, usually of the stimulant type, suppositories or enemas may be needed in addition to advice on diet and fluid intake (see Chapters 5 and 62).

Improvement of residual sphincter dysfunction

Most patients will lose all incontinence after rectopexy but, in those where it persists, a postanal sphincter repair may be required. As the muscles of the pelvic floor exhibit a neuro-myopathy [35], attempts at improving sphincter function with physiotherapy, faradic stimulation or electronic sphincters are usually unsuccessful.

Descending perineum syndrome

The descending perineum syndrome describes a condition found in patients with various anal symptoms who, when asked to strain, show marked descent of the perineum with loss of the anorectal angle [33]. The patients' symptoms can include anorectal bleeding, discharge of mucus, a feeling of incomplete rectal evacuation with obstruction to outflow, a constant bearing down sensation, discomfort and even anal pain. There is usually a long history of straining at stool which may lead to mucosal prolapse. The patient interprets this as a stool awaiting evacuation and responds

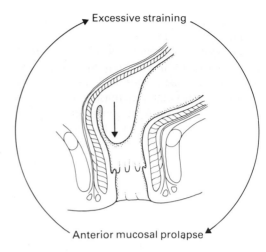

Fig. 66.16. The 'vicious circle' theory for the aetiology of rectal prolapse.

by further straining efforts—thus a vicious circle is created (Fig. 66.16). Finally incontinence develops.

Aetiology

It is thought this condition is caused by a traction neuropathy, which involves the nerve supply to the levator ani and external anal sphincter muscles. This may be caused by excessive defecatory straining or by damage at the time of childbirth.

Treatment

This is directed at avoiding straining at stool with bowel regulation and correction of any mucosal prolapse. Incontinence is best treated by a postanal repair [20]. It is also important to explain the nature of the problem to the patient. Clinicians unaware of the true nature of the diagnosis may attribute the symptoms to a psychosomatic problem.

Solitary ulcer syndrome

The solitary ulcer syndrome is also associated with excessive straining at stool [27].

The fundamental difference from the descending perineum syndrome is that during straining there is contraction, rather than relaxation, of the external anal sphincter and puborectalis. The mucosal changes, which may include ulceration, are thought to be caused by trauma to the mucosa against the contracting mucle [38].

The patient may complain of the passage of mucus and blood, with an inability to evacuate the rectum and excessive straining at stool. This latter symptom sometimes necessitates self-digitation which may aggravate the condition.

Sigmoidoscopic examination

This usually reveals reddening of the rectal mucosa with, in most patients, a pale ulcerated area in its centre. The ulceration may be present only on the anterior wall, in those with mucosal prolapse, or it may be circumferential in those with internal intussusception. On palpation the lesion may easily be confused with a carcinoma of the rectum and biopsy is essential—the typical appearances of traumatic proctitis should be present with smooth muscle fibres growing into the lamina propria.

Management

This can be very difficult. An explanation of the cause of the symptoms is important, as is advice on bowel regulation. It has recently been reported that healing is improved if the patient takes at least 30–40 g of dietary fibre per day [5]. Local treatment with steroid retention enemas or suppositories may reduce the amount of bleeding and discharge but seldom result in healing. Several surgeons have reported improvement after rectopexy.

Incontinence (Table 66.9) [43]

Faecal continence is normally maintained through a number of factors. These include sustained contraction of the internal (smooth muscle) and external (striated

Table 66.9. The causes of incontinence.

Normal sphincter	Severe diarrhoea
	Faecal impaction
Abnormal sphincter	Congenital abnormality
	Trauma
	Lower motor neuron lesions
	Complete rectal prolapse
	Idiopathic

muscle) sphincters, keeping the anal canal closed; the puborectalis muscle maintaining a normal (<90°) anorectal angle and the anterior rectal wall covering the anal canal as a 'flap valve' (Fig. 66.17).

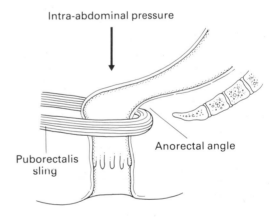

Fig. 66.17. The acute 'anorectal' angle created by the puborectalis sling. It is an important mechanism for faecal control.

Incontinence with a normal sphincter is usually due to **severe diarrhoea**, caused by an infection or inflammatory bowel disease, which may overwhelm the normal sphincter mechanism leading to incontinence. Alternatively, **faecal impaction**, sometimes called physiological incontinence, causes distension of the rectum which invokes a

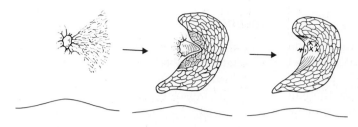

Fig. 66.18. The technique for an 'overlap' repair of the anal sphincter.

rectosphincteric relaxation reflex of the internal sphincter with incontinence.

Incontinence with an abnormal sphincter may be due to a larger range of problems.

Congenital abnormalities of the anal sphincter usually present in infancy and may be corrected by operative reconstruction by an experienced paediatric surgeon (see Chapters 62 and 77).

Trauma may distrupt the sphincter ring. Pelvic fractures, impalement, anal operations and obstetric injuries are the main causes. The gap in the sphincter ring can usually be detected clinically but electromyography will provide further useful information. An overlap repair (Fig. 66.18) is a relatively simple operation, although it requires temporary faecal diversion while healing occurs. Complete restoration of continence is achieved in 78% and significant improvement in a further 13% [7].

Lower motor neuron lesions affecting the anal sphincter mechanism are rare (< 2% in most series) and are mainly due to cauda equina tumours or trauma [41].

Complete rectal prolapse is associated with incontinence in approximately two-thirds of patients.

Idiopathic faecal incontinence is probably the commonest cause. There is now evidence that the muscle dysfunction is due to a localized neuropathy [35, 41] and is associated with the descending perineum syndrome. Because the muscle is defective, secondary to the neuropathy, physical and electrical methods of treatment are rarely successful. However continence may be restored by performing the operation of **post-anal sphincter repair** [20, 21, 33]. In this operation the external sphincter, puborectalis and levator ani are exposed by dissection in the intersphincteric space and are then darned loosely together with monofilament nylon, to lengthen the anal canal and restore the anorectal angle. Satisfactory continence is restored in approximately 80% of those operated upon in this way [8].

References

1 ALEXANDER-WILLIAMS J. Causes and management of anal irritation. *Br Med J* 1983;**287**:1528.

2 AMBROSE NS, HARES MM, ALEXANDER-WILLIAMS J, KEIGHLEY MRB. Prospective randomised comparison of photocoagulation and rubber band ligation in treatment of haemorrhoids. *Br Med J* 1983;**286**:1389–1391.

3 AMBROSE NS, MORRIS D, ALEXANDER-WILLIAMS J, KEIGHLEY MRB. A randomized trial of photocoagulation or injection sclerotherapy for the treatment of first- and second-degree hemorrhoids. *Dis Colon Rectum* 1985;**28**:238–240.

4 BOULOS PB, STRYKER SJ, NICHOLLS RJ. The long-term results of polyvinyl alcohol (Ivalon) sponge for rectal prolapse in young patients. *Br J Surg* 1984;**71**:213–214.

5 BRANDT-GRADEL VAN DEN, HUIBREGTSE K, TYTGAT GNJ. Treatment of solitary rectal ulcer syndrome with high-fibre diet and abstention of straining at defaecation. *Dig Dis Sci* 1984;**29**:1005–1008.

6 BRODEN, B, SNELLMAN B. Procidentia of the rectum studied with cineradiography; a contribution to the discussion of causative mechanisms. *Dis Colon Rectum* 1968;**11**:330–347.

7 BROWNING GGP, MOTSON RW. Results of Parks' operation for faecal incontinence after anal sphincter injury. *Br Med J* 1983;**1**:1873–1875.

8 BROWNING GGP, PARKS AG. Postanal repair for neuropathic faecal incontinence: correlation of clinical result and anal canal pressures. *Br J Surg* 1983;**70**:101–104.

9 COOPER PH, MILLS SE, ALLEN MS JR. Malignant melanoma of the anus. Report of 12 patients and

analysis of 255 additional cases. *Dis Colon Rectum* 1982;**25**:693–703.

10 GARTELL PG, SHERIDAN RJ, McGINN FP. Out-patient treatment of haemorrhoids: a randomised clinical trial to compare rubber-band ligation with phenol injection. *Br J Surg* 1985;**72**:478–479.

11 GOLDBERG SM. Closed haemorrhoidectomy. In: Todd, IP, FIELDING LP. *Rob and Smith's Operative Surgery*. 4th ed. London: Butterworths, 1983:489–494.

12 GOLIGHER JC. *Surgery of the Anus, Rectum and Colon*. 4th ed. London: Bailliere Tindal, 1980.

13 GOUGH MJ, LEWIS A. The conservative treatment of fissure-in-ano. *Br J Surg* 1983;**70**:175–176.

14 GRACE RH, HARPER IA, THOMPSON RG. Anorectal sepsis: microbiology in relation to fistula-in-ano. *Br J Surg* 1982;**69**:401–403.

15 GREENALL MJ, QUAN SHQ, STEARNS MW, URMACHER C, DeCOSSEE JJ. Epidermoid cancer of the anal margin. Pathological features, treatment and clinical results. *Am J Surg* 1985;**149**:98–101.

16 HANCOCK BD. Lord's procedure for haemorrhoids: a prospective anal pressure study. *Br J Surg* 1981;**68**:729–730.

17 JAMES RD, POINTON RS, MARTIN S,. Local radiotherapy in the management of squamous carcinoma of the anus. *Br J Surg* 1985;**72**:282–285.

18 JEFFREY PJ, RITCHIE JK, PARKS AG. Treatment of haemorrhoids in patients with inflammatory bowel disease. *Lancet* 1977;**i**:1084–1085.

19 JENSEN SL. Comparison of podophyllin application with simple surgical excision in clearance and recurrence of perianal condylomata acuminata. *Lancet* 1985;**ii**:1146–1148.

20 KEIGHLEY MRB. Postanal repair for faecal incontinence (review). *J R Soc Med* 1984;**77**:258–288.

21 KEIGHLEY MRB, FIELDING JWL. Management of faecal incontinence and results of surgical treatment. *Br J Surg* 1983;**70**:463–468.

22 KEIGHLEY MRB, FIELDING JWL, ALEXANDER-WILLIAMS J. Results of Marlex mesh abdominal rectopexy for rectal prolapse in 100 consecutive patients. *Br J Surg* 1983;**70**:229–232.

23 LEACH RD, EYKYN SJ, PHILLIPS A, *et al*. Anaerobic axillary abscesses. *Br Med J* 1979;**2**:5–7.

24 LEWIS AAM, ROGERS HS, LEIGHTON M. Trial of maximal anal dilatation, cryotherapy and elastic-band ligation as alternatives to haemorrhoidectomy in the treatment of large prolapsed haemorrhoids. *Br J Surg* 1983;**70**:54–56.

25 LOCK MR, THOMSON JPS. Fissure-in-ano: the initial management and prognosis. *Br J Surg* 1977;**64**:355–358.

26 McDONALD P, DRISCOLL AM, NICHOLLS RJ. The anal dilator in the conservative management of acute anal fissure. *Br J Surg* 1983;**70**:25–26.

27 MADIGAN MR, MORSON BC. Solitary ulcer of the rectum. *Gut* 1969;**10**:871–881.

28 MANN CV. Open haemorrhoidectomy (St Mark's ligation/excision method). In: Todd IP, Fielding LP, eds. *Rob and Smith's Operative Surgery*, 4th ed. London: Butterworths, 1983:495–502.

29 MORSON BC, DAWSON IMP. *Gastrointestinal Pathology*. 2nd ed. Oxford: Blackwell Scientific Publications, 1979.

30 MURIE JA, SIM AJW, MACKENZIE I. Rubber band ligation versus haemorrhoidectomy for prolapsing haemorrhoids: a long-term prospective clinical trial. *Br J Surg* 1982;**69**:536–538.

31 PARKS AG. Haemorrhoidectomy. In: Todd IP, Fielding LP, eds. *Rob and Smith's Operative Surgery*. 4th ed. London: Butterworths, 1983:480–488.

32 PARKS AG, GORDON PH, HARDCASTLE JD. A classification of fistula-in-ano. *Br J Surg* 1976;**63**:1–12.

33 PARKS AG & PERCY J. Postanal pelvic floor repair for anorectal incontinence. In: Todd IP, Fielding LP, eds. *Rob and Smith's Operative Surgery*. 4th ed. London: Butterworths, 1983:433–438.

34 PARKS AG, PORTER NH, HARDCASTLE J. The syndrome of the descending perineum. *Proc R Soc Med* 1966;**59**:477–482.

35 PARKS AG, SWASH M, URICH H. Sphincter denervation in anorectal incontinence and rectal prolapse. *Gut* 1977;**18**:656–665.

36 PYPER PC, PARKS TG. The results of surgery for epidermoid carcinoma of the anus. *Br J Surg* 1985;**72**:712–714.

37 QUINN TC, COREY L, CHAFFEE R, *et al*. The etiology of anorectal infections in homosexual men. *Ann Intern Med* 1981;**71**:395–406.

38 RUTTER KRP, RIDDELL RH. The solitary ulcer syndrome of the rectum. *Clin Gastroenterol* 1975;**4**:505–530.

39 SALMON RJ, FENTON J, ASSELAIN B, *et al*. Treatment of epidermoid anal canal cancer. *Am J Surg* 1984;**147**:43–48.

40 SOUTHAM JA. Haemorrhoids treated by cryotherapy: a critical analysis. *Ann R Coll Surg Engl* 1983;**65**:237–239.

41 SWASH M. The neuropathology of idiopathic faecal incontinence. In: Smith WT, Cavenagh JB, eds. *Recent Advances in Neuropathology*. London: Churchill Livingstone, 1982:243–270.

42 TEMPLETON JL, SPENCE RAJ, KENNEDY TL, PARKS TG, MACKENZIE G, HANNA WA. Comparison of infrared coagulation and rubber-band ligation for first and second degree haemorrhoids: a randomised prospective clinical trial. *Br Med J* 1983;**286**:1387–1389.

43 THOMSON JPS. Anal sphincter incompetence. In: Russell RCG, ed. *Recent Advances in Surgery* No. 12. London: Churchill Livingstone 1986:155–178.

44 THOMSON JPS, GRACE RG. Perianal and anal condylomata acuminata. In: Todd IP, Fielding LP, eds. *Rob and Smith's Operative Surgery*. 4th ed. London: Butterworths, 1983:538–541.

45 THOMSON JPS, PARKS AG. Contemporary surgery:

anal abscesses and fistulas. *Br J Hosp Med* 1979;21:413–435.

46 THOMSON WG. Proctalgia fugax. *Dig Dis Sci* 1981;26:1121–1124.

47 THOMSON WHF. The nature of haemorrhoids. *Br J Surg* 1975;62:542–545.

48 THOMSON WHF. The real nature of 'perianal haematoma' *Lancet* 1975;i:467–468.

49 TRAYNOR OJ, CARTER AE. Cryotherapy for advanced haemorrhoids: a prospective evaluation with a 2 year follow-up. *Br J Surg* 1984;71:287–289.

50 WARD MWN, ROMANÒ G, NICHOLLS RJ. The surgical treatment of anorectal malignant melaenoma. *Br J Surg* 1986;73:68–69.

51 WATTS JD, ROTHERNBERGER DA, BULS JG, GOLDBERG SM, NIVATVONGS S. The management of procidentia: 30 years' experience. *Dis Colon Rectum* 1985;28:96–102.

52 WRIGHT JE. Inhaled salbutamol for proctalgia fugax. *Lancet* 1985;ii:659–660.

SECTION XI

FUNCTIONAL DISORDERS OF THE GUT

Chapter 67
Irritable Bowel Syndrome

C. D. HOLDSWORTH

Organic disease cannot be found in up to 60% of out-patients presenting with either abdominal pain or bowel disturbance. Although the nature and severity of the symptoms in such patients vary considerably, in the majority there are sufficient common features to enable the recognition of a syndrome [15]. For much of this century the condition has been called 'spastic colon' or 'irritable colon' syndrome. It is now recognized that in these patients symptoms can arise from virtually any part of the gastrointestinal tract and the term irritable bowel syndrome has become generally accepted [20, 24, 32].

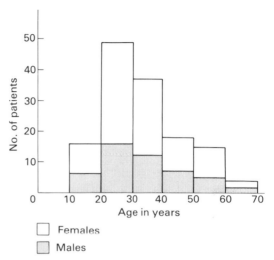

Fig. 67.1. Age and sex distribution of a consecutive series of patients with irritable bowel syndrome [7].

Prevalence

It is not possible to collect comparative international statistics for a condition that has no pathology, no mortality, no diagnostic tests and normally does not cause admission to hospital. It is certainly universal in Western and may be as common in other cultures.

In patients presenting to hospital out-patient clinics the condition is commoner in women than men, with a ratio approximately 2:1 in most recent series. The age distribution shown in Fig. 67.1 is typical—the maximal incidence is in women during their reproductive years. It is much less common for symptoms to develop for the first time over the age of 40. Patients presenting over this age require particularly careful investigation to exclude organic disease.

The prevalence of irritable bowel

syndrome in the community has been little studied, but it has been suggested [34] that one or more symptoms of the syndrome occur in about 30% of normal non-complaining adults. It may well be that only the more neurotic of such individuals report their symptoms to a doctor and are referred to hospital, or that those individuals with symptoms only report to their doctors when they are under stress, or coincidentally develop depression [21, 33]. This may account for the high proportion of neuroticism and depression in patients who present as hospital out-patients with the irritable bowel syndrome (see Chapter 68).

Aetiology

Abnormal smooth muscle activity is demonstrable in the irritable bowel syndrome and is doubtless responsible for many of its manifestations. For example, pain can be correlated with colonic spasm or distension, and diarrhoea is associated with rapid small and large bowel transit. These pathophysiological correlates of symptoms will be discussed later, but it is likely that they are in most patients largely secondary to the psychiatric abnormalities, rather than due to any intrinsic abnormality of smooth muscle.

Personality

There is general agreement amongst clinicians that most patients with the irritable bowel syndrome have an increased number of abnormal personality traits. All objective psychological studies have confirmed this long-held clinical impression. All objective psychological studies have confirmed this long-held clinical impression. There is no specific personality profile, and the severity of psychiatric disability correlates poorly with severity of bowel symptoms. In general, patients with irritable bowel syndrome are more anxious, depressed and neurotic than controls [30, 37, 41].

Depression is common. In one of the earliest objective studies, 70% of the women were judged as depressed, some to the extent of being suicidal [10]. Another series reported a 45% incidence of depression with a total prevalence of psychiatric illness of 72%, compared to 18% in controls [41]. Attempts to correlate specific psychiatric abnormalities with specific symptoms have met with mixed success. Esler & Goulston [6] claimed greater scores of anxiety, neuroticism and introversion in 'diarrhoea predominant' irritable bowel patients, but only high scores for neuroticism in patients with 'predominant pain'. Whitehead, Engel & Schuster [38] could not find personality traits that correlated particularly with diarrhoea or constipation, but confirmed significantly increased abnormal personality

traits, in particular anxiety, abnormal interpersonal sensitivity, depression, hostility and somatization of affect.

The irritable bowel syndrome may, therefore, be largely attributable to psychological factors [37]. It is certainly an everyday clinical observation that, in susceptible individuals, stress often provokes or exacerbates the symptoms. It is not clear, however, why some patients with a personality disorder develop bowel symptoms and others do not, and it remains a possibility that in some patients the abnormal personality traits are secondary to the symptoms rather than their cause. It may be that there is also some as yet unidentified genetic predisposition to disordered function of bowel muscle.

Food intolerance

An abnormal reaction to a particular food has often been suggested as an aetiological factor, but is difficult to prove. A group of patients with diarrhoea as the main manifestation, had symptoms that remitted on elimination diets, but recurred when certain specific foods such as wheat, corn, dairy products, tea or coffee were re-introduced [1]. In a few patients symptoms were reproduced and rectal production of prostaglandin E_2 increased when the suspect food was introduced in a double-blind fashion by nasogastric tube [1].

There seems to be little doubt that food intolerance is a true entity, but its frequency as a cause of irritable bowel syndrome remains to be established. This type of food intolerance is quite distinct from the rare food allergies which cause immediate bowel symptoms, often with a rash (see Chapter 75).

Other aetiological factors

In some patients the syndrome is provoked by dysentery or gastroenteritis and may then persist for months, years, or permanently. Surgery may be blamed by patients for initiating the symptoms, but a scrutiny of their records usually shows that symptoms were present before operation. A fibre-deficient diet has also been blamed for the condition, but studies have failed to show any difference in fibre intake between patients with irritable bowel and age and sex-matched controls [7]. In some there is a history of purgative abuse, but this was far more common in the past; often the purgatives have been prescribed for the symptoms.

Clinical features

As can be seen from Table 67.1, possible symptoms are legion, and permutations infinite. Although in any one individual the pattern of symptoms tends to remain the same, during exacerbations new symptoms may arise, necessitating further investigation.

The commonest symptoms are undoubtedly abdominal pain, disturbance of bowel habit and abdominal distension or 'wind'. When all these symptoms are present (particularly if they are of long standing), are associated with psychiatric manifestations, and occur in a woman aged between 20 and 40 years, it may be possible to make a clinical diagnosis with a fair degree of certainty. However, differentiation from organic disease can be difficult and may at times require extensive investigation.

Abdominal pain

This can be anywhere in the abdomen (Fig. 67.2) but is most commonly in the right or

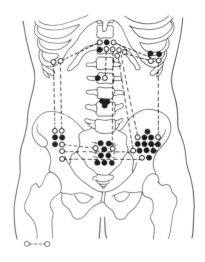

Fig. 67.2. Distribution sites of abdominal pain in 38 patients with irritable bowel (29 ●; nine ○ ---- ○). ● = single site of pain; ○ ---- ○ = multiple sites of pain in the same patient [36].

left iliac fossa, or both. It can be of any degree of severity. Most often it is described as an ache or, much less commonly, as colic. Its colonic origin may be obvious if it is relieved, even temporarily, by defaecation or passing wind. In a minority the pain is worse following defaecation. Association of

Table 67.1. Symptoms of irritable bowel syndrome.

Common G.I. symptoms	Other G. I. symptoms	Non G.I. symptoms
Abdominal pain	Nausea	Dysmenorrhoea
Bowel disturbance (including urgency and incontinence)	Vomiting	Dyspareunia
	Heartburn	Urinary frequency
Passage of mucus	Dyspepsia	Loin pain
Sense of incomplete evacuation	Globular hystericus	Pain in back, thighs
Abdominal distension		Psychiatric
'Wind'		

Chapter 67

Table 67.2. Mean small bowel transit time, determined by breath hydrogen technique, and total bowel transit time, determined by radio-opaque markers, in 44 patients with irritable bowel syndrome, compared with 53 matched control subjects [4].

Mean daily stool weights are shown separately for the 12 males and nine females with diarrhoea, and 21 females with constipation.

	Control	Irritable bowel syndrome	
		Diarrhoea ($n=21$)	Constipation ($n=23$)
Small bowel transit (h)	4.2 ± 0.2	3.3 ± 0.3	5.4 ± 0.3
Total bowel transit (50% markers) (h)	53 ± 4	35 ± 5	78 ± 13
Daily stool weight (g) (Females) (Males)	112 ± 12 166 ± 20	128 ± 25 230 ± 21	61 ± 17 —

Mean $\pm$ SEM

the pain with the gastrointestinal tract may also be obvious if pain follows eating, either immediately, or with a delay of up to two or three hours. If pain is unrelated to eating or defaecation, the differential diagnosis can be more difficult. This is particularly true if, as in many women, the intensity of discomfort varies with the menstrual cycle, or is worse on sexual intercourse. In some patients pain occurs at a particular time of the day, often the evening or, less commonly, at night.

Pain can also occur at sites not shown in Fig. 67.2, for example, in the left side of the chest, left shoulder, back, or down the thigh.

Constipation and diarrhoea

Some disturbance of bowel habit exists in 75% or more of patients. 'Constipation predominant' or 'diarrhoea predominant' cases do occur, but most patients have a variable bowel habit.

Constipation in the irritable bowel syndrome is almost always confined to females. **Diarrhoea** occurs in both sexes and can often be distinguished from that due to organic disease, by a careful history and by observation of stool at sigmoidoscopy or in a bed pan. The stools may be fluid and, especially if associated with mucus, may mimic those of inflammatory bowel disease. More often they are pellety, like sheep droppings, or normal in consistency. Stool weights also reflect this, being not very much greater than normal, even if stool frequency is much increased (Table 67.2). It is **stool frequency**, urgency of defaecation and sometimes minor **incontinence** that characterize the diarrhoea of the irritable bowel syndrome. Particularly common is a **'morning rush syndrome'**, in which the patient on arising and soon after breakfast passes several small, bitty stools, and even then has a sense of incomplete evacuation of the bowels. **Mucus** may accompany the stools in constipation or diarrhoea; indeed, the 'diarrhoea' sometimes consists solely of frequent passage of small amounts of mucus, normal or constipated stools being passed only occasionally and independently. Fifty years ago much was written of this 'mucous colitis', patients being reported to pass coagulated mucus in considerable quantities. This is now rarely seen, and was probably due to the widespread use of purgatives.

Unfortunately, stool frequency, urgency, the 'morning rush syndrome' and mucus may also occur with many types of organic diarrhoea.

Abdominal distension or 'wind'

This very frequent symptom can occur in patients whose other major complaint is either pain, constipation or diarrhoea. It is often described as swelling of the lower abdomen, particularly in the evening. The swelling may be so severe that clothing has to be loosened to provide comfort. The distension is usually largely subjective, being a source of considerable distress to the patient when not even discernible on physical examination.

Being 'full of wind' is often associated with 'distension', but most patients using this term are also describing a definite sensation of gas being trapped in their bowel. They may hear borborygmi and see or feel movement of gas in the bowels with relief of discomfort when the gas is passed *per anum*. Flatus is usually passed in normal, but occasionally, excessive amounts. Belching may occur, but is usually clearly due to aerophagy. In some patients gas appears to the patient to be consistently trapped at the same site; if this is in the left hypochondrium, the condition has been graced by the term 'splenic flexure syndrome'. In others gas appears to be trapped in the caecum.

Non-gastrointestinal symptoms [40]

Gynaecological symptoms are common; dysmenorrhoea is frequent, but more puzzling and very frequent is dyspareunia. This may be due to lower abdominal tenderness on external pressure, or there may be an internal dyspareunia causing immediate pain and aching, which persists after intercourse. In addition, the bowel symptoms may themselves be more prominent at certain stages of the menstrual cycle.

Urinary frequency, urinary urgency, and sometimes pain on micturition is frequent, mainly in females. As colonic pain can be referred to the loin, renal disease can be closely mimicked.

Back pain can occur and, as colonic pain can be referred to the thigh, orthopaedic or neurological conditions may also be suspected. **Migraine and headache** are commoner in children than adults.

Psychiatric symptoms are as variable as the somatic manifestations. Depressive symptoms, such as fatigue, lowering of mood, and sleep disturbance are frequent. They are difficult to assess, as any chronic and painful disorder can induce similar depressive symptoms, but the depression is far more frequent than in organic disorders such as Crohn's disease, which can cause comparable, or far greater discomfort and disability [17]. Over half of the patients recognize that symptoms have been made worse by stress. In others, the source of the stress is not admitted at the time but is recognized much later when symptoms are found to have remitted—for example, improvement after the dissolution of an unhappy marriage. For a full discussion of the psychiatric aspects of alimentary symptoms see Chapter 68.

Previous history of abdominal surgery

There is often a history of appendicectomy, cholecystectomy, laparotomy 'to divide adhesions' or laparotomy for suspected endometriosis. In retrospect it may be clear that the surgery was misguided, as symptoms have persisted and were clearly due to the irritable bowel syndrome. Appendicectomy for chronic right iliac fossa pain is rarely successful [2]. Studies of patients with irritable bowel published 20 years or more ago report previous appendicectomy in as many as 36% [27], but in a recent personal series of 68 patients, only 10 (15%) had undergone an appendicectomy, suggesting that surgeons have learned to be more cautious than in the past when faced with the problem of chronic abdominal pain. With modern, more accurate diagnostic techniques, exploratory laparotomies for the irritable bowel syndrome are fortunately becoming less common.

Common symptom patterns

Although the clinical picture is diverse, three main types can usefully be distinguished.

Patients with predominant pain

If the pain is associated with bowel symptoms, categorization is straightforward. If the pain is present in an unusual site (e.g. the back, or left upper leg), diagnosis is more difficult. Sometimes only observation and investigation over a period of time, or the development of other symptoms make diagnosis possible.

Patients with predominant constipation

Constipation as an isolated symptom is best considered separately but, if associated with pain or alternating with diarrhoea, the 'spastic colon' variant of the irritable bowel syndrome can again be diagnosed after appropriate investigation (see Chapters 5 and 65).

Patients with predominant chronic diarrhoea

This is the least common symptom pattern. Patients with chronic diarrhoea who experience little pain are perhaps better labelled as having nervous or functional diarrhoea, rather than an irritable bowel. If, as is more often the case, there is also abdominal pain, the more appropriate label is diarrhoea-predominant irritable bowel syndrome.

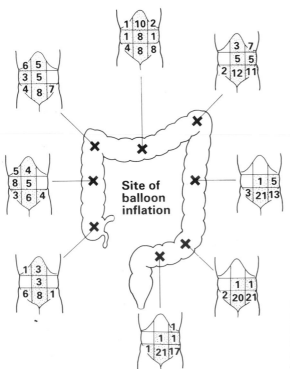

Fig. 67.3. The distribution of abdominal pain induced by balloon inflation in 48 patients investigated for abdominal pain apparently due to irritable bowel syndrome [31].

Pathophysiology of symptoms

Many of the symptoms can be explained in terms of disordered smooth muscle activity or of enhanced visceral sensation [16, 29]. Ritchie [26] clearly demonstrated that a significantly higher proportion of irritable bowel patients than controls complain of pain when a balloon within the sigmoid colon is inflated. Abdominal pain in any site can be reproduced in most irritable bowel patients by a balloon inflated somewhere within the colon or small intestine (Fig. 67.3); the pain from colonic distension in these patients could also be felt in the back, lower ribs, shoulder, groin, thigh or perineum [14, 29]. Others have shown that gas infused into the small intestine of irritable bowel patients produces more discomfort and subjective distension than similar gas infusions into normal subjects [18]. Motility studies have consistently shown increased colonic contractions in response to food and to psychological stress. Small bowel as well as large bowel transit is faster in irritable bowel patients with diarrhoea than in normal subjects (Table 67.2). This may be a manifestation of stress, as stress in normal subjects can speed bowel transit. Abnormal bowel motility has also been shown in psychoneurotic subjects with no abdominal complaints [19]. It may be that patients with irritable bowel syndrome have a bowel that is in some way more sensitive, or 'irritable' than normal subjects, which renders them prone to abdominal symptoms when under stress, or when they develop depression, or other psychiatric illness.

Differential diagnosis

In total this is vast, as the irritable bowel syndrome can mimic so many disorders, but certain conditions are particularly liable to cause confusion [25].

Inflammatory bowel disease: Ulcerative colitis is only occasionally mistaken for the irritable bowel syndrome and vice-versa, as sigmoidoscopy and rectal biopsy usually distinguish the two [33]. Crohn's disease is more commonly initially misdiagnosed as irritable bowel, because both cause abdominal pain and bowel disturbance and often begin in young adults. Should weight loss, or any systemic disturbance develop in a patient thought to have an irritable bowel, reinvestigation by small bowel radiology, barium enema, or colonoscopy should be undertaken. Conversely, the irritable bowel syndrome is such a common disorder that it may coexist with inflammatory bowel disease. Diarrhoea in a patient with ulcerative colitis is sometimes inappropriately treated with corticosteroids when it is really due to a coexisting irritable bowel, or even self-purgation.

Amoebic or bacillary dysentery need exclusion by appropriate tests, specify particularly in endemic areas. Symptoms of an irritable bowel may first develop after dysentery and lead to frequent but negative re-investigation. **Giardiasis** can be an elusive diagnosis.

Diverticular disease of the colon causes left iliac fossa pain and bowel disturbance, and it may coexist with an irritable bowel. Symptoms due to diverticular disease are unusual below the age of 40, whereas the initial onset of an irritable bowel is usually earlier.

Carcinoma of the colon may be missed in patients with a pre-existing irritable bowel. New symptoms in patients with known irritable bowel (for example, the passing of blood) often need a further barium enema or colonoscopy.

Chronic pancreatitis and carcinoma of the pancreas cause abdominal pain, with initial investigations that are often normal.

Malabsorption causing diarrhoea is sometimes misdiagnosed as irritable bowel. The presence of true diarrhoea, as opposed to frequent pellety stools, is an indication for estimation of faecal fat.

Alactasia can also cause diarrhoea, but is so common that it may be an incidental and irrelevant finding in a patient with the irritable bowel syndrome. A trial of dietary exclusion of milk is often worthwhile; this is often more useful and certainly more convenient than a diagnostic test for alactasia, although improvement of symptoms may also occur in the rare allergy to milk as well as in alactasia.

Peptic ulcer and reflux oesophagitis may be mimicked by an irritable bowel [33]. Equally, they may be found during investigation, but not be the cause of the main disability. Usually peptic ulcer will respond to medical treatment and residual symptoms after ulcer healing can then be distinguished as due to an irritable bowel. In the fit patient coincidental gallstones may lead to cholecystectomy to prevent future morbidity, but the patient should be warned that the symptoms may continue after operation.

Physical examination

Thorough general physical examination is essential in any patient with suspected irritable bowel syndrome, as it is in any patient with abdominal symptoms, in order to exclude any endocrine or systemic disorder that may be causing abdominal pain or bowel symptoms. The physical accompaniments of anxiety or depression will often be obvious; it is claimed that cool, clammy hands and neurodermatitis are both present in more than 50% of these patients [13].

Abdominal tenderness is frequently present and it can be elicited anywhere along the colon, although most often in the left iliac fossa. Rebound tenderness can occur and at times mislead a surgeon into the diagnosis of local peritonitis. Deep tenderness on rectal examination is striking in a few patients and can be similarly misleading. Excessive borborygmi are audible in some patients. Occasionally colon in spasm can be felt as a tender hard cord, and the rare patient may have visible colonic contractions.

Sigmoidoscopy is particularly useful, and should be an essential part of the physical examination in a patient with a suspected irritable bowel syndrome. Essentially sigmoidoscopic appearances are normal: the mucosa may be somewhat duskier than usual; this hyperaemia with loss of the normal vessel pattern (a common non-specific finding in any patient with diarrhoea) can cause the unwary to diagnose ulcerative colitis. Rectal biopsy should be done if there is the slightest suspicion of abnormality—some would say in all cases, as on rare occasions biopsy of normal-looking mucosa reveals inflammatory bowel disease. Sigmoidoscopy also provides a valuable opportunity to inspect colonic contents; pellety stools with a little mucus are typical of the irritable bowel, although there can also be a true fluid diarrhoea. The pale yellow, sticky stools of steatorrhoea, or the presence of blood obviously indicate some other diagnosis. An empty or full rectum and the nature of the stool, help in the assessment of constipation. Some observers claim that a hypermotile sigmoid colon (the 'winking colon' sign) is usually present. Reproducing the patient's pain by inflation of air into the sigmoid colon is useful for diagnosis and for explanation to the patient of the nature of his or her symptoms.

Investigation and diagnosis

Investigations, by definition, in patients with the irritable bowel syndrome are normal. Tests may even be misleading by revealing common conditions such as gallstones, colonic diverticular disease, hiatus hernia or gastro-oesophageal reflux, or even peptic ulcer, which are not causing the patient's symptoms.

Most patients need only to have a full blood count and perhaps a barium enema, but occasionally investigation has to be much more extensive. How extensive depends on the nature and duration of the symptoms, the age of the patient and, it must be admitted, on the personal bias and experience of the investigator. Should, for example, a constipated young woman in perfect health, but with right iliac fossa pain, be subjected to the incovenience, expense and irradiation involved in colonic and small intestinal radiology merely because there is a slight possibility of Crohn's disease—a condition in which early diagnosis in any case will not affect prognosis? Over the age of 40 years any new symptoms, even if associated with stress and very suggestive of an irritable bowel, should be investigated as organic disease is likely.

The nature, extent and sequence of investigations, apart from simple tests such as a blood count, ESR and microscopy of urine, depend upon the presenting symptoms.

A barium enema is usually necessary, but not invariably so, particularly in the young person. In experienced hands, in addition to excluding organic disease, it is claimed that there may be characteristic findings, such as reduced diameter, increased haustral markings and areas of spasm which relax with relief of pain on injection of an anticholinergic drug, or glucagon [22, 27].

The patient with true diarrhoea, rather than the commoner increased bowel frequency, will often require estimation of 24-hour stool fat, thyroid function, stool culture and microscopy, radiological examination of large and small intestine and perhaps jejunal biopsy, the exclusion of alactasia by a suitable technique, and estimation of urine 5-hydroxyindoleacetic acid. Concealed purgative taking may need exclusion. Upper abdominal symptoms often need endoscopy, and exclusion of gallbladder or pancreatic disease, lower abdominal pain may require laparoscopy usually by the gynaecologist. Incontinence may need ano-rectal manometry for clarification.

Management

There is no specific treatment for the irritable bowel syndrome, and it is often a chronic, perhaps life-long disorder. Management demands the establishment of a satisfactory therapeutic relationship between doctor and patient, as this is a prerequisite for the explanation and reassurance which are fundamental in the treatment of this condition. This is emphasized in Table 67.3, which outlines a suggested order of management.

Table 67.3. Management of irritable bowel syndrome.

History and physical examination
Provisional diagnosis and reassurance
Investigation
Further explanation and reassurance
Dietary advice; drug treatment (Table 67.4)

The worst possible approach to such patients is to investigate their symptoms in an impersonal manner and then confront them with the fact that the investigations show nothing wrong—implying that they must be emotionally disturbed and imagining their symptoms. The patient will depart resentful and probably demand an urgent second opinion.

History and physical examination

The taking, in a sympathetic manner, of a careful and detailed history with a subsequent physical examination is an essential prerequisite to establishing a therapeutic relationship. Although the stress and personality factors may well emerge during questions about family relationships and occupation, detailed questions to probe these aspects should not be asked until the patient's confidence has been won by showing interest and concern for the abdominal symptoms. Leading questions about common symptoms not spontaneously volunteered, such as abdominal swelling and distension, pellety stools and, in patients with diarrhoea, urgency and incontinence, produce relief which is obvious in the patient's face, as he or she appreciates that they have found someone who understands their condition. During sigmoidoscopy this impression will be reinforced if trouble is taken to ask if inflation of air reproduces their pain.

Provisional diagnosis and reassurance

At this stage, on first interview, it is often possible to make a diagnosis, and to reassure the patient that organic disease is unlikely. Explanation that this is 'the commonest disorder I see' often relieves the patient, particularly if he or she has previously had the 'there is nothing wrong, it's all in the mind' approach. It may also be useful to state at this stage that the symptoms can be helped, but perhaps not cured. Then the patient can be told that, to be completely certain, some investigations will be done and the situation re-assessed.

Further explanation and reassurance

After investigation, if normal, a further explanation of the symptoms in physiological terms may be appropriate. Spasm, or muscle cramp are terms understood by most patients and analogies with asthma or migraine can be helpful. A detailed psychiatric history is often more acceptable to the patient at this stage, particularly seeking depressive symptoms which may affect the choice of drug therapy. Referral to a psychiatrist is necessary only if there is severe depression, if suicide is threatened, or if a complicated situation is revealed or suspected. The patient may then welcome

a psychiatric consultation, but in others any hint of this will arouse unnecessary hostility and loss of confidence. Relaxation techniques using biofeedback or hypnosis may be helpful [9, 39].

Dietary advice

Patients usually ask for dietary advice. They may volunteer that certain foods upset them—lettuce, tomatoes and onions are frequently blamed—and it is reasonable to agree with the patient that these should be excluded. Excessive coffee or tea should be discouraged in patients with diarrhoea. If food intolerance is suspected and the patient is sufficiently motivated, exclusion diets can be tried, with subsequent introduction of other foods [1].

High fibre diet or supplementary bran is often recommended as if this was a universal panacea—such a diet is undoubtedly valuable for constipation. For other symptoms it may be no better than a placebo [4]. Sufficient fibre can be recommended to prevent the formation of hard stools, the amount being increased until the motions are semi-formed. Increase of dietary fibre intake should be gradual, as sudden changes may provoke abdominal distension and flatus.

Drug treatment

The main types of drugs used are listed in Table 67.4.

Table 67.4. Types of drugs used in treatment of irritable bowel syndrome [11].

Antidiarrhoeal agents
Anticholinergic drugs
Other antispasmodics
Stool bulking agents
Tranquilizers
Antidepressants

Antidiarrhoeal drugs

Traditional remedies for acute diarrhoea, such as kaolin, are not useful, but the three antidiarrhoeal agents (codeine phosphate 30 mg, diphenoxylate 2.5 mg with atropine, or loperamide 2 mg) are valuable. They decrease not only stool frequency but, what is more important to the patient, also help urgency and incontinence [27]. The dose should be tailored in amount and timing to the patient's symptoms. Side-effects are least common with loperamide, but for many patients the other two are as satisfactory. Codeine phosphate does, however, have mild potential for addiction and its long-term use is best avoided.

Antispasmodic drugs

Most of these are anticholinergic drugs. Examples include mebeverine (Colofac), dicyclomine hydrochloride (Merbentyl), and mepenzolate bromide (Cantil). They can help some patients, mainly relieving pain, but in the irritable bowel syndrome any drug can evoke a placebo response, and few placebo-controlled double-blind studies have been done [12].

Stool bulking agents

Some constipated patients, who are upset by a high wheat-fibre diet or bran, find that other vegetable fibre products provide useful relief. These differ not only chemically, but also in their metabolism by colonic bacteria and it is worth trying more than one. Ispaghula may be tried first (Isogel, Fybogel, Regulan), then sterculia (Normacol Special), or methylcellulose (Celevac, Cologel). Purgatives should be avoided.

Tranquillizers

These have been widely recommended and do often produce temporary benefit, but for a chronic condition such as the irritable bowel syndrome there is a danger in encouraging dependence on a benzodiazepine drug, such as diazepam. They should only be prescribed for short-term use if there is an acute exacerbation related to a particular stress.

Antidepressant drugs

These should always be tried if there is any suggestion of associated depression, even if the patient is adamant that the depression is secondary to the intractable abdominal pain. They should be used more frequently than tranquillizers, but careful explanation is required about likely initial side-effects and the delay before therapeutic response can be expected. They may make constipation worse. Amitriptyline or dothiepin 25–75 mg at bedtime will help many patients, without causing excessive daytime sedation [41].

Combination therapy

Not infrequently patients find themselves taking more than one drug, for example, a stool bulking agent, an antidepressant and an anticholinergic drug. Most clinicians still prefer to tailor treatment to the patient and avoid multiple drug therapy.

Other drugs

In patients with functional dyspepsia as part of the syndrome, antacids and metoclopramide may be helpful, although nausea can unfortunately be particularly intractable.

Prognosis

There is no suggestion of any important morbidity, or progression to carcinoma or ulcerative colitis, and patients are often relieved to learn this [8]. Unfortunately there is also little evidence that treatment really affects the course of the condition. In one study, after one year of follow-up only six out of 50 patients were symptom-free, 18 showed some clinical improvement, 25 were unchanged, but only one was worse [36]. These and other authors suggest that follow-up in a clinic has therapeutic value, but the condition is so common that a sympathetic gastroenterologist would soon find himself completely occupied with such patients. Some skill and tact is necessary to encourage these patients to survive without frequent medical consultations, but to attend for re-investigation should symptoms alter or weight loss occur.

Post-dysenteric irritable bowel syndrome patients have a more favourable prognosis [5], but in others prognosis only seems to be improved if some change for the better occurs in the patient's social or family circumstances.

References

1 ALUN JONES V, SHORTHOUSE M, McLAUGHLAN P, WORKMAN E, HUNTER JO. Food intolerance: a major factor in the pathogenesis of irritable bowel syndrome. *Lancet* 1982;ii:1115–1117.

2 ALVAREZ WC. When should one operate for 'chronic appendicitis'? *JAMA* 1940;114:1301–1306.

3 CANN PA, READ NW, BROWN C, HOBSON N, HOLDSWORTH CD. Irritable bowel syndrome: relationship of disorders in the transit of a single solid meal to symptom patterns. *Gut* 1981;24:405–411.

4 CANN PA, READ NW, HOLDSWORTH CD. What is the benefit of coarse wheat bran in patients with the irritable bowel? *Gut* 1984;25:168–173.

5 CHAUDHARY NA, TRUELOVE SC. The irritable colon syndrome. A study of the clinical features predisposing causes and prognosis in 130 cases. *Q J Med* 1962;31:307–322.

6 ESLER MD, GOULSTON KJ. Levels of anxiety in colonic disorders. *N Engl J Med* 1973;288:16–20.

7 FIELDING JF. The irritable bowel syndrome. Part I: Clinical Spectrum. TP Almy, JF Fielding, eds. *Clin Gastroenterol* 1977;6:3:607–622.

8 HASTRUP SVENDSEN J, MUNCK LK, ANDERSEN JR. Irritable bowel syndrome—prognosis and diagnostic safety. A 5-year follow-up study. *Scand J Gastroenterol* 1985;20:415–418.

9 HEALTH AND PUBLIC POLICY COMMITTEE. Biofeedback for gastrointestinal disorders. *Ann Int Med* 1985;103:291–293.

10 HISLOP IG. Psychological significance of the irritable colon syndrome. *Gut* 1971;12:452–457.

11 HOLDSWORTH CD. Drug treatment of irritable bowel syndrome. In: Read NW ed. *Irritable bowel syndrome*. London: Grune & Stratton, 1985:223–232.

12 IVEY KJ. Are anticholinergics of use in the irritable colon syndrome? *Gastroenterology* 1975;68:1300–1306.

13 KEELING PWN, FIELDING JF. The irritable bowel syndrome. A review of 50 consecutive cases. *J of the Irish Colleges of Physicians & Surgeons* 1975;4:91–94.

14 KINGHAM JGC, DAWSON AM. Origin of chronic right upper quadrant pain. *Gut* 1985;26:783–788.

15 KRUIS W, THIEME C, WEINZIER IM, SCHUSSLER P, HOLL J, PANHIS W. A diagnostic score for the irritable bowel syndrome. *Gastroenterology* 1984;87:1–7.

16 KUMAR D, WINGATE DL. The irritable bowel syndrome: a paroxysmal motor disorder. *Lancet* 1985;ii:973–977.

17 LANCET. An irritable mind or an irritable bowel? *Lancet* 1984;ii:1249–1250.

18 LASSER RB, BOND JH, LEVITT MD. The role of intestinal gas in functional abdominal pain. *N Engl J Med* 1975;293:524–526.

19 LATIMER P, SARNA S, CAMPBELL D, LATIMER M, WATERFALL W, DANIEL EE. Colonic motor and myoelectrical activity: a comparative study of normal subjects, psychoneurotic patients, and patients with irritable bowel syndrome. *Gastroenterology* 1981;80:893–901.

20 LENNARD JONES JE. Functional gastrointestinal disorders. *N Engl J Med* 1983; 308:431–435.

21 LIPSITT DR. Through the sigmoidoscope brightly. *Gastroenterology* 1984;87:433–40.

22 LUMSDEN K, CHAUDHARY NA, TRUELOVE SC. The irritable colon syndrome. *Clin Radiol* 1963;14:54–63.

23 PALMER KR, CORBETT CL, HOLDSWORTH CD. Double blind cross over study comparing loperamide, codeine and diphenoxylate in the treatment of chronic diarrhoea. *Gastroenterology* 1980;79:1272–1275.

24 READ NW. *Irritable bowel syndrome*. London: Grune & Stratton, 1985.

25 RICKERT RR. The important 'impostors' in the differential diagnosis of inflammatory bowel disease. *J Clin Gastroenterol* 1984;6:153–163.

26 RITCHIE JA. The irritable bowel. Part II: manometric and cineradiographic studies. *Clin Gastroenterol.* 1977;3:622–631.

27 RYLE JA. Chronic spasmodic affections of the colon. *Lancet* 1928;ii:1115–1119.

28 SANDLER RS, DROSSMAN DA, NATHAN HP, McKEE DC. Symptom complaints and health care seeking behaviour in subjects with bowel dysfunction. *Gastroenterology* 1984;87:314–318.

29 SARNA SK. Cyclic motor activity; migrating motor complex: 1985. *Gastroenterology* 1985;89:894–913.

30 SVEDLUND J, SJODIN I, DOTEVALL G, GILLBERG R. Upper gastrointestinal and mental symptoms in the irritable bowel syndrome. *Scand J Gastroenterol* 1985,20:598–601.

31 SWARBRICK ET, BAT T, HEGARTY JE, WILLIAMS CB, DAWSON AM. Site of pain from the irritable bowel. *Lancet* 1980;ii:443–446.

32 THOMPSON WG. The irritable bowel. *Gut* 1984;25:305–320.

33 THOMPSON WG. Gastrointestinal symptoms in the irritable bowel compared with peptic ulcer and inflammatory bowel disease. *Gut* 1984;25:1089–1092.

34 THOMPSON WG, HEATON KW. Functional bowel disorders in apparently healthy people. *Gastroenterology* 1980;79:283–288.

35 TREACHER DP, CHAPMAN JR, NOLAN DJ, JEWELL DP. Irritable bowel syndrome: is barium enema necessary? *Clin Rad* 1986;37:87–88.

36 WALLER SL, MISIEWICZ JJ. Prognosis in the irritable bowel syndrome. *Lancet* 1969;ii:753–756.

37 WELCH GW, HILLMAN LC, POMARE EW. Psychoneurotic symptomatology in the irritable bowel syndrome: a study of reporters and non-reporters. *Br Med J* 1985;291:1382–1384.

38 WHITEHEAD WE, ENGEL BT, SCHUSTER MM. Irritable bowel syndrome. Physiological and psychological differences between diarrhoea-predominant and constipation-predominant patients. *Dig Dis Sci* 1980;25:404–413.

39 WHORWELL PJ, FARAGHER EB, PRIOR A. Controlled trial of hypnotherapy in the treatment of severe refractory irritable-bowel syndrome. *Lancet* 1984;2:1232–1234.

40 WHORWELL PJ, McCALLUM M, CREED FW, ROBERTS CT. Non-colonic features of irritable bowel syndrome. *Gut* 1986;27:37–40.

41 YOUNG SJ, ALPERS DH, NORLAND CC, WOODRUFF RA. Psychiatric illness and irritable bowel syndrome: Practical implications for the primary physician. *Gastroenterology* 1976;70:162–166.

Chapter 68
Psychiatric Illness and the Gut

E. STONEHILL

Physical symptoms frequently accompany emotional disturbance and psychological symptoms often accompany organic disease. Many of the physical symptoms associated with psychiatric disturbances are the same as those found in physical disease. Such symptoms referable to the gastrointestinal system include abdominal discomfort, pain, bloating, wind, constipation, diarrhoea, nausea, vomiting, anorexia and weight loss. Thus, it is often impossible to exclude organic disease on the history alone.

It is therefore not surprising to learn that an organic cause cannot be found for the symptoms of about half the patients attending gastroenterology clinics, even after thorough clinical and laboratory investigations. There is, however, no substitute for taking a full and detailed case history which should include the mental state and psychosocial background. Further investigations may be necessary to exclude organic disease but in some cases, such as primary anorexia nervosa, the diagnosis should be made on the history and not by a process of exclusion of other disease.

It is not known why some patients somatize emotional conflict while others do not. The explanation of possible mechanisms was dominated until recently by psychoanalytical theory. Alexander [1] in his specificity theory, postulated a causal link between a specific constellation of unconscious conflicts, of psychological modes of dealing with them and their emotional and physical correlations on the one hand and the development of one of several

organic diseases including duodenal ulcer and ulcerative colitis, on the other. This theory was tested in an elegant prospective study of duodenal ulcer [32, 39]. In recent years it has become more fashionable to adopt a psychosomatic or holistic approach to all disease. One fundamental assumption of this approach is that the mind and the body should not be regarded as being independent from each other.

Psychoanalytic theory regards the defence mechanism of denial as important in the production of psychosomatic symptoms. Emotional conflict, which is too painful to face, becomes repressed in the unconscious mind and replaced by emergent somatic symptoms. The concept of alexithymia, or *pensée operatoire*, has also been put forward to explain the presence of somatic rather than psychological symptoms. This postulates a constitutional inability to be aware of inner feelings. More recently much interest has been directed to psychophysiological and psychoendocrinological mechanisms and their relationship to feeling states, life events and psychodynamic factors.

Depression and anxiety are the two most common psychiatric disturbances; both form part of universal experience as feeling states. They are commonly severe enough in intensity and duration to result in complaints to the doctor, and hence a clinical diagnosis.

Depression

A life-time risk of about one in ten has been described in several studies concerned with the epidemiology of depression [10, 38]. During the child-bearing period of life women suffer twice as often as men [27]. Depression heads the list of mental illnesses necessitating admission to psychiatric hospital and between 1954 and 1969 the numbers admitted annually in England and Wales per 100,000 of the population ranged between 79–88 for men and 152–167 for women [14]. Depression is also the commonest psychiatric disorder to accompany physical illness, affecting about a quarter of medical in-patients and usually improving with physical recovery [21].

The principal manifestation of depression is a lowering of mood, the intensity of which may range from sadness to increasing gloominess, blackness and utter despair. There are frequently biological or vegetative accompaniments to depressive illness; in severe depression these often include diurnal variation of mood which is worse in the morning, loss of energy and libido, sleep disturbance in the form of early waking, and anorexia associated with loss of weight.

Pain can also be an accompaniment of depressive illness. Changes in psychomotor activity can occur, which may be increased with agitation or reduced with retardation. The symptoms complained of by the patient may be focused on the disturbance of bodily function rather than the mood. Thus he or she may present complaining of weight loss, abdominal pain or constipation. The mechanism of constipation may have its origin in anorexia resulting in reduced consumption of food. In addition decreased intestinal motility may be associated with generalized psychomotor retardation. Finally, the anticholinergic activity of many antidepressant drugs, especially the tricyclics, can contribute to constipation. In very severe depression of psychotic intensity, constipation may form the seed of a somatic delusional belief that the bowels are permanently blocked—the patient may be convinced that this is caused by a malignant tumour.

It is not difficult to make a diagnosis of depression if depressed mood is a focus of complaint, but it may be much more difficult to diagnose if the mood component is not part of the initial presentation [30]. The term 'masked depression' has been used to describe such cases [26]. A variety of mechanisms may underlie such atypical presentation—sometimes feelings of depression are felt to be signs of weakness and therefore resented; a physical complaint may be much more acceptable to the patient or the doctor than a psychiatric complaint; in some severe cases the feelings may be so different from the normal experience of despondency that it is difficult for the patient to equate them as such. Certain personalities tend to somatize and express distress by atypical symptoms. Thus some African and Asian cultures express depression predominantly in somatic symptoms, and indeed their languages may have no word clearly expressing depression [22].

It is not uncommon for a patient who has been attending the gastroenterology department with organic disease to develop depression, which becomes incorporated in a complaint of exacerbation of the physical symptoms. The physician's 'mental set' has already been tuned to the patient's physical illness and the emergent state of depression may be missed.

Case Report

Mrs C.R., a 66-year-old married woman, had a long history of gastrointestinal complaints. She had presented to the gastroenterology department 25 years earlier complaining of persistent diarrhoea with mucus and a diagnosis of proctitis was made. Three years previously she presented again with a short history of episodes of pain in the right hypochondrium associated with acid regurgitation—cholecystitis was suspected, but not confirmed. A few weeks later she was seen again with rectal bleeding which was attributed to constipation. During the following year she developed increasing dysphagia with regurgitation and heartburn. She was noticed to be dishevelled in her appearance. Investigations showed a small sliding hiatus hernia, a deformed duodenal cap and a Shatzki ring of the lower oesophagus. Her symptoms became worse, she refused endoscopy and was noted to be a 'difficult personality'. She lost 10 kg in weight over the course of a year and persisted in vomiting all solid food in spite of repeated endoscopic dilatation. When it was finally noted that she was also tearful she was referred to a psychiatrist. At psychiatric interview she acknowledged feeling depressed which she attributed to her physical illness. She reported having no energy and being unable to cope with her domestic duties which her husband had now taken over. Her husband recounted that he had noticed that the patient displayed a gradually increasing loss of vitality over the previous three years. She had become withdrawn and dishevelled because she showed no interest in herself. On questioning she reported disturbance of sleep with initial insomnia and early waking, but no diurnal variation in mood.

Her husband, a forceful character, was obliged to retire from his own business four years previously when he developed bilateral cataracts for which he underwent successful surgery. He subsequently suffered from a myocardial infarction and then remained at home with the patient, whose illness started at about this time.

She was treated with a tricyclic antidepressant, as well as supportive psychotherapy which included her husband, and she started to improve within two weeks. Six months later she reported feeling cheerful in her mood, had regained the lost weight and was no longer vomiting. Although she reported some persistent retching in the morning and retrosternal burning, this no longer greatly worried or preoccupied her.

Anxiety

Anxiety, unlike many other emotions, is a fundamental biological drive. At low levels it improves performance, but at high and pathological levels performance falls off rapidly. This is the Yerkes-Dobson Law (Fig. 68.1).

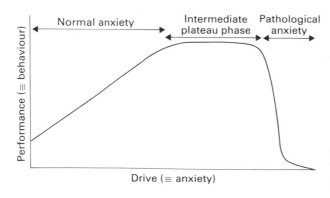

Fig. 68.1. Yerkes-Dobson Law— The relationship between anxiety and performance.

The emotion of anxiety may range from apprehension, through fear, to panic and terror. It has psychological and bodily manifestations. Anxiety states are common disorders with a 2–5% prevalence in the general population, and between six and 27% in psychiatric practice [18]. However, most patients can be managed as out-patients and less than 1% of psychiatric in-patients suffer from anxiety neurosis.

A distinction is usually made between anxiety which appears to have no constant or predictable stimulus—so-called free-floating anxiety, and anxiety that only occurs in certain situations, which is described as phobic anxiety. Amongst the commonest physical symptoms of anxiety are dryness of the mouth, nausea, abdominal churning, and increased bowel frequency. Some patients emphasize their somatic symptoms and minimize the affective component. Conversely, organic disease such as thyrotoxicosis and Crohn's disease, may mimic anxiety. Hence the need to exclude a physical cause in some patients presenting with somatic symptoms—indeed, the coexistence of physical illness and anxiety is common. Furthermore, patients with neurotic disorders of sufficient severity to need hospital admission, die earlier than non-neurotic individuals, even allowing for such causes of death as suicide and accidents [31].

Case Report

Miss R.P., aged 18, was referred by her general practitioner to the gastroenterology department with a history of excessive bowel frequency. A history of urgency of defaecation and of a sensation of incomplete evacuation of the bowels was obtained. She reported the need to go to the lavatory 10 times a day, but would only pass a motion on three or so occasions. Her motions were described as normal, with no blood or mucus. Examination and investigations did not show an organic cause for her symptoms and a psychiatric referral was made.

It became apparent that her symptoms had conferred a state of agoraphobia upon her, as she was reluctant to travel anywhere where it might be difficult to get to a lavatory because of a fear of faecal incontinence. The problem stemmed from childhood, following one episode of bowel incontinence about which she had been teased, but had been much worse since leaving home for university.

She was judged to be a shy and anxious girl, excessively dependent on her mother, who found the demands of adolescence and increasing independence very difficult to cope with. To this extent the symptoms conferred a degree of safety and protection for her.

She was treated with an intensive two-day in-patient behavioural programme which included anxiety management control techniques and biofeedback, as well as frank discussion of her problems about which she had been very ambivalent. Subsequent follow-up showed considerable symptomatic improvement.

Treatment of anxiety or depression

The treatment of underlying anxiety and depression involves making a diagnostic formulation based on a full case history. The weight of constitutional, psychodynamic, biological and social factors can only then be evaluated and a treatment programme planned. Such treatment may involve psychotherapy, which can be supportive or insight-orientated. Behaviour therapy includes the techniques of desensitization and flooding, as well as more recently described cognitive behaviour therapy.

There are a large number of antidepressant drugs of several different chemical groups. They are most effective in depressed patients who display biological accompaniments of depression. Minor tranquillizers are often effective in relieving the symptoms of anxiety but the problems of tolerance, dependency and withdrawal should be considered. Other drugs, such as beta-blockers also have a role in anxiety when vegetative symptoms predominate. If the measures of simple support and perhaps first-line psychotropic medication are not successful, the gastroenterologist should consider referring the patient for psychiatric assessment.

Personality disorders

A personality disorder can be said to exist when the character of an individual differs markedly from types found within the normal population. Personality disorder is a developmental abnormality which may take many or several forms, but a feature common to all is a recurrent disturbance of relationships with other people.

The poor ability to initiate, or sustain healthy interpersonal relationships can contribute to the development of symptoms of a psychoneurotic or psychosomatic nature. These symptoms may then become incorporated within the individual's strategy for coping with life and its problems. The symptoms may be mobilized as a focal point in human relationships, which in turn may serve to perpetuate the symptoms. Functional abdominal pain often arises in this context.

Such symptoms, which may initially evoke the concern and sympathy of others and appear to justify the patient's restricted life style, are usually regarded as respectable if labelled as organic, but may cause considerable loss of credibility and hence self-esteem, if labelled as functional. Thus, the change of diagnosis from a physical to psychological is often resisted, as it may pose a considerable threat to the patient, with consequent anger and resentment.

Case report

Mrs A.D., aged 34, was referred for a second gastroenterological opinion. She gave a 12-year history of severe constipation with no sense of wanting to pass a motion. She described abdominal distension and pain, and transient weight loss. No definitive cause was found and she continued using regular laxatives and enemas until she underwent a partial colectomy two years earlier.

The operation failed to produce any improvement and her complaint of generalized abdominal pain, with acute exacerbation of lower abdominal colic became more pronounced. Her husband repeatedly called the emergency doctor because of the pain. She remained preoccupied with her complaint of inability to pass a normal motion more frequently than once every few weeks. Further investigations failed to show an organic cause for her symptoms and a psychiatric opinion was obtained.

The psychiatric interview revealed that she had received no affection from her parents, of whom she was afraid as a child. Her mother, who wanted a second son, favoured the patient's brother, with whom the patient compared herself unfavourably. She developed as a socially isolated girl, nervous and unable to make friends. She met her husband at work and her symptoms developed soon after their marriage. He has been concerned and sympathetic in relation to her ill-health, but their relationship was emotionally distant.

The patient and her husband had little sexual contact and no social life outside the family. There were two children aged 9 and 11 years. The husband, who was also a homosexual, administered enemas to the patient and performed digital rectal evacuation. It is probable that the patient's continuing symptoms played an important part in maintaining the stability of the marital relationship. It was concluded that the patient, and probably her husband as well, had a personality disorder. He refused to attend a psychiatric interview and the patient declined psychiatric admission.

Anorexia nervosa [12]

Anorexia nervosa is characterized by over-determined dieting behaviour with avoidance of carbohydrate (Fig. 68.2). The central feature is that of a phobia of normal weight; the subject feels fat even though he or she is underweight (Fig. 68.3). The physical accompaniments of rapid loss of weight may include delayed gastric emptying [20], bradycardia, hypotension, restlessness associated with early morning waking, peripheral vasoconstriction, disturbance of thermo-regulatory control mechanisms, lowered basal metabolic rate and the growth on the body of fine downy hair, called lanugo hair [2]. Secondary amenorrhoea supervenes early [9] and is associated with reduced gonadotrophin production and a prepubertal response to LH/FSH-RH [24].

The illness occurs most commonly in teenage girls; less than 10% of patients are male. The disorder may last for only a few months, but can span several decades. The typical patient is not depressed, has a bland affect and does not complain of weight loss. He or she may minimize or even deny any problems. For example, the only complaint of a championship tennis player who weighed 35 kg was that her forehand drive had lost its power. The patient is usually accompanied by a concerned and worried parent.

The term anorexia is a misnomer— usually, in common with most people on weight-reducing diets, the patient has not in fact lost his or her appetite. Indeed, it is likely that he or she is controlling a voracious appetite and that he or she has become deeply preoccupied with thoughts of body weight, food and calories. Some patients who give in to their hunger and overeat may then induce vomiting and/or purging behaviour in order to avoid gaining weight. This may result in metabolic abnormalities and electrolyte imbalance. The goal of the anorectic patient is the pursuit and maintenance of thinness. As the diet usually predominantly involves carbohydrate restriction, severe hypoproteinaemia is rare.

There has been a striking increase in the prevalence of this disorder in the last two decades and it occurs more commonly in the higher social classes [33]. A state of premorbid overweight is a constitutional predisposing factor.

The disorder can be construed in psychological terms as a phobic avoidance response invoked in adolescence, which unconsciously meets the patient's own emotional needs at that time, enabling the patient to regress and thus escape from conflicts that are faced in growing up [3]. The regression is biological as well as psychological; it confers upon the patient a feeling of greater safety.

Adolescent conflicts are, of course, universal and there are many factors that determine whether an individual needs to resort to a pathological mechanism to deal with them. One factor is the support and strength of the family and an adolescent may be more vulnerable if there is parental conflict. Such conflict may be covert, for the patient may unite the parents through their joint concern over his or her illness which then temporarily cements the marriage. The diagnosis of anorexia nervosa should be made at the initial interview when the

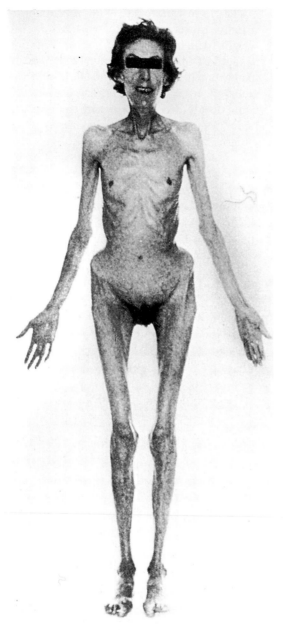

Fig. 68.2. A patient with severe and chronic anorexia nervosa. Note the blandness of facial expression. She weighed 26 kg on admission and discharged herself from hospital weighing 34 kg. She died two months later.

patient attends with one, or both parents. It is not a diagnosis to be made by exclusion of other organic disease. It is also important to attempt to formulate a view of the psychodynamic background at this time.

Treatment needs to be directed at concurrently restoring the patient's weight to a normal level, and helping the patient and his or her family to cope with the underlying emotional problems. This usually requires a period of in-patient treatment which may last three to four months. The patient is treated with bed rest and refeeding with a 3,000 calorie normal diet, to

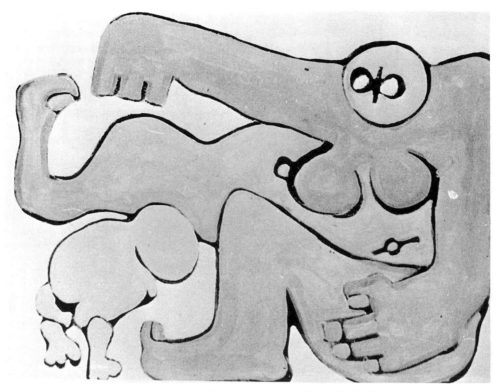

Fig. 68.3. A painting by an in-patient with anorexia nervosa whose body weight had been restored to normal but who painted herself as grossly obese, ugly, angry and sexual [3].

enable weight gain of 1.5–2 kg/week until the matched population mean weight is reached. During this time regular psychotherapeutic help is provided for the patient and his or her family. A contract including agreement of the target weight should be established at the outset. Treatment is best carried out in a specialized unit. These

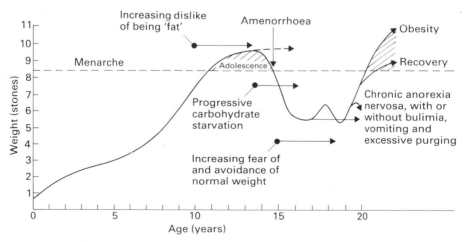

Fig. 68.4. The evolution of anorexia nervosa [2].

patients, who may often be quite manipulative, do better with experienced staff. In such circumstances it is never necessary to tube feed patients. About 40% of patients with severe anorexia nervosa, who come to treatment, recover. The remainder may develop chronic anorexia nervosa at low body weight, with a pattern of abstention or purging and vomiting. Some go on to develop obesity and, if they induce vomiting, may subsequently be diagnosed as suffering from bulimia nervosa (Fig. 68.4). Approximately 5% of chronically ill patients die prematurely, often from suicide. Patients with anorexia nervosa have a decreased bone mass due to osteoporosis, but a high level of physical activity may protect their skeletons [28, 37].

Bulimia nervosa [12]

Mild periodic bulimic, or binge, eating is a common neurotic response to emotional stress that occurs frequently in normal teenage girls. This is separated by degree from bulimia nervosa [23, 29]. The patients may be of normal weight or overweight and can be divided into two populations—those who have previously suffered from anorexia nervosa and those who have not. The first group, comprising 15–30% of ex-anorexia nervosa patients, continue to display a phobia of normal weight [4]. The second group, who suffer from a range of psychological problems including depression and personality disorder, do not display a morbid fear of being fat although they declare a normal female preoccupation with weight and shape.

In contrast to the anorexia nervosa patients, who abstain from eating and maintain a low body weight, those with bulimia nervosa may continue to menstruate and are often sexually active. Indeed, their sexual behaviour may be as impulsive as their eating behaviour. In contrast with abstaining anorectics they are often extrovert. Alcohol and drug-dependence, self-poisoning, stealing or depression are common complications. Balanced and regular meals are avoided by this group; carbohydrate intake is low except in a binge when carbohydrate foods are usually selected. Electrolyte imbalance, in particular hypokalaemia, is common. Bizarre eating patterns can result in the development of hypercarotinaemia [7]. Dental decay is common [15].

A period of in-patient treatment, aimed at helping the patient to reach her matched population mean weight and to eat normally, may be helpful in the group who stem from an anorectic population. Concurrent psychotherapy is also important.

Bulimic patients who do not have a history of anorexia nervosa have been regarded as having a number of characteristics in common with patients who have massive obesity. However they have thwarted the development of severe obesity by mechanisms of abstention from food—self-induced vomiting or laxative abuse, the consumption of appetite suppressants [35] or diuretic drugs, or a combination of these methods [16]. An out-patient treatment programme aimed at this group has recently been described [17]. Patients are treated for 10 weekly, half-day sessions in individual and group therapy. The outcome of this approach has been very encouraging.

Massive obesity [12]

Obesity is widespread in the general population affecting up to 50% of middle-aged women in social class 5. It has a multifactorial aetiology and constitutional factors are very important. There is no good evidence to suggest that psychological factors necessarily play a major aetiological role in mild obesity and such subjects in the general population report a low degree of psychoneurotic complaint [5].

As the state of obesity usually starts early

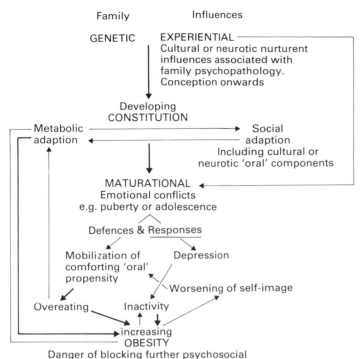

Family Influences

GENETIC EXPERIENTIAL
Cultural or neurotic nurturent
influences associated with
family psychopathology.
Conception onwards

Developing
CONSTITUTION

Metabolic adaption ← → Social adaption
Including cultural or
neurotic 'oral' components

MATURATIONAL
Emotional conflicts
e.g. puberty or adolescence

Defences & Responses

Mobilization of comforting 'oral' propensity   Depression

Worsening of self-image

Overeating   Inactivity

increasing OBESITY

Danger of blocking further psychosocial
maturation with increasing investment in
established circular neurotic and
psychosomatic defences

Fig. 68.5. Some mechanisms evident in patients with massive obesity attending a psychiatric clinic.

in life in patients with massive obesity, it would be surprising if this state did not incorporate some neurotic components during childhood and adolescence. In adulthood, the state of massive obesity may provide a mechanism, both psychophysiological and symbolic, for dealing defensively with problems of life. In such patients the psychological problems may emerge if the individual is stripped of his or her obese state [8]. Fig. 68.5 displays some of the mechanisms and their interactions, evident in patients with massive obesity attending the psychiatric clinic.

The irritable bowel syndrome (see Chapter 67)

Psychiatric abnormality can be detected in most patients with the irritable bowel, although this may sometimes be attributed to symptoms of the disorder rather than a cause [30, 36, 40].

If psychological factors are thought to be important, a full psychiatric history should be taken. A misdiagnosis of the irritable bowel syndrome may sometimes be made in a patient presenting with an affective illness in which the somatic symptoms are emphasized. In such a case treatment should be directed at the underlying disorder [34]. Although patients with the irritable bowel syndrome report a moderate degree of psychoneurotic symptoms, which fall half-way between matched psychoneurotic out-patients and controls, they nevertheless display a high degree of autonomic arousal as measured by basal forearm blood flow [25]. In common with other psychosomatic populations, this group has a propensity to somatize emotional conflict.

As in other chronic relapsing conditions,

the physician needs to pay particular attention to the doctor–patient relationship. A positive and continuing relationship with a doctor who can provide support, encouragement and discussion is often very important. The physician needs to guard against his own feelings of frustration and failure which may be expressed in aggression towards, or even rejection of, the patient who fails to improve. In difficult and intractable cases a combined approach by the gastroenterologist, psychiatrist and the general practitioner is encouraged. Finally, therapeutic techniques such as relaxation training and biofeedback, which have not yet been adequately evaluated in the irritable bowel syndrome, should not necessarily be discounted [11, 19].

Psychogenic vomiting

Frequent vomiting in the absence of other disease is quite common among females. The prevalence was found to be 3.2% among secondary schoolgirls [6]. Such behaviour is usually not the reason for complaint, but severe vomiting with associated cachexia and loss of weight may result in hospital admission. Severe vomiting, in the absence of other organic or psychological disease, is often involuntary. The patient is usually female and hypokalaemia is a frequent accompaniment. The psychodynamic background often shows the patient to be living with a person to whom she feels great antipathy, but from whom she feels unable to get away [13]. The symptoms usually remit in hospital only to relapse on returning home, unless the underlying conflicts can be resolved.

Case report

O.N., aged 38, is Irish Catholic and for 12 years has been the common-law wife of a wealthy Anglo-Indian entrepreneur. He has two children by a previous marriage and the patient has three children by him. He is divorced from his first wife, but he and the patient are not married although she has taken his surname by deed poll. She comes from a close-knit, religious family that believes that she is legally married. The common-law husband, a generous, energetic but egocentric man, comes from a family in which his grandfather had four wives. Throughout the relationship he has had frequent extramarital affairs which he has only thinly attempted to disguise. The patient failed to confront him earlier in the relationship and has always been unable to mobilize any aggressive feelings towards him. She maintains an intensely ambivalent relationship with him.

She suffered from recurrent episodes of severe vomiting, requiring hospital admission on several occasions. Her symptoms remit on each occasion, but they relapse immediately on returning home. On the last admission she had lost 10 kg in weight and had a plasma potassium of 2.1 mmol/l. Other physical investigations were normal.

The patient and her husband were interviewed at length separately and also in a series of conjoint marital interviews. The husband appeared defensive, but acknowledged his promiscuous behaviour; he gave lip service to changing his ways. The patient, who talked of leaving him, was quite unable to do so. She returned home and subsequently relapsed once more.

References

1 ALEXANDER F. *Psychosomatic medicine: its principles and application.* London: George Allen and Unwin, 1952.
2 CRISP AH. Anorexia nervosa. *Hosp Med* 1967;1:713–718.
3 CRISP AH. *Anorexia nervosa: Let me be.* London: Academic Press, 1980.
4 CRISP AH. Anorexia nervosa at normal body

weight I. The abnormal normal weight control syndrome. *Int J Psychiatry Med* 1981;**11**:203–233.

5 CRISP AH, McGUINNESS B. Jolly fat: relation between obesity and psychoneurosis in the general population. *Br Med J* 1976;**i**:7–9.

6 CRISP AH, PALMER RL, KALUCY RS. How common is anorexia nervosa? A prevalence study. *Br J Psychiatry* 1976;**128**:549–554.

7 CRISP AH, STONEHILL E. Hypercarotinaemia as a symptom of weight phobia. *Postgrad Med J* 1967;**43**:721–725.

8 CRISP AH, STONEHILL E. Treatment of obesity with special reference to seven severely obese patients. *J Psychosom Res* 1970;**14**:327–345.

9 CRISP AH, STONEHILL E. Relationship between aspects of nutritional disturbance and menstrual activity in primary anorexia nervosa. *Br Med J* 1971;**3**:149–151.

10 ESSEN-MOLLER E, HAGNELL O. The frequency and risk of depression within a rural community in Scania. *Acta Psychiatr Scand [Suppl]* 1961;**162**:37.

11 HEALTH AND PUBLIC POLICY COMMITTEE. Biofeedback for gastrointestinal disorders. *Ann Int Med* 1985;**103**:291–293.

12 HERZOG DB, COPELAMD PM. Eating disorders. *N Engl J Med* 1985;**313**:295–303.

13 HILL OW. Psychogenic vomiting and hypokalaemia. *Gut* 1967;**8**:98–101.

14 HMSO. Hospitals selected psychiatric illness. *Social Trends* 1972;**3**:Table 63.

15 JACOBS MB, SCHNEIDER JA. Medical complications of bulimia: a prospective evaluation. *Q J Med* 1985;**214**:177–182.

16 LACEY JH. The bulimic syndrome at normal body weight: reflection on pathogenesis and clinical features. *Int J Eating Disorders* 1982;**ii**:59–66.

17 LACEY JH. Bulimia nervosa, binge-eating and psychogenic vomiting: a controlled treatment study and long term outcome. *Br Med J* 1983;**286**:1609–1613.

18 LADER M, MARKS I. *Clinical anxiety.* London: Heinemann, 1971.

19 LEADING ARTICLE. An irritable mind or an irritable bowel? *Lancet* 1984; **ii**:1249–1250.

20 McCALLUM RW, GRILL BB, LANGE R, PLANKY M, GLASS EE, GREENFELD DG. Definition of a gastric emptying abnormality in patients with anorexia nervosa. *Dig Dis Sci* 1985; **30**:713–722.

21 MOFFIC HS, PAYKEL ES. Depression in medical inpatients. *Br J Psychiatry* 1975;**126**:346–353.

22 NDETEI DM, MUHANGI J. The prevalence and clinical presentation of psychiatric illness in a rural setting in Kenya. *Br J Psychiatry* 1979;**135**:269–272.

23 PALMER RL. Dietary chaos syndrome: a useful new term? *Br J Med Psychol* 1979;**52**:187–190.

24 PALMER RL, CRISP AH, MacKINNON PCB, FRANKLIN M, BONNAR J, WHEELER M. Pituitary sensitivity to 50 g LH/FSH-RH in subjects with anorexia nervosa in acute and recovery stages. *Br Med J* 1975;**i**:179–182.

25 PALMER RL, STONEHILL E, CRISP AH, WALLER SL, MISIEWICZ JJ. Psychological characteristics of patients with the irritable bowel syndrome. *Postgrad Med J* 1974;**50**:416–419.

26 PAYKEL ES, NORTON KRW. Masked depression. *Br J Hosp Med* 1982;**28**:151–157.

27 POLLITT J. CROWN S, ed *The management of depression in practical psychiatry. Vol 1.* London: Northwood Books 1981:30–33.

28 RIGOTTI NA, NUSSBAUM SR, HERZOG DB, NEER RM. Osteoporosis in women with anorexia nervosa. *N Engl J Med* 1984;**311**:1601–1606.

29 RUSSELL GFM. Bulimia nervosa: an ominous variant of anorexia nervosa. *Psychol Med* 1979;**9**: 429–448.

30 SANDLER RS, DROSSMAN DA, NATHAN NP, McKEE DC. Symptom complaints and health care seeking behaviour in subjects with bowel dysfunction. *Gastroenterology* 1984;**87**:314–318.

31 SIMS ACP. Mortality in neurosis. *Lancet* 1973;**ii**:1072–1076.

32 STONEHILL E. Reading about psychosomatics. *Br J Psychiatry* 1980;**136**:302–304.

33 STONEHILL E. Anorexia nervosa; a disorder of affluent and Westernized socieities. *The Listener* 1985;**113**:11–12.

34 STONEHILL E, MISIEWICZ G. The irritable bowel syndrome — a psychiatric view. *Medicine* 1980;**36**:1850–1853.

35 SULLIVAN AC, GRUEN RK. Mechanisms of appetite modulation by drugs. *Fed Proc* 1985;**44**:139–144.

36 SVEDLUND J, SJODIN I, DOTEVALL G, GILLBERG R. Upper gastrointestinal and mental symptoms in the irritable bowel syndrome. *Scand J Gastroenterol* 1985;**20**:595–601.

37 SZMUKLER GI, BROWN SW, PARSON V, DARBY A. Premature loss of bone in chronic anorexia nervosa. *Br Med J* 1985;**290**:26–27.

38 WATTS CHA. *Depressive disorders in the community.* Bristol: Wright, 1966.

39 WEINER H, THALER M, REISER MF, MINSKY IA. Aetiology of duodenal ulcer. I. Relation of specific psychological characteristics to rate of gastric secretion (serum pepsinogen). *Psychosom Med* 1957;**19**:1–10.

40 WELCH GW, HILLMAN LC, POMARE EW. Psychoneurotic symptomatology in the irritable bowel syndrome: a study of reporters and non-reporters. *Br Med J* 1985;**291**:1382–1384.

SECTION XII
OTHER GASTROINTESTINAL PROBLEMS

Chapter 69
Ischaemia of the Gut

A. MARSTON

The mesenteric circulation, which comprises about a quarter of the blood volume and a fifth of the cardiac output, supplies the gut via three large vessels: the coeliac axis, the superior mesenteric artery, and the inferior mesenteric artery. The superior mesenteric artery is the most important of these vessels as it is an end-artery that nourishes the entire midgut, from the duodenojejunal flexure to the mid-transverse colon. Blood returns to the liver via the portal vein.

At the upper and lower ends of the abdomen there are extra-coelomic connections that protect against falls in blood flow. If the coeliac axis is occluded, the deficiency is quickly made up from diaphragmatic, intercostal and oesophageal vessels. In the same way, because the pelvic organs have a rich supply from the internal iliac artery, the inferior mesenteric system is, within certain limits, 'disposable'. Ischaemic problems in the stomach and rectum are so rare as to be clinically unimportant.

Chronic occlusion of the superior mesenteric artery is, on the whole, well-tolerated due to the build-up of a collateral circulation. Sudden interruption is not tolerated because of the potentially infective nature of the bowel contents. The gut lives in equilibrium with its luminal bacterial population; any reduction of viability due to ischaemia will immediately result in bacterial invasion, with an inflammatory response causing an enteritis or colitis. An infarct of the kidney or myocardium can heal cleanly by fibrosis. The same does not apply to the bowel where necrosis always leads to gangrene and to death of the patient, unless action is taken. When the balance between bacterial challenge and mucosal defence is upset, an abrupt series of changes takes place, the consequence of which can vary between mild inflammation and fatal infarction.

Classification of gut ischaemia

In the past, gut ischaemia was thought of in terms of morbid anatomy, and was classified as being due to acute or chronic arterial obstruction (embolus or thrombosis), inflammatory disease, 'non-occlusive infarction', and venous disorders. In fact the situation is more complex.

Mesenteric embolus, classically a complication of rheumatic heart disease, is now almost unknown. However, it is of scientific interest because it is the only clinical parallel of the standard laboratory model of intestinal ischaemia—the abrupt occlusion of blood supply to the mid-gut loop of an animal with normal vessels. Most patients who die from intestinal infarction do not have emboli—some have atheromatous lesions at the origins of their visceral arteries, but in one-third of fatal cases of gut necrosis no vascular occlusion is found at autopsy. Conversely, stenosis, plaques and even complete occlusion of the mesenteric vessels can be found in completely asymptomatic patients [3].

Mesenteric thrombosis can no longer be considered a direct cause of acute intestinal ischaemia, because of the uncertain relationship between the vascular lesion and what occurs in the gut. There is circumstantial evidence, however, that a person with an atheromatous plaque on a visceral artery may sustain an infarction if for some reason the pressure across this lesion is reduced [11].

A better classification of mesenteric vascular disease, which fits the observed clinical pattern, is as follows:

Acute small intestinal ischaemia
    with arterial occlusion
    without arterial occlusion
Chronic arterial obstruction
    of the small bowel
Focal ischaemia
    of the small bowel or colon

Acute small intestinal ischaemia

Acute small intestinal ischaemia occurs when the metabolic needs of the small intestine outrun its blood supply, resulting in threatened or complete necrosis.

Clinical picture

The classic description of acute ischaemia is of a sudden onset of extremely severe abdominal colic, followed by the passage of blood and mucus and *per rectum*, with peripheral circulatory collapse within a few hours. The colicky pain may be so severe that intravenous narcotics fail to relieve it. The initial colic is quickly superseded by a dull, generalized abdominal pain with ileus and peritonitis. Death occurs within one or two days if nothing is done.

Such striking symptoms are easily recognized but, in fact, few patients are diagnosed early because the classically-described clinical picture is far from typical. Very often a major infarct presents with mild cramps which are dismissed as a gastrointestinal infection; in addition, the general condition of a patient with severe intestinal damage may remain deceptively normal for hours or days.

It is well-established experimentally that the result of occluding a normal superior mesenteric artery is intense spasm of the small intestine [12, 13]; this accounts for the severe colicky pain at the onset, and for the fact that a patient seen at this stage may have no abdominal signs, apart from exaggerated bowel sounds. Later, the spasm relaxes and the bowel becomes immobile, although without much in the way of peritoneal reaction; the patient now presents typically with a moderately distended silent abdomen and tenderness in the right iliac fossa. As necrosis proceeds outwards to the serosa there is a peritoneal reaction; the clinical picture becomes that of a desperate illness with gross distension and ileus, exquisite tenderness with a characteristic odour on the breath. Abdominal pain and distension further interferes with respiratory movements, resulting in anxiety, restlessness, air-hunger and cyanosis. Urine output falls off as dehydration and hypotension develop; lowered tissue perfusion and metabolic acidosis compound the gross physiological disturbance. Eventually restlessness gives place to stupor and frank coma.

The clinical picture will obviously be modified by the administration of antibiotics and fluids. However it remains true that, by the time that florid physical signs appear, the point of recovery has probably passed.

X-ray and laboratory investigations

These are disappointing, tending to confirm a clinical impression rather than add materially to the precision of diagnosis.

Plain films of the abdomen show gas-filled loops of small bowel with multiple fluid levels (Fig. 69.1); these appearances are non-specific. Bubbles of gas in the mesenteric veins are virtually pathognomonic of small bowel infarction, but indicate a late and probably irrecoverable stage in the disease.

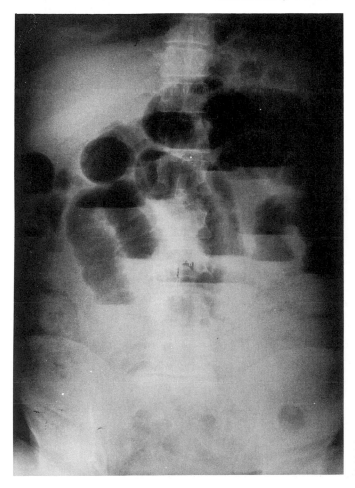

Fig. 69.1. Plain abdominal X-ray in acute small intestinal ischaemia.

Laboratory tests have little to offer. The leucocyte count rises very rapidly after the acute onset of pain: a white blood count of $20–30 \times 10^9/l$, especially if the abdominal signs are unimpressive, should prompt the suspicion of acute intestinal ischaemia.

Another helpful feature may be a markedly elevated packed cell volume without any obvious explanation. Serum transaminase and amylase concentrations vary in an inconstant and unhelpful pattern. However a rise in the level of inorganic phosphate does correlate with the degree of ischaemic damage, perhaps due to the liberation of alkaline phosphatase from the bowel [6].

Emergency aortography

Immediate aortography has been recommended for the diagnosis of bowel infarction [1], but this advice should be questioned. As already mentioned, varying degrees of visceral arterial occlusion are commonly found in apparently healthy older subjects: the presence of a blocked mesenteric artery does not inevitably lead to a diagnosis of acute ischaemia in a patient with undiagnosed abdominal pain. Furthermore, an open intestinal circulation seen on X-ray does not exclude infarction.

The main advantage of an aortogram is the possible demonstration of a mesenteric

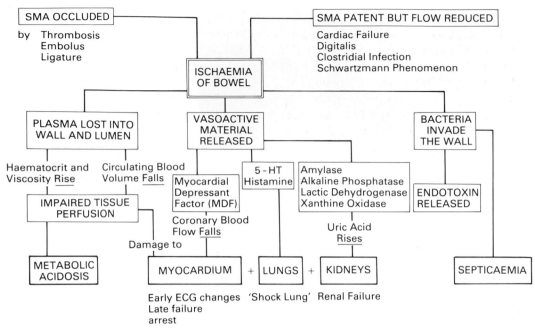

Fig. 69.2. Physiological effects of acute small intestine ischaemia.

embolus providing a precise preoperative diagnosis. However, delaying surgery may allow time for irrevocable ischaemic damage.

Boley *et al.* [1] have reported encouraging results in cases of non-occlusive intestinal infarction, treated by injection of vasodilator drugs directly into the superior mesenteric artery via an aortic catheter [1], but there is a danger of less experienced clinicians being misled by a 'normal' aortogram into missing a surgically correctable peritonitis.

Medical management

Death of the intestine leads to a complex disturbance the main features of which are fluid loss and the effects of bacterial invasion (Fig. 69.2). Both these life-threatening processes require correction. The initial loss is of water, electrolytes and protein with a rise of haematocrit and blood viscosity, and a fall in circulating blood volume leading to

impaired tissue blood flow in the gut wall and the rest of the body.

Intravenous fluid replacement is monitored by serial measurements of the haematocrit, central venous pressure and urine output. Depending on the patient's cardiac status and reserve, liberal quantities of balanced salt solutions (Hartmann or Ringer-lactate) or plasma expanders (purified protein fraction, albumin or medium molecular weight dextran) are given, until the haematocrit falls to below 45% and the central venous pressure rises to +5–10 cm of saline.

Bacterial invasion and toxaemia indicate a need for **antibiotics**. Laboratory studies suggest that such agents mitigate the effects of intestinal ischaemia, but whether they work in the clinical context is difficult to assess. Blood cultures are almost always sterile. The chosen drugs (given intravenously) usually will be an aminoglycoside, combined with metronidazole and a broad-spectrum penicillin or cephalosporin.

Perhaps their main use is to combat anastomotic breakdown and wound infection.

Full heparinization prevents extension of thrombus in the mesenteric vessels and gut wall and, perhaps more importantly, counteracts disseminated intravascular coagulation. This is achieved by the immediate intravenous injection of 10,000 units supplemented by 1,000 units/hour by continuous infusion. Accentuation of bleeding from the haemorrhagic infarct is the theoretical objection to heparin therapy, but in practice this is not a problem.

Metabolic acidosis is brought about by the combination of low tissue perfusion, haemoconcentration and absorption of the products of bacterial and gut necrosis. To this is added a respiratory component due to interference with respiratory movement and increased blood viscosity with intrapulmonary sludging. Measurements of the base excess, pCO_2 and arterial pH will guide the amount of **sodium bicarbonate** therapy required. With reasonably normal pulmonary and renal function, restoration of the circulating blood volume will be enough to correct acid-base equilibrium if the arterial pH is greater than 7.

Laboratory evidence suggests that **alpha-adrenergic blocking agents**, such as phenoxybenzamine, and beta-stimulators, such as isoprenaline, may increase mesenteric blood flow and help to preserve viability. There is no controlled clinical information about their use. It is somewhat doubtful if, in the presence of a mesenteric vascular occlusion, or a massive shut-down of the mesenteric blood supply, any drug is capable of penetrating to the gut wall. Additionally, the fall in blood pressure caused by phenoxybenzamine may be difficult to control. In contrast, vasoconstrictor agents, such as metaraminol or noradrenaline, should obviously be avoided. There is no controlled evidence concerning the use of dopamine or glucagon for the management of the acutely ischaemic small bowel.

Massive doses of **corticosteroids** may help patients with endotoxaemic shock [9].

Digoxin constricts the mesenteric vessels and hence it is a possible cause of intestinal failure [15, 20]. Its cautious use may nonetheless be justified for the control of fast atrial fibrillation or congestive cardiac failure.

Surgical management

When the patient has been resuscitated, the decision regarding surgery can be made. Bearing in mind that untreated complete infarction of the mid-gut is usually lethal, exploration should always be carried out if there is the remotest hope of success.

Under light general anaesthesia with intubation and muscular relaxation, the abdomen is opened through a long right paramedian incision. The situation is obvious immediately because of ischaemic small bowel's characteristic 'musty' smell—impossible to describe but unforgettable when once experienced. There is generally a small quantity of lightly blood-stained ascites. Total full-thickness necrosis with perforation is rare.

About one-third of patients with acute mid-gut ischaemia have no demonstrable block in any major artery. The mortality in these patients is very high; non-occlusive ischaemia is not surgically correctable. If no arterial occlusion can be demonstrated and the ischaemic gut is still viable, the correct course is to inject liberal quantities of local anaesthetic into the coeliac and mesenteric plexuses, supplemented perhaps by papaverine into the superior mesenteric artery, and to close the abdomen. The mortality remains very high [1, 15, 19].

If an embolus is found and the origin of the superior mesenteric artery is accessible, the vessel is opened and cleared with a Fogarty catheter [15]. If the embolus is removed quickly, the bowel becomes pink and healthy with pulsation in the arcade vessels. There is a tendency at this stage for oedema and haemorrhage to occur; the loops of the intestine must be handled very gently. Unless there are areas of frank gangrene, no resection should be undertaken, because it is difficult to judge the extent of possible recovery and suture lines are liable to break down. Successful revascularization is usually followed by a sharp fall in blood pressure. This is due partly to 'washout' of vaso-active material from the damaged bowel into the portal and systemic circulation, but is mainly the result of blood and fluid loss. The damaged small vessels of the bowel wall rupture and bleed when subjected to arterial pressure; replacement of three or four units of blood may be necessary at this stage, and in the post-operative period.

The post-operative course is likely to be stormy, and complicated by renal, respiratory or circulatory problems, quite apart from the prolonged period of malabsorption which follows revascularization of the ischaemic gut [7, 21]. The policy of routine re-exploration of the abdomen 24 hours later, virtually regardless of the state of the patient, is strongly recommended. Success or failure of revascularization can then be assessed, and any gangrenous area of bowel resected.

If the patient is seen late, when there is already massive necrosis of the mid-gut, a primary resection of dead bowel is carried out, and the ends exteriorized. With modern techniques of intravenous alimentation, it is quite a simple matter to cope with the large fluid losses issuing from a high-level fistula. Over the next few days the patient can then be allowed to recover to a normal metabolic state. Continuity of the gut is then restored electively—the main problem being the medical management of the patient with a short bowel (see Chapter 46).

Vasculitis of the bowel (see Chapter 74)

Extensive necrosis of small and large intestine are well-recognized complications of such conditions as systemic lupus, polyarteritis nodosum, and rheumatoid arthritis. The appearances are distinctive: the whole gut is not involved but there is patchy gangrene with intervening segments of healthy well-vascularized bowel (Fig. 69.3). Such patients always require massive resection with later restoration of continuity, if feasible.

Results

The results of treatment for acute small intestinal ischaemia are dismally bad. Complete success is confined to those patients where there is a definite vascular occlusion. The reasons for the enormous mortality will be apparent from Fig. 69.2 which illustrates the physiological disturbance caused by ischaemia of the mid-gut. Furthermore, the condition usually affects elderly patients who may already have some failure of the myocardium, lungs or kidneys. Small intestinal ischaemia is often a complication of central or peripheral circulatory collapse, and is thus more a mode of dying than a cause of death.

Much of the study of acute small intestinal ischaemia has been made in the post-mortem room. Autopsy reveals a massive infarction which was quite unsuspected during life; the pathologist then extrapolates backwards to the clinical events leading up to it. The high preponderance of autopsy studies naturally skews the mortality figures. Common sense would suggest that milder forms of the illness occur, and pass unrecognized; they either resolve spontaneously or else respond to simple supportive measures.

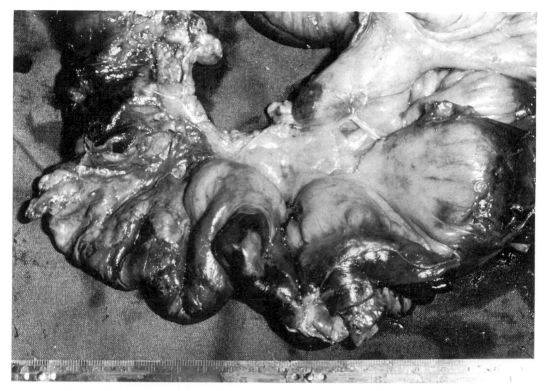

Fig. 69.3. Necrotizing vasculitis of the bowel complicating rheumatoid arthritis.

Chronic arterial obstruction

The concept of peristaltic pain in the intestine felt in response to food intake, analogous to angina pectoris and stemming from obstruction to the arterial supply, is attractive—especially to vascular surgeons. 'Cures' of such chronic abdominal pain, achieved by reconstruction of the visceral arteries, have been reported.

The situation is not that simple, and doubt has been cast on whether 'intestinal angina' is a real clinical entity. Stenosis, even to the point of complete occlusion of the main vessels, is a common autopsy finding in people who have had no alimentary symptoms during life [3]. Patients with this sort of arteriographic abnormality have been investigated very carefully [4, 15] and, because such lesions are easily reproduced in animals, there is also a thorough back-up of laboratory experience [14]. However, no-one has succeeded in demonstrating a structural or functional abnormality of the intestine which can be reliably correlated with a diminution of the blood supply, unless there is infarction. In other words, it is an all-or-nothing situation—the intestine remains normal to our present (admittedly insensitive) tests, until the point is reached when its cells can no longer metabolize or resist bacterial challenge.

The fact remains that many patients who die from fatal intestinal necrosis give a prodromal history of abdominal pain. If it were possible to identify those at risk, lives could be saved.

History and physical signs

The symptoms that constitute the syndrome of intestinal angina have been defined as pain coming on shortly after eating a meal (sometimes described as 'food fear'), weight loss, and disturbance of bowel habit. Study of the literature shows that these complaints are very variable—some patients having no pain at all, others no weight loss, while the bowel disturbance may be either profuse diarrhoea or obstinate constipation. There is really no such thing as the 'classical' patient. A background of cardiovascular disease, with a history of claudication, myocardial infarction, or stroke, provides circumstantial evidence that an obscure abdominal pain may be due to arterial insufficiency.

Physical signs are frequently absent, and the diagnosis must be made by exclusion. An audible arterial bruit in the epigastrium gives no diagnostic clue, because this often arises from atheroma in the aorta rather than the mesenteric trunks, and such bruits can often be heard in fit young individuals with no symptoms [5, 8].

Investigations

Every effort must be made to exclude common and potentially treatable causes of the patient's symptoms: peptic ulcer, oesophagitis, gallstones, chronic pancreatitis, upper abdominal cancer, and (most importantly) myocardial pain referred to the abdomen. A careful medical history and complete physical examination, followed by endoscopy and ultrasound scanning, will exclude most of these diagnoses.

The final decision to operate must be made following aortography. In order to demonstrate the first few centimetres of the arteries, which is where the lesion is almost always to be found, it is necessary to have both free and selective studies on anteroposterior and lateral views. Only in this way can the extent of the arterial pathology be assessed and, most importantly, the degree to which it is compensated by cross-circulation from other vascular territories [15].

Treatment

If the patient's general cardiovascular status appears to permit major surgery, reconstruction of the stenosed visceral arteries can be considered [16]. There are various ways of achieving this, which are illustrated in Fig. 69.4. Most require a thoraco-abdominal approach, which gives full and safe access to the origins of all three visceral arteries.

Results

Our experience at The Middlesex Hospital is shown in Fig. 69.5—100 patients were investigated for suspected intestinal angina, of whom 22 were subjected to arterial reconstruction with three postoperative deaths. Fifteen of the patients have been symptomatically improved, two are unchanged, and one is symptomatically worse. It should be pointed out that this small number represents the 22-year experience of a unit actively interested in the problem, underlining the rarity of the condition.

The right patient for successful surgery is hard to identify, but certainly the rescue of an emaciated pain-racked individual by a timely revascularization of the gut is a most satisfying surgical exercise. Additionally, although this is hard to quantify, such an operation may forestall a fatal intestinal infarction.

Focal ischaemia

Infarction is a matter of degree. Ischaemia in a loop of gut may lead to total necrosis, to a transient inflammatory response, or to the formation of a fibrous stricture. All these processes are well-recognized by the pathologist, and can be reproduced in the experimental animal [15]. It is likely, though impossible to prove, that many unexplained episodes of abdominal pain

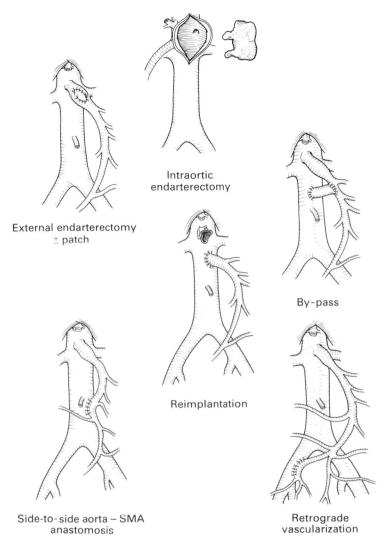

External endarterectomy
± patch

Intraortic
endarterectomy

By-pass

Reimplantation

Side-to-side aorta – SMA
anastomosis

Retrograde
vascularization

Fig. 69.4. Techniques for the surgical correction of chronic occlusion of the superior mesenteric artery.

occurring in patients with vascular disease are in fact minor infarcts.

The small intestine

The following are the more important causes of focal ischaemia of the small intestine:

1 Strangulation by hernia or adhesions.
2 Trauma to the abdomen, particularly when there is a longitudinal tear of the mesentery.
3 Vascular occlusion by embolus or thrombosis.
4 Inflammatory disease of the intestinal arteries.
5 Radiation injury (see Chaspter 70).
6 Action of enteric-coated potassium tablets or other irritants on the mucosal circulation.

The patient who develops a fibrous small intestinal stricture presents with the typical symptoms of subacute small intestinal obstruction—colicky pain occurring after a

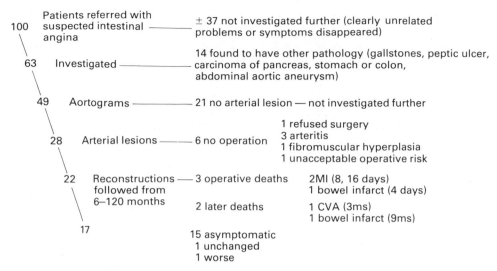

Fig. 69.5. Chronic arterial obstruction—experience at the Middlesex Hospital, London 1962–1984.

meal, accompanied by eructations, vomiting, and distenion (see Chapter 72). This usually continues for a few weeks or months and then regresses, to return later with more intensity. Untreated, the condition leads to either frank perforation of the bowel wall or complete obstruction.

Physical examination is frequently normal, but it may reveal visible peristalsis with exaggerated bowel sounds, indicating obstruction. Laboratory tests are unhelpful. X-ray examination will confirm the presence of dilated loops of jejunum with occasional fluid levels. A small bowel meal may define the position of the stricture.

The management of a focal ischaemic lesion obviously depends on the patient's symptoms, but excision and primary anastomosis of such strictures usually gives a good result.

The large intestine

Because of the poorer collateral circulation and the presence of pathogenic bacteria, focal ischaemia is more likely to occur in the colon than in the small bowel. The clinical effects vary according to the mag-

nitude and duration of the ischaemia. The two basic types of presentation are either gangrene of the colon (which presents as a fulminating, undiagnosable, abdominal catastrophe) or a milder non-gangrenous form of the disease (which usually clears spontaneously but may go on to the formation of a fibrous stricture, which usually affects the splenic flexure). It is the latter, relatively common, condition which is now referred to as ischaemic colitis. Since it was originally described in 1966 [18], ischaemic colitis has been extensively documented and the condition has been reproduced in the experimental animal [10].

Gangrene of the colon

This occurs through the same mechanisms as acute small intestinal ischaemia, and the clinical picture and management are identical. The abdomen is opened following appropriate resuscitation: a variable length of bowel, usually in the region of the splenic flexure, is found to be frankly necrotic; perforation is not unusual. The safest course is immediate resection of the affected segment with a generous margin of apparently normal bowel at either end, followed by exteriorization. Primary anastomosis under these circumstances is unwise. The mortality is high.

Ischaemic colitis

The majority of patients present with milder degrees of ischaemia. Typically there is acute pain in the left iliac fossa, fever and a moderate amount of dark rectal bleeding. Examination suggests a localized left-sided peritonitis and the usual provisional diagnosis is of acute diverticulitis of the colon, although the degree and quality of rectal bleeding is a distinguishing feature. Sigmoidoscopy usually shows a normal rectal mucosa without ulceration or inflammation (thus excluding 'colitis') but it may show submucosal oedema and a cyanotic appearance if the upper rectum is involved in the ischaemic process. A polymorphonuclear leucocytosis is found in patients seen at an early stage.

Without surgery the acute illness rapidly subsides, but there may be transient episodes of bleeding over the following few weeks. The illness may then take one of two forms: either the symptoms disappear completely and the X-ray returns to normal, or a stricture develops in the bowel, which leads to a permanent abnormality on the barium enema. Most of these strictures are asymptomatic and do not require treatment.

The changes of ischaemic colitis seen on a barium enema are typical and diagnostic. Naturally, they depend on the timing of the examination. 'Thumb-printing' is the earliest change, and has been reported as early as three days after the onset of symptoms [15]. It consists of a series of blunt semi-opaque projections into the bowel lumen. Although seen most frequently in the region of the splenic flexure, they can occur anywhere from the caecum to the recto-sigmoid (Fig. 69.6). The changes may

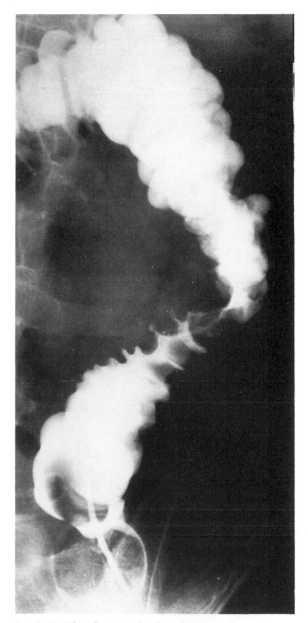

Fig. 69.6. 'Thumbprinting' in the ischaemic colon.

disappear rapidly, persist for a few weeks or progress to the more mature changes of ulceration, narrowing of the bowel, and the formation of a local stricture (Figs 69.7–9). Strictures are usually permanent, but some do resolve completely after surprisingly long intervals.

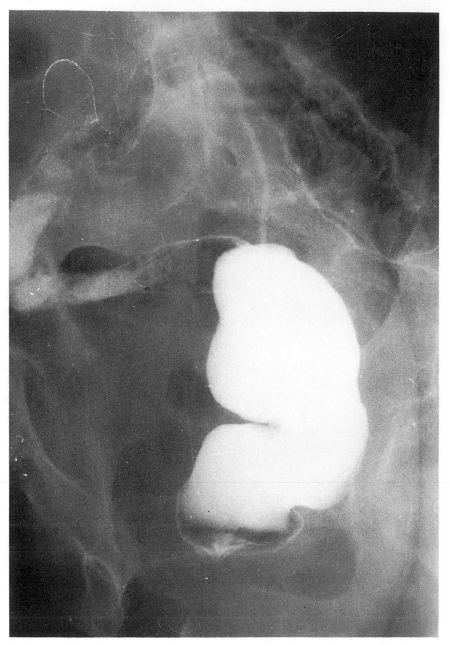

Fig. 69.7. Ischaemic colitis—barium enema showing ulceration and narrowing (the patient had undergone aortic resection six months previously).

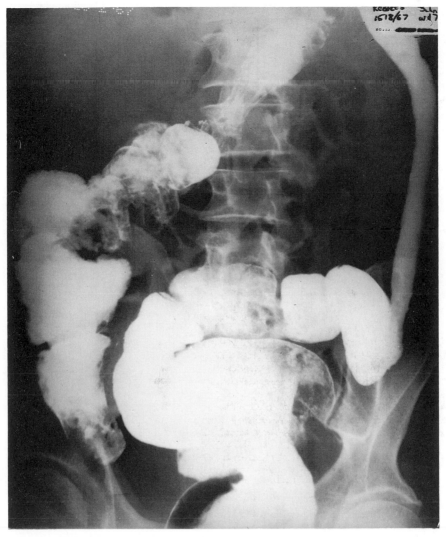

Fig. 69.8. Ischaemic colitis—a long stricture in the splenic flexure (courtesy of Dr M. Lea Thomas).

Initial management consists of making the diagnosis by ordering an early barium enema. It seems that this examination is completely safe, except in the presence of gangrene where the patient's condition would obviously preclude it. Thereafter, treatment is conservative and the majority of patients show steady spontaneous improvement. Progression from ischaemic colitis to frank gangrene is practically unknown [15]. The only indications for surgery are persistent obstructive symptoms or the presence of a short stricture which cannot be distinguished from a neoplasm.

The differential diagnosis, in the acute phase, is from perforated diverticular disease, and later on from inflammatory bowel disease. The main differentiating features are in Table 69.1.

It is possible to produce venous lesions in the colon which closely resemble ischaemic colitis [10, 15, 16] and this may have some

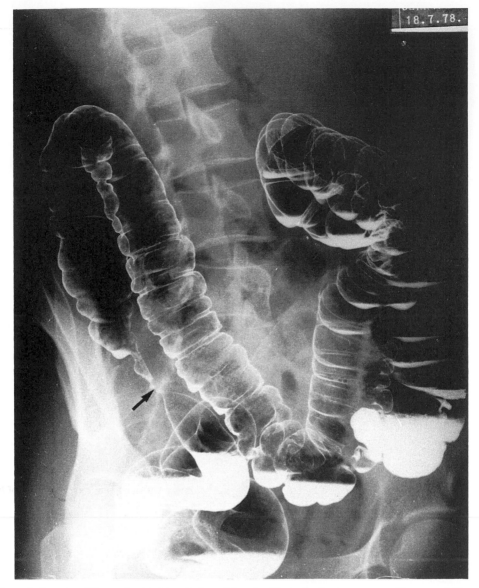

Fig. 69.9. Ischaemic colitis—a short stricture in the pelvic colon (the patient was a 24-year-old woman taking an oral contraceptive).

clinical relevance. Certainly, ischaemic (possibly venous) lesions in premenstrual women seem to have a close association with the use of oral contraceptives [2], though the evidence is entirely circumstantial (Fig. 69.9).

Conclusions

The frequency of vascular accidents in the intestinal circulation is far less than that observed in the heart, brain or limbs. Perhaps the lethal effect of such lesions has had a selective influence on the evolution

Table 69.1. Differential diagnosis of ischaemia and inflammatory bowel disease.

	Ischaemic colitis	Ulcerative colitis	Crohn's disease
Age of onset	Elderly	Any age	Any age
Presentation	Always acute	Acute or chronic	Usually chronic
Segment involved	Splenic flexure (rectum rare, anus never)	Left-sided or total (rectum always)	Anywhere (rectum usual, anus commonly)
Radiology	Thumbprints, stricture	Shortening, ulceration, megacolon	Spicules, skip lesions, obstruction
Pathology	Fibrosis, haemosiderosis	Mucosal loss, crypt abscesses	Fissures, granuloma
Associated conditions	Claudication, angina, stroke	Iritis, arthritis, erythema nodosum	Enteric fistulae, oral involvement, failure of B_{12} absorption

of the splanchnic blood supply. Mid-gut necrosis is almost always fatal, and survival figures have not improved despite advances in resuscitation and operative technique. Chronic arterial stenosis of true clinical importance is hard to find though radiological lesions are common. Focal ischaemia, particularly in the colon, occurs quite frequently, and should be considered in the differential diagnosis of an enterocolitis of unexplained origin.

References

1 BOLEY SJ, SPRAYREGAN S, SIGELMAN SS, VEITH FJ. Initial results from an aggressive surgical approach to acute mesenteric ischaemia. *Surgery* 1977;**82**: 845–855.

2 COTTON PB, THOMAS ML. Ischaemic colitis and the contraceptive pill. *Br Med J* 1971;ii:27–29.

3 CROFT RJ, MENON GP, MARSTON A. Does intestinal angina exist? A critical study of obstructed visceral arteries. *Br J Surg* 1981;**68**:316–318.

4 DELMONT JP. L'insuffisane artérielle dans les territoires du tronc céliaque et des mésenteriques supérieure et inférieure. *J Chir (Paris)* 1979;**101**: 213–236.

5 EDWARDS AJ, HAMILTON JD, TAYLOR GW, DAWSON AM. Experience with the coeliac axis compression syndrome. *Br Med J* 1970:i:342–345.

6 JAMIESON WG, MARCHOK S, ROLDSOM J, DURAND D. The early diagnosis of massive intestinal ischaemia. *Br J Surg* 1982;**69**:552–553.

7 JOSKE RA, SHAMM'A MH, DRUMMEY GD. Intestinal malabsorption following temporary occlusion of the superior mesenteric artery. *Am J Med* 1958;**25**:449–454.

8 JULIUS S, STEWART BH. Diagnostic significance of abdominal murmurs. *N Engl J Med* 1967;**276**:1175–1178.

9 LILLEHEI RC, LONGERBEAM JK, MANNAX WG. The nature of irreversible shock. *Ann Surg* 1964;**160**:682–710.

10 MARCUSON RW, STEWART JO, MARSTON A. Experimental venous lesions of the colon. *Gut* 1972;**13**:1–7.

11 MARSTON A. The bowel in shock. *Lancet* 1962;**2**:365–370.

12 MARSTON A. Causes of death in mesenteric arterial occlusion. *Ann Surg* 1963;**158**:952–969.

13 MARSTON A. Patterns of intestinal ischaemia. *Ann R Coll Surg Engl* 1964;**35**:151–181.

14 MARSTON A. Diagnosis and management of intestinal ischaemia. *Ann R Coll Surg Engl* 1972;**50**:29–44.

15 MARSTON A. *Intestinal ischaemia.* London: Edward Arnold, 1977.

16 MARSTON A, CLARKE JMF, GARCIA J, MILLER AL. Intestinal function and intestinal blood supply: a 20 year surgical study. *Gut* 1985;**26**:656–666.

17 MARSTON A, MARCUSON RW, CHAPMAN M, ARTHUR JF. Experimental study of devascularization of the colon. *Gut* 1969; **10**:121–130.

18 MARSTON A, PHEILS MT, THOMAS ML, MORSON BT. Ischaemic colitis. *Gut* 1966;**7**:1–10.

19 OTTINGER LW. Non-occlusive mesenteric infarction. *Surg Clin North Am* 1974;**54**:689–698.

20 PAWLIK W, JACOBSEN ED. The effect of digitalis on the mesenteric circulation. *Cardiovasc Res Cent Bull* 1974;**12**:80–84.

21 RUIS X, EXCALANTE JF, LLAVRADO JM, JOVER J, PUIG LA, CALLE J. Mesenteric infarction. *World J Surg* 1979;**3**:4.

Chapter 70
Radiation Damage to the Gut

B. T. JACKSON

Therapeutic X-rays directed to the pelvis or abdomen may cause undesirable side-effects on the gut [51]. This was first recognized only two years after X-rays had been discovered, when Walsh [60] described a case of acute enteritis in a research worker who had irradiated his own abdomen for two hours a day over a period of several weeks.

During the early part of the twentieth century the use of radiation as a treatment for cancer was extensively studied and both systemic and intestinal side-effects became increasingly well-defined. Experimental irradiation of the intestine in animals by Warren and Whipple [62] and by Martin and Rogers [36] produced both the early acute effects of ulceration and diarrhoea and the later more serious effects of stricturing and obstruction.

Clinical accounts of radiation damage to the human gut were either single case reports or very small series until Warren and Friedman [61] reported a series of 38 patients. The 20 years after super-voltage therapy was introduced in the 1950s witnessed an enormous increase in the published literature as the various presentations became increasingly common due to higher and higher therapeutic doses of radiation being given for an increasingly wide range of pathology. The literature is now immense. Even so, while the acute manifestations of diarrhoea, abdominal colic and nausea are well known, the diagnosis of chronic radiation injury to the gut is often delayed for an excessively long time after presentation. The management remains both controversial and difficult with high morbidity and mortality rates.

Epidemiology

The majority of patients who develop chronic radiation injury to the gut are young or middle-aged women who have been treated for pelvic malignancy. A mean age of 52 years was reported in an unusually large series of 100 patients [11]. Ninety-five were women, of whom 84% had been treated for either carcinoma of the cervix or the endometrium. Other authors have reported similar findings [13, 18]. Intestinal injury may occur in any patient who has undergone radiotherapy to the abdomen or pelvis—it is well-recognized in elderly men with carcinoma of the prostate [15] and adolescents treated for testicular tumours [47].

The reported incidence varies widely in different series and is difficult to assess. Some papers do not distinguish between large and small bowel injury and others give an incidence relating only to those complications requiring surgical treatment. It is likely that the true incidence lies between 2% [46] and 12% [11] of those patients at risk, but such figures are not strictly comparable as radiotherapeutic regimens vary in different centres.

Aetiology

Ionizing radiation preferentially damages intermitotic cells with short reproductive cycles. Thus the whole of the gut is radio-sensitive, especially the small bowel with its rapid enterocyte turnover cycle [48]. Immediate radiation effects on the gut range from minor degenerative changes in the mucosal epithelium to massive necrosis of the bowel wall, depending on the total radiation dose and the fractionation scheme.

The chronic effects of intestinal irradiation are associated with a progressive ischaemia of the gut caused by an obliterative vasculitis [9]. These ischaemic changes may take several years to develop and have been studied experimentally in animals using angiography [5]. Electron microscopy has shown that irradiation causes an early reversible spasm of gut arterioles and venules [17]. This is later replaced by irreversible thrombosis and narrowing of the vessel lumen.

The reason why only a minority of patients undergoing therapeutic irradiation develop such chronic ischaemic changes is unclear. Although there is a loose association between the development of severe acute radiation enteritis at the time of treatment and the late development of chronic symptoms, the absence of acute effects gives no assurance that late complications will not develop. In a study of 410 patients receiving pelvic radiation, 41% of the 34 patients developing late bowel complications had been without symptoms during treatment [31].

It is accepted that the likelihood of chronic gut injury is directly related to the total radiation dose. Strockbine, *et al.* [54] studied a series of 831 patients with carcinoma of the cervix and found the incidence of chronic gut complications to increase in linear fashion with higher doses of radiation, confirming the earlier findings of Gray and Kottmeier [25]. It has also been shown that the greater the volume of gut irradiated, the greater the likelihood of late gut complications [44,65]. These studies all showed a much higher incidence of gut injury when patients with pelvic malignancy underwent irradiation to the para-aorta lymph nodes in addition to the pelvis, thus exposing a larger volume of bowel to the radiation. Most published series of chronic gut injury include a small number of patients who have received an exceptionally high total dose of radiation, given either deliberately for advanced disease or in error, and those who have had an unusually large volume of bowel irradiated. However, in the majority of patients, neither of these factors apply.

Despite a keen awareness by radiotherapists of possible gut complications resulting from treatment and a consequent care with dose calculation, fractionation and shielding, a minority of patients still develop these complications while the majority, treated in identical fashion, do not. Why should this be so?

Various factors have been incriminated but none are agreed; the many accounts are confusing. Graham and Villalba [24] suggested that patients with a history of previous abdominal operation or pelvic sepsis are at special risk of small bowel injury because they are likely to have adhesions that anchor loops of small bowel in the pelvis and thus within the irradiated field. Although both Joelsson and Raf [29] and Schmitz *et al.* [50] confirmed these associations, Maruyama *et al.* [37] were unable to demonstrate any association with previous abdominal operations but agreed that sepsis might be important. DeCosse *et al.* [11] found the opposite—while previous abdominal hysterectomy seemed to be a factor, there was no association with pelvic sepsis.

Similarly, hypertension and diabetes mellitus have both been suggested as a factor by some [58] but denied by others [18]. Arteriosclerosis was considered important by DeCosse *et al.* [11] but not by Galland and Spencer [18]. While somatotype was incriminated by Graham and Villalba [24] it was denied by DeCosse *et al.* [11]. Some authors suggest that concomitant chemotherapy at the time of irradiation may increase the risk of late bowel complications—actinomycin-D [14] 5-fluorouracil

[39] and adriamycin [7] have all been implicated, but the vast majority of patients who develop chronic gut injury have not had chemotherapy. In short, not one of these factors can confidently be asserted as the cause of chronic gut radiation injury—the aetiology in most patients remains elusive.

Pathology

The progressive ischaemia which underlies chronic radiation injury of the gut may take many years to develop and may affect any part of the gut from duodenum [6] to anus [63]. The ileum and rectosigmoid region of the large bowel are the areas most commonly damaged.

The macroscopic changes in radiation-damaged bowel vary somewhat according to the interval after exposure. There is more oedema and fibrinous peritonitis in cases occurring shortly after radiation with more fibrosis and rigidity in those of late onset. In general there is an obvious colour change in the bowel which has a matt white appearance in contrast to its normal pink sheen. The bowel wall is markedly thickened and indurated. The serosa may

also have a mottled, red and white, roughened appearance (Fig. 70.1).

Narrowing of the lumen is usual and frank stenosis may occur, in which case there will be distension of the bowel proximal to the stricture (Fig. 70.2). Adherence to adjacent structures is common, especially in the pelvis, and fistulae may be present. Mucosal ulceration may be observed within the lumen of the bowel. The macroscopic abnormalities are rarely discrete and almost always merge surreptitiously into the non-injured bowel, making it difficult or impossible to tell with certainty where the junction lies. This causes difficulty for the surgeon as the anastomosis of occultly damaged intestine is likely to result in anastomotic breakdown and leakage. An added, fairly frequent finding is the presence of multiple segments of damaged bowel interposed with relatively normal segments.

There is a wide variety of microscopic abnormality [4]. Consistently, the submucosa is severely damaged showing gross thickening by fibrosis (Fig. 70.3) in which there are scattered bizarre fibroblasts with abnormal nuclei. Venous and lymphatic ectasia is prominent. Throughout the bowel wall, arterioles and small arteries show an obli-

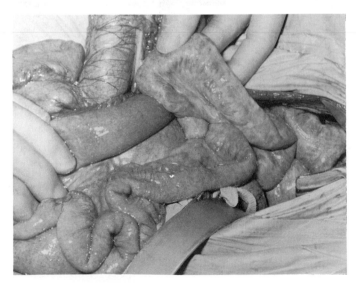

Fig. 70.1. Radiation damaged terminal ileum held adjacent to a normal segment of jejunum in a 51-year-old woman treated $2\frac{1}{2}$ years earlier for a carcinoma of cervix. The serosal colour change and narrowed lumen are clearly seen.

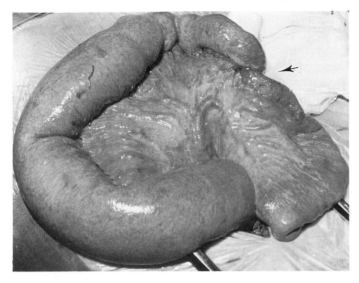

Fig. 70.2. Localized radiation stricture of small intestine (arrowed) showing proximal dilation of bowel in a 73-year-old woman eight years after irradiation of a carcinoma of cervix.

terative vasculitis leading on to sclerosis. Venules may also show obliterative changes. The mucosa is usually flat and often ulcerated, while the muscularis mucosa is thicker than normal as a result of both muscular hypertrophy and fibrosis. The serosa is always thickened by collagen and is usually infiltrated with lymphocytes and bizarre fibroblasts.

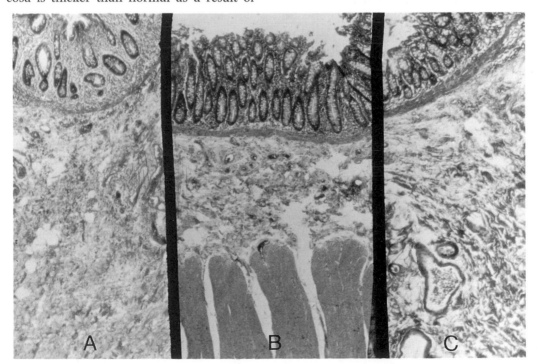

Fig. 70.3. Photomicrograph showing greatly increased submucosal fibrosis in a section of colon damaged by irradiation (A), contrasted with the normal appearance of colon (B) and the appearance of ischaemic colitis (C) (by permission of *Br J Surg*) [63].

Clinical features

A variety of clinical presentations may occur depending on the site and severity of the underlying pathology. Thus, the presenting features could be principally those of large bowel pathology, such as a change in bowel habit or alternatively those of small bowel pathology, such as malabsorption. Not infrequently, large and small bowel disease co-exist and the presentation is somewhat ill-defined.

Strictures will cause partial **intestinal obstruction**. Colicky abdominal pain associated with abdominal distension, nausea and occasional vomiting are typical of small bowel obstruction but large bowel strictures more commonly cause a change in bowel habit. Characteristically, these symptoms are intermittent, a feature which may lead to delay in diagnosis. Necrosis of the intestine may cause free **perforation** into the peritoneal cavity with sudden onset of peritonitis but, alternatively, may cause a fistula, especially to the vagina. A localized perforation of the terminal ileum sometimes becomes sealed by omentum with resulting symptoms and signs similar to those of an appendix mass. Ulceration of the mucosa may be associated with **haemorrhage** which can be severe, intermittent, or more often occult and recognized only by the development of an iron-deficiency anaemia. Small bowel **malabsorption** can result in differing presentations—diarrhoea and steatorrhoea are the most common, but megaloblastic anaemia, hypocalcaemia, hypomagnesaemia or hypoproteinaemia may also occur. Weight loss and clinical evidence of **malnutrition** to the point of cachexia may also occur—these features may incorrectly be ascribed to recurrence of the original malignancy.

Radiation injury to the rectum causes a decrease in rectal capacity and compliance, which corelates with the frequency and urgency of defecation [59].

In addition to symptoms and signs caused by gut damage, there is often associated damage to the urinary bladder with symptoms such as frequency of micturition, dysuria or haematuria. On occasions, the pelvis may become grossly indurated with radiation fibrosis and a 'frozen pelvis' may be palpable on rectal or vaginal examination. This must not be confused with recurrence of the tumour.

The time interval between the course of radiotherapy and the onset of symptoms is very variable, and is no diagnostic guide. DeCosse *et al.* [11] reported a mean interval of 6.5 years (range 1 month to 31 years) between radiation and symptoms, which is similar to the author's experience [28]. Once it develops, radiation injury to the gut is typically progressive with one feature following another over a period of many years. No patient should ever be considered wholly cured, for he or she always at risk from further problems.

Investigations

The diagnosis of radiation injury to the gut should be considered in every patient who presents with abdominal symptoms after a past history of pelvic or abdominal irradiation. In many instances, this diagnosis will be wrong but, unless radiation damaged bowel is suspected and appropriate investigations performed, the true explanation of the patient's symptoms may easily be missed.

Laboratory studies by and large, are less helpful than radiology and endoscopy. Blood analysis may show evidence of malabsorption of iron, calcium, magnesium or vitamin B_{12} while stool analysis may show steatorrhoea [16, 57]. The Schilling test has been used to show subclinical malabsorption of vitamin B_{12} after pelvic radiation [35] and C^{14} bile-acid breath testing has also been suggested as a useful test of subclinical ileal damage [30, 41]. Recently it

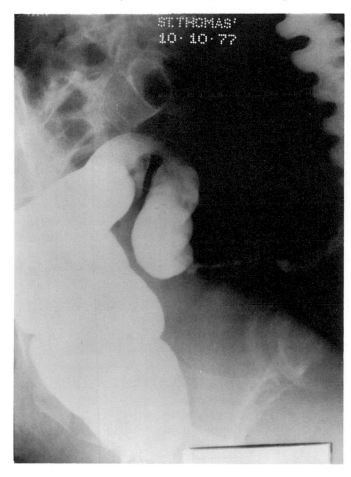

Fig. 70.4. Radiation sigmoid stricture in a 35-year-old woman treated four years earlier for a carcinoma of cervix.

has been shown that patients with radiation gut injury have a high platelet count and this may be useful as a diagnostic aid [8].

Contrast radiology is the mainstay of investigation. Although plain abdominal radiographs may show dilated loops of intestine, with or without fluid levels, these are usually normal and barium contrast studies of both large and small bowel are necessary. Single, or multiple, strictures (Fig. 70.4), transverse barring (Fig. 70.5), rose thorn fissures, nodular filling defects and fistulae (Fig. 70.6) all may be observed, often in combination. These changes, while not radiologically specific for radiation injury [23], are virtually diagnostic when combined with history and physical signs. Misleadingly, however, contrast studies of the damaged bowel are sometimes normal and should unhesitatingly be repeated if symptoms continue and clinical suspicion persists. Gentle **sigmoidoscopy** should alway precede the barium enema and this may show a mucosal abnormality or stricturing.

Fibreoptic colonoscopy is often helpful in the diagnosis of colonic damage, showing abnormalities such as shallow ulceration or mucosal haemorrhage which were not shown on barium radiography.

Intravenous urography and cystoscopy should also be performed if urinary symptoms are present.

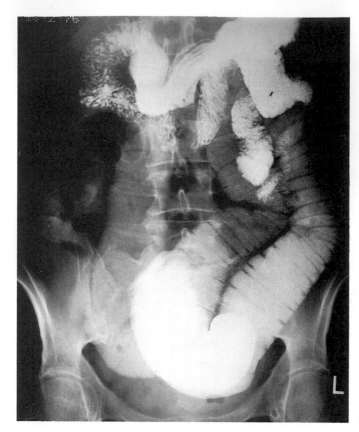

Fig. 70.5. Distended small bowel showing transverse barring in a 56-year-old woman treated 12 years earlier for a carcinoma of ovary.

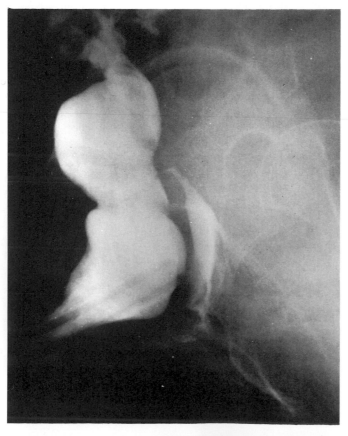

Fig. 70.6. Rectovaginal fistula in a 62-year-old woman treated 28 years earlier with radiotherapy for menorrhagia.

Differential diagnosis

The keynote of diagnosis is to have a high index of suspicion and to actively think of radiation damage as a possible explanation for the patient's symptoms. All too often the correct diagnosis is delayed for many months as a result of the clinician wrongly ascribing the clinical features to an alternative cause, especially that of **recurrent tumour**. This error is especially likely if the pelvis is fibrotic as a result of the radiation, and vaginal palpation demonstrates woody-hard induration in the pouch of Douglas. Although recurrent tumour and radiation injury to the gut may coexist, this is not the case in the majority of patients. Most patients presenting with gut radiation injury are tumour-free.

Another common diagnostic mistake is to ascribe the sometimes rather non-specific abdominal symptoms as being caused by the **irritable bowel syndrome** or even as **psychogenic** in origin. Investigation is then delayed and the true diagnosis may not be made until a fistula develops or the bowel perforates many months later [28].

Prevention

When the radiotherapist plans treatment for pelvic or abdominal malignancy, a balance is made between the giving of optimal cancer therapy and the risk of unacceptable side-effects caused by an excessive dose of radiation. These two factors should be balanced as a conscious exercise for each and every patient. A very high dosage should only be given after considered judgement.

Some radiotherapists recommend that pelvic radiation should be performed with the patient in the head-down position, to displace the small bowel as far away from the pelvis as is possible [26]. In this way the incidence of ileal damage may be lessened. Small bowel may also be excluded from the pelvis by the insertion of a silastic prosthesis, when it is known that high dosage pelvic radiotherapy is indicated [55].

Experimentally, the use of sulphonamides [52], salicylates [38] or antiproteases [45] have been shown to reduce acute radiation enteritis, but none of these agents have found a place in clinical practice and there is no evidence that they reduce the likelihood of chronic gut injury.

Management

The management of the radiation injured gut is difficult, protracted and often dangerous. All too often complication follows upon complication, especially after surgical operation. Long-term follow-up is essential. Although the mainstay of treatment is surgical resection of the diseased intestine, supportive medical treatment is also necessary. In as much as the clinical presentations may vary widely, the management will clearly vary in detail from patient to patient.

Medical treatment

Not all patients are sufficiently ill to require surgical operation, while many who have undergone an operation require active and long-lasting medical care. Watery diarrhoea may be associated either with radiation damage to the terminal ileum or to surgical resection, especially if the ileocaecal valve is removed. In part, this is caused by bile salts entering the colon. Vitamin B_{12} malabsorption may also occur. Large resections of the ileum may be associated with steatorrhoea, while diffuse disease or removal of the jejunum may cause deficiency of folate, lactose, iron, calcium and magnesium. Medical treatment of small bowel disease is therefore principally directed towards the correction of these abnormalities (see Chapter 46).

A low fat diet should be encouraged

although compliance may be poor. Cholestyramine should reduce diarrhoea if bile
salts are irritating the colon, while drugs
such as codeine phosphate, diphenoxylate
or loperamide slow intestinal transit time.
Regular vitamin B_{12} injections should be
given if the terminal ileum is diseased, or
has been resected and care must be taken
that the patient does not insidiously develop
folate, calcium or other deficiency. Smooth
muscle relaxants are often prescribed but
are of uncertain value. Other less widely
used medical measures that have been suggested include medium-chain-triglyceride
supplements [14], a gluten-free diet [27],
sulphonamides [22], steroids [40] or a low
residue, high calorie liquid diet [3].

The medical treatment of large bowel disease is largely the treatment of diarrhoea or
bleeding caused by radiation-induced
proctocolitis. Topical steroids are usually
given although their efficacy is not proven
and sulphasalazine may also be prescribed.
Iron-deficiency anaemia caused by chronic
bleeding should be corrected.

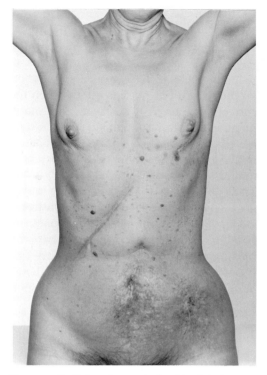

Fig. 70.7. Radiation changes in the skin of the
anterior abdominal wall in a 56-year-old woman
treated 29 years earlier for a soft tissue sarcoma of
the retroperitoneum.

Surgical treatment

The indications for operation are intestinal
obstruction, fistula formation, perforation,
haemorrhage or long continued abdominal
symptoms, especially pain, which are uncontrolled by medical treatment.

Energetic preoperative management is
necessary for many patients. Rehydration,
correction of electrolyte imbalance and correction of anaemia are essential. If the
patient is chronically malnourished, parenteral nutrition may be necessary.

Intravenous metronidazole and a broad-
spectrum antibiotic are given at the time of
anaesthetic induction. Prophylaxis against
deep-vein thrombosis is given routinely and
a generous incision is made to get good exposure and access to the entire peritoneal
cavity. The incision should avoid any skin
which has obviously been damaged by

radiation (Fig. 70.7). A full laparotomy is
performed in order to exclude the presence
of metastatic tumour or local tumour recurrence. Sometimes the irradiated pelvic
contents are hard and fixed, but these
changes should not be mistaken for infiltrating tumour. If in doubt, a biopsy and
frozen tissue section may be performed.
Deep pelvic dissection must be avoided at
all costs as the risk of damage to surrounding organs, especially the bladder and ure-
ters, is considerable.

Both small and large bowel are carefully
examined throughout, with special reference to the ileum and rectosigmoid junction. Occasionally, the radiation damage
will macroscopically be confined to a localized segment of intestine but usually there
is no clear line of demarcation between nor-

mal and abnormal bowel and the surgeon is faced with uncertainty as to how much to resect; too little may result in a leaking anastomosis, while too much may lead to the development of the 'short bowel syndrome'. This problem has led some authors to suggest that side-to-side bypass of damaged small bowel is less dangerous than resection [12, 56]. This view is challenged by others [34, 42]. Sterns *et al.* [53] stressed that bypass operations do not ent perforation of the bypassed bowel, reporting this complication with death of a patient. Massive haemorrhage has occurred from bypassed intestine six years after the surgery [49].

That there are risks to resection and anastomosis cannot be denied—one retrospective review reported five patients with radiation damage to the small bowel who underwent a total of 11 anastomoses with a leakage rate of 100%—all five patients died [64]. Another series of 17 patients had a mortality rate of 53% and an anastomotic leak rate of 65% [56]. Despite these depressing results most writers agree that resection is the treatment of choice. Although it has been suggested that frozen tissue section examination of the cut ends of the bowel should be performed before anastomosis in order to exclude radiation changes [33], meticulous surgical technique with careful attention to detail is probably more important. The anastomosis should be performed without clamps to avoid jeopardizing an already precarious blood supply; the anastomosis should be tension free; a pulsatile blood supply should be visible at the cut ends of the bowel; small bites of tissue should be taken and the sutures not inserted too tightly; the anastomosis should be wrapped in omentum; and if there is any vestige of doubt about the viability of the anastomosis, a temporary loop stoma above the anastomosis should be performed without hesitation.

Resection of the damaged rectosigmoid or upper rectum poses special problems, for the risk of anastomotic breakdown when using conventional operative techniques is especially high [32]. This has led to the suggestion that a simple defunctioning colostomy is safer than resection [2]. Increasing experience with a staged sleeve colo-anal anastomosis technique [43] is very encouraging, and is now probably the operation of choice [10, 21]. By this means a permanent colostomy can be avoided. It is important to ensure that the proximal colon used for the anastomosis is non-irradiated [19].

Radiation-induced fistulae may also be treated by sleeve colo-anal anastomosis [43], but some authors prefer exclusion techniques [1, 20].

Prognosis

A reading of the references quoted in this review will confirm that the average patient with radiation injury of the gut has a grim prognosis. Firstly, the diagnosis may be delayed allowing complications to develop. Secondly, when the diagnosis is made and surgical operation performed, the outcome may all too often be death or long-term morbidity as a result of the operation itself. Thirdly, recurrence of radiation injury is not uncommon as the disease is often progressive. In few fields of gastroenterology are the problems and difficulties of management more challenging.

References

1 AITKEN RJ, ELLIOT MS. Sigmoid exclusion: a new technique in the management of radiation-induced fistula. *Br J Surg* 1985;72:731–732.
2 ANSELINE PF, LAVERY IC, FAZIO VW, JAGELMAN DG, WEAKLEY FL. Radiation injury to the rectum. *Ann Surg* 1981;194:716–724.
3 BEER WH, FAN A, HALSTED CH. Clinical and nutritional implications of radiation enteritis. *Am J Clin Nutr* 1985;41:85–91.
4 BERTHRONG M, FAJARDO LF. Radiation injury in surgical pathology. *Am J Surg Path* 1981;5:153–178.

5 BOSNIAK MA, HARDY MA, QUINT J, GHOSSEIN NA. Demonstration of the effect of irradiation on canine bowel using in vivo photographic magnification angiography. *Radiology* 1969;**93**:1361–1368.

6 BURN JI. Radiation duodenitis. *Proc R Soc Med* 1971;**64**:395–396.

7 BYFIELD JE, WATRING WG, LEMKIN SR, *et al*. Adriamycin; a useful drug for combination with radiation therapy. *Proc Am Assoc Cancer Res* 1975;**16**:253.

8 CARR ND, HOLDEN D, HASLETON PS, SCHOFIELD PF. Platelet count in radiation bowel disease: an aid to diagnosis. *Brit J Surg* 1985;**72**:287–288.

9 CARR ND, PULLEN BR, HASLETON PS, SCHOFIELD PF. Microvascular studies in human radiation bowel disease. *Gut* 1984;**25**:448–454.

10 COOKE SAR, DE MOOR NG. The surgical treatment of the radiation-damaged rectum. *Br J Surg* 1981;**68**:488–492.

11 DeCOSSE JJ, RHODES RS, WENTZ WB, REAGEN JW, DWORKEN HJ, HOLDEN WD. The natural history and management of radiation induced injury of the gastrointestinal tract. *Ann Surg* 1969;**170**:369–384.

12 DENCKER H, JOHNSSON JE, LIEDBERG G, TIBBLIN S. Surgical aspects of radiation injury to the small and large intestines. *Acta Chir Scand* 1971;**137**:692–695.

13 DEVENEY CW, LEWIS FR, SHROCK TR. Surgical management of radiation injury of the small and large intestine. *Dis Colon Rectum* 1976;**19**:25–29.

14 DONALDSON SS, JUNDT S, RICOUR C, SARRAZIN D, LEMERLE J, SCHWEISGUTH O. Radiation enteritis in children. *Cancer* 1975;**35**:1167–1178.

15 DUGGAN FJ, SANFORD EJ, ROHNER TJ. Radiation enteritis following radiotherapy for prostatic carcinoma. *Br J Urol* 1975;**47**:441–444.

16 DUNCAN W, LEONARD JC. The malabsorption syndrome following radiotherapy. *Q J Med* 1965;**34**:319–329.

17 FONKALSRUD EW, SANCHEZ M, ZERUBAVEL R, MAHONEY A. Serial changes in arterial structure following radiation therapy. *Surg Gynecol Obstet* 1977;**145**:395–400.

18 GALLAND RB, SPENCER J. Radiation-induced gastrointestinal fistulae. *Ann Roy Coll Surg Eng* 1986;**68**:5–7.

19 GALLAND RB, SPENCER J. Surgical aspects of radiation injury to the intestine. *Br J Surg* 1979;**66**:135–138.

20 GALLAND RB, SPENCER J. Surgical management of radiation enteritis. *Surgery* 1986;**99**:133–138.

21 GAZET JC. Parks' coloanal pull-through anastomosis for severe, complicated radiation proctitis. *Dis Colon Rectum* 1985;**28**:110–114.

22 GOLDSTEIN F, KHOURY J, THORNTON JJ. Treatment of chronic radiation enteritis and colitis with salicylazosulfapyridine and systemic corticosteroids. *Am J Gastroenterol* 1976;**65**:201–208.

23 GOLDSTEIN HM. Small bowel and colon. In Libschitz HI, ed. *Diagnostic Roentgenology of Radiotherapy Change*. Baltimore, Williams & Wilkins Company: 1979;85–100.

24 GRAHAM JB, VILEALBA RJ. Damage to the small intestine by radiotherapy. *Surg Gynecol Obstet* 1963;**116**:665–668.

25 GRAY MJ, KOTTMEIER HL. Rectal and bladder injuries following radium therapy for carcinoma of the cervix at the Radiumhemmet. *Am J Obstet Gynecol* 1957;**74**:1294–1303.

26 GREEN N, IBA G, SMITH WR. Measures to minimise small intestine injury in the irradiated pelvis. *Cancer* 1975;**35**:1633–1640.

27 HADDAD H, BOUNOS G, TAHAN WT, DEVROEDE G, BEAUDRY R, LAFOND R. Long-term nutrition with an elemental diet following intensive abdominal irradiation. *Dis Colon Rectum* 1974;**17**:373–376.

28 JACKSON BT. Bowel damage from radiation. *Proc R Soc Med* 1976;**69**:683–686.

29 JOELSSON I, RAF L. Late injuries of the small intestine following radiotherapy for uterine carcinoma. *Acta Chir Scand* 1973;**139**:194–200.

30 KINSELLA TJ, BLOOMER WD. Tolerance of the intestine to radiation therapy. *Surg Gynecol Obstet* 1980;**151**:273–284.

31 KLINE JC, BUCHLER DA, BOONE ML, PECKHAM BM, CARR WF. The relationship of reactions to complications in the radiation therapy of cancer of the cervix. *Radiology* 1972;**105**:413–416.

32 LEDDA P, SHAW JFL, EVERETT WG. Surgical treatment of irradiation injury to the large bowel. *J R Coll Surg Edinb* 1981;**26**:348–356.

33 LOCALIO SA, PACHTER HL, GOUGE TH. The radiation-injured bowel. In: Nyhus LM ed, *Surgery Annual*. New York: Appleton-Century-Croft, 1979;181–205.

34 LOCALIO SA, STONE A, FRIEDMAN M. Surgical aspects of radiation enteritis. *Surg Gynecol Obstet* 1969;**129**:1163–1172.

35 McBRIEN MP. Vitamin B$_{12}$ malabsorption after cobalt teletherapy for carcinoma of the bladder. *Br Med J* 1973;**1**:648–650.

36 MARTIN CL, ROGERS FT. Roentgen-ray cachexia. *Am J Roentgen* 1924;**11**:280–286.

37 MARUYAMA Y, VAN NAGELL JR, UTLEY J, VIDER ML, PARKER JC. Radiation and small bowel complications in cervical carcinoma therapy. *Radiology* 1974;**112**:699–703.

38 MENNIE AT, DALLEY VM, DINEEN LC, COLLIER HOJ. Treatment of radiation induced gastrointestinal distress with acetylsalicylate. *Lancet* 1975;**ii**:942–943.

39 MOERTEL CG, CHILDS DS, REITEMEIER RJ, COLBY MY, HOLBROOK MA. Combined 5-fluorouracil and supervoltage radiation therapy of locally unresectable gastrointestinal cancer. *Lancet* 1969;**ii**:865–867.

40 MORGENSTERN L, THOMPSON R, FRIEDMAN NB. The

modern enigma of radiation enteropathy: sequelae and solutions. *Am J Surg* 1977;**134**:166–172.

41 NEWMAN A, KATSARIS J, BLENDIS LM, CHARLESWORTH M, WALTER LH. Small intestinal injury in women who have had pelvic radiotherapy. *Lancet* 1973;**ii**:1471–1473.

42 PALMER JA, BUSH RS. Radiation injuries to the bowel associated with the treatment of carcinoma of the cervix. *Surgery* 1976;**80**:458–464.

43 PARKS AG, ALLEN CLO, FRANK JD, McPARTLIN JF. A method of treating post-irradiation rectovaginal fistulas. *Br J Surg* 1978;**65**:417–421.

44 PIVER MS, BARLOW JJ. High dose irradiation to biopsy confirmed aortic node metastases from carcinoma of the uterine cervix. *Cancer* 1977;**39**:1243–1246.

45 RACHOOTIN S, SHAPIRO S, YAMAKAWA T, GOLDMAN L, PATIN S, MORGENSTERN L. Potent anti-proteases derived from *Ascaris lumbricoides*: efficacy in amelioration of post-radiation enteropathy. *Gastroenterology* 1972;**62**:796.

46 REQUARTH W, ROBERTS S. Intestinal injuries following irradiation of pelvic viscera for malignancy. *Arch Surg* 1956;**43**:682–688.

47 ROSWIT B, MALSKY SJ, REID CB. Severe radiation injuries of the stomach, small intestine, colon and rectum. *Am J Roentgen* 1972;**114**:460–475.

48 RUBIN P, CASARETT GW. Clinical radiation pathology as applied to curative radiotherapy. *Cancer* 1968;**2**:767–778.

49 SCHMITT FH, SYMMONDS RE. Surgical treatment of radiation induced injuries of the intestine. *Surg Gynecol Obstet* 1981;**153**:896–900.

50 SCHMITZ RL, CHAO JH, BARTOLOME JS. Intestinal injuries incidental to irradiation of the cervix of the uterus. *Surg Gynecol Obstet* 1974;**138**:29–32.

51 SCHOFIELD PF. Bowel disease after radiotherapy. *J Roy Soc Med* 1983;**76**:463–466.

52 SPRATT JS, HEINBECKER P, SLATZSTEIN SL. The influence of succinylsulfathiazole (sulfasuxidine) upon the response of canine small intestine to irradiation. *Cancer* 1961;**14**:862–874.

53 STERNS EE, PALMER JA, KERGIN FG. The surgical significance of radiation injuries to bowel. *Can J Surg* 1964;**7**:407–413.

54 STROCKBINE MF, HANCOCK JE, FLETCHER GH. Complications of 831 patients with squamous cell carcinoma of the intact uterine cervix treated with 2000 rad or more whole pelvis irradiation. *Am J Roentgen* 1970;**108**:293–304.

55 SUGARBAKER PH. Intrapelvic prosthesis to prevent injury of the small intestine with high dose pelvic irradiation. *Surg Gynaecol Obstet* 1983;**157**(3):269–271.

56 SWAN RW, FOWLER WC, BORONOW RC. Surgical management of radiation injury to the small intestine. *Surg Gynecol Obstet* 1976;**142**:325–327.

57 TANKEL HI, CLARK DH, LEE FD. Radiation enteritis with malabsorption. *Gut* 1965;**6**:560–569.

58 VAN NAGELL JR, MARUYAMA Y, PARKER JC, DALTON WL. Small bowel injury following radiation therapy for cervical cancer. *Am J Obstet Gynecol* 1974;**118**:163–167.

59 VARMA JS, SMITH AN, BUSUTTIL A. Correlation of clinical and manometric abnormalities of rectal function following chronic radiation injury. *Br J Surg* 1985;**72**:875–878.

60 WALSH D. Deep tissue traumatism from Roentgen ray exposure. *Br Med J* 1897;272–273.

61 WARREN S, FRIEDMAN NB. Pathology and pathologic diagnosis of radiation lesions in the gastrointestinal tract. *Am J Path* 1942;**18**:499–513.

62 WARREN SL, WHIPPLE GH, Roentgen ray intoxication. *J Exp Med* 1922;**35**:187–202.

63 WELLWOOD JM, JACKSON BT. The intestinal complications of radiotherapy. *Br J Surg* 1973;**60**:814–818.

64 WELLWOOD JM, JACKSON BT, BATES TD. Breakdown of small bowel anastomoses after pelvic radiotherapy. *Ann R Coll Surg Eng* 1974;**54**:306–308.

65 WHARTON JT, JONES HW, DAY TG, RUTLEDGE FN, FLETCHER GH. Preirradiation celiotomy and extended field irradiation for invasive carcinoma of the cervix. *Obstet Gynecol* 1977;**49**:333–338.

Chapter 71
Diseases of the Peritoneum

G. H. HUTCHINSON

The peritoneum is the endothelial lining of the abdominal cavity and forms one of the largest of the serous sacs of the body. Like the pleura and pericardium it is formed of a parietal and visceral layer separated by a thin film of lubricating fluid. It is a closed sac apart from the opening of the fallopian tubes in women.

The peritoneum is a tough layer of elastic areolar tissue lined by pavement epithelium with a deeper, loose connective tissue layer. Electron microscopy reveals numerous microvilli projecting from the mesothelial surface. Most of the visceral peritoneum receives a blood supply from the splanchnic circulation and is drained by the portal venous system.

The parietal peritoneum derives its nerve supply from the segmental spinal nerves that innervate the overlying muscle layers while most of the nerve supply to the visceral peritoneum is derived from the autonomic nerves of the abdominal cavity. The one exception is the diaphragmatic peritoneal covering, which receives its nerve supply through the phrenic nerve—which explains why inflammation in this area produces pain in the shoulder tip.

The peritoneum acts as a semipermeable membrane with a surface area approaching that of the skin ($2\,m^2$). It accounts for a significant exchange of water, electrolytes, peptides and similar molecules (up to 5,000 daltons in size). In addition to passive osmotic and hydrostatic forces, there is also intracellular and transcellular active transport—property used in peritoneal dialysis. However endogenous and exogenous toxic substances, such as bacterial toxins in faecal peritonitis, are also readily absorbed to produce systemic effects. Particulate materials ($<10\,\mu m$), such as erythrocytes and bacteria, are taken up by phagocytic cells or are absorbed through stomata on the peritoneal surface of the diaphragm into lymph channels, assisted by respiratory movements of the diaphragm.

Peritonitis is an inflammation of part or all of the parietal and visceral surfaces of the abdominal cavity. It may be acute or chronic, infective or sterile, localized or diffuse, and primary or secondary. When 'peritonitis' is used without qualification it generally implies acute suppurative bacterial peritonitis.

Acute suppurative peritonitis

Pathogenic organisms may reach the peritoneal cavity:

1 By perforation, suppuration or ischaemia of the gastrointestinal or biliary tract.
2 Via the female genital tract (salpingitis or puerperal infection).
3 Through a penetrating abdominal injury (gunshot or stabbing).
4 Via the blood supply ('primary' peritonitis).

The interaction of host defences and microbacterial features governs the natural history of acute bacterial peritonitis.

Host factors

The peritoneal cavity is well-adapted to combat infection. More than 80 years ago

1056

MacCallum demonstrated clearance of bacteria from the peritoneal cavity via the diaphragmatic lymphatics acting as a front-line defence mechanism [40]. This operates within a few minutes of the contamination and is accompanied by a brisk inflammatory response. The peritoneal membrane becomes hyperaemic and oedematous with local vascular congestion; this is followed by production of an exudate rich in polymorphs, phagocytes and antibodies (and antibiotics, if already in the circulation). The number of polymorphs increases with time and is directly correlated with the number and virulence of the bacteria, many of which activate the alternative complement pathway resulting in opsonic and chemotactic enhancement of bacterial clearance [7].

The exudate is fibrinous and this glues together the bowel and omentum to seal off any inflamed focus. The way in which the greater omentum migrates to the source of the inflammation is ill-understood but this mechanism ('abdominal policeman') is of great value in localizing infection within the abdominal cavity [1]. In children the omentum is short and fragile and peritonitis is more often diffuse with a higher morbidity [29]—supporting the strategic role of the omentum in controlling contamination.

Anatomical factors also tend to localize spread [44]. Three barriers divide the peritoneal cavity into four potential compartments:

1 A longitudinal barrier—formed by the vertebrae, aorta, inferior vena cava and mesentery—separating right and left infracolic spaces.

2 An upper transverse barrier—formed by the transverse colon and its mesentery—separating supra- and infra-colic compartments.

3 A lower transverse barrier—formed by the pelvic brim, iliac vessels and psoas muscles—delineating a pelvic compartment.

Microbial factors

The severity and progression of suppurative peritonitis depends on the type and virulence of the organism(s) and the magnitude of the inoculum. Most intra-abdominal sepsis is polymicrobial with a mixture of aerobes, facultative anaerobes and strict anaerobic bacteria in 70% of cultures (Table 71.1).

An infection is established by fewer bacteria if a synergistic combination of aerobic and anaerobic organisms are present (for example, *Escherichia coli* and *Bacteroides fragilis*) [46]. It is thought that the facultative bacteria serve to lower the partial pressure of oxygen in the tissues, promoting the growth of obligate anaerobes. Experimental studies have also shown different elimination patterns from the peritoneum of *B. fragilis* (granulocyte mobilization) and *E. coli* (requires opsonization to be more readily phagocytosed), indicating a likely difference in bacterial surface characteristics [45].

Coliform organisms produce endotoxins which are readily absorbed through the inflamed peritoneum. These can produce systemic effects. Other substances (such as blood, bile, urine, faeces, gastric mucin, necrotic tissue and barium) can enhance microbial virulence and reduce bacterial clearance.

Clinical features and pathophysiology

The effects of peritonitis are superimposed upon those of the causative lesion (for example, acute appendicitis, pancreatitis, diverticulitis, perforation, etc.) whose specific clinical features are detailed in other sections. Briefly, if a viscus ruptures or perforates, pain is often severe over the site of leakage, becoming diffuse unless defence mechanisms contain the spillage to one site.

With generalized peritonitis the patient is anorexic, pyrexial and motionless with a painful rigid abdomen. Abdominal disten-

Table 71.1. Bacterial flora of secondary peritonitis.

Gram-positive	Gram-negative	
Aerobic		
Streptococcus faecalis	*Escherichia coli*	
Streptococcus	*Klebsiella*	'Aerobacter
Non-haemolytic		Coliforms'
Alpha-haemolytic	*Enterobacter* species	
Beta-haemolytic		
Streptococcus milleri		
Staphylococcus aureus	*Pseudomonas* species	
Staphylococcus albus	*Proteus* species	
Anaerobic		
Peptostreptococcus species	*Bacteroides fragilis*	
Clostridium species	*Fusobacterium* species	
Peptococcus species	*Bifido* bacterium species	
	Lactobacillus species	

sion and pain produce rapid, shallow respiration, often followed by basal atelectasis. Peritoneal irritation produces vasoconstriction, tachycardia and sweating.

The pain may decrease as the exudate dilutes the infection. However a copious exudate, together with fluid sequestration within the adynamic intestine (ileus) and vomiting, may lead to a severe hypovolaemia. This may be compounded by the effects of an endotoxaemia. Lipopolysaccharide endotoxins, produced by many of the coliform organisms, cause dilatation of arterioles and venules with loss of endothelial integrity. This can result in a rapid expansion of the venous and capillary compartments leading to irreversible septic shock. Endotoxaemia produces an initial picture of vasodilatation (warm shock) until the effects of hypovolaemia predominate when hypothermia ensues (especially in children). Poor tissue perfusion also leads to a shift towards anaerobic metabolism and the development of lactic acidosis.

Hypovolaemia stimulates aldosterone and anti-diuretic hormone secretion leading to enhanced renal conservation of sodium and water, increased potassium loss and a diminished urine output—which may end in renal failure.

Types of secondary peritonitis

Infective

This is the commonest form of peritonitis, complicating such conditions as appendicitis, cholecystitis, colonic perforation or infection, intestinal ischaemia and acute salpingitis.

Sterile (chemical)

This develops when sterile but irritant material soils the peritoneal cavity. Examples include blood, bile, gastric or pancreatic juices, chyle, foreign bodies and barium.

Blood (for example from a ruptured ectopic pregnancy) or urine (from a ruptured bladder) may evoke only a mild inflammatory reaction, but superadded infection significantly increases morbidity. Although all contamination stemming from the gastrointestinal tract will eventually become infected (often within 12 hours), cultures taken at operation after gastric or duodenal perforation are often sterile. Small bowel perforations from, for example, fish bones are also often sterile although those that occur in association within intestinal obstruction are always infected.

Meconium peritonitis occurs through intra-uterine intestinal perforation, usually secondary to obstruction or atresia. The meconium is sterile but contains digestive enzymes that evoke an intense peritoneal reaction leading to the characteristic calcification within the peritoneal cavity. Meconium ileus is seen in 5–10% of cystic fibrosis patients and the inspissated plugs of meconium may cause ileal perforations with a poor prognosis [39].

Postoperative

Postoperative peritonitis is more lethal than other forms of peritonitis [8]. A bile leak after biliary surgery, or a gastroduodenal leak after gastric surgery, may be initially sterile but it inevitably becomes infected. Leakage from a large bowel anastomosis will cause either local or diffuse faecal peritonitis with an appropriate outcome (Table 71.2).

Investigations

The diagnosis of peritonitis is largely clinical—history and, in particular, abdominal examination. A definitive diagnosis often leads to an immediate laparotomy and clinical judgement holds sovereignty over laboratory investigations. Computer-aided diagnosis has been shown to improve the accuracy of clinical assessment [15, 16].

A **full blood count** may demonstrate a leucocytosis but this may be absent in elderly or debilitated patients, or in advanced peritonitis where 'trapping' of neutrophils in the exudate or abscesses occurs. Neutropenia is an ominous sign.

Biochemical investigations should include urea and electrolytes to assess hydration and a serum amylase to exclude acute pancreatitis (see Chapter 35).

An **erect chest X-ray** may reveal free gas under the diaphragm, basal atalectasis, or may exclude an early basal pneumonia. **Plain abdominal radiographs**, erect and supine, may show features of an ileus (local or generalized) varying from one or two 'sentinel' loops of dilated small bowel with fluid levels in localized peritonitis to widespread dilatation of the whole gut in severe advanced generalized peritonitis. A massive pneumoperitoneum usually implies a perforation of an obstructed colon although it has been described in gastric perforations when associated with aerophagy [28].

Four-quadrant **paracentesis** has been advocated in the diagnosis of intra-abdominal haemorrhage, pancreatitis or postoperative peritonitis. However a single

Table 71.2. The mortality of different types of peritonitis.

Aetiology of peritonitis	Mortality (%)
Perforated appendicitis	5 (maximal at extremes of age)
Gastroduodenal perforation	10 (gastric twice as lethal as duodenal perforation)
Perforated colon localized contamination generalized faecal peritonitis	15–25 75
Small bowel pathology	15
Postoperative peritonitis	50–70

peritoneal tap at the point of maximal tenderness, or insertion of a peritoneal dialysis catheter into the pelvis, may prove equally effective [19] particularly if a saline intraperitoneal lavage is performed when the tap is dry.

Treatment

Analgesia

Pain relief is often demanded but the premature use of analgesia may hamper proper evaluation of the patient; analgesia should therefore be withheld until a diagnosis or decision to operate has been made. If pain is severe small, repeated doses of an intravenous narcotic are preferred to the traditional large intramuscular dose, especially in patients who are unstable or in shock.

Drip and suck

The correction of hypovolaemia is an essential prerequisite to further management. Surgery should not be undertaken until this is well in hand. Crystalloid solutions are often satisfactory, with appropriate potassium supplements, but colloid solutions (such as purified protein fraction) may be needed if peritoneal exudate is considerable. With serious 'septic shock', it is advisable to monitor urine osmolarity, central venous pressure and blood gases; the patient may require inotropic drugs and ventilatory support.

Gastric decompression lessens the risk of inhalation of vomit and helps relieve discomfort by preventing intestinal distension. Fluid and gas should be aspirated frequently and the tube placed on free-drainage.

Antibiotics

Every patient with generalized peritonitis must be considered a candidate for bacter-aemia and therefore merits treatment with antibiotics. To provide effective cover against likely pathogens (a mixture of aerobic and anaerobic bacteria) a triple combination of an aminoglycoside, metronidazole and ampicillin (or cephalosporin) is recommended [34]. Irrigation of the peritoneal cavity with an antibiotic solution (for example tetracycline) has been advocated [34] which may also reduce the risk of subsequent wound infection [62].

Surgical principles

Peritonitis may spread by errors of omission as well as by errors of commission. The essential objective is to control the source of peritoneal contamination—by resection, suture, drainage, or thorough peritoneal debridement [27]. Bacteriology swabs should always be taken and sent for both aerobic and anaerobic culture.

Intraoperative peritoneal lavage (using saline, hydrogen peroxide in saline, iodine preparation, noxythiolin or antibiotic solution) is a popular adjunct. Mechanical cleansing may be enhanced by postoperative peritoneal irrigation via a dialysis catheter [42,48], but advantages over thorough intra-operative lavage are disputed [3, 34].

Non-operative treatment is indicated for certain well-localized peritoneal collections (for example appendix mass). This conservative regimen requires careful monitoring and progression of symptoms or enlargement of the mass warrants surgical intervention. Surgery is also held in reserve where the diagnosis is considered to be pancreatitis, salpingitis, post-partum peritonitis or blood-borne peritonitis.

Mortality and morbidity

The mortality of generalized peritonitis remains unacceptably high (Table 71.2). Mortality is highest at the extremes of age and when other organ system failures intervene (for example renal failure in this situation has a mortality of 70% despite haemodialysis).

The high mortality of postoperative peritonitis requires additional comment. Delayed diagnosis and treatment worsens the prognosis and in up to 15% of patients with peritonitis the diagnosis is only made at post-mortem [8].

There is also a substantial morbidity associated with pulmonary, renal or hepatic complications, as well as wound infections (>40% of wounds) and intra-abdominal abscesses (around 30% of patients).

Intra-abdominal abscesses

Host factors encourage purulent collections to localize at certain sites within the abdomen [2]. An abscess is composed of an outer collagen wall, an inner band of intact polymorphs and a central area of necrotic debris containing a viable polymicrobial flora [7].

The symptoms characteristically appear after a latent interval, sometimes several days after apparent resolution of the peritonitis. A swinging pyrexia, malaise, anorexia, rigors, sweating attacks and a prolonged ileus are often present—although the prior use of antibiotics may modify this picture making the diagnosis more difficult. The time-honoured aphorism 'pus somewhere, pus nowhere, pus under the diaphragm' still holds true with this diagnosis being reached when all other sites of suppuration have been excluded.

Special investigations

Ultrasound, computerized tomography, combined liver and lung isotope scans and gallium^{67} imaging have all been used to localize intra-abdominal collections, but no single technique is clearly superior to the others [31]. Indium-labelled autologous leukocyte scanning has also been employed and early reports are encouraging [11, 33] but this technique is not available in most centres and it is very costly.

Treatment

Because antibiotics often obscure the diagnosis it is often preferable to discontinue them, when a residual abscess is suspected, and to rely upon direct efforts to locate the collection [3, 12, 25]. The principle is to provide open drainage at an early stage when the site of the abscess has been identified—unless a pelvic abscess appears likely to discharge spontaneously *per rectum*. X-ray or ultrasound-guided percutaneous drainage may occasionally be indicated, particularly in the critically-ill postoperative patient [41].

Primary peritonitis

Primary peritonitis is a monomicrobial infection of the peritoneum unrelated to intra-abdominal disease. Before the advent of antibiotics it accounted for up to 10% of all abdominal emergencies in children [21] but now it is rare. Accurate bacteriology is essential.

Pneumococcal peritonitis

This results either from direct infection from the exterior, via the genital tract in the female aged 5–10 years or from a pneumococcal septicaemia. Marked hyperaemia with exudate is initially confined to the pelvis but may spread rapidly and diffusely, associated with a high fever and toxaemia. Laparotomy is often performed to exclude appendicitis. An emergency Gram-stain of the pelvic pus confirms the presence of the characteristic oval Gram-positive diplococci, arranged in pairs. Penicillin is curative—it must be given intravenously.

Pneumococcal peritonitis in adults is

normally the result of blood-spread from a pulmonary primary focus. As in other forms of primary peritonitis, the patient's resistance may be lowered due to malnutrition, immunosuppression or cytotoxic therapy for malignancy.

Haemolytic streptococcal peritonitis

This can occur through blood-spread from a primary streptococcal infection of the middle ear, pharynx, tonsil or erysipelas. It can also complicate scarlet fever. *Streptococcus pyogenes* produces the enzymes streptokinase and hyaluronidase which encourage the rapid and diffuse spread of the infection. This form of peritonitis is almost confined to children and usually responds to penicillin treatment.

Staphylococcal peritonitis

This is a very rare but lethal complication of a generalized staphylococcal septicaemia. A primary cutaneous or bony infection may be present. At operation there is either a diffuse, thick, creamy pus or loculated abscesses between loops of bowel extending into the perinephric spaces. Treatment consists of appropriate anti-staphylococcal antibiotics with drainage of localized collections.

Fungal or parasitic peritonitis

Candida and other yeast-like organisms are ubiquitous in the intestine and occasionally become pathogenic. *Candida albicans* may become a serious disseminated infection in patients with impaired cell-mediated immunity, especially if receiving antibiotics and/or steroids [9]. Treatment requires adequate drainage and systemic or intraperitoneal amphotericin (maximum 1.5 mg/kg.day) or flucytosine (maximum 200 mg/kg.day).

Coccidioides immitis causes granulomatous peritonitis in 1–2% of patients with disseminated coccidiodomycosis. The spherical fungus is found in wet mounts of ascitic fluid or peritoneal biopsies. Coccidiodal peritonitis is usually self-limiting and amphotericin is indicated only in patients with acute peritonitis, disseminated infection or persistently elevated complement-fixation titres [53].

Cryptococcus neoformans and *Histoplasma capsulatum* rarely involve the peritoneum but may appear in the ascites of immunosuppressed patients.

The parasites *Schistosoma mansoni* and *Enterobius vermicularis* may give rise to a granulomatous peritonitis which mimics tuberculosis or carcinomatosis. *Strongyloides stercoralis* and *Entamoeba histolytica* can cause fulminant peritonitis and ascites by spread across the gut wall. Peritoneal signs may be minimal but the patients are severely ill with ascites, pain, distension and diarrhoea. The amoebocide metronidazole (400 mg six-hourly) or thiabendazole (50 mg/kg.day) for strongyloidiasis should be started before surgical intervention is considered.

Peritoneal dialysis and ventriculo-peritoneal shunts

Since the late 1970's continuous ambulatory peritoneal dialysis has gained popularity for the treatment of renal failure [49]. Peritonitis is a major complication of this procedure. The clinical signs are a cloudy dialysate or increased neutrophils in the returned fluid. A Gram-stain and culture usually reveals a monomicrobial infection (Gram-positive cocci, usually *S. aureus* or *S. albus*). Anaerobes are rarely cultured and usually indicate intestinal perforation, sometimes caused by erosion of the Tenckhoff catheter through the bowel wall.

The patient normally responds to the installation of the appropriate antibiotic with an increased frequency of dialysis exchange over the next few days. A sterile eosinophilic exudative peritonitis has also been described [20], often being asymptomatic and resolving spontaneously. However it is not known if recurring episodes of sterile or bacterial peritonitis will have long-term detrimental effects on the peritoneal transport characteristics.

Staphylococcal peritonitis (and sometimes ventriculitis) can complicate ventriculoperitoneal shunts used in the treatment of hydrocephalus. Infection occurs in around 25% of these patients and often requires the removal of the shunt.

Spontaneous bacterial peritonitis in cirrhosis

Crossley and Williams have reviewed this topic [13], emphasizing that spontaneous bacterial peritonitis is an often-overlooked fatal complication of cirrhosis. Its prevalence approaches 25%. A monomicrobial infection is found in most cases, with Gram-negative bacilli present in 70% of isolates (principally *E. coli*).

Although fever and abdominal pain occurs in most patients, approximately one-third have no signs referable to the abdomen. A rising creatinine or temporary resistance of ascites to diuretics is often an early sign, with later deterioration in hepatic function with increasing ascites and encephalopathy. With mortality rates of 48–70%, early diagnosis and treatment are imperative. An ascitic fluid polymorphonuclear cell count of greater than 250/ml appears to be the best index for the diagnosis of spontaneous bacterial peritonitis before bacterial culture results are available. A triple antibiotic regimen of ampicillin (or a cephalosporin), an aminoglycoside and metronidazole intravenously is recommended, although monitoring of the blood concentration of the aminoglycoside is required to prevent nephrotoxicity and ototoxicity. Nutritional support is also important.

Granulomatous peritonitis

The peritoneal reaction in this group of diseases is characterized by granuloma formation and adhesions.

Tuberculous peritonitis

Tuberculous peritonitis may be primary, due to blood spread, or secondary to intra-abdominal tuberculosis [59]. The **wet phase** refers to an early ascitic stage, while the **dry phase** occurs during later resolution and is associated with extensive matted adhesions. The clinical features and treatment are detailed in Chapter 47.

Sarcoidosis

This disease very rarely affects the peritoneum causing a granulomatous peritonitis and ascites. It is a diagnosis of exclusion, with negative fungal and mycobacterial cultures, a positive Kveim test and a lack of response to anti-tuberculous treatment. Despite the presence of non-caseating granulomas, and a good response to steroids if the diagnosis is uncertain, it is probably wise to treat the patient with anti-tuberculous treatment.

Crohn's disease

A miliary form of Crohn's disease has been described [14] with serosal nodules (non-caseating granulomas) and only minimal changes of the gut wall. At laparotomy it is easily confused with tuberculous peritonitis.

Foreign bodies (iatrogenic)

A number of foreign bodies may stimulate a granulomatous hypersensitivity reaction in the peritoneum—the most common being the **starch** used as a lubricant for surgical gloves [23]. This may present two to six weeks after a laparotomy as malaise, anorexia, pyrexia, non-specific abdominal pain, abdominal distension, tenderness, ascites, or intestinal obstruction (in 25% of cases). Unless the diagnosis is suspected a second laparotomy may be undertaken. At operation, up to two litres of straw-coloured fluid may be found with numerous peritoneal nodules mimicking carcinomatosis. Adhesions between bowel loops occur, some obstructing the bowel. If the diagnosis is considered, a paracentesis with microscopy of the fluid will reveal the typical Maltese Cross-shaped starch crystals, when the examination is performed under polarized light [66]. Skin testing will prove starch hypersensitivity [24]. If a second laparotomy is avoided, treatment is supportive (intravenous fluids and nasogastric suction) until the obstruction resolves. Steroids or indomethacin may decrease morbidity, but the prognosis is usually good with no specific treatment. Pathologically the lesions consist of granulomas with epithelioid cells, giant cells and an intense mononuclear infiltrate. A similar picture is seen with other glove lubricants (such as talc, lycopodium, mineral oil), and with cellulose from disposable gauze pads, towels and gowns.

If **barium** escapes into the peritoneal cavity a granulomatous peritoneal reaction occurs with microabscesses forming persisting foci of sepsis. The examination should be terminated at the first sign of a perforation and residual barium within the gut should be aspirated to reduce further spillage. Laparotomy is recommended to close the perforation and to lavage the abdominal cavity. It is virtually impossible to remove all of the barium crystals.

Familial mediterranean fever (Recurrent polyserositis; periodic peritonitis) [68]

'Benign paroxysmal peritonitis' was first described in 1945 as a feature of familial mediterranean fever [58]. Familial mediterranean fever is a rare inherited disorder of unknown aetiology characterized by recurrent, unprovoked, painful attacks of polyserositis (peritonitis, pleuritis, synovitis) often with fever. The disease is largely confined to certain ethnic groups of the Middle East, especially Sephardic Jews, Armenians and Levantine Arabs. Most studies suggest that it is of autosomal recessive inheritance [54]. A recent hypothesis suggests that familial mediterranean fever is the result of an inborn error of catecholamine metabolism [5].

Clinical features

The onset of this disease is often in infancy—90% of patients presenting before 20 years of age [60]. At irregular intervals, varying from one week to several months, patients become pyrexial (38–40°C) with occasional prodromal lethargy or mild abdominal discomfort. Rigors may occur. Although fever may be the sole manifestation of an attack, it is often accompanied by symptoms and signs typical of peritonitis. Laparotomy is often undertaken in error. Less often, pleuritic chest pain with shoulder tip radiation occurs. Normally an attack lasts for two to three days. Any serosal surface can be involved and joint pains are prominent symptoms in some patients. During any one attack peri-articular swelling usually occurs in a single large joint and is often associated with an erysipeloid rash around the ankles. Rarely pericarditis and meningitis occur.

A major complication, in Israel and Turkey, is amyloidosis, which may cause splenomegaly or nephrotic syndrome. Amyloidosis is probably a second phenotype of familial mediterranean fever. Amyloid nephropathy may result in progressive renal failure and death. Renal failure may also be precipitated by renal vein thrombosis [52].

Pathology

The pathogenesis remains obscure. At laparoscopy or laparotomy, the visceral and parietal peritoneum appears hyperaemic with discrete petechiae and fibrinous strands. Biopsy reveals that the muscular layers of the gallbladder, appendix and bowel are normal while serosal surfaces show a polymorphonuclear infiltration, vascular dilatation and oedema. Synovial biopsies show non-specific inflammation and culture of the synovial fluid is sterile. Between the attacks the peritoneum invariably returns to normal, though rarely fibrinous adhesions form.

The pattern of amyloidosis is unusual. Heavy amyloid deposits are found in the kidneys, spleen and adrenals but the heart, liver, tongue and other organs commonly involved in primary amyloidosis are spared. In addition the amyloid displays a characteristic perireticular distribution in arterioles throughout the body, with deposition of serum amyloid A protein in the intima of arterioles spreading into the media.

Investigations

Until recently the diagnosis was one of exclusion in the ethnic groups affected. During febrile attacks there may be an elevated leucocyte count, ESR, fibrinogen and C-reactive protein. Serum proteins are usually normal, unless amyloidosis is present. Deficiency of serum complement activity or complement inhibitor has been found in some patients, but not in unaffected relatives [51]. Rectal biopsies may reveal amyloid deposits in the inner coat of small blood vessels. X-rays may show a non-obstructive ileus or pleural effusion.

A recent report from Kuwait suggests a high specificity and sensitivity for the metaraminol provocation test [5]. A challenge with the sympathomimetic agent metaraminol (10 mg in 500 ml normal saline given intravenously over 3–4 hours) induced a short mild attack in all 21 patients studied, leaving healthy subjects unaffected.

Treatment

It is vital to explain to patients with familial mediterranean fever that their disease is normally a benign, self-limiting condition, not requiring surgical exploration. Many patients will, however, undergo appendicectomy before the disease is diagnosed.

Long-term treatment with oral colchicine (0.5 mg two to three times daily) appears to reduce the frequency and severity of attacks [22]. The mechanism remains obscure but colchicine appears to correct the suppressor cell deficiency found in such patients [30]. Prophylactic colchicine therapy may prevent, reverse or impede the progression of amyloidosis [68]. Colchicine may cause diarrhoea and the risk of chromosomal nondisjunction and azoospermia must be considered in patients in their reproductive years. Prolonged low-dose reserpine has also suppressed attacks [6].

Empirical use of antibiotics, antihistamines, corticosteroids and dietary manipulation have all proved ineffective. Analgesics are required during the acute attack and addiction to narcotics is sometimes a problem.

Peritoneal tumours

Secondary carcinoma (carcinoma peritonei)

Secondary malignancy is the most common form of neoplastic involvement of the peritoneum. The majority are adenocarcinomas secondary to primary tumours of the stomach, pancreas, ovary, colon, lung or breast. However peritoneal involvement by sarcomas, lymphomas, leukaemia and multiple myeloma can also occur.

Patients with peritoneal carcinomatosis

present with ascites (usually blood-stained), diffuse abdominal pain, weight loss and occasionally nausea or vomiting. Barium studies may show indentations of the intestine, or angulation, fixation or displacement of bowel loops.

Spread occurs in three ways—by direct extension, by transcoelomic spread (for example from papillary cystadenomas of the ovary, or Krukenberg tumours of the ovary from a gastric primary) and by blood or lymphatic dissemination.

The diagnosis and prognosis are discussed in the section dealing with the treatment of malignant ascites (p. 1069).

Pseudomyxoma peritonei [38]

Pseudomyxoma peritonei is a rare condition in which masses of mucinous gelatinous material are found within the peritoneal cavity. It occurs following serosal implantation of mucigenic columnar cells. Most cases result from rupture of a well-differentiated, mucin secreting adenocarcinoma of the ovary or appendix, or of a mucocele or mucigenic cystadenoma of the appendix [26, 55, 61].

Other causes include ovarian teratomas and fibromas, carcinoma of the uterus or common bile duct, mucinous intestinal adenocarcinomas and cystadenoma/adenocarcinoma of the vitello-intestinal duct remnant and urachal cysts [26, 38].

Clinical features

Pseudomyxoma presents with a gradual onset of painless abdominal distension, mimicking ascites, but without shifting dullness. Though computerized tomography and ultrasound scanning may detect loculated cystic masses [56], a preoperative diagnosis is often difficult and bacterial infection may complicate attempts at paracentesis.

Treatment

Aggressive surgery with removal of all gross tumour and ascites provides the best results. The organs of origin, such as both ovaries, appendix and greater omentum, should be removed [18, 61]. Recurrence is common even when surgery is combined with radiotherapy and/or intracavity thiotepa.

Mesothelioma [50]

Primary peritoneal mesotheliomas are rare tumours arising from the epithelial and mesenchymal elements of the peritoneum. They can consist of a spreading mass covering large areas of the visceral and parietal peritoneum or may form discrete nodules or plaques of tumour. Superficial capsular invasion of organs and lymph node involvement can be found but metastases are rare. Concomitant pleural involvement is seen in up to three-quarters of the patients.

Epithelial elements predominate in 70% of patients with tubular, papillary, sheet-like or solid nest-like patterns. In the remainder there is a marked fibromatous component with spindle cells. The pathologist's task is difficult and misdiagnosis of mesothelioma is common [67].

As with pleural mesothelioma, occupational or indirect exposure to asbestos dust has been implicated but, as up to half of the general population have pulmonary asbestos bodies and only one-third of patients with peritoneal mesothelioma have asbestos fibres present in the tumour, the role of asbestos remains uncertain.

Mesotheliomas are commoner in males. Patients present with abdominal pain, ascites, nausea and weight loss. Prognosis is poor, most patients being dead within two years of diagnosis. Peritoneal involvement and mesenchymal patterns fare worse than pleural tumours and epithelial varieties. Intraperitoneal or systemic chemotherapy and radiation are rarely helpful in providing tumour pain relief or longer survival.

Ascites [57]

The term ascites describes an accumulation of excessive fluid in the peritoneal cavity. Ascites results when the balance between fluid formation and absorption is upset. Factors contributing to the pathogenesis include:

1 Increases in peritoneal capillary permeability, in inflammatory or neoplastic disorders.
2 A low plasma colloid osmotic pressure as with hypoproteinaemia.
3 An increased hepatic sinusoidal hydrostatic pressure in cirrhosis, hepatic or inferior vena caval obstruction, congestive heart failure, etc.
4 Lymphatic obstruction, in congenital or aquired chylous ascites.
5 Secondary hyperaldosteronism and increased ADH activity, which serve to maintain rather than to initiate ascitic formation.

Broadly, therefore, the causes may be classified as peritoneal and non-peritoneal. In Western societies the major causes are intra-abdominal malignancy and cirrhosis.

Clinical features

The patient may have no symptoms or be aware only of a slowly distending abdomen. With marked ascites there may be abdominal discomfort, pressure symptoms and breathlessness.

Large ascites (> 1 litre) are detectable clinically through shifting dullness, flank dullness and a fluid thrill. Smaller volumes may be detectable by placing the patient in the knee-elbow position and demonstrating peri-umbilical dullness. When the ascites is massive the abdominal skin becomes tight and shiny, the heart is displaced upwards, the umbilicus is everted and inferior venal

caval compression leads to scrotal and lower limb oedema.

The 'five F's' remain a useful *aide-memoire* for the differential diagnosis (fat, fluid, flatus, faeces or foetus). A grossly distended bladder may be excluded by catheterization but a large ovarion cyst may cause more difficulty. Usually this can be diagnosed by the presence of central abdominal dullness and resonance in the flanks.

A rectal and/or pelvic examination is mandatory and is easier after tapping of the ascites. After paracentesis, organomegaly may be discernable or plaques of tumour may be palpable.

A low grade fever is common in both carcinomatosis and progressive cirrhosis. The release of pyrogens from necrotic cells may be responsible. A spike of temperature may indicate infection of the ascitic fluid.

Investigations

For all patients it is important to know the results of a full blood count, ESR, plasma urea and electrolytes and liver function tests including serum albumin. Other special blood tests may include serum amylase, clotting studies, alpha-foetoprotein and hepatitis B antigen.

ASCITIC FLUID EXAMINATION

Paracentesis is performed under local anaesthesia by insertion of a needle or cannula in the mid-line 5 cm below the umbilicus or in an iliac fossa, after emptying the bladder. Only 50 ml of ascitic fluid is required for diagnostic purposes. The fluid is analysed as follows:

Biochemistry

By custom the fluid is designated as either exudate or transudate (see Table 71.3) depending on this analysis. An exudate typifies the ascites found in inflammatory dis-

Table 71.3. Characteristics of ascitic fluid.

	Exudate	Transudate
Colour	turbid (occ. haemorrhagic)	clear/amber (bilirubin may approach serum levels)
Specific gravity	high (>1.015)	low (1.005–1.015)
Total protein	high (>30 g/l)	low (<25 g/l)
Protein electrophoresis	as in plasma	almost all albumin
Fibrin	present (clots spontaneously)	absent
Cells	inflammatory cells governed by aetiology (eg. polymorphs or lymphocytes)	rare (endothelial cells ± macrophages)

orders or malignancy. Transudates occur in hypoalbuminaemia and cirrhosis. However there is often a mixed picture [65].

Microbiology

Ascitic fluid should always be subjected to Gram stain and bacterial culture. A sample of fluid can be added conveniently to a blood culture bottle.

Cytology

Blood-stained ascitic fluid suggests malignancy. A white cell count of greater than 250 cells/ml, with mainly polymorphs, suggests bacterial peritonitis; a high mononuclear count suggests neoplasia or tuberculosis. Cytological smears of the centrifuged deposit allow examination of exfoliated peritoneal cells and malignant cells. Cytology provides a positive diagnosis of malignancy in 60–90% of ascites of malignant tumour origin.

Ultrasound and X-ray

Gross ascites produces a characteristic picture on plain abdominal X-ray, with loss of density and detail. Ultrasound can demonstrate much smaller volumes of free perito-neal fluid and can distinguish between free and loculated collections.

Laparotomy and laparoscopy

Laparoscopy and peritoneal biopsy has a limited role in malignant ascites but may be very useful in hepatic ascites. Laparotomy is often of greater value in establishing the cause and determining the prognosis.

Treatment [37]

Ascites due to cirrhosis

As ascites often resolves with improvement of hepatic function, and paracentesis may precipitate encephalopathy, there is an argument for ignoring the ascites unless it is severe [17]. However, the high rate of spontaneous bacterial peritonitis dictates that ascites should be treated promptly [13].

Sodium restriction consists of a diet with no added salt and no salty foods aiming at an intake of around 50 mmol per day.

Diuretics should be potassium-sparing (spironolactone, amiloride, triamterene). Spironolactone is given in doses ranging from 50 to 200 mg per day. Occasionally a loop diuretic (such as frusemide) may also be required.

Mechanical removal is best avoided as it can precipitate renal failure and encephalopathy due to loss of protein. To avoid this problem the ascites may either be recycled through a filter system returning the protein to the blood or via a peritoneal-venous shunt (LeVeen or Denver shunt). These methods are reserved for ascites which prove resistant to diuretics.

Malignant ascites

Patients with malignant ascites have a very gloomy prognosis but they merit palliative treatment to improve the quality of their lives [35].

Paracentesis

Survival times after initial paracentesis average less than four months, but may occasionally be longer than 12 months. Repeated paracenteses cause protein depletion and require hospitalization. Operative and malignant adhesions with fibrosis increase the risk of visceral injury. Spironolactone (100–400 mg/day) may help to prevent reaccumulation.

Intracavity radiocolloids

Most experience has been gained using intraperitoneal injections of colloidal chromic phosphate (P^{32}). This isotope emits beta radiation with a maximum tissue penetration of 8 mm and a half life of 14 days. As the penetration is limited, little effect is seen with large tumours. The full therapeutic effect of P^{32} occurs within three months and only about half of the patients show a slowing of fluid reaccumulation.

Intracavity chemotherapy

Talc has been used in an attempt to sclerose the peritoneal cavity with little benefit. The cytotoxic agent **bleomycin** has been recommended and complete or partial responses can be expected in around one-third of patients. **Thiotepa, adriamycin** and **5 fluorouracil** can produce comparable results but with more side-effects.

Immunotherapy

This involves an attempt to stimulate (non-specifically) the host's immune system. Three out of five patients may be expected to respond for a few weeks to weekly intraperitoneal injections of the **streptococcal preparation OK-432**. During treatment serum proteins increase and the peripheral blood T-cell count rises. The patient's response to skin testing with recall antigens (for example Mantoux testing) also increases, as a measure of immunostimulation. The best responses are achieved in those patients with a large number of malignant cells in their ascitic fluid before treatment. Intraperitoneal, heat-inactivated **Corynebacterium parvum** has also been shown to diminish the reaccumulation of ascites.

Peritoneovenous shunting (LeVeen or Denver)

These shunts may be used to make a terminal illness less uncomfortable. Survival is not increased and there is a theoretical danger of disseminating the tumour.

Before undertaking the procedure one should have determined that reaccumulation of ascites is rapid after paracentesis and that the ascitic fluid is sterile on culture. The procedure is contraindicated if the prothrombin time is prolonged (> 4 seconds over control), if the serum bilirubin is high or rising, and if the patient is in incipient heart failure. Diuretics and prophylactic antibiotics should be given to cover the procedure.

Palliation is poor if the ascitic fluid is high in protein, if it contains large numbers of cells, or if it is loculated—as the shunt tends to block at an early stage. It has been claimed that the Denver shunt is less liable to block under these circumstances.

Miscellaneous peritoneal disorders

Peritoneal vasculitis [43]

The multi-system collagen disorders share a common pathogenesis—that of vasculitis. It is not surprising that one in five patients with systemic lupus erythematosis, polyarteritis nodosum, scleroderma and dermatomyositis develop acute abdominal problems (ulceration, haemorrhage, perforation, obstruction or infarction). However an isolated peritonitis, resulting from arteritis of the subserosal arteries, occurs in less than 1% of patients. The peritoneum is usually affected after the gut wall is diseased.

A vasculitic peritonitis most commonly occurs in systemic lupus causing a typical acute peritonitis with ascites. This will respond to steroids but often laparotomy is undertaken to exclude a surgically correctable cause.

Whipple's Disease

The spectrum of Whipple's disease is discussed in Chapter 47. However a few patients may first present with peritoneal manifestations. The features mimic tuberculous peritonitis with weight loss, low-grade fever, ascites and multiple peritoneal nodules. The nodules consist of chronic inflammatory cells with periodic acid-Schiff positive material in macrophages. Long-term penicillin or tetracycline leads to resolution of the peritoneal disease and ascites.

Sclerosing peritonitis

A rare form of peritonitis came to light in the mid-1970s following the use of the beta-adrenergic-blocking drug practolol [10]. Less than 200 cases have been collected world-wide [32]. Of 26 patients reported from two United Kingdom centres, the mean age was 61 years and the average duration of exposure to the drug was 30 months. Nine of these patients developed this condition after practolol had been discontinued. In addition most patients have practolol-associated psoriasis-like skin lesions and conjunctivitis—the oculomucocutaneous syndrome.

These patients usually present with the signs and symptoms of intestinal obstruction and in more than 60% of patients a mass is palpable. Weight loss is often profound. Laparotomy findings are striking—the small intestine is caught up in a dense white adhesive membrane surrounding the bowel like a cocoon. Histologically there is a non-specific inflammation, fibrinous exudation and a peculiar laminated fibrosis.

Treatment involves careful dissection of this membrane from the intestine.

Peritoneal (mesenteric) cysts

Small (1–2 cm) to large (up to 20 cm) cystic masses are occasionally found within the mesenteries or attached to the parietal peritoneum. If large enough they may be palpable as abdominal masses, creating a diagnostic problem [61].

Peritoneal cysts arise from:
1   Embryonic multipotential cells.
2   Pinched-off enteric diverticula.
3   The urogenital ridge or derivatives.
4   Walled-off infections (pseudocysts).
5   Rarely, a neoplastic origin—such as a pseudomyxoma.

Usually the cysts are single but occasionally multiple cysts are found either attached or dispersed (loose bodies) throughout the abdominal cavity. The fluid is serous, mucinous or occasionally turbid. Torsion on a pedicle may cause symptoms.

Blood-filled 'chocolate' cysts of endometriosis may involve the bowel wall and cause ascites, although peritoneal involvement alone is rare.

Hydatid disease

Rupture of a hydatid cyst into the peritoneal cavity may cause peritonitis or occasionally an acute anaphylactic reaction which can rapidly lead to death.

Echinococcus granulosa and *Echinococcus multilocularis* are the most important cestodes producing serious disease in man, because of the size and location of their larval form (hydatid cyst). The definitive host for these small adult tape worms is the dog—man, sheep and cattle acting as intermediate hosts. The tapeworm passes its eggs in the dog faeces and the intermediate host becomes infected through ingestion of contaminated water or vegetables (flies). Gastric juice dissolves the chitinous envelope and the eggs (oncospheres with six hooks) penetrate the gut wall and circulate to the liver and other organs where they multiply and form adult cysts.

The presentation may be as a palpable mass, or because of pain due to pressure. Eosinophilia, calcification in cysts and ultrasound are helpful. Skin testing (Casoni) is not as reliable as complement fixation tests.

Treatment consists of excision of the cysts, where possible, taking care to avoid spillage (1% iodine can kill the scolices). Albendazole may control the growth of cysts [36].

Chylous ascites

In rare circumstances (Table 71.4) lipid-rich lymph may accumulate as chylous ascites. Paracentesis recovers a sterile milky fluid with a high concentration of triglycerides. The fluid also contains lymphocytes. Chylomicrons separate from the fluid on standing.

Chyloperitoneum is rarely present at

Table 71.4. Aetiology of chylous ascites.

	%
Congenital (1%)	
Congenital malformation	39
Idiopathic	31
Inflammation	15
Neoplastic	3
Miscellaneous	12
e.g. obstruction	
malrotation	
Acquired (99%)	%
Traumatic (including surgery)	12
Neoplastic	30
Idiopathic	
Lymphangiectasia	23
Inflammatory	35
e.g. pancreatitis	
mesenteric adenitis	
TB	
pulmonary fibrosis	
filariasis	
syphilis	
cirrhosis	
nephrotic syndrome	

birth and usually develops after the first few days or weeks of life [63].

Investigations should exclude a correctable underlying cause. Lymphangiograms may disclose lymphatic obstruction, intraperitoneal leakage or reflux into the intestine. Laparotomy is often the definitive investigation. When no cause is found paracentesis may improve the condition. Resting the gastrointestinal tract proves effective in stemming the production of chyle. The introduction into the diet of short- or medium-chain triglycerides may also control the ascites. Internal drainage procedures or parenteral re-infusions of chyle are not helpful. Acute or idiopathic cases often resolve spontaneously.

References

1 AIRD I. Peritonitis. In: *A companion in surgical studies* 2nd ed. Edinburgh: Churchill Livingstone, 1958:850.
2 ALTEMEIER WA, CULBERTSON WR, FULLEN WD, SHOOK CD. Intra-abdominal abscesses. *Am J Surg* 1973;**125**:70–79.
3 ANONYMOUS. Peritonitis today. *Br Med J* 1980;**6222**:1095–1096.

4 BAILEY H. In Clain A, ed. *Hamilton Bailey's demonstration of physical signs in clinical surgery* 15th ed. Bristol: John Wright, 1973:249.

5 BARAKAT MH, EL-KHAWAD AO, GUMAA KA, EL-SOBKI NI, FENECH FF. Metaraminol provocative test: a specific diagnostic test for familial Mediterranean fever. *Lancet* 1984;i:656–657.

6 BARAKAT M, GUMAA KA, EL-KHAWAD A, MENON K, BADAWI A. Suppression of familial Mediterranean fever by reserpine therapy. *J Kwt Med Ass* 1981;15:3–6.

7 BARTLETT JG. The pathophysiology of intra-abdominal sepsis. In: McKwatts J, McDonald PJ, O'Brien PE, Marshall UR, Finlay-Jones, JJ, eds. *Infections in surgery: Basic and clinical aspects.* Edinburgh: Churchill Livingstone, 1981:47.

8 BOHNEN J, BOULANGER M, MEAKINS JL, McLEAN APH. Prognosis in generalized peritonitis: Relation to cause and risk factors. *Arch Surg* 1983;118:285–290.

9 BOYER AS, BLUMENKRANTZ MJ, MONTGOMERIE JZ, GALPIN JE, COBURN JW, GUZA LB. Candida peritonitis. *Am J Med* 1976;61:823–840.

10 BROWN P, BADDELY H, READ AE, DAVIES, JD, McGARRY J. Sclerosing peritonitis, an unusual reaction to a beta adrenergic blocking drug (practolol) *Lancet* 1974;ii:1477–1481.

11 COLEMAN RE, BLACK RE, WELCH DM, MAXWELL JG. Indium-111 labelled leukocytes the evaluation of suspected abdominal abscesses. *Am J Surg* 1980;139:99–104.

12 CONDON RE, MALANGONI MA. Peritonitis and intra-abdominal abscesses. In: Schwartz SI, ed, *Principles of surgery* 4th ed. New York: McGraw-Hill, 1984:1410–1413.

13 CROSSLEY IR, WILLIAMS R. Spontaneous bacterial peritonitis. *Gut* 1985;26:325–331.

14 DAUM F, BOLEY SJ, COHEN MI. Miliary Crohn's disease. *Gastroenterology* 1974;67:527–530.

15 DeDOMBAL FT. Computers and the surgeon—a matter for decision. In: Nyhus L, ed. *Surgery Annual* New York: Appleton Croft, 1979:33–57.

16 DeDOMBAL FT. Diagnosis of acute abdominal pain—what the computer teaches us. *Tidsskr Nor Laegeforen* 1980;100:1852–1855.

17 ELIAS E. Management of ascites in patients with liver disease. *Prescribers J* 1985;25:26–30.

18 FERNANDEZ RN, DALY JM. Pseudomyxoma peritonei. *Arch Surg* 1980;115:409–414.

19 GJESSING J, OSKARSSON BM, TOMLIN PJ, BROCK-UTNE J. Diagnostic abdominal paracentesis. *Br Med J* 1972;1:617–619.

20 GOKAL R, RAMOS JM, WARD MK, KERR DNS Eosiniphilic peritonitis in continuous ambulatory peritoneal dialysis (CAPD) *Clin Nephrol* 1980;15:328–330.

21 GOLDEN GT, SHAW A. Primary peritonitis. *Surg Gynecol Obstet* 1972;135:513–516.

22 GOLDFINGER SE. Colchicine for familial Mediterranean fever. *N Engl J Med* 1972;287:1302.

23 GOODACRE RL, CLANCY RL, DAVIDSON RL, et al. Cell-mediated immunity to corn starch in induced granulomatous peritonitis. *Gut* 1976;17:202–205.

24 GRANT JBF, DAVIES JD, ESPINER HJ, ELTRINGHAM WK. Diagnosis of granulomatous starch peritonitis by delayed hypersensitivity skin reactions. *Br J Surg* 1982;69:197–199.

25 HARLEY HRS. Subphrenic Abscess. In Keen G, ed. *Operative surgery and management* Bristol: Wright, 1981:255–260.

26 HIGA E, ROSAI J, PIZZIMBOND CA, WISE L. Mucosal hyperplasia, mucinous cystadenoma and mucinous cystadenocarcinoma of the appendix: a re-evaluation of appendiceal 'mucocele'. *Cancer* 1973;32:1525–1541.

27 HUDSPETH AS. Radical surgical debridement in the treatment of advanced generalized bacterial peritonitis. *Arch Surg* 1975;110:1233–1236.

28 HUTCHINSON GH, ALDERSON DM, TURNBERG LA. Fatal tension pneumoperitoneum due to aerophagy. *Postgrad Med J* 1980,56:516–518.

29 HUTCHINSON GH, PATEL BG, DOIG CM. A double-blind controlled trial of metronidazole suppositories in children undergoing appendicectomy. *Curr Med Res Opin* 1983;8:441–445.

30 ILFELD D, KUPERMAN O. Correction of a suppressor cell deficiency in 4 patients with familial Mediterranean fever by 'in-vitro' or 'in-vivo' colchicine. *Clin Exp Immunol* 1982;50:99–106.

31 ISIKOFF MB, GUTER M. Diagnostic imaging of the upper part of the abdomen. *Surg Gynecol Obstet* 1979;149:161–167.

32 JACKSON B. Sclerosing peritonitis. *Adhesions—the problems.* 15–21. *Proc Symp R Coll Obstet Gynecol.* Michael Bungey Medical.

33 KNOCHEL JQ, KOEHLER PR, LEE TG, WELCH DM. Diagnosis of abdominal abscesses with computerised tomography, ultrasonography and In¹¹¹ leucocyte scan. *Radiology* 1980;137:425–432.

34 KRUKOWSKI ZH, MATHESON NA. Peritonitis. *Surgery (Oxford)* 1984;1:260–267.

35 LACY JH, WIEMAN TJ, SHIVELEY EH. Management of malignant ascites. *Surg Gynecol Obstet* 1984;159:397–412.

36 LANCET LEADER. Albendazole: worms and hydatid disease. *Lancet* 1984: ii:675–676.

37 LANCET LEADER. Treatment of refractory ascites. *Lancet* 1985;ii:1164–1165.

38 LONG RT, SPRATT JS, DOWLING E. Pseudomyxoma peritonei. *Am J Surg* 1969;117:162–169.

39 LORIMER WS JR, ELLIS DG. Meconium peritonitis. *Surgery* 1966;60:470–475.

40 MacCALLUM WG On the mechanism of absorption of granular materials from the peritoneum. *Bull John Hopkins Hosp* 14:105–115.

41 MacERLEAN DP, OWENS AP, HOURIHANE JB. Ultrasound guided percutaneous abdominal abscess drainage. *Br J Radiol* 1981;54:394–397.

42 McKENNA JP, CURRIE DJ, MacDONALD JA, MAHONEY

LJ, FINLAYSON DC, LANSKAIL DJ. The use of continuous postoperative peritoneal lavage in the management of diffuse peritonitis. *Surg Gynecol Obstet* 1970;130:254–258.

43 MATOLO NM, ALBO D. JR. Gastrointestinal complications of collagen vascular diseases. *Amer J Surg* 122:678–682.

44 MITCHELL GAG. The spread of acute intraperitoneal effusions. *Br J Surg* 1941;28:291–313.

45 NYSTROM P-O, SKAU T. Elimination patterns of Escherichia coli and Bacteroides fragilis from the peritoneal cavitiy. *Acta Chir Scand* 1983;149:383–388.

46 ONDERDONK AB, BARTLETT JG, LOUIE T, SULLIVAN-SEIGLER N, GORBACH SL. Microbial synergy in experimental intra-abdominal abscess. *Infection and Immunity* 1976;13:22–26.

47 PETERS RS, LEHMAN TJA, SCHWABE AD. Colchicine for familial Mediterranean fever—observations associated with long-term treatment. *West J Med* 1983;138:43–46.

48 POLK HC, FRY DE. Radical peritoneal debridement for established peritonitis. *Ann Surg* 1980;192:350–355.

49 POPOVICH RP, MONCRIEF JW, NOLPH KD, GHODS AJ, TWARDOWSKI ZJ, PYLE WK. Continuous ambulatory peritoneal dialysis. *Ann Intern Med* 1978;88:449–456.

50 RAPTOUPOULES V. Peritoneal mesothelioma. *CRC Crit Rev Diagn Imaging* 1985;24:293–328.

51 REIMANN HA, COPPOLA ED, VILLEGAS GR. Serum complement defects in periodic diseases. *Ann Intern Med* 1970;73:737–740.

52 REUBEN A, HIRSCH M, BERLYNE GW. Renal vein thrombosis as the major cause of renal failure in familial Mediterranean fever. *Q J Med* 1977;46:243–258.

53 SAW EC, SHIELDS SJ, COMER TP, *et al.* Granulomatous peritonitis due to *Coccidioides immitis*. *Arch Surg* 1974;108:369–371.

54 SCHWABE AD, PETERS RS. Familial Mediterranean fever in Armenians: An analysis of 100 cases. *Medicine (Baltimore)* 1974;53:453.

55 SCULLY RE. Common epithelial tumours of borderline malignancy (Carcinoma of low malignant potential). *Bull Cancer (Paris)* 1982;69:228–238.

56 SESHUL MB, COULAM CM. Pseudomyxoma peritonei: computed tomography and sonography. *Am J Radiol* 1981;136:803–806.

57 SHERLOCK S. Ascites. *Diseases of the liver and biliary system.* Oxford: Blackwell Scientific Publications, 1985;117–134.

58 SIEGEL S. Benign paroxysmal peritonitis. *Ann Intern Med* 1945;23:1–3.

59 SINGH MM, BHARGAVA AN, JAIN KP. Tuberculous peritonitis. *N Engl J Med* 1969;281:1091–1094.

60 SOHAR E, GAFNI J, PRAS M, HELLER H. Familial Mediterranean Fever: a survey of 470 cases and review of the literature. *Am J Med* 1967;43:227–253.

61 SPRATT JS, WALD H, ADCOCK BS. Pseudomyxoma peritonei. In: Spratt JS, ed. *Neoplasma of the Colon, Rectum and Anus; mucosal and epithelial* Philadelphia: W. B. Saunders, 1984:316–330.

62 STEWART DJ, MATHESON NA. Peritoneal lavage in appendicular peritonitis. *Br J Surg* 1970;65:54–56.

63 UNGER SW, CHANDLER JG. Chylous ascites in infants and children. *Surgery* 1983;93:455–461.

64 VANEK VW, PHILLIPS AK. Retroperitoneal, mesenteric and omental cysts. *Arch Surg* 1984;119:838–842.

65 WALTER JB, ISRAEL MS. *General Pathology* 4th ed. Edinburgh: Churchill-Livingstone, 1974:491.

66 WARSHAW AL. Diagnosis of starch peritonitis by paracentesis. *Lancet* 1972;ii:1054–1056.

67 WILLIS RA. Metastasis. In: *Pathology of Tumours* 4th ed. London: Butterworths, 1967:181.

68 ZEMER D, PRAS M, SOHAR E, MODAN M, CABILI S, GAFNI J. Colchicine in the prevention and treatment of the Amyloidosis of Familial Mediterranean fever. *New Engl J Med* 1986;314:1001–1005.

Chapter 72
Intestinal Obstruction

S. T. D. McKELVEY

Acute intestinal obstruction is a life-threatening condition which requires urgent medical and surgical management. The decline in the mortality rate in the past 50 years, from 25% to less than 10%, is largely attributable to a recognition of the need for correction of fluid and electrolyte deficits, and for early surgical relief. When obstruction is complicated by strangulation the mortality rate, even today, is 30%.

Clinical features

Intestinal obstruction exists when transit through the bowel is arrested by mechanical blockage or failure of peristaltic activity. The syndrome presents with abdominal pain, distension, vomiting and constipation. These features vary in severity in order of onset, according to the level and type of obstruction. It is dangerous to await the development of all of them before considering the possibility of obstruction.

Pain

Mechanical obstruction causes vigorous contraction of the bowel proximal to the lesion, in an attempt to overcome the impasse. Occurring at intervals of a few minutes, these peristaltic waves cause crampy abdominal pain and high-pitched gurgling bowel sounds which are sometimes audible without the use of a stethoscope. In thin patients the contracting loops of bowel are often visible through the abdominal wall.

Pain is the first major symptom of distal small bowel obstruction. Crampy central abdominal pain should always suggest this possibility and prompt a search for herniae, abdominal scars, or other cause for an obstruction. The patient is often anxious and restless; during attacks the knees may be drawn up, followed by good relief of pain between attacks. Pain is obscured by analgesics. If strangulation of a loop of bowel supervenes, the pain becomes continuous and is associated with tenderness. Incomplete obstruction causes less dramatic and less frequent pain, which may be tolerated for days or weeks before its cause is recognized.

Obstruction of the left colon causes pain referred to the lower abdomen, presenting as lower abdominal cramps. Chronic large bowel symptoms, such as altered bowel habit or blood in the stool, frequently precede the onset of obstructive symptoms and are important indicators of the source of the trouble.

Distension

When the distal bowel, especially the left colon, is obstructed, the accumulation of gas and faeces readily causes abdominal distension which is tympanitic on percussion. High pressures can develop in the colon, if the ileocaecal valve is competent, leading to a serious risk of perforation of the caecum with faecal peritonitis (Fig. 72.1). Obstruction of the ileum causes abdominal distension which is central in position, but this may not be visible in obese patients until the obstruction is advanced.

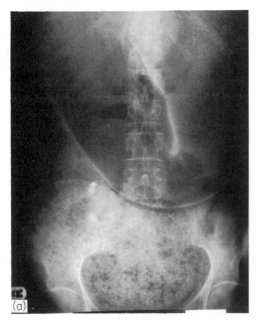

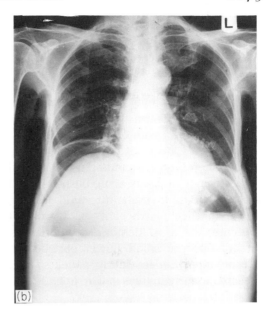

Fig. 72.1. (a) a 70-year-old female developed obstruction of the colon because of a malignant stricture at the splenic flexure. (b) caecal perforation occurred causing collapse of the right colon and intraperitoneal liquid stool is seen throughout the abdominal cavity. Free gas under the diaphragm is visible on the chest X-ray. The patient survived an emergency two-stage resection.

Vomiting

Vomiting is the major and often only feature of proximal gut obstruction. In the adult it is frequently caused by pyloric stenosis (Fig. 72.2). Dehydration and acid-base disturbances develop rapidly. If the obstruction is high in the jejunum, for example obstruction of the efferent loop after Pólya's gastrectomy or gastroenterostomy, the vomitus is heavily bile-stained and the fluid and electrolyte loss is enormous. Lesions of the ileum can cause vomiting, though often only as a later feature; in colonic obstruction it may be absent. If stasis in the bowel is not relieved, bacterial activity causes profound changes in the small bowel contents leading to the vomiting of faeculent material. This indicates advanced obstruction and is an adverse prognostic sign.

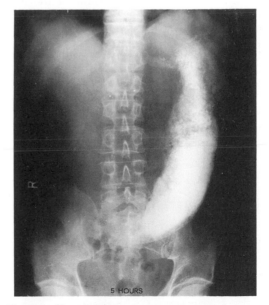

Fig. 72.2. Chronic pyloric stenosis causes severe dilatation of the stomach. In this patient the greater curvature is outlined below the pelvic brim on the five-hour film after a barium meal.

Constipation

Peristaltic activity may continue distal to a mechanical obstruction with passage of stool or flatus until the unobstructed portion of bowel is empty. Only in obstruction of the left colon is constipation an early feature. In patients with a previously regular bowel habit, the development of absolute constipation for faeces and flatus for several days strongly suggests acute obstruction of the colon. Paradoxically, intestinal obstruction may cause diarrhoea if the obstruction is incomplete, as in Richter's type of hernia, or in subacute small bowel obstruction. Faecal impaction in elderly patients often presents with symptoms of diarrhoea.

Radiological investigations

When the cause of the obstruction is obvious, as in incarcerated groin hernia (Fig. 72.3), X-ray investigation is unimportant. In most other cases plain films of the ab-

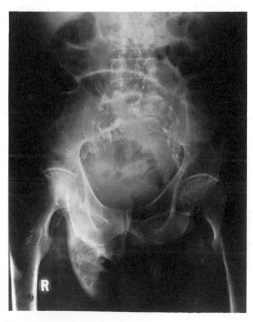

Fig. 72.3. Incarcerated inguinal hernia is a common cause of intestinal obstruction and is normally diagnosed without radiology.

domen, taken in the erect and supine positions, are helpful in determining the site and severity of the obstruction. A chest X-ray should also be taken as it frequently reveals chest lesions or subphrenic signs relevant to the diagnosis and management of the patient (see Fig. 72.1).

Ileal obstruction produces a step-ladder effect on the erect film caused by multiple fluid levels extending from the right iliac fossa obliquely towards the left upper quadrant; supine films show central abdominal loops distinguished by the complete transverse markings of the valvulae conniventes (Fig. 72.4). Sometimes obstructed bowel contains no air and may be easily missed on plain X-ray [22]—in such cases ultrasound may be helpful [17]. Obstructed jejunum is usually seen in the left upper abdomen. The valvulae conniventes produce indentations at the margin of the bowel, except when it is grossly distended. In patients with subacute or chronic obstruction, contrast radiology using Gastrografin or dilute barium with administration of metoclopramide may define the site of the lesion (Fig. 72.5).

Colonic obstruction is recognized by distension of the bowel in the flanks and right iliac fossa. The incomplete markings of the haustra help to distinguish transverse colon from jejunum when both small and large bowel are distended (Fig. 72.6). A sharp cut-off point for the colonic gas may indicate the site of the obstructing lesion, although it is often more distally placed and separated from the gas by a column of liquid stool (Fig. 72.7). When doubt about the existence, or level, of a large bowel obstruction then a barium enema should be performed (Fig. 72.7)—this may obviate the necessity for a full laparotomy as the initial step of a three-stage procedure.

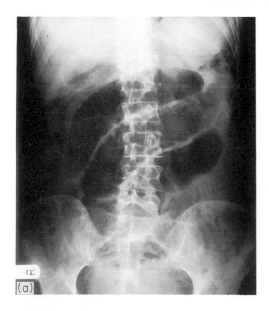

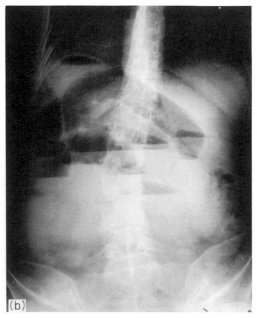

Fig. 72.4. Band obstruction of the terminal ileum. On the supine film the central position of the small bowel loops with the transverse markings of the valvulae conniventes is shown. The erect film shows the step-ladder effect of fluid levels extending obliquely towards the left upper quadrant.

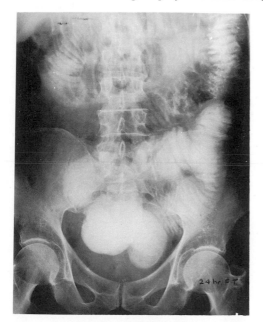

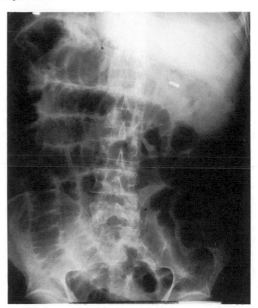

Fig. 72.5. This patient had symptoms suggesting sub-acute obstruction of the small bowel. A 24 hour follow-through study using metoclopramide, barium and Gastrografin confirmed the presence of obstruction in the ileum, which was caused by an adhesion.

Fig. 72.6. A case of malignant obstruction of the left colon affecting small and large bowel because of incompetence of the ileocaecal valve.

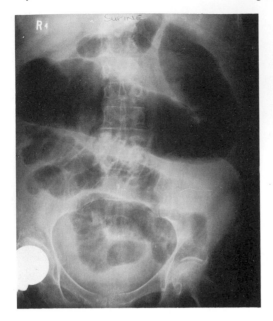

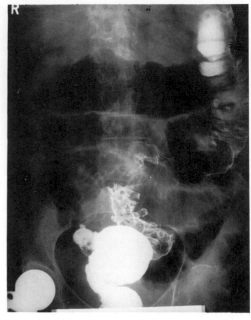

Fig. 72.7. The plain film suggests that the colon is obstructed at the splenic flexure because the gas is separated from the stricture in the sigmoid colon by a column of liquid stool.

Aetiology

Mechanical obstruction

External herniae, band adhesions and malignant strictures of the colon account for 75% of cases of mechanical intestinal obstruction. A wide variety of lesions are responsible for the remainder—they may arise in the lumen of the bowel, or be caused by intrinsic disease of the bowel or extrinsic compression.

Occlusion of the bowel lumen

Ingested **foreign bodies** may cause obstruction, the patients often having a psychiatric disorder or mental subnormality. In the majority of patients the ingested object, having successfully negotiated the pylorus of the stomach, will continue its onward progress to be passed in the stool (Fig. 72.8). Surgical intervention is only needed for removal of large or sharp objects which

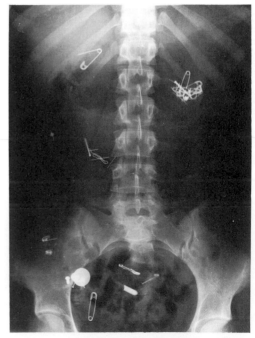

Fig. 72.8. Foreign bodies which negotiate the cardia will usually pass spontaneously, although sharp or pointed objects are liable to cause perforation. This patient lived in a psychiatric institution.

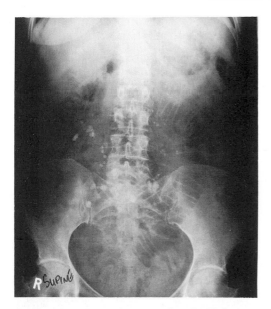

Fig. 72.9. Small bowel obstruction by a food bolus. This patient underwent vagotomy and pyloroplasty many years previously. Recently her dentures were causing discomfort so she stopped using them.

are causing signs of obstruction or penetration of the bowel wall.

Bolus obstruction, caused by undigested food should be suspected in patients who have undergone a Pólya's gastrectomy, gastroenterostomy, or pyloroplasty especially if the patient is edentulous (Fig. 72.9). Poorly masticated orange pith is a common cause, but dried fruit which swells on rehydration in the bowel, or nuts, have a similar effect. Gross dietary indiscretion in young healthy people, for example ingestion of large amounts of coconut, may also cause impaction. Drug-filled condoms, swallowed to avoid Customs' detection, can cause spectacular (and potentially lethal) obstruction. Conservative treatment should be tried initially and if surgery is required it is often possible to milk the obstructing material through the ileum into the colon.

Gallstone ileus is a misnomer for mechanical occlusion of the intestine by a large stone which has entered the bowel, usually the duodenum, by ulceration through the

wall of an adherent inflamed gallbladder creating a cholecystenterostomy fistula. Over 80% of such patients are female and most are old [1]. The stone usually impacts in the terminal ileum causing partial or complete obstruction. Less commonly, the jejunum is occluded and occasionally recurrence of the syndrome is caused by the passage of further stones [15]. The clinical features of small bowel obstruction are confirmed on the plain abdominal film and, if gas is seen in the biliary tree or a large calcified stone is present in the lower abdomen, the diagnosis is confirmed. Often the onset is subacute, the clinical and X-ray signs of obstruction are indefinite and the gas in the biliary tree is easily overlooked. In such patients the diagnosis may be made by contrast radiology (Fig. 72.10). Delay in

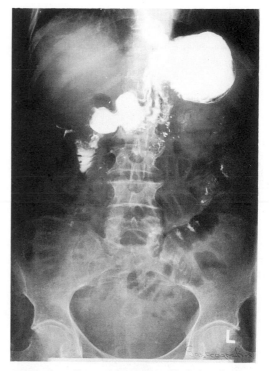

Fig. 72.10. Gallstone ileus. In this elderly female the cause of the small bowel obstruction was not clear on the plain films. Contrast studies showed a fistula between the gall bladder and the duodenum and a gallstone in the terminal ileum.

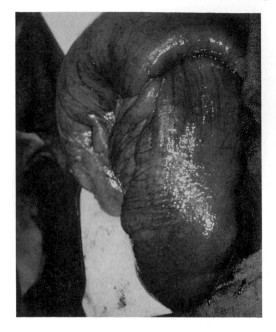

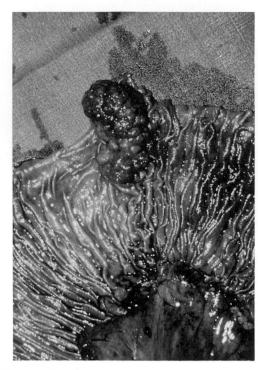

Fig. 72.11. Small bowel intussusception in the adult caused by a simple polyp.

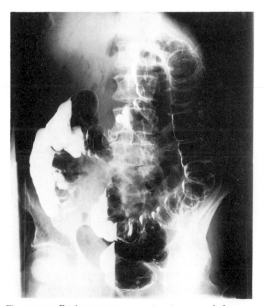

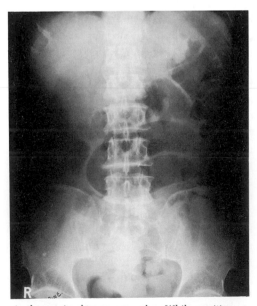

Fig. 72.12. Barium enema examination revealed a carcinoma in the proximal transverse colon. While awaiting elective surgery the patient developed obstruction caused by intussusception of the tumour.

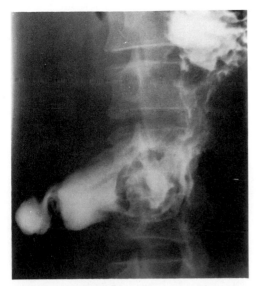

Fig. 72.13. Intussusception of the afferent loop following gastroenterostomy; the picture mimics that of a polypoidal tumour. This is one cause of failure of the stomach to empty after surgery.

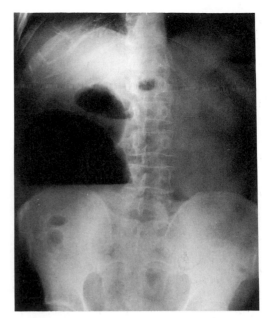

Fig. 72.14. Obstruction of the right colon with a competent ileocaecal valve carries a high risk of caecal perforation.

performing a laparotomy and the fraility of the patient adversely affect prognosis.

Intussusception, in the adult, is uncommon and is usually caused by an abnormality of the bowel wall. Benign tumours such as lipoma, Peutz–Jegher hamartoma or polyp are the usual precipitating factors in small bowel intussusception (Fig. 72.11). Adenocarcinoma is the main cause of colonic intussusception (Fig. 72.12). Many other rare causes, such as Meckel's diverticulum, secondary melanoma, typhoid enteritis, amoebic dysentery and invaginated appendix stump, have been described [8]. Episodes of intussusception may produce relapsing symptoms for some time before an acute obstruction develops. Intussusception of the afferent loop of a gastroenterostomy is an important cause of malfunction of the stomach in the early postoperative period (Fig. 72.13).

Intrinsic bowel lesions

Carcinoma of the colon frequently causes intestinal obstruction. This complication of malignant stricture occurs more readily in the left colon where the stool is formed; about 40% of patients with carcinoma of the left colon have obstructive symptoms on presentation [10]. In the right colon, where the fluid stool passes more easily through the stricture, only 20% have obstruction on clinical presentation. Tumours of the caecum may encroach on the ileocaecal valve and present as obstruction of the ileum. In the ascending colon, obstruction may cause a large fluid level in the caecum (Fig. 72.14), sometimes the tumour is outlined by air and diagnosed on the plain film (Fig. 72.15).

Diverticular disease is an uncommon cause (4%) of acute obstruction of the sigmoid colon [4], though subacute obstructive symptoms are common. Frequently it is difficult to distinguish from malignant obstruction on both clinical and radiological signs; the exact nature of the lesion may only emerge when a resection is performed.

Small intestinal strictures account for

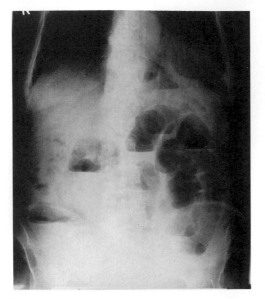

Fig. 72.15. The cause of the small bowel obstruction is indicated by the fluid level in the caecum and the gas outlining the malignant stricture just distal to it.

only a few cases of acute obstruction. Crohn's disease causes narrowing of the lumen and may lead to episodes of subacute obstruction that usually settle with conser-

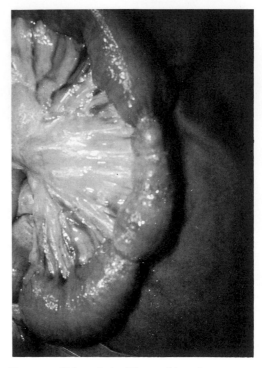

Fig. 72.17. Tuberculosis of the small bowel may result in multiple fibrous strictures which cause subacute obstruction.

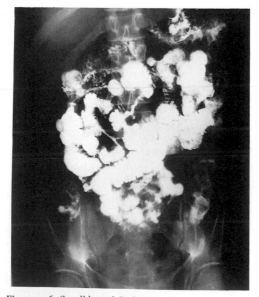

Fig. 72.16. Small bowel Crohn's disease causing multiple strictures and sub-acute symptoms of obstruction.

vative treatment (Fig. 72.16); only rarely is there an acute obstruction needing emergency surgery. Similarly, ileocaecal tuberculosis, which is more prevalent in Asian immigrants, may cause subacute rather than acute occlusion at the ileocaecal region. Tuberculous strictures of the small bowel are often multiple (Fig. 72.17). Malignant strictures, mainly lymphosarcoma, adenocarcinoma and carcinoid tumours, are uncommon and when they present as small bowel obstruction the diagnosis is usually only made at laparotomy. Iatrogenic factors may also cause small bowel narrowing—these include irradiation, haematoma following anticoagulation, potassium chloride tablets or ischaemic narrowing after failure to resect an obstructed and partially ischaemic loop of bowel [5] (Fig. 72.18).

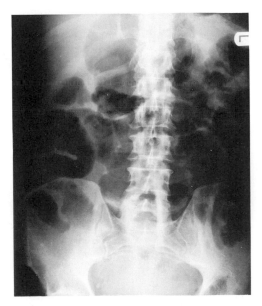

Fig. 72.18. Ischaemic stenosis of the small bowel devloped in this patient several weeks after release of an obstructed hernia containing dusky bowel.

Extrinsic compression of the bowel

Adhesions develop following surgery or peritonitis and serve an important role in the repair of damaged tissue. As healing is completed most of the adhesions contract and regress. In so doing, short bands may form which sometimes tether and entrap a loop of bowel, which is almost always small intestine. Intestinal obstruction may follow and, if not relieved, the loop of bowel is liable to strangulate. The problem often arises in the early postoperative period when it may be confused with paralytic ileus. in other patients the interval from surgery is frequently many months or years. the incidence of this problem has grown with the increased frequency of abdominal operations; currently it accounts for approximately one-third of all cases of intestinal obstruction and 60% of all strangulations.

An **inguinal hernia** may become irreducible and intestinal obstruction follows; the entrapped loop may strangulate if not

relieved by surgery. The incidence of these serious hernia complications has declined in developed countries where elective surgery for herniae is common. A **femoral hernia** carries a greater risk of strangulation because of the rigidity of the walls of the canal. The hernia is often small and easily overlooked in an elderly obese patient with a dependent abdominal wall. **Paraumbilical** and **incisional herniae** are more likely to obstruct and strangulate if the abdominal wall defect is small; they may be difficult to recognize in elderly obese patients. **Internal herniae** into the paraduodenal or paracaecal fossae and obturator herniae are rare and usually diagnosed first at laparotomy.

Volvulus of the sigmoid colon is a common cause of obstruction in developing countries accounting for 30–40% of cases, compared to 3–5% in the West (Fig. 72.19). The sigmoid colon is usually excessively long with a narrow base to its long mesentery. The distal limb of the sigmoid shows hypertrophy and dilatation which extends into the rectum. Patients are usually middle-

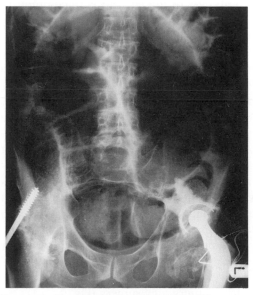

Fig. 72.19. The typical appearance of sigmoid volvulus with the inverted U-shaped loop extending obliquely towards the right upper quadrant.

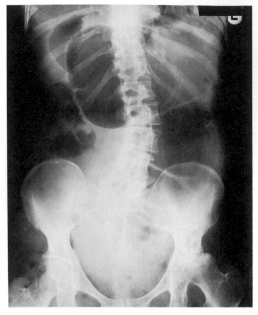
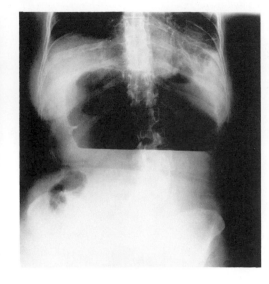

Fig. 72.20. In caecal volvulus the abnormally mobile caecum rotates into the upper abdomen.

aged or elderly and often have a history of mental illness. Subacute episodes of abdominal pain frequently precede the final acute attack.

Volvulus of the caecum is uncommon in Western countries and is associated with an abnormally mobile right colon and terminal ileum (Fig. 72.20). Adhesions, pelvic tumour, or pregnancy may precipitate the twist which may present as recurrent subacute attacks or as an acute obstruction. **Volvulus of the splenic flexure** is a rare cause of obstruction [2] (Fig. 72.21). **Volvulus of the small bowel** is an important surgical problem in neonates but is uncommon in adults in developed countries. **Volvulus of the stomach** is usually associated with eventration of the diaphragm or a large paraoesophageal hernia—chronic cases often have only mild symptoms, but in acute cases obstruction usually presents with severe epigastric pain and retching, requiring emergency surgery (Fig. 72.22).

An unusual cause of extrinsic small bowel obstruction is **compression of the**

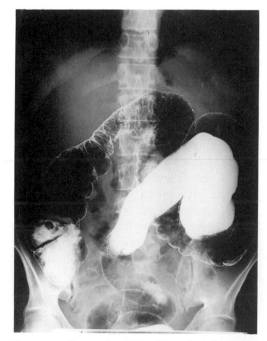

Fig. 72.21. Abnormal mobility of the splenic flexure predisposes to an uncommon form of large bowel volvulus.

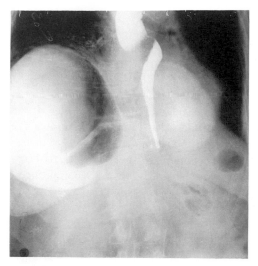

Fig. 72.22. Acute volvulus of the stomach in an elderly patient. The twisted fundus of the stomach lies to the right of the barium column and the distended body and antrum to the left side.

duodenal jejunal flexure by the superior mesenteric vessels (Fig. 72.23). Some clinicians deny that this is a cause of symptoms.

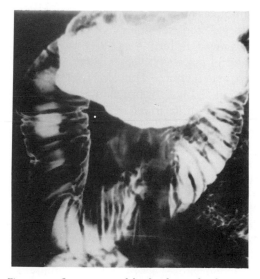

Fig. 72.23. Compression of the duodenum by the superior mesenteric vessels in a patient subject to recurrent episodes of vomiting. This finding is frequently incidental and unrelated to the patient's symptoms.

Ileus

Following laparotomy motor activity in the gastrointestinal tract is temporarily inhibited. Motility in the small intestine recovers rapidly [16], usually within 24 hours, whereas the stomach and colon [23] may take several days to recover.

Rupture of abdominal viscera causing spillage of intestinal contents may lead to ileus but it is important to recognize that bowel sounds frequently persist until severe peritonitis is established.

Retroperitoneal lesions such as pancreatitis, haemorrhage (especially if associated with spinal fracture) or urinary tract obstruction are commonly associated with an ileus. **Surgical operations** to the renal tract, the great vessels or for lumbar sympathectomy have a similar effect. Severe **metabolic disturbances**, such as renal failure, diabetic coma or depletion of potassium may also be complicated by ileus.

Infarction of the small intestine leads to paralytic ileus and gas may be seen in the portal system in the terminal stages (Fig.

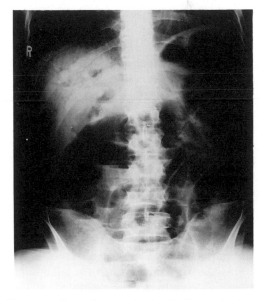

Fig. 72.24. Gas in the portal system in the terminal stages of small bowel infarction.

72.24). Focal intestinal ischaemia may cause a fibrous small intestinal stricture.

The differential diagnosis of paralytic ileus from mechanical obstruction is important as surgery should be avoided in ileus. Vomiting (or large gastric aspirates), abdominal distension and absolute constipation are common to both. If the abdomen is silent and cramps are absent, a diagnosis of ileus may be acceptable—provided that resolution occurs within a few days. If distension persists, or passage of flatus commences and ceases again, the development of a mechanical obstruction should be suspected and investigated by further radiology or laparotomy.

Pseudo-obstruction of the bowel

Pseudo-obstruction of the colon frequently causes problems in diagnosis because the clinical and radiological features closely mimic those of an organic obstructon. Crampy lower abdominal pain, absolute constipation, abdominal distension and obstructive bowel sounds suggest a malignant stricture in the left colon and the plain films may support this diagnosis (Fig. 72.25(a)) although there may be a paucity of fluid levels on the erect film (Fig. 72.25(b)). Barium enema examination is often helpful in resolving the problem (Fig. 72.25(c)).

An important feature of colonic pseudo-obstruction is the frequent association with extracolonic disease. In younger women it may complicate pregnancy, caesarean section or pelvic surgery [19]. In older patients myocardial infarction, cardiac failure or pneumonia may precede the obstruction; this should prompt the diagnosis and alert the clinician to the hazards of performing an unnecessary laparotomy. Abdominal inflammation such as an empyema of the gallbladder or pancreatitis, or a generalized illness (alcoholism, disseminated malignancy, metabolic disturbance, myxoedema or severe burns) may precipitate the

syndrome. Drugs in the phenothiazine group, tricyclic antidepressants and some antihypertensive agents have all been incriminated. In a quarter of patients no cause is found.

Conservative management is indicated while the associated disease is treated. If the colon becomes grossly distended and caecal perforation is anticipated, it may be necessary to decompress the bowel by caecostomy or colostomy [9]. Decompression using a colonoscope has also been advocated [12].

Pseudo-obstruction of the small intestine is uncommon and may be associated with raised prostaglandin levels [14]. Aperistalsis of the oesophagus with incomplete relaxation of the cardia is common [20] and a familial form has been described [13].

Pathophysiology

Small bowel obstruction

Fluid and gas accumulate in the obstructed bowel causing distension, which in turn stimulates further secretion of fluid [18]. The gas consists mainly of nitrogen from swallowed air but, in addition, bacterial activity in stagnant loops synthesizes hydrogen and methane [7]. The volume of gas present in ileal obstruction may be large and account for much of the abdominal distension which, by splinting the diaphragm, restricts ventilation.

Fluid loss is the most important consequence of simple small bowel obstruction. High small bowel obstruction causes severe vomiting with loss of water, sodium, potassium, chloride and hydrogen; dehydration, hypokalaemia, hypochloraemia and metabolic alkalosis develop. Ileal obstruction causes less vomiting initially, so that hydrogen ion is conserved and alkalosis avoided. The fluid and electrolyte deficit is nonetheless serious in ileal obstruction because of sequestration of secretions in the

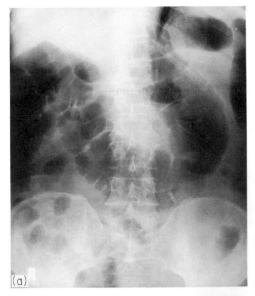

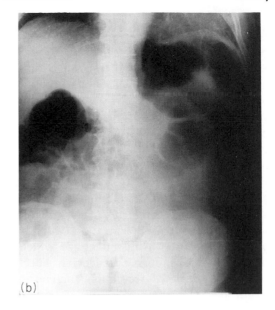

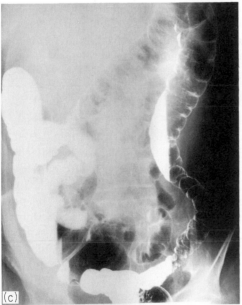

Fig. 72.25. A 75-year-old man had taken debrisoquine for hypertension for several years before developing the clinical features of large bowel obstruction. The supine film suggests obstruction of the large bowel (a), although the erect film shows few fluid levels (b). Emergency barium enema failed to reveal any obstructing lesion thus confirming colonic pseudo-obstruction (c).

dilated loops. Without treatment the venous pressure falls and oliguria develops, this is accompanied by a rapid and thready pulse and can be followed by circulatory collapse.

Normally the bacterial flora of the small bowel is scant. Obstruction and stasis of the small intestine allows bacterial proliferation [21] with a faeculent appearance of the contents. Vomiting of this material is distressing for the patient and indicates a prolonged obstruction.

Patients with far-advanced abdominal malignant disease, causing intestinal obstruction, can usually be managed medically [2].

Strangulated obstruction

Impairment of the circulation to an en-trapped loop of bowel will result in stran-gulation. Postoperative adhesions account for the majority of such cases in Western countries. A whole loop of bowel may be incarcerated in an inguinal hernia and ex-tensive portions of bowel may be involved in a volvulus. In contrast, a Richter's her-nia may strangulate only a small knuckle of bowel. Increasing intraluminal pressure occludes the venous return causing conges-tion and haemorrhagic infiltration. Mucosal breakdown results in haemorrhage which may be severe enough to adversely affect the already depleted circulation. Increasing turgor occludes the arterial circulation to the loop and gangrene ensues. Bacterial ac-tivity in the presence of infarcted tissue and stagnant fluid, forms a highly toxic and in-fective mixture which can permeate through the necrotic bowel wall. Perfora-tion of the bowel follows and rapidly re-leases the fluid causing severe peritonitis if it escapes into the peritoneal cavity. Endo-toxic shock and renal failure will follow and the prognosis becomes grave.

The consequences of strangulation are best avoided by early surgical intervention following correction of the fluid deficit. In subacute small bowel obstruction from ad-hesions, it is sometimes justified to per-severe with conservative management if there have been previous episodes, but this carries the risk of missing the onset of stran-gulation. Abdominal pain, which changes to a continuous pattern, and tenderness on percussion are important indicators for ur-gent laparotomy. A rising pulse rate is also an important sign and other constitutional signs such as fever and leucocytosis may be present. Frequently the clinical picture is indistinguishable from that of simple ob-struction.

Colonic obstruction

Closed obstruction of the colon occurs if the ileocaecal valve is competent. Progressive gaseous distension impairs mucosal blood flow and causes stretching of the serosa. The caecum, being the widest and most spherical part of the colon, is vulnerable to serosal tearing leading to caecal perforation if the obstruction is not urgently decom-pressed. Copious spillage of fluid stool after caecal perforation rapidly leads to faecal peritonitis and a deteriorating prognosis. An obstructing carcinoma in the left colon may also perforate, although the presenta-tion is usually less dramatic.

When incompetence of the ileocaecal valve is present obstruction of the colon presents as combined small and large bowel obstruction. The risk of colonic perforation is much less but there is a greater tendency to develop fluid and electrolyte imbalance.

Treatment of intestinal obstruction

Surgical relief of intestinal obstruction should be carried out as soon as it is safe. Exceptions to this policy are justified in cases of subacute obstruction caused by Crohn's disease, disseminated intra-abdomi-nal tumour [2] or adhesions in the post-operative period [24]. Surgery for sigmoid volvulus is postponed to advantage if en-doscopic decompression is successful; in in-tussusception of infancy, surgery may be avoided if hydrostatic reduction can be achieved.

Selection of the optimum time to operate is governed by the severity of the fluid and electrolyte deficit and the presence of other acute medical conditions. These factors must be balanced against the risk of stran-gulation which is difficult to assess with ac-curacy. Obstruction complicated by gan-grene has a mortality rate of 30%.

Resuscitation

The extent of the deficit of fluid and electrolytes cannot be estimated accurately at the bedside. Elevation of the blood urea, together with a fall in plasma sodium, potassium and chloride, indicate a major loss. Arterial blood gas estimation will quantify metabolic alkalosis if vomiting is severe. A rising pulse rate proceeding to falling blood pressure is seen in severe cases. On the assumption that several litres of fluid are required, it is appropriate to commence infusion of one litre of 0.9% saline at a brisk pace through a peripheral venous line. The response to treatment is then monitored by measuring the central venous pressure and the hourly output of urine. If there is a urinary output, potassium is added to the infusion which is continued at a brisk rate until the central venous pressure is stabilized as a normal level. Blood transfusion is required if strangulation of bowel has caused a substantial blood loss.

Nasogastric suction relieves the distressing symptoms of nausea and vomiting, and reduces abdominal distension minimizing the risk of inhalation during induction of anaesthesia. It can decompress the upper small bowel, although the more distal loops may require decompression at laparotomy if they are grossly distended.

The patient's general medical condition requires careful assessment. Intestinal obstruction has an adverse effect on conditions such as diabetes mellitus, chronic chest disease or chronic renal failure. Medication for cardiac conditions may have lapsed or not been absorbed for several days. Systemic treatment of these secondary problems, in consultation with a physician and the anaesthetic team, should be undertaken vigorously while resuscitation is in progress.

Operative treatment

Small bowel obstruction

External herniae, which are causing obstruction, are approached by the same incision as is used for uncomplicated herniae. The sac should be opened and the entrapped bowel secured before relieving the constriction. This avoids the possibility of non-viable bowel and infected fluid escaping into the peritoneal cavity.

Laparotomy for small bowel obstruction is normally performed through a vertical incision. The obstructive lesion is at first obscured by loops of distended bowel and may be located by finding a collapsed loop and following it retrogradely. More than one site of obstruction may be present, particularly where adhesions, metastatic tumour or tuberculous strictures are the cause.

The viability of released bowel is sometimes difficult to predict. Preservation of the serosal sheen and improving colour are propitious signs, whereas persisting duskiness with lack of peristalsis and loss of sheen indicates the need for resection. Placing the bowel in a warm saline pack for 15 minutes may restore the bowel to a satisfactory appearance. Doppler ultrasound assessment can be valuable in assessing long segments of bowel of doubtful viability [6]. If doubt persists, it is better to resect than risk gangrenous perforation or ischaemic stricture. Occasionally, where a long, possibly ischaemic, segment is present, it may be justified to close the abdomen and perform a second laparotomy after 24 hours.

If the bowel is sufficiently distended to make closure of the abdomen difficult or to restrict movement of the diaphragm it should be decompressed by passing a sucker through an enterotomy and 'feeding' the loops of bowel onto it. Alternatively it may be possible to milk the small bowel contents backwards into the stomach to allow aspiration through the nasogastric tube [20].

Large bowel obstruction

Obstruction of the right colon is best managed by emergency right hemicolectomy. Distension of the ileum facilitates the anastomosis without causing an adverse effect on its blood supply. If the lesion proves to be an inoperable carcinoma or if secondary deposits in the liver are extensive, a side-to-side ileotransverse colostomy provides adequate palliation.

Malignant strictures causing obstruction of the transverse colon may also be managed by extended right hemicolectomy to provide an immediate one-stage solution to the problem. If the patient is ill or frail and the tumour is to the left of the spine, a transverse colostomy and staged resection may be a safer policy.

In the left colon, acute or acute-on-chronic obstruction is usually caused by a carcinoma and carries a mortality rate of 30%. Immediate resection and anastomosis is difficult and hazardous because of impairment of the blood supply to the mucosa of the proximal distended colon. The traditional method of management is to perform a laparotomy to assess the lesion and then a transverse loop colostomy to provide decompression. After the patient has recovered a second laparotomy is performed for resection of the tumour. A month later the colostomy is closed and the three-stage procedure is complete.

Elderly patients frequently do not complete this arduous three-stage procedure and alternative policies have been used. Immediate resection of the tumour is technically feasible, though more difficult in the presence of obstructed distended bowel; the proximal end is brought out alongside the distal end if it is sufficiently mobile (Paul-Mikulicz procedure), but often it is necessary to oversew the distal bowel and return it to the abdomen (Hartmann's operation). When the patient has recovered a second operation is required to restore intestinal continuity. This two-stage policy is recommended for the management of an acute sigmoid volvulus if endoscopic decompression is not successful. Some surgeons are prepared to perform an initial anastomosis following resection with, or without, a temporary caecostomy to relieve pressure on the anastomosis. This remains a controversial mode of management although it does avoid the need for further surgery in an elderly or ill patient.

In poor-risk patients a simple policy for initial relief is achieved by immediate barium enema examination to confirm the presence of the malignant stricture. A transverse loop colostomy is then performed through a transverse rectus-cutting incision, which also allows palpation of the lesion and confirmation that small bowel is not adherent and tethered by it. By avoiding a full laparotomy, recovery is rapid and resection two weeks later is possible.

More details about ileostomy and colostomy surgery can be found in Chapter 55.

The X-ray illustrations in this chapter were selected with the help of Dr J. O. Manton Mills, FRCR.

References

1 ANDERSSON A, ZEDERFELT B. Gallstone ileus. *Acta Chir Scand* 1969;**135**:713–717.
2 BAINES M, OLIVER DJ, CARTER RL. Medical management of intestinal obstruction in patients with advanced malignant disease: a clinical and pathological study. *Lancet* 1985;ii:990–993.
2 BLUMBERG NA. Volvulus of the splenic flexure. *Br J Surg* 1958;**46**:292–295.
4 CAMPBELL JA, GUNN AA, McLAREN IF. Acute obstruction of the colon. *J R Coll Surg Edinb* 1956;1:213–239.
5 CHERNEY LS. Intestinal stenosis following strangulated hernia: review of the literature and report of a case. *Ann Surg* 1958;**148**:991–994.
6 COOPERMAN M, MARTIN EW, CAREY LC. Evaluation of ischemic intestine by Doppler ultrasound. *Am J Surg* 1980;**139**:73–77.
7 DUTHIE HL. Intestine. In: Irvine WT, ed. *The Scientific Basis of Surgery*. London: Churchill Livingstone, 1972:82.
8 ELLIS H. *Intestinal Obstruction*. New York: Appleton-Century-Crofts, 1982:321–342.

9 GIERSON ED, STORM FK, SHAW W, COYNE SK. Caecal rupture due to colonic ileus. *Br J Surg* 1975;**62**:383–386.

10 GOLIGHER JC, SIMIDDY FG. The treatment of acute obstruction or perforation with carcinoma of the colon and rectum. *Br J Surg* 1957;**45**:270–274.

11 JONES PF, MATHESON NA. Operative decompression in intestinal obstruction. *Lancet* 1968;**i**:1197.

12 KUKORA JS, DENT TL. Colonoscopic decompression of massive non-obstructive cecal dilation. *Arch Surg* 1977;**112**:512–517.

13 LEADING ARTICLE. Intestinal pseudo-obstruction. *Lancet* 1979;**i**:535.

14 LUDERER JR, DEMERS LM, BONNEM EM, SALEEM A, JEFFRIES GH. Elevated protoglandin E in idiopathic pseudo-obstruction. *N Engl J Med* 1976;**295**:1179.

15 ROGERS FA, CARTER R. Recurrent gallstone ileus. *Am J Surg* 1958;**96**:379–386.

16 ROSS B, WATSON BW, KAY AW. Studies on the effect of vagotomy on small inestinal motility using the radiotelemetring capsule. *Gut* 1963;**4**:77–81.

17 SCHEIBLE W, GOLDBERGER LE. Diagnosis of small bowel obstruction: the contribution of diagnostic ultrasound. *AJR* 1979;**133**:685–688.

18 SHIELDS R. The absorption and secretion of fluid and electrolytes by the obstructed bowel. *Br J Surg* 1965;**52**:774–779.

19 SPIRO IA, RODRIGUES R, WOLFF WI. Pseudo-obstruction of the colon. *Am J Gastroenterol* 1976;**65**:397–408.

20 SULLIVAN MA, SNAPE WJ, MATARZZO SA *et al.* Gastrointestinal myoelectric activity in idiopathic intestinal pseudo-obstruction. *N Engl J Med* 1977;**297**:233–238.

21 SYKES PA, BOULTER KH, SCHOFIELD PF. The microflora of the obstructed bowel. *Br J Surg* 1976;**63**:721.

22 WILLIAMS JL. Fluid-filled loops in intestinal obstruction. *AJR* 1962;**88**:677–686.

23 WILSON JP. Postoperative motility of the large intestine in man. *Gut* 1975;**16**:689–692.

24 WOLFSON PJ, BAUER JJ, GELERNT IM, KREEL I, AUFSES AH JR. Use of the long tube in the management of patient with small-intestinal obstruction due to adhesions. *Arch Surg* 1985;**120**:1001–1006.

Chapter 73
Pneumatosis Cystoides Intestinalis

M. EASTWOOD & J. GILLON

Pneumatosis cystoides intestinalis is a rare condition where gas-filled cysts are found in the subserosa or submucosa of the small intestine or colon.

Epidemiology

Relatively few physicians have recognized or treated this condition. The disease used to be considered three times more prominent in males than females [15], but more recent reports suggest that males and females are affected with approximately equal frequency. Small bowel disease used to be relatively common [12], largely due to its association with pyloric stenosis and other conditions of the upper gastrointestinal tract, but in the past 20 years most reports have suggested that colonic disease is more common.

Aetiology

Pneumatosis cystoides intestinalis usually occurs as a primary idiopathic condition. There are secondary forms of the disease which may occur in association with a variety of conditions (Table 73.1).

In infants pneumatosis occurs as a com-

Table 73.1. Conditions associated with pneumatosis cystoides.

Obstructive airways disease
Pseudomembranous colitis
Diverticular disease
Duodenal ulcer
Pyloric stenosis
Jejunoileal by-pass
Instrumentation of the colon
(Necrotizing enterocolitis in infants)

plication of acute necrotizing enterocolitis, and is a potentially dangerous condition in these circumstances, with the risk of massive dissection of gas causing loss of vasculature and mucosal sloughing. This enterocolitis is undoubtedly the result of bacterial infection, and overwhelming sepsis may result from the absorption of toxic intraluminal material (see p. 1161). It is not the same disease as primary pneumatosis in the adult.

In adults the condition is usually benign and the cysts may be either submucosal or subserosal. There is usually no obvious infection, and various pathogenic mechanisms have been proposed. Of these, neoplasia, dietary deficiency and biochemical abnormalities may be dismissed as their proponents have failed to provide substantiating evidence. The debate about aetiology has revolved largely around the mechanical and bacterial theories.

The mechanical theory of the disease arose from its undoubted association with chronic obstructive airways disease [1, 11]. It was suggested that, during severe bouts of coughing, air from a ruptured alveolus could track along the major arteries, through the mediastinum and diaphragm, to the mesentery and subserosal plane. This theory was supported by experiments in which gas was introduced under pressure into the mediastinum of animals; the tracking of such gas to the bowel was demonstrated. However, the proponents of this theory have failed to explain how the cysts, once formed, can remain unchanged for many years.

The possibility that the gas cysts result from bacterial activity has been considered by most physicians studying this condition. Pneumatosis occurs in pigs in an epidemic form [15]. The association of pneumatosis with necrotizing enteritis, pseudomembranous enterocolitis and diverticulitis is well established [14]. Pneumatosis has been produced in rats by innoculating the peritoneal cavity with various bacteria—pneumatosis arising most frequently with *C. perfringens* and *C. tertium* [18]. Nevertheless, attempts to culture organisms from the cysts themselves have invariably proved negative, and stool cultures from pneumatosis patients have revealed only a normal pattern of faecal flora [8].

There are, however, sound theoretical reasons for believing that a constant source of gas is necessary to prevent reabsorption of the cysts [13]. The composition of the gas within the cysts is variable, but it is different from that of air with a hydrogen content of up to 20% (Table 73.2). Patients with pneumatosis have been shown to excrete hydrogen in the breath in abnormally large quantities, even when fasting, suggesting that there is constant gas production by intestinal bacteria [6, 16]. It is probable that bacterial gas production is the major aetiological factor in the production of the cysts. This is supported by the finding

Table 73.2. Approximate composition of cyst gas in pneumatosis cystoides.

Nitrogen	70%
Oxygen	10–20%
Hydrogen	20%
Methane	trace
Carbon dioxide	trace

of pneumatosis in the by-passed small bowel of patients who have undergone jejunoileal by-pass for morbid obesity. This complication is more likely if there is any obstruction to the drainage of the loop, suggesting that raised intraluminal pressure may also play a part. The disease has also been reported in association with sigmoid volvulus [4].

Pathology

Pneumatosis may be found anywhere along the gastrointestinal tract. Most commonly it affects the left side of the colon, although the rectum is rarely involved [7]. Pneumatosis of the small bowel is relatively uncommon. The cysts may be subserosal or submucosal, varying in size from the microscopic to several centimetres. Large mesenteric gas cysts are sometimes seen. Spontaneous pneumoperitoneum may occur as a result of subserosal cyst rupture.

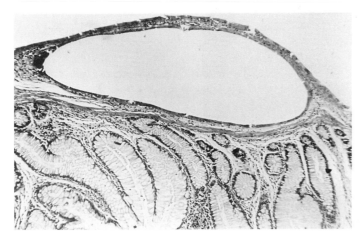

Fig. 73.1. Histological section of a submucosal gas cyst in the large intestine.

Histologically the lesions are seen to consist of thin-walled cysts lined by endothelial cells and separated from each other by connective tissue; a variable inflammatory infiltrate may be present (Fig. 73.1). It has been suggested that the cysts arise from lymphatic channels but this has been difficult to substantiate. Bacteria are rarely seen in the cysts [18].

Clinical features

The presentation is very variable. Often the condition is symptomless and may be found by chance at radiology or at laparotomy. Alternatively patients may present with intestinal obstruction, intermittent rectal bleeding, diarrhoea, excess flatus or mucus in the stool. In these circumstances misdiagnosis is common, and pneumatosis is often mistaken for ulcerative colitis.

Patients with small bowel pneumatosis may present with malabsorption.

When the disease occurs in association with other pathological conditions (see Table 73.1) it may be difficult to ascertain the exact cause of symptoms. In this case, however, treatment of the primary condition is appropriate and usually curative.

Primary pneumatosis is a benign condition which may persist for long periods without causing great disability. Occasional complications can arise, the most significant being haemorrhage and pneumoperitoneum. Inappropriate surgical intervention is an additional hazard for these patients.

Investigations

The cysts may be recognized at sigmoidoscopy although they are often initially

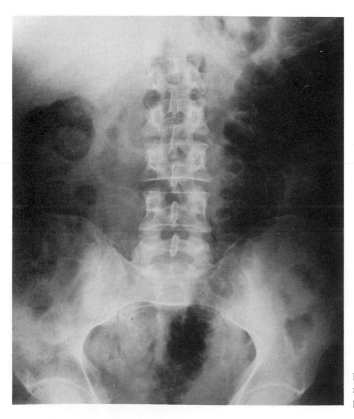

Fig. 73.2. Plain abdominal radiograph showing extensive pneumatosis of the left colon.

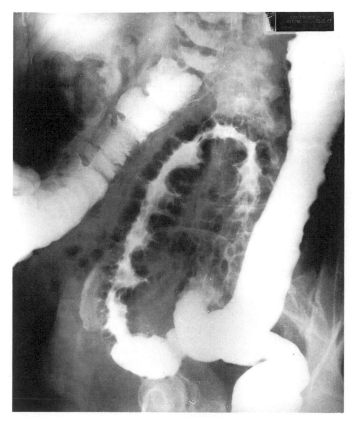

Fig. 73.3. Colonic pneumatosis seen on barium enema in a 94-year-old man.

mistaken for tumours, lymphoid hyperplasia, multiple polyps, or colitis with pseudopolyp formation. They look like white, shiny, thin-walled submucosal blebs—gas-filled cysts! The condition may be recognized on plain abdominal X-rays (Fig. 73.2). Barium studies show the gaseous line between the contrast medium and the outer limits of the intestinal wall (Fig. 73.3).

Differential diagnosis

It is important to differentiate pneumatosis from other life-threatening conditions in order to avoid inappropriate surgery. It is also important to recognize when pneumatosis is merely a complication of some other primary lesion which may be amenable to treatment. The main differential diagnoses are neoplasia or inflammatory bowel disease (Table 73.3).

Table 73.3. Differential diagnosis of pneumatosis cystoides.

Pseudo-polyps of ulcerative colitis
Multiple polyposis
Carcinoma
Colitis profunda cystica
Lymphoma—benign or malignant
Lipomata

Treatment

The treatment of secondary pneumatosis cystoides is that of the underlying condition. Management of uncomplicated primary disease is conservative. When symptoms demand some therapeutic intervention the first line of treatment should be intermittent high-flow oxygen therapy, aiming to provide an oxygen concentration of 70% almost continuously for five days by nasal catheters or mask [39]. This treatment appears to work by altering the partial pressures of gases within the blood. It almost invariably provides successful resolution of cysts, but unfortunately most patients relapse within a year of successful treatment [9].

It has been shown that the cysts may resolve with antibiotic treatment using either ampicillin [10] or metronidazole [2]. In the absence of controlled trials antibiotics should only be used with caution or where high-flow oxygen is contraindicated by pulmonary disease, since the response to antibiotics is variable and deterioration on treatment with metronidazole has been described [5]. Maintenance treatment with sulphasalazine 3 g/day may be helpful.

If the bacterial theory of the causation of pneumatosis is correct, dietary treatment designed to alter the carbohydrate substrates available in the colon should provide an alternative form of therapy. A preliminary report suggests that a period of treatment with an elemental diet can lead to resolution of the cysts [17].

Surgical treatment

Resection of primary pneumatosis may be necessary when complications, such as bleeding or volvulus, arise but recurrence of the disease may occur even when surgical removal of the cysts has been successful.

Prognosis

Primary pneumatosis cystoides is a benign condition which is only life-threatening in the presence of complications or when treated by inappropriate surgery.

References

1 Doub HP, Shea JJ. Pneumatosis cystoides intestinalis. *JAMA* 1960;**172:**1238–1242.

2 Ellis BW. Symptomatic treatment of primary pneumatosis coli with metronidazole. *Br Med J* 1980;**1:**763–764.

3 Forgacs P, Wright PH, Wyatt AP. Treatment of intestinal gas cysts by oxygen breathing. *Lancet* 1973;**i:**579–582.

4 Gillon J, Holt S, Sircus W. Pneumatosis coli and sigmoid volvulus: a report of 4 cases. *Br J Surg* 1979;**66:**802–805.

5 Gillon J, Logan RFA, Sircus W, Heading RC. Symptomatic treatment of primary pneumatosis coli with metronidazole. *Br Med J* 1980;**280:**1087.

6 Gillon J, Tadesse K, Logan RFA, Holt S, Sircus W. Breath hydrogen in pneumatosis cystoides intestinalis. *Gut* 1979;**20:**1008–1011.

7 Hirzel LF jr., Hahne OH. Pneumatosis cystoides intestinalis of the rectum. *Am J Proctol* 1976;**27(5):**29–31.

8 Holt S, Gillon J, Heading RC, Sircus W. Pneumatosis coli. *Gut* 1979;**20:**448.

9 Holt S, Gilmour HM, Buist TAS, Marwick K, Heading RC. High flow oxygen therapy for pneumatosis coli. *Gut* 1979;**20:**493–498.

10 Holt S, Stewart IC, Heading RC, MacPherson AIS. Resolution of primary pneumatosis coli. *J R Coll Surg Edinb* 1978;**23:**297–300.

11 Keyting WS, McCarver RR, Kovarick JL, Daywitt AL. Pneumatosis intestinalis: a new concept. *Radiology* 1961;**76:**733–741.

12 Koss LG. Abdominal gas cysts (pneumatosis cystoides intestinorum hominis): an analysis with a report of a case and a critical review of the literature. *Arch Pathol* 1952;**53:**523–549.

13 Levitt MD, Bond JH. In: *Scientific foundations of gastroenterology.* London: Wm. Heinemann, 1980.

14 McKenzie EP. Pneumatosis intestinalis. *Paediatrics* 1951;**7:**537–549.

15 Nitch CAR. Cystic pneumatosis of the intestinal tract. *Br J Surg* 1924;**11:**714–735.

16 Van der Linden W, Hoflin F. Pneumatosis cystoides coli recurs after oxygen treatment. A clue to pathogenesis? *Eur Surg Res* 1978;**10:**225–229.

17 Van der Linden W, Marsell R. Pneumatosis cystoides coli associated with high H_2 excretion. Treatment with an elemental diet. *Scand J Gastroenterol* 1979;**14:**173–174.

18 Yale CE, Balish E. Pneumatosis cystoides intestinalis. *Dis Colon Rectum* 1976;**19:**107–111.

Chapter 74
Systemic Illness and the Gut

G. NEALE & R. J. DICKINSON

A great many systemic disorders may disturb gastrointestinal function. In some cases the gut disorder is an integral part of the pathological process, such as the dysphagia of systemic sclerosis or the abdominal pain of Schönlein-Henoch purpura; in other diseases the manifestations of gastrointestinal involvement are rarely encountered and may be difficult to distinguish from the effects of an unrelated coexistent pathology—this might be true of gastrointestinal bleeding in a patient with systemic lupus erythematosus or of diarrhoea in a patient with psoriasis. Thus the gastroenterologist has not only to be aware of the possible associations between systemic illnesses and gastrointestinal dysfunction, but must also be wary of accepting a simple or clever explanation without firm proof of a causal relationship.

The information on the relation of systemic disease, or of its treatment, and gastrointestinal dysfunction is not only very considerable but also spread through a wide range of journals. Much of it is in the form of interesting case reports—anecdotes by general physicians to tease the specialists. In this chapter we have worked through general medicine on a systematic basis and have tried to identify the problems on which the gastroenterologist may be asked to advise.

Systemic disorders capable of producing significant gastrointestinal disease, are listed according to the symptoms in Tables 74.1–74.7.

Table 74.1. Systemic disorders that may cause dysphagia.

Candidiasis

Infiltrations, e.g. amyloidosis, sarcoidosis (rarely)

Neurological disorders
  Upper motor neuron disease, e.g. cerebrovascular disease
  Lower motor neuron disease, e.g. toxic neuropathy (rare)
  Parkinson's disease
  Myaesthenia gravis*
  Chagas' disease*

Muscular diseases
  Muscular dystrophy (rare)
  Polymyositis

Rheumatology/connective tissue disorders
  Systemic sclerosis*
  Rheumatoid arthritis
  Systemic lupus erythematosus

*Dysphagia may be the presenting feature of these conditions.

Table 74.2. Systemic disorders and peptic ulceration.

Chronic respiratory disease

Chronic renal failure

Alcoholism

Rheumatology/connective tissue disorders especially as a result of treatment with non-steroidal anti-inflammatory drugs, steroids

Hyperparathyroidism

Systemic mastocytosis

Table 74.3. Systemic disorders that may cause bleeding from the gut.

Renal failure

Alcoholism*

Rheumatological/connective tissue disorders
  In association with therapy (steroids, non-steroidal
    anti-inflammatory drugs)
  Vasculitis
  Polyarteritis

Disorders that usually present with dermatological
    lesions
  Telangiectasia
  Neurofibromatosis
  Pseudoxanthoma elasticum*
  Ehlers-Danlos disease*
  Blue rubber bleb naevus
  Kaposi's sarcoma

Haematological disorders
  Leukaemias
  Bleeding disorders with mucosal pathology*
  Thrombotic conditions (e.g. polycythaemia,
    thrombotic thrombocytopenic purpura)
  Haemolytic-uraemic syndrome*

Dysproteinaemias*

---

* In these disorders gastrointestinal bleeding may be the presenting feature.

Table 74.4. Intestinal perforation as a manifestation of systemic disease.

Vasculitides
  Polyarteritis
  Polymyositis
  Systemic lupus erythematosus/Rheumatoid disease
  Fabry's disease

Behçet's syndrome

Ehlers-Danlos syndrome

Neurofibromatosis

Leukaemias

Treatment with non-steroidal anti-inflammatory drugs

Malnutrition

The intestinal mucosa has a rapid turnover of epithelial cells, thus it is vulnerable to nutritional deficiencies.

General malnutrition

In protein-energy malnutrition the mucosa of the small intestine is often abnormal with varying degrees of villous atrophy and infiltration with inflammatory cells. In most patients, however, there is an associated pathology such as parasitic infestation, bacterial overgrowth or viral infection. Thus it is difficult to be sure to what extent the observed changes are due to nutritional deficiency. The pathological changes appear to be most severe in patients with kwashiorkor [40]. They may be associated with impaired cell-mediated immunity and bacterial overgrowth in the small intestine. In children lactose intolerance, diarrhoea and steatorrhoea are common.

The structural and functional changes are non-specific, and in many cases not dissimilar to those found in patients with tropical malabsorption syndromes. After nutritional rehabilitation clinical recovery is rapid, with a complete recovery of intestinal structure. However, lactase activity often remains depressed [46].

Deficiency of specific nutrients

Zinc

Severe zinc deficiency causes pustular skin lesions around the body orifices and on the extremities accompanied by diarrhoea, hence the term acrodermatitis enteropathica. It occurs as an inherited disease in children (presumably due to a specific defect of zinc absorption) and as an acquired disease in adults [28, 132]. Cases have been reported in association with severe Crohn's disease, jejuno-ileal by-pass surgery, alcoholic cirrhosis, alcoholic pancreatitis and during the course of total parenteral nutrition. The small intestinal mucosa may show non-specific histological changes. Ultrastructural damage of the enterocyte has been demonstrated in experimental animals [57].

Table 74.5. Systemic disorders with diarrhoea as an associated feature.

Malnutrition	Protein/energy malnutrition Zinc deficiency Niacin deficiency (pellagra)
Immunodeficiency syndromes*	Viral, bacterial and parasitic diseases of the gut Mucosal enteropathies
Infiltrative disorders	Amyloidosis* Eosinophilic gastroenteritis
Endocrine disease	Diabetes Thyrotoxicosis* Addison's disease
Metabolic disease	Uraemic enterocolitis Systemic mastocytosis
Alcoholism*	
Rheumatological/connective tissue disorders	Polyarteritis Behçet's disease
Dermatological disorders	Dermatitis herpetiformis Dermatogenic enteropathy, e.g. eczema, psoriasis
Leukaemia	
	Bacterial overgrowth Leukaemic infiltration Drug-induced diarrhoea

* Disorders in which diarrhoea is not uncommonly the presenting complaint.

Table 74.6. Systemic disorders causing intestinal malabsorption (steatorrhoea).

Nutritional deficiencies	Folate, niacin, zinc
Immuno-deficiencies	Associated enteropathies Associated gluten sensitivity Bacterial overgrowth
Chronic granulomatous disease	
Infiltrative disorders	Amyloidosis* Eosinophilic gastroenteritis
Neurogenic disorders	causing pseudo-obstruction*
Endocrine/metabolic disorders	Diabetes (rarely)* Hypoparathyroidism Abetalipoproteinaemia
Rheumatological/connective tissue disorders	Systemic sclerosis* rarely with rheumatoid/systemic lupus erythematosus
Dermatology	Dermatitis herpetiformis/coeliac disease

* Conditions in which bacterial overgrowth is described.

Fig. 74.1a and b. Acrodermatitis
enteropathica:
Skin lesions responding to
treatment with oral zinc.
(Photographs by courtesy of Dr
Neil Walker, Addenbrooke's
Hospital.)

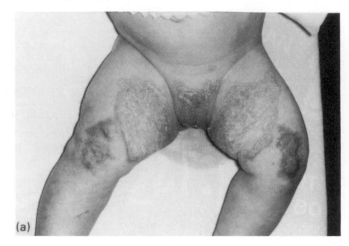

(a)

Table 74.7. Enterocolitis in association with systemic
disease.

Immune deficiency (occasional)
   e.g. Nezelof's syndrome
      Wiskott-Aldrich syndrome

Renal failure

Arteritides and vasculitis
   Rarely in rheumatoid/systemic lupus erythematosus
      syndromes—beware effect of drugs, e.g. gold
   Polyarteritis
   Haemolytic-uraemic syndrome*

Circulatory failure
   Ischaemic enterocolitis

Behçet's disease

Leukaemic disorders*

---

* May present as an enterocolitis.

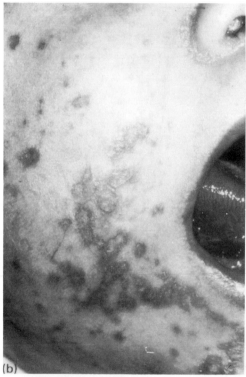

(b)

Treatment with zinc leads to rapid clearing of the skin lesions and resolution of the
diarrhoea. The gastroenterologist must be
careful not to confuse the skin lesions of the
glucagonoma syndrome with those of zinc
deficiency [93].

Iron

Gastrointestinal disorders frequently cause
iron deficiency which in turn may adversely
affect gut function. Chronic iron deficiency
causes epithelial metaplasia of the buccal
and oesophageal mucosa sometimes with
glossitis and occasionally with the development of an oesophageal web. Gastric mucosal atrophy with hypochlorhydria is common and there may be minor changes in
the epithelial surface of the small intestine
[215].

Niacin

Pellagra is usually caused by a diet deficient in niacin (vitamin B₃). Protein deficiency may be a contributory cause because the essential amino acid l-tryptophan provides a proportion of the body's requirements for niacin. In developed countries pellagra is most commonly seen in alcoholics. Niacin deficiency may also occur in conditions allowing bacterial overgrowth of the small intestine [207] and in carcinoid disease [206].

The classical clinical triad of dermatitis, dementia and diarrhoea is rarely fully expressed [198]. Diarrhoea occurs in 50% of cases, occasionally with steatorrhoea. Histology of the small intestinal mucosa is often unexciting and may merely reflect co-existing disease [144]. Effective treatment leads to a rapid regression of symptoms.

Vitamin B₁₂ and folic acid

The synthesis of DNA is impaired in patients with deficiency of vitamin B₁₂ or folic acid. Epithelial cells show megaloblastic changes with a reduced number of mitoses. Intestinal villi are shorter than normal and there may be an increase in round cell infiltration [63]. A sore tongue and diarrhoea are common symptoms in patients with prolonged deficiencies.

Vitamin A

Vitamin A deficiency is also associated with epithelial changes. Goblet cells become less prominent and cell proliferation is impaired [159, 176]. The functional significance of these changes is uncertain.

Disorders of the immune system

The gut has important defence mechanisms with a specialized immune system [52]. Defects in humoral and cell-mediated systems may lead to major disturbances of gastrointestinal function. Rather surprisingly, however, many immunodeficient patients are free of associated gastrointestinal disorders.

The pattern of gastrointestinal disease is very variable (Table 74.8). **Hypogammaglobulinaemia** is associated with an increased incidence of parasitic (e.g. *Giardia*), bacterial (e.g. *Salmonella*) or chronic viral (e.g. ECHO) infection [70]. Proliferation of colonic-type bacteria in the small intestine may also occur particularly if there is an associated achlorhydria. Unfortunately in many case reports the concentration of immunoglobulins in secretions is not stated, thus it is not possible to correlate disorders of the gut with the function of the local immune system. Curiously most patients with IgA deficiency are symptom-free whereas a proportion of subjects with severe immunoglobulin deficiencies develop a mucosal enteropathy with villous atrophy. This condition may be due to sensitivity to a dietary protein, particularly gluten and less commonly cow's milk.

In contrast, patients with **T cell deficiencies** are prone to fungal infections, especially candidiasis. Giardiasis does not seem to occur [96] but chronic rotavirus infection is described [180]. Hyperinfestation with *Strongyloides stercoralis* is a problem in tropical countries.

Paradoxically the hypogammaglobulinaemias appear to be associated with diseases, such as pernicious anaemia and coeliac disease, which are normally regarded as immune-mediated. A variety of malignancies have been reported in patients with IgA deficiency but there is no good evidence of a causal association. There is an increased risk of malignancy (especially lymphomas) in patients with panhypogammaglobulinaemia [114, 122] and in patients with long-standing deficiency of cell-mediated immunity.

Table 74.8. The gastrointestinal manifestations of B- and T-lymphocyte disorders.

B-Lymphocyte disorders	Gastrointestinal manifestations

IgA deficiency (prevalence 1:700) [25, 86, 118]	Majority symptom free
	Associated gastrointestinal disorders
	  Gluten sensitive enteropathy
	  Crohn's disease
	  Cow's milk intolerance
	  Giardiasis
	  Disaccharidase deficiency
	  Post-vagotomy diarrhoea

Secretor piece deficiency [201]	Diarrhoea Intestinal candidiasis

Congenital hypogammaglobulinaemia (X-linked)—rare [4, 180]	Infants present with respiratory disorders.
	  Later may develop:
	    Diarrhoea
	    Giardiasis
	    Chronic viral infection (especially
	      ECHO)

Common variable hypogammaglobulinaemia (Prevalence: 1.5 per 10^5 males; 0.4 per 10^5 females) [23, 88, 194, 219]	Gastro-intestinal disorders more common
	  than in congenital variety
	Include:
	  Pernicious anaemia
	  Gastric carcinoma
	  Chronic diarrhoea (majority)
	  Steatorrhoea:
	    Gluten sensitive enteropathy
	    Idiopathic mucosal enteropathy
	    Pancreatic insufficiency
	    Bacterial contamination of small
	      intestine
	    Giardiasis
	    Cryptosporidiosis
	  Infectious diarrhoea:
	    Shigella
	    Salmonella
	    Campylobacter
	    Viral enteritis

T-Lymphocyte disorders	**Gastrointestinal manifestations**

Congenital thymic aplasia
  (Di George syndrome)
  Absent T-cell function
  Cardiovascular anomalies
  Hypoparathyroidism
	Oesophageal atresia
	Chronic candidiasis
	Watery diarrhoea

Chronic mucocutaneous candidiasis (autosomal recessive)	Chronic oesophageal moniliasis Oesophageal stricture
Combined B- and T-cell defects	**Gastroentestinal manifestations**
Severe combined immunodeficiency disease (*SCID*) (inherited defect of adenosine deaminase is a well-defined entity in this group of disorders) [96]	Recurrent severe infection especially respiratory Diarrhoea, malabsorption Failure to thrive

Table 74.8.—*contd.*

Combined B- and T-cell defects	Gastrointestinal manifestations
	Jejunal mucosa may contain PAS-positive macrophages in stunted villi Candidiasis, Systemic BCG-itis, Chronic rotavirus infection [180]
T-cell deficiency with variable B-cell defect (Nezelof's syndrome) [124]	Similar changes to those occurring in SCID but less severe. Candidiasis and enterocolitis may occur

Combined immune deficiency	Gastrointestinal manifestations
Ataxia telangiectasia (T-cell deficiency and serum IgA deficiency with cerebellar ataxia and oculo-cutaneous telangiectasia) [4]	Minor gastrointestinal symptoms B_{12} malabsorption
Wiskott-Aldrich syndrome Thrombocytopenia, eczema (atopic) and partial combined immune deficiency X-linked recessive [4]	Gastrointestinal manifestations rare but may appear as immune function declines with age Steatorrhoea and colitis described [4]

Secondary immuno-deficiency	Gastrointestinal manifestations
Causes of hypogammaglobulinaemia Severe nephrotic syndrome Protein-losing enteropathy (with lymphocytopenia if lymphatics severely affected) Protein-calorie malnutrition *Causes of suppressed cell-mediated immunity* ($\pm$ *hypogammaglobulinaemia*) Malignancies Treatment with steroids and cytotoxic drugs Acquired immuno-deficiency syndrome (AIDS) [60] (see chapter 57)	Often remarkably good response to infection. But spectrum very wide and opportunistic infection common in severe cases. Gastrointestinal disorders may occur as a result of: Recurrent viral infection especially Herpes, CMV, E-BV Pathogenic bacterial infection of gut Invasive bacterial infection, e.g. Mycobacteria intracellulare Bacterial overgrowth of small intestine Chronic fungal infection, e.g. Candidiasis Protozoan infection of gut, e.g. Cryptosporidiosis Parasite hyper-infestation, e.g. Strongyloidiasis Kaposi's sarcoma

Chronic granulomatous disease

Deficient neutrophil NADPH oxidase activity leads to a failure of oxygen-dependent bactericidal systems. This disorder is characterized by an inability to kill catalase-positive organisms and leads to a clinical syndrome of recurrent infection with multifocal abscesses affecting skin, lymph nodes, liver, bone and intestine. Intestinal mucosal biopsies show pigmented lipid laden macrophages with granulomatous changes [4]. Patients are prone to episodes of steatorrhoea and malabsorption and may develop a colitis [222]. Salmonellosis is common and may cause death [143].

C1-esterase inhibitor deficiency

Disorders of the complement system are rare. Of the recognized defects only C1 esterase inhibitor deficiency causes prominent gastrointestinal symptoms. Affected patients present with recurrent episodes of angioedema of the extremities, face and pharynx. They also suffer attacks of colicky abdominal pain often with diarrhoea and vomiting caused by intestinal oedema. The primary form of this condition has an autosomal dominant pattern of inheritance with two phenotypes—more commonly the amount of circulating enzyme is much reduced; less commonly there is a normal amount of enzyme protein that is functionally inactive [110]. The condition may be acquired by patients with malignancy (especially lymphoid) or with a dysproteinaemia. In these conditions there is excessive consumption of the enzyme protein by C1 which itself is rapidly cleared from the circulation.

The production of C1-esterase inhibitor is increased by treatment with androgens. Danazol (200 mg/day) or stanozol (2 mg twice a week) will prevent attacks of angioedema [218]. Injections of purified C1-esterase inhibitor have been used successfully to abort attacks, whereas the use of fresh frozen plasma gives variable results presumably because it contains the substrate C1 [67].

Cryoglobulinaemia

Cryoglobulinaemia occurs either as an essential disorder or as one that may complicate a number of conditions in which there are circulating immune complexes. The associated vasculitis can cause patchy ischaemia of the intestine with repeated attacks of abdominal pain, nausea and vomiting. Pyrexia is a common feature of these attacks [173].

Waldenström's macroglobulinaemia

The hyperviscosity of the blood in Waldenström's macroglobulinaemia sometimes leads to diffuse mucosal bleeding. In addition the abnormal protein may be deposited in the lamina propria, obstructing lymphatics, impairing absorption and causing a protein-losing enteropathy [27].

Infiltrative disorders

Systemic amyloidosis

Amyloid is an extra-cellular scleroprotein (protein-polysaccharide complex) consisting of two basic components. The fibrils are polypeptide structures with recognizable sequences of amino acids. In multiple myeloma they are similar to light chains; in some of the familial amyloidoses they are akin to pre-albumin; and in the amyloid of chronic inflammatory disease (including familial mediterranean fever) they are described as amyloid A substance. The fibrils are associated with a glycoprotein which behaves as an $\alpha 1$-globulin and is termed amyloid P substance. This appears to be derived from a circulating polypeptide (serum amyloid P), which is structurally related to C-reactive protein, although it is not an acute phase reactant [61].

Amyloid damages tissues by infiltration and direct pressure. In the gastrointestinal tract perivascular infiltration causes patchy ischaemic damage which may lead to perforation, bleeding or protein-losing enteropathy; peri-neural deposits affect intestinal motility occasionally to the point of pseudo-obstruction; and submucosal deposits are associated with malabsorption and, rarely, true intestinal obstruction [107]. Nevertheless even widespread amyloidosis of the gut may be asymptomatic [121].

Histological examination of involved tissue is necessary for the diagnosis of

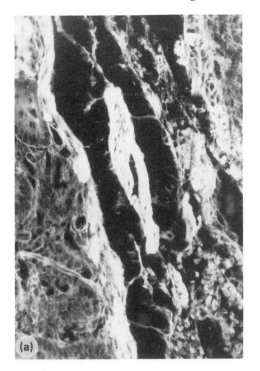

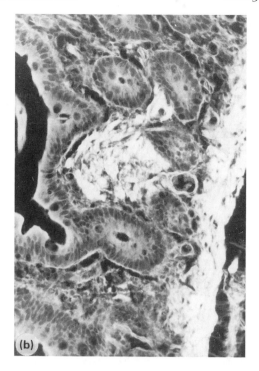

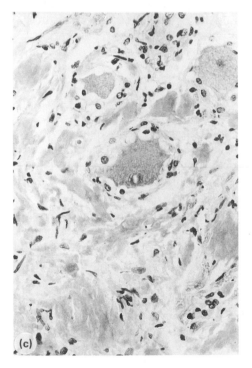

Fig. 74.2. Familial amyloidosis (Portuguese-Andrade variety). (a), small intestine, submucosal deposits of amyloid (Thioflavin T × 266); (b), small intestine, perivascular amyloid (Thioflavin T × 266); (c), small intestine, ganglion cell (Congo Red × 266). (Photomicrographs by courtesy of Dr Aled Jones, Hope Hospital, Manchester).

amyloidosis. Rectal biopsy is the most convenient available means and provides a diagnosis in more than 80% of patients with diffuse disease [121]. Peroral endoscopic biopsy of stomach or small intestine may provide positive results in some cases with a negative rectal biopsy [47].

Patients with amyloidosis may have difficulty in eating because of macroglossia or infiltration of the temporo-mandibular joints [187]. Dysphagia due to oesophageal dysmotility is uncommon. Involvement of the stomach may simulate gastric carcinoma or pyloric obstruction [51]. More often however symptoms are associated with intestinal damage. Diarrhoea, steatorrhoea, and protein-losing enteropathy are seen with infiltration of the jejunum and ileum; and constipation, megacolon and faecal incontinence with colonic involvement [121]. Gastrointestinal bleeding may occur at any level and nodular lesions may obstruct the intestine [35].

The prognosis of systemic amyloidosis is poor (mean survival less than two years) although it may be improving with more vigorous cytotoxic regimens for plasma cell dyscrasias and improved forms of treatment for chronic inflammatory disease. There are reports of the resorption of amyloid deposits although this is probably unusual, even if the progress of the underlying disorder is arrested.

Most patients with systemic amyloidosis die of cardiac or renal failure. Nevertheless gastrointestinal disease may dominate the clinical picture. It is seen in its most intractable form in the Andrade type of heredo-familial amyloidosis for which there is no effective teatment. Enterostomy may help some patients with colonic pseudo-obstruction [56].

Sarcoidosis

The gut is rarely involved in sarcoidosis. Hilar lymphadenopathy may cause dys-phagia and infiltration of the stomach is described as leading to changes indistinguishable from linitis plastica [119]. Direct damage of the wall of the intestine is extremely uncommon [117] but involvement of the mesenteric lymphatic system may cause protein-losing enteropathy [169].

Eosinophilic infiltration

Infiltration of the wall of the gut with eosinophils occurs rarely and usually without apparent cause. In some cases there is good evidence of an allergic response either to parasites [77] or to food antigens [36] but mostly this is not so. **Eosinophilic gastroenteritis** occurs mainly in young adults and other organs may be affected especially bladder, prostate and gallbladder [108].

Clinically it may present predominantly as a mucosal disease with diarrhoea as the prime symptom. Circulating eosinophils are increased and a patchy eosinophilia is found in biopsies of the gastrointestinal mucosa. It is important to exclude parasitic disease, atypical Crohn's disease, lymphoma and the arteritides. The condition usually responds well to oral corticosteroids although relapses may occur if the patient is treated for only a few weeks.

More often the gut wall is diffusely involved and this leads to nausea, vomiting and abdominal pain as predominant symptoms. Affected gut wall becomes rigid and often there is irregular narrowing of the lumen of the gut. The antrum is affected most frequently. Again there is usually a good response to treatment with corticosteroids although severe diffuse disease may be progressive and fatal [135].

Occasionally only the serosa is involved. Patients present with ascites that contain large numbers of eosinophil leucocytes. The ascites clears promptly on treatment with corticosteroids [116].

Multifocal eosinophilic granuloma (histiocytosis X) appears not to involve the gut although the common bile duct may be affected [109]. On the other hand most patients with the **hypereosinophilia syndrome** have gastrointestinal symptoms. This is a multisystem disorder, of which the principal features are endomyocardial fibrosis and thrombo-embolic disease [199].

Plasma cell infiltration

In **multiple myeloma** amyloid may be deposited in the gastrointestinal tract (p. 1104). The gut is also a site for the development of **plasmacytomas** which produce polypoid masses or obstructive lesions at any level from oesophagus to rectum. Twenty-five percent of plasmacytomas are part of a generalized myeloma [74].

Infiltration of the submucosa of the small intestine with sheets of round cells is seen in **alpha heavy chain disease** (see Chapter 47) which is a common form of lymphoma in countries of the eastern Mediterranean. **Gamma heavy chain disease** is a less well documented and presumably much more uncommon condition. The clone of plasmacytoid cells responsible for the excessive production of heavy chains may present as a tumour of the stomach [163].

Secondary malignant infiltration

The gastrointestinal tract is frequently involved by lymphomatous and leukaemic cells. In addition many non-gut epithelial cancers may involve the gastrointestinal tract mainly as serosal implants [2]. Infiltrating masses occur most frequently in association with cancer of the breast, cancer of the bronchus and malignant melanoma. These tumours may cause pain, bleeding, obstruction and perforation of the intestine [115].

Cardiorespiratory disorders

Patients with serious cardiorespiratory disorders, especially those with right-sided failure (constrictive pericarditis, tricuspid incompetence or cor pulmonale), frequently have impaired gastrointestinal function. Organs are under-perfused, often with poorly oxygenated blood. The central venous pressure is elevated causing congestion of the liver and, in extreme cases, ascites. Even without ascites there is frequently generalized fluid retention and marked hypoproteinaemia. Tissues including the gut are not only poorly perfused but also waterlogged. As a result appetite is often markedly depressed and digestive-absorptive function impaired. In severe cases this leads to cardiac cachexia [89, 167].

The congested liver and the waterlogged splanchnic circulation provide an excessive flow of lymph. In some cases this flow is reduced because the raised central venous pressure causes a functional obstruction of the thoracic duct. The lymphatics distend and the increased pressure may then be transmitted to the lacteals. This causes lymphangiectasia and the loss of protein and lymphocytes into the gut [72, 120].

Stress ulceration is common in patients with cardiorespiratory failure undergoing intensive care and may cause life-threatening haemorrhage [83]. The incidence of stress ulceration is reduced by giving prophylactic antacids or H_2-receptor antagonists.

Non-occlusive intestinal infarction occurs in the elderly with severe low output cardiac failure especially after vigorous treatment with digoxin, diuretics and vaso-constrictor drugs. In all patients with severe cardiorespiratory disease it is important to try to maintain the supply of oxygen to the tissues. In this context it is necessary to remember the possible adverse effects of vaso-constrictor agents (given to maintain the blood pressure) and of intravenous glucose leading to hypophosphataemia, which in turn may enhance infection by depressing polymorph function and impairing the delivery of oxygen to the tissues by shifting the oxyhaemoglobin dissociation curve [26].

The commonly quoted association between chronic obstructive airways disease and peptic ulceration is not very marked and smoking may be the common factor [195].

Neuromuscular disorders

Disorders of the central nervous system

Damage of the motor pathways to the pharynx, oesophagus and stomach may lead to dysphagia and gastric atony. In practice dysphagia is the most significant symptom in a range of disorders which include cerebro-vascular insufficiency, pseudobulbar palsy and motor neurone disease, syringo-bulbia, bulbar polio and disseminated sclerosis. The dysphagia may relate to oro-pharyngeal dyscoordination or to failure of relaxation of the oesophageal sphincter. Various abnormal swallowing patterns may be recognized cine-radiographically [62, 84, 175, 191]. In some instances crico-pharyngeal myotomy may be of value in relieving symptoms [125, 160].

Parkinson's disease

This can cause dysphagia as a result of tongue tremor and difficulties in initiating swallowing. Sphincter disturbances have also been described [84, 191].

Peripheral neuropathy

Damage to the pharyngeal nerves may occur following a variety of toxic stimuli of which the most important is alcohol [228].

Swallowing disorders may also occur in diabetic neuropathy (p. 1109).

Damage to the sacral nerves may cause not only loss of perianal sensation but also faecal incontinence if the autonomic component is involved.

Myasthenia gravis

Dysphagia is a common presenting complaint in myasthenia. With cine-radiology one may see the characteristic ballooning of the pharynx that occurs with muscle fatigue [62, 162, 191].

Autonomic nervous system

In *Herpes zoster* affecting the sacral nerve roots sphincter disturbances can lead to incontinence through damage to the autonomic nerve supply to the bladder and rectum [106].

After **spinal cord injury** faecal impaction is the major problem [202].

Familial autonomia (Riley-Day syndrome) is a rare disease in which aspiration pneumonia secondary to swallowing disorders is the commonest cause of death [12, 138].

Autonomic function is also compromised by diseases that affect the myenteric plexus. These include **Chagas' disease**, which causes oesophageal dysfunction and dilatation [20], and those forms of **intestinal pseudo-obstruction** that are related to myenteric plexus nerve damage either separately or as part of a generalized neurological disorder [14, 184, 185, 196].

Primary muscular diseases

Of the muscular dystrophies the rare **oculopharyngeal muscular dystrophy** is most commonly associated with dysphagia although this may also occur in patients with **dystrophia myotonica** [98, 154]. Abnormalities of smooth muscle may be found at autopsy in patients with **Duchenne dystrophy** but gastrointestinal symptoms are rare [100, 154].

In addition, some cases of intestinal pseudo-obstruction appear to be caused by a widespread disorder of intestinal smooth muscle [61, 186].

Stiffness of the pharyngeal muscles due to generalized muscle disease may also cause dysphagia in the **'stiff man' syndrome** [204] and **trichinosis** [101]. Inflammatory diseases of muscle causing dysphagia are considered elsewhere (p. 1114).

Endocrine disorders

This section is concerned with endocrine disorders in which the major hormonal effects are remote from the gastrointestinal tract. Disease due to disorders of the apud system are described in Chapter 39.

Diabetes mellitus

In patients with poorly-controlled diabetes dysphagia is not uncommon as a result of oral sepsis or oropharyngeal candidiasis. Cine-radiographic studies have demonstrated oesophageal motor abnormalities in most patients with diabetic neuropathy, although clinical symptoms are unusual [9, 94, 200]. The motor defect results in dilatation and tertiary contractions; the lower oesophageal sphincter appears to function normally.

Gastric complications include acute dilatation of the stomach, which may occur with ketoacidosis, and chronic atony in patients with insulin-dependent diabetes. The cause of the gastric atony is unclear although both vagal damage and disordered antral motor activity may contribute [9, 32, 175, 182]. Usually gastric atony is asymptomatic but it may sometimes cause symptoms that include vomiting and abdominal distension. Diabetic gastric stasis is associated with poor diabetic control, weight loss and the formation of bezoars [131]. Treatment with metoclopramide is of proven value [197], but surgical procedures rarely give permanent relief of symptoms.

There are data to show that diabetics are more liable to gastric atrophy and pernicious anaemia [6, 102], but most diabetics have normal maximal acid production [97]. There is some dispute concerning the incidence of peptic ulcers in diabetics, but overall this is much the same as that of the general population—although duodenal ulcer may be less common because of vagal denervation and atrophic gastritis [9].

A small minority of diabetics suffer from chronic diarrhoea. Often it is particularly troublesome at night. It almost invariably occurs in the presence of evidence of a widespread neuropathy [136] and may be associated with steatorrhoea. It is usually assumed to occur as a result of motility disturbances although the precise site of the lesion has not been defined [9]. Other factors may contribute—small bowel contamination occurs [182] and coincident coeliac disease is described [217]. Furthermore there may be differences in gallbladder function and bile composition [71, 151], and coincident pancreatic insufficiency. It is important to recognize and treat associated disorders but most patients with this unpleasant disorder can be helped only by simple symptomatic treatment and improved control of blood sugar levels.

Constipation is also common in patients with diabetes and may be due to an impaired gastrocolic reflex [16].

Thyroid disorders

Sub-clinical gastritis and dysphagia have been reported in **thyrotoxicosis** [147, 148] but diarrhoea is the only common symptom. It appears to be due to enhanced gastrointestinal motility. There is no evidence of malabsorption from the small intestine

[147]. Mild steatorrhoea has been described because of an increased consumption of fat secondary to hyperphagia [210].

In **myxoedema** constipation is common. Occasionally the condition presents as an acute ileus [1, 221]. In Hashimoto's disease atrophic gastritis and other autoimmune diseases may coexist with the thyroid disorder.

Medullary carcinoma of the thyroid is associated with a high volume watery diarrhoea in the absence of significant steatorrhoea. The mechanism is humoral because the diarrhoea improves with removal of the tumour. It is not certain which humoral agent is responsible, although calcitonin has been shown to affect fluid absorption in the distal small bowel [49, 104].

Parathyroid disorders

In **hyperparathyroidism** nausea, vomiting, constipation or diarrhoea have all been described as presenting features [69]. Peptic ulcer is also common particularly if the hyperparathyroidism is a manifestation of multiple endocrine neoplasia type 1, when it is associated with the development of gastrinoma. The symptoms associated with hyperparathyroidism are largely those of the hypercalcaemia, but the symptoms of peptic ulcer or pancreatitis may be superimposed.

Gastrointestinal symptoms are uncommon in **hypoparathyroidism** except in the congenital form in which widespread candidiasis can cause dysphagia. Steatorrhoea has also been described [128, 152, 166].

Adrenal disorders

In **Addison's disease** gastrointestinal complaints are common and include nausea, vomiting and diarrhoea. Gastroenteritis may be erroneously diagnosed and, if the patient has abdominal pain, it may be sufficiently severe to mimic an acute abdomen [102].

Patients with **phaeochromocytoma** may develop abdominal pain during a hypertensive crisis [76, 150] and constipation, diarrhoea, nausea and vomiting or gastrointestinal bleeding may occur [99]. Ileus caused by autonomic inhibition and symptoms of intestinal ischaemia as a result of splanchnic vaso-constriction are also described [50, 177].

Renal disorders

Gastrointestinal symptoms are common in patients with **uraemia**. Nausea and vomiting invariably complicate severe uraemia and are relieved by dialysis. Dysphagia results from the associated stomatitis, which in advanced cases leads to xerostomia [105]; parotitis is common in these circumstances. Gastrointestinal bleeding is common in unrelieved uraemia. Peptic ulceration, gastric erosions and mucosal petechiae are frequent endoscopic findings. Clotting defects, hyperparathyroidism and hyperchlorhydria due to hypergastrinaemia are possible contributory factors [203].

In the small intestine, duodenal polyposis secondary to Brunner's gland hypertrophy [164, 232], bacterial overgrowth [149] and alterations in the concentrations of intra-luminal bile acids [75] are described. Diarrhoea may herald the onset of uraemic enterocolitis secondary to poor mucosal perfusion [10]. Ileus and intestinal obstruction or perforation have also been reported [27, 48, 178].

Uraemic colitis is probably not a distinct entity but there is an increased incidence of non-specific (stercoral) ulceration and of perforation of diverticula [27, 182]. Colonic intussusception has been described [231]. Pancreatitis also occurs more commonly than would be expected, although this may be missed during life [11].

Kidney transplantation does not eliminate the risk of gastrointestinal complications in association with chronic renal disease. Bleeding from peptic ulcer is common [78] and in some centres prophylactic vagotomy and drainage procedures were performed to avoid this complication [79, 129] before the widespread use of prophylactic H_2-blockade. Small bowel perforations, intestinal bleeding and malabsorption have all been described [78, 146]. Suppression of immunity also leads to an increased risk of Kaposi's sarcoma which may involve the gut and thereby provide another cause of gastrointestinal bleeding [82]. Patients with a renal transplant suffer acute abdominal catastrophes more often than control subjects—the causes include ruptured sigmoid diverticula, acute pancreatitis and hyperinfestation with *Strongyloides stercoralis* [146].

Metabolic disorders

In **Wolman's disease** and **cholesterol ester storage disease** there is a deficiency of acid lipase. Cholesterol esters accumulate throughout the body including the gut. Wolman's disease is the more severe form. Patients often present with vomiting and diarrhoea and do not survive beyond infancy. In patients with cholesterol ester storage disease the intestine is also involved, but gastrointestinal symptoms are unusual—abdominal pain and gastrointestinal bleeding have, however, been described [8].

Esterified cholesterol also accumulates in macrophages in the gastrointestinal tract, lymph nodes and liver of patients with **Tangier disease** (familial high density lipoprotein deficiency). Apolipoprotein A levels are extremely low possibly because of abnormal metabolism of chylomicra [73]. Patients suffer diarrhoea and peripheral neuropathy. The liver and spleen enlarge and the tonsils are streaked with yellow deposits of cholesterol.

Triglyceride droplets accumulate in the intestinal mucosa of patients with **abetali-**poproteinaemia and in **homozygous hypobetalipoproteinaemia**. In abetalipoproteinaemia the absence of apolipoprotein B is associated with acanthocytic erythrocytes, atypical retinitis pigmentosa, ataxia, and mild steatorrhoea (p. 1177).

Hyperlipoproteinaemia may also be associated with abdominal symptoms. In familial hyperchylomicronaemia (type I hyperlipidaemia) patients may suffer recurrent febrile episodes with abdominal pain, peritonitis or pancreatitis. Rather similar attacks may also occur with hyperbetalipoproteinaemia (type IV hyperlipidaemia) and in this condition there is an increased incidence of gallstones and cholecystitis.

In **Fabry's disease** (alpha-galactosidase A deficiency) glycolipid metabolism is disordered causing deposits of ceramide trihexosides in tissues. This leads to vascular damage with characteristic angiokeratoma and associated dysfunction of renal, pulmonary, cardiovascular, central nervous and gastrointestinal systems. Episodic diarrhoea occurs and small bowel perforation has also been described [29]. Involvement of autonomic ganglion cells may impair gastrointestinal motility and allow bacterial overgrowth in the small intestine [65, 155].

In **systemic mastocytosis** (and basophilic granulocytic leukaemia) hyperchlorhydria may cause peptic ulceration and probably accounts, at least in part, for the accompanying diarrhoea [5, 90, 158]. Diarrhoea has also been explained on the basis of coexistent coeliac disease [188]. There are data to suggest that high tissue levels of histamine are responsible for the gastrointestinal symptoms since hyper-histaminaemia is not invariable [5].

In **idiopathic recurrent urticaria** gastric acid secretion may also increase during an attack [123] but the abdominal pain and diarrhoea which sometimes occur are believed to be due to urticarial lesions of the intestinal mucosa. There is also an increased incidence of gallbladder disease and curiously the tendency to urticate may disappear after cholecystectomy [30].

Familial polyserositis (**familial mediterranean fever**) is an inherited disease which is believed to have a metabolic basis. Abdominal pain frequently occurs as a manifestation of episodic peritonitis [190]. The condition is not confined to families of Mediterranean stock and has been described in the United Kingdom [226].

Alcoholism may conveniently be considered in the context of the metabolic diseases. Alcohol has widespread effects on gastrointestinal function. It increases the incidence of oesophagitis, dysphagia due to oesophageal myoneuropathy and also carcinoma of the oesophagus [213, 225, 228]. Gastritis is common and the resulting nausea and vomiting are often presenting features of the disease [214]. Weight loss and specific nutritional deficiencies in the alcoholic are not caused solely by an inadequate diet. Malabsorption also occurs [211]. This may be related in part to the effects of folate deficiency but alcohol also has a direct toxic action on the small intestine [80, 179]. Ultrastructural abnormalities are described [179] and intestinal permeability is increased [23].

Iron overload from whatever cause (haemochromatosis, transfusional haemosiderosis and even excess intake of iron) predisposes to infection with *Yersinia enterocolitica*. Systemic Yersiniosis should be suspected in patients who develop signs of septicaemia [41, 174].

Rheumatological disorders

Gastrointestinal disease is common in patients with rheumatological disorders. The commonly used drugs have important side-effects. Corticosteroids are associated with peptic ulceration, pancreatitis and an increased risk of infection. Non-steroidal anti-inflammatory agents damage the gastroduodenal mucosa, alter intestinal permeability and occasionally cause diarrhoea. Gold by injection may predispose to entero-colitis [223] and by mouth almost invariably causes diarrhoea [18].

In some rheumatological conditions the underlying pathological process also has an effect on the gastrointestinal tract. Often this is the result of an associated vasculitis (as in rheumatoid disease and systemic lupus) but there may be direct involvement of submucosal tissues as in scleroderma and dermatomyositis. Finally, long-continued inflammation may cause amyloidosis (p. 1104).

Systemic lupus erythematosus

Gastrointestinal symptoms are common in systemic lupus. Anorexia and weight loss affect more than 50% of patients with active disease. Polyserositis is a well-recognized feature. Peritoneal involvement may cause abdominal pain and is occasionally associated with an exudate of protein-rich fluid. In fact systemic lupus can present with ascites. More often, there is focal peritonitis with perihepatitis or perisplenitis.

Difficulty in swallowing, diarrhoea, vomiting and gastrointestinal bleeding are more common features and may occur in about one-third of patients with lupus although the reported incidence is very variable [54, 92]. Disorders of motility may occur in the oesophagus (causing dysphagia), stomach (causing outlet obstruction), and small intestine (causing pseudo-obstruction).

Most of the serious complications are related to lupus vasculitis affecting the gut, the pancreas or the liver. Vasculitis in the intestine may cause submucosal bleeding (pseudotumours) or ischaemic necrosis. Ulcers present with bleeding [54] or occasionally perforate especially in the colon [232]. Lymphadenopathy may cause intussusception [87] and venular inflammation may lead to malabsorption [17] with or without protein-losing enteropathy [220].

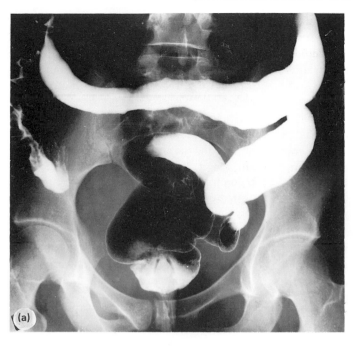

(a)

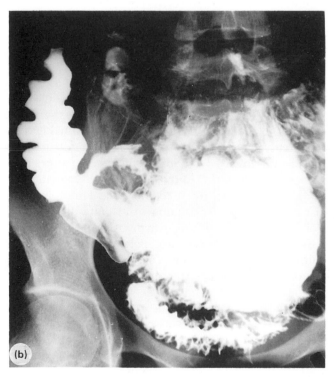

(b)

Fig. 74.3. Gold enterocolitis. Patient presented with severe diarrhoea 6 weeks after starting treatment with Myocrisin (total dose 86 mg). (a), barium enema: pan colitis with effacement of mucosa and loss of haustral folds; (b), barium follow-through: abnormal ileal mucosa with possible ulceration. The patient remained very ill and apparently unresponsive to treatment for 6 weeks. She then made a spontaneous and complete recovery.

The management of abdominal pain in systemic lupus requires sound clinical judgement. Long-continued mild to moderate pain is more likely to be due to intercurrent disease or to the side-effects of drugs than to lupoid inflammation. Radiological studies may be useful and the value of isotope scans has yet to be fully evaluated. Active inflammatory disease, cutaneous vasculitis and positive radiological findings in the patient with lupus who has obscure abdominal pain will favour a diagnosis of lupus-related vasculitis affecting the splanchnic circulation. A short course of corticosteroids in high dosage may help resolve the problem. Decisions are more difficult in the patient with systemic lupus who develops an acute abdomen. Perforation of a viscus, intestinal necrosis and acute pancreatitis should be managed in a conventional manner. In the absence of positive indications of focal pathology it may be reasonable to give high doses of prednisolone (60–100 mg per day) and antibiotics. If the patient does not improve within 24 hours, it is probably best to advise an exploratory laparotomy [92].

Rheumatoid disease

Patients with rheumatoid disease often have gastrointestinal symptoms. Usually these are mild but because they are often drug-related they may compromise medical management.

Some weight loss is common and this may be due in part to difficulties in eating and swallowing. Inflammation of the tempero-mandibular joint occurs in 85% of severely affected patients and impairment in oesophageal motility may be equally common although often asymptomatic [205]. Peptic ulceration occurs at some stage in up to 30% of patients with rheumatoid disease undergoing active treatment. Men and women are affected equally and the usual complications may occur

(see Chapter 21). Antacids, H_2-receptor antagonists and mucosal protective agents are of considerable help in managing the patient who develops gastroduodenal symptoms during treatment for rheumatoid arthritis.

Rheumatoid disease affects tissues other than joints. Vasculitis is the common denominator. In the intestine this may cause pathology similar to that described for systemic lupus. It occurs especially in patients with long-standing sero-positive arthropathy who have well developed subcutaneous nodules [21, 81]. The pathology and associated symptoms are usually mild and subacute. Rarely segmental or diffuse necrosis of the intestine occurs usually with fatal consequences [212]. As with systemic lupus, malabsorption and protein-losing enteropathy have been described but this is rarely of much clinical importance [168].

Dermatomyositis (Polymyositis)

Polymyositis with or without skin involvement is a rare disease. It may be associated with a generalized vasculitis and collagen changes similar to those seen in scleroderma. Widespread degeneration of Type I and Type II muscle fibres with hyalinization is the primary pathological process. Later features include muscle atrophy, fibrosis and ectopic calcification. The skin may be involved and in chronic cases changes may be similar to those seen in scleroderma. An underlying malignancy is found in 25% cases of dermatomyositis but only rarely in uncomplicated polymyositis [31].

Patients with polymyositis commonly present with a progressive proximal muscle weakness. The involvement of facial, pharyngeal and upper oesophageal muscles causing difficulties in mastication and in swallowing is associated with a poor prognosis [165]. In such patients weight loss and aspiration pneumonitis are important features of the disease. Most patients respond to treatment with corticosteroids. The inflammatory process resolves to a variable degree and usually becomes quiescent within months although may persist for two to three years. Abnormalities of the distal oesophagus are common in patients who respond slowly to treatment [95]. In many cases these abnormalities occur in the absence of proximal oesophageal dysfunction and are functionally similar to the changes occurring in systemic sclerosis. In most cases coming to necropsy there is no evidence of smooth muscle atrophy nor of fibrosis and the functional disturbance is ascribed to a neuronal disorder [145].

The stomach and small intestine may also be affected [95]. Hypomotility is the principal feature leading to delayed emptying of the stomach and dilatation of the small intestine with the formation of pseudo diverticula [127]. Intestinal perforation is a serious complication. This may occur insidiously causing submucosal pneumatosis or a chronic pneumo-peritoneum [153]. Involvement of the colon also causes dilatation and sacculation. The anal sphincter may be damaged with selective involvement of the external component which comprises striated muscle. As a result patients suffer post-prandial discomfort with abdominal distension and constipation with overflow.

The vasculitis which may be associated with polymyositis can affect the gastrointestinal tract. Mucosal ulceration and haemorrhage or focal ischaemic necrosis are serious complications [227].

Systemic sclerosis (scleroderma)

In primary systemic sclerosis fibrous connective tissue may replace smooth muscle in the gut. The oesophagus is affected most commonly (80%) (see Chapter 10), the stomach only occasionally; the duodenum in 50% [24] and the colon rather rarely. Extensive gut involvement may occur with minimal changes in the skin.

Patients often have difficulty in eating. The skin around the mouth becomes tight, the buccal mucosa thins and the tongue papillae may atrophy. The loss of taste sensation, the difficulties with mastication and the dysphagia associated with oesophageal involvement leads to a reduced intake of food. Many patients become markedly wasted.

Involvement of the small intestine increases the patient's misery and exacerbates the tendency to malnutrition. Transit time through the gut is markedly delayed with abdominal bloating, nausea and occasional vomiting. Radiologically prominent jejunal valvulae conniventes are characteristic of this condition. Later pseudo-diverticula may form. In severely affected patients the whole small intestine becomes distended and presents the picture of 'pseudo-obstruction'. Malabsorption is common (see Chapter 44). In many cases it is exacerbated by bacterial overgrowth which can be controlled by orally administered antibiotics.

Damage to the colon appears to be found only in patients with widespread involvement of gut. The haustral pattern disappears and the colon dilates with formation of saccules. The patient becomes severely constipated with impaction which may lead to overflow diarrhoea or large bowel obstruction. Pneumatosis cystoides is a rare complication (see Chapter 73). The smooth muscle component of the anal sphincter may also be damaged. As a result the internal sphincter fails to relax with distension of the rectum. This exacerbates the constipation.

Vasculitis is common in systemic sclerosis. Thus the gastrointestinal mucosa usually appears normal apart from an increase of inflammatory cells. Ulceration and bleeding rarely occur except in association with inspissation and impaction of intestinal contents to form faecoliths.

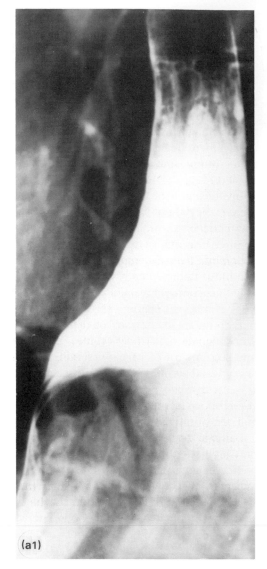

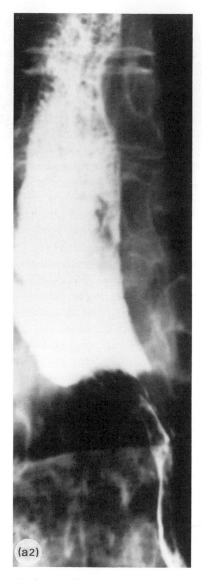

Fig. 74.4. Systemic sclerosis. (a), oesophagus may simulate achalasia (1) but usually does not show a tapering tail (2). These are radiographs taken at the same examination; (b), small intestine shows dilated loops often with prominent folds ('wire spring' effect); (c), large intestine has largely lost its haustra and may show wide-necked pseudo-diverticula.

Sjögren's syndrome

This condition is characterized by dry eyes (keratoconjunctivitis sicca) and dry mouth (xerostomia) in association with rheumatoid disease, systemic lupus erythematosus, primary biliary cirrhosis and other disorders with an autoimmune component. Affected tissues (especially the lacrimal gland, salivary glands and pancreas) are infiltrated with lymphocytes.

The excessive dryness of the eyes, the mouth and the pharynx is the major cause of discomfort suffered by those affected.

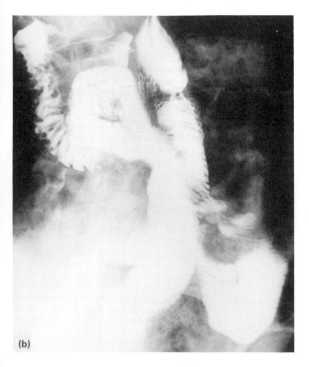

(b)

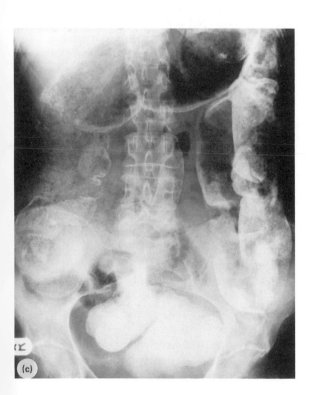

(c)

Associated disorders include sterile and suppurative parotitis [44], dysphagia [171], atrophic gastritis with lymphocyte infiltrates [208] and pancreatic dysfunction [53].

Polyarteritis nodosa and associated disorders

Polyarteritis is an inflammatory disorder of medium- and small-sized blood vessels with focal fibrinoid necrosis. Abdominal symptoms are prominent in about 50% of cases. Nausea, vomiting, abdominal pain, weight loss and diarrhoea are common whereas the more dramatic symptoms of steatorrhoea, focal infarction of the intestine, acute cholecystitis, haemorrhagic pancreatitis, ulcerative enterocolitis and intraperitoneal haemorrhage occur rarely [33, 130]. In abdominal polyarteritis nodosa a chronic wasting syndrome resembling diffuse malignancy has been described [34].

Polyarteritis appears to be one of a cluster of disorders characterized by primary inflammation of vessels, eosinophilia and granulomatous changes affecting tissues. The hypereosinophilic syndrome may also involve the gastrointestinal tract [20] whereas Wegener's granulomatosis (midline granuloma) only rarely affects the gut with an associated necrotizing arteritis [45].

Behçet's syndrome

Behçet's syndrome is an uncommon, poorly understood, multi-system disorder. The pathological changes are non-specific although vasculitis and venous thrombosis are prominent features. There are interesting associations with several HLA antigens suggesting a genetic susceptibility. Recently parts of the Herpes virus genome have been found transcribed in peripheral blood mononuclear cells [55]. Several immunological abnormalities (for example, circulating

Table 74.9. Diagnostic criteria for Behçet's syndrome.

U.S.A. [156]
   3 out of 6 criteria (including 2 out of 3*)

	Approx. incidence (%)
Aphthous stomatitis*	99
Genital ulcers*	80
Uveitis*	66
Dermal vasculitis	66
Arthritis	55
Meningo-encephalitis	22

Japan and Europe
   3 major or 2 major and 2 minor criteria

Japan [111]	*U.K.* [142]
Major: Aphthous stomatitis	Major: Aphthous ulceration
Genital ulceration	Genital ulceration
Ocular involvement	Eye lesion
Positive prick test	Skin lesion
Minor: Arthritis	Minor: Arthritis
Vasculitis	Thrombophlebitis
Intestinal ulceration	GI lesions
Neurological involvement	CNS lesions
Respiratory disease	Cardiovascular involvement
	Family history

---

* Aphthous ulceration and vulvitis in young women is usually self-limited and should not be labelled as Behçet's syndrome.

immune complexes and tissue specific antibodies) have also been described, but at present a pathogenetic role cannot be ascribed with certainty to any of these findings.

The diagnosis of Behçet's syndrome remains clinical. The key features are orogenital ulceration, ocular inflammation and skin lesions (major criteria) together with a wide range of other disorders (minor criteria). This makes classification difficult (Table 74.9). The disorder is most common in Japan and the Middle East. In these areas HLA-B5 (BW51 split of B5) increases the relative risk thirteen-fold. In the West the prevalence is about 0.5 per 100,000 [39, 156]. HLA-B5 is associated only with the ocular form of the disease; DR7 with ocular and neurological types; and B12 and/or DR2 with muco-cutaneous or arthritic types [126]. Recurrent oral ulceration is usually the first symptom. Diagnosis at this stage is impossible because in control studies the overall prevalence of oral ulcers is about 10%. Treatment of major ulceration is unsatisfactory although topical steroids used early in the course of the disease together with careful oral and dental hygiene may be helpful (see Chapter 7).

Dysphagia occurs if aphthous ulcers extend to the oesophagus. Rarely stricture or perforation of the oesophagus may occur and there is a single case report of ganglion cell degeneration leading to achalasia [7].

In the Western world and Near East intestinal involvement in Behçet's syndrome is rare, whereas in Japan it is common with at least 50% of patients complaining of abdominal symptoms [13]. In a detailed study from Guy's Hospital 19/69 patients with Behçet's syndrome had gastrointestinal symptoms mostly not severe and only one had an ulcer in the small intestine [192]. No gastrointestinal involvement was found in 41 Israeli patients with Behçet's syndrome [37].

In contrast Japanese patients suffer attacks of anorexia, nausea and vomiting, abdominal pain and diarrhoea. Barium studies reveal dilated loops of intestine sometimes with thickened folds or ulcers [161]. Behçet's ulcers may occur from oesophagus to rectum. In one study of over 100 cases coming to surgery ulcers were distributed as follows—stomach 1%, duodenum 2%, small intestine (excluding terminal ileum) 4%, terminal ileum 45%, ileo-caecal region 35%, caecum 10%, colon 3%. Patients coming to surgery usually have long-standing Behçet's syndrome. Commonly there is an area of marked tenderness in the right iliac fossa associated with a mass in 20% and severe bleeding in 20%. Japanese surgeons recommend a wide resection (at least 100 cm of intestine) to try to prevent recurrent ulceration which in one series was as high as 65% over six months [111].

The pathology of the intestinal Behçet's syndrome is unexciting. There is deep ulceration with non-specific inflammation. Granulomas are not seen. Perivascular inflammation is usual but this may be secondary to the ulceration and not a primary disorder. The distinctive Japanese enteropathy has been described on several occasions in Europe and the U.S.A. but is distinctly uncommon. Rather more often a gastrointestinal disorder indistinguishable from non-specific inflammatory bowel disease is seen in association with Behçet's syndrome [39, 157].

The involvement of major blood vessels in Behçet's syndrome may also cause intra-abdominal pathology including that due to arterial or venous occlusion in the splanchnic circulation. The Budd-Chiari syndrome has also been described [134].

Dermatological disorders

Several gastrointestinal disorders have dermatological manifestations such as the acanthosis nigricans of gastrointestinal malignancies; the pigmentation and papillomata associated with the polyposis syndromes; the dysplastic changes of hair, skin and nails which occur in association with malnutrition secondary to severe malabsorption; and the skin lesions which may occur during the course of inflammatory bowel disease. These disorders and their associations are discussed elsewhere. Here we are concerned with the gastrointestinal complications of disorders which are primarily dermatological.

The mouth and pharynx are affected in **pemphigus, pemphigoid** and **lichen planus** [139]. More dramatic lesions occur with **Stevens-Johnson syndrome** which includes severe buccal ulceration and which often allows candida to colonize the upper gastrointestinal tract. Oesophageal lesions also occur in **epidermolysis bullosa**. These may lead to stricture formation and severe dysphagia.

Gastrointestinal bleeding is common in patients with **hereditary haemorrhagic telangiectasia** (Osler-Rendu-Weber disease) but usually is not troublesome until after the age of 40 years. Gastrointestinal bleeding may also complicate **blue rubber** bleb naevi [64], **pseudo xanthoma elasticum** [42] and the **Ehlers-Danlos syndrome.** Ehlers-Danlos syndrome is associated with intestinal diverticulosis and perforation of the small intestine may occur [19].

Gastrointestinal bleeding, small bowel obstruction and perforation have also been described in patients with **disseminated neurofibromatosis** [137]. Abdominal pain may occur in **urticaria** in a manner analogous to that in hereditary angioedema.

A contemporary problem is gastrointestinal bleeding from systemic **Kaposi's sarcoma**—whereas this lesion is usually superficial and circumscribed, in the African and the immunosuppressed it may disseminate widely and death from gastrointestinal haemorrhage can occur [68, 82,

209]. Disseminated Kaposi's sarcoma is now being increasingly recognized in homosexual patients with the acquired immune deficiency syndrome [66] (see Chapter 57).

Malabsorption syndromes can also occur in association with skin diseases. The association of **dermatitis herpetiformis** and **coeliac disease** is well recognized and this in turn renders the patient at increased risk of gastrointestinal malignancies [139]. More controversial is the entity of 'dermatogenic enteropathy'—the association of severe skin diseases with alterations in small intestinal function in the absence of any significant alterations in villous architecture [140]. The precise cause of the malabsorption, which has been documented as steatorrhoea, is not known but it is well documented in some cases of **severe psoriasis** and **eczema,** and it resolves with the resolution of the skin disease [141].

Haematological disorders

Leukaemia

Leukaemic involvement of the gastrointestinal tract occurs in 5–10% of untreated patients. It used to be seen most commonly in chronic lymphatic leukaemia affecting especially the stomach and ileum. Any part of the gastrointestinal tract could be involved although the oesophagus was nearly always spared. Infiltration of the mucosa led to the development of plaques or polypoid masses which could ulcerate and bleed, or even intussuscept. Nevertheless in the period before effective cytotoxic therapy most cases of leukaemia were free of gastrointestinal symptoms and diarrhoea was uncommon.

Today few patients escape gastrointestinal disease. The use of cytotoxic drugs, steroids and antibiotics has brought a wide range of gastrointestinal lesions including oesophageal moniliasis, peptic ulceration, haemorrhagic necrosis of the intestine, entero-colitis and severe anorectal lesions. Moreover prolongation of life has allowed infiltration of the gastrointestinal tract in a much higher percentage of patients than formerly. This development may occur during apparent remission of the leukaemic process. An acute abdomen may occur in 5–10% of leukaemic patients with a wide range of underlying pathologies—appendicitis, caecitis, intussusception, intestinal obstruction, perforation of the intestine, pancreatitis and intra-abdominal abscesses [58]. Graft-versus-host disease following bone marrow transplantation causes profound gastrointestinal symptoms with mouth ulceration, abdominal pain and diarrhoea [133, 191].

The mouth

Patients with acute leukaemia may present with oral lesions especially focal ulceration of the gums, palate and buccal surfaces and gingival hypertrophy with bleeding. Stomatitis is an almost universal concomitant of treatment with cytotoxic drugs and may be associated with secondary bacterial or fungal infection.

The oesophagus

Moniliasis occurs in many patients undergoing treatment for acute leukaemia. It causes dysphagia, substernal pain and occasionally may completely obstruct the oesophagus. Treatment with nystatin is usually effective. Systemic moniliasis may occur and is treated with amphotericin B.

The stomach

Lesions of the stomach (gastritis and peptic ulceration) are often secondary to treatment but leukaemic infiltrates may occur. They simulate gastric cancer or diffuse polyposis and the diagnosis is made by endoscopic biopsy.

The intestine

Most patients undergoing treatment for leukaemia will suffer diarrhoea. In many instances this appears to be no more than a simple enteritis induced by a combination of the effects of cytotoxic drugs [193] and antibiotics [15]. All patients should be carefully studied because of the wide spectrum of pathology. Leukaemic infiltration may be localized causing bleeding, obstruction or perforation. More rarely, it is sufficiently diffuse to cause protein-losing enteropathy [43]. In the immunosuppressed patient steatorrhoea may occur as a result of bacterial overgrowth in the small intestine and in the patient with severe agranulocytosis necrotizing colitis is a fairly common complication.

It is important to examine stools repeatedly for pathogenic organisms and especially to recognize *Clostridium difficile* and its enterotoxin. Pseudo-membranous colitis is the most common disorder of the colon and usually responds well to treatment with vancomycin or metronidazole. Occasionally patients develop a diffuse ischaemic colitis. They do poorly and may have to face the hazard of proctocolectomy. A third colitic disorder occurs only in the presence of neutropaenia and involves primarily the right side of the colon where there are localized erosions with bacterial invasion. This disorder may be due to *Clostridium septicum* which has been cultured from blood and demonstrated locally in the ulcers [113].

Ano-rectal lesions

Perianal infiltration with the development of nodular lesions is an uncommon manifestation of leukaemia. On the other hand, abscess formation, ulceration and proctitis may be troublesome features during the course of active treatment.

Gastrointestinal bleeding

Patients with leukaemia frequently bleed. Lesions in the stomach and colon are well characterized and have already been described. Haemorrhagic necrosis of the small intestine is less well recognized. Three forms have been described: thrombocytopenia with a haemorrhagic diathesis and diffuse mucosal bleeding may occur without evidence of ulceration; in other patients diffuse haemorrhage is associated with superficial erosions and probable bacterial or fungal invasion; finally, bleeding may occur from overt ulceration which is often multifocal, and may perforate the wall of the intestine. It is suggested that some ulcers are caused by microthrombi which form in the presence of thrombocytosis [112].

Bleeding disorders and the gastrointestinal tract

Many bleeding disorders may cause gastrointestinal disease including the thrombocytopenic purpuras, the haemophiliac disorders, anticoagulant therapy and the leukaemias. In the absence of intestinal ulceration or mucosal erosion, bleeding occurs primarily into the wall of the intestine or into retroperitoneal tissues. Submucosal bleeding causes acute abdominal pain and the lesions may be recognized radiologically. Surgery should be avoided as the lesions normally regress with control of the bleeding tendency and simple conservative measures. Retroperitoneal haematomas cause severe pain often associated with an intestinal ileus. The diagnosis can be confirmed by CT scanning.

If a patient with a bleeding disorder bleeds heavily into the lumen of the intestine, there is nearly always associated mucosal pathology. This may be caused

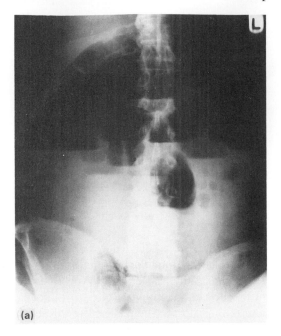

(a)

Fig. 74.5. Intestinal ileus secondary to retroperitoneal bleeding following trauma to right kidney. (a), erect, (b), supine.

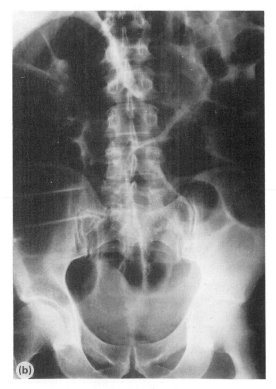

(b)

by microvascular occlusion, as occurs in thrombotic thrombocytopenic purpura and in the thrombocytosis of some myeloproliferative disorders.

The **haemolytic-uraemic syndrome** occurs most commonly in children. Anaemia, thrombocytopenia and renal failure dominate the clinical picture. But most cases present with what appears to be an entero-colitis and in the later phases of the disorder ischaemic bowel disease may provide an added complication [224]. The syndrome merges with that of **thrombotic thrombocytopenia purpura**. This is a serious but uncommon disorder of young adults characteristically presenting with bleeding, haemolysis, renal failure and variable neurological signs. Abdominal pain occurs in about 10% of cases and bleeding into the gut is common. It is postulated that patients with both illnesses lack a plasma factor needed to stimulate the production of PGI_2 (prostacyclin) which inhibits the aggregation of platelets [85, 172]. The infusion of plasma, with or without exchange transfusion, appears to provide effective treatment for many patients with this serious condition.

References

1 ABBASI AA, DOUGLASS RC, BISSELL GV, CHEN Y. Myxedema ileus. *JAMA* 1975;**234**:181–183.

2 ABRAMS HL, SPIRO R, GOLDSTEIN N. Metastases in carcinoma: analysis of 1000 autopsied cases. *Cancer* 1950;**3**:74–85.

3 AMENT ME, OCHS HD. Gastro-intestinal manifestations of chronic granulomatous disease. *N Engl J Med* 1973;**288**:382–387.

4 AMENT ME, OCHS HD, DAVIS SD. Structure and function of the gastro-intestinal tract in primary immunodeficiency syndromes: a study of 39 patients. *Medicine* 1973;**52**:227–248.

5 AMMAN RW, VETTER D, DEYHLE P, TSCHEN H, SULSER H, SCHMID M. Gastro-intestinal involvement in systemic mastocytosis. *Gut* 1976;**17**:107–112.

6 ANGERVALL L, DOTERALL G, LEHMANN KE. The gastric mucosa in diabetes mellitus: functional and histopathological study. *Acta Med Scand* 1961;**169**:339–349.

7 ARMA S, HABIBULLA KS, PRICE JJ. Dysphagia in Behçet's syndrome. *Thorax* 1971;**26**:155–158.

8 ASSMANN G, FREDRICKSON DS. Acid lipase deficiency: Wolman's disease and cholesterol ester storage disease. In: Stanbury JB, Wyngaarden JB, Fredrickson DS, Goldstein JL, Brown MS, eds. *The metabolic basis of inherited disease.* 5th ed. New York: McGraw-Hill, 1983:803–819.

9 ATKINSON M, HOSKING DJ. Gastro-intestinal complications of diabetes mellitus. *Clin Gastroenterol* 1983;**12**(3):633–650.

10 AUBIA J, LLOVERAS J, MUNNÉ A, *et al.* Ischemic colitis in chronic uremia. *Nephron* 1981;**29**:146–150.

11 AVVAM MM. High prevalence of pancreatic disease in chronic renal failure. *Nephron* 1977;**18**:68–71.

12 AXELROD FB, ABULARRAGE JJ. Familial dysautonoma: a prospective study of survival. *J Pediatr* 1982;**101**:234–236.

13 BABA S, MARUTA M, ANDO K, TATSUO T, ENDO I. Intestinal Behçet's disease: report of five cases. *Dis Colon Rectum* 1976;**19**:428–440.

14 BANNISTER R, HOYES AD. Generalised smooth-muscle disease with defective muscarinic-receptor function. *Br Med J* 1981;**282**:1015–1018.

15 BARTLETT JG. Antibiotic-associated pseudomembranous colitis. *Rev Infect Dis* 1979;**1**:530–539.

16 BATTLE WM, SNAPE WJ, ALAVI A, COHEN S, BRAUNSTEIN S. Colonic dysfunction in diabetes mellitus. *Gastroenterology* 1980;**79**:1217–1221.

17 BAZINET P, MANN GA. Malabsorption in systemic lupus erythematosus. *Am J Dig Dis* 1971;**16**:460–466.

18 BEHRENS R, DEVEREAUX M, HAZLEMAN B, SZAZ K, CALVIN J, NEALE G. Investigation of Auranofin-induced diarrhoea. *Gut* 1986;**27**:59–65.

19 BEIGHTON P, HORAN F. Surgical aspects of the Ehler's-Danlos syndrome: a survey of 100 cases. *Br J Surg* 1969;**56**:255–259.

20 BETTARELLO A, PINOTTI HW. Oesophageal involvement in Chagas' disease. *Clin Gastroenterol* 1976;**5**:103–117.

21 BIENENSTOCK M, MINICK P, ROGOFF B. Mesenteric arteritis and intestinal infarction in rheumatic disease. *Arch Int Med* 1967;**119**:359–364.

22 BISCHEL MD, REESE T, ENGEL J. Spontaneous perforation of the colon in a haemodialysis patient. *Am J Gastroenterol* 1980;**74**:182–184.

23 BJARNASON I, WARD K, PETERS TJ. The leaky gut of alcoholism: possible route of entry for toxic compounds. *Lancet* 1984;**i**:179–181.

24 BLUESTONE R, MacMAHON M, DAWSON J. Systemic sclerosis and small bowel involvement. *Gut* 1969;**10**:185–191.

25 BLUM PM, HONG R, STIEHM ER. Spontaneous recovery of selective IgA deficiency. *Clin Pediatr* 1982;**21**:77–80.

26 BONE RC. Acute respiratory failure and chronic obstructive lung disease: recent advances. *Med Clin North Am* 1981;**65**:563–579.

27 BRANDT LJ, DAVIDOFF A, BERSTEIN LH, BIEMPICA L, RINDFLEISCH B, GOLDSTEIN ML. Small intestinal involvement in Waldenström's macro-globulinaemia. *Dig Dis Sci*, 1981;**26**:174–179.

28 BRAZIN SA, JOHNSON WT, ABRAMSON LJ. The acrodermatitis enteropathica-like syndrome. *Arch Dermatol* 1979;**115**:597–599.

29 BRYAN A, KNAUFT RF, BURNS WA. Small bowel perforation in Fabry's disease. *Ann Intern Med* 1977;**86**:315–316.

30 BUSHKELL LL. Chronic urticaria and gall bladder disease: clearing after cholecystectomy. *Arch Dermatol* 1979;**115**:638.

31 CALLE JP. Dermatomyositis and malignancy. *Clin Rheum Dis* 1982;**8**:369–381.

32 CAMPBELL IW, HEADING RC, TOTHILL P, BUIST TA, EWING DJ, CLARKE BF. Gastric emptying in diabetic autonomic nuropathy. *Gut* 1977;**18**:462–467.

33 CARRON DB, DOUGLAS AP. Steatorrhoea in vascular insufficiency of the small intestine. 5 cases of polyarteritis nodosum and allied disorders. *Q J Med* **34**:331–340.

34 CASE RECORDS OF THE MASSACHUSETTS GENERAL HOSPITAL. *N Engl J Med* 1979;**300**:243–251.

35 CASE RECORDS OF THE MASSACHUSETTS GENERAL HOSPITAL. Case 5. *N Engl J Med* 1980;**302**:336–344.

36 CELLO JP. Eosinophilic gastroenteritis—a complex disease entity *Am J Med* 1979;**67**:1097–1104.

37 CHAJEK T, FAINARU M. Behçet's disease: Report of 41 cases and a review of the literature. *Medicine* 1975;**54**:179–196.

38 CHAMBERLAIN MA. Behçet's in 32 patients in Yorkshire. *Ann Rheum Dis* 1977;**36**:491–499.

39 CHAMBERLAIN MA. Behçet's syndrome as seen in England. *Haematologica* 1980;**65**:384–389.

40 CHANDRA RK. Nutritional deficiency and susceptibility to infection. *Bull WHO* 1979;**57**:167–177.

41 CHIU HY, FLYNN DM, HOFFBRAND AV, POLITIS D. Infection with *Yersinia enterocolitica* in patients with iron overload. *Br Med J* 1986;**292**:97.

42 COCCO AE, GRAYER DI, WALKER BA, MARTIN LJ. The stomach in pseudo-xanthoma elasticum. *JAMA* 1969;**210**:2381–2382.

43 COCKINGTON RA. Leukemic infiltration of the gastro-intestinal tract. An unusual cause of protein-losing enteropathy. *Med J Aust* 1975;**1**:103–105.

44 COHEN M, BANKHURST AD. Infectious parotitis in Sjögren's syndrome: A case report and review of the literature. *J Rheumatol* 1979;**6**:185–188.

45 CONN P. Wegener's granulomatosis presenting with intestinal perforation. In Booth CC, Neale G, eds. *Disorders of the small intestine*. Oxford: Blackwell Scientific Publications, 1985:339–340.

46 COOK GC, LEE FD. The jejunum after Kwashiorkor. *Lancet* 1966;**ii**:1263–1267.

47 COUGHLIN GP, REINER RG, GRANT AK. Endoscopic diagnosis of amyloidosis. *Gastrointest Endosc* 1980;**26**:154–158.

48 COONEY DR. Small bowel obstruction and ileal perforation: complications of uremia. *J Indiana State Med Assoc* 1976;**69**:781–784.

49 COX TM, FAGAN EA, HILLYARD CJ, ALLISON DJ, CHADWICK VS. Role of calcitonin in diarrhoea associated with medullary carcinoma of the thyroid. *Gut* 1979;**20**:629–633.

50 CRUZ SR, COLWELL JA. Phaeochromocytoma and ileus. *JAMA* 1972;**219**:1050–1051.

51 DASTUR KJ, WARD JF. Amyloidoma of the stomach. *Gastrointest Radiol* 1980;**5**:17–21.

52 DOE WF, HAGEL AJ. Intestinal immunity and malabsorption. In: Sleisinger M, ed. *Clin Gastroenterol* 1983;**12**:415–435.

53 DREILING DA, SOTO JM. The pancreatic involvement in disseminated 'collagen' disorders. *Am J Gastroenterol* 1976;**66**:546–549.

54 DUBOIS FL, TUFFANELLI DL. Clinical manifestations of systemic lupus erythematosus. *JAMA* 1964;**190**:104–111.

55 EGLIN RP, LEHNER T, SUBAK-SHARPE JH. Detection of RNA complementary to Herpes-simplex virus in mononuclear cells from patients with Behçet's syndrome and recurrent oral ulcers. *Lancet* 1982;**ii**:1356–1361.

56 EK BO, HOLMLUND DE, SJÖDIN JG, STEEN LE. Enterostomy in patients with primary neuropathic amyloidosis. *Am J Gastroenterol* 1978;**70**:365–370.

57 ELMES ME, JONES JG. Ultrastructural changes in the small intestine of zinc-deficient rats. *J Pathol* 1980;**130**:37–43.

58 EVELBY PR. Management of the acute abdomen in children with leukemia. *Cancer* 1975;**35**:826–829.

59 FALCK HM, MAURY CP, TEPPO AM, WEGELIUS O. Correlation of persistently high serum amyloid A protein and C-reactive protein concentrations with rapid progression of secondary amyloidosis. *Br Med J* 1983;**286**:1391–1393.

60 FAUCI S. Acquired immunodeficiency syndrome (NIH Conference). *Ann Int Med* 1984;**100**:92–106.

61 FAULK DL, AMURAS S, GARDNER GD, MITROS FA, SUMMERS RW, CHRISTENSEN J. A familial visceral myopathy. *Ann Intern Med* 1978;**74**:922–931.

62 FISCHER RA, ELLISON GW, THAYER WR, SPIRO HM, GLASER GH. Esophageal motility in neuromuscular disorders. *Ann Intern Med* 1965;**63**:229–248.

63 FOROOZAN P, TRIER JS. Mucosa of the small intestine in pernicious anemia. *N Engl J Med* 1967;**277**:553–559.

64 FRETZIN DP, POTTER B. Blue rubber bleb nevus. *Arch Int Med* 1965;**116**:924–929.

65 FRIEDMAN LS, KIRKHAM SF, THISTLETHWAITE JR, PLATIKA D, KOLODNY EH, SCHUFFLER MD. Jejunal diverticulosis with perforation as a complication of Fabry's disease. *Gastroenterology* 1984;**86**:558–563.

66 FRIEDMAN-KIEN AE, LAUBENSTEIN IJ, RUBINSTEIN P, et al. Disseminated Kaposi's sarcoma in homosexual men. *Ann Intern Med* 1982;**96**:693–700.

67 GADEK JE, HOSCA SW, GELFORD JA, et al. Replacement therapy in hereditary angioedema. *N Engl J Med* 1980;**302**:542–546.

68 GANGE RW, WILSON-JONES E. Kaposi's sarcoma and immuno-suppressive therapy: an appraisal. *Clin Exp Dermatol* 1978;**3**:135–146.

69 GARDNER EC, HERSH T. Primary hyperparathyroidism and the gastro-intestinal tract. *South Med J* 1981;**74**:197–199.

70 GEDDES AM, ELLIS CJ. Infection in immunocompromised patients. *Q J Med* 1985;**216**:5–14.

71 GITELSON S. Gallbladder dysfunction in diabetes mellitus. The diabetic neurogenic gallbladder. *Diabetes* 1963;**12**:308–312.

72 GLEICH G. Cardiomyopathy, heart failure and protein-losing enteropathy. *Chest* 1973;**64**:417–418.

73 GLICKMAN RM, KILGORE A, KHORANA J. Chylomicron apoprotein localisation within rat intestinal epithelium: studies of normal and impaired lipid absorption. *J Lipid Res* 1978;**19**:260–268.

74 GOEGGEL-LAMPING C, KAHN SP. Gastrointestinal polyposis in multiple myeloma. *JAMA* 1978;**239**:178–182.

75 GORDON SJ, MILLER LJ, HAEFFNER LJ, KINSEY MD, KOWLESSAR OD. Abnormal intestinal bile acid dis-

tribution in azotemic man: a possible role in the pathogenesis of uremic diarrhea. *Gut* 1976;**17**:58–67.

76 GREATOREX RA, RAFTERY AT. Intra-peritoneal rupture of a phaeochromocytoma. *J R Soc Med* 1984;77.513.

77 GREENBERGER N, GRYBOSKI JD. *Allergic disorders of the intestine and eosinophilic gastroenteritis in gastrointestinal disease.* Philadelphia: W. B. Saunders & Co. 1978:1128.

78 HADJIYANNAKIS EJ, EVANS DB, SMELLIE WAB, CALNE RY. Gastrointestinal complications after renal transplantation. *Lancet* 1971;**ii**:781–784.

79 HAFFNER JFW, JAKOBSEN A, FLATMARK AL. Upper gastrointestinal bleeding in renal transplant recipients: the role of prophylactic gastric surgery. *World J Surg* 1983;**7**:738–742.

80 HALSTED CH, ROBLES EA, MEZEY E. Intestinal malabsorption in folate-deficient alcoholics. *Gastroenterology* 1973;**64**:526–532.

81 HART FD. Rheumatoid arthritis: Extra-articular manifestations I. *Br Med J* 1969;**iii**:131–136.

82 HARWOOD AB, OSOBA D, HOFSTADER SL, *et al.* Kaposi's sarcoma in recipients of renal transplants. *Am J Med* 1979;**67**:759–765.

83 HASTINGS PR, SKILLMAN JT, BUSHNELL S. Antacid titration in the prevention of acute gastro-intestinal bleeding: a controlled randomized trial in 180 critically ill patients. *N Engl J Med* 1978;**298**:1041–1045.

84 HELLEMANS J, AGG HO, PELEMANS W, VANTRAPPEN G. Pharyngoesophageal swallowing disorders and the pharyngoesophageal sphincter. *Med Clin N Am* 1981;**65**(6):1149–1171.

85 HENSBY CN, LEWIS PJ, HILGARD P, MUFTI GJ, HOWS J, WEBSTER J. Prostaglandin deficiency in thrombotic thrombocytopenic purpura. *Lancet* 1979;**2**:748.

86 HEREMANS JF, CRABBE PA. IgA deficiency: general considerations and relation to human disease. In: Good RA, Bergstra D, eds. *Immunologic deficiency diseases in man. Birth Defects.* 1968;**4**:116–121.

87 HERMANN G. Intussusception secondary to mesenteric adenitis. *JAMA* 1967;**200**:74–75.

88 HERMANS PE, DIAZ-BUXO JA, STOBO JD. Idiopathic late-onset immunoglobulin deficiency. Clinical observations in 50 patients. *Am J Med* 1970;**61**:221–237.

89 HEYMSFIELD SB, SMITH J, REDD S, WHITWORTH HB JR. Nutritional support in cardiac failure. *Surg Clin North Am* 1981;**61**:635–652.

90 HIRSCHOWITZ BI, GROARKE JF. Effect of cimetidine on gastric hyper-secretion and diarrhoea in systemic mastocytosis. *Ann Int Med* 1979;**90**:769–771.

91 HOCHBERG FH, DASILVA AB, GALDABINI J, RICHARDSON FP. Gastro-intestinal involvement in von Recklinghausen's neurofibromatosis. *Neurology (Minneap)* 1974;**24**:1144–1151.

92 HOFFMAN BI, KATZ WA. The gastrointestinal manifestations of systemic lupus erythematosus: a review of the literature. *Semin Arthritis Rheum* 1980;**9**:237–247.

93 HOITSMA MFW, CUESTA MA, STARINK MA. Zinc deficiency syndrome versus glucagonoma syndrome. *Arch Chir Neu* 1979;**31**:131–135.

94 HOLLIS JB, CASTELL DO, BRADOM RL. Oesophageal function in diabetes mellitus and its relation to peripheral neuropathy. *Gastroenterology* 1977;**73**:1098–1102.

95 HOROWITZ M, MCNEIL JD, MADDERN GJ, COLLINS PJ, SHEARMAN DJC. Abnormalities of gastric and esophageal emptying in polymyositis and dermatomyositis. *Gastroenterology* 1986;**90**:434–439.

96 HOROWITZ S, LORENZSOM VW, OLSEN WA, *et al.* Small intestinal disease in T cell deficiency. *J Pediatr* 1974;**85**:457–462.

97 HOSKING DJ, MOODY F, STEWART IM, ATKINSON M. Vagal impairment of gastric secretion in diabetic autonomic neuropathy. *Br Med J* 1975;**2**:588–590.

98 HURWITZ AL, NELSON JA, HADDAD JK. Oropharyngeal dysphagia: Manometric and cine-oesophago-gastric findings. *Am J Dig Dis* 1975;**20**:313–324.

99 HUSTON JR, STEWART WR. Hemorrhagic phaeochromocytoma with shock and abdominal pain. *Am J Med* 1965;**39**:502–505.

100 HUVOS AG, PRUZANSKI W. Smooth muscle involvement in primary muscle disease. II. Progressive muscular dystrophy. *Arch Pathol* 1967;**83**:234–240.

101 IMPERATO PJ, HARVEY RP, SHOOKHOFF HB, CHAVES AD. Trichinosis among Thais living in New York City. *JAMA* 1974;**227**:526–529.

102 IRVINE WJ, SCARTH L, CLARKE BF, CULLEN DR, DUNCAN LJ. Thyroid and gastric auto-immunity in patients with diabetes mellitus. *Lancet* 1970;**ii**:163–168.

103 IRVINE WJ, TOFT AD. Diagnosing adrenocortical insufficiency. *Practitioner* 1977;**218**:539–545.

104 ISAACS P, WHITTAKER SM, TURNBERG LA. Diarrhoea associated with medullary carcinoma of the thyroid. Studies of intestinal function in a patient. *Gastroenterology* 1974;**67**:521–526.

105 JASPERS MT. Unusual oral lesions in a uremic patient. *Oral Surg* 1975;**39**:934–944.

106 JELLINEK EH, TULLOCH WS. Herpes zoster with dysfunction of bladder and anus. *Lancet* 1976;**ii**:1220–1222.

107 JOHNSON DH, GUTHRIE TH, TEDESCO FJ, GRIFFIN JW, ANTHONY HF JR. Amyloidosis masquerading as inflammatory bowel disease with a mass lesion simulating a malignancy. *Am J Gastroenterol* 1982;**77**:141–145.

108 JOHNSTONE JM, MORSON BC. Eosinophilic gastroenteritis. *Histopathology* 1978;**2**:335–348.

109 JONES MB, VOET R, PAGANI J, LOTYSCH M, O'CONNELL T, KORETZ RL. Multifocal eosinophilic granuloma involving the common bile duct: histologic and cholangiographic findings. *Gastroenterology* 1981;**80**:384–389.

110 KAPLAN AP. Angioedema. *N Engl J Med* 1984;**310**:1662–1663.

111 KASAHARA Y, TANAKA S, NISHINO M, UMEMURA H, SHIRAHA S, KUYAMA T. Intestinal involvement in Behçet's disease. *Dis Colon Rectum* 1981;**24**:103–106.

112 KAWAMURA S, SAWADA Y, FUJIWARA S, KAWATSU S, CHIBA Y, YOSHIDA Y. Clinical pathologic studies of gastrointestinal haemorrhage in acute leukemia. *Tohoku J Exp Med* 1979;**127**:345–352.

113 KING A, RAMPLING A, WIGHT DGD, WARREN RE. Neutropenic enterocolitis due to Clostridium septicum infection. *J Clin Path.* 1984;**37**:335–343.

114 KIRKPATRICK CH. Cancer and immunodeficiency diseases. *Birth defects* 1976;**12**:61–78.

115 KLEIN MS, SHERLOCK P. Gastric and colon metastases from breast cancer. *Am J Dig Dis* 1972;**17**:881–886.

116 KLEIN NC, HARGROVE RI, SLEISENGER MH, JEFFERIES GH. Eosinophilic gastroenteritis. *Medicine* 1970;**49**:299–319.

117 KOHN NN. Sarcoidosis of the colon. *J Med Soc NJ* 1980;**77**:517–523.

118 KOISTINEN J. Selective IgA deficiency in blood donors. *Vox Sang* 1975;**29**:192–202.

119 KORSAGER S. Sarcoidosis of the stomach. A case report. *Scand J Resp Dis* 1979;**60**:24–27.

120 KUMPE DA, JAFFE RB, WALDMANN TA, WEINSTEIN MA. Constrictive pericarditis and protein-losing enteropathy: an imitator of intestinal lymphangiectasis. *Am J Roentgenol Radium Ther Nucl Med* 1975;**124**:365–373.

121 KYLE RA, BAIRD ED. Amyloidosis: Review of 236 cases. *Medicine* 1975; **54**:271–299.

122 LAMERS CB, WAGENER T, ASSMANN KJ, VAN TONGEREN JH. Jejunal lymphoma in a patient with primary adult-onset hypogammaglobulinaemia and nodular lymphoid hyperplasia of the small intestine. *Dig Dis Sci* 1980;**25**:553–557.

123 LASS N, DORON O, GILAT T. Gastric acid secretion in cold urticaria. *Dig Dis Sci* 1980;**25**:526–528.

124 LAWLOR GJ, AMMANN AJ, WRIGHT WC, LA FRANCHI SH, BILSTROM D, STIEHM FR. The syndrome of cellular deficiency with immunoglobulins. *J Pediatr* 1974;**84**:183–192.

125 LEBO CP, SANG UK, NORRIS FH. Cricopharyngeal myotomy in amyotrophic lateral sclerosis. *Laryngoscope* 1976;**86**:862–865.

126 LEHNER T, BATCHELOR JR. Classification and an immunogenetic basis of Behçet's syndrome. In: Lehner T, Barnes CG, eds. *Behçet's syndrome: Clinical and immunological features.* New York: Academic Press, 1979;13–32.

127 LEVESQUE M, FAUCK C, MORNET P, BARSAMIAN I, LECRONIER M, VITAL C. Manifestations digestives de la dermatomyosite. *J Radiol* 1981;**62**:13–18.

128 LEWIN IG, PAPAPOULOS SE, TOMLINSON S, HENDY GN, O'RIORDAN JL. Studies of hypoparathyroidism and pseudohypoparathyroidism. *Q J Med* 1978;**47**:533–548.

129 LINDER MM, KÖSTERS W, RETHEL R. Prophylactic gastric operations in uremic patients prior to renal transplantation. *World J Surg* 1979;**3**:501–503.

130 LOPEZ LR, SHOCKET AL, STANFORD RE, CLAMAN HN, KOHLER PF. Gastrointestinal involvement in leucoclastic vasculitis in polyarteritis nodosa. *J Rheumatol* 1980;**7**:677–684.

131 LOO FD, PALMER DW, SOERGEL KH, KALBFLEISCH JH, WOOD CM. Gastric emptying in patients with diabetes mellitus. *Gastroenterology* 1984;**86**:485–494.

132 MCCLAIN C, SOUTOR C, ZIEVE L. Zinc deficiency: a complication of Crohn's disease. *Gastroenterology* 1980;**78**:272–279.

133 MCDONALD GB, SHULMAN HM, SULLIVAN KM, SPENCER GD. Intestinal and hepatic complications of human bone marrow transplantation. Part I. *Gastroenterology* 1986;**90**:460–477.

134 MCDONALD GS, GAD-AL-RAB J. Behçet's syndrome with endocarditis and the Budd Chiari syndrome. *J Clin Pathol* 1980;**33**:660–669.

135 MALE PJ, DE TOLEDO F, WINDGREN S, DE PAYER R, BERTHOUD S. Pseudotumoral enterocolitis and massive eosinophilia. *Gut* 1983;**24**:345–350.

136 MALINS JM, MAYNE N. Diabetic diarrhoea. A study of 13 patients with jejunal biopsy. *Diabetes* 1969;**18**:858–866.

137 MANLEY KA, SKYRING AP. Some heritable causes of gastrointestinal disease. *Arch Int Med* 1961;**107**:182–203.

138 MARGULIES SI, BRUNT PW, DONNER MW, SILBIGER ML. Familial dysautonomia. A cineradiographic study of the swallowing mechanism. *Radiology* 1968;**90**:107–112.

139 MARKS J. The relationship of gastrointestinal disease and the skin. *Clin Gastroenterol* 1983;**12**(3):693–712.

140 MARKS J, SHUSTER S. Small intestinal mucosal abnormalities in various skin diseases—fact or fancy? *Gut* 1970;**11**:281–291.

141 MARKS J, SHUSTER S. Intestinal malabsorption and the skin. *Gut* 1971;**12**:938–947.

142 MASON RM, BARNES CG. Behçet's syndrome with arthritis. *Ann Rheum Dis* 1969;**28**:95–103.

143 MATAMOROS N, NORTH ME, CIRIA I, WEBSTER ADB. Chronic granulomatous disease with normal neutrophil glutathione peroxidase activity in a brother and sister. *Acta Paediatr Scand* 1982;**71**:327–328.

144 MEHTA SK, KAUR S, AVASTNI G, WIG NN, CHUTTANI PN. Small intestinal deficiency in pellagra. *Am J Clin Nutr* 1979;**25**:545–549.

145 DE MERIEUX P, VERITY MA, CLEMENTS PJ, PAULUS HE. Esophageal abnormalities and dysphagia in polymyositis and dermatomyositis. *Arthritis Rheum* 1983;**26**:961–968.

146 MEYERS WC, HARRIS N, STEIN S, *et al.* Alimentary tract complications after renal transplantation. *Ann Surg* 1979;**190**:535–542.

147 MIDDLETON WR. Progress report: Thyroid hormones and the gut. *Gut* 1971;**12**:172–177.

148 MING RH, DREOSTI IM, TIM IO, SEGAL I. Thyrotoxicosis presenting as dysphagia: a case report. *S Afr Med J* 1982;**61**:554–555.

149 MITCH WE. Nitrogen metabolism in patients with chronic renal failure. *Am J Clin Nutr* 1978;**31**:1594–1600.

150 MODLIN IM, FARNDON JR, SHEPHERD A, *et al.* Phaeochromocytomas in 72 patients: clinical and diagnostic features, treatment and long term results. *Br J Surg* 1979;**66**:456–465.

151 MOLLOY AM, TOMKIN GH. Altered bile in diabetic diarrhoea. *Br Med J* 1978;**2**:1462–1463.

152 MORSE WI, COCHRANE WA, LANDRIGAN P. Familial hypoparathyroidism with pernicious anaemia, steatorrhoea and adrenocortical insufficiency. *N Engl J Med* 1961;**264**:1021–1025.

153 MUELLER CF, MOREHEAD R, ALTER AJ. Pneumatosis intestinales in collagen disorders. *Am J Roentgenol Radium Ther Nucl Med* 1972;**115**:300–305.

154 NOWAK TV, IONASESCU V, ANURAS S. Gastrointestinal manifestation of the muscular dystrophies. *Gastroenterology* 1982;**82**:800–810.

155 O'BRIEN BD, SHNITKA TK, McDOUGALL R, *et al.* Pathophysiologic and ultrastructural basis for intestinal symptoms in Fabry's disease. *Gastroenterology* 1982;**82**:957–962.

156 O'DUFFY JD. Prognosis in Behçet's syndrome. *Bull Rheum Dis* 1978;**29**:977–979.

157 O'DUFFY JD, CALNEY JA, DEODHAR S. Behçet's disease. Report of 10 cases, 3 with new manifestations. *Ann Int Med* 1971;**75**:561–570.

158 OLINGER EJ, McCARTHY DM, YOUNG RC, GARDNER JD. Hyperhistaminaemia and hyperchlorhydria in basophilic granulocytic leukemia. *Gastroenterology,* 1976;**71**:667–669.

159 OLSON JA, ROJANAPO W, LAMB AJ. The effect of vitamin A status on the differentiation and function of goblet cells in the rat intestine. *Ann NY Acad Sci* 1981;**359**:181–191.

160 ORRINGER MB. Extended cervical oesophagomyotomy for oropharyngeal dysfunction. *J Thorac Cardiovasc Surg* 1980;**80**:669–678.

161 OSHIMA Y, SHIMIZU T, YOKOHARI R, *et al.* Clinical studies on Behçet's syndrome. *Ann Rheum Dis* 1963;**22**:36–43.

162 OSSERMAN KE, GENKINS G. Studies in myasthenia gravis: Review of a twenty year experience in over 1200 patients. *Mt Sinai J Med* 1971;**38**:497–537.

163 PAPAC RJ, ROSENSTEIN RW, RICHARDS F, YESNER R. Gamma heavy chain disease seen initially as gastric neoplasm. *Arch Intern Med* 1978;**138**:1151–1155.

164 PAIMELA H, TALLGREN LG, STENMAN S, NUMERS HV, SCHEININ TM. Multiple duodenal polyps in uraemia. a little known clinical entity. *Gut* 1984;**25**:259–263.

165 PEARSON CM. In: McCarty DJ, ed. *Arthritis and allied conditions: a textbook of Rheumatology.* Philadelphia: Lea & Febiger, 1979:740–761.

166 PISANTY S, GARFUNKEL A. Familial hypoparathyroidism with candidiasis and mental retardation. *Oral Surg* 1977;**44**:374–383.

167 PITTMAN JG, COHEN P. The pathogenesis of cardiac cachexia. *N Engl J Med* 1964;**271**:403–408.

168 PLANTIN LO, STRANDBERG O. Gastrointestinal protein loss in rheumatoid arthritis studied with ^{51}Cr-chromic chloride and ^{125}I albumin. *Scand J Rheumatol* 1974;**3**:169–174.

169 POPOVIC OS, BRKIC S, BOJIC P, *et al.* Sarcoidosis and protein losing enteropathy. *Gastroenterology* 1980;**78**:119–125.

170 POWELL RW, MOSS JP, NAGAR D, *et al.* Strongyloidiasis in immuno-suppressed hosts. Presentation as massive lower gastro-intestinal bleeding. *Arch Intern Med* 1980;**140**:1061–1063.

171 RANIREZ-MATA M, PENA-ANCIRA FF, ALARCON-SEGOVIA D. Abnormal oesophageal motility in primary Sjögren's syndrome. *J Rheumatol* 1976;**3**:63–69.

172 REMUZZI G, MISIANI R, MECCA G, DE GEATANO G, DONATI MB. Thrombotic thrombocytopenic purpura—a deficiency of platelet factors regulating platelet-vessel wall interaction? *N Engl J Med* 1978;**299**:311.

173 REYA MJ, BENNET ER, POPS M, GOLDBERG LS. Internal vasculitis in essential mixed cryoglobulinaemia. *Ann Intern Med* 1974;**81**:632–637.

174 ROBINS-BROWNE MA, RABSON AR, KOORNHOF HJ. Generalised infection with yersinia enterocolitica and the role of iron. *Contrib Microbiol Immunol* 1979;**5**:277–282.

175 ROCK E, MALMUD L, FISHER RS. Motor disorders of the stomach. *Med Clin North Am* 1981;**65**(6):1269–1290.

176 ROJANAPO W, LAMB AJ, OLSON JA. The prevalence metabolism and migration of goblet cells in rat intestine following the induction of rapid synchronous Vitamin A deficiency. *J Nutr* 1980;**31**:103–110.

177 ROSATI LA, AUGUR NA. Ischemic enterocolitis in pheochromocytoma. *Gastroenterology* 1971;**60**:581–585.

178 RUBENSTEIN RB. Uremic ileus. Uremia presenting as colonic obstruction. *NY State J Med* 1979;**79**:248–249.

179 RUBIN E, RYBAK BJ, LINDENBAUM J, GERSAN CD,

WALKER G, LIEBER CS. Ultrastructural changes in the small intestine induced by ethanol. *Gastroenterology* 1972;**63**:810–814.

180 SAULSBURY FT, WINKELSTEIN JA, YOLKEN RH. Chronic rotavirus infection in immunodeficiency. *J Paediatr* 1980;**97**:61–65.

181 SCARPELLO JHB, BARBER DC, HAGUE RV, CULLEN DR, SLADEN GE. Gastric emptying of solid meals in diabetics. *Br Med J* 1976;**2**:671–673.

182 SCARPELLO JHB, HAGUE RV, CULLEN DR, SLADEN GE. The ^{14}C-glycocholate test in diabetic diarrhoea. *Br Med J* 1976;**2**:673–675.

183 SCHEFF RT, ZUCKERMAN G, HARTER H, DELMEY J, KOEHLER R. Diverticular disease in patients with chronic renal failure due to polycystic kidney disease. *Ann Intern Med* 1980;**92**:202–204.

184 SCHUFFLER MD. Chronic intestinal pseudo-obstruction syndromes. *Med Clin North Am* 1981;**65**(6):1331–1358.

185 SCHUFFLER MD, BIRD TD, SUMI SM, COOK PA. A familial neuronal disease presenting as intestinal pseudo-obstruction. *Gastroenterology* 1978;**75**:889–898.

186 SCHUFFLER MD, LOWE MC, BILL AH. Studies of idiopathic intestinal pseudo-obstruction. I. Hereditary hollow visceral myopathy. Clinical and pathological studies. *Gastroenterology* 1977;**73**:327–338.

187 SCHWARTZ Y, TANISE A, KISSIN F, SHANI M. An unusual case of temporo-mandibular joint arthropathy in systemic amyloidosis. *J Oral Med* 1979;**34**:40–42.

188 SCOTT BB, HARDY GJ, LOSOWSKY MS. Involvement of the small intestine in systemic mast cell disease. *Gut* 1975;**16**:918–924.

189 SEROTA FT, ROSENBERG HK, ROSEN J, *et al.* Delayed onset of gastro-intestinal disease in the recipients of bone marrow transplants. A variant graft-versus-host reaction. *Transplantation* 1982;**34**:60–64.

190 SIEGAL S. Familial paroxysmal polyserositis. Analysis of 50 cases. *Am J Med* 1964;**36**:893–918.

191 SILBIGER ML, PIKIELNEY R, DONNER MW. Neuromuscular disorders affecting the pharynx: cineradiographic analysis. *Invest Radiol* 1967;**2**:442–448.

192 SLADEN GE, LEHNER T. Gastrointestinal disorders in Behçet's syndrome. In: Lehner T, Barnes CG, eds. *Behçet's syndrome: Clinical and immunological features.* New York: Academic Press, 1979:151–158.

193 SLAVIN RE, DIAS MA, SAVAL R. Cytosine arabinoside induced gastro-intestinal toxic alterations in sequential chemotherapeutic protocols. A clinicopathologic study of 33 patients. *Cancer* 1982;**42**:1747–1759.

194 SLOPER KS, DOURMASHKIN RR, BIRD RB, SLAVIN G, WEBSTER ADB. Chronic malabsorption due to cryptosporidiosis in a child with immunoglobulin deficiency. *Gut* 1982;**23**:80–82.

195 SMOKING AND HEALTH: A report of the Surgeon General. Chapter 3: Morbidity. No. 79-50066 US Dept of HEW:1979.

196 SNAPE WJ. Pseudo-obstruction and other obstructive disorders. *Clin Gastroenterol* 1982;**11**(3)593–608.

197 SNAPE WJ, BATTLE WM, SCHWARTZ SS, BRAUNSTEIN SN, GOLDSTEIN HA, ALAVI A. Metoclopramide to treat gastroparesis due to diabetes mellitus: a double-blind controlled trial. *Ann Intern Med* 1982;**96**:444–446.

198 SPIVAK JL, JACKSON DL. Pellagra: an analysis of 18 patients and review of the literature. *Johns Hopkins Med J* 1977;**140**:295–309.

199 SPRY CJ, DAVIES J, TAI PC, OLSEN EG, OAKLEY CM, GOODWIN JF. Clinical features of fifteen patients with the hypereosinophilic syndrome. *Q J Med* 1983;**52**:1–22.

200 STEWART IM, HOSKING DJ, PRESTON BJ, ATKINSON M. Oesophageal motor changes in diabetes mellitus. *Thorax* 1976;**31**:278–283.

201 STROBER W, KRAKAUER R, KLAEVEMAN HL, REYNOLDS HY, NELSON DL. Secretory component deficiency. A disorder of the IgA immune system. *N Engl J Med* 1976;**294**:351–356.

202 SUGARMAN B. Medical complications of spinal cord injury. *Q J Med* 1985;**54**:3–18.

203 SULLIVAN SN, TUSTANOFF E, SLAUGHTER DN, LINTON AL, LINDSAY RM, WATSON WC. Hypergastrinaemia and gastric acid hypersecretion in uremia. *Clin Nephrol* 1976;**5**:25–28.

204 SULWAY MJ, BAUM PE, DAVIS E. Stiff-man syndrome presenting with complete oesophageal obstruction. *Am J Dig Dis* 1970;**15**:79–84.

205 SUN DCH, ROTH SH, MITCHELL CS, ENGLAND DWW. Upper gastrointestinal disease in rheumatoid arthritis. *Am J Dig Dis* 1974;**19**:405–410.

206 SWAIN CP, TAVILL AS, NEALE G. Studies of tryptophan and albumin metabolism in a patient with carcinoid syndrome, pellagra and hypoproteinaemia. *Gastroenterology* 1976;**71**:484–489.

207 TABAQCHALI S, PALLIS C. Reversible nicotinamide deficiency encephalopathy in a patient with jejunal diverticulosis. *Gut* 1970;**11**:1024–1028.

208 TAKASUGI M, HAYAKAWA A, KIRAKATA H. Gastric involvement in Sjögren's syndrome simulating early gastric cancer. *Endoscopy* 1979;**4**:263–266.

209 TAYLOR JF, TEMPLETON AC, VOGEL CL, ZIEGLER JL, KYALWAZI SK. Kaposi's sarcoma in Uganda: a clinical pathologic study. *Int J Cancer* 1971;**8**:125–135.

210 THOMAS FB, CALDWELL JH, GREENBERGER NJ. Steatorrhoea in thyrotoxicosis. Relation to hypermotility and excessive dietary fat. *Ann Int Med* 1973;**78**:669–675.

211 THOMSON AD, MAJUMDAR SK. The influence of ethanol on intestinal absorption and utilisation of

nutrients. *Clin Gastroenterol* 1981;10(2):263–293.

212 TSAI JT. Perforation of the small bowel with rheumatoid arthritis. *South Med J* 1980;73:939–940.

213 TUYNS AJ. Epidemiology of alcohol and cancer. *Cancer Res* 1979;39:2840–2843.

214 VALENCIA-PARPARCEN J. Alcoholic gastritis. *Clin Gastroenterol* 1981;10(2):389–399.

215 VYAS D, CHANDRA RK. Functional significance of iron deficiency. In: Stekel A, Guesry P, eds. *Iron deficiency in infancy and childhood.*

216 WALDMANN TA, STROBER W. Metabolism of immunoglobulins. *Prog Allergy* 1969;13:1–110.

217 WALSH CH, COOPER BT, WRIGHT AD, MALINS JM, COOKE WT. Diabetes mellitus and coeliac disease: a clinical study. *Q J Med* 1978;47:89–100.

218 WARIN AP, GREAVES MW, GATECLIFF M, WILLIAMSON DM, WARIN RP. Treatment of hereditary angioedema by low dose attenuated androgens: dissociation of clinical response from levels of CI esterase inhibitor and C4. *Br J Dermatol* 1980;103:405–409.

219 WEBSTER ADB, SLAVIN G, SHINER M, PLATT-MILLS TAE, ASHERSON GL. Coeliac disease with severe hypogammaglobulinaemia. *Gut* 1981;22:153–157.

220 WEISER MM, ANDRES GA, BRENTJENS JR, EVANS JT, REICHLIN M. Systemic lupus erythematosus and intestinal venulitis. *Gastroenterology* 1981;81:570–579.

221 WELLS I, SMITH B, HINTON M. Acute ileus in myxoedema. *Br Med J* 1977;1:211–212.

222 WERLIN SL, CHUSID MJ, CAYA J, DECHLER HW. Colitis in chronic granulomatous disease. *Gastroenterology* 1982;82:328–331.

223 WHITE RF, MAJOR GA. Gold colitis. *Med J Aust* 1983;19:174–175.

224 WHITINGTON PF, FRIEDMAN AL, CHESNEY RW. Gastrointestinal disease in the hemolytic-uremic syndrome. *Gastroenterology* 1979;76:728–733.

225 WIENBECK M, BERGES W. Oesophageal lesions in the alcoholic. *Clin Gastroenterol* 1981;10(2):375–388.

226 WILLIAMSON LM, HULL D, MEHTA R, REEVES WG, ROBINSON BHB, TOGHILL PJ. Familial Hibernian Fever. *Q J Med* 1982;51:469–480.

227 WINKELMANN RK. Dermatomyositis in childhood. *Clin Rheum Dis* 1982;8:353–368.

228 WINSHIP DH, CAFLISCH CR, ZBORALSKE F, HOGAN WJ. Deterioration of oesophageal peristalsis in patients with alcoholic neuropathy. *Gastroenterology* 1968;55:173–178.

229 WYATT RA, YOUNOSZAI K, ANURAS S, MYERS MG. Campylobacter fetus septicaemia and hepatitis in agammaglobulinaemia. *J Pediatr* 1977;91:441–442.

230 YOLKEN RH, BISHOP CA, TOWNSEND TR, *et al.* Infectious gastroenteritis in bone marrow transplant recipients. *N Engl J Med* 1982;306:1010–1012.

231 YOUNG R, BRYK D. Colonic intussusception in uremia. *Am J Gastroenterol* 1979;71:229–232.

232 ZIZIC TM, SHULMAN LE, STEVENS MB. Colonic perforations in systemic lupus erythematosus. *Medicine* 1975;54:411–426.

233 ZUKERMAN GR, MILLS BA, KOEHLER RE, SIEGEL A, HARTER HR. Nodular duodenitis. Pathologic and clinical characteristics in patients with end-stage renal disease. *Dig Dis Sci* 1983;28:1018–1024.

Chapter 75
Allergy and the Gut

M. H. LESSOF

Public interest in food allergy has increased rapidly [9, 13, 22, 25, 32], and those who believe themselves to have this disease often embark on complex, self-imposed dietary restrictions [2]. Patients who present with this self-diagnosis therefore need to be examined critically, for they include those who are psychiatrically ill and who may have an obsessional aversion to a variety of foods [29, 30]. In such cases, the diagnosis of food allergy is easily disproved by the absence of reproducible symptoms of intolerance after specific foods are ingested [8]. Exclusion of this diagnosis may thus be relatively simple. A more positive diagnosis of food allergy may, however, be extremely difficult.

The demonstration of a reproducible intolerance to a specific food does not necessarily indicate that the cause is allergic (Table 75.1). In order to justify the diagnosis of food allergic disease, it is necessary to demonstrate both that there is a specific food intolerance and that the patient's adverse reaction is associated with an abnormal immunological response. Food allergic disease may involve immediate allergic reactions, in which there is an immunoglobulin E (IgE) antibody response, but can also involve late responses in which IgE mechanisms play little or no part. At their most severe, these late reactions are associated with villous atrophy and well-marked enteropathy, of which by far the most common example is coeliac disease (see Chapter 42).

Epidemiology

Of those who believe, for whatever reason, that they have food-related symptoms, perhaps two or three out of every 10 can be shown to have a true food intolerance. Perhaps one in 10 will prove to have food allergic disease. Epidemiological data on prevalence can be almost impossible to

Table 75.1. Causes of food intolerance.

Type of intolerance	Causative agents
Local irritants	Curries Very hot drinks
Toxic	Hexachlorbenzine (seed wheat dressing)
Pharmacological	Caffeine in strong coffee or tea Tyramine in fermented cheese Histamine release (canned fish or rotten mackerel)
Enzyme defects	Alactasia
Altered bacterial flora	Broadspectrum antibiotics
Immunological	Food allergy

obtain. Published estimations of the prevalence of cow's milk protein intolerance vary from 0.3 to 12% [2]. Furthermore, cow's milk intolerance may have a variety of causes, including the hypolactasia which, in Nigeria and in several other countries, can affect up to 50% of the population.

The incidence of true food allergy remains unknown. In adult life, the position is obscured by the lack of diagnostic criteria. M. L. Burr of the M.R.C. Epidemiology Unit in Cardiff has noted that among 475 Welsh citizens picked at random from the electoral register, 23% held food to be responsible for a variety of symptoms, from fainting to sore throat. The commonest were major abdominal symptoms—vomiting, diarrhoea, pain—reported by 9% of these subjects. A further 7% blamed certain foods for headaches and various types of skin rash. Symptoms caused by fruit, onion, garlic and cheese ranged from the trivial to the severe. The difficulties inherent in this type of population survey proved to be formidable.

Aetiology

In food allergy, as in all allergic diseases, genetic factors play an important part. This is particularly evident in infancy, when the protective mechanisms are immature and may fail to distinguish adequately between harmful micro-organisms, on the one hand, and the proteins of a regularly ingested food. During this vulnerable, neonatal period it has been suggested that a heavy antigenic load can sometimes provoke an allergic reaction, regardless of the nature of the antigen.

Those with a family history of atopy may lack IgA antibodies in their mucous secretions in the early weeks of life. It has been suggested [34] that, when cow's milk or mixed feeding are introduced very early in infancy, this greatly increases the risk that food allergy will develop. Since IgA is present in breast milk and is resistant to digestion, breast feeding may not only reduce the risk of swallowing infected material but may provide a useful source of protective antibodies. Furthermore, if no other antigenic foods are given, this allows time for the baby's own protective mechanisms to mature before mixed feeding is introduced. At this age, it is clear that both genetic and environmental factors are important.

An increased susceptibility to bowel disorders can arise, not only as the result of a precocious exposure to foreign antigens, but also when the integrity of the mucosal barrier is disturbed, as has been shown to occur in some patients with eczema [15]. It is possible that this may help to explain the increased incidence of allergic disorders in patients with fibrocystic disease. When the bowel wall is once affected by an immunological reaction, it becomes more permeable to other macromolecules, and further sensitization may then occur [3]. There are also deficiencies which increase the tendency to develop allergic reactions, including inherited deficiencies of complement components such as C2 [35] and also defects in leucocyte phagocytosis [34]. There are thus a variety of ways in which a defect in the defence mechanisms can encourage the development of sensitivity reactions, whether that defect is immunological or based in the integrity of the mucous barrier, the permeability of the cell membrane, or the response to submucosal intra-epithelial and mast cells.

In those with the most clear-cut allergic reactions, there is often an urticarial or asthmatic response, a high serum IgE level, and there are IgE antibodies to the appropriate food. Where the main reaction to food is a late one, however, even highly atopic subjects may have no obvious evidence of an IgE response—at least, as far as skin tests or circulating IgE antibodies are concerned. It has been suggested that IgG4 or other subclasses of IgG antibody can sometimes cause allergic reactions [11, 28], and it is also possible that some reactions to foods containing tartrazine or other colouring agents may be mediated by IgD [26]. Laboratory investigations that seek to establish the cause of late reactions of this kind are still, however, of little diagnostic value.

Pathology

Histological changes in the bowel can provide useful information. Infants with cow's milk allergy have abnormally blunted villi in the small bowel [37]. Soy protein, fish, chicken and rice can cause similar but usually less marked changes [1, 36]. Since the appearances resemble those seen in coeliac disease, it seems likely that cow's milk protein intolerance and coeliac disease are both part of a wider spectrum of food-induced enteropathy. Cow's milk intolerance may be a cause of infantile colitis [12, 16].

The pathogenesis of these mucosal changes remains uncertain, however. Despite the evidence of an IgE response in some infants with cow's milk allergy, this is an inconstant finding. While the histological resemblance to coeliac disease has been thought to indicate an immune complex reaction, there are also clear points of difference in cow's milk protein intolerance, of which the most obvious is the frequent association with florid allergic reactions in other organs. More than one type of response may therefore occur in the same patient, involving both early and late, local and more generalized immunological responses, with the release of prostaglandins [5] and other complex pathophysiological sequelae which vary from patient to patient. Indeed, in some conditions, it is not certainly known whether the changes that occur are a cause of the inflammatory reactions or a consequence—for example, the

mild mucosal damage seen in atopic eczema [24].

Negative skin tests, or negative IgE-dependent blood tests, do not necessarily exclude a local IgE response within the gut. For example, patients with haemorrhagic proctitis have an excess of IgE-containing cells in the rectum, even when systemic evidence of allergy is lacking [31]. Eosinophilic gastroenteritis may also be associated with a striking sensitivity to food, even in the absence of evidence of an immunological response elsewhere in the body [19].

Clinical features

Cow's milk protein intolerance is the most studied food allergic syndrome—it usually presents with recurrent vomiting and diarrhoea but can also manifest itself through the insidious changes of eczema, which are sometimes unaccompanied by a bowel disorder. The symptoms commonly begin within a few weeks of starting cow's milk, usually at about the age of two months. Other manifestations include urticaria, wheezing and asthma. Occasionally, acute anaphylaxis may even cause death [14]. The symptoms may occur transiently after an acute attack of gastroenteritis, and in such patients cow's milk restriction is needed only for a matter of days or weeks. Even in well-established cases, the majority recover tolerance to cow's milk after a period of dietary restriction lasting six months to one year.

The reasons for considering cow's milk protein intolerance in more detail are that it is relatively common, and that it exemplifies the wide range of reactions which are also seen with other foods. Abdominal pain and constipation may occur, steatorrhoea is not unknown, and temper tantrums and irritability may indicate a non-specific reaction to ill health. In addition, those who are most severely affected can develop iron deficiency and retarded growth [4, 38].

Table 75.2. Clinical features of food allergy.

Gastrointestinal reactions
Early
    swelling of lips
    tingling of mouth and throat
    vomiting, diarrhoea
    pain, bloating
Late
    constipation
    steatorrhoea
    protein loss*, blood loss*

Remote effects
Rhinorrhoea, urticaria, angioedema, headache,
    migraine
Anaphylaxis, asthma, eczema
Joint pains*

* Relatively uncommon but well-documented.

In older children and adults, foods such as egg, fish, nuts and protein may also provoke gastrointestinal symptoms or a variety of remote effects (see Table 75.2). While non-immunological causes of food intolerance are relatively common, food allergy is by no means rare and classical allergic symptoms such as urticaria, asthma, or even anaphylaxis leave the diagnosis in little doubt. Exceptionally, haemorrhagic proctitis may be food-induced [20], and there have been occasional patients in whom cow's milk ingestion has caused an exacerbation in pre-existing rheumatoid arthritis, in steroid-sensitive nephrotic syndrome, and even in thrombocytopenia [21]. Although it seems possible that a rise in circulating immune complexes after a milk feed might have a non-specific adverse effect in such cases, this does not fully explain why cow's milk should so often be the involved food.

Differential diagnosis

Where symptoms are provoked by cow's milk and are confined to the gastrointestinal tract, a lactose tolerance test may be needed to exclude lactase deficiency. In older patients, assuming the psychiatric causes of food aversion have been eliminated (if necessary, by assessing the response to a placebo-controlled challenge in a disguised form), the differential diagnosis includes conditions that range from the pharmacological effects of caffeine to the fat intolerance which is noted by patients with gallstones (Table 75.1).

Investigation

In terms of diagnosis, it is first necessary to establish the relationship between taking a specific food and the onset of symptoms. In case of doubt, the patient is asked to keep a food diary, recording the diet on one side of the page and symptoms on the other. Asthmatics who are given an elimination diet should also be asked to record peak expiratory flow readings at regular intervals. If the symptoms disappear, or if the peak flow readings rise, suspicion may fall on one or more foods.

Where correlations between symptoms and the ingestion of specific foods are suspected but not proven, it may then be necessary to arrange an 'elimination diet' and challenge tests [13]. The starting diet either removes an individual suspect food or, in cases of uncertainty, begins with an empirical diet which omits several common food allergens. The main exclusions are milk and dairy products, egg, fish and nuts, together with artificial preservatives and colouring agents. In addition, gluten-free bread is prescribed, a prescription which may be of particular importance in patients with the irritable bowel syndrome [17]. A simple exclusion diet is presented in Table 75.3.

Challenge tests

A challenge test can then be carried out, giving the suspect food openly in the first instance and then repeating this challenge, preferably on a double-blind basis with a

Table 75.3. Simple exclusion diet (modified from a diet used at Northwick Park Hospital [6]).

1. Permitted (weeks 1–2)	2. Alternative to 1 (weeks 3–4)	Major exclusions
Lamb or mutton	Beef or chicken	Other meat and poultry. Fish
Gluten free bread, rice (and Rice Krispies)	Rye cripsbread, maize (and cornflakes). Tapioca	Other bread, cakes, biscuits, pasta, cereals
Tomor or Golden Rose margarine	No change	Milk, butter and dairy products. Eggs
Fresh fruit and vegetables	Exclude citrus fruits, apples, beans, peas, soya	Strawberries, nuts, preserves and commercially frozen food
Tea, coffee, sugar, fresh fruit juice	Water or spring water	Wines and spirits
Barley sugar	Corn syrup	Confectionary
Olive oil	Corn oil, sunflower seed oil or cotton seed oil	Other cooking oils

placebo control [7]. The food and 'control' are made up in a similarly flavoured form, and should also be made to be of similar appearance (for example, by adding tomato). Oral challenge is to be preferred to a nasogastric tube, which is unpleasant and may by-pass some important receptor areas [7].

Where there is objective evidence of allergy—for example, in patients who develop urticaria promptly after eating fish or processed food—dietary elimination procedures and food challenge tests can be carried out openly. In other cases, if the patient remains symptom-free on an elimination diet, the omitted foods are reintroduced at three-day intervals until either a satisfactory diet is achieved, or until symptoms recur necessitating the return to a simpler diet. Lack of response to an elimination diet within two to three weeks usually means that food allergy can be excluded. In a few patients it may be justifiable to introduce further empirical dietary changes (Table 75.3) or an even more restricted diet (for example, lamb, pears and spring water).

In life-threatening illness—severe angioedema or eosinophilic gastroenteritis—the use of an 'elemental' diet can be given under hospital supervision, using preparations of the Vivonex type together with bottled water which is presumed to be free of plasticizers. The need for this type of regimen is rare. It should be noted that even these preparations used may not be free from chemical contamination.

One-third of patients with urticaria have a sensitivity to food additives [18]. While it is relatively uncommon for gastrointestinal symptoms to be due to food additives, the possibility needs to be borne in mind. There is a wide range of additives in processed foods and even in what appear to be 'natural foods'—including most types of butter, most bottled or canned drinks, and apparently natural products such as vegetable oil or meats that have been 'tenderized' with papain.

The help of a dietician can be of great value in any dietary approach to investigation or treatment, especially when a 'fresh food only' diet is attempted in patients whose symptoms include urticaria. When urticaria remits on such a diet, attempts should be made to provoke a recurrence by giving capsules containing dyes such as tartrazine (5, 10 or 50 mg), preservatives such as butylated hydroxytoluene or hydroxyanisole (1, 10 or 50 mg), powdered yeast (three B.P. tablets), 0.5 mg penicillin G or—as a control—10 mg lactose. An appropriate interval between different doses of the same substance is 60–90 minutes, which may allow cumulative effects to develop in some patients. When—as frequently happens—urticaria subsides on an elimination diet but then fails to reappear on challenge, the part played by food remains unproven.

Challenge tests do not always induce gastrointestinal symptoms. Nor do they invariably reproduce asthma or other symptoms, even in allergic subjects. Children who are known to wheeze after a cola drink often have no obvious response to challenge in the somewhat artificial environment of a hospital. If however the response to inhaled histamine is measured both before and after the drink is given, an increased sensitivity to histamine can provide useful diagnostic confirmation [39].

Immunological investigations

The simplest, cheapest and most rapid tests for allergy involve pricking antigenic solutions into the skin and measuring the size of the wheals which develop. Their value is limited by the difficulty in standardizing antigenic extracts for this purpose, but nevertheless a number of useful extracts are now available. These include extracts of grass pollen, dust mites, cat protein and other inhaled allergens, as well as certain venoms and a small number of food extracts derived from egg, fish, nut, yeast, soy and chocolate.

The other useful test for IgE-mediated actions is the radioallergosorbent test (RAST) which is more expensive and cumbersome but offers a useful cross-check in patients with equivocal skin test results. Of those patients who have a reproducible adverse reaction to egg, nut or fish, it has been estimated that approximately three-quarters have a positive skin test or RAST [23]. By way of contrast, only 14 out of 46 patients (30%) with milk intolerance or milk allergic symptoms are reported as giving positive skin or radioallergosorbent tests for IgE antibody.

Allergy tests, apart from their ability to confirm the presence of a specific allergy, can also be of value in identifying atopic subjects who have a high total serum IgE concentration or who react to one or more of the commonly inhaled antigens. It is of interest that in one study two-thirds of patients with diarrhoea associated with the irritable bowel syndrome have had their symptoms reproduced during double-blind food challenges [17]. Nevertheless, the serum IgE level was not raised in these patients and no immunological abnormality was found. While this does not exclude an IgE reaction that is confined to the gut, it is notable that the foods that appeared to be responsible for the irritable bowel syndrome include some (wheat, corn, dairy products) that are known to be capable of initiating an immunological reaction—and others (coffee, tea and citrus fruits) for which an immunological role is less certain. IgE or other immunological responses must be regarded as unproven in such patients.

The search for diagnostic laboratory tests continues. While there has been some interest in tests for circulating immune complexes after food challenge, it should be emphasized that these are of research interest but not of diagnostic value. Any discussion of other laboratory tests is largely a catalogue of disappointed hopes. The 'cytotoxic test', which depends on changes in the white cells when whole blood is incubated with an appropriate food, produces highly variable results which are of no value for clinical purposes. Complement activation and lymphocyte transformation tests are no more useful [10], but rises of plasma histamine concentration have been shown to follow food challenge in children with atopic dermatitis [33].

Management

Diet

In cow's milk protein intolerance, the problems of feeding a baby a balanced and well tolerated diet are considerable. While goat's milk may be useful, it is deficient in folate and has the additional disadvantage that it may itself cause sensitization. In difficult cases, oral cromoglycate may, however, provide some additional protection. The use of boiled or evaporated cow's milk or UHT ('Long Life') milk is useful in some subjects, but not when heat-resistant proteins such as beta-lactalbumin or casein are involved. In such patients, casein hydrolysates are well-tolerated but are costly. Soya products are good substitutes but may provoke allergic manifestations. Human milk remains the most effective source of nutrition.

For many adults with food intolerance, simple avoidance of those articles of diet which provoke symptoms is all that is required. An exclusion diet, followed by food challenge, provides the basis to plan dietary treatment. There is, however, the additional problem that a restricted diet requires careful analysis by a dietician to ensure that it is nutritionally adequate.

Drugs

It may also be necessary to provide symptomatic treatment with antispasmodics or to treat manifestations outside the gastrointestinal tract. Drugs and diet sometimes reinforce each other in the treatment of food intolerance or allergy. Those who react to artificial colours or preservatives may not infrequently have an associated intolerance to aspirin and similar drugs. Those who tolerate aspirin, however, sometimes find this drug useful in the symptomatic treatment of diarrhoea or other gastrointestinal reactions. Since cyclo-oxygenase inhibitors can relieve a variety of other types of diarrhoea, the effect is presumably non-specific.

A practical point concerns the need to avoid coloured antihistamine tablets or other pills in patients who are sensitive to artificial colours or preservatives. Useful antihistamines which are not coloured include brompheniramine (Dimotane), mebhydrolin (Fabahistin), hydroxyzine (Atarax), azatadine (Optimine) and terfenadine (Triludan).

Oral sodium cromoglycate has also been claimed to be of value when given prophylactically in patients with relatively mild symptoms [27]. Its use has stimulated interest in other mast cell stabilizing drugs which have still to be fully evaluated.

Prognosis

Milk allergy in the infant is usually a transient disorder, and there is in general a tendency for food allergy which develops in early childhood to remit within one to two years. A relic of the childhood problem can sometimes be found in adults in the form of a persisting skin test reactivity to a food such as egg in a patient who has a past history of food reactions which have long ceased to occur.

In adult life, the development of intolerance to one food is sometimes followed by the acquisition of intolerance to other substances. This is not necessarily associated with evidence of an IgE-mediated reaction, and it is possible that local changes in the intestinal mucosa are responsible for these further developments. It is tempting to see a parallel with bronchial asthma, in which the effects of allergy and of bronchial hyper-reactivity may potentiate one another, but in which the non specific control of bronchial hyper-reactivity offers the most practical method of controlling symptoms. If, like asthma, gastrointestinal reactions to food depend on both allergy and local tissue hypersensitivity, the most practical approach may once again depend on non-specific measures to suppress the hyper-reactive response.

Despite the lack of formal evidence that remissions can be induced by non-specific measures, patients who avoid the foods to which they are intolerant and confine their therapy to drugs that control bowel symptoms not infrequently find that they can gradually extend their diet without provoking fresh symptoms. While there is no evidence, in the form of clinical trial results, which would support this approach, it is worth bearing in mind that it is less obtrusive than the alternatives which include attempts at desensitization, either with food drops or injections. While many claims have been made for these alternative approaches to treatment, there is no acceptable evidence in their favour.

References

1 AMENT ME, RUBIN CE. Soy protein—another cause of the flat intestinal lesion. *Gastroenterology* 1972;**62**:227–234.

2 BAHNA SL, HEINER DC. Cow's milk allergy. *Adv Pediatr* 1978;**25**:1–37.

3 BRANDTZAEG P, TOLO K. Mucosal permeability enhanced by serum-derived antibodies. *Nature* 1977;**266**:262–263.

4 BUISSERET PD. Common manifestations of cow's milk allergy in children. *Lancet* 1978;**i**:304.

5 BUISSERET PD, YOULTEN LJF, HEINZELMANN DI, LESSOF MH. Prostaglandin-sythetase inhibitors in prophylaxis of food intolerance. *Lancet* 1978;**i**:906–908.

6 DENMAN AM. Diagnostic methods and criteria. In: Coombs RAA, ed. *Proceedings of the First Food Allergy Workshop.* Oxford: Medical Education Services, 1980: 47–55.

7 EGGER J, CARTER CM, WILSON J, TURNER MW, SOOTHILL JF. Is migraine food allergy? *Lancet* 1983;**ii**:865–868.

8 FARAH DA, CALDER I, BENSON L, MACKENZIE JF. Specific food intolerance: its place as a cause of gastrointestinal symptoms. *Gut* 1985;**26**:164–168.

9 FERGUSON A. Food-allergic disorders. In: Booth CC, Neale G, eds. *Disorders of the small intestine.* Oxford: Blackwell Scientific Publications, 1986:118–134.

10 FREED DLJ. Laboratory diagnosis of food intolerance. In: Brostoff J, Challacombe SJ, eds. *Food allergy.* London: WB Saunders, 1982:181–203.

11 GYNN CM, INGRAM J, ALMOUSAUR T, STANWORTH DR. Bronchial provocation tests in atopic patients with allergen-specific IgG4 antibodies. *Lancet* 1982;**i**:254 256.

12 HODGSON HJF. Inflammatory bowel disease and food intolerance. *J R Coll Phys* 1986;**20**:45–48.

13 HUNTER JO, JONES VA. Eds. *Food and the gut.* London: Ballière Tyndall, 1985.

14 HUTCHINS P, WALKER-SMITH JA. The gastrointestinal system. In: Brostoff J, Challacombe SJ, eds. *Food allergy.* London: WB Saunders, 1982:43–76.

15 JACKSON PG, LESSOF MH, BAKER RWR, FERRETT J, MACDONALD DM. Intestinal permeability in patients with eczema and food allergy. *Lancet* 1981;**i**:1285–1287.

16 JENKINS HR, PINCOTT JR, SOOTHILL JF, *et al.* Food allergy: the major cause of infantile colitis. *Arch Dis Child* 1984; **59**:326–329.

17 JONES VA, MCLAUGHLIN P, SHORTHOUSE M, WORKMAN E, HUNTER JO. Food intolerance: a major factor in the pathogenesis of irritable bowel syndrome. *Lancet* 1982;**ii**:1115–1117.

18 JUHLIN L. Recurrent urticaria: clinical investigation of 330 patients. *Br J Dermatol* 1981;**104**:369–381.

19 KLEIN NC, HARGROVE RJ, SLESINGER MH, JEFFRIES GH. Eosinophilic gastroenteritis. *Medicine (Baltimore)* 1970;**49**:299–319.

20 LEADER. Infantile bloody diarrhoea and cow's milk. *Lancet* 1984;**i**:1159–60.

21. LESSOF MH. Food intolerance and allergy. *Q J Med* 1983;**52**:111–119.

22 LESSOF MH ed. *Clinical reactions to food.* Chichester: John Wiley and Sons, 1983.

23 LESSOF MH, WRAITH DG, MERRETT TG, MERRETT J, BUISSERET PD. Food allergy and intolerance in 100 patients in local and systemic effects. *Q J Med* 1980;**49**:259–271.

24 MCCALLA R, SAVILANTI E, PERKKIO M, KUITUNEN P, BACKMAN A. Morphology of the jejunum in children with eczema due to food allergy. *Allergy* 1980;**35**:563–571.

25 METCALFE DD, KALINER MA. 'What is food to one ...' *N Engl J Med* 1984;**311**:399–400.

26 Miller K. Sensitivity to tartrazine. *Br Med J* 1982; **285**:1597–1598.

27 Monro J, Carini C, Brostoff J. Migraine is a food-allergic disease. *Lancet* 1984:**ii**:719–721.

28 Parish WE. Evidence for human IgG antibodies anaphylactically sensitizing man. In: Bach MK, ed. *Immediate hypersensitivity, modern concepts and developments.* New York: Marcel Dekker, 1978:277–279.

29 Pearson DJ. Pseudo food allergy. *Br Med J* 1986;**292**:221–222.

30 Pearson DJ, Rix KJB, Bentley SJ. Food allergy: how much in the mind? *Lancet* 1983;**i**:1259–1261.

31 Rosenkrans PCM, Meijer CJLM, Van der Wal AM, Lindeman D. Allergic proctitis, a clinical and pathological entity. *Gut* 1980;**21**:1017–1023.

32 'RCP report 1984'. Food intolerance and food aversion. *A joint report of the Royal College of Physicians and British Nutrition Foundation. J R Coll Physicians,* London 1984;**18**:83–123.

33 Sampson HA, Jolie PL. Increased plasma histamine concentrations after food challenges in children with atopic dermatitis. *N Engl J Med* 1984;**311**:372–376.

34 Soothill JL. Some intrinsic and extrinsic factors predisposing to allergy. *Proc R Soc Med* 1976;439–442.

35 Turner MW, Mowbray JF, Harvey BAM, Brostoff J, Wells RS, Soothill JL. Defective yeast opsonization and C2 deficiency in atopic patients. *Clin Exp Immunol* 1978;**34**:253–259.

36 Vitoria JC, Camarero C, Sojo A, Ruiz A, Rodriguez-Soriano J. Enteropathy related to fish, rice and chicken. *Arch Dis Child* 1982;**57**:44–48.

37 Walker-Smith J, Harrison M, Kilby A, Phillips A, France N. Cow's milk-sensitive enteropathy. *Arch Dis Child* 1978;**53**:375.

38 Wilson FJ, Heiner DC, Lahey ME. Milk-induced gastrointestinal bleeding in infants with hypochromic microcytic anaemia. *JAMA* 1964;**189**:568.

39 Wilson N, Vickers H, Taylor G, Silverman M. Objective test for food sensitivity in asthmatic children: increased bronchial reactivity after cola drinks. *Br Med J* 1982; **284**:1226–1228.

Chapter 76
Congenital Malformations of the Gut

J. WAGGET

Congenital diaphragmatic hernia

Congenital diaphragmatic hernias are commoner on the left than the right; they have
an incidence of approximately one in 2,500
live births. The congenital defect of the diaphragm may, if very large, amount to the
complete absence of a hemidiaphragm.

Symptoms of respiratory distress usually
develop within 24 hours of birth. Survival
depends not upon the size of the defect, but
upon the degree of pulmonary hypoplasia.
Distension of the intestinal tract with swallowed air can further reduce the cardiorespiratory reserve by pressing on the lungs
and heart.

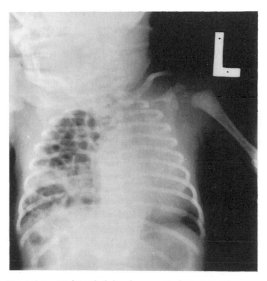

Fig. 76.2. Right-sided diaphragmatic hernia with
multiple gas filled loops of small intestine in right
chest, heart displaced to the left.

In general, the earlier the onset of symptoms the worse is the prognosis. A chest
radiograph is taken to confirm the diagnosis
(Figs 76.1 and 76.2). On-the-spot emergency treatment includes passage of a nasogastric tube (FG 8, if possible), aspirating
it regularly and leaving it to free drainage
between aspirations. Oxygen is given by
face mask. If the baby's condition stabilizes
with this simple treatment, artificial ventilation and intubation are withheld. The decision whether or not to give artificial ventilation is extremely difficult—ventilation by
endotracheal tube may cause a pneumothorax, but ventilation by face mask carries
the added danger of further intestinal distension.

Immediate transfer to a neonatal surgical

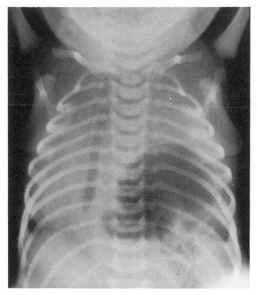

Fig. 76.1. Left-sided diaphragmatic hernia with large
gastric air shadow; air in displaced oesophagus, heart
and mediastinum to the right.

service is necessary where surgery is performed without delay. Reduction of the bowel from the chest and repair of the defect are performed best through a high oblique abdominal incision, which can be extended into an intercostal space if necessary. The abdominal approach also allows correction of a commonly-associated intestinal malrotation. Postoperative problems include tension pneumothorax, bilateral pneumomediastinum, pulmonary hypertension, pulmonary interstitial emphysema and paradoxical movements of the affected diaphragm, especially if a patch has been required to close the defect [42]. Most babies will require intermittent positive pressure ventilation following surgery.

The hypoplastic lung does grow to a limited extent in the weeks following operation. Follow-up investigations have shown there is decreased perfusion of the affected lung but, if the children survive the newborn period, most are able to lead normal active lives [6].

Oesophageal atresia with tracheo-oesophageal fistula

Oesophageal atresia with tracheo-oesophageal fistula, and upper intestinal atresia, are the commonest treatable foetal causes of polyhydramnios. The diagnosis can be made antenatally by ultrasound, which identifies amniotic fluid in the dilated proximal oesophageal blind pouch.

Tracheo-oesophageal fistula occurs in one out of 3,500 live births. Associated congenital abnormalities occur in about one-third of patients, the commonest being heart disease, other atresias of the intestinal tract including imperforate anus and urinary tract abnormalities [20, 27].

Some maternity units screen for tracheo-oesophageal fistula by passing a nasal catheter into the pharynx at birth—the catheter is held up in the blind upper pouch of the oesophagus. If this diagnosis

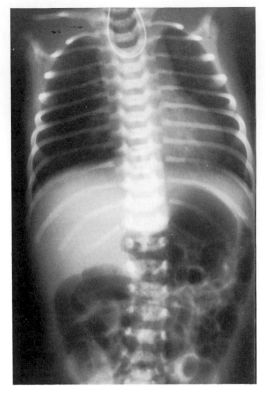

Fig. 76.3. Erect radiograph with radio-opaque catheter in blind upper oesophageal pouch.

is suspected, continuous pharyngeal suction must be started immediately, preferably with a double-lumen Replogle tube (Argyle, Sherwood Medical). The next investigation is an erect chest and abdominal X-ray, with a lateral view of the chest. The catheter has a radio-opaque line; it is pushed gently downwards while the radiograph is being taken (Fig. 76.3). Air in the intestinal tract below the diaphragm will indicate the presence of a fistula from trachea to lower oesophagus; the catheter curled in the upper pouch will give an indication of the length of the upper oesophageal segment.

Oesophageal atresia with a tracheo-oesophageal fistula accounts for approximately 95% of cases (Fig. 76.4). End-to-end anastomosis is usually possible—the operation is best performed with an extraplural approach through a right thoracotomy at

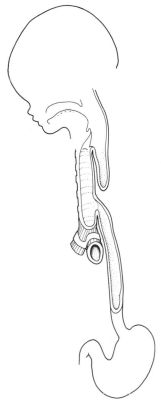

Fig. 76.4. Diagram of the commonest form of oesophageal atresia with tracheo-oesophageal fistula.

tension on the suture line—most surgeons use a single layer of fine, interrupted non-absorbable sutures to complete this anastomosis. The tension can be eased by circular myotomies on the upper pouch (Fig. 76.5) and even on the lower segment; they are best performed before the anastomosis is started. A myotomy does not adversely affect later oesophageal function [5, 24, 36].

Early complications include pneumonia (often secondary to aspiration before surgery), leak from the anastomosis, recurrent fistula and stricture. All patients have disordered motility of the oesophagus which is worse in the distal segment; gastro-oesophageal reflux is common [26]. The 'brassy' cough is often mistakenly treated as a respiratory infection. Respiratory infections, however, are frequent in the early years and may be related to aspiration secondary to disordered motility or to gastro-oesophageal reflux. Tracheal instability causing apnoea and cyanotic attacks may need tracheopexy [10, 14]. The less common varieties of oesophageal atresia may need staged surgery for successful repair [11, 17, 21, 45].

the fourth or fifth interspace. The fistula is divided and the tracheal end sutured. During the operation the surgeon has to balance the problems of blood supply versus

Gastroschisis and exomphalos

Gastroschisis and exomphalos are congenital defects of the abdominal wall which

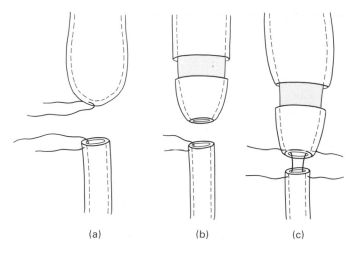

(a)   (b)   (c)

Fig. 76.5. Circular myotomy on upper oesophageal pouch to decrease tension on suture line [29]; (a) holding sutures on upper and lower segments; (b) myotomy performed; (c) sutures drawing two ends together passing through all layers of oesophageal wall.

have major implications for the intestinal tract. They are obvious at birth, but some cases have been diagnosed during intrauterine life following screening for neural tube defects. The amniotic-fetoprotein concentration is raised, as is cholinesterase activity [13].

Purists may argue over differentiation between the two conditions, but from the practical point of view the surgical management is very similar. In **gastroschisis** the intestines prolapse alongside the umbilical ring, and the umbilical cord is usually to the left of the prolapsed bowel. In **exomphalos**, which represents a failure of closure of the umbilical ring, the bowel is usually covered with a membrane formed by the stretched-out base of the umbilical cord. In gastroschisis and exomphalos which has ruptured the intestines are coated with a thick membrane which gives them a rubbery consistency. There is usually an element of malrotation of the mid-gut in both conditions; atresias of the intestinal tract occur in approximately 10% of patients with gastroschisis. Exomphalos is also associated with other congenital abnormalities, such as congenital heart disease; it is also a major element in the Beckwith-Weiderman syndrome [39].

The emergency care of such babies is to prevent hypothermia, to prevent kinking of the bowel and liver over the edge of the defect and to prevent vomiting or aspiration. The intestines, and especially the liver, must be kept from kinking acutely over the edge of the defect—even if this means that one person is solely responsible for holding them in place. If blood becomes trapped within the liver it can swell enormously, taking blood from the general circulation and making reduction of the liver back into the abdominal cavity extremely difficult. For transport, sterile dressings are packed round the abdominal viscera and an intestinal bag, Vi-drape (Parke Davis) or a clear polyethylene bag is drawn over the lower part of the baby up to the axillae. A nasogastric tube is placed to prevent vomiting and aspiration, using the largest tube that can be passed reasonably through the baby's nose. The baby is wrapped in insulating foil and transported in an incubator to a specialist neonatal surgical unit.

The treatment of choice is to reduce the bowel and liver back into the peritoneal cavity at the primary operation. The defect is closed primarily, or with a patch, and skin is then mobilized and closed in a separate layer. Primary closure must neither compromise blood supply to the abdominal contents nor splint the diaphragm so as to prevent breathing. It must also not impair venous return from the legs. If closure cannot be obtained without these complications, the contents may be reduced in stages by closure with either skin alone or a silastic silo (Fig. 76.6). Recently, chemically-dehydrated human dura [16] has been used to close the defect with or, as in the illustrated patient (Fig. 76.7), without skin closure over the repair.

It may be necessary to carry out nasotracheal intubation and intermittent positive pressure ventilation postoperatively. Nutrition is maintained intravenously until the baby can take adequate enteral feeds—normally up to three weeks [33].

Duodenal atresia and stenosis

Duodenal atresia presents in the first few hours of life with bile-stained vomiting, usually without abdominal distension. The atresia may be present in various forms and an aberrant pancreas may surround the duodenum as part of the anomaly. It may also coexist with malrotation, oesophageal atresia, vertebral defects, imperforate anus and congenital heart disease. There is also a strong association with Down's syndrome.

A plain erect radiograph of the abdomen is usually all that is necessary to confirm

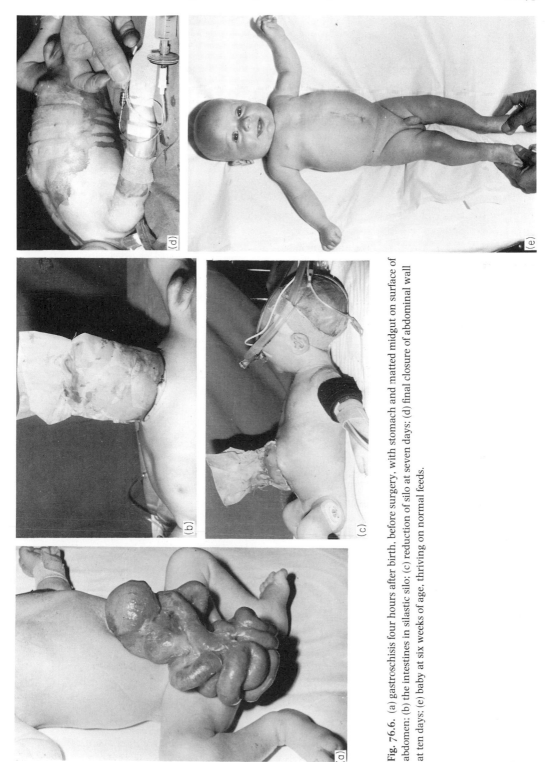

Fig. 76.6. (a) gastroschisis four hours after birth, before surgery, with stomach and matted midgut on surface of abdomen; (b) the intestines in silastic silo; (c) reduction of silo at seven days; (d) final closure of abdominal wall at ten days; (e) baby at six weeks of age, thriving on normal feeds.

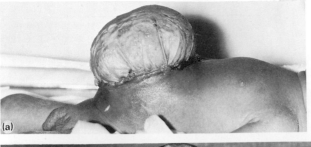

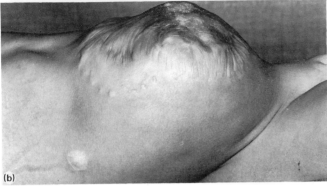

Fig. 76.7. (a) human dura closing
large exomphalos which had
ruptured following skin closure.
New blood vessels invading dural
patch. (b) abdominal wall at one
year, following human dura
closure of abdominal wall. Seen
from right side of patient, who is
thriving.

the diagnosis. The typical 'double bubble',
with air-fluid levels in stomach and dilated
duodenum, confirm the diagnosis (Fig.
76.8).

A nasogastric tube is passed as soon as
the diagnosis is suspected, aspirated and left
to free drainage. The baby is transferred to
a neonatal surgical service. Vitamin K 1 mg
is given by intramuscular injection. Blood
is cross-matched and a laparotomy carried
out immediately.

The treatment of choice is anastomosis
by the most direct method. A duodenoduo-
denostomy is preferable to a duodenojejunostomy, with suture lines such that there
is no encroachment on the ampullary area.

Intravenous nutrition is preferable to a
trans-anastomotic feeding tube, as the anastomosis does not become functionally patent for 10 to 14 days.

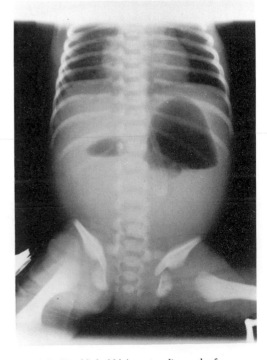

Fig. 76.8. 'Double bubble' erect radiograph of
duodenal atresia.

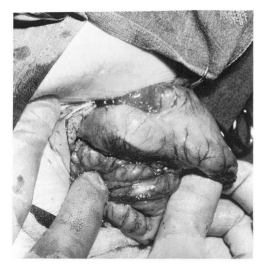

Fig. 76.9. Pyloric 'tumour' of hypertrophicpyloric stenosis exposed at operation.

Infantile hypertrophic pyloric stenosis

Pyloric stenosis in early life has an incidence of approximately 3 per 1,000 live births (male:female ratio 5:1). It is familial, involving both genetic and environmental factors [8]. Studies of plasma gastrin concentration have produced conflicting evidence [38,41]; concentrations of motilin, gastric inhibitory peptide, enteroglucagon and neurotensin are all low [9]. Hypertrophic pyloric stenosis is associated with gastro-oesophageal reflux, and anomalies of the genitourinary tract [1]. The muscle of the pyloric canal becomes hypertrophied and oedematous causing obstruction of the outlet of the stomach (Figs 76.9 and 76.10).

The peak incidence of presentation is about six weeks of age, but it has been reported in the first few days of life and up to

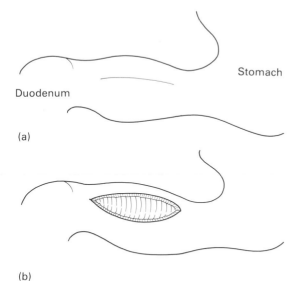

Duodenum

Stomach

(a)

(b)

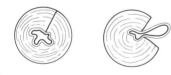

(c)

Fig. 76.10. (a) diagram of Fig. 76.9 with incision along upper border area of least vascularity; (b) Split in circular muscle with mucosa pouting; (c) Transverse section of pylorus, before and after myotomy.

the age of three months. The presenting symptom is non-bilious vomiting. At first the baby is hungry and will retake a feed immediately after vomiting if one is offered. Sooner or later the vomiting becomes projectile. Some babies have a small 'coffee ground' haematemesis due to gastritis; most are constipated. The infant soon becomes dehydrated, wasted and lethargic. There is a metabolic alkalosis, due to the loss of gastric acid with potassium depletion.

The physical findings in the abdomen are visible gastric peristalsis, and a palpable pyloric tumour which softens and hardens as peristalsis passes through it. The tumour is most easily felt during a test feed. If the tumour cannot be felt a barium meal with a small amount of barium (5 ml) will outline the elongated and narrowed pyloric canal. Delayed gastric emptying alone is not diagnostic.

The baby who is dehydrated and alkalotic may require 24 to 48 hours preoperative fluid therapy to rehydrate and correct the metabolic abnormalities. Operation is best performed under general anaesthesia, but local anaesthesia is still used in some centres [7].

Pyloromyotomy is curative, dividing all the circular muscle of the pyloric canal. Occasionally the mucosa at the duodenal end of the myotomy is perforated but, if this is recognized and closed with fine interrupted sutures, it does not give rise to further problems. Wound infection and more serious wound dehiscence are the main postoperative complications. Vomiting is not uncommon in the build-up to normal postoperative feeds. It may be due to gastritis or an associated hiatus hernia with gastro-oesophageal reflux. The infant can be fed six hours following operation with a dextrose feed, building up to full strength feeds at normal volumes within about 48 hours.

Duplications

Accessory enteric formations include duplications, vitelline remnants and dorsal enteric remnants [2, 15, 40].

Duplications are tubular or cystic segments of the intestinal tract, which are in contiguity with the normal bowel sharing a common blood supply [19]. Cystic duplications do not usually communicate with the intestinal tract, unlike the tubular forms. The dividing wall may be complete or a double layer of epithelium; the epithelium may contain ectopic gastric mucosa. They are uncommon, may be multiple, and are associated with vertebral abnormalities. Most present in childhood, but they can present even in the elderly [30].

Duplications cause problems by increasing in size causing obstruction, ulceration and volvulus and by peptic ulceration due to gastric ectopic mucosa. They occur at any site in the intestinal tract, but are commonest in the small bowel, presenting as a mass, distension, vomiting or rectal bleeding.

In the abdomen, where technically feasible, complete resection of the contiguous bowel with the duplication is the treatment of choice. In other sites total excision is also preferable as remaining ectopic gastric mucosa may cause ulceration [35]. In a few instances submucosal resection may be feasible [12].

Case reports

A baby girl had one episode of blood *per rectum* at the age of six months. Seven months later, dark blood was mixed with the stool in every nappy. A technetium scan showed rapid appearance of radioactivity in the right lower quadrant. Histology of the specimen (Fig. 76.11) showed areas of ectopic gastric mucosa lining the duplication, with a peptic ulcer

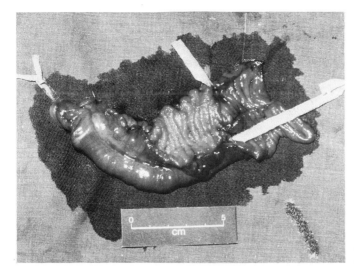

Fig. 76.11. Photograph of resected specimen with tape through normal lumen, opened at distal end when it is joined by the tubular duplication which is partly lined by gastric mucosa. A 0.5 cm penetrating peptic ulcer lies at the junction of the mucosa, indicated by the smaller tape.

penetrating deep into the intestinal wall. The duplication was resected with the contiguous small bowel and an end-to-end anastomosis performed. The child made an uneventful recovery.

A five-week-old baby had a three-day history of progressive bilious vomiting with abdominal distension. X-rays showed small bowel obstruction. A laparotomy revealed a cystic duplication (Fig. 76.12) which was causing a volvulus of the distal ileum. The duplication was lined in part with gastric epithelium. The overlying bowel was resected with an end-to-end anastomosis. The baby made an uneventful recovery.

Malrotation

Malrotation of the midgut results from a failure of normal rotation and peritoneal fixation when the intestines return from the physiological hernia to the abdominal cavity in the tenth week of intrauterine life [4]. The normal peritoneal folds and attachments, which hold the superior mesenteric pedicle of vessels across a broad base on the posterior abdominal wall, do not occur. The ascending and descending colon are normally not mobile, being held in place by peritoneal reflections. In malrotation the whole of the midgut is highly mobile—the normal curve of the third and fourth parts of duodenum is absent; the caecum is often

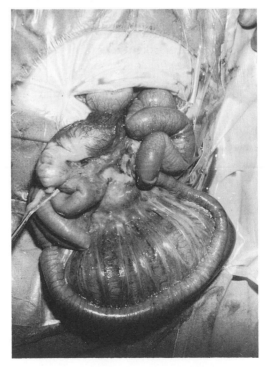

Fig. 76.12. Cystic duplication of terminal ileum which caused a volvulus.

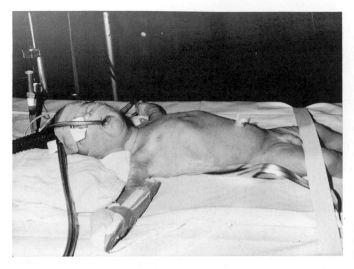

Fig. 76.13. Malrotation and volvulus, presenting with scaphoid abdomen.

high and to the left of the duodenum; adhesions running across the front of the duodenum from the caecum may kink and obstruct it.

Patients may present with intermittent abdominal pain and vomiting, or with vomiting and bleeding *per rectum*. Some patients present as failure to thrive with vomiting [22], but normal rotation with non-fixation of the mudgut may cause the same clinical picture [23].

Volvulus of part or all of the midgut is a serious complication of malrotation that may occur at any time, but has its peak incidence in the first week of life. The new-born infant develops bile-stained vomiting after a few days of normal feeding and may have had changing stools. The abdomen is not distended and may even be scaphoid (Fig. 76.13). The diagnosis must be suspected on these few symptoms and signs—urgent investigation and laparotomy are necessary. In the later stages of volvulus the baby may vomit blood or pass blood *per rectum*, developing abdominal distension due to blood accumulating in the twisted bowel. These signs indicate that infarction of the intestines is already taking place.

Once the diagnosis is suspected, erect and supine radiographs (Fig. 76.14 (a)(b)) often show air-fluid levels in the stomach, but a paucity of gas in the rest of the intestinal tract. A small amount of barium sulphate passed into the stomach will demonstrate the misshapen duodenal loop (Fig. 76.14(c)).

Surgery must not be delayed as one cannot forecast when infarction will take place. Laparotomy is carried out through a transverse incision—all the midgut is delivered onto the surface, dividing adhesions to free the duodenum. There is sometimes considerable oozing from the adhesions, and blood transfusion may be necessary. The mesenteric pedicle is widened and the colon lies on the left, as shown in Fig. 76.15. Appendicectomy is performed as the caecum usually lies in the left lower quadrant. Fixation of the intestines in the non-rotated position is unnecessary [43].

Atresia of the small intestine

Polyhydramnios is often present during pregnancy. The clinical features are bilious vomiting, abdominal distension and the failure to pass meconium. A plain radiograph in the erect and supine positions will confirm the diagnosis. A large nasogastric

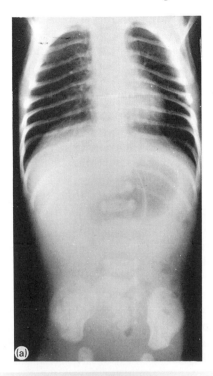

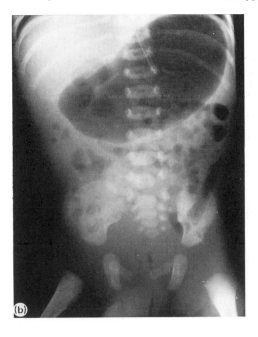

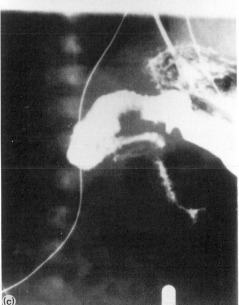

Fig. 76.14. (a) malrotation and volvulus—erect X-ray of five-day-old 1.2 kg baby who had bile-stained vomiting, but normal stools. No fluid levels on this film. (b) radiograph of same baby three days later when flecks of blood had been noted in stools. (c) barium meal showing abnormal loop and obstruction of duodenum. Laparotomy later that day confirmed malrotation with volvulus with viable midgut.

tube is passed and the child is transported to a neonatal surgical unit. Laparotomy is carried out through an upper abdominal transverse incision. A check is made for multiple atresias—it may be necessary to perform several anastomoses to preserve a minimum length of small intestine for survival. This minimum length is probably about 40 cm, but there is difficulty in assessing the exact minimum length as other factors, such as the presence of the ileocaecal valve and terminal ileum, are important. The proximal anastomosis is often very oblique, due to disparity in size between proximal and distal bowel. This does not usually become functional for about two weeks following surgery, so intravenous nutritional support is necessary until full feeds can be established [33]. If there is a very short length of the intestine, the nutritional support may have to be continued for several months, to allow time for intestinal growth and adaptation.

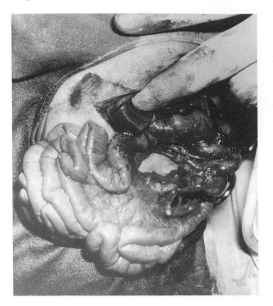

Fig. 76.15. Malrotation with pedicle widened at operation prior to appendicectomy. Large bowel on left. The duodenum lies fairly straight down from underneath the liver on the right.

Case reports

A female child weighed 2.5 kg at birth. Polyhydramnios was present during pregnancy. At laparotomy there were multiple atresias with a gap in the mesentery and an 'apple peel bowel' of the distal small intestine (Fig. 76.16). An adequate length of intestine was present, but intravenous feeding was needed postoperatively for three weeks before the child could take full oral feeds. She began to thrive properly at nine weeks of age.

A male child, born at 38 weeks gestation, weighed 3 kg. Polyhydramnios was present during pregnancy. He was noted to be distended shortly after birth and vomited bile-stained fluid. A plain X-ray of the abdomen suggested a duodenal obstruction, but on clinical examination there was a visible and palpable loop of bowel (Fig. 76.17). Laparotomy revealed a malrotation with duodenal obstruction caused by adhesions and a jejunal atresia with disparity of the lumen between proximal and distal bowel (Fig. 76.18). Resection and end-to-end anastomosis (Fig. 76.19) were performed, the malrotation corrected and an appendicectomy was carried out. He was discharged home at two weeks, feeding well, and has thrived normally since then.

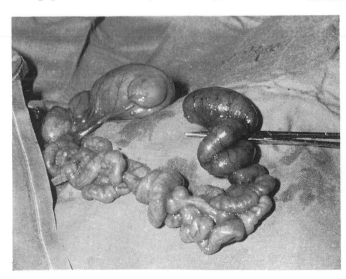

Fig. 76.16. Multiple small bowel atresia with loss of bowel and mesentery, and 'apple peel' bowel spiralling round blood vessels.

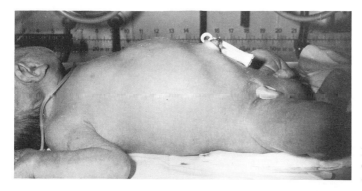

Fig. 76.17. Upper abdominal distension caused by jejunal atresia.

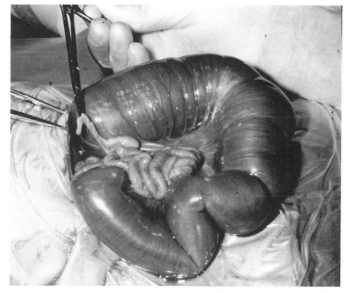

Fig. 76.18. Operative findings with a single atresia without loss of intestinal length, but great disparity in lumen.

Anorectal anomalies

Anorectal anomalies result from the failure of proper descent of the urorectal septum and its failure to fuse with the cloacal membrane, together with excessive fusion of the skin developed from the anal tubercles [4]. There is usually a fistula from the bowel to the genitourinary tract. Attempts have been made to agree on an international classification [25, 44].

There is a high incidence of other congenital abnormalities of the intestinal tract, such as oesophageal atresia, tracheo-oesophageal fistula and duodenal atresia. Cardiac abnormalities and genitourinary tract abnormalities are also very common. Some of the children may already have damage to the urinary tract, especially the female with a cloaca who already may have serious hydronephrosis and hydroureter at birth, secondary to obstruction caused by the accumulation of faeces and urine in the cloaca [18]. Sacral agenesis is not uncommon and carries a bad prognosis for future continence.

If there is no perineal opening or fistula (Figs 76.20 and 76.21) or vulval opening in the female, a right transverse colostomy must be performed. An exception may be in cloaca where it may be preferable to detach the bowel from the cloaca and bring this to

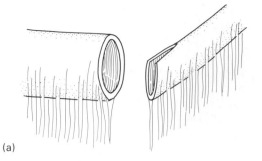

(a)

Fig. 76.19. Technique of 'end-to-back' anastomosis, with inversion of proximal bowel.

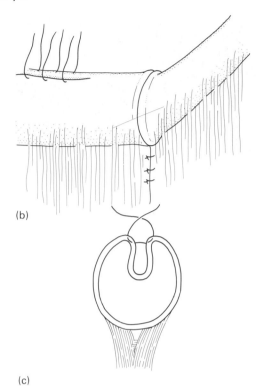

(b)

(c)

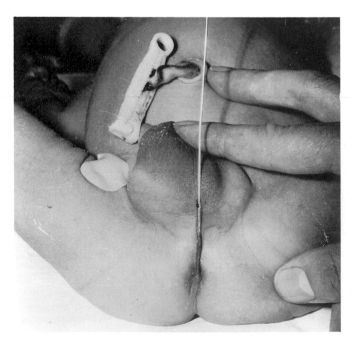

Fig. 76.20. The reward for careful physical examination in an anorectal anomaly—one that can be dealt with from below. Fine eye-probe in fistula.

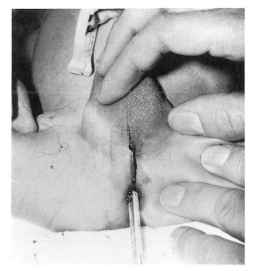

Fig. 76.21. Perineal fistula opened up and anal canal exposed.

the surface as an end colostomy. Plain radiographs have little value preoperatively in making the decision as to whether the anomaly requires a colostomy. It is important, when planning definitive surgery, to obtain a retrograde vaginogram, cloacogram or urethrogram (Fig. 76.22). An intravenous pyelogram is carried out in the first six months to check on the anatomy of the urinary tract.

Definitive surgery is carried out when the infant weighs about 10 kg—at this size the pelvic anatomy is big enough to allow access for surgery, which can in most cases be completed through a sacroperineal approach. The rectum can be dissected from behind, off the back of the vagina or urethra, with minimal trauma. A 'cone' dissection, limiting the dissection close to the rectal wall, avoids damage to other pelvic structures, such as the nerves to the bladder. It is extremely important to detach urethral fistulae as close to the urethra as possible to avoid the serious complication of a urethral diverticulum or a recurrence of the

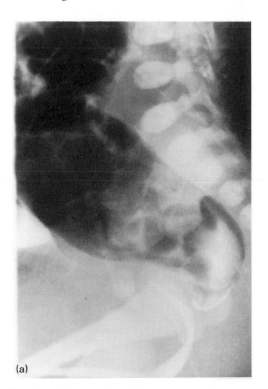

(a)

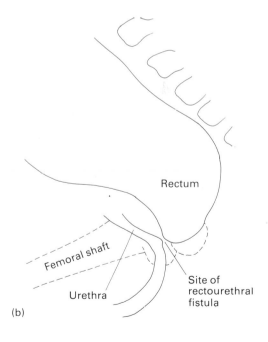

Rectum

Femoral shaft

Urethra

Site of rectourethral fistula

(b)

Fig. 76.22. Retrograde urethrogram in a male infant with contrast in urethra and distal rectum.

fistula. Both of these complications are extremely difficult to deal with at secondary operations [46].

From the sacroperineal approach the levator sling can be identified carefully and bowel brought down to the perineum anterior to this muscle without damage. A posterior approach dividing the levator in the mid-line has been described [34]. Early reports of follow-up suggest that this direct approach, with tailoring of the rectum, may be at least as satisfactory in the long-term. The child is usually about one year of age when the definitive surgery is undertaken; this gives time for colostomy closure about two months later and a long period for bowel training to become effective before the child needs to start at school. Entrance to school is an important fixed landmark and, although continence will never be 'normal', a 'learned continence which is socially acceptable' [31] can usually be obtained. These children lack normal anorectal sensation—the fine discrimination between faeces, fluid and flatus is lacking.

Just as important as the surgery is the careful follow-up, preferably by the same team at regular intervals. The results are closely related to the understanding and support given to the child throughout the early years by family and professionals. They can be helped by encouraging regular bowel actions with firm faeces. In later childhood the use of bio-feedback has also proved helpful to increase the child's awareness of his levator function [32].

Abdominal situs inversus

This is a rare condition that is frequently associated with serious congenital cardiac anomalies [28] and congenital asplenia. The cardiac anomalies are more likely to cause symptoms than the situs inversus of the abdominal viscera.

References

1 ATWELL JD, LEVICK P. Congenital hypertrophic pyloric stenosis and associated abnormalities in the genitourinary tract. *J Pediatr Surg* 1981;**16**:1029–1035.

2 BENTLEY JFR, SMITH JR. Developmental posterior enteric remnants and spinal malformations. *Arch Dis Child* 1960;**35**:76–86.

3 BILL AH. Malrotation of the intestine. In: Ravitch MM, Welch KJ, Benson CD, Abereeen E, Randolph JG, eds. *Pediatric Surgery*. 3rd ed. Chicago, London: Year Book Medical Publishers, 1979:912–923.

4 BILL AH, JOHNSON RJ. Failure to migration of the rectal opening as the cause for most cases of imperforate anus. *Surg Gynecol Obstet* 1958;**106**:643–651.

5 BOOS D, HOLLWORTH M, BAUER H. Endoscopic esophageal anastomosis. *J Pediatr Surg* 1982;**17**:138–143.

6 BRAY RJ. Congenital diaphragmatic hernia. Review Article. *Anaesthesia* 1979;**34**:567–577.

7 BRISTOL JB, BOLTON RA. The results of Ramstedt's operation in a District General Hospital. *Br J Surg* 1981;**68**:590–592.

8 CARTER CO, EVANS KA. Inheritance of congenital pyloric stenosis. *J Med Genet* 1969;**6**:233–254.

9 CHRISTOFIDES ND, MALLET E, GHATEI MA, LEE Y, BLOOM SR. Plasma enteroglucagon and neuro tension in infantile pyloric stenosis. *Arch Dis Child* 1983;**58**:52–55.

10 COHEN D. Tracheopexy—aorto-tracheal suspension for severe trancheomalacia. *Aust Paediatr J* 1981;**17**:117–121.

11 COHEN DH, MIDDLETON A, FLETCHER J. Gastric tube oesophagoplasty. *J Pediatr Surg* 1974;**9**:451–460.

12 COOKSEY G, WAGGET J. Tubular duplication of the rectum treated by mucosal sleeve resection. *J Pediatr Surg.* 1984;**19**(3):318–319.

13 DALE G, ARCHIBALD A, BONIIAM JR, LOWDON P. Diagnosis of neural tube defects by estimation of amniotic fluid acetyl cholinesterase. *Br J Obstet Gynecol* 1981;**88**:120–125.

14 FILLER RM, ROSSELO PJ, LEBOWITZ RL. Life threatening anoxic speels caused by tracheal compression after repair of oesophageal atresia: correction by surgery. *J Pediatr Surg* 1976;**11**:739–748.

15 FORSHALL I. Duplications of the intestinal tract. *Postgrad Med J* 1961;**37**:570–589.

16 GAUGER JU, WILLITAL GH. The use of solvent dehydrated dura in surgery. *Munch Med Wochen* 1979;**121**:603–604.

17 GOUGH MH. Esophageal atresia—use of an anterior flap in the difficult anastomosis. *J Pediatr Surg* 1980;**15**:310–311.

18 HENDREN WH. Further experience of reconstructive surgery for cloacal anomalies. *J Pediatr Surg* 1982;**17**:695–717.

19 HOCKING M, YOUNG DG. Duplications of the alimentary tract. *Br J Surg* 1981;**68**:92–96.

20 HOLDER TM, ASHCRAFT KW. Developments in the care of patients with esophageal atresia and tracheo-oesophageal fistula. *Surg Clin North Am* 1981;**61**:1051–1061.

21 HOWARD R, MYERS NA. Esophageal atresia: A technique for elongating the upper pouch. *Surgery* 1965;**58**:725–727.

22 HOWELL DG, VOZZA F, SHAW S, *et al.* Malrotation, malnutrition and ischemic bowel disease. *J Pediatr Surg* 1981;**17**:469–473.

23 JANIK JS, EIN SH. Normal intestinal rotation with non-fixation; a cause of chronic abdominal pain. *J Pediatr Surg* 1979;**14**:670–674.

24 JANIK JS, FILLER RM, EIN SH, SIMPSON JS. Longterm follow-up of circular myotomy for esophageal atresia. *J Pediatr Surg* 1980;**15**:835–841.

25 JAPAN STUDY GROUP OF ANO-RECTAL ANOMALIES. A group study of the classification of ano-rectal anomalies in Japan with comments to the International Classification, 1970. *J Pediatr Surg* 1982;**17**:302–308.

26 JOLLEY SG, JOHNSON DG, ROBERTS CC, *et al.* Patterns of gastroesophageal reflux in children following repair of esophageal atresia and distal tracheo-oesophageal fistula. *J Pediatr Surg* 1980;**15**:857–862.

27 KLUTH D. Atlas of esophageal atresia. *J Pediatr Surg* 1976;**11**:901–919.

28 KUENZLER R. Positional anomalies of the heart. In: Graham G, Ross R, eds. *Heart Disease in Infants and Children.* Edward Arnold: London, 1980:387–393.

29 LIVATIDIS A, RADBERG L, ODENSJO G. Esophageal end to end anastomosis: reduction of anastomotic tension by circular myotomy. *Scand J Thorac Cardiovasc Surg* 1972;**6**:206–214.

30 MAIR WSJ, ABBOTT CR. Perforation of an ileal duplication in old age. *Br Med J* 1976;**2**:621.

31 NIXON HH. Congenital abnormalities of the gut. *Br J Hosp Med* 1977;**18**:202–219.

32 OLNESS K, McPARLAND FA, PIPER J. Biofeedback: a new modality in the management of faecal soiling. *J Pediatr* 1980;**96**:505–509.

33 PANTER-BRICK M, WAGGET J, DALE G. In: Karran SJ, Alberti KGMM, eds. *Practical nutritional support.* Pitman Medical: Tunbridge Wells, 1980:261–274.

34 PENA A, DEVRIES PA. Posterior sagittal anorectoplasty: important technical considerations and new applications. *J Pediatr Surg* 1982;**17**:796–811.

35 RANGECROFT L, WAGGET J. Gastric duplication cyst of neck: case report. *Zeit Kinderchir* 1977;**22**:173–175.

36 RÉHBEIN F, SCHEDER N. Reconstruction of the oesophagus without colon transplantation in cases of atresia. *J Pediatr Surg* 1971;**6**:746–752.

37 RICKETTS RR, LUCK SR, RAFFENSBERGER JG. Circular esophagomyotomy for primary repair of long-gap esophageal atresia. *J Pediatr Surg* 1981;**16**:365–369.

38 RODGERS BM, DIX PM, TALBERT JL, *et al.* Fasting and postprandial serum gastrin in normal human neonates. *J Pediatr Surg* 1978;**13**:13–16.

39 SMITH DW. Recognisable patterns of human malformation. In: *Major problems in clinical pediatrics* Vol. VII, 3rd ed. Philadelphia: W B Saunders 1982.

40 SMITH JR. Accessory enteric formations: a classification and nomenclature. *Arch Dis Child* 1960;**35**:87–89.

41 SPITZ L, ZAILE SS. Serum gastrin level in congenital hypertrophic pyloric stenosis. *J Pediatr Surg* 1976;**11**:33–35.

42 SROUJI MN, BUCK B, DOWNES JJ. Congenital diaphragmatic hernia: deleterious effects of pulmonary interstitial emphysema and tension extra-pulmonary air. *J Pediatr Surg* 1981;**16**:45–54.

43 STAUFFER UG, HERMANN P. Comparison of late results in patients with corrected intestinal malrotation with and without fixation of the mesentery. *J Pediatr Surg* 1980;**15**:9–12.

44 STEPHENS FD, SMITH ED. *Ano-rectal malformations in children.* Chicago: Year Book Medical Publishers, 1971.

45 WATERSON D. Colonic replacement of esophagus (intra thoracic). *Surg Clin North Am* 1964;**44**:1441–1447.

46 WISEMAN NE, DECTER A. The Kraske approach to the repair of recurrent recto-urethral fistula. *J Pediatr Surg* 1982;**17**:342–346.

Chapter 77
Gastrointestinal Disease in Children

R. NELSON

The common gastrointestinal diseases of children are closely related to age. In the neonate there are problems related to birth, and congenital or inherited disorders. Infants predominantly suffer from malabsorption syndromes or infection, and school children tend to present with functional disorders. During adolescence the commoner diseases of young adults need to be considered.

Periods of rapid growth and development are periods of increased vulnerability to growth retardation and malnutrition; the effects of gastrointestinal disease and its treatment must be monitored carefully.

Gastrointestinal disease related to age

The neonatal period

This is the first four weeks of life, when medical problems often arise from mishaps involving the hazardous processes of birth and adaptation to extrauterine life. Neonatal necrotizing enterocolitis is of unknown aetiology, but it is strongly associated with prematurity, neonatal asphyxia, and the introduction of enteric feeding.

After birth there is a sudden change from continuous intravenous placental nutrition to intermittent enteral nutrition. The complex interrelated functions of the gut vary considerably in their state of maturity and readiness for the normal processes of ingestion, digestion, absorption and elimination. Compared with older individuals, normal full-term and particularly preterm neonates have significant malabsorption [37]. These features of the new-born gastrointestinal tract need consideration during the feeding of neonates, particularly extremely premature infants in whom optimum growth rates are difficult to achieve by enteral feeding. The age of maturation of different gut functions varies considerably. For example, digestive enzyme secretion by the exocrine pancreas is not fully developed until several months after birth, but the activity of the small intestinal brush-border enzymes such as the disaccharidases reach full maturity by term. Some aspects of postnatal gastrointestinal maturation may depend upon oral feeding and may be initiated by the surge of gastrointestinal hormone secretion that follows the initial feeds after birth [39].

The neonate is also influenced after birth by the persistent effects of maternal metabolism—for example, maternal gastrin hypersecretion in late pregnancy produces an increased gastric parietal cell mass and acid hypersecretion in the new-born infant, which is occasionally associated with peptic ulceration.

Congenital malformation (see Chapter 76) and inborn errors of metabolism are individually rare, but collectively fairly common. Many such disorders involving the alimentary system will present with clinical features shortly after birth and the introduction of enteral feeding—for example, gastrointestinal obstruction or congenital glucose-galactose malabsorption. Cystic fibrosis is the commonest recessively-inherited disorder, and it can now be detected by neonatal screening tests.

Infancy and the early pre-school period

Infancy is a period of very rapid growth, when many babies increase their weight by 200% and their length by 50%. Compared with older individuals, the infant's calorie, protein, mineral and water requirements are high relative to its size. The effects of acute and chronic gastrointestinal disease are typically more dramatic than in later life— for example water and electrolyte depletion during gastroenteritis is more common in young infants.

Table 77.1. Coeliac disease—variation in clinical picture at different ages.

Age	Clinical features
Early infancy (first six months)	Early weaning—usually before one month old. Acute vomiting and diarrhoea. Dehydration and severe malnutrition. Secondary sugar and protein intolerance.
Late infancy or early childhood	Vomiting—often projectile. Diarrhoea and steatorrhoea. Severe anorexia and failure to thrive. Lethargy and muscular hypotonia. Abdominal distension.
Middle childhood	Chronic malabsorption. Anaemia and vitamin deficiencies. Moderate abdominal distension. Growth failure.
Late childhood or adolescence	Growth failure. Anaemia—iron and folate deficiency. Delay in sexual development. Bowels may be normal. Abdominal distension minimal.
Adulthood	Anaemia—iron and folate deficiency. Anorexia and loss of energy. Symptoms may be mild or almost absent. Symptoms or crisis may develop during another illness e.g. gastrointestinal infection, pregnancy. Risk of malignancy.

Small infants are probably more able to survive severe metabolic disorders, malnutrition and extensive tissue damage than older people. They can survive severe dehydration and hypernatraemia. Intensive therapy of serious problems such as neonatal necrotizing enterocolitis (Fig. 77.1) and intractable diarrhoea (Fig. 77.2) are sometimes surprisingly rewarding.

Malabsorption is not uncommon during infancy—cystic fibrosis, coeliac disease and post-gastroenteritis syndromes are the most frequent causes. Malnutrition and abdominal distension are often severe whatever the cause (Fig. 77.3)—more so than in malabsorption presenting in older children (Figs 77.4 and 77.5). The presentation of coeliac disease varies with age (Table 77.1).

Infants are most susceptible to infections. Some gastrointestinal infections, such as Rotavirus or *E. coli* enteritis, are largely confined to this age group.

Enteropathies of the small intestine are probably commoner in infancy than in other ages (Table 77.2). The post-gastroenteritis syndrome is increasingly uncommon beyond the age of three months. The confident diagnosis of coeliac disease in children depends upon the demonstration that an abnormal intestinal mucosal biopsy is related to gluten ingestion—repeated biopsies, or reliable tests of gastrointestinal function such as sugar permeability [48] are necessary following dietary gluten withdrawal and challenge.

Congenital disorders can be diagnosed during infancy if their clinical presentation is related to either milk feeding (glucose-galactose malabsorption) or to a mixed solid diet (sucrose-isomaltase deficiency).

Late pre-school and early school period

Major organic gastrointestinal problems are diagnosed less frequently in this age group. Gastrointestinal symptoms are very common and are often related to functional

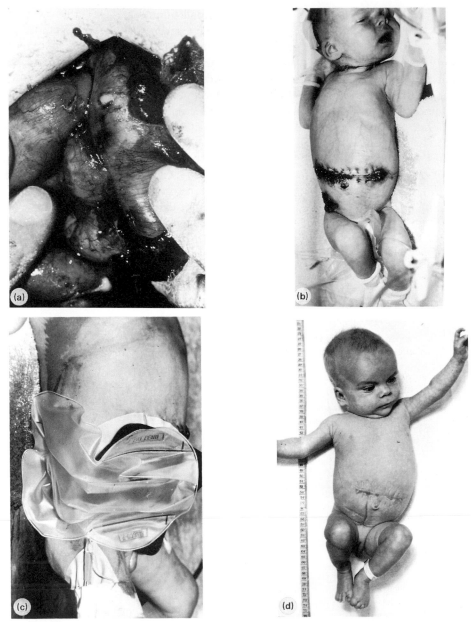

Fig. 77.1. Neonatal necrotizing enterocolitis. (a) findings at laparotomy—extensive bowel necrosis and peritonitis. (b) three days after laparotomy—abdominal wall necrosis and sepsis. Breakdown of abdominal incision. (c) six days after laparotomy—complete breakdown of abdominal incision. Abdominal contents contained within plastic bag. Total parenteral nutrition continued. (d) three months after laparotomy. Abdominal wall repaired and healed. Tolerating oral nutrients.

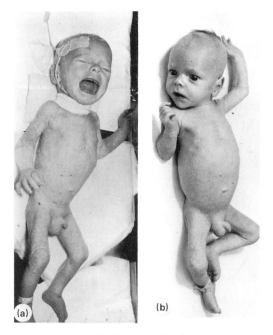

Fig. 77.2. Intractable diarrhoea of infancy (a) malnourished infant with intractable diarrhoea. Parenteral feeding maintained through central venous catheter. (b) parenteral nutrition discontinued after three weeks. Oral feeding with Pregestemil tolerated.

disorders, where no organic pathology is demonstrable (Table 77.3). For instance, recurrent abdominal pains affect about 10% of school children [1]. The basic aetiology of such disorders may be psychological problems affecting the patient and his family, or less frequently a dietary problem such as insufficient fibre. Some are related to minor variations of gastrointestinal physiology, where explanation and reassurance is all that is required (for example, many patients with toddler diarrhoea). Most children with functional disorders have a good long-term prognosis, but psychological and physiological problems can persist into adulthood following severe encopresis or anorexia nervosa. Approximately one-third of all children with recurrent functional abdominal pains continue to have symptoms during adult life.

Late school period and adolescence

Some of these common gastrointestinal disorders of adult life, such as peptic ulcer and inflammatory bowel disease, affect older

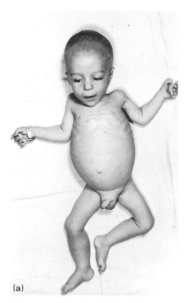
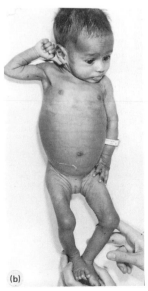
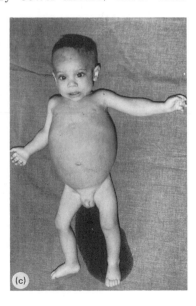

Fig. 77.3. Malabsorption during infancy. Severe malnutrition and abdominal distension. (a) cow's milk protein intolerance. (b) post-gastroenteritis malabsorption syndrome. (c) intestinal lymphangiectasia.

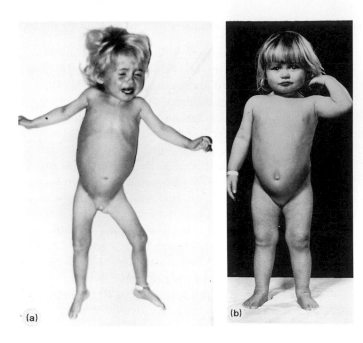

(a)

(b)

Fig. 77.4. Coeliac disease in late infancy. (a) abdominal distension; malnutrition and muscle wasting; miserable and hypotonic. (b) six months on gluten-free diet.

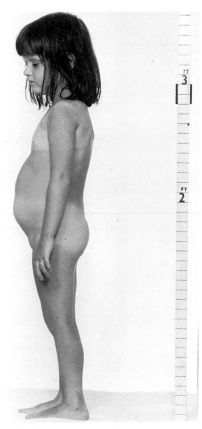

Fig. 77.5. Coeliac disease in middle childhood. Short stature, iron-deficiency anaemia, mild malnutrition and mild abdominal distension.

children. They demonstrate specific features within the paediatric age group.

Peptic ulceration has a different clinical picture and is less common than in adults (Table 77.4) [12, 32, 50]. The relationship of pain to food intake and fasting is much less apparent among children than adults. Peptic ulcer is difficult to diagnose from the very common functional disorders which cause vomiting and abdominal pains. A clinical suspicion is confirmed by radiology or by gastroduodenoscopy, which is well-tolerated by children over eight years of age. Treatment is not significantly different from that of adults.

Adolescence is also a period of accelerated growth rate. Inflammatory bowel disease, particularly Crohn's disease, is increasing in incidence in most developed countries. Children of all ages can be affected, but it is commonest among adolescents who are particularly susceptible to growth failure. This may precede the clinical onset of Crohn's disease by several years [40], but it demands urgent correction to prevent permanent stunting [35, 46]. Growth failure is much more common in the child with Crohn's disease. It is related to the activity of the inflammatory bowel disease, which may not only aggravate a prolonged inadequate intake of protein and calories, but also be associated with complications due to strictures or fistulae. Growth failure is treated by suppression of disease activity, using corticosteroids or immunosuppression, and improved nutritional intake (at least 1.6 g protein and 80 calories/kg.day) using enteral or parenteral nutrition.

Specific gastrointestinal disorders of children

Neonatal necrotizing enterocolitis

The basic aetiology of the widespread patchy necrosis of the large and small

Table 77.2. Disorders of childhood associated with abnormal small intestinal histology.

Non-specific histological changes (villous atrophy)
Coeliac disease
Post-gastroenteritis syndrome
Immune deficiency states
Dietary protein intolerance (e.g. cow's milk protein)
Tropical sprue
Protein-calorie malnutrition
Severe iron deficiency
Drugs, e.g. neomycin, methotrexate

Specific histology

Disorder	Histological features
Abetalipoproteinaemia	Fat filled enterocytes over upper part of the villi
Intestinal lymphangiectasia	Dilated intestinal lymphatics in affected areas
Chronic infections and infestations e.g. Giardiasis	Trophozoites may be seen close to the enterocyte luminal surfaces
Whipple's disease (very rare in childhood)	Foamy macophages with P.A.S. positive granules within the lamina propria

Table 77.3. Gastrointestinal functional disorders of infancy and childhood.

Infantile vomiting
Intracranial haemorrhage or tumour, oesophageal reflux and pyloric stenosis must be excluded.

Infantile abdominal colic

Diarrhoea shortly after infancy
'Toddler diarrhoea'.

Recurrent rectal prolapse
Seldom seen beyond the age of four years. Need to exclude cystic fibrosis and underlying constipation.

Encopresis
Chronic constipation and faecal incontinence. Constipation from time of 'potty training'. Often psychological and behaviour problems.

Recurrent abdominal pain
Extremely common among school children.

Anorexia nervosa
Characteristically affects adolescent girls and young women.

Table 77.4. Clinical features of chronic peptic ulcer in childhood.

Early infancy
Vomiting—diagnosis often missed.
Haematemesis and perforation.
Rise in gastric acid output during first 48 hours after
  birth.

Early childhood (rare)
Recurrent vomiting.
Abdominal pain less frequent than later in life.

Late childhood and adolescence
Probably increasing in incidence and recognition.
Recurrent abdominal pains—the site of the pain and
  relationship to meals is less specific than in adults.
Over 50% have positive family history.
Nocturnal pain—useful feature to differentiate from
  the very common functional abdominal pains of
  childhood.

intestine in neonatal necrotizing enteritis is unknown.

Epidemiology and aetiology

The overall incidence is impossible to evaluate, because of wide variation at different times and in different locations. The clinically recognizable onset is normally

Table 77.5. Neonatal necrotizing enterocolitis.

Strongly associated factors
Low birth weight—less than 1500 g.
Prematurity—usually less than 33 weeks gestation.
Neonatal asphyxia and/or shock—resuscitation often
  required with Apgar score less than 6.
Oral feeding—volume of initial feeds.
              —size of volume increments.
              —osmolality of feeds.

Weakly associated factors
Umbilical vein and artery catheterization.
Congenital heart disease e.g. patent ductus arteriosus.
Respiratory distress syndrome.
Acidosis.
Hypoglycaemia.
Prolonged maternal rupture of membranes.
Intravenous hypertonic injections—e.g. glucose,
  bicarbonate, calcium and antibiotics.
Exchange transfusions.
Commoner in developed societies and in neonatal
  intensive care units.

within ten days of birth. Both sexes are equally affected. Factors associated with its occurrence are shown in Table 77.5.

Pathology

Fig. 77.6 illustrates the sequence of pathological events which have been observed in necrotizing enterocolitis. Progression

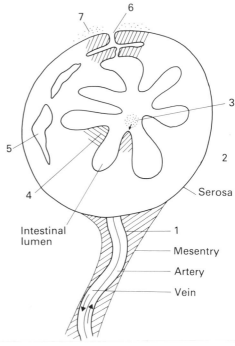

Cross–section of intestine

**Fig. 77.6. Neonatal necrotizing enterocolitis—
sequence of pathological events.** 1. Localized and
widespread vascular impairment. Possible aetiological
factors: a. vascular response to anoxia, hypotension,
etc. b. thrombosis, embolization and vasospasm. c.
intestinal permeability to macromolecules (?immune
complex vasculitis) d. local and systemic enteric
bacterial infection (endotoxaemia). 2. Intestinal
mucosal necrosis. Any area of the intestine but distal
ileum and proximal colon most common. 3. Enteric
bacteria penetrate the necrotic mucosal lesion.
Klebsiella, E. coli, Pseudomonas and various species of
Clostridia have been isolated. 4. Deeper layers of
intestinal necrosis. 5. Cystic spaces containing gas
and bacteria. 6. Full thickness necrosis of the
intestine and perforation. 7. Localized and
generalized peritonitis.

through all the stages does not always occur. Intestinal involvement may be widespread, sometimes with skip lesions.

Clinical features

The mortality and the need for surgery are reduced by early diagnosis and introduction of specific medical treatment, if possible when the signs are non-specific. These include recurrent apnoea, bradycardia, unstable body temperature, lethargy or irritability, poor feeding or vomiting.

Neonatal necrotizing enterocolitis should always be considered whenever a neonate develops gastric retention, diarrhoea (particularly if there is blood, mucus or melaena), or abdominal distension. Shock, gastrointestinal haemorrhage or peritonitis will develop later, depending upon the severity and the extent of intestinal necrosis. Massive gastrointestinal bleeding, intestinal perforation, and ecchymosis or necrosis of the abdominal wall (see Fig. 77.1) are the most serious local complications. Thrombocytopenia and disseminated intravascular coagulation are the major systemic problems. Approximately 60% of patients have demonstrable sepsis [9].

Most infants who recover have no long-term adverse sequelae [62]. However, intestinal strictures (sometimes multiple), malabsorption and the short bowel syndrome can be a problem; internal fistulae are rare [55, 62].

Investigations

Whatever the patient's condition, a full-blood picture and platelet count, clotting studies, glucose, urea and electrolyte measurements are required as well as bacteriological examination of blood, urine, C.S.F. and stool. Proctoscopy may assist the early diagnosis [19].

Repeated abdominal X-rays are important to diagnose and assess the progress of

Table 77.6. Radiological features of neonatal necrotizing enterocolitis.

Early suspicious changes
Mild to moderate small intestinal distension.

Later definitive changes
Large bowel distension with/without small bowel distension.
Pneumatosis intestinalis—localized intramural gas collections.
　　　　　　　　—diffuse linear stripes of intramural gas.
　　　　　　　　—ring translucencies, where intramural gas outlines the bowel end-on.
Persistent separation of small bowel loops.
Unchanging areas of bowel distension.

Changes of advanced disease with a poorer prognosis
Gas within the portal venous system.
Pneumoperitoneum.

necrotizing enterocolitis. Seriously ill patients may require abdominal X-rays routinely every four to six hours (Table 77.6). Abdominal ultrasound can assess the progression of peritonitis or intra-abdominal abscesses.

Because of the risk of strictures, barium studies should be performed shortly after clinical recovery and before final surgery [57].

Differential diagnosis

The early differential diagnosis includes hypoglycaemia, sepsis, electrolyte disturbance, central nervous system haemorrhage or infection, and intestinal obstruction. Haemorrhagic disease of the new-born, secondary to hypothrombinaemia, was a more common cause of gastrointestinal haemorrhage before the routine administration of vitamin K to compromised infants.

Medical treatment

All oral intake should be stopped, nasogastric aspiration started, and the neonate supported by warmth, oxygen and parenteral feeding. The neonate should be given broadspectrum antibiotics—for example, benzyl penicillin, gentamicin and metronidazole.

Medical management should be maintained for at least two weeks before the reintroduction of enteric feeding. A cautious return to normal nutrition is best using a lactose-free, low-osmolar formula containing medium chain triglycerides—for example, Portagen.

Surgical treatment

Surgery is required for a minority of infants with necrotizing enterocolitis. Perforation is the sole absolute indication for surgery. Peritonitis does not necessarily indicate that a perforation has occurred.

At operation, any peritoneal free fluid should be cultured. Only perforated, or unquestionably necrotic, bowel should be divided or resected. Stomas are less hazardous than a primary anastomosis of potentially damaged inestine. If possible the ileocaecal valve should be preserved. Repeated operations may be necessary.

Medical treatment and oral fasting should continue for at least two weeks post-operatively. Final surgery may be required to close stomas, and to resect areas of stenosis.

Prognosis

Prognosis has improved with earlier recognition and treatment, particularly effective antibiotic treatment of anaerobic sepsis with metronidazole. However, 10–30% of patients with necrotizing enterocolitis die.

Acute gastroenteritis

Acute gastroenteritis is a clinical syndrome of acute vomiting with diarrhoea, sometimes accompanied by fever and constitutional symptoms.

Viruses are the commonest cause of gastroenteritis, particularly in developed countries. In Britain, Rotavirus infection accounts for approximately 80% of infant admissions to hospital with gastroenteritis. It rarely causes clinical disease beyond the age of two years. The proportion of infections due to bacteria varies throughout the world—in underdeveloped societies E. coli frequently causes gastroenteritis among children, whereas in Europe Campylobacter is a more common pathogen than E. coli.

In 1975 it was estimated that three to five billion episodes of gastroenteritis occurred throughout the world with five to eighteen million deaths, mainly in infants and the elderly, in the debilitated and malnourished peoples of Africa, Asia and South America.

Aetiology

E. coli infections cause gastroenteritis by three distinct pathogenic mechanisms—E. coli subtypes are either enteropathogenic, enterotoxigenic or enteroinvasive (Table 77.7). The O antigenic types were found to be virulent on epidemiological data, and their recognition in stool culture is still the standard method of identification. In England, less than 1% of E. coli gastroenteritis is due to enterotoxigenic bacteria[18]—the majority are from enteropathogenic E. coli. Adherence factors probably enable E. coli to colonize the upper small intestine[41]—both enterotoxigenicity and adherence are plasmid related.

Rotavirus was first recognized in epithelial cells of the duodenum by electron microscopy[6]. Electron microscopy of the stools shows the virus to have a diameter of 65–70 nm. They cause endemic gastroenteritis in young children with a marked seasonal variation—in most regions peak incidence is during the cooler or winter months[43].

Epidemic viral gastroenteritis, among

Table 77.7. *Escherichia coli* and acute gastroenteritis [51].

E. coli subtypes	Enteropathogenic	Enterotoxigenic	Enteroinvasive
Pathogenic mechanism	Unknown. Probably a toxin ? cytotoxin. Adhesive factor [41].	Enterotoxins. Heat labile toxin. Secretion via increased cellular cyclic A.M.P. Heat stable toxin. ? increased cellular cyclic G.M.P. Adhesive factor.	Epithelial cell invasion and multiplication. Demonstrated by Guinea pig eye model (Sereny test). Dysentery-like illness [16].
Susceptible age groups	Infants. Rarely adults	Infants and children. Adult travellers.	All ages.
Geographic distribution	Worldwide	Mainly developing countries of Africa, Asia and South America.	Worldwide.
Associated O antigenic types	26, 55, 86, 111, 114, 119, 125, 126, 127, 128, 142.	6, 8, 15, 25, 27, 63, 78, 148, 159.	28ac, 112ac, 124, 136, 143, 144, 152, 164.

children and adults, is associated with **Parvovirus** or **Norwalk agent** infection. These viruses cause short-lasting infections, rarely requiring hospitalization. They have a diameter of 28–30 nm, and require specialized techniques for identification in stool specimens [8].

Pathology

Histological damage to the upper small intestine has been observed following infections with enteropathogenic *E. coli*, Rotavirus and Norwalk agent. This probably accounts for the occasional development of the chronic post-gastroenteritis syndromes.

The toxin produced by enterotoxigenic *E. coli* is similar to that of cholera, causing cyclic A.M.P.-mediated intestinal secretion of water and electrolyte, without any disturbance of intestinal morphology or absorptive function [20].

Clinical features

The major symptoms are vomiting and diarrhoea. Clinically, it is rarely possible to diagnose the infective agent except during epidemics. There is considerable variation

between individual patients with the same infection. Table 77.8 outlines the clinical features of the more common bacterial and viral infections.

Dehydration is the most important early complication, and is a major cause of mortality in underdeveloped countries. Isotonic dehydration occurs frequently throughout the world, but hyponatraemia (and hypokalaemia) are more common in the Third World. Hypernatraemia was common in Europe, causing convulsions, with long-term brain damage and epilepsy. The high incidence of hypernatraemia during the 1950s and 1960s has fallen during the past decade due to improved feeding practices, better management of acute gastroenteritis, and the introduction of low sodium infant milks [49].

Severe dehydration may cause temporary renal impairment and rare renal tubular necrosis. Most cases of haemolytic-uraemic syndrome develop shortly after an acute, presumably infective, diarrhoeal illness [30].

Recovery of normal gastrointestinal function is occasionally delayed because of post-gastroenteritis malabsorption. Several varieties of this problem exist—secondary

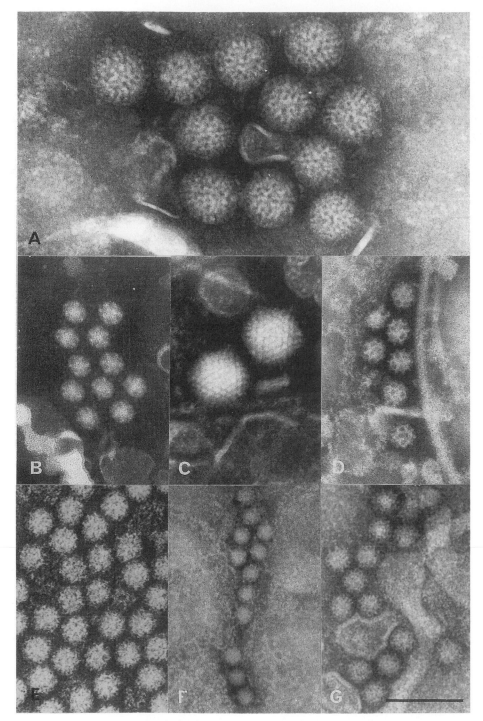

Fig. 77.7. Viruses associated wih infantile diarrhoea which are detectable by electron microscopy. A. Rotavirus. B. Astrovirus. C. Adenovirus. D. Calicovirus. E. Norwalk virus. F. Small round virus (S.R.V.). G. Small round structured virus (S.R.S.V.). All negatively stained from stool extracts. Scale bar = 100 nm. (Microscopy of Norwalk virus reproduced from [33] by permission of the editor. Other micrographs reproduced by permission of Professor C. R. Madeley).

Table 77.8. Clinical features of the common viral and bacterial forms of acute gastroenteritis.

Infecting agent	Enteropathogenic *E. coli*	*Campylobacter*	Endemic viruses (e.g. Rotavirus)	Epidemic viruses (e.g. Norwalk Agent, Parvo-like viruses)
Susceptible age groups	Under 2 years	All ages	Under 2 years.	All ages. Epidemics in schools etc.
Incubation period	24–48 hours.	2–5 days.	48–72 hours.	14–24 hours.
Vomiting	Sometimes present.	Occasionally present.	Prominent. Onset before diarrhoea.	Prominent but may be absent.
Diarrhoea	Watery diarrhoea without blood.	Variable. Lasts 2–3 days. From insignificant to severe with blood.	Watery diarrhoea without blood.	May be absent. Dehydration mild.
Fever	Absent.	Sometimes high fever.	Fever common.	May be low-grade pyrexia.
Constitutional and other symptoms	Rare.	Abdominal pain common. About 50% have nausea, exhaustion, headache, myalgia, and dizziness. Symptoms less severe in children.	Respiratory symptoms e.g. cough and otitis media are common.	Abdominal pain, myalgia, headaches, nausea, anorexia, and malaise are common.
Duration of illness	Usually 1–2 weeks.	Usually 1–2 weeks. Sometimes up to 6 weeks.	From 5–21 days. Usually 8–11 days.	1–3 days.

mono- or di-saccharide intolerance, secondary cow's milk protein intolerance, or intractable diarrhoea of infancy.

Investigations

Infants admitted to hospital require measurement of the plasma urea and electrolytes to help assess the approximate degree of dehydration.

Faeces should be cultured for bacterial pathogens such as the O antigen types of *E. coli*, *Campylobacter* etc.

Faeces can be examined by electron microscopy when negatively-stained faecal extracts may identify Rotaviruses [22]. This technique is less time-consuming than immune electron microscopy and, being non-specific, allows the identification of several viral species (see Fig. 77.7) [11, 66, 67].

Differential diagnosis

In infants, gastroenteritis cannot be differentiated clinically from other local or systemic infections which may present as an acute gastrointestinal disturbance. Upper respiratory infections, such as otitis media, urinary infections and the serious infections (septicaemia, meningitis or pneumonia), must be excluded.

At all ages, it is important that patients with acute surgical problems such as hypertrophic pyloric stenosis, intussusception, acute appendicitis or intestinal obstruction are not erroneously diagnosed to have gastroenteritis.

Prevention

In addition to its lower risk of contamination, breast feeding confers active resistance to infantile gastroenteritis. Colostrum and human milk contain numerous factors which are potentially protective against gastrointestinal infection. No satisfactory vaccines against either Rotavirus or *E. coli* infections have been developed.

Treatment

Vomiting and diarrhoea will usually cease using an oral regimen of clear fluids, without milk or solids. The composition in terms of osmolality, glucose (or sucrose), and electrolyte concentration of an ideal clear fluid is unknown. Glucose will enhance the absorption of sodium and water in secretory diarrhoea due to enterotoxigenic *E. coli* infections or cholera, but it may increase the diarrhoea in temporary or persistent monosaccharide intolerance [36].

In underdeveloped countries and the USA, where hyponatraemia occurs frequently, WHO/UNICEF recommended solutions of sodium 90 mmol/l, and potassium 20–30 mmol/l are widely used. Low sodium

concentrations of 25–43 mmol/l (for example, in the commercial preparations Electrosol and Dioralyte) are routinely used in the UK, because of the risk of hypernatraemia which can develop on oral clear fluids of excessive osmolality and sodium concentrations [10, 53]. Most patients can start partial oral feeding within two to four days. Repeated relapses of diarrhoea or vomiting on refeeding suggests the development of a post-gastroenteritis syndrome.

In patients with severe dehydration, intravenous fluid and electrolyte transfusion is required for resuscitation, to correct disturbances of water, electrolyte and acid/base homeostasis, and to supply maintenance needs during fasting. Estimation of the fluid volume replacement depends upon the patient's age, the clinical severity of the diarrhoea, and the plasma electrolyte (especially sodium) concentration [14].

Antiemetic, antidiarrhoeal drugs and sedatives are usually of little help during the management of acute gastroenteritis [54]. Their use in domiciliary treatment is

Table 77.9. Milk formulae used for therapy of chronic gastrointestinal disorders. Indications for formula: 1 lactose intolerance; 2 disaccharide intolerance; 3 monosaccharide intolerance; 4 cow's milk protein intolerance; 5 soy bean protein intolerance.

Proprietary milk	Principle carbohydrate	Protein source	Fat	Indications for formula
Galactamin 17	Glucose	Cow's milk	Long chain triglyceride (LCT) (Full cream)	1, 2
Galactamin 18	Glucose	Cow's milk	LCT Half cream	1, 2
Galactamin 19	Fructose	Cow's milk	LCT	3
Sobee Prosobee Velactin Wysoy	Sucrose	Soy bean	LCT	1, 4
Nutramigen	Sucrose	Hydrolysed cow's milk	LCT	1, 4, 5
Pregestemil	Glucose polymers	Hydrolysed cow's milk	Medium chain triglycerides (MCT)	1, 2, 3, 4, 5
Cow & Gate MCT Formula 1	Lactose	Cow's milk	MCT	Selected cases of malabsorption syndrome

unfortunately commoner than the more effective oral clear fluids [44].

Even in *E. coli* infections, antibiotics are not indicated unless septicaemia is suspected. Their use does not alter the natural history of the disease, and may prolong the diarrhoea and carrier state.

Most post-gastroenteritis disorders involve intolerance of carbohydrate and/or protein, which may require an elimination diet. Medium chain triglycerides may also be useful if there is steatorrhoea. Numerous special milk formulae have been developed for the treatment of primary and secondary dietary intolerances—a selection is listed in Table 77.9, with the clinical applications of the individual preparations. In the most severe post-gastroenteritis problems, several weeks of partial or total parenteral nutrition is sometimes necessary.

Prognosis

During the 1970s, a marked improvement in the prognosis of infantile gastroenteritis has occurred in most developed countries [65].

Malabsorption in infancy and childhood

There are numerous reasons why infants or children may fail to derive nutritional benefit from a normal diet. Some involve the maldigestion or malabsorption of individual nutrients—fat in abetalipoproteinaemia, neutral aminoacids in Hartnup disease, vitamin B_{12} in familial megaloblastic anaemia or zinc in acrodermatitis enteropathica. Malabsorption involving multiple nutrients is caused by a variety of congenital and acquired problems.

In early infancy the clinical effects of malabsorption may be extremely serious, the most severe illness being called the intractable diarrhoea of infancy (Fig. 77.2) [3]. Conversely, in older children the effects of

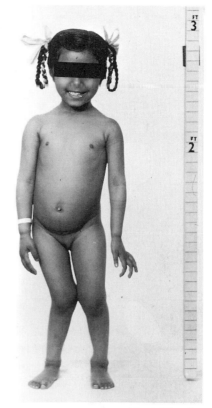

Fig. 77.8. Coeliac disease in middle childhood.

malabsorption may be less obvious (Figs 77.8 and 77.9).

Disorders of carbohydrate digestion and absorption

These are a fairly common problem in children. There are several inherited defects of the digestion and absorption of individual sugars (Table 77.10). A variety of insults, such as gastroenteritis, damage to small intestinal enterocyte and loss of their brush-border enzymes produces a temporary, secondary sugar intolerance.

The main dietary carbohydrates are the polysaccharides (starch), and the disaccharides (lactose from milk and sucrose mainly from fruits). Disorders of the digestion and absorption of sugars results in a characteristic clinical picture with watery diarrhoea.

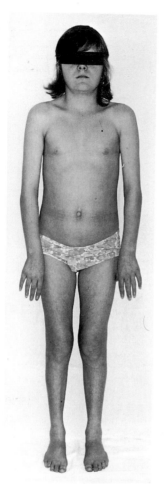

Fig. 77.9. Coeliac disease in adolescence. Short stature, delayed puberty and menarche, iron-deficiency anaemia, normal stools, no malnutrition or abdominal distension.

Epidemiology and aetiology

Table 77.10 illustrates the inheritance and the different racial distribution of the primary causes of sugar malabsorption, all of which are characterized by normal small bowel morphology.

Secondary sugar malabsorption is an uncommon complication of gastroenteritis but, because infantile gastroenteritis is so common, it is seen quite frequently, particularly in infants under three months old. Lactase activity is more susceptible to

brush-border damage than other disaccharidases, and recovers more slowly. Secondary disaccharide intolerance also occurs in coeliac disease, giardiasis, cow's milk protein intolerance and protein-calorie malnutrition.

Secondary monosaccharide malabsorption has been classified into two types—a *transient* form following gastroenteritis, and a more severe *prolonged form* of unknown aetiology in which all monosaccharides are malabsorbed, which can follow neonatal surgery, kwashiorkor, Rotavirus or idiopathic gastroenteritis, or immune deficiency [64].

Clinical features

These are similar whatever disorder of carbohydrate absorption. The major symptoms are water, fermentative diarrhoea with intestinal and abdominal gaseous distension and perianal excoriation. Adults and older children may experience cramp-like abdominal pains on ingestion of the offending sugars.

Investigations

Numerous investigations have been used to diagnose the underlying metabolic defect and the specific sugars responsible for the symptoms. The more popular tests are shown in Table 77.11. The hydrogen breath test is a sensitive method of investigating sugar malabsorption, and methods for collecting end-expired air from infants and young children have been developed [24]. However, after gastroenteritis [60] or antibiotic therapy [25] there may not be sufficient bacteria in the colon to synthesize hydrogen from the malabsorbed sugars—it is therefore not a completely reliable method for the investigation of post-gastroenteritis sugar malabsorption.

Table 77.10. Inherited disorders of digestion and absorption of carbohydrate.

Basic defect	Pancreatic amylase deficiency (Temporary developmental problem)	Deficiency of brush-border sucrase and isomaltase	Deficiency of brush-border lactase	Loss of brush-border lactase after infancy	Defect of active absorption of monosaccharide by enterocytes
Genetics	Autosomal dominant (?)	Autosomal recessive	Autosomal recessive (?)	Autosomal dominant	Autosomal recessive
Age of onset	Late infancy. Immediately after first exposure to starch.	Late infancy. After exposure to sucrose.	Early infancy or neonatal period.	Beyond age of two years.	Usually early infancy but may be later.
Dietary treatment	Starch restriction until age of two to three years.	Sucrose-free diet.	Lactose-free diet.	Symptoms unusual on normal milk intake of adults and older children.	Glucose-Galactose free diet. Fructose is absorbed normally.
Prevalence	Very rare	Uncommon, except in 10% of Eskimos in Greenland	Extremely rare	Over 90% in some non-Caucasian ethnic groups.	Rare

Table 77.11. Investigations useful for the diagnosis of gastrointestinal sugar intolerance.

Test stools for reducing sugars and pH [34]
Less reliable beyond infancy.
Over 0.5% sugar concentrations significant during infancy; over 1% in neonates [64].
N.B. Sucrose is not a reducing sugar. Drugs which can give false positive reactions include ascorbic acid, nalidixic acid, cephalosporins and probenecid.

Sugar chromatography of stools
Very sensitive and will detect normal small amounts of faecal sugars.

Oral sugar tolerance tests
Flat blood glucose/galactose curve indicates sugar malabsorption but not necessarily intolerance. Blood glucose curves are unreliable, with many falsely abnormal results.
Demonstration of typical symptoms by dose of test sugar.
Demonstration of symptoms plus reducing sugar in the watery stools is even more reliable.

Hydrogen breath tests
A rise in breath hydrogen excretion is demonstrated following an oral sugar load.

Problems of collecting end expired breath from young children [24].
Breath hydrogen can be measured by gas chromatography or rapidly by an electrochemical method using a polarographic cell [4].
Also useful for detecting small bowel bacteria contamination, and for measuring small intestinal transit, using lactulose as the ingested sugar.

Barium-sugar radiology
Non-absorbed sugar produces dilatation and distortion of the small bowel barium follow-through—a subjective test.

Disaccharidase assay of small bowel biopsy
Mainly useful for diagnosing isolated primary enzyme defects associated with normal small bowel morphology. Other brush-border enzyme activities should be normal.

Treatment

This is by elimination of the offending sugar from the diet. Special milk formulae are available (Table 77.9). In the primary disorders, the need for dietary restriction is life-long. With increasing maturity, some reduction in the clinical sensitivity to sugar ingestion can be expected. This is particularly helpful in glucose-galactose malabsorption, allowing some easing of the very restrictive fructose-only diet.

Secondary sugar intolerances vary considerably in duration but a normal diet can be resumed within three months in over 60% of patients and within six months in over 90% [64].

Intractable diarrhoea of infancy

This term was first used in 1968 [3] to describe infants with severe persistent diarrhoea, unresponsive to medical treatment and of unknown aetiology. These infants had severe malnutrition and a high mortality. More recently, improvements in treatment and prognosis have occurred, but our understanding of its aetiology is incomplete.

Epidemiology

This is almost solely a problem of young infants—over 90% are under three months old.

Aetiology

There are probably a variety of underlying causes, mostly unknown. Some cases have a genetic component, with a positive family history. One recently described inherited disorder of enterocyte microvillus morphology is associated with this problem [13].

Intractable diarrhoea can follow a wide variety of gastrointestinal insults during infancy—gastroenteritis, neonatal surgery, coeliac disease in crisis, immune deficiency, necrotizing enterocolitis, or primary monosaccharide intolerance. The mechanism of this uncommon reaction to these conditions is unknown.

Clinical features

The main symptom is severe watery diarrhoea leading to dehydration and acidosis. Diarrhoea may continue during fasting, but

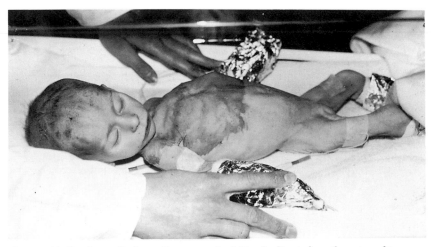

Fig. 77.10. Intractable diarrhoea of infancy. Extreme malnutrition leading to hypothermia and to hypoglycaemia.

it is more commonly dependant upon oral feeding. As enteric feeding is impossible, malnutrition develops rapidly with a high mortality due to the malnutrition or secondary infection (Fig. 77.10).

Investigations

Defects of T and B lymphocyte function indicate a primary immune deficiency in some patients, and the secondary effect of malnutrition in others. Defective yeast opsonization has been described[10]. Nonspecific changes of the small intestinal biopsy are common[59], but are not helpful in the primary diagnosis. On recovery, small bowel histology may remain abnormal for up to three years.

Treatment

Partial or total parenteral nutrition is associated with a rapid improvement in some patients allowing a resumption of oral elemental feeding (e.g. Pregestimil) within three weeks, and a normal diet within six months or more.

Other forms of therapy may also be helpful. These include plasma transfusions[10], oral cholestyramine[63] or oral loperamide[54].

Prognosis

There is still an appreciable mortality despite recent advances in treatment. A poor prognosis is suggested by onset at birth; a family history of intractable diarrhoea, especially in siblings; diarrhoea persisting during oral feeding or after three weeks of parenteral nutrition; persistent monosaccharide intolerance; or primary immune deficiency.

Cystic fibrosis

Cystic fibrosis is an inherited disorder of exocrine glands. Despite much experimental effort, the molecular basis of the disease is unknown. The clinicopathological features are numerous and varied, principally affecting the gastrointestinal tract and the lungs. The classical picture is one of steatorrhoea and chronic bacterial bronchial infection. Recent advances in management have improved the prognosis, with some centres predicting an 80% survival into adulthood.

Epidemiology and aetiology

Cystic fibrosis is the commonest serious disease inherited in Caucasians by a single abnormal autosomal recessive gene. Among affected races, the incidence is approximately one in every 1,600 births, indicating that one in 20 of the population is a heterozygous carrier of the gene.

Most of the recognized pathological changes are related to the abnormal physical properties of mucus, which is thicker and more tenacious than normal. It obstructs narrow passages such as the ductules of the exocrine pancreas, the bronchioles and bronchi. In cystic fibrosis all the exocrine gland secretions have an increased solute concentration and the mucus has a higher sodium content than normal.

Clinical features

Most, not all, patients with cystic fibrosis are diagnosed by the age of two years. To some extent, the clinical presentation varies according to the age of diagnosis.

Cystic fibrosis may present in the neonatal period with meconium ileus, or be diagnosed by routine screening of new-born infants by the measurement of blood immunoreactive trypsin[15]. Similarly, affected siblings of known patients with cystic fibrosis can be identified by screening in infancy or early childhood.

Sporadic cases of cystic fibrosis may present in infancy or early childhood because of pancreatic exocrine deficiency,

chronic pulmonary infection, rectal prolapse, or rarely as obstructive jaundice of
infancy. Cystic fibrosis may also rarely
present due to hypoproteinaemia causing
oedema, especially in infants fed with soy
or human milk[21]. In older children or
adults, cystic fibrosis may also present with
recurrent abdominal pain or portal hypertension due to multinodular biliary cirrhosis. Hepatocellular failure and ascites
are less common.

Neonatal intestinal obstruction or meconium ileus occurs in about 10% of new-
born infants with cystic fibrosis. The lumen
of the distal ileum is obstructed *in utero* by
mucus and meconium. Shortly after birth,
signs of intestinal obstruction develop with
bile-stained vomiting, delay in passing meconium, and abdominal distension.

There are several possible causes for recurrent **abdominal pain** in a child with cystic fibrosis. Rare ileal obstruction in older
patients is called meconium ileus equivalent. It causes recurrent abdominal pain,
and usually there is a palpable abdominal
mass. Bulky stools may cause faecal impaction obstructing the lower colon. Patients
with minimal pancreatic damage may develop recurrent pancreatitis[58]. Duodenal
ulceration can be related to low pancreatic
bicarbonate output.

Deficiency of the exocrine pancreas is an
acquired complication of cystic fibrosis
causing steatorrhoea in approximately 90%
of patients. The internationally accepted
name of the disease 'Cystic Fibrosis (of the
pancreas)' describes the fibrotic and cystic
damage to the gland that results from the
mucus obstruction of the ducts. Maximum
pancreatic damage develops *in utero* and
during early infancy. Cystic fibrosis is the
commonest cause of pancreatic exocrine
failure in children (Table 77.12).

Patients with pancreatic steatorrhoea
pass pale, greasy, bulky and extremely offensive stools. Growth and weight gain are
unsatisfactory despite a large appetite. De-

Table 77.12. Recognized causes of chronic exocrine pancreatic deficiency of children.

Primary disease	Means of inheritance
Total pancreatic involvement [27].	
Cystic fibrosis (95% of childhood pancreatic disease).	Single autosomal recessive gene.
Shwachman-Diamond syndrome. Congenital pancreatic hypo-plasia. Neutropenia or pancytopenia. Growth retardation and metaphysial dysostosis etc.	Single autosomal recessive gene.
Pancreatic insufficiency with congenital abnormalities [56]. Aplastic ala nasi, aplasia cutis. Deafness. Growth and developmental retardation.	Not inherited.
Chronic pancreatitis (usually familial). Recurrent abdominal pains rather than malabsorption.	Autosomal dominant.
Isolated enzyme defects (extremely rare) [27].	
Isolated lipase deficiency.	Autosomal recessive.
Isolated amylase deficiency. (?delayed development).	?Autosomal dominant.
Isolated trypsinogen deficiency.	Autosomal recessive.
Intestinal enterokinase deficiency (defective pancreatic zymogen activation).	Autosomal recessive.

ficiency of fat soluble vitamins A, E and K
are common.

Chronic pulmonary infection—Virtually
all patients develop chronic lung disease by
adolescence, with a chronic cough producing purulent sputum and varying severity of respiratory handicap.

Other complications include collapse
during hot weather, due to excessive sweat
electrolyte loss, which can be prevented by
oral salt supplements. Nasal polyps and
chronic otitis media are common. Diabetes
mellitus is usually non-ketotic and responds
to oral hypoglycaemics. Infertility affects
both sexes—males have aspermia or hypo-

spermia and thickened spermatic cords. Female infertility is probably related to inpenetrable mucus at the uterine cervix.

Investigations

Sweat test

The diagnosis depends upon the demonstration of increased electrolyte concentrations in the sweat. Sweat is collected after stimulation by pilocarpine iontophoresis. It is notoriously difficult to maintain consistent accuracy of sweat test results. Sweat sodium and chloride concentrations above 60 mmol/l are found in children with cystic fibrosis. Normal sweat electrolyte concentrations increase with age, and, therefore, in adults with cystic fibrosis, sodium and chloride results should be above 80 mmol/l.

Young infants produce small volumes of sweat, and sweat tests below the age of three months may be less accurate than later. At all ages cystic fibrosis should only be diagnosed on the basis of consistent, repeatedly abnormal sweat test results.

Tests of pancreatic disease (see Chapter 34)

Approximately 10% of patients have no steatorrhoea and do not require pancreatic enzyme supplements. A useful clinical screening test for pancreatic steatorrhoea is examine a specimen of stool stirred with water or Sudan III on a microscope slide. Many more than six fat globules of undigested triglyceride per high power field supports the presence of steatorrhoea (Fig. 77.11).

Tests for faecal tryptic activity are unreliable and are no longer used.

Formal tests of pancreatic exocrine function by duodenal intubation are not usually required for the diagnosis or management of cystic fibrosis, but they have provided interesting information about the basic genetic defect. On stimulation by intravenous pancreozymin and secretin, all children with cystic fibrosis show a reduced volume output, with increased viscosity, increased chloride output and reduced bicarbonate output—which are therefore primary defects. Only children with steatorrhoea, and presumably more severe secondary pancreatic damage, show a reduced output of digestive enzymes [28].

The simpler-to-perform Lundh test shows that all children with cystic fibrosis, with or without steatorrhoea, produce low concentrations of trypsin in the duodenal aspirate following test meal stimulation of the pancreas.

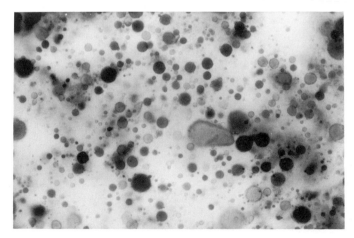

Fig. 77.11. Cystic fibrosis. Microscopy of stool in severe pancreatic steatorrhoea. Numerous fat globules per high power field stained with Sudan III.

Investigation of neonatal intestinal obstruction

All neonates suspected to have intestinal obstruction should have erect and supine abdominal X-rays, and signs of ileal obstruction should also indicate the possibility of meconium ileus. On X-ray, an uneven distension of the upper small intestinal loops, a paucity of air-fluid levels, and granula 'small soap bubble' areas of the intestinal lumen are related to the increased viscosity of the intestinal contents of cystic fibrosis with meconium ileus.

A Gastrografin enema may support this diagnosis by demonstrating a previously unutilized microcolon. It may also be therapeutic.

Investigation of the nutritional status

Despite long-term dietary treatment and pancreatic enzyme supplementation, many patients with cystic fibrosis became deficient in vitamins A, E, K and B_{12}. Deficiencies of these nutrients may occasionally produce specific clinical problems and may effect long-term prognosis and resistance to infection [47, 61].

Medical treatment

Total correction of the steatorrhoea can only be achieved by the combined use of oral pancreatic enzymes and by elemental dietary supplements, including medium chain triglycerides, which have to be continued long-term and are unpalatable [17]. Pancreatic enzyme supplements should be taken before and during every meal or snack. Bicarbonate or cimetidine (3 mg/kg, in 3–4 doses 30 minutes before meals) may protect enzyme supplements from destruction by gastric acid [31]. Fat-soluble vitamin supplements should maintain double the normal daily intake. In many patients, satisfactory growth and weight gain is maintained despite continuing steator-

rhoea. A later deterioration in growth and weight gain may herald the onset of advanced pulmonary infection.

Meconium ileus

A variety of detergent and mucolytic solutions have been administered rectally to dislodge the material obstructing the terminal ileum. Gastrografin is currently the most popular. Within the intestine, its hyperosmolality causes a flow of water into the lumen, washing the ileal contents into the colon. Hydration must be maintained during the procedure.

Meconium ileus equivalent, or partial ileal obstruction in older patients, can usually be treated medically by an oral mucolytic agent (N acetyl cysteine 10% solution flavoured with Coca-Cola. The usual dose is 5 ml q.d.s. for two weeks, reducing the dose by 5 ml daily every two weeks; 5 ml daily may need to be continued for long-term maintenance); an increase in oral pancreatic supplements; and an occasional Gastrografin enema for resistant patients. However, surgery is required occasionally [42].

Surgical treatment

The indications for the surgical treatment of meconium ileus are failure of medical treatment to relieve the obstruction, failure to differentiate meconium ileus from other forms of intestinal obstruction, or suspicion of complicating intestinal atresia or perforation. Surgery consists of resection of the most distended bowel above the obstruction and a double-barrelled ileostomy (Fig. 77.12).

Differential diagnosis

Wide variations in the presentation of cystic fibrosis makes a comprehensive outline of the differential diagnosis difficult. The main

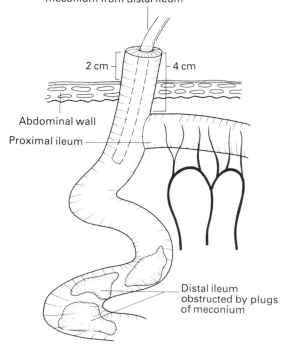

Catheter instilled with acetyl cysteine or Gastrografin to dislodge obstructing meconium from distal ileum

2 cm — 4 cm

Abdominal wall

Proximal ileum

Distal ileum obstructed by plugs of meconium

Fig. 77.12. Surgical treatment of neonatal meconium ileus. Bishop-Koop form of double-barrelled ileostomy.

disorders for differentiation are the various malabsorption syndromes and chronic pulmonary diseases of infants and children, including allergic asthma which may exist with cystic fibrosis in the same patient.

Prognosis

This has improved considerably during the past three decades. The majority of patients with cystic fibrosis now survive into adult life, some with little respiratory problems. Survival beyond the fourth decade is unusual. With prolonged survival certain complications are increasing in incidence, particularly portal hypertension and diabetes mellitus. Infertility creates problems for the adult with cystic fibrosis.

Abetalipoproteinaemia

Epidemiology and aetiology

Abetalipoproteinaemia is a rare inborn error of metabolism inherited by an abnormal autosomal recessive gene, characterized by a failure of chylomicron formation, and an accumulation of dietary fat within enterocytes [29]. Betalipoprotein is an essential component of chylomicrons, without which long-chain triglycerides cannot, following absorption, be transported from the enterocytes into the thoracic duct lymph [26].

Pathology

Histology of the upper small intestine is characteristic but not pathognomonic. The enterocytes of the upper half of the villi are fat filled, and have a vacuolated appearance on haemotoxylin and eosin staining.

Clinical features

The condition presents during infancy with symptoms of steatorrhoea and failure to thrive. During later childhood neurological complications develop with an atypical retinitis pigmentosa with macular involvement and an ataxic neuropathy, because of degeneration of the posterior columns, pyramidal and the cerebellar pathways of the central nervous system.

Investigations

The definitive investigation is the demonstration of absent serum betalipoprotein by electrophoresis, immunoelectrophoresis, or ultracentrifugation.

Very low serum phospholipid and cholesterol (less than 60 mg/100 ml) strongly suggests the condition, as does the demonstration of distorted red cells (acanthocytes) on blood film and the characteristic abnormality on small bowel biopsy [38].

Treatment

Steatorrhoea is effectively treated by a low fat diet adequately supplemented by medium-chain triglycerides. Adequate supplements of essential fatty acids (linoleic acid) and fat-soluble vitamins A and E are needed. Long-term treatment with large oral doses of vitamin E (100 mg/kg.day) appears to preserve normal neurological function [5, 45].

Differential diagnosis

Abetalipoproteinaemia requires differentiation from other causes of infantile steatorrhoea and failure to thrive.

Heterozygous carriers of the abnormal recessive gene may have low serum cholesterol and betalipoprotein concentrations, but no clinical manifestations. Familial hypobetalipoproteinaemia [23] is inherited by an abnormal autosomal dominant gene. It is characterized by low serum cholesterol (below 75 mg/100 ml) and betalipoprotein concentrations. There are no gastrointestinal symptoms, but there may be a risk of a long-term neurological damage due to vitamin E deficiency.

References

1 APLEY J. *The child with abdominal pain.* Oxford: Blackwell Scientific Publications, 1975.
2 ATERMAN K. Duodenal ulceration and fibrocystic pancreatic disease. *Am J Dis Child* 1960;**10**:210–215.
3 AVERY GB, VILLAVICENCIO O, LILLY JR. Intractable diarrhoea in early infancy. *Pediatrics* 1968;**41**:712.
4 BARTLETT K, DOBSON JV, EASTHAM EJ. A new method for the detection of hydrogen in breath and its application to acquired and inborn sugar malabsorption. *Clin Chim Acta* 1980;**108**:189–194.
5 BIERI JG, CORASH L, HUBBARD VS. Medical uses of vitamin E. *N Engl J Med* 1983;**308**:1063–1070.
6 BISHOP RF, DAVIDSON GP, HOLMES IH, RUCK BJ. Virus particles in epithelial cells of duodenal mucosa from children with non-bacterial gastroenteritis. *Lancet* 1973;**ii**:1281–1283.
7 BISHOP HC, KOOP CE. Management of meconium ileus. resection, roux en Y anastomosis and ileostomy irrigation with pancreatic enzymes. *Am Surg* 1957;**145**:410–414.
8 BLACKLOW NR, CUKOR G. Viral gastroenteritis. *N Engl J Med* 1981;**304**:396–406.
9 BROWN EG, SWEET AY. *Neonatal necrotizing enterocolitis: monographs in neonatology.* London: Grune and Stratton, 1980.
10 CANDY DCA, LARCHER VF, TRIPP JH, HARRIES JT, HARVEY BAM, SOOTHILL JF. Yeast opsonization in children with chronic diarrhoeal states. *Arch Dis Child* 1980;**55**:189–193.
11 CUKOR G, VERRY MK, BLACKLOW NR. Simplified radioimmunoassay for detection of human rotavirus in stools. *J Infect Dis* 1978;**138**:906–910.
12 CURCI MR, LITTLE K, SIEBER WK, KIESWETTER W. Peptic ulcer disease in childhood re-examined. *J Pediatr Surg* 1976;**11**:329–335.
13 DAVIDSON GP, CUTZ E, HAMILTON JR, GALL DG. Familial enteropathy. A syndrome of protracted diarrhoea from birth, failure to thrive and hypoplastic villous atrophy. *Gastroenterol* 1978;**75**:783–790.
14 DELL RB. Pathophysiology and dehydration. In: Winters RW, ed. *The body fluids in pediatrics.* Boston: Little Brown and Co., 1973:134–154.

15 Dodge JA, Ryley HC. Screening for cystic fibrosis. *Arch Dis Child* 1982;**57**:774–780.

16 Dupont HL, Formal SB, Hornick RB, *et al.* Pathogenesis of *E. coli* diarrhoea. *N Engl J Med* 1971;**285**:1–9.

17 Durie PR, Newth CJ, Forstner GG, Gall DG. Mal absorption of medium chain triglycerides in infants with cystic fibrosis —correction with pancreatic enzyme supplements. *J Pediatr* 1980;**96**:862–864.

18 Evans N. Pathogenic mechanisms in bacterial diarrhoea. *Clin Gastroenterol* 1979;**8**:599–623.

19 Fenton TR, Walker-Smith JA, Harvey DR. Proctoscopy in infancy with reference to its use in necrotizing enterocolitis. *Arch Dis Child* 1981;**56**:121–124.

20 Field M. Intestinal Secretion: Effect of cyclic A.M.P. and its role in cholera *N Eng J Med* 1971;**184**:1137–1144.

21 Fleischer DS, Di George AM, Barness LA, Cornfeld D. Hypoproteinaemia and oedema in Infants with cystic fibrosis of the pancreas. *J Pediatr* 1964;**64**:341–348.

22 Flewett TH, Davies H, Bryden AS, Robertson MJ. Diagnostic electron microscopy of Faeces. II. Acute gastroenteritis associated with Reovirus-like particles. *J Clin Pathol* 1974;**27**:608–614.

23 Fosbrooke A, Choksey S, Wharton E. Familial hypobetalipoproteinaemia. *Arch Dis Child* 1973;**48**:729–732.

24 Gardiner AJ, Tarlow MJ, Sutherland IT, Sammons HG. Collection of breath for hydrogen estimation. *Arch Dis Child* 1981;**56**:125–127.

25 Gilat T, Ben-Hur H, Gelman-Malachi E, Tardiman R, Peled Y. Alterations of the colonic flora and their effect on the hydrogen breath test. *Gut* 1978;**19**:602–605.

26 Glickman RM, Green PHR, Lees RS, Lux SE, Kligre A. Immunofluorescence studies of apolipoprotein B in intestinal mucosa. *Gastroenterology* 1979;**76**:288–292.

27 Haddin B. The exocrine pancreas. In: Anderson CM, Burke V. *Paediatric gastroenterology.* Oxford: Blackwell Scientific Publications, 1975.

28 Hadorn B, Zoppi G, Schmerling DH, Prader A, McIntyre I, Anderson CM. Quantitative assessment of exocrine pancreatic function in infants and children. *J Pediatr* 1968;**73**:39–50.

29 Herbert PN, Assmann G, Grotto AM Jr, Fredrickson DS. Familial lipoprotein deficiency: abetalipoprotein, hypobetalipoproteinamie and Tangier disease. In: Stanbury JB, Wyngaarden JB, Fredrickson DS, Goldstein JL, Brown MS, eds. *The Metabolic Basis of Inherited Disease.* 5th ed. New York: McGraw-Hill Book Co.,1983:589–621.

30 Herdman RC, Urigar RE. Hemolytic uremic syndrome. In: Rubin MI, Barret, MT, eds. *'Pediatric Nephrology'.* Baltimore: Williams and Williams Co., 1975:196–204.

31 Hubbard VS, Dunn, GD and Lester LA. Effectiveness of cimetidine as an adjunct to supplemental pancreatic enzymes in patients with cystic fibrosis. *Am J Clin Nutr.* 1980;**33**:2281–2286.

32 Johnston D, L'Heureux P, Thompson T. Peptic ulcer disease in early infancy. Clinical presentation and roentgenographic features. *Acta Paedatr Scand.* 1980;**69**:753–760.

33 Kapikian AZ, Wyatt RG, Dolin R, Thornhill TS, Kalica AR, Chanock RM. Visualization by Immune electron microscopy of a 27 nm. particle associated with acute infectious non-bacterial gastroenteritis. *J Virol* 1972;**10**:1075–1081.

34 Kerry KR, Anderson CM. A ward test for sugar in faeces. *Lancet* 1964;**i**:981–982.

35 Kirschner BS, Vionchet O, Rosenberg IH. Growth retardation in inflammatory bowel disease. *Gastroenterology* 1978;**75**:504–511.

36 Kjellman J, Ronge E. Oral Solutions for gastroenteritis—optimum glucose concentration. *Arch Dis Child* 1982;**57**:313–315.

37 Lebenthal E, Lee PC, Heitlinger LA. Impact of development of the gastrointestinal tract on infant feeding. *J Pediatr* 1983;**102**:1–9.

38 Lloyd JK. Disorders of the serum lipoproteins. *Arch Dis Child,* 1968;**43**:393–403.

39 Lucas A. Endocrine aspects of enteral nutrition. In *New aspects of Clinical Nutrition.* Basel: Karger AG, 1983:581–594.

40 McCaffrey TD, Nasi K, Lawrence AM, Kirsner JB. Severe growth retardation in children with inflammatory bowel disease. *Pediatrics* 1970;**45**:386–393.

41 McNeish AS, Turner P, Fleming J, Evans N. Mucosal adherence of human enteropathogenic *E. coli. Lancet,* 1975;**ii**:946–948.

42 Mateshe JW, Go VLW, Di Magno EP. Meconium ileus equivalent complicating cystic fibrosis in postneonatal children and young adults: report of 12 cases. *Gastroenterology,* 1977;**72**:732–736.

43 Middleton PJ, Szymanski MT, Petric M. Viruses Associated with acute gastroenteritis in young children. *Am J Dis Child* 1977;**131**:733–737.

44 Morrison PS, Little TM. How is gastroenteritis treated? *B Med J,* 1981;**283**:1300.

45 Muller DPR, Lloyd D. Effect of large oral doses of vitamin E on the neurological sequelae of patients with abetalipoproteinaemia. *Ann NY Acad Sci* 1982;**77**:133–144.

46 Nelson R, Eastham EJ. Parenteral nutrition in inflammatory bowel disease in children. *New Aspects of Clinical Nutrition.* Basel: Karger, AG. 1983:650–661.

47 Park RW, Grand RJ. Gastrointestinal manifestations of cystic fibrosis. A review. *Gastroenterology,* 1981;**81**:1143–61.

48 Pearson ADJ, Eastham EJ, Laker MF, Craft AW, Nelson R. Intestinal permeability in children with

Crohn's disease and coeliac disease. *B Med J*, 1982;**285**:20–21.

49 PULLAN CR, DELLAGRAMMATIKAS H, STEINER H. Survey of gastroenteritis in children admitted to hospital in Newcastle upon Tyne in 1971–5. *B Med J*, 1977;1:619–621.

50 ROLTER JI. The genetics of peptic ulcer. More than one gene, more than one disease. *Prog Med Genet* 1980;**4**:1–18.

51 ROWE B. The role of *E. coli* in gastroenteritis. *Clin Gastroenterol* 1979;**8**:625–644.

52 SALT, HB, WOLFF DH, LLOYD, JK, FOSBROOKE AS, CAMERON AH, and HUBBLE DV. On having no beta-lipoprotein, A syndrome comprising abetalipo-proteinaemia, acanthocytosis and steatorrhoea. *Lancet*, 1960;**ii**:325–329.

53 SANDHU BK, JONES BJM, BROOK CGD, and SILK DBA. Oral rehydration in acute infantile diarrhoea with a glucose-polymer electrolyte solution. *Arch Dis Child* 1982;**57**:152–160.

54 SANDHU BK, TRIPP JH, MILLA PJ, HARRIES JT. Loperamide in severe protracted diarrhoea. *Arch Dis Child*, 1983;**58**:39–43.

55 SCHULINGER JN, MOLLITT DL, VINOIUR CD, SANKILTI TV, DRISCOLL JM JR. Neonatal necrotizing enterocolitis. survival, management, and complications. A 25 year study. *Am J Dis Child*, 1981;**135**:612–614.

56 SCHUSSHEIN A, SOOK JC, SILVERBERG M. Exocrine pancreatic insufficiency with congenital abnormalities. *J Pediatr*, 1976;**89**:782–784.

57 SCHWARTZ MZ, HAYDEN KC, RICHARDSON JC, TYSON KRT, THORN EL. A Prospective evaluation of intestinal stenosis following necrotizing enterocolitis. *J Pediatr Surg* 1982;17:764–770.

58 SHWACHMAN H, LEBENTHAL E, KHAW KT. Recurrent Acute pancreatitis in patients with cystic fibrosis with normal pancreatic enzymes. *Pediatrics*, 1975;**55**:86–95.

59 SHWACHMAN H, LLOYD-SMITH JD, KHAW KT, ANTONOWICZ I. Protracted diarrhoea of infancy treated by intravenous alimentation II. Studies of small intestinal biopsy results. *Am J Dis Child*, 1978;**125**:365–368.

60 SOLOMONS NW, GARCIA R, SCHNEIDER R, VITERI FE, VON KAENEL VA. H₂-breath tests during diarrhoea. *Acta Paediatr Scand*, 1979;**68**:171–172.

61 SOLOMONS NW, WAGONFELD JB, RIEGE C, JACOB RA, BOLT M, HORST JV. *et al.* Some biochemical indices of nutrition in treated cystic fibrosis patients. *Am J Clin Nut.* 1981;**34**:462–474.

62 STEVENSON DK, KERNIER JA, MALACHOWSKI N, SUNSHINE P. Late morbidity among survivors of necrotizing enterocolitis. *Pediatrics*, **66**:925–927.

63 TAMER AMA, SANTORA RT, SANDBERG DH. Cholestyramine therapy for intractable diarrhoea. *Pediatrics*, 1974;**53**:217–220.

64 WALKER-SMITH J. *Diseases of the Small Intestine in Childhood.* Tunbridge Wells: Pitman Medical, 1979.

65 WHARTON BA. Gastroenteritis in Britain. Management at home. *B Med J* 1981;**383**:1277–1278.

66 WOLF JL., SCHRIEBER DS. Viral gastroenteritis. *Med Clin North Am*, 1982;**66**:575–595.

67 YOLKEN RH, KIM HW, CLEM T. *et al.* Enzyme-linked immunosorbent assay (ELISA) for detection of human reovirus-like agent of infantile gastroenteritis. *Lancet*, 1977;**ii**:263–266.

Chapter 78
Enteral and Parenteral Nutrition

D. B. A. SILK

Twenty to 50% of hospitalized patients have some evidence of protein-calorie malnutrition [5, 16] yet awareness of the nutritional status of ill patients is a neglected area of clinical management.

Assessment of protein-calorie malnutrition

Few problems arise in recognizing the grossly malnourished patient when weight loss is marked, hypoproteinaemic oedema present, muscle wasting extreme and the serum albumin concentration is less than 25 g/l. Problems may arise however, in reaching the diagnosis in the fitter-looking patient who at first sight may even look obese (Fig. 78.1). During the last few years a battery of clinical, biochemical, haematological and immunological tests have been described to help diagnose protein-calorie malnutrition (Table 78.1).

Clinical history

A routine clinical history usually neglects the nutritional intake, yet patients requiring enteral nutrition often have had a markedly reduced nutritional intake for as long as three weeks before nutritional

Table 78.1. Diagnosis of protein-calorie malnutrition [64].

Parameter	Values suggesting protein–calorie malnutrition
Clinical and dietary history	
Clinical examination	
Body weight	Loss $> 10\%$ normal weight
Anthropometric measurements	
Mid-arm circumference	< 23 cm ♂; < 22 cm ♀
Mid-arm muscle circumference	< 19 cm ♂; < 17 cm ♀
Measurements of protein stores	
24 hour urinary creatinine	
Creatinine-height index	Not in general use
3-methyl histidine excretion	
Circulating hepatic proteins	
Albumin	< 35 g/l
Transferrin	< 2 g/l
Prealbumin	< 200 mg/l
Retinol-binding protein	< 100 mg/l
Immunology	
Lymphocyte count	$< 1.2 \times 10^9$/l

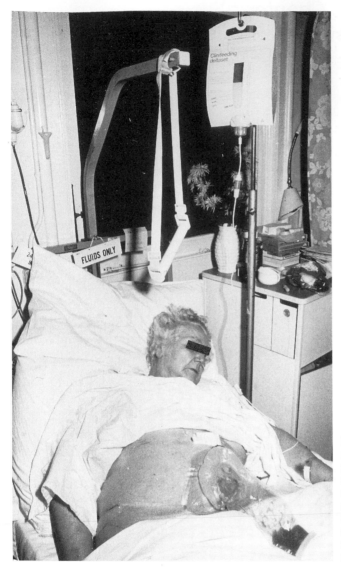

Fig. 78.1. Severe protein-calorie malnutrition in a woman aged 65 years. Wound dehiscence and enterocutaneous fistula following second laparotomy for recurrent small bowel obstruction. Note apparent obesity, but serum albumin 24 g/l. Patient is receiving nutritional support via the enteral route.

support is considered [20, 27]. When performing any estimate of nutritional intake, the possibility of malabsorption must also be considered.

Clinical examination

Many nutritional deficiencies are unaccompanied by physical signs, but clinical examination should always be carried out. Angular stomatitis, increased capillary fra-gility, anaemia, muscle wasting and oedema signify severe nutritional deficiency. Loss of body weight may provide the first clue that a patient is malnourished, particularly a loss of more than 10% of normal body weight.

Anthropometric measurements

Anthropometric measurements, such as mid-arm muscle circumference, triceps skinfold thickness and derivatives of these arm measurements provide a simple means of assessing the protein and fat reserves of hospitalized patients. An assessment of muscle mass can be obtained by measurement of the mid-arm circumference (MMC), which is calculated from the mid-arm circumference and triceps skinfold thickness, using the formula: MMC = mid-arm circumference − (π × triceps skinfold thickness). Erroneous measurements can be obtained in oedematous patients, and correlations between change in body nitrogen and mid-arm muscle circumference are not exact [7].

Although of limited value in obese patients and those with peripheral oedema, body fat content can be estimated simply using Harpenden skin callipers to measure skinfold thickness at four sites: triceps, biceps, subscapular and suprailiac [18]. The sum of the four skinfolds should be greater than 40 mm.

Measurement of protein stores

Malnutrition is associated with a decrease of total body protein content and, in clinical practice, measurements of muscle mass have been regarded as relatively sensitive measures of total body protein. Measurement of the mid-arm muscle circumference is the simplest available method. Other methods for assessing protein stores (24 hour urinary creatinine excretion, the creatinine-height index, neutron activation analysis for whole body nitrogen, whole body counts of potassium, urinary 3-methyl histidine [47] and isotope techniques for measuring total exchangeable potassium and water content) have not found a place in routine clinical practice [64].

Indirect measurements of protein synthesis

Numerous claims have been made that measurement of circulating hepatic proteins provides useful information about nutritional status and response to nutritional support. In the absence of parenchymal liver disease and proteinuria, the serum albumin concentration provides useful information about the nutritional state, values below 30 g/l indicating moderate-to-severe malnutrition. Although claims have been made of its value in monitoring the response to treatment, albumin has a long half-life and it shows a poor response to short-term nutritional support [20, 62].

Transferrin has a half life of eight days, shorter than albumin, and the plasma concentration is reduced in protein-calorie malnutrition. Its usefulness in clinical practice is limited by increased synthesis due to either coexisting iron deficiency or as part of the 'acute phase' protein response to infection or stress. Thyroxine-binding prealbumin and retinal binding protein are two other hepatic proteins whose plasma concentrations are also lowered in obvious protein-calorie malnutrition [17].

Immunology

Protein-calorie malnutrition has been shown to be associated with impaired immunocompetence [36]—for example, a decrease in total peripheral lymphocyte count to below 1.2×10^9/l.

Negative skin tests with ubiquitous antigens have been reported in patients with protein-calorie malnutrition and skin testing has been proposed as a practical aid to its diagnosis [50]. However, effective nutritional support is not always associated with reversal of the anergic state, and the use of skin tests has now been abandoned.

Indications for providing nutritional support

To be aware of protein-calorie malnutrition is the most important key to improving the nutritional care of the hospitalized patient. Practical management should be to take a clinical and dietary history, examine and weigh the patient, measure the mid-arm circumference and skinfold thickness, and measure the serum albumin and circulating lymphocyte count.

One of the major roles of nutritional support is to prevent the development of protein-calorie malnutrition. Consequently, any decision whether to institute nutritional support is now influenced more by previous dietary history and the natural history of the primary disease process in respect of future nutritional intake, than by measurements of nutritional parameters.

In surgical circles there is growing enthusiasm for vigorous nutritional support of malnourished patients about to undergo major surgery [14]. This argument is based on the unproven premise that malnourished patients have more postoperative complications or even an increased risk of death. However, clinical nutrition trials have often included large numbers of normally or near-normally nourished, rather than malnourished patients, which have

Table 78.2. General indications for nutritional support.

Obvious gross malnutrition—albumin < 30 g/l; marked weight loss; muscle wasting; oedema.

Nutritional parameters suggesting protein-calorie malnutrition, or dietary history showing impaired nutrient intake for one week or more.

Medical and surgical disorders likely to result in protein-calorie malnutrition if nutritional support witheld.

made the interpretation of any benefits of nutritional support virtually impossible. Finally, when differences are noted between treatment and control groups it can be a matter of opinion whether they are clinically significant; for example, decreasing hospital in-patient stay after surgery by

a short period can hardly be cited as a clinically significant benefit of nutritional support.

Guidelines for assessing the indications for providing nutritional support are summarized in Table 78.2.

Clinical problems

It has been traditional to categorize those clinical conditions that may be frequently associated with protein-calorie malnutrition and to imply that patients with these conditions are likely to require nutritional support. Such an approach, however, is a gross

Table 78.3. Specific indications for nutritional support.

Definite benefit
Management of short bowel syndrome.
Intestinal fistulae—without distal obstruction.
Intra-abdominal sepsis.
Major burns.
Major sepsis.
Multiple injuries involving viscera.
Pancreatic abscess/pseudocyst/trauma/fistula.

Possible benefit
Acute pancreatitis.
Inflammatory bowel disease.
Preoperatively—major cancer surgery.
Postoperatively—major surgery and complications.

over-simplification of the problems that arise when deciding whether or not to institute nutritional support, because almost *all* medical and surgical conditions *can* be accompanied by protein-calorie malnutrition.

Despite the difficulties that exist in defining the indications for nutritional support, clinical trials and clinical experience have highlighted a number of areas where clear benefits have been obtained (Table 78.3). Inflammatory bowel disease and pancreatitis are of particular interest.

Inflammatory bowel disease (see Chapters 50 and 53)

There is much literature on the influence that nutritional support has had on the short- as well as long-term management of inflammatory bowel disease. With a few exceptions, it is almost impossible to evaluate the results critically because of the absence of control groups.

Five conclusions can be deduced from the available information [64]:
1. Nutritional support, administered either by the enteral or parenteral route, in combination with medical therapy, frequently results in an improvement of the nutritional status of patients with inflammatory bowel disease [55, 56]. There appears no specific reason, however, to advocate parenteral rather than enteral nutrition and there is no evidence to suggest that the so-called 'chemically-defined elemental diets' are in any way superior to the cheaper whole-protein containing polymeric diets.
2. The immediate outcome of patients with acute colitis, due either to Crohn's disease or ulcerative colitis, is uninfluenced by parenteral nutrition [8, 41].
3. A recommendation for surgery in a malnourished patient with small intestinal Crohn's disease should not be made until efforts have been made to improve the patient's nutritional status. There is a strong suggestion from uncontrolled studies that surgery may be rendered unnecessary in a significant proportion of such patients by nutritional support [10, 49, 55, 68, 69].
4. Abnormal growth patterns in children with Crohn's disease may be restored by means of short- or long-term enteral nutrition using either elemental or polymeric diets in combination with medical therapy [34, 46].
5. There is now a suggestion based on the results of two controlled trials that acute exacerbations of Crohn's disease in adults

may be managed in the short-term as effectively with a pre-digested, chemically-defined elemental diet as with corticosteroids [48].

Acute pancreatitis (see Chapter 35)

Seventy to 80% of patients with acute pancreatitis run a limited course and, after the abdominal pain and ileus resolve, introduction of oral feeding is usually possible within about five days. These patients do not require nutritional support.

In about 20% of patients [11] the pancreatitis persists for longer, or the patient develops haemorrhagic or post-necrotic pancreatitis, or the pancreatitis is complicated by abscess or pseudocyst formation. Nutritional support is mandatory in these patients, since they are hypermetabolic with nitrogen losses often in excess of 15 g/day. Due to the fact that there is often an underlying ileus, and because a significant proportion will come to surgery, the parenteral rather than enteral route is preferred.

Metabolic responses to starvation or injury

The aim of nutritional therapy is to achieve an input of nitrogen and calories in excess of output. Patients requiring nutritional support have usually either undergone a period of starvation or have been subjected to injury in the form of trauma, burns, sepsis or surgery. It must be appreciated from the outset that the metabolic responses to starvation and injury differ, and that these differences markedly affect the nutritional requirements of the two groups of patients. The metabolic rate falls in response to **starvation**, and the body's adaptive changes are geared towards keeping the losses of essential constituents to a minimum. In contrast, after **injury** the basal metabolic rate and energy expenditure rise; weight loss may be

Table 78.4. Factors affecting energy expenditure
(+ increases; − decreases).

Factors	Change in energy expenditure
Starvation	−
Sepsis	+
Physical activity	+
Paralysis	−
Core temperature rise	+ 13% per °C
Heat losses	
Low ambient temperature	+
Burns	+
Low humidity	+
Diminished body mass	−
Injury	
Elective uncomplicated surgery	+ 10%
Major elective surgery	+ 15–20%
Multiple fractures	+ 10–20%
Septicaemia/peritonitis	+ 20–50%
Large area burns	+ 30–125%

pronounced and nitrogen losses high. The basic nutritional requirements of the injured patients are, therefore, far greater than those of the starved patient. The common factors affecting energy expenditure are summarized on Table 78.4.

Starvation

In the earliest stages of starvation small increases in catecholamines (the so-called catabolic hormones) and glucagon mobilize stored glycogen. There is a rapid fall in weight during the first 48–72 hours due to losses of sodium and water, but these are retained later and may cause oedema. A fall of insulin production allows lipolysis and the mobilization of protein-bound amino acids from muscle. Amino acids are then either converted to glucose or used for the hepatic synthesis of albumin and acute phase proteins. Resting metabolic expenditure falls steadily and nitrogen losses fall from initial values of 8–10 g/24 hours to 2–4 g/24 hours over a period of two weeks. In

time, more and more energy is derived from fat until more than 95% is supplied by that source.

Injury

The rise in metabolic rate following injury may be marked—up to 100% after burns. Catecholamines, glucagon and cortisol predominate over the anabolic hormone insulin; the output of insulin is often raised but the patients are often insulin resistant.

The resultant substrate changes maintain the necessary energy for the increased metabolic requirements. In contrast to starvation, fat stores provide only a maximum of 80% of total energy requirements, the remainder being derived from body protein. The net result is a rapid release of amino acids from muscle protein with concomitant muscle wasting. The amino acids in the muscle are deaminated and the carbon fragments are transported to the liver via glutamine and alanine. In the liver the carbon moieties are resynthesized to glucose, and the amino groups incorporated into urea. Net nitrogen loss occurs not only because of breakdown of injured tissue protein, but also from the protein mass as a whole. Moreover, recent studies also indicate that there is reduced protein synthesis in postoperative patients and this will also contribute to the negative nitrogen balance.

Assessment of nutritional requirements

Any attempt to correct the nutritional deficits in undernourished or injured patients must include the provision of a readily utilized energy substrate, as well as nitrogen for protein synthesis. In general the response to injury is governed by the severity of the injury (Table 78.4)—although the response is decreased, for any given injury size, by prior starvation. As many patients undergoing major surgery have experienced a period of preoperative malnutrition it is quite difficult to assess nutritional requirements without direct measurement. Ideally, nitrogen output should be estimated by direct measurement of nitrogen in urine and stools. In practice the methods are cumbersome, time consuming and costly. With the exception of patients with protein-losing enteropathies or fistulae, reliable estimations of nitrogen losses in g/24 hours can be calculated from the formula:

nitrogen losses

$= $ (mmol urinary urea/24 h × 0.028) + 2

where the factor of 2 is added to take into account constant non-urea urinary nitrogen as well as faecal and skin losses. Simple corrections for proteinuria and rising blood urea values in renal failure patients have been described [37, 38].

Specific nutritional requirements

Energy and nitrogen

There is a close relationship between energy and nitrogen balances, so the two requirements can be considered together. In a normal active man, positive nitrogen balance is achieved with a nitrogen intake of 8–9 g/24 hours. Non-protein energy requirements are in the region of 1338 kj/g (320 kcal/g) of nitrogen.

As the metabolic expenditure of a starved, re-feeding patient is low, nitrogen equilibrium can be attained with a nitrogen intake of 8–10 g/day, with a non-protein energy requirement of 960 kj/g (200 kcal/g) of nitrogen.

When the metabolic rate is increased after injury or during febrile illness nitrogen requirements often rise markedly and this rise is greater than the increased requirement for energy (Table 78.5).

Table 78.6. A guide to the daily nutritional requirements for enteral and parenteral nutrition.

Nitrogen	8–24 g
Energy	7,500–16,500 kJ
	(1,600–3,500 kcal)
Electrolytes and trace elements	
Sodium	70–150 mmol
Chloride	70–220 mmol
Potassium	50–100 mmol
Calcium	5–10 mmol
Magnesium	5–20 mmol
Fluoride	50 μmol
Manganese	2–4 mg
Copper	1.5–3.0 mg
Zinc	10–20 mg
Iron	10–15 mg
Selenium	100–200 μg
Iodine	10–200 μg
Chromium	5–10 μg

Electrolytes

Attention should be paid to correcting electrolyte imbalance in all patients receiving nutritional therapy; the values shown in Table 78.6 can be considered only as a

Table 78.5. Approximate daily requirements for energy and nitrogen.

	Non-catabolic	Intermediate	Catabolic
Nitrogen			
g/24 h	8–10	12–14	16–24
Energy			
kJ/24 h	7,680–9,600	9,120–11,040	10,750–16,130
kcal/24h	1,600–2,000	1,900–2,300	2,240–3,360
Non-protein Energy			
kJ/g of nitrogen	960	754	658
kcal/g of nitrogen	200	160	140

guide to requirements. Potassium losses occur in a fixed ratio to nitrogen losses, so at least 5 mmol potassium should be administered with each gram of nitrogen.

As a general principle, biological fluids should be collected from appropriate orifices of sick patients (for example, gastric aspirates, fistulae and drain effluents, urine, diarrhoeal faeces) and analysed for electrolyte content. Hypophosphataemia is a common complication of parenteral (intravenous) nutrition, and at least 30 mmol phosphate must be administered daily.

Minerals

Mineral deficiences in patients receiving long-term nutritional support have been well-documented. Unfortunately the minimal daily requirements of most minerals are not known with any certainty, so the values for manganese, copper, zinc and selenium given in Table 78.6 are, at best, approximate. Further research will almost certainly indicate that additional trace metals should be added to this list.

Vitamins

Vitamins are necessary for the utilization of nutritional components. Vitamin deficiencies can occur rapidly in the debilitated state and supplements should be given as soon as nutritional support is started.

Objectives of nutritional support

The objectives vary according to the underlying metabolic status of each patient. Ideally, nutritional status should be maintained in the normally-nourished patient and improved in the nutritionally-depleted patient. At the very least, the reduction of protein and energy resources should be minimized.

In practice however, the achievement of the ideal objectives is limited by a number

Table 78.7. Factors limiting achievement of nutritional objectives.

Most common
Sepsis
Trauma
  Severe fractures
  Major visceral injury
  Major burns
  Major operations
Immobility
  Bedbound
  Splintage of fractures
  Neurological causes
  Muscle relaxant drugs in intensive care
  Pain

Common
Technique
  Insufficient energy supply
  Insufficient nitrogen supply
  Insufficient co-factors for nitrogen utilization
Fluid balance
  Inability to tolerate volume required for nutritional support

Unusual
  Hyperglycaemia unresponsive to insulin
  Hyponatraemia due to inappropriate anti-diuretic hormone secretion
Occult losses of protein
Low ambient temperature

of factors (Table 78.7); again there are differences between injury and starvation. Nutritionally-depleted starving patients, particularly children, can be expected to show marked improvements in lean body mass and can even go into positive nitrogen balance when sufficient protein is given, despite low calorie intake; malnourished patients, suffering the catabolic response to injury or sepsis, do not show significant gains in lean body mass during nutritional therapy until the catabolic response ceases and the anabolic phase commences.

Table 78.7 lists the factors that, together with poor feeding techniques and various specific nutritional deficiencies, are associated with a delay in the onset of the anabolic phase and thus go against the achievement of net protein synthesis.

During the catabolic phase, therefore, all

that can be expected of nutritional support is the maintenance of lean body mass at its pre-therapy value, such that subsequent anabolism starts in the least malnourished state that is possible.

Methods of providing nutritional support

It is important to emphasize that, when gastrointestinal function is normal, attempts should be made to use enteral rather than parenteral (intravenous) nutrition. Ideally the patient should be fed orally, either with whole food, or with the addition of palatable supplements. If this is not possible, liquid feeds can be administered via a nasoenteric tube. Some patients requiring nutritional therapy have a gastrostomy or jejunostomy and nutrition can be administered via these routes. Only if these methods fail should nutrients be provided intravenously.

In general, too many patients are managed unnecessarily via the parenteral route, which is far more expensive and carries a higher morbidity. In addition, the expertise and back up services required for its correct administration are considerable compared with those required for enteral nutrition. However, the two methods should be thought of as complementary and not as competitive.

Enteral nutrition

Once the decision is made to provide nutritional support using the enteral route, the best formulation to meet the nutritional needs of the individual patient must be selected. There are many commercially available enteral diets in the United Kingdom with important differences in their nutritional components.

Diet formulation

Diets for patients with normal gastrointestinal function

Patients with normal gastrointestinal function can assimilate whole protein and unhydrolysed triglyceride. Enteral diets for these patients should therefore contain whole protein as the nitrogen source, and a mixture of triglycerides and carbohydrate as the energy source. High molecular weight glucose polymers are the most suitable carbohydrate energy source [19]. The inclusion of small quantities of lactose in these diets does not predispose patients to gastrointestinal side effects, if the diets are administered by continuous gravity infusion [26]. Controversy exists as to what constitutes the optimum non-protein energy to nitrogen ratio of these diets— since the nitrogen and energy requirements of different patients vary (see Table 78.5), a ratio of 150 kcal/gN would appear a reasonable compromise. Enteral diets for patients with normal gastrointestinal function should contain sufficient electrolytes, trace elements and vitamins to satisfy nutritional requirements.

Diets for patients with impaired gastrointestinal function

In a small group of patients, nutrient assimilation may be impaired either on account of insufficient hydrolysis of luminal nutrients, or because the functional absorptive capacity of the intestine is so decreased that it cannot cope with the quantities of nutrients presented for absorption. In these circumstances nutrients should be presented to the gut in a predigested form, to ensure maximal possible absorption.

Conditions in which luminal nutrient hydrolysis is severely impaired include severe exocrine pancreatic insufficiency, obstructive jaundice and the short bowel

Table 78.8. Indications for use of predigested 'elemental' diets.

Impaired luminal nutrient digestion
Severe exocrine pancreatic insufficiency
Total pancreatectomy
Carcinoma of pancreas
Severe chronic pancreatitis
Short bowel syndrome
Intestinal resections
Intestinal fistulae

Reduced functional absorptive capacity
Intestinal resections
Intestinal fistulae
Severe untreated coeliac disease*
Severe active Crohn's disease*

*rare

---

syndrome. The functional absorptive capacity of the intestine may be severely decreased in the short bowel syndrome and in clinical conditions characterized by a severe and extensive mucosal lesion—for example, very severe, untreated coeliac disease with jejunal and ileal involvement or very severe Crohn's disease (Table 78.8). The old term 'elemental diet' is a misnomer—used initially to describe the early free amino acid- and glucose-containing diets, it was used later to describe all the other diets containing predigested nutrients that were far from 'elemental' in design.

The use of 'elemental' diets has been advocated in a variety of other clinical conditions [59] but there are little controlled data to support any of these claims [35]. Indeed, there is no evidence for the superiority of 'elemental' diets over polymeric diets containing whole protein as the nitrogen source, in the management of malnourished patients with normal gastrointestinal function [20, 22].

The ideal pre-digested chemically-defined 'elemental' diet

Results of recent basic physiological intestinal perfusion and protein turnover studies suggest that the nitrogen source of these pre-digested diets should consist of **oligopeptides** rather than free amino acids [22, 33]. Purified partial enzyme hydrolysates of whole protein containing peptides of 2–3 amino acid residues have recently been shown to provide the most suitable peptide-based nitrogen source [52].

As **high molecular weight carbohydrate polymers** can be assimilated efficiently even in the absence of luminal amylase activity [18], they should probably constitute the carbohydrate fraction of the energy source.

Since these diets are indicated in conditions where luminal fat digestion is impaired, they should not contain large amounts of a long chain length triglyceride-based energy source. It is not clear in the clinical setting how efficiently medium chain triglycerides are absorbed in the absence of luminal hydrolysis, so they should probably not be included in these diets. The diet should contain at least 4% of their total energy content as **linoleic acid**, in the hopes of preventing essential fatty acid deficiency.

Recent research indicates that these diets should contain at lest 70–90 mmol of **sodium** per litre, which is far in excess of the sodium content of most currently available diets [65]. The diet should also contain sufficient **trace elements and vitamins** to satisfy the requirements of the average malnourished patient.

Enteral feeding—modern techniques

ORAL FEEDING

When the patient is able to swallow but still unable to eat normal food (for example,

Table 78.9. Proprietary polymeric enteral diets, all of which have a whole protein nitrogen content.

	Flavouring necessary	Presentation	Osmolality mosmol/kg	Non-protein energy/nitrogen ratio (kcal/gN)
*Polymeric diet**				
Build up (Carnation)	No	Powder	575	100
Clinifeed 400 (Roussel)	No	Liquid	426	142
Clinifeed Favour (Roussel)	No	Liquid	403	142
Clinifeed Iso (Roussel)	No	Liquid	321	200
Ensure (Abbott)	No	Liquid	430	154
Fortison Standard (Cow and Gate)	No	Liquid	300	131
Fortison Energy-Plus (Cow and Gate)	No	Liquid	410	167
Isocal (Mead Johnson)	Yes	Liquid	350	170
Nutrauxil (Kabivitrum)	No	Liquid	386	140
Trisorbon (BDH)	No	Powder	400	130
Chemically defined (elemental diets)				
Flexical (Mead Johnson)	Yes[†]	Powder[‡]	580	256
Nutranel (Roussel)	Yes[†]	Powder[‡]	550	131
Vinox HN (Eaton)	Yes[†]	Powder[×]	830	121

* All have whole protein as nitrogen source.
† in the opinion of the author.
‡ Oligopeptate nitrogen source.
× Free amino acid nitrogen source.

because of a fractured jaw or an oesophageal stricture), a liquid diet can be provided from any hospital diet kitchen. The large volume of fluid required to liquidize whole food may make this type of supplement unacceptable to some patients and as a consequence liquidized food is now seldom used. The next five years will see a rapid growth in the quantity and quality of specially formulated palatable liquid nutritional supplements for such patients.

The 'palatable' proprietary enteral diets are listed in Table 78.9 and are theoretically suitable for oral feeding, either as a means of supplementing an inadequate intake of normal food or as the sole means of nutritional support. The point should be made, however, that most patients find these diets less palatable and acceptable than the manufacturers claim. The exception seems to be the 'elemental diet' now used in the group of exceptional motivated patients with acute exacerbations of Crohn's disease [48]. 'Elemental diets' should only be used in pre-ference to the standard polymeric enteral diet, if positive indications for their use are present (see Table 78.6).

If it is planned to use the proprietary enteral diets as the sole means of nutritional support, it is best to administer the diets using a nasoenteric tube, because it is easier to control intake precisely and, as mentioned, most patients find that these diets are not palatable and excessive nursing time is taken up encouraging patients to drink the desired quantities.

TUBE FEEDING

Hospital tube feeds

Before the recent resurgence of interest in enteral nutrition, those patients with normal gastrointestinal function who did receive nutritional support were fed with tube feeds prepared in the hospital dietetic department. Although these tube feeds are cheap, their preparation places a significant burden on the workload of the diet kitchen. Problems with infection have been well-documented with such diets and there are controlled data to show that the incidence of diarrhoea is higher when 'home brew' rather than commercial, diets are used for enteral feeding [6, 25].

Proprietary enteral diets

Some of the more widely-used polymeric and predigested 'elemental diets' are listed in Table 78.9.

Nasogastric tube feeding

Patients who cannot swallow, or who will not tolerate oral feeding, can be fed using a nasogastric tube [58].

The time-honoured method of tube feeding has been to place a large-bore Ryles tube into the stomach and instil intermittently up to 200 ml of liquid feed, having

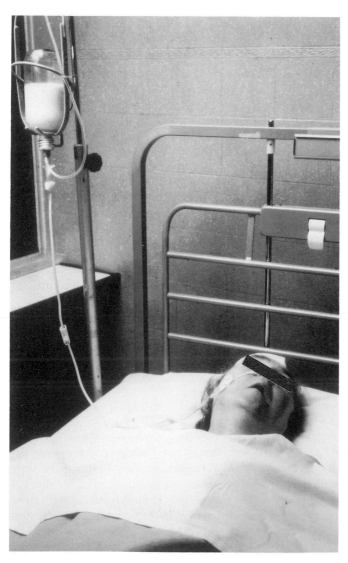

Fig. 78.2. Enteral feeding of a patient following neurosurgery. The patient is intubated nasogastrically with a fine-bore feeding tube, and receiving an enteral diet by constant gravity infusion from a 500 ml glass container using a standard giving set.

first aspirated the gastric residue. This method is probably responsible for the poor reputation of enteral feeding, as the incidence of side-effects (diarrhoea, aspiration pneumonia and oesophageal ulceration) is unacceptably high.

Major new developments have taken place in this field and most of these problems have been circumvented. Enteral feeds (Fig. 78.2) can be administered from containers by gravity infusion using narrow-bore feeding tubes, most of which are inserted into the stomach using an introducer. These fine-bore tubes are more comfortable than the older wide-bore tubes and their use has not so far been associated with oesophageal erosions, ulcers or strictures. Although easy to pass, the final position should be checked radiologically, or by insufflating 5 ml air while listening over the epigastrium, to ensure that the feeding tube has been positioned in the stomach and not the bronchial tree.

Types of feeding tubes

There are now many different fine-bore nasogastric feeding tubes on the market which are of two main types—either tubes with an unweighted or weighted tip. The limitations and drawbacks of both types of fine-bore feeding tube have been defined [28]. Controlled trials have shown that incorporating a weight in the tip does not improve clinical performance [31, 53], polyurethane is preferred to polyvinyl chloride. The results of the author's latest trial favours the use of a polyurethane tube incorporating a specially moulded unweighted distal aspiration port [53]. There are three clinical areas, however, where there appears to be distinct advantages using a weighted tube [32]:
1. Nasogastric intubation of patients already intubated with an endotracheal tube.
2. Intubation of patients with oesophageal strictures in whom endoscopic intubation with an unweighted tube has failed.
3. Nasoenteric feeding.

Endoscopic tube placement

Although nasogastric tube placement is usually easy, difficulties do arise when attempts are made to perform intubation in patients with oesophageal strictures or gastric atony. In the first group of patients, irrespective of whether the stricture is malignant or benign, intubation is usually required either during diagnostic endoscopy or immediately following endoscopic dilatation [30]. In the second group, despite claims to the contrary [9, 45] feeding tubes rarely pass through the pylorus spontaneously and have to be placed in the jejunum or duodenum at endoscopy.

Nasoenteric feeding

In certain patients with neurological disorders of swallowing (for example, motor neuron disease, pseudobulbar palsy) or gastric atony, regurgitation or aspiration of feeds necessitates the cessation of nasogastric feeding. Theoretically, these problems should be circumvented by direct duodenal or jejunal feeding, after endoscopic intubation with one of the longer weighted tubes.

Early postoperative nasoenteral feeding

The recognition that small bowel motility returns earlier in the postoperative period than gastric emptying, has lead to the concept of early postoperative enteral feeding using either a fine needle catheter jejunostomy or nasoenteric tubes positioned at the time of laparotomy [61]. On theoretical grounds, this would appear to represent an ideal means of providing nutritional support in the early postoperative period, but clinical benefit remains unproven [72].

Techniques of administration

Enteral diets are best administered from feed reservoirs using a giving set and feeding

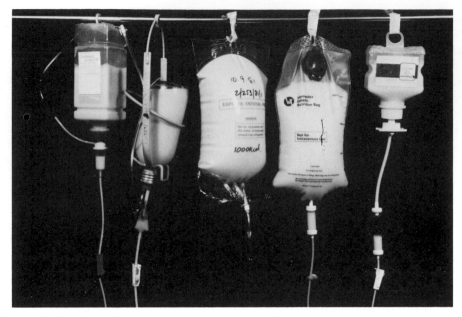

Fig. 78.3. A selection of enteral feeding bags and reservoirs. From left to right: (1) Roussel Clinifeeding System 3 (1.3 l); (2) Re-useable DHSS Winchester container (0.5 l); (3) Express enteral feeding bag (2 l); (4) Viomedex enteral feeding bag (1.5 l); (5) Boots Flow Fusor enteral feeding bottle (0.5 l).

tube which passes directly into the stomach, duodenum or jejunum (Fig. 78.2). There has been a proliferation of delivery systems (Fig. 78.3) and debate exists as to the ideal volume of the feed reservoirs.

Feeds which are mixed in the diet kitchen are subject to significant bacterial contamination [3]. During administration of the these feeds further bacterial multiplication occurs, so they should not be prepared in volumes of more than 0.5 l. No significant bacterial contamination of presterilized enteral feeds appears to occur during filling of reservoirs using a 'no touch' technique so, if these diets are used, reservoirs of up to 1–2 l volume can be used.

Prescribing the regimen

As one of the main objectives of nutritional support is, wherever possible, to place patients in positive nitrogen balance, the first aim of any treatment programme is to determine nitrogen losses. Positive nitrogen balance can only be achieved if daily nitrogen intake is approximately 4 g in excess of output. As it is difficult to increase muscle mass and body weight in an immobilized patient, aggressive physiotherapy and exercising is encouraged whenever possible.

Use of a starter regimen

Upper abdominal symptoms (distension, discomfort and colicky pains, as well as diarrhoea) are said to occur frequently if full-strength enteric feeding is introduced too quickly [63]. These side-effects can be due to intolerance of a high osmotic load, lactose intolerance, use of contaminated feeds, or coincidental antibiotic therapy [29, 64]. It is generally believed that the incidence of these side-effects can be minimized by gradually introducing full-strength enteral feeds over three to four days by means of a 'starter regimen' (Table 78.10).

Starter regimens are, however, usually unnecessary in patients with normal

Table 78.10. A starter regimen for enteral feeding.

Day	Strength	Volume (litres)
Normal gastrointestinal function		
1	Half	2
2	Three-quarter	2
3	Full	2
4	Exact composition modified according to nitrogen balance studies conducted over previous 3 days (nitrogen input = output + 4 g/day).	
Impaired gastrointestinal function		
1	Quarter	1
2 8	Strength and volume should be cautiously increased over 5–7 days.	

Table 78.11. Complications of enteral nutrition.

Tube related problems
Oesophagitis
Oesophageal erosions
Oesophageal stricture
Tube misplacement
Tube withdrawal

Gastrointestinal side-effects
Diarrhoea
Abdominal distension
Abdominal pain
Intussusception

Metabolic complications
Hyperglycaemia
Hypokalaemia
Hypomagnesaemia
Hypocalcaemia
Hypophosphataemia
Zinc deficiency
Low red cell folate

Abnormalities of liver function

Intravenous administration of enteric feeds

Regurgitation and aspiration

gastrointestinal function fed with polymeric diets by constant gravity infusion [29], but their use has been found to be necessary when chemically defined 'elemental' diets are used in patients with acute exacerbations of inflammatory bowel disease [54]. Over 85% of patients can be fed successfully by simple gravity infusion using the giving set clamp to control the infusion rate [21]. The use of an enteral feeding pump is, however, beneficial for patients with impaired gastrointestinal function who develop diarrhoea during enteral feeding, and may save up to 30 minutes nursing time per patient, per day [21].

Complications of enteral nutrition (Table 78.11)

Tube-related problems

Complications associated with wide-bore Ryles tubes (oesophageal erosions, haemorrhage and strictures) have not been reported with the fine-bore nasogastric tubes. The fine-bore tubes can be passed into the trachea rather than into the oesophagus, especially in comatose patients, so care must be taken to ensure correct positioning

before enteric feeding is started. A common problem with the fine-bore feeding tube is the ease with which the tube rides up into the oesophagus, or is removed completely by the patient; many patients on enteral feeding regimens require more than one intubation [28]. Intravenous administration of an enteric feed has been reported, but this complication should not occur if feeding tubes and giving sets are used with reversed luer locks.

Gastrointestinal side-effects

Diarrhoea, abdominal distension and abdominal pain are common side-effects, occurring at some stage during the treatment in up to 25% of patients receiving enteral nutrition [20]. As the most likely cause is coincidental antibiotic therapy antibiotics should be stopped if clinically possible. If not, symptomatic treatment with imodium or codeine phosphate is often effective, if diarrhoea is the main problem.

Metabolic complications

Hyperglycaemia may occur during enteral feeding, caused by excessive sugar intake or insulin resistance associated with trauma and injury. Initially, frequent urine testing for glucose or blood glucose measurements should be performed. Electrolyte abnormalities, particularly hypokalaemia, commonly occur during enteral nutrition and are related not only to the feeding regimen, but also to the underlying medical or surgical disorder. Low blood concentrations of calcium, magnesium, zinc and phosphate can also occur, and supplements may be required.

Abnormalities of liver function

Minor, intermittent elevations of hepatocellular enzymes are common, and of uncertain aetiology.

Parenteral nutrition

Parenteral nutrition is indicated only when malnourished patients cannot be given nutritional support by the enteral route. It must satisfy the full nutritional requirements of the patient and wherever possible provide a positive nitrogen balance. Parenteral nutrition can be more hazardous than enteral nutrition, and it requires obsessional attention to detail if the patient is to avoid trouble.

The catheter

Silicone rubber catheters are preferred as they cause less intravascular trauma and venous thrombosis than polyethylene, polyvinyl or Teflon catheters [71]. The author now routinely uses a 35 cm long silicone feeding catheter (Vygon Nutricath S, code 2180.20) with a 25 cm long multipurpose extension tube (Vygon, code 220.02).

Catheter entry site

Infusion solutions for parenteral nutrition have high osmolalities and are sclerosant if given through a short catheter into peripheral veins. Similarly, infusion through a long plastic catheter, threaded through an antecubital vein and terminating in the superior vena cava, is a notorious cause of thrombophlebitis [23].

One of the safest methods of introducing these solutions is directly into the superior vena cava, using subclavian vein catheterization. In this way solutions with a concentration of 1500 mOsmol/l can be infused through a short catheter at a rate of 2–3 ml/minute, while being diluted a thousand-fold by a blood flow of 2–3 l/minute. The entry site of the catheter is a large vein, which decreases the likelihood of thrombophlebitis. The route of choice is the infraclavicular approach to the subclavian vein, through the pectoral skin below the clavicle. This is an excllent place to keep clean and dress because it is flat, relatively immobile and does not collect perspiration or other secretions. Moreover, the patient's arm and neck remain free for normal activity.

In patients with clotting disorders, recent cervical surgery or severe obstructive airways disease, the subclavian approach should be avoided and the internal jugular vein should be used instead.

Catheter placement

Catheter placement should be performed by an experienced clinician, under aseptic conditions, preferably in an operating theatre [60]. Parenteral nutrition is never an emergency procedure, and the complication rate of catheter placement is inversely proportional to the experience of the inserter; it is usually high in emergency catheterizations.

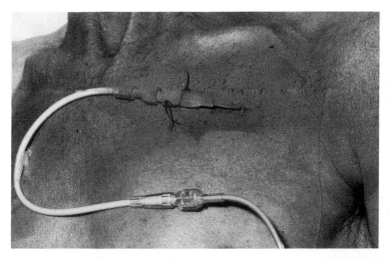

Fig. 78.4. Silicone intravenons feeding catheter in place. Note the separation of the infraclavicular venous entry incision from the site of exit of the feeding catheter from the subcutaneous skin tunnel. To avoid 'tugging' forces exerted by the infusion apparatus on the feeding catheter, the extension tube is connected to the feeding catheter and the infusion apparatus to this.

Skin tunnelling (Fig. 78.4)

One of the major complications of parenteral nutrition is catheter sepsis as a result of introduction of organisms through the catheter or at the venous entry site [70]. When a short catheter is used, the infusion apparatus is attached close to the entry site. By contrast, if a long catheter is used, the end point of the catheter can be tunnelled subcutaneously, so that junction between catheter and infusion apparatus is separated from the venous entry site. There is a lower incidence of catheter-related sepsis in patients whose feeding catheter is tunnelled subcutaneously, compared to those whose infusion apparatus is attached directly to the catheter close to the venous entry site [27].

Dressing

After insertion of the catheter, the venous entry site incision and the skin tunnel exit sites are sprayed with iodine and Opsite skin spray. The skin tunnel exit site is then covered with semipermeable adhesive dressing (Steripad 12.5 × 10 cm, Johnson & Johnson, Slough).

Although it has been traditional nursing practice to re-dress the catheter entry site every 48 hours recent experience suggests that this is wrong—these dressings should only be taken down if there are clinical suggestions or signs of catheter-related sepsis [51].

Catheter-related sepsis

Catheter-related sepsis is a common complication of parenteral nutrition and has an incidence up to 30% depending on the technique used, the type of patient and the operator's experience. Whenever a pyrexia develops in a patient on parenteral nutrition, it is important to exclude all other causes of sepsis. The feeding line should be removed only when no other apparent site of infection can be identified. After removing an infected feeding line, the pyrexia usually settles within 24–48 hours and antibiotics are seldom indicated. The commonest organism isolated from cultures of blood, 'through-line' fluid, catheter tip and skin entry site are *Staphylococcus epidermidis*, *S. aureus*, coliforms and *Candida albicans*. It is important to remember that acute bacterial endocarditis or distant infection (for example, lung or brain abscess) may result from failure to recognize catheter-related sepsis.

Low doses of heparin [2] have been reported to reduce the incidence of catheter-related sepsis—heparin 1000u should be added to each 3 litre delivery bag. Scrupulous nursing care, ideally by a trained nutrition nurse, also decreases the incidence of catheter-related sepsis [27].

Administration technique

The position of the catheter should always be checked radiologically before a hypertonic parenteral infusion is commenced. The major components of the parenteral nutrition regimen should be infused simultaneously. Until recently, infusion was from individual containers connected to the feeding catheter by a two or three line giving set. Sepsis rates, nursing time and insulin requirements can be reduced if all constituents of the regimen, including additives, are mixed together in a 3 litre bag. This

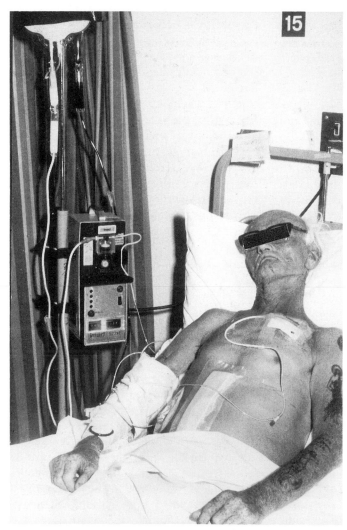

Fig. 78.5. Parenteral nutrition delivery system: the parenteral fluids are mixed together in the 3l bag (Travenol B 7992 3l empty parenteral nutrition container) and delivered via the single lead giving set (Travenol C 2071 sterile administration set) by means of an Imed 922 columetric infusion pump.

should be done aseptically by a pharmacist, using a laminar flow cabinet, and infused using a single line giving set into the feeding catheter. The complete parenteral nutrition delivery system is shown in Fig. 78.5.

Mixtures of amino acids, hypertonic dextrose, electrolytes and trace metals are compatible, and *in vitro* studies also indicate that fat emulsions may be safely mixed with the above nutrients, but only stored for up to four days [13]. Ideally such mixtures should be used within 36 hours of preparation.

The intravenous nutrition regimen

Nitrogen source

Pure L-amino acid solutions provide the source of nitrogen (Table 78.12). It is generally agreed that the essential amino acids should comprise approximately 40% of the total amino acid content by weight. There is considerable controversy, however, as to whether glycine, present in comparatively large proportions in some of the solutions (for example, Aminoplex 12 and 14), acts as an efficient precursor for synthesis of other amino acids or is effectively utilized as an energy source via gluconeogenesis.

The energy source

Glucose is the most commonly used carbohydrate energy source. Because of possible hyperglycaemia (necessitating the administration of insulin, sometimes in large quantities because of coexisting 'insulin resistance') alternative carbohydrate energy sources such as xylotol, sorbitol, fructose, maltose and ethanol have been proposed. None has proved to be as effective as glucose and all cause side-effects [37].

Lipid is an alternative energy source, but opinion is still divided about the relative merits of glucose versus lipid [1, 39, 40]. Most regimens use a mixture of glucose and fat as the energy sources and the consensus from most recent studies suggests that 30–50% of the non-protein energy source should be provided in the form of a fat emulsion.

The energy and nitrogen requirements of each patient are closely linked. They can be determined by assessing the caloric requirements and then administering amino acids to give 672–960 kJ of non-protein energy/g of nitrogen (140–200 kcal of non-protein energy/g of nitrogen) depending upon the degree of catabolism indicated by the metabolic rate. A useful working figure of 25 kcal/kg·day satisfies the basal metabolic requirements for normal adults and recent estimated requirements in disease states suggest a figure of 35–45 kcal/kg·day [15]. Allowances are then made for the factors shown in Table 78.4 and nitrogen requirements matched according to the standard values in Table 78.5. Alternatively, nitrogen losses can be assessed in the urine, faeces, fistulas or drain fluids. In practice, this often can be achieved by measurement of urinary urea excretion alone.

Electrolytes

No single preparation is adequate and close monitoring is required especially in catabolic patients to avoid deficiency or excess (Table 78.13).

The basic regimen

The two basic regimens for the 3 litre bag delivery system used at Central Middlesex Hospital (Table 78.14) are based on the use of Synthamin 14 and Synthamin 17 as the nitrogen source, and a mixture of dextrose and Intralipid as the energy sources. Regimen I has a non-protein energy to nitrogen ratio (kcal/gN) of 157:1 and regimen II has a ratio of 133:1.

Table 78.12. Some amino acid solutions used in the United Kingdom.

Preparation	Manufacturer	Nitrogen g/litre	Energy kJ/litre	Electrolytes mmol/litre					Other components/litre
				K^+	Na^{2+}	Mg^{2+}	$Acet^-$	Cl^-	
Aminofusin L Forte	Merck	15.2	1700	30	40	5	10	27.5	vitamins
Aminoplasmal L5	Braun	8.03	850	25	48	2.5	59	31	$H_2PO_4^-$ 9 mmol, malate 7.5 mmol
Aminoplasmal L10	Braun	16.06	1700	25	48	2.5	59	62	$H_2PO_4^-$ 9 mmol, malate 7.5 mmol
Aminoplex 12	Geistlich	12.44	1300	30	35	2.5	5	67	malic acid 4.6 g
Aminoplex 14	Geistlich	13.4	1400	30	35	–	–	79	vitamins, malic acid 5.36 g
FreAmine III 8.5%	Boots	13.0	1400	–	10	–	72	<3	HPO_4^{2-} 10 mmol
FreAmine III 10%	Boots	15.3	1650	–	10	–	88	<2	HPO_4^{2-} 10 mmol
Synthamin 9	Travenol	9.1	1000	60	73	5	100	70	$H_2PO_4^-$ 30 mmol
Synthamin 14	Travenol	14.0	1000	60	73	5	130	70	$H_2PO_4^-$ 30 mmol
Synthamin 14 without electrolytes	Travenol	14.0	1600	–	–	–	68	34	
Synthamin 17	Travenol	16.5	1900	60	73	5	150	70	$H_2PO_4^-$ 30 mmol
Vamin 9	KabiVitrum	9.4	1000	20	50	1.5	–	55	Ca^{2+} 2.5 mmol
Vamin 14	KabiVitrum	13.5	1400	50	100	8	135	100	Ca^{2+} 2.5 mmol, SO_4^{2-} 8 mmol

Table 78.13. Recommended daily electrolyte and trace element requirements and some available preparations [64].

	Na^+ (mmol)	K^+ (mmol)	Mg^{2+} (mmol)	Ca^{2+} (mmol)	Zn^{2+} (µmol)	Mn^{2+} (µmol)	Fe^{3+} (µmol)	Cu^{2+} (µmol)	Cl^- (mmol)	PO_2^{3-} (mmol)	F^- (µmol)	I^- (µmol)	Cr^{2+} (µmol)	Se^{2+} (µmol)	Mo^{2+} (µmol)
Recommended daily requirement	70–220	60–120	5–20	5–10	50	7	70	5	70–220	20–40	50	1	0.2	0.4	0.2
Addamel N (KabiVitrum) per 10 ml ampoule	–	–	–	–	100	5	20	20	13	–	50	1	0.2	0.4	–
Nutracel 400¹ (Travenol) per 500 ml	–	–	9	7.5	40	40	–	–	33	–	–	–	–	–	–
Nutracel 800¹ (Travenol) per 1 l	–	–	9	7.5	40	40	–	–	33	–	–	–	–	–	–
Glucoplex 1600² (Geistlich) per 500 ml	25	15	1.25	–	23	–	–	–	33.5	9	–	–	–	–	–
Glucoplex 1000³ (Geistlich) per 500 ml	25	15	1.25	–	23	–	–	–	33.5	9	–	–	–	–	–

¹ Dextrose 20%
² Dextrose 40%
³ Dextrose 25%

Table 78.14. Breakdown of parenteral nutrition regimen I and II (units are mmol unless other stated).

	V*	E*	N*	Ratio*	Na+	K+	Cl−	PO4^3−	Ca2+	Mg2+	Zn2+	Mn2+
Regimen I												
Synthamin 14	1000	–	14.0		73	60	70	30	–	5	–	–
Intralipid 20%	500	1000	–		–	–	–	7.5	–	5	–	–
Nutracel 400	500	400	–		–	–	33	–	75	9	40	40
Dextrose 20%	1000	800	–		–	–	–	–	–	–	–	–
Total	3000	2200	14.0	157:1	73	60	103	37.5	75	14	40	40
Regimen II												
Synthamin 17	1000	–	16.5		73	60	70	30	–	5	–	–
Intralipid 20%	500	1000	–		–	–	–	7.5	–	–	–	–
Nutracel 400	500	400	–		–	–	33	–	7.5	9	40	40
Dextrose 20%	1000	800	–		–	–	–	–	–	–	–	–
Total	3000	2200	16.5	133:1	73	60	103	37.5	75	14	40	40

*V = volume (ml); E = non-protein energy (kcal); N = nitrogen (g); Ratio = non-protein energy to nitrogen ratio (kcal/gN).

Table 78.15. Vitamin solutions for intravenous infusion.

	Recommended daily intake	Multibionta	Parenterovite IVHP ampoule 1	ampoule 2	Solivito	Vitlipid adult	Intralipid 20% (500 ml)
Thiamine (mg)	1.4	50	250	–	1.2	–	–
Riboflavin (mg)	2.1	7.29	4.0	–	1.8	–	–
Pyridoxine (mg)	2.1	15	50	–	2.43	–	–
Cyanocobalamin (µg)	2.0	–	–	–	2.0	–	–
Nicotinamide (mg)	14	100	–	160	10	–	–
Biotin (mg)	0.35	–	–	–	0.3	–	–
Pantothenic acid/dexpanthenol (mg)	14	25	–	–	10	–	–
Folic acid (mg)	2	–	–	–	0.2	–	–
Ascorbic acid (mg)	35	500	–	500	30	–	–
Calciferol (IU)	100	–	–	–	–	120	–
Phytylmenaquinone (µg)	140	–	–	–	–	150	–
Rentinol (IU)	700	10,000	–	–	–	2,500	–
Tocopheryl acetate (IU)	30	5	–	–	–	–	30

Vitamin and trace element additives (see Tables 78.13 and 78.15)

The fat-soluble vitamin requirements are satisfied by adding one vial of Vitlipid (Table 78.15) to each 3 litre bag.

The water-soluble vitamins are provided by adding one vial of Solivito, one vial of Multibionta, and ampoules 1 and 2 of Parentrovite IVHP in rotation on a daily basis. B vitamins are adversely affected by sunlight, so the 3 litre bag should be covered by an opaque plastic bag.

Nutracel 400 and 800 are 20% dextrose containing minerals and trace elements (Table 78.13). One vial of Addamel N is added daily hoping to satisfy additional trace element requirements (Table 78.13). Supplementary trace elements are probably not necessary for periods of less than one week, unless nutritional depletion has occurred prior to starting parenteral nutrition.

If hyperglycaemia develops insulin can either be added to the container, administered subcutaneously, or given intravenously by an insulin infusion pump.

Complications of parenteral nutrition
(Table 78.16)

Complications are mainly due to catheter insertion (including catheter-related sepsis) or metabolic problems.

Glucose intolerance

Injured or septic patients may have high plasma concentrations of insulin and also insulin antagonists (adrenocorticotrophin, glucagon, growth hormone and catecholamines). Such patients may develop marked hyperglycaemia leading to hypernatraemic, hyperosmolar dehydration, and even coma when receiving 20 or 50% dextrose without insulin. Insulin must therefore be given to most catabolic patients fed with

Table 78.16. Complications of parenteral nutrition.

Complications of catheter insertion
Pneumothorax
Haemothorax
Hydrothorax (intrapleural infusion)
Chylothorax (thoracic duct damage)
Haemo/hydropericardium and tamponade
Arrhythmias (line on tricuspid valve)
Tracheal puncture
Arterial puncture
Air embolism
Major venous thrombosis
   superior vena cava
   obstruction, axillary vein
   thrombosis, pulmonary
   embolus, right atrial thrombi
Haematoma
Nerve injury
   phrenic nerve, branchial plexus,
   recurrent laryngeal nerve
Catheter-related sepsis
Metabolic complications
Hyperglycaemia
Rebound hypoglycaemia and hyperkalaemia
Deficiencies of:
   Potassium
   Sodium
   Phosphate
   Zinc
   Magnesium
   Other trace metals
   Folate
   Essential fatty acids
   Vitamins
Osteomalacia
Hypercalcaemia with osteomalacia*
Metabolic acidosis
   Excess amino acids
   Fructose
Increased carbon dioxide production with high glucose
   loads
Hyperammonaemia
Hepatic disturbances
Elevated liver enzymes
Jaundice
Intrahepatic cholestasis
Biliary sludging
Fatty infiltration
Periportal lymphocytic infiltration
Increased gastric acid secretion†

---

* Long-term parenteral nutrition
† There is no evidence of increased erosive gastritis or haemorrhage.

hypertonic dextrose. By contrast, starved nutritionally-depleted patients seldom require added insulin.

Intracellular ion deficiencies

During the catabolic phase on injury, loss of intracellular protein carries with it associated losses of intracellular ions. Failure to supplement regimens appropriately can result in deficiency states which usually become overt when the catabolic phase gives way to anabolism. Thus, serum concentrations of potassium, phosphate, zinc, magnesium and folate can fall dangerously low. Hypophosphataemia can result in rapid onset of dysarthria, paraesthesiae, disorientation, coma and asthenia (including impairment of respiratory muscle function). Decreases of red cell 2,3-diphosphoglycerate shift the oxygen dissociation curve to the left and red cell ATP may fall to 15% of normal.

Zinc deficiency

Although low serum zinc concentrations do not necessarily imply a total body or intracellular deficiency, falling concentrations should be covered by increased zinc supplements. Zinc deficiency causes diarrhoea, impaired insulin responses, leucocyte dysfunction and delayed wound healing. In addition a positive nitrogen balance cannot be achieved. Cutaneous manifestations resemble perioral and perineal candidiasis and also include stomatitis, alopecia, increased pigmentation and an acrodermatitis entropathica-like dermatitis.

Magnesium deficiency

Magnesium deficiency may induce muscular fibrillation and should be suspected in patients with prolonged diarrhoea (for example, Crohn's disease), or resistant hypocalcaemia.

Other mineral deficiencies

Copper deficiency results in anaemia and leucopenia and chromium deficiency may cause impaired glucose tolerance. Other trace elements (cobalt, selenium, manganese, iron, fluoride and iodine) are also necessary, but knowledge of their requirements during parenteral nutrition is limited.

Vitamin deficiencies

Vitamin deficiencies tend to occur under similar circumstances to intracellular ionic deficiencies. Thiamine deficiency in alcoholics may be unmasked by carbohydrate infusions, thus precipitating acute Wernicke's encephalopathy with coma. In the absence of folate supplementation, depletion occurs rapidly in catabolic patients during parenteral nutrition and may lead to acute pancytopenia, jaundice or impaired protein synthesis by interference with methionine metabolism. Vitamins A and K should be given, but the position of vitamin D is currently a subject of review. Unless vitamin D deficiency is present before parenteral nutrition is started, supplements of this vitamin are not indicated during short-term parenteral nutrition.

Hepatic disturbance

Abnormal liver function tests frequently occur during parenteral nutrition [66]. A cholestatic picture tends to predominate, with rises of alkaline phosphatase and bilirubin. Elevations in serum transaminases may, however, also be seen. Liver biopsies performed in such patients show histological evidence of fatty infiltration, periportal lymphocytic infiltration with bile duct proliferation and intrahepatic cholestasis, or biliary sludging resulting in extrahepatic obstruction. A great deal of speculation surrounds the causes of these biochemical and histological abnormalities [44, 57].

It is important to remember that coexisting medical or surgical problems, rather than parenteral nutrition, may be responsible for the liver function test changes. If, however, a patient on parenteral nutrition becomes jaundiced and extrahepatic obstruction due to biliary sludging is thought to be responsible, cyclical (nocturnal) parenteral nutrition should be tried [42].

Patient monitoring

A full clinical, biochemical, haematological and immunological assessment of nutritional status should be performed before any form of nutritional support is instituted. The recommendations shown in Table 78.17 are guidelines. If electrolyte or other

abnormalities occur, measurements should be made at more frequent intervals. Careful monitoring is important to ensure early identification of the possibly serious complications of parenteral nutrition.

References

1 ASKANAZI J, CARPENTIER YA, ELWYN DH, *et al.* Influence of total parenteral nutrition on fuel utilisation in injury and sepsis *Ann Surg* 1980;191:40–46.
2 BAILEY MJ. Reduction of catheter-associated sepsis in parenteral nutrition using low dose intravenous heparin *Br Med J* 1979;1:1671–1673.
3 BASTOW MD, ALLISON SP, GREAVES P. Study of microbial contamination of nasogastric feeds. In: *Proceedings 3rd European Congress on Parenteral and Enteral Nutrition,* 1981:75.
4 BASTOW MD, GREAVES P, ALLISON SP. Microbial

Table 78.17. Patient monitoring in enteral and parenteral nutrition.

Parameters	Before treatment	Daily	Twice weekly	Weekly
Weight	x	x		x
Mid triceps skin fold thickness	x			x
Arm muscle circumference	x			x
Albumin†	x		x	
Transferrin†	x			x
Lymphocyte count	x			x
Candida—skin tests for PPD (tuberculin) Streptokinase Streptodornase	x			
Full blood picture, ESR	x		x	
Iron†	x			x
Folic acid†	x			x
Vitamin B$_{12}$†	x			x
Prothrombin time	x		x	
Electrolytes and urea†	x	x		
Blood—glucose	x	x		
Phosphate†	x		x	
Calcium, magnesium*	x		x	
Liver function tests	x		x	
Zinc†	x			x
24 hours urinary urea excretion* (for nitrogen balance estimations)	x	x		

*It is our practice to perform daily estimations (recommended definitely for one week to estimate nitrogen requirements). Twice weekly thereafter will usually be sufficient, unless the clinical condition of patient changes.
† serum or plasma.

contamination of enteral feeds. *Human Nutr Appl Nutr* 1982;**36A**:213–217.

5 BRISTIAN BR, BLACKBURN GL, HALLOWELL E, HEDDLE R. Protein status of general surgical patients. *JAMA* 1974;**230**:858–860.

6 CASEWELL MW. Nasogastric feeds as a source of *Klebsiella* infection for intensive care patients. *Research Clinical and Forums* 1979;**1**:101–105.

7 COLLINS JP, McCARTHY ID, HULL GL. Assessment of protein nutrition in surgical patients—the value of anthropometrics. *Am J Clin Nutr* 1979;**32**:1527–1530.

8 DICKINSON RJ, ASHTON MG, AXON ATR, SMITH RC, YOUNG CK, HILL GL. Controlled trial of intravenous hyperalimentation and total bowel rest as an adjunct to the routine therapy of acute colitis. *Gastroenterology* 1980;**79**:1199–1204.

9 DOBBIE RP, BUTTERVICH OD. Continuous pump/tube enteric hyperalimentation—use in oesophageal disease. *JPEN* 1977;**1**:100–104.

10 FISCHER JE, FOSTER GS, ABEL RM. Hyperalimentation as primary therapy for inflammatory bowel disease. *Am J Surg* 1973;**125**:165–175.

11 GLIEDMAN ML, BOBOKI H, ROSEN RG. Acute pancreatitis. *Curr Probl Surg*, 1970:1–52.

12 GRIMBLE GK, REES RG, HALLIDAY D, FORD C, SILK DBA. Are peptides better utilised than free amino acids in the short bowel syndrome? *JPEN* 1986;**10**:155–160.

13 GRIMBLE, GK, REES RG, PATIL DH, *et al.* Administration of fat emulsions with nutritional mixtures from the 3-litre delivery system in total parenteral nutrition. *JPEN* 1985;**9**:456–460.

14 HILL GL. Do malnourished patients need nutritional therapy before major surgery? *Med J Austr* 1979;**2**:464.

15 HILL GL, CHURCH J. Energy and protein requirements of general surgical patients requiring intravenous nutrition. *Br J Surg* 1984;**71**:1–9.

16 HILL GL, BLACKETT RL, PICKFORT I, YOUNG GA. Malnutrition in surgical patients. An unrecognised problem. *Lancet* 1977;ii:689–692.

17 INGENBLEEK Y, VAN DEN SHRIEK HG, DE NAYER P, DE BISSCHER M. Albumin, transferrin and thyroxine binding prealbumin/retinol binding protein (TBPA/RBP) complex in assessment of malnutrition. *Clin Chim Acta* 1975;**63**:61–67

18 JAMES WPT. The assessment of nutritional status. *Medicine International* 1982;**15**:663–667.

19 JONES BJM, BROWN BE, GRIMBLE GK, SILK DBA. The formulation of energy dense enteral feeds—the use of high molecular weight glucose polymers. In: *Proceedings 3rd European Congress on Parenteral and Enteral Nutrition*, 1981:75.

20 JONES BJM, LEES R, ANDREWS J, FROST P, SILK DBA. Comparison of an elemental and polymeric enteral diet in patients with normal gastrointestinal function. *Gut* 1983;**24**:78–84.

21 JONES BJM, PAYNE S, SILK DBA. Indications for

pump assisted enteral feeding *Lancet* 1980;i:1057–7.

22 JONES DC, RICH AJ, WRIGHT PD, JOHNSTON IPA. Comparison of proprietary elemental and whole-protein diets in unconscious patients with head injury. *Br Med J* 1980;1:493–495.

23 JONES BJM, SILK DBA. Parenteral nutrition. *Medicine International* 1982;**15**:674–678.

24 KAMINSKI M.V. Enteral hyperalimentation. *Surg Gynecol Obstet* 1976;**143**:12–16.

25 KEIGHLEY MRB, MOGG B, BENTLEY S, ALLAN C. 'Home brew' compared with commercial preparations for enteral feeding. *Br Med J* 1983;1:163.

26 KEOHANE PP, ATTRILL H, JONES BJM, BROWN I, FROST P, SILK DBA. Influence of lactose and *Cl. difficile* in the pathogenesis of enteral feeding associated diarrhoea. *Clin Nutr* 1983;1:259–64.

27 KEOHANE PP, ATTRILL H, JONES BJM, NORTHOVER J, CRIBB A, SILK DBA. Significance of tunnelling and a nutrition nurse in TPN catheter sepsis—a controlled trial. *Lancet* 1983;ii:1388–1390.

28 KEOHANE PP, ATRILL H, JONES BJM, SILK DBA. Limitations and drawbacks of fine bore nasogastric feeding tubes. *Clin Nutr* 1983;**2**:85–86.

29 KEOHANE PP, ATTRILL H, LOVE M, FROST P, SILK DBA. Relation between osmolarity of diet and gastrointestinal side effects in enteral nutrition. *Br J Med.* 1984;**288**:678–680.

30 KEOHANE PP, ATTRILL H, SILK DBA. Endoscopic placement of fine bore nasogastric and nasoenteric feeding tubes. *Clin Nutr* 1983;1:245–247.

31 KEOHANE PP, ATRILL H, SILK DBA. Clinical effectiveness, weighted and unweighted 'fine bore' nasogastric feeding tube in enteral nutrition—a controlled trial. 1986 (in press).

32 KEOHANE PP, SILK DBA. Indications for use of mercury tipped nasogastric feeding tubes. *Clinic Nutr* 1983;**2**:27–28.

33 KEOHANE PP, SILK DBA. Peptides and free amino acids. In: Robeau JL, Caldwell MD, eds. *Enteral and Tube Feeding*. Philadelphia: W.B. Saunders Co., 1984:44–59.

34 KIRSCHNER BS, KLICH JR, KALMAN SS. Reversal of growth retardation in Crohn's disease with therapy emphasising oral nutritional restitution. *Gastroenterology* 1981;**80**:10–15.

35 KORETZ RL, MEYER JH. Elemental diets—facts and fantasies. *Gastroenterology* 1980;**78**:393–410.

36 LAW DK, DUDRICK SJ, ABDON NI. Immunocompetence of patients with protein calorie malnutrition. Effects of nutritional repletion. *Ann Intern Med* 1973;**79**:545–550.

37 LEE HA. Parenteral nutrition. In: Dickenson WT, Lee HA, eds. *Nutrition in the Clinical Management of Disease*. London: Edward Arnold, 1978;349–376.

38 LEE HA, HARTLEY TF. A method of determining daily nitrogen requirements. *Postgrad Med J* 1975;**51**:441–445.

39 LONG JM, WILMORE DW, MASON AD. Fat carbo-

hydrate interaction. Effects on nitrogen sparing in total intravenous feeding. *Surg Forum* 1974; **25**:61–63.

40 MACFIE J, SMITH RC, HILL GL. Glucose or fat as a non-protein energy source? A controlled trial in gastroenterological patients requiring parenteral nutrition. *Gastroenterology* 1981;**80**:103–107.

41 MCINTYRE PB, POWELL-TUCK J, WOOD SR, *et al.* Controlled clinical trial of bowel rest in the treatment of severe colitis. *Gut* 1986;**27**:481–485.

42 MATUCHANSKY C, MORICHAU-BEAUCHANT M, DRUART F, TAPIN J. Cyclic (nocturnal) total parenteral nutrition in hospitalised adult patients with severe digestive diseases. Report of a prospective study. *Gastroenterology* 1981;**81**:433–437.

43 MEAKINE JL, PIETSCH JB, BUBEWICK O. Delayed hypersensitivity: indicator of acquired failure of host defences in sepsis and trauma. *Ann Surg* 1977;**186**:241–250.

44 MESSING B, BORIES C, KUNSTILINGER F, BERNIER JJ. Does parenteral nutrition induce a lithogenic gallbladder bile? *JPEN* 1982;**5**:560.

45 METZ G, DILAWARI J, KELLOCK TD. Simple technique for naso-enteric intubation. *Lancet* 1978;ii:454–455.

46 MORIN CL, ROULET M, ROY CC, WEBER A. Continuous elemental enteral alimentation in children with Crohn's disease and growth failure. *Gastroenterology* 1980;**79**:1205–1210.

47 MUNRO H. Biological limiting factors to parenteral amino acid feeding. In: Johnston IBA. ed. *Advances in Parenteral Nutrition*. Lancaster: MTP Press 1978:107–118.

48 O'MORAIN C, SEGAL AUS LEVI AJ. Elemental diet as primary treatment of acute Crohn's disease: a controlled trial. *Br. Med J* 1984;**288**:1859–1862.

49 OSTRO MJ, GREENBERG GR, JEEJEEBHOY KN. Total parenteral nutrition and bowel rest in Crohn's disease. *JPEN* 1985;**9**:280–287.

50 PIETSCH JB, MEAKINS JL, MACLEAN LD. The delayed hypersensitivity response: application in clinical surgery. *Surgery* 1977;**82**:349–355.

51 POWELL-TUCK J, NIELSEN T, FARWELL JA, LENNARD-JONES JE. Team approach to long-term intravenous feeding in patients with gastrointestinal disorders. *Lancet* 1978;ii:825–828.

52 REES RG, GRIMBLE GK, KEOHANE PP, CARTWRIGHT T, DESREUMAUX M, SILK DBA. The effect of peptide chain length on the absorption of egg protein by hydrolysis in human jejunum. *Gastroenterology* 1986 (in press).

53 REES RG, KEOHANE PP, ATTRILL H, QUINN DG, SILK DBA. Improved design of nasogastric feeding tubes. *JPEN* 1986;**10**:205–210.

54 REES RG, KEOHANE PP, GRIMBLE GK, FROST PG, ATRILL HA, SILK DBA. Tolerance of elemental diet administered without starter regimen. *Br Med J* 1985;**290**:1869–1870.

55 REILLY J, RYAN JA, STROLE W, FISCHER JE. Hyper-alimentation in inflammatory bowel disease *Am J Surg* 1976;**131**:192–200.

56 ROCCHIO MA, CHA CJM, HAAS KF, RANDALL MT. Use of chemically defined diets in the management of patients with acute inflammatory bowel disease. *Am J Surg* 1974;**127**:469–475.

57 ROWLANDS BJ, DUDRICK SJ. Gallbladder bile composition during intravenous hyperalimentation in dogs. *JPEN* 1982;**5**:577.

50 RUPPIN H, SAILER D. Nasoenteral nutrition: technical procedures and follow-up. *Hepatogastroenterology* 1983;**30**:161–169.

59 RUSSELL RI. Elemental diets. *Gut* 1975;**16**:68–79.

60 RYAN JA. Complications of total parenteral nutrition. In: Fischer JE, ed. *Total Parenteral Nutrition* Boston: Little Bown, 1976:55.

61 SAGAR S, HARLAND P, SHIELDS R. Early postoperative feeding with elemental diet. *Br Med J* 1979;1:293–295.

62 SHETTY PS, WATRASIEWICZ KE, JUNG RT, JAMES WPT. Rapid-turnover transport proteins: an index of subclinical protein energy malnutrition. *Lancet* 1978;ii:230–232.

63 SILK DBA. Enteral nutrition. *Hosp Update* 1980;**6**:761–765.

64 SILK DBA. *Nutritional Support in Hospital Practice.* Oxford: Blackwell Scientific Publications, 1983.

65 SILK DBA. Formulation of enteral diets. *Gut* 1986 (in press).

66 SITGES-CREUS A, CANADAS E, VILAR L. Cholestatic jaundice during parenteral alimentation in adults. In: Johston IDA, ed. *Advances in Parenteral Nutrition*. Lancaster: MTP Press, 1978:461–469.

67 SPANIER AH, PIETSCH JB, MEAKINS JL. Relationship between immune competance and nutrition. *Surg Forum* 1976;**27**:332.

68 VOGEL CM, CORWIN TR, BANE AE. Intravenous hyperalimentation in the treatment of inflammatory diseases of the bowel. *Arch Surg* 1974;**108**:460–467.

69 VOITK AK, ECHAVE V, FELLER JH, BROWN RA, GURD FN. Experience with elemental diet in the treatment of inflammatory bowel disease. *Arch Surg* 1973;**107**:329–333.

70 WALTER CW. Bacterial contamination of intravenous infusion due to faulty technique. In: Johnston IAD, ed. *Advances in Parenteral Nutrition* Lancaster: MTP Press, 1978:325.

71 WELCH GW, MCKELL DW, SILVERSTEIN P, WALKER HL. The role of catheter composition in the development of thrombophlebitis. *Surg Gynecol Obstet* 1974;**138**:421–424.

72 YEUNG CK, YOUNG GA, HACKETT AF, HILL GL. Fine needle catheter jejunostomy—an assessment of a new method of nutritional support after major gastrointestinal surgery. *Br J Surg* 1979;**66**:727–732.

Index